NATURAL HEALING WISDOM & KNOW-HOW

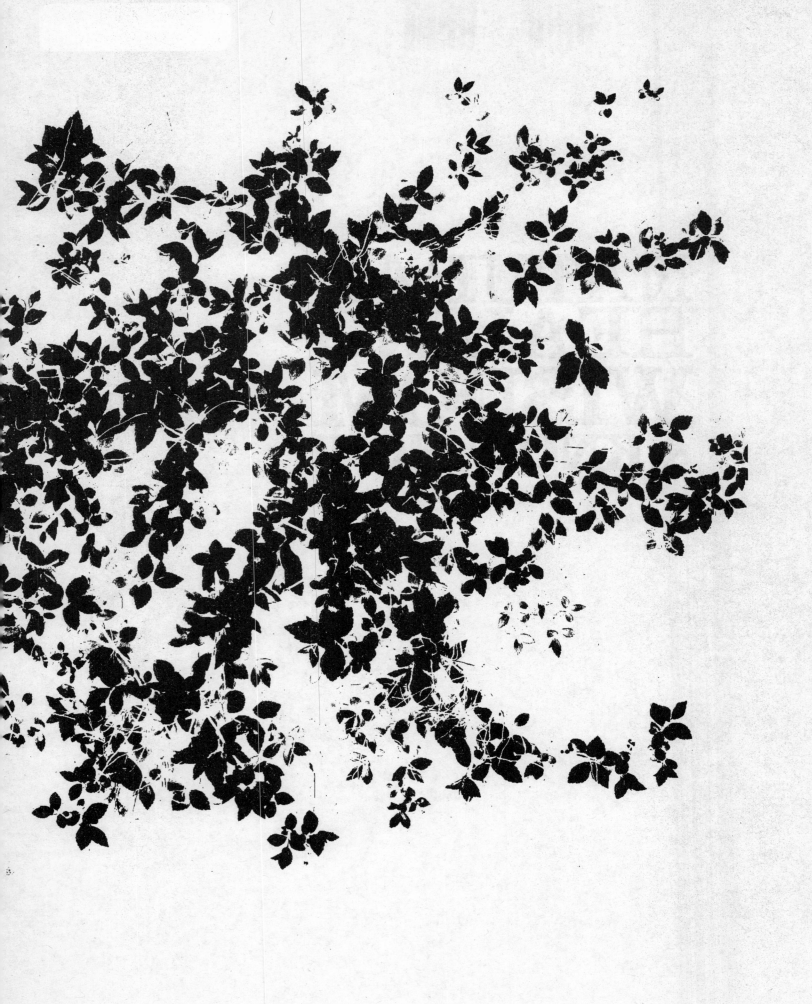

NATURAL HEALING WISDOM & KNOW-HOW

Useful Practices, Recipes, and Formulas for a Lifetime of Health

Compiled by Amy Rost

BLACK DOG
& LEVENTHAL
PUBLISHERS
NEW YORK

Published by

Black Dog & Leventhal Publishers, Inc.

151 West 19th Street

New York, NY 10011

Distributed by

Workman Publishing Company

225 Varick Street

New York, NY 10014

Manufactured in the United States of America

Cover and interior design by Ohioboy Design

Cover illustration © Ken Krug

The materials contained in this work are originally published and copyrighted by
Celestial Arts and Crossing Press and used by permission of the publishers.

ISBN-13: 978-1-57912-800-5

k j i h g

Library of Congress Cataloging-in-Publication Data available on file.

Contents

COMPLETE INDEX OF AILMENTS & CONDITIONS

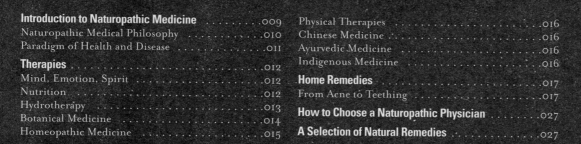

Naturo-pathy

INTRODUCTION TO NATUROPATHIC MEDICINE

Judith Boice, N.D.

Naturopathic medicine relies for its healing knowledge on the vast repository of wisdom innate in the Earth. When you begin working with naturopathic medicine, you will be using the oldest, most clinically researched medicine available—natural therapeutics that have been applied effectively for tens of thousands of years—combined with the best of contemporary research and technology.

Naturopathic medicine is a system of classical medicine defined by its philosophy. The term *classical* more fully captures the essence of naturopathic medicine than do the terms *alternative* or *complementary*. The roots of naturopathic medicine reach back to classical times, when physicians studied the processes of health as well as the processes of disease. Those roots extend even deeper into the soil of time, to an era when humans understood the healing power in their own bodies, as well as in the plants and elements that surround them. This innate healing power, or natural intelligence, directs the body to regenerate and rebalance.

Many techniques or healing modalities fit under the umbrella of naturopathic medicine. The philosophy of naturopathic medicine provides the link

that unifies this group of diverse practices. A core aspect of this philosophy, outlined more fully below, is that treatment must be individualized to meet the needs of a particular patient. Naturopathic medicine treats diseases by treating people. Ten people with similar cold or flu symptoms may walk into my office, and those ten patients probably will walk out with ten different treatment plans, each tailored to suit a particular set of needs.

This diversity in treatment methods makes naturopathic medicine difficult for some people to understand. Legislative bodies understand other healing modalities—acupuncture, for example—more readily because the method of healing is consistent from patient to patient. Acupuncturists use needles. Chiropractic physicians administer "force" or "nonforce" methods of adjustment. Medical doctors prescribe pharmaceutical drugs and surgery.

A naturopathic physician, however, has a vast array of potential treatments from which to choose. Naturopathic medical students study all of the medical sciences, including clinical and physical diagnosis, pathology, anatomy (with dissection lab), biochemistry, physiology, pharmacology, and specialty areas such as pediatrics, gynecology, and cardiology—in short, all of the courses taught at any medical school. In addition, we spend several hundred hours studying courses that have disappeared from most medical school curricula, including counseling, nutrition, exercise therapeutics, home-

opathy, botanical medicine, hydrotherapy, and physical therapies.

Like any physician, a naturopathic physician takes medical histories, performs physical exams, orders lab tests, and makes diagnoses. A naturopathic doctor differs from other physicians only in how she treats the diagnosed illness, in what she does with the information gathered. A treatment plan may include nutritional counseling, a homeopathic prescription, and a discussion of how a specific exercise program will benefit the patient's health. The discussion may cover job or family pressures and how they are impacting the patient's life. If indicated, an office visit may include some form of physical therapy. Occasionally, a condition requires minor surgery, e.g., removal of skin tags or closure of a laceration. Finally, in certain situations a naturopathic physician may choose to prescribe pharmaceutical drugs.

As a naturopathic physician, I am not completely opposed to the use of drugs and surgery. I do have certain drugs available to me as part of my formulary. For patients with certain conditions, I believe surgery is a viable, even necessary, option. Conventional medicine excels in its treatment of catastrophic conditions, e.g., major bodily injury after a car accident, or removal of large cancerous growths. When the "big guns" are required, conventional medicine responds with reassuring aggression and swiftness. When a body requires ongoing treat-

Continued ➨

ment for a chronic illness, conventional medicine has little to offer.

Even "simple" acute conditions have few treatments in the conventional medical system. A college friend, recently graduated from conventional medical school, acknowledged his helplessness in treating common colds. "I mean, I don't even know what to do for myself," he confided. "What can I tell my patients?" I was as surprised by his lack of knowledge as I was by his honesty. I can think of at least half a dozen treatments to resolve a cold, and several therapies to abort a cold in its early stages.

In jettisoning the wisdom of classical medicine, the conventional medical system has lost invaluable resources. Gone is the knowledge of supporting the body and working with the healing power innate in the human body. Largely gone is a true understanding of investing in health as a means of prevention. Unfortunately, the big guns of conventional medicine have provided people with a false sense of security. Many people assume that they can continue to eat lifeless food, avoid exercise, smoke, and drink to excess, then be "saved" from illness later in life by the wonders of modern medicine. Half a century after the introduction of the pharmaceutical wonder drugs, we are learning that drug miracles are temporary, not permanent, phenomena. Bacteria and viruses mutate and become resistant to antibiotics. Chemotherapy and antihypertensive medications have serious and sometimes irreversible side effects. Such "miracles" exact as many payments as they offer rewards, and the borrowing margin is the health and vitality of our bodies.

Naturopathic medicine relies on the body's innate strength for its miracles. Its wonder drugs are reliable plant and elemental sources that have been used effectively since the dawn of the healing arts.

Naturopathic Medical Philosophy

Vis Medicatrix Naturae: The Healing Power of Nature

Both our human bodies and the Earth's body have an innate wisdom that governs the cycles of birth, growth, maturation, and decay. Bodily health is supported by moving and living in harmony with these natural cycles. Many healing tools come directly from the Earth. Hydrotherapy, for example, relies on the healing qualities of water. Botanical medicines derive their restorative properties from plants. Mineral, plant, and animal substances provide the foundation for homeopathic medicines. Each of these medications has a native intelligence that interacts with the body's healing wisdom to bring about health, balance, and harmony. Health is a result of balance, which may be maintained by what appear to be destructive forces, e.g., fever or inflammation, that ultimately restore the health and vitality of our bodies (see "Paradigm of Health and Disease," page 011).

Tolle Causum: Identify and Treat the Cause

Illness does not occur without cause. The body, in its elegant wisdom, always whispers before it shouts. Informed health care means learning to listen to the body and its early warning signs. Body symptoms are metaphors—or, perhaps more accurately, markers—of shifts and changes in life processes. Symptoms usually are the result of the body's trying to rebalance itself. Identifying the cause requires seeking the psychic, social, and spiritual roots of the problem, as well as the physical causes of disease. Symptomatic treatment rarely addresses the underlying disturbance. In fact, symptomatic treat-

ment may suppress the illness and make the cause more difficult to identify. Treating the cause requires addressing the body as a whole.

Chinese medicine refers to the treatment principles of ben and biao, the "roots" and "branches" of disease. The skillful physician learns to differentiate between the deep-seated causes (roots) and the peripheral manifestations (branches) of a disease. "When considering the root (ben) and manifestation (biao)," writes Maciocia in The Foundations of Chinese Medicine, "it is important to understand the connection between the two. They are not separate entities, but two aspects of a contradiction, like yin and yang. As their names suggest, they are related to one another, just as the roots of a tree are connected to its branches, the former under the ground and invisible, the latter above the ground and visible. The same relation exists between the root of a disease and its clinical manifestations: they are indissolubly related, and they are from two aspects of the same entity."

Treating the cause means addressing the roots of an illness, not just the stems and leaves that symbolize signs and symptoms in the body. The root imbalance may manifest as a group of symptoms. Sometimes several damaged roots manifest as one symptom, e.g., shortness of breath may be a symptom related to several concurrent illnesses such as congestive heart failure, pulmonary edema, chronic bronchitis, and/or emphysema. A guiding principle in both Chinese and naturopathic medicine is, "To treat a disease, find the root."

"First Do No Harm"

Classical, natural therapeutics aim to rebalance the body with the least invasive treatments possible. In my practice, I always begin with the simplest treatments (generally dietary changes and hydrotherapy) before adding more complex, and more expensive, treatments. I will prescribe a well-balanced herbal formula before recommending a bag full of supplements. "Doing no harm" also includes implementing therapies that nourish and strengthen the body. Both Western and Eastern classical medical traditions employ "tonics," herbs and other formulas that strengthen the body. These tonics generally are prescribed after births (for the mother) and after long-term illnesses, and for preventive care. The Chinese, for example, often drink special teas and eat certain foods at the change of each season to prepare the body for new environmental conditions.

Doctor as Teacher

The word docere means "to teach." The physician's primary function is to provide information, thus empowering people to regulate their own health. A great deal of time in a naturopathic physician's practice is spent educating patients. Once a patient has applied the information and achieved improved levels of health, the physician serves as a source of further information for emergencies, or as a coach for reaching even higher levels of health.

Unfortunately, some patients do not want such information. They want to be fixed like a car in an auto service center. After my spending nearly an hour coaching a patient on diet, exercise changes, and stress reduction, trying to explain why her (mostly junk food) diet was intimately linked with her fatigue, the patient gave me an exasperated look. "Can't you just give me some pills?" she said. "I mean, the last naturopathic physician I went to gave me some tablets, and I felt better as long as I was taking them. Can't you just give me something to take?"

Reluctantly, I prescribed some antioxidants, knowing that I was offering a Band-Aid for a much bigger problem. In addition to poor diet and lack of

exercise, the patient worked a very stressful job and nursed her terminally ill mother in the evenings. She was overwhelmed at the prospect of making any significant changes in her life. She wanted her health to improve without charging any of the conditions that were contributing to her illness.

Many people continue to operate in a paradigm engendered by the conventional medical system: "I'm hurting. Give me a pill to take away the pain so I can continue on with my life." The problem with this paradigm is that sometimes the patient's lifestyle is the cause of the pain. Simply taking away the pain with a "magic bullet" will not empower that patient. Even some naturopathic physicians are content to prescribe for quick symptomatic relief and hope the patient will return one day to address the underlying condition.

Perhaps in the situation I have described, I needed to spend more time in the educative process. And perhaps the patient, at this time in her life, was not ready for a medical model that required her participation. Not every patient is interested in health or empowerment. For such patients, drugs and surgery may be valid choices.

Prevention

Preventive care requires studying health as closely as one studies the processes of disease. Most conventional medical practices focus on disease, returning patients from prone to a standing position (crisis intervention). Classical medicine likewise can return patients from prone to standing, and can also help them to walk, run, and, finally dance in their physical forms. Conventional medicine aims for survival; classical medicine aims for optimal health.

True preventive medicine requires making daily investments in our health—eating foods that nourish our body, exercising, developing loving relationships and supportive communities, contributing to the health of the Earth. Healthy people live in healthy environments. Preventive medicine means working for clean air, land, and water. Human health is inseparable from the health of the planet.

Treat the Whole Person

The cause of disease is almost always multifactorial; hence, the treatment must be multifaceted. Usually I ask a patient, "What is going on in your life? Why do you think you are ill right now?" Some are surprised. They are not used to having a physician consider anything but physical symptoms and the results of lab tests in the diagnostic workup. Many already know the cause of their illness. Others need coaching and cajoling to understand that their physical body is intimately linked with their mental, emotional, and spiritual lives.

I do not mean to imply that every physical disturbance can be traced to an emotional, mental, or spiritual cause. At one time, I was convinced that all illness was due to an "issue" or "issues" the patient was manifesting through physical illness. Identifying and changing emotional/mental patterns would resolve the physical illness. Over time, my thinking has changed. Sometimes people do create diseases to work through "issues." Other times people have an iron deficiency because they have an iron deficiency, not because they have some great cosmic lesson to learn. Letting go of the need to find a "metaphysical" cause for every illness has allowed me to be much less judgmental, and much more understanding of the complexities of health and disease. Abandoning my certainty about the causes of disease has provided much more room for the great mystery of health and disease to express itself.

Continued ➔

The healing process often causes unresolved wounds from the past to resurface. Such wounding may have occurred on the physical, mental, emotional, or spiritual level. Focusing on healing any aspect of the self can restimulate past hurts as well. The body has enough energy to "clean house"—to bring forth, examine, and discharge past garbage. Clearing emotional pain, for example, may be accompanied by the return of a skin rash that plagued the patient during childhood. Healing the rash may be followed by the realization of an unworkable relationship pattern that he or she is ready to change. The path by which someone returns to wholeness is unique to each individual, although certain patterns of healing may typify that path. The template of healing outlined below is common to both naturopathic and homeopathic medicines:

THE LAWS OF CURE

Healing occurs

- from inside to outside (internal organs first, skin last)
- from top to bottom (from the head region down to the feet)
- from most recent to most distant (recent symptoms recur first, followed by older symptoms—in other words, in reverse chronological order)
- from least important to most important organs

Paradigm of Health and Disease

Each healing art operates within a particular framework that elucidates the causes of illness and outlines methods for returning to a state of health. The therapies section will explore some of the major healing systems that fall under the umbrella of naturopathic medicine.

Outlined below is a basic paradigm that explains the development of disease from a naturopathic perspective. The model also suggests how to reverse the disease process and return to a state of health.

Keep in mind that a model is not necessarily the "truth." An enlightened teacher once said that we entertain ourselves with models until the truth reveals itself. Although the following paradigm may not represent absolute truth, I have seen this model function very effectively in clinical practice. The outline provides a simple, elegant understanding of health, illness, and healing that is a major source of guidance for me in my practice.

Most of us begin life in a state of optimal health. Through the course of living, we are exposed to conditions that disturb our equilibrium, that challenge the body beyond its ability to compensate. The body responds by generating inflammation (*rubor, dolor, calor,* and *tumor*—redness, pain, heat, and swelling). Fever is one of the most common inflammatory responses.

Inflammation is the body's way of discharging a disturbance from the body. If the body is allowed to complete the inflammatory response, the disturbance is discharged, and the body returns to optimal health:

> Optimal Health → Disturbance → Inflammation → Discharge → Optimal Health

Natural therapeutics, when properly applied, can speed up the discharge phase and hasten the return to health. Unfortunately, most people attempt to stop the inflammatory response before it has a chance to discharge the disturbance from the body. Stopping or suppressing the inflammation can drive the disturbance deeper into the body, causing chronic irritation. If chronic irritation continues long enough, the body tissues begin to degenerate (atrophy, tumors, necrosis).

> Optimal Health → Disturbance → Inflammation → Supression → Chronic Inflammation → Tissue Degeneration

A classic example of suppression, recognized by conventional as well as naturopathic medicine, is applying cortisone cream to eczema rashes. Cortisone stops inflammation by suppressing the activity of the immune system. Patients with eczema who apply cortisone creams often notice that asthma develops (or worsens) as the eczema clears. In essence, the cortisone cream suppresses the eczema and drives the inflammation deeper into the body, in this case to the lungs. Patients often notice that, as their asthma improves, the eczema returns, the body has strengthened to the point of pushing the inflammation to the surface (skin) once again (see the "Laws of Cure," left). They reapply the cortisone cream, the eczema improves, and the asthma worsens. This chronic cycle of suppression and improvement may continue for years before the body becomes too weary to push the inflammation to the surface any longer. At that point, the eczema diminishes to a low-grade irritation as the asthma becomes a more deep-seated, chronic condition.

Natural therapeutics, when improperly applied, can also cause suppression of inflammation and irritation. Although suppression is less likely with natural therapeutics, a practitioner of hydrotherapy, herbs, and homeopathics must be mindful of his or her prescriptions and watch carefully for any signs of suppression. In the example given above, asthma is a "chronic irritation" of the lung tissue caused by suppressing a surface irritation. From a naturopathic perspective, the surface irritation (eczema) is a less serious condition than chronic inflammation in a vital organ (asthma). If the chronic inflammation continues long enough, degeneration of tissues will occur.

Generally the body will not develop measurable signs of damage until the disease has reached the "chronic inflammation" or "degeneration" level. Taking a biopsy of an acutely infected sinus, for example, and examining the tissue under a microscope usually will not reveal major tissue changes. A chronically infected sinus, however, will show signs of irritation at the cellular level. Long-term irritation may cause degeneration of the tissues. Necrosis is a late-stage manifestation of tissue degeneration.

The model for returning to health is a reversal of the disease process.

> Degeneration → Chronic Inflammation → Inflammation → Discharge → Optimal Health

From a naturopathic perspective, the healing process is stimulated first through the digestive system, by two central methods—proper nutrition and hydrotherapy. The digestive system is absolutely essential for the regeneration of any body tissue. The alimentary tract is responsible for absorption of all nutrients and disposal of most wastes in the body. If the digestive system is functioning optimally, the body has a fighting chance of receiving all the nutrition available in the food we eat, and disposing of all the wastes generated by the body during the natural processes of maintenance and repair.

Constitutional hydrotherapy—a specific hydrotherapy treatment designed to stimulate the immune system and increase circulation in the digestive system, is the simplest, most powerful, least expensive method to support healing of the digestive tract.

Dietary changes and constitutional-hydrotherapy treatments also stimulate something that our current medical terminology has no tool to measure, the body's own innate healing ability. As the body strengthens, the disease process begins to reverse itself. Degeneration improves to the level of chronic irritation, and then chronic irritation becomes acute—the body finally has enough energy to "clean house," to bring the acute inflammation that was suppressed back to the surface. Often the acute inflammation returns in the form of a low-grade fever, or a cold or flulike illness, that lasts for a couple of days. Sometimes the housecleaning, also referred to as the "healing crisis," manifests as the return of an old illness. In contrast to earlier episodes, however, the healing crisis usually is much briefer and less intense than the original occurrence.

If allowed to run its course, the acute inflammation allows the body to discharge the original disturbance, and the body returns once again to a state of optimal health. When the body finally mounts an acute inflammation after a long, chronic illness, remember that the inflammation must be allowed to run its course without any further suppression (e.g., no cortisone or aspirin).

In addition to nutrition and hydrotherapy, many other treatments stimulate the body's innate healing ability. Homeopathy, botanical medicines, stress reduction, acupuncture, and physical therapies all may support the body in its healing journey. Inner work, meditation, and counseling address the roots of some illnesses. Choosing a particular modality requires both skill and intuition—a practitioner needs a solid knowledge of his or her subject, and a well-honed intuition to select the method or methods that will most benefit a patient. Often I tell patients that we will be doing some "detective work," discovering what treatments will be most catalytic for them. Of course, the response depends in part on the skill of the practitioner, and on his or her ability to utilize a particular healing tool.

This marriage of knowledge and intuition is paramount for application of these principles at home. Learn everything you can about the modalities you find most useful, or to which you feel most drawn. Consult local practitioners, read, and study. Practice what you are learning. Information becomes living knowledge when you apply the information in your life. Learn to listen to your intuition, the "natural intelligence" that guides the application of knowledge. Remember that each person is different, and that what affects one person may not affect another. As you become more familiar with your own and your family's bodies, you will make better and better selections based on your healing knowledge.

—From *Pocket Guide to Naturopathic Medicine*

Progression of Disease

- OPTIMAL HEALTH
- DISTURBANCE (emotional or physical trauma, overwork, etc.)
- INFLAMMATION
- CHRONIC INFLAMMATION
- DEGENERATION (tissue atrophy, tumors, necrosis)

Discharge and resolution of acute inflammation

Restoration of Health

Continued →

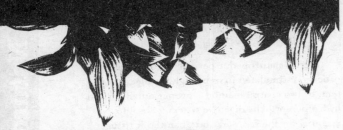

THERAPIES

Judith Boice, N.D.

So, you've decided to improve your health and reap the rewards of increased energy, flexibility, concentration, and creativity. You've begun to walk down the aisles of the whole-foods store and the public library searching for resources to help you fulfill your dreams of improved health.

Choosing a therapeutic approach can be the most exciting, frustrating, rewarding, and baffling search for anyone interested in the healing arts. Take a deep breath. Know that over time you probably will explore several healing modalities. Some paths will reward you; others will meander or dead-end before you decide to explore other byways.

Each healing modality has an important role to play. The art of working with natural therapeutics is matching your needs with the natural intelligence invested in each therapeutic method. What works well for you may be anathema for a neighbor or your spouse. Respect your differences. What works well for one person may not necessarily work for another. Your body also may respond to different methods at different times—keep listening to your body's needs and note its responses over time.

If you are fortunate to have a naturopathic physician in your community, you may be able to bypass some of the trial-and-error tactics involved in discovering the therapeutics that work best for you. Together with your naturopathic physician you can do the "detective work" needed to identify the most supportive treatment methods for you. You also will benefit from his or her expertise in applying the most appropriate healing modalities in your specific situation. To become a gifted homeopathic prescriber, for example, may require a lifetime of study. You can bypass some of the frustration of investing in books and remedies and obtaining marginal results by working with someone who already has studied a particular modality. Best of all, find a physician who offers classes in how to apply natural therapeutics in your daily life.

The following is an outline of the chief healing modalities employed by naturopathic physicians, including brief descriptions of other major systems of medicine that share a common philosophy with naturopathic medicine. When working with a new patient, I consider potential treatments in a particular order, based on what I know of how the body heals. The following list of therapeutics reflects that order. In addition to describing the therapy, I've included information on how and when to consider using a specific treatment. My hope is that this information will assist you in deciding when to choose a particular treatment.

Mind, Emotion, Spirit

No amount of physical therapy or herbs can take the place of companionship in the life of a lonely person. The "perfect" acupuncture treatment cannot compensate for a soul-draining job or an emotionally toxic home environment. In these and other situations, therapeutic methods offer, at best, a means of supporting someone until he or she is ready to make the kinds of life changes that will engender overall health.

I hesitate to place this at the top of the list, again for fear of falling into the trap of identifying a "spiritual imbalance" or "emotional issue" at the root of every illness. Keep in mind that people with a profound spiritual connection and a rich, positive emotional life still can manifest disease in their body. Too many malnourished, overworked women (and sometimes men) have been told that their illnesses are in their head, that they should quit complaining and get on with their life. Clearly, their illnesses are *not* all in their head. Recovery involves the physical body as well as the patient's mental or emotional state.

When illness develops, a simple way of utilizing the therapy of mind, emotions, and spirit is to ask yourself the following questions:

- What is going on in my life now?
- What are the biggest concerns, the major stressors, in my life now?
- Am I working too much? Too little? Does my work bring me satisfaction?
- Is my lifestyle sustainable, i.e., can I complete everything I need to complete and still remain healthy?
- Are my relationships supporting me? Am I investing time and attention in the major relationships in my life?

Twylah Nitsch, a Seneca elder, poses the following questions:

- Am I happy with what I'm doing?
- Is what I'm doing adding to the confusion?
- What am I doing to bring about peace and contentment?
- How will I be remembered when I'm gone?

Keep in mind that these questions are a *beginning*. They are meant to invoke insight, not provide fodder for self-destructive thoughts (i.e., don't beat yourself up if you discover some challenging areas). Illnesses can offer the opportunity to slow down and reevaluate our lives, to make new choices based on our greatest dreams, our deepest joys.

These questions may serve as a good reality check as well. When humans endure a certain intensity or number of stresses, the body is more likely to develop an illness. One of my current patients has struggled with depression for almost three years. Reviewing her life shortly before the onset of the depression provided some obvious clues about the cause of her depression: within the space of six months, she lost five family members and two close friends. Further history revealed that she was adopted and shared a pattern common to many adopted children—she felt profoundly abandoned when significant people exited from her life. We continue to pursue supportive therapies in conjunction with counseling, with an understanding that true healing probably will require deep emotional work to resolve her primary experience of loss and abandonment.

Nutrition

A healthy digestive system is vital to overall health. The digestive system is responsible for the absorption of the majority of our nutrients and for the removal of most waste from the body. Even the most nutritious food and the best supplements will not be fully utilized if the digestive system is unable to absorb the nutrients and dispose of waste.

The body has two nervous systems running simultaneously, the sympathetic and parasympathetic. They both function at all times, but one always predominates. When the sympathetic nervous system is more active, the body is in "fight or flight" mode, geared up to protect us from danger. The body responds to outside stress in the same way whether the "predator" is a hungry tiger or an irritated boss. Norepinephrine (adrenaline) dumps into the bloodstream, increasing the heart and respiratory rates. The vascular system responds by shunting blood away from the internal organs toward the peripheral muscles to prepare for quick movement. The digestive system begins to "shut down" with reduced gastric secretions and peristalsis.

Many people in today's culture live continuously on low levels of adrenaline, with the sympathetic nervous system predominating. In this situation, the digestive system receives very little blood flow. Food sits in the digestive tract for long periods of time without adequate supplies of gastric juices to digest it. The digestive tract cannot adequately absorb nutrients or expel wastes.

The parasympathetic nervous system predominates when we are relaxed, favoring regeneration of body tissues and increased activity in the digestive tract. You may have noticed that your stomach and intestines gurgle when you are relaxed and happy. This gurgling (not to be confused with the growls of hunger) is a good sign, indicating that the digestive system is working well.

If the digestive system is not functioning optimally, even the healthiest foods and the most potent nutritional supplements will not be utilized fully by the body. In addition, one nutritionist noted that Americans have the most expensive urine in the world: we swallow pills that cannot be utilized by the body because the digestive system has a difficult time breaking down the pills. The body can use only a certain amount of water-soluble vitamins at any one time; within a short period, unused vitamins are dumped into the urine for removal.

Proper nutrition starts with identifying any foods that may cause irritation in the digestive tract. Many lab tests exist to identify food allergies, irritants, and sensitivities. One such test checks for constitutional food intolerances—foods the body fundamentally does not digest well. If the body is repeatedly exposed to these foods over a long period of time, the gut becomes irritated. Eventually the irritation causes a breakdown of the intestinal mucosa. "Leaky gut" syndrome develops, and larger molecules of food cross the gut mucosa. The immune system, unused to seeing these large molecules, may develop antibodies to fight the presumed "foreign" invaders.

Avoiding food allergens and sensitivities can help to resolve innumerable symptoms; however, simply avoiding foods will not cause the gut to heal, nor will it help to identify the *primary* foods that caused the gut disturbance in the first place. Identifying constitutional food intolerances satisfies one part of the equation—removing the root cause of irritation in the gut. In addition to taking away the primary disturbance, the body requires support to encourage regeneration of healthy gut mucosa.

Constitutional hydrotherapy is the simplest, most powerful method to support healing of the digestive tract. See the following "Hydrotherapy" section for specific instructions for the constitutional hydrotherapy treatment.

Basic Guidelines for Better Nutrition

1. Eat foods as close as possible to their natural state. A baked potato, for example, contains more nutrition (and fewer additives) than potato chips. Whole, fresh apples contain more roughage and nutrients than apple juice.
2. Eat local foods, which generally contain the nutrients that are best for the local population.

Continued ➡

In the Pacific Northwest, for example, wild salmon have high levels of essential fatty acids, which help prevent hormonal swings associated with "seasonal affective disorder," a common malady in Oregon and Washington. Eating local foods also reduces fossil fuel consumption by eliminating the need to truck or fly foods long distances.

3. Buy organic foods. Recent studies show that organic foods have at least 70 percent more nutrients than their conventionally grown counterparts. In addition, organic food are free of petroleum-based pesticides and herbicides. The chemical residues tend to concentrate in our reproductive organs and fatty tissues, causing decreased fertility, breast cancer, and a host of other degenerative diseases. In the long run, organic agriculture contributes to soil fertility and overall ecosystem health, while reducing our reliance on fossil fuels.

4. Choose foods low on the food chain. In words, choose grains, legumes, and vegetables more frequently than fish or meat. The following are general guidelines for nutrition based on calorie intake. Keep in mind, however, that each individual varies radically in her or his nutritional needs.

   • 70 percent grains and legumes
   • 20 percent fruits and vegetables
   • 10 percent meat, cheese, eggs, tofu, and other concentrated protein sources

Most Americans eat far too much concentrated protein. The processing of excess protein metabolites by the kidneys can weaken organ function over a period of time. All food sources, including plant foods, contain protein. The World Health Organization recommends eating 50 grams of protein per day, with increased amounts for pregnant or lactating women.

5. Ideal fat content in the diet is 10–15 percent of the daily caloric intake. The type of fat or oil is as important as the quantity. Altered fats (rancid or hydrogenated fats and oils) should be eliminated entirely from the diet. These include margarines and shortenings, whether they are used fresh, or included in processed and deep-fried foods. Keep saturated animal fats to a minimum. Include cold-pressed, properly stored oils in your daily diet. Keep all oils, including olive oil, in the refrigerator: heat, light, and air cause oils to become rancid.

6. Take time to chew. Some sources recommend chewing every bite of food as many as fifty times. This first step in the digestive process grinds food into smaller pieces and mixes saliva with the food. Saliva contains many enzymes that begin the process of carbohydrate digestion before the food ever leaves the mouth. Following this simple advice can eliminate a host of digestive complaints.

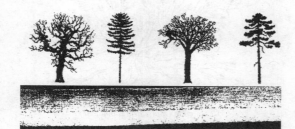

Hydrotherapy

Earth is a water planet, bestowed with a blue-green vastness of liquid life. Our bodies are 70 percent water—we left the amniotic support of the sea by learning to contain it within our skin. Humans can survive for weeks without food. Without water, we perish within days, even hours in an arid desert climate.

For thousands of years water has been used to treat disease and trauma, with various revivals punctuating its long history. At his mountain sanitarium, Vincent Priessnitz (1799–1852) championed the most recent European rediscovery of water's healing properties. In the United States, John Harvey Kellogg, M.D. (1852–1943) was a major proponent of water cures. His Battle Creek Sanitarium combined water treatments with sine-wave, massage, and dietary therapies. (His method of pressing whole grains into "flakes" survives today in the Kellogg cereal industry.) Kellogg kept meticulous records and conducted scientific research in his sanitarium. The data gathered became the foundation for *Rational Hydrotherapy* (1901), still the definitive textbook on the subject.

Hydrotherapy involves the use of hot and cold water in specific treatments to stimulate the immune system and alter blood circulation to particular areas of the body. Outlined below are five specific hydrotherapy treatments that can be used to treat a wide range of conditions.

General Caution: Diabetic patients should never apply heat to the feet. This also applies to anyone with compromised circulation in the extremities (e.g., Raynaud's syndrome). Instead, apply a large fomentation (towels wrung out in very warm water) to the groin area.

CONSTITUTIONAL HYDROTHERAPY TREATMENT

The constitutional hydrotherapy treatment increases immune-system function, improves digestion, and promotes detoxification. It can be used to treat almost any acute or chronic condition. In a trained hydrotherapist's clinic, the treatment would include the use of a sine-wave machine to further stimulate the digestive tract. The following instructions are for home application.

When not to apply this treatment: in acute cases of asthma, acute bladder infection, or low body temperature (below 97°F oral temperature). Be careful to avoid drafts or chills during the treatment. Apply a hot-water bottle to the feet and add more blankets if you feel chilly.

Equipment

   • shower or bath
   • one towel
   • two blankets
   • one sheet

Directions

1. Spread the blankets lengthwise on a bed with the sheet over them.

2. Wet the towel with cold water and wring out excess water. The towel should be damp, not dripping.

3. Take a hot bath or shower, as hot as you can comfortably stand it, for 5–10 minutes. You should feel warm after the bath or shower; if not, postpone the treatment until you are feeling warmer.

4. Get out of the shower and dry off.

5. Wrap the cold towel all the way around your trunk.

6. Lie down on the blankets and sheet prepared earlier.

7. Wrap the sheets and blankets snugly around you.

8. Sleep, rest, meditate, or listen to quiet music for 25–30 minutes, or until your body has warmed the toweling.

Note: The greater the contrast between hot and cold applications, the stronger the treatment. You can increase the effect of the treatment by placing the cold, wet towel in the freezer for 5–10 minutes before applying.

SALT-WATER LAVAGE AND GARGLE

This treatment helps to eliminate excessive mucous from the nose and throat. Salt water soothes inflamed mucosal tissue *and* acts as an anti-microbial. Viruses and bacteria cannot survive in a concentrated saline solution. The difference in osmotic pressure between the salt solution and their own cellular-fluid concentration causes the viruses and bacteria literally to explode.

Begin gargling with salt water at the first sign of a sore throat. Repeat every 3–4 hours until the symptoms resolve. Use the nasal lavage technique when nasal congestion develops, or after exposure to irritating inhalants (e.g., dust, air pollution, mold).

Equipment

   • tall glass or large cup
   • water, as warm as you can comfortably tolerate
   • 1 1/2 teaspoons of sea salt (noniodized)

Directions

1. Add sea salt to glass of warm water.

2. For gargle, take one mouthful of salt water at a time. Some physicians recommend swallowing the salt water after gargling. Do not swallow the salt water if you have hypertension or diabetes.

3. For nasal lavage, pour salt water into your cupped hand. Gently inhale the salt water, then gently blow the water from the nostrils. This is best done over a sink. At the end of the treatment, be sure to blow any excess water from the nose. You may notice increased nasal and sinus drainage after the treatment.

Note: Too much or too little salt or cool water may cause nasal tingling and discomfort. Adjust the water temperature or amount of salt if you experience nasal discomfort.

WET-SOCKS TREATMENT

This simple, powerful treatment stimulates the production and activity of white blood cells and draws congestion away from the upper body. The wet-socks treatment speeds resolution of an upper-respiratory infection. If used when the very first symptoms begin, the treatment can even abort a cold.

Equipment

   • foot bath (a plastic dishpan works well, or sit on the edge of a bathtub and soak feet in hot, shallow water)
   • towel
   • one pair of cotton ankle-high socks
   • one pair of wool socks

Directions

1. Soak feet in water as hot as you can comfortably tolerate for 5–10 minutes. Add more hot water if necessary.

2. Dry feet.

3. Wet cotton socks in cold tap water. Wring out thoroughly. (Socks should be damp, not dripping.)

Continued ➡

4. Get in bed. Put on the damp cotton socks. Immediately cover with the wool socks.

5. Go to sleep.

Note: This treatment is best done right before bedtime. In most cases, the socks will be dry by morning.

HOT FOOT BATH

A hot foot bath can treat a wide variety of ailments, from simple tension headaches, to upper-respiratory infections, to menstrual cramps.

Equipment

- plastic dishpan, tub, or bowl large enough to soak the feet

- towel for drying feet.

Directions

1. Fill the pan with enough water to cover the ankles. The water should be as hot as you can comfortably stand it.

2. Soak the feet for 5–10 minutes maximum. More than ten minutes of heat exposure promotes congestion more than circulation.

For a more powerful treatment, alternate between hot-water and cold-water baths.

1. Soak the feet in hot water for five minutes.

2. Soak the feet in cold water for one minute.

3. Repeat this cycle at least three times.

4. Always end with cold water.

ALTERNATING HOT AND COLD APPLICATIONS

Alternating hot and cold applications to a local area increases circulation and decreases congestion. From a Chinese perspective, congestion or "stagnation" causes pain. This simple method can be employed to reduce pain and swelling associated with acute injuries, ear infections, headaches, and other conditions.

In general, the greater the contrast in temperature between the hot and cold applications, the stronger the treatment. For children, the elderly, and severely debilitated people (e.g., terminal cancer, late stages of AIDS or emphysema), moderate the temperature extremes.

Equipment

- two towels

- a large pan of hot water, or a microwave

- a pan of cold water, with ice cubes (if tolerated)

- a plastic sheet (or an old shower curtain), if needed to protect bedding

Directions

1. Always begin with a 3–5-minute hot application. This can be a towel wrung out in hot water (as hot as you can stand it) or a wetted towel placed in a microwave for 3–4 minutes. If the towel is too hot, shake it back and forth for a couple of moments—towels cool quickly. Apply the towel to the affected area.

2. Apply a cold application (towel wrung out in cold tap water or ice water) to the affected area for one minute.

3. Repeat this cycle at least three times.

4. Always end with a cold application.

General Advice

- Make sure an area is warm before applying a cold towel. If someone is severely chilled, or if the body temperature is below 98°F, warm the body with a hot bath or shower before applying cold towels.

- For acute earaches, a 40-watt lightbulb can be substituted for a hot, wet towel. Sit 6–8 inches away from the lightbulb, close enough to feel

heat, but not close enough to burn the skin. To reduce pain associated with earache, use heat alone for up to 30 minutes.

- A hot-water bottle can substitute for a hot, wet towel.

- For a small area, frozen peas in a plastic bag can be substituted for a cold, wet towel.

Botanical Medicine

The plant realm provides an astounding array of medicines. Botanical medicines, or herbs, are available in several forms. Consider growing your own medicinal herbs—you will learn much more about their healing properties, and you will have a steady supply of medicines.

Outlined below are some basic preparation techniques and dosage instructions. Please follow the recommended dosages for the different types of herbs to achieve maximum benefit while minimizing potential side effects from overdosage.

A Note on Dosages

The following is a general rule of thumb for dosing herbs:

- For acute illnesses, take two dropperfuls of tincture, or two capsules of dried herb, every 2–4 hours, depending on the severity of the condition.

- *Six years old:* take half the adult dosage (i.e., one dropperful every 2–4 hours)

- *Three years old:* take one-fourth the adult dosage.

- *One year old:* take one-sixth the adult dosage.

A Few Definitions

Infusion (steeped tea): For leafy herbs, use one ounce of herbs per pint of water. Bring water to a boil and pour over the herbs. Steep for 10–15 minutes, strain, and drink.

Decoction (simmered tea): Roots, berries, and thick leaves require more than infusing to release the healing constituents of the plant. Bring a pint of water to a boil, then add two tablespoons of dried herb to the water. Simmer for 10–15 minutes. If you are adding leaves to the herbal formula, add them to the decoction after simmering, remove the pan from the burner, and allow the herbs to steep for another ten minutes.

Tincture: Tinctures are made by soaking herbs in a solvent—generally food-grade alcohol or vinegar—to produce a concentrated herbal medicine. The constituents released, which will vary depending on the solvent and the herb, are similar to those found in botanical infusions and decoctions, albeit in a more concentrated form.

Essential Oils

Essential oils are extremely concentrated herbal preparations. An ounce of essential oil represents several pounds of dried plant material. Use the oils respectfully.

Inhalations: Steam inhalations are very effective for breaking up lung and sinus congestion. Steam also deep-cleans the skin. Pour boiling water into a large bowl or pan. Add two or three drops of essential oil. Make a "tent" by draping a towel over the head and edges of the basin. Lean over the hot water and inhale the steam. End the treatment by rinsing the face with cold water.

Internal use: For stomach upset, add one drop of essential oil of peppermint to a glass of warm water. Never take more than one or two drops of essential oil internally. Some essential oils (e.g., sandalwood) are toxic and should never be taken internally.

External use: Add four to five drops of essential oil to a cup of vegetable oil for a soothing massage or after-bath oil. Oils of peppermint, eucalyptus, clove, and/or tea tree added to vegetable oil or petroleum jelly make a soothing chest rub for coughs and colds. If the essential oil causes a skin rash even when diluted in vegetable oil, discontinue use.

Caution: Applying essential oils directly to the skin can cause irritation and skin rash. Never apply to the area around the eyes or genitals, where essential oils can cause tissue damage.

Baths

The skin and muscles especially benefit from herbal baths. Place herbs in a soft, loosely woven cloth (muslin is ideal), gather the edges in at the center, and tie with a string or ribbon. Tie the herbal pouch below the water spigot so that warm bath water runs through it as you fill the tub. *Alternative method:* steep herbs as for an herbal infusion and add the strained tea to the bath water.

Granules

Chinese herbs are sometimes prepared in granular form. The granules are made from evaporated herbal teas.

Basic Herbs for the Home Medicine Chest

Alfalfa (*Medicago sativa*) leaves—Alfalfa has an overall tonifying effect on the body, making it an ideal herb to help rebuild after a major illness. Encourages healthy teeth and gum tissue.

Chamomile (*Matricaria chamomile*) flowers—Chamomile contains high levels of calcium, making it an excellent nerve and muscle relaxant. Chamomile soothes upset stomach, and encourages sleep if taken 1–2 hours before bedtime.

Dandelion (*Taraxacum officinalis*) root and leaf—Dandelion leaf acts as a diuretic, potent enough to affect even congestive heart failure. Dandelion root is a liver tonic, increasing bile production and encouraging detoxification.

Echinacea (*Echinacea angustafolia* or *purpurea*) flowers—Echinacea's antimicrobial action is excellent for upper-respiratory infections. As a general immune

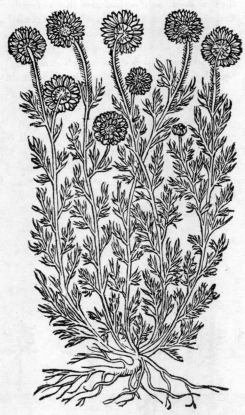

Chamomile (Matricaria chamomile)

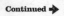

Continued ➡

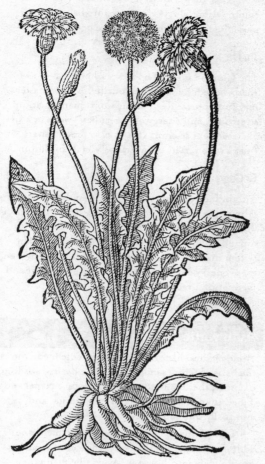

Dandelion (Taraxacum officinalis)

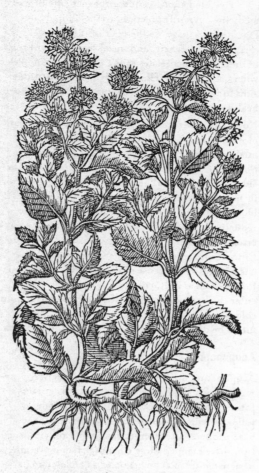

Mint (Mentha piperita)

stimulant, echinacea increases white blood cell activity.

Ginger (*Zingiber officinalis*) root—Ginger is a warming carminative, soothing digestive function. Ginger also acts as a diaphoretic, inducing sweating.

Goldenseal (*Hydrastis Canadensis*) root—Goldenseal is antimicrobial and tonic for both the digestive and circulatory systems. Helpful for chronic stomach problems, sinusitis, colds, and coughs.

Note: Goldenseal also kills helpful intestinal bacteria. After taking a course of goldenseal, encourage repopulation of normal gut flora by eating fresh sauerkraut, yogurt, kefir, or Korean *kim chee* (cabbage pickled in garlic and chile).

Mint (*Mentha piperita*) leaves and essential oil—Mint leaves can be brewed into a tea for upset stomach, or taken at the beginning of a cold. One or two drops of essential oil in a bowl of hot water makes a wonderful vapor inhalation for a cough or cold. Mint has the ability to increase oxygenation, thereby helping to stop bacterial and viral lung infections.

Nettles (*Urtica urens*) leaves—Nettle leaves are a powerful spring tonic, particularly beneficial for the kidneys.

Oatstraw (*Avena sativa*) straw and seed chaff—Oatstraw is soothing and nourishing for the nerves. Also excellent for stress, anxiety, and mild insomnia.

Red raspberry leaf (*Rubus ideus*) leaves—This uterine tonic helps normalize menstrual periods and supports uterine tone during pregnancy.

Yarrow (*Achillea millefolium*) flowers—Yarrow stanches bleeding and acts as a diaphoretic, inducing sweating and mild temperature elevation. As a urinary antiseptic, yarrow can help stop urinary-tract infections if taken in the early stages.

Note: All leafy herbs (e.g., mint leaves) should be replaced annually. If kept longer, the herbs lose their essential oils and other healing constituents. Root herbs may be kept for two seasons if stored in a cool, dry place.

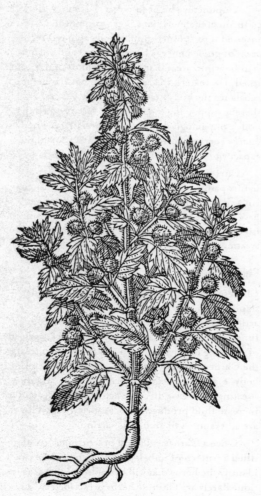

Nettles (Urtica urens)

Homeopathic Medicine

Homeopathy, which literally means "study of similars," is a medical science that shares a common healing philosophy with naturopathic medicine. Both aim to stimulate the body's innate healing capacity to bring about a "cure." Developed by Samuel Hahnemann, a late-nineteenth-century German physician, the science of homeopathy grew out of Hahnemann's years of medical-text translations. Discouraged by the medical practices of his day, Hahnemann turned to translating medical texts in part to support his large family, and also in hopes of discovering, or rediscovering, certain universal laws of healing that seemed to be missing in contemporary medical practice.

While translating a *material medica*, Hahnemann noted an explanation that quinine cured malaria because of its astringent properties. To test the assertion, Hahnemann took four drams (one-half ounce), or about fifteen doses, of quinine every morning and evening. Within four days he developed the symptoms of malaria in his formerly healthy body. When Hahnemann stopped taking the quinine, the symptoms disappeared.

With this experiment, Hahnemann confirmed the "law of similars," an ancient healing principle of using like to cure like. In other words, a substance that produces symptoms in a healthy person can be used to treat the same symptoms in an ailing person. Hahnemann—and, later, a large following of students—began a series of experiments to test the effects of various plant and mineral extracts on healthy subjects. Hahnemann himself tested and meticulously recorded the effects of many substances before his death in 1843 at the age of eighty-eight.

During his years of research, Hahnemann discovered another basic truth: the more dilute the medicine, the more potent its effect. His discovery ran contrary to the practices of his day, an era when doctors used large doses of mercury, sulfur, coal oil, and other toxic compounds to produce violent, cathartic effects in the body.

Homeopathic remedies are prepared by diluting one drop of base tincture, prepared from the whole plant, in either ten ("x" potencies) or 100 ("c" potencies) drops of water. This mixture is "secussed" (banged or shaken a specific number of times) to potentize the remedy. Next, one drop of the 1x (1:10) or 1c (1:100) solution is placed in a vial with another ten or 100 drops of water. The process is repeated until the solution is the desired potency, or dilution.

Many physicians have dismissed the effects of homeopathic remedies, declaring them placebos. Voluminous clinical studies, however, have demonstrated the efficacy of homeopathic medicines. Recent double-blind research also conclusively demonstrates the effectiveness of homeopathic remedies in treating particular diseases.

Despite positive test results, all double-blind studies of homeopathic treatments share a common weakness: the same homeopathic remedy is given to different subjects suffering with the same disease. In contrast to this procedure, the homeopathic method of prescribing involves assessing the complete symptom picture and choosing a remedy that best suits the individual. One person with a cold, for example, may have severe chills, sensitivity to light, and extreme irritability, while another patient reports having a fever, desiring cold air, and wanting company to console her. For the first patient, the homeopath might prescribe *Nux vomica*; for the second, *Pulsatilla*. In a double-blind study, she would be required to give both patients the same remedy.

Continued ➔

Using a double-blind study to test homeopathic medicines is like using a yardstick to measure the pitch of a sound—the instrument is inappropriate for the task. The homeopath's great strength is his or her ability to focus first on the human being and secondarily on the disease.

Physical Therapies

Physical therapies include a broad range of techniques and therapeutic approaches. Again, different patients respond best to different techniques. Therapies range from osseous (bone) manipulation and deep-tissue work, to more subtle approaches such as cranio-sacral or Bowen work. The therapies generally address musculoskeletal ailments, although the chiropractic profession has demonstrated quite definitively that a wide range of acute and chronic internal conditions will respond to osseous manipulation.

Chinese Medicine

Balance is the hallmark of Chinese medicine. In a state of health, our bodies are constantly shifting, elegantly balanced organisms. "Balance" by no means implies "static" within the Chinese healing paradigm. A healthy body constantly shifts and changes to maintain a dynamic state of equilibrium. The Chinese refer to the balance of *yin* and *yang*, which encompasses all of the opposites one could imagine—e.g., light/dark, hot/cold, dry/wet, interior/exterior. The Chinese understand that an extreme of any one condition inevitably leads back to its opposite, like the snake curling to bite its own tail. The classic yin/yang symbol contains a spot of light within the dark half, and a spot of dark within the light half, hinting at the understanding that each condition or quality carries the seed of its opposite within itself.

Traditional Chinese medicine aims to address the whole person. Like naturopathic physicians, a practitioner of Chinese medicine will ask questions about a person's constitution, lifestyle patterns, and general physical symptoms. This information allows the practitioner to identify patterns of health or imbalance. Such patterns, or "syndrome pictures," guide the practitioner to the most supportive treatments for a particular patient, treatments that will help restore the balance of the body so that it can return to optimal health.

Traditional Chinese medicine includes four major treatment areas: acupuncture, Chinese herbs, *tui na* (body work), and *qi gong* (movement and meditation). An office visit might include one or more of these four major treatment methods.

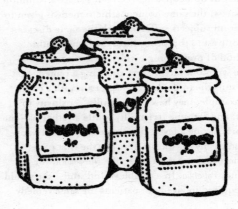

"Five Elements" is another branch of Chinese medicine currently practiced in the United States. Practitioners diagnose the relationships between earth, fire, water, air, and metal in the body. Each of these elements relates to the others in a complex, synergistic pattern. The Five Elements practitioner aims to rebalance the five elements and thus restore health to the body.

Note: Chinese medicine often describes conditions more poetically than does our objective Western medical terminology. A Chinese medical practitioner, for example, might diagnose someone with "blood deficiency." The patient does not necessarily have a blood imbalance that would show up on a blood test (e.g., anemia), but rather a qualitative reduction of the blood's moistening, cooling properties that might manifest as dry skin and hair. The Chinese also refer to "external pernicious influences" (EPI's) as a cause of disease. These external forces—such as heat, cold, wind, and damp—can enter the body and cause acute illnesses. A common cold with sore throat and headache, for example, might be diagnosed as an invasion of wind and heat.

Acupuncture

Acupuncture works with the body's own energy currents, which are measurable as electromagnetic forces. This magnetic force, or "river of energy," follows predictable patterns in the body. Chinese practitioners, after centuries of study and observation, have mapped these currents of energy and designated them as "meridians" correlated to particular organs and systems in the body.

Acupuncture helps to direct the energy flow, or *qi*, through the meridians. Very thin needles inserted into "points" on the body help redirect areas of pooled energy ("stagnation") and encourage *qi* to flow into areas that are deficient or undernourished. Ultimately, the acupuncture needles help to rebalance the body's electromagnetic currents, thereby supporting the internal organs and all the body's physiological systems. Redirecting the body's energy currents through acupuncture also has the capacity to restore mental and emotional balance.

Currently, acupuncture is covered under a naturopathic physician's license only in Connecticut and Arizona. Some naturopathic physicians also have a degree in Oriental medicine and can administer acupuncture in addition to other naturopathic treatments.

Chinese Herbs

Chinese herbal medicine relies on a deep understanding of herbs from the perspective of their actions as "simples" (single herbs), as well as their function in combination with other herbs. Instead of focusing on what illness a particular herb treats, the Chinese consider the general effects on the body, e.g., does the herb warm the body? Cause sweating? Increase digestive action? Does it tend to increase fluid production? Cause dryness? These are all examples of an herb's "actions."

Once a Chinese medical practitioner has identified a pattern of imbalance in the body, she can identify the herbs that will best address the situation. Rarely are Chinese herbs prescribed as "simples"; instead, they are combined to create a powerful synergistic blend. Formulas include secondary herbs to balance potential side effects of the major herbs in the formula. A combination of herbs to stop a fever, for example, may contain a small amount of warming herb along with the cooling herbs. The single warming herb moderates the strong cooling action of the other herbs, thereby protecting the body from harsh extremes in temperature. Other herbs may amplify the effects of

one of the major herbs in a formula. The herbal combinations always aim to restore balance, or physiological equilibrium, in the body.

Tui Na

The Chinese form of body work known as *tui na* is a richly varied therapeutic modality. A *tui na* master may incorporate deep-tissue work, manipulation, stretching, and energy or "meridian" work in a single treatment session. Gifted *tui na* practitioners treat a wide variety of musculoskeletal conditions.

Qi Gong

This branch of Chinese Medicine applies the wisdom of the body's "subtle energies" in conjunction with the universal life energy. *Qi gong* masters expand upon the understanding of the meridian system in the body and teach students to strengthen these energy currents through daily movement and meditation practices.

Ayurvedic Medicine

Some medical historians cite Ayurvedic medicine as the basis of Chinese medicine. The healing wisdom of India, they contend, moved first into Nepal and Tibet, then gradually filtered into China, and eventually into Japan as well.

Like Chinese medicine, Ayurvedic medicine addresses balance in the body. Instead of focusing on five elements, however, Ayurvedic medicine focuses on three: fire (*pitta*), earth (*kapha*), and air (*vatta*). Ayurvedic diagnosis involves evaluating a patient's constitution according to the predominance of one or more of these elements, or *doshas*. In reality, the *doshas* constantly fluctuate in the body, maintaining a dynamic equilibrium from moment to moment. An Ayurvedic practitioner prescribes treatment according to the patient's constitution. In addition, he or she may include treatments to rectify acute imbalances.

A complete Ayurvedic therapeutic program may include diet, exercise, herbs, meditation, breathing, and physical therapy recommendations. The physical therapies encompass a broad range of treatments, including massage, sound and color therapy, and detoxification techniques.

Indigenous Medicine

Indigenous Earth-based cultures the world over possess a profound knowledge of healing. One Chippewa (Ashnabe) teacher described three types of healers in his culture: those who heal with their hands, those who heal with herbs, and those who heal with their mind, through teaching. His path was the last one, although he also had an impressive knowledge of herbs. When a woman approached him for information about a particular plant and its healing properties, he gave her a mystified look. "You're a two-legged, just like me," he said. "Why don't you go ask the plant?"

Many Western scientists assume that indigenous peoples developed their healing methods strictly through trial and error. In reality, most indigenous cultures employ a higher form of investigative science. They know the plants and animals in their locale as intimately as they do their own children. They watch ailing animals to see what they do to heal themselves. Through dreams, they are guided to new plant allies. In quiet moments, they are inspired to use therapies involving minerals, water, air, and fire. Most indigenous peoples have perfected the art of "deep listening," stilling the

Continued ➔

mind's chatter enough to make room for the quieter, subtler voices of the Earth's inhabitants. This ability to listen deeply has developed healers and therapeutic techniques that sometimes defy scientific explanation.

Many indigenous healers know, for example, that a plant acts more powerfully when one gives thanks and honors its spirit. Distractedly throwing mint in a teapot and brewing an after-dinner tea has a less potent effect than skillfully growing the herb, gathering it with prayer, offering thanks to the Creator, and invoking the healing capacities of that plant ally. This attitude of reverence evokes a different response, a deeper resonance, and a profound opportunity for healing. One's relationship to a plant or element greatly affects its healing power. Western technology has no means of measuring, and thereby justifying, such qualitative differences in administering a healing method.

Native cultures have a deep understanding of "right relationship" with all life forms. Right relationship begins with self and Creator, and circles outward to include one's family, community, and world. "Community" includes all aspects of creation, and relating rightly within that community also includes considering the generations yet to come.

Most indigenous cultures strengthen this weave of Creator, self, community, and world through *ceremony*. Each indigenous culture develops a ceremonial cycle that reflects its relationship with the land and the seasons. If a people must migrate because of famine or invasion, they retain their essence as a culture while adopting the ceremonial cycle of their new home. Ceremonies are specific to different parts of the Earth. Cacti grow well in the desert but not in the rain forest; similarly, ceremonies of the Eastern woodlands do not necessarily make sense in the Southwestern pueblos, even though the indigenous peoples share compatible spiritual concepts.

Ceremony can be a powerful healing tool, encouraging people to reconnect with themselves and their communities. Ceremonies mark individual life transitions as well as the revolving wheel of the seasons. Prayer and ritual can invoke profound healings. Through ceremony we are rooted in place and time, which allows us to expand outward to greet and honor the larger circle of life.

—From *Pocket Guide to Naturopathic Medicine*

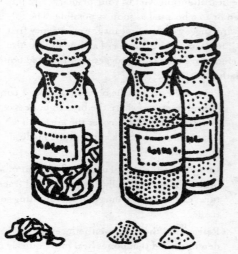

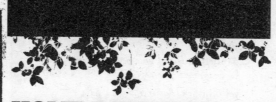

HOME REMEDIES

Judith Boice, N.D.

The body is wise in its response to changes in the internal and external environment. Symptoms we may regard as nuisances may be the body's way of trying to restore balance in a system that is off-kilter. The home remedies mentioned in this section are meant to stimulate the body's ability to restore balance, rather than merely eradicate symptoms.

Keep in mind that treatments must be individualized to address the needs of a particular person. The following suggestions are not intended as one-size-fits-all prescriptions, but as general guidelines to approaching an acute illness or accident. Please incorporate the suggestions in concert with your own intuition and, when necessary, with the guidance of a physician. (Most of the sections below contain information on "When to consult a physician.")

Once the body's equilibrium is disturbed, whether by overwork, emotional upset, or physical injury, the body will attempt to restore balance. The body's most common response to a disturbance is to generate an inflammatory reaction. Fever, for instance, is an inflammatory response to an overgrowth of a bacteria or virus. The body, in its wisdom, knows that bacteria and viruses can survive only in a very narrow temperature range. Elevating the core body temperature by as little as one or two degrees can make the body completely inhospitable to the invading organisms. Clinical studies show that even virulent spirochetes like syphilis cannot endure temperatures above 106°F. Fever therapy, in this case, would entail slowly elevating, maintaining, and then reducing the body temperature over several hours in a clinical setting. Generally the therapeutic range for a fever is 99°–102°F. Please refer to the section of this chapter on "Fevers" for more information on how to work with fevers to restore health.

When a virus takes hold, we say we have "caught a cold." In reality, we are surrounded by viruses and bacteria all the time. As one friend, a devoted bus rider, says, "Riding a public bus in winter is like riding in a petri dish." The bus is a concentrated microcosm of the larger environment. In truth, the Earth as a whole is a "petri dish" teeming with microorganisms that are both harmful and beneficial to human life.

At least two major factors determine whether or not someone "comes down with a cold" or other illness while riding in the "petri dish." One is the strength of the virus. Some pathogens are more virulent than others. The second factor is the strength of the human being (or, more precisely, the condition of the human being's immune system). Someone who eats well, enjoys work, has a loving family environment, and exercises regularly will probably be less susceptible to a virus than someone who eats fast food, works thirteen hours a day, sleeps four hours a night, hates his or her job, and argues incessantly with her mate.

What are the basic principles that support health? Four major areas contribute to overall health and well-being:

· nutrition
· exercise
· mental/emotional health
· trust in and connection with "divinity," i.e., a supportive force larger than oneself

All these factors function synergistically to strengthen health. Restoring health may involve addressing one or more of these factors. Making changes in one area almost certainly will bring about changes in another area. One friend notes that her tendency to overeat diminishes when she meditates twenty minutes before going to sleep at night (mind/spirit affecting body). I notice that I am calmer and more patient when I exercise aerobically at least twenty minutes per day (body affecting mind/spirit).

The newly emerging field of psychoneurimmunology explores this interconnectedness of mind and body, which occurs through the actions of the endocrine, nervous, and immune systems. As Westerners, we are learning what Easterners and indigenous peoples have known for thousands of years: we are "webbed," interconnected within ourselves and with the larger pattern of Creation on this planet. The content of our mind affects our body, just as surely as our physical state affects our mental and emotional well-being.

The best home care is preventive care. Investing in good food, in time for exercise and relaxation, and in loving communication with friends and family will repay you many times over. The suggestions that follow are meant to support you when, despite your best efforts, you are unable to maintain health. Ideally, these treatments will help speed the healing process and quicken the return from inflammation to optimal health (see "Paradigm of Health and Disease"). The aim is to support, not suppress, the body's attempts to heal.

Agatha Thrash, M.D. and Calvin Thrash, M.D. have devoted their lives to administering natural therapeutics for a wide range of illnesses. Their book, *Home Remedies*, is packed with wisdom and therapeutic suggestions. They remind readers that

the natural remedies require time to apply and a simple skill that demands carefulness more than expertise. Because few are willing to give the time and care, the natural remedies are dying out from among us. It is not that natural remedies are less effective than drug remedies, but drug administration makes personal nursing care much less necessary. Simple remedies are not as dramatic, but are generally more effective, and they have far fewer side effects.

From Acne to Teething

Acne

Skin eruptions can be painful, irritating, and embarrassing. Recalling "Laws of Cure," skin irritations and eruptions are less serious than internal-organ diseases because they are closer to the surface of the body. (Try telling that to a teenager getting ready for the prom!) Treating acne requires persistence and a willingness to make lifestyle changes.

Nutritional therapy: From a Chinese perspective, an accumulation of dampness and heat causes acne. Foods that increase dampness in the body include cold foods (ice cream and iced drinks), raw foods, fatty foods (nuts, corn chips, fatty meats, cheese), and sweets. Foods that cause heat accumulation include meat (chicken is the most warming), seafood, and spicy foods.

Generally, include more whole grains, fruits, and vegetables in the diet. These foods are high in fiber and help stimulate elimination of toxins from the body. When the digestive system is overburdened and cannot discharge waste, the body pushes out waste products through the skin.

Eat foods that support the liver. Skin health is

Continued ➡

intimately linked with the liver, which is responsible for removal of many toxins from the body. Liver-supporting foods include beets (root and greens), olive oil, garlic, and lemon juice. Drink plenty of filtered water, at least two to three quarts per day. Water flushes toxins from the body and moisturizes the skin.

Nutritional supplements:

- Vitamin A reduces sebum secretion from the oil glands and encourages tissue healing. This vitamin must be taken at high doses for at least three months to produce an effect. Unfortunately, high doses of vitamin A have potentially toxic side effects. Signs of toxicity include headache, fatigue, constipation, dry or scaly skin, mouth fissures, brittle nails, hair loss, nausea, and vomiting. Vitamin A therapy should be followed by liver screening tests. **Note:** Consult a physician before beginning vitamin A therapy.
- Beta carotene is the precursor to vitamin A and can be taken at high doses (up to 150,000 IU) without risk of side effects. Unfortunately, beta carotene does not have the effect of reducing sebum production but will encourage healing of skin tissue.
- Vitamin E also encourages skin healing and acts as an antioxidant, preventing lipid oxidation and cell damage. Take 400 IU per day.
- Zinc stimulates immune function, promotes skin healing, and acts as an antioxidant. Take 30–60 mg per day.
- Vitamin C has many functions, chief among them being antioxidant activity and connective-tissue healing. Only three mammals—guinea pigs, primates, and humans—do not produce their own vitamin C internally and must rely on their food supply to obtain it. Most humans need far more than the 40 mg of vitamin C that is listed as the Recommended Daily Allowance. For acne treatment, take at least one gram of vitamin C three times per day. Gradually build up to taking nine grams of vitamin C (three grams, three times per day). The body begins to use up more C if a steady supply is available. You cannot take too much—any unused amount of this water-soluble vitamin is passed in the urine. **Caution:** If you have a history of kidney stones, be sure to drink plenty of water with vitamin C therapy, at least two to three quarts of filtered water per day. Whether or not you have kidney stones, use buffered vitamin C supplementation. Instead, gradually reduce your dosage over at least two weeks.

Physical therapies:

- Avoid harsh soaps and ointments that contain sulfur. These cause excessive drying and can irritate the skin.
- Wash the face at least twice per day with a washcloth to stimulate the removal of dead skin.
- Alternate hot and cold applications to the face to stimulate circulation and encourage healing (see "Hydrotherapy" section). Add *Calendula succus* (fresh plant extract) to the cold-water application.
- Avoid picking at the pimples and blackheads. Squeezing and picking can cause scarring and further tissue irritation.

Botanical medicines: The following herbal tea encourages liver health and skin healing. Drink 3–4 cups of herbal tea per day, or two dropperfuls of tincture four times per day.

Combine:

> dandelion root (*Taraxacum officinalis*), 2 parts, by weight
>
> yellow dock (*Rumex crispus*), 1 part
>
> red clover blossoms (*Trifolium pratens*), 1 part
>
> Oregon grape root (*Berberis aquafolium*), 1 part
>
> nettles (*Urtica urens*), 1 part
>
> licorice (*Glycerrhiza glabra*), 1/2 part

Homeopathic remedies: Consult with a homeopathic practitioner to determine the best remedy for you. Generally, a constitutional remedy is more helpful than a prescription based on acute acne symptoms.

When to consult a physician:

- If acne persists, despite following the preceding therapeutic guidelines for at least three months.
- If acne scars the face.
- If acne appears after adolescence, or persists after twenty years of age.

Allergic Reactions, Hay Fever

Hay fever is a relatively mild, although very uncomfortable form of allergic reaction. Treatment of hay fever should begin at least half a year before the onset of allergy season. Supportive therapies may include dietary changes, nutritional supplements, herbal preparations, and stress reduction so that the body's immune system is in optimal condition when hay-fever season arrives.

Mild to moderate allergic reactions may manifest in a variety of ways, from minor headaches or digestive disturbances, to itchy, blotchy skin rashes. Severe allergic reactions, called "anaphylactic shock," cause swelling of the airways. Sufferers often gasp and wheeze, trying to get air through the swollen passageways. In very severe cases, the airway can become completely blocked, causing respiratory arrest.

The following suggestions are for hay fever and mild to moderate allergic reactions:

- Nettles, in freeze-dried capsules, two capsules, every two hours. In freeze-dried form, nettles have been shown to benefit 50 percent of patients suffering hay-fever symptoms.
- Eliminate food and inhalant sensitivities, if known.
- For hay-fever symptoms, reduce or eliminate foods that encourage mucus formation, e.g., dairy products, sugar, and alcohol.

Homeopathic remedies: 30c potency, to be taken every 30–60 minutes during an acute attack, or twice per day during an ongoing allergy reaction. Stop the remedy once you notice signs of improvement.

- *Apis*—for edema, swelling, and blotching of the skin.
- *Carbo veg*—for "air hunger," wants to be fanned.
- *Arsenicum*—for allergic reaction to food; vomiting and diarrhea, burning pains, wants small sips of warm water.

Boils

A boil is caused by a staphylococcus infection localized in a hair follicle. The body's immune system attempts to contain the infection by "walling off" the infected area, leading to increased pressure and pain. Often a boil will cause sharp, even excruciating pain before it comes to a head and releases its pus and blood. The suggestions below are intended to abort the boil, if caught in its early stages, or to speed the resolution and healing of a ripening boil.

- The skin is the largest organ of elimination in the body. When other elimination systems (chiefly the liver, colon, bladder, and lungs) become overburdened, the body will throw off

waste products through the skin. Boils often occur when someone is tired and rundown; the immune system is overburdened, and the organs of elimination cannot process water intake to at least two quarts per day. Eat more whole grains, steamed vegetables, and other fiber-rich foods that will encourage elimination through the colon rather than the skin.
- From a Chinese medical perspective, boils are caused by an accumulation of dampness and heat in the body. Boils are more common in hot, damp climates and occur more frequently during hot, humid summers. When boils begin to form, avoid foods and activities that will increase dampness and heat. Dampness-forming foods include sugar, dairy products (especially ice cream), and greasy foods. Heating foods include alcohol, meat, and hot spices. Living in a damp basement or a damp climate can increase dampness in the body. Saunas, sweat lodges, and steam baths can increase heat in the body.

Homeopathic remedies: 30c potency. Take the remedy 3–4 times per day until the pain and swelling resolve (early stages), or until the boil erupts and discharges (later stage).

- *Belladonna*—for early stage, when the area is red, swollen, and painful.
- *Hepar sulph*—for later stage, when the boil begins to develop a pocket of pus. *Hepar sulph* will cause the coil to discharge or resolve.
- *Silica*—will encourage the boil to discharge. *Silica* also can speed the healing of a boil that is slow to resolve after discharge.

Hydrotherapy: you can increase circulation to the affected area, thus encouraging the boil to come to a head, by alternating hot and cold wet towels to the area. Cover the area with a hot wet towel for five minutes, followed by a cold wet towel for one minute. Alternate the towels at least three times. Always end with a cold application. Repeat the treatment in the morning and evening. The hot towels will increase circulation and soften the skin to encourage discharge from the boil. To avoid spreading the infection, be sure to wash the towels after each treatment. Do not share towels with any household members during the time you are treating the boil.

When to consult a physician:

- If a boil develops near the eyes or nose—the infection can spread to the brain via the facial artery.
- If the boil does not resolve within 4–5 days.
- If the boil erupts but does not heal.

Broken Bones

Broken bones are serious injuries that require medical attention. Get to your primary-care physician or to a hospital as soon as possible. The following suggestions are meant for emergency first aid, to decrease the trauma of a bone break. Also included are home-care suggestions to speed bone healing.

- Protect the area of the bone break. For a compound fracture (where the broken bone has penetrated the skin), cover the area with a clean, soft cloth. Seek appropriate medical attention.
- Immobilize the area. Further movement of a broken bone, especially of a compound fracture, can increase damage to surrounding soft tissue.
- Research in the early twentieth century demonstrated that bones heal more quickly if

Continued ➡

they are bandaged and allowed to move, rather than being immobilized in a cast, because the stress of movement and weight-bearing stimulates healing in the bone. Although you may not be able to convince your physician to eliminate the cast, you can move the limb as much as possible within the constraints of the cast and request a walking cast for a broken fibula or tibia (lower leg).

Homeopathic remedies: 30c potency

- *Arnica*—for acute pain, swelling, trauma to bone and soft tissues. Take one dose every 15–30 minutes as needed for the first 3–4 hours after injury. Continue taking Arnica as needed for the first 36–48 hours after injury.
- *Eupatorium*—specific for bone pain. Begin taking after acute swelling and trauma have passed.
- *Symphytum*—stimulates bone healing.
- *Calcarea phosphorica*, helps reduce bone pain. *Calc phos* is also available as a cell salt, usually in 6x potency.
- *Hypericum*—for shooting, nerve-like pain.
- *Ruta*—stimulates healing of the periosteum (surface layer of the bone). *Ruta* will encourage the final stages of healing, e.g., resolve pain that persists after a cast is removed.

Hydrotherapy can increase circulation and encourage healing. Apply alternating hot (five minutes) and cold (one minute) wet towels to the limb *opposite* the one that is broken. Increasing circulation in one limb reflexively increases circulation in the opposite limb. This method is especially helpful if the limb is bandaged or in a cast.

Note: Never apply heat or cold to a cast or splint.

Bruises

Cayenne liniment: add one tablespoon cayenne pepper to one cup apple-cider vinegar. Allow to sit for a week. Apply the liniment to bruised areas to increase circulation.

Caution: Apply to unbroken skin only. Avoid contact with the eyes.

Homeopathic remedies: 30c potency

- *Arnica*—is the principle remedy, especially for injuries to the head. Take every 30–60 minutes immediately following injury, then 2–3 times per day until you note improvement. Taking Arnica immediately after an injury may stop bruising and swelling completely.
- *Hypericum*—for injuries to highly enervated areas (e.g., eyeball, hands, feet, genitals) or in case of nerve damage or bruising.
- *Aconite*—for hot, throbbing, no discoloration; patient is anxious.
- *Belladonna*—if discolored, throbbing, hot.

Hydrotherapy: alternating hot and cold applications to increase blood circulation.

When to consult a physician:

- If you see red streaks developing around the bruise (usually moving from the site of injury toward the heart), a sign of possible infection.
- If the area continues to swell.
- If a bruise persists for more than 7–10 days.
- If you bruise frequently and easily (a possible sign of bioflavonoid deficiency, clotting disorder, diabetes, or other condition).

Burns

Minor burns respond well to home treatment. The sooner you treat the burn, the less damage will occur and the quicker the healing will take place.

Caution: Do not apply butter or any kind of oil-based cream to the burn. Putting fat or oil on a burn is like throwing fat on a fire—it will intensify the effect of the burn.

Hydrotherapy: Immerse the burned area in cold water as soon as possible.

Homeopathic remedies: 30c potencies. Repeat one dose (three pellets) of the remedy every 2–3 hours until pain and inflammation diminishes, then stop the remedy.

First-degree burn (pain, inflammation, redness)

- *Cantharis*—for burning pain that improves with cold applications. Also for second-degree burn with blister formation.
- *Hypericum*—for extremely tender, painful burns; shooting, nerve-like pain.
- *Apis*—for stinging, itching pain.

Second-degree burn (inflammation, redness and blistering of the skin)

- *Cantharis*—for burning pain that improves with cold applications.

Third-degree burn (charring of the skin, tissue damage)

- *Cantharis*—for burning pain that improves with cold applications. Blister formation.
- *Causticum*—for severe burns, including chemical burns.

Botanical treatments:

- *Aloe vera*, soothes burns and encourages healing. The best, and cheapest, source is fresh leaves from the aloe plant. Open the leaves and use the gel-like substance inside. (The skin of the aloe leaf is not effective for treating burns.) The second best source is bottled aloe vera, available in health food stores. Look for a product without preservatives. Beware of oil-based creams and lotions, which will worsen the effects of the burn.

- *Hypericum* (St. John's Wort)—encourages healing of burns. Use crushed fresh blossoms in a poultice. You also can apply diluted Hypericum tincture to the burn. (Dilute one part of the tincture in ten parts water.) Hypericum oil may be used to *prevent* burns if applied hourly to the skin during sun exposure. For sun-sensitive, fair-skinned people, use Hypericum oil as an emergency backup only. Hypericum is not as strong as a sunblock, but can be helpful if you are stranded somewhere without any other form of protection.

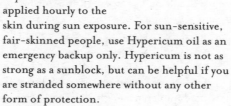
Aloe vera

Caution: Do not use oil of Hypericum *on* burns.

When to consult a physician:

- If you have a second- or third-degree burn (blistering and/or charring of the skin).
- If the burn becomes infected.
- If pain and swelling associated with the burn has not resolved within 4–5 days. (The actual burn, especially with blistering, may take longer to heal, but the pain should stop within 1–2 days.)
- If the burn covers more than 10–15 percent of the body.

Colds

A cold is a healing reaction, the body attempting to regain balance after having been affected by physical or emotional stresses. Fever and mucus discharges are a way of ridding the body of external pernicious influences (such as wind, cold, and heat—see "Chinese Medicine") and built-up waste. Colds do not require treatment; they *are* the treatment. You can speed up the healing process, however, by encouraging the body to discharge the disturbance and return to optimal health (see "Paradigm of Health and Disease").

How To Catch a Cold

Go to a relative's house for Thanksgiving. Eat everything in sight, until you are well beyond pleasantly full. Get into an argument with the brother you haven't seen for three years. Relive every childhood pattern you thought you had outgrown. Stand in the doorway, saying good-bye, without buttoning your coat, for at least twenty minutes. Get in the car, drive home, and watch football on TV. When dinnertime arrives, eat more even though you're not hungry. (Besides, you deserve something delicious because your team lost again in the Kumquat Bowl.)

General recommendations for a cold:

- Rest! Get in bed as soon as possible, and continue to rest for at least twenty-four hours after the symptoms resolve.
- Stop eating for at least one full day, and drink plenty of fluids. Digesting food requires energy that the body might better utilize fighting a viral or bacterial overgrowth. Increasing fluids will thin mucus, making it easier to expel. Fluids also will help prevent dehydration if you have a fever.
- Wet-socks treatment (see "Hydrotherapy" section) before going to sleep. Begin the treatment with the very first symptoms, and you may completely abort the cold. Continue the treatment every night until the symptoms resolve.
- Encourage sweating to push out what the Chinese call "external pernicious influences" (EPIs), such as an invasion of wind, heat, or cold. Simmer a tablespoon of fresh ginger in two cups of water for ten minutes, or steep a tablespoon of yarrow blossom tea in two cups boiling water for ten minutes. Draw a hot bath. Sip the tea while relaxing in the bath. Once you begin to sweat, get out of the bath, towel dry, and get into bed. Wrap up in warm blankets and allow yourself to sweat. Make sure that you are not exposed to drafts or chills during the treatment. Your pores are open, and therefore more susceptible to drafts and chills. In the morning, take a shower to rinse off the sweat and excreted toxins.

Caution: Sweating therapy can further weaken someone who is debilitated (elderly persons, or those with long-term chronic illnesses). Also, children often do not need such aggressive therapy.

- *Tin qiao san*—a Chinese patent medicine for "wind heat invasion." Symptoms include sore throat, feeling more feverish than chilled, slight headache, and yellowish mucus discharge. Do not take the remedy if you feel more chills than fever and have no sore throat, the formula is very cooling. *Tin qiao san* is meant to cause sweating to help push out wind and heat. Make sure to avoid drafts and chills after taking the remedy. Take three tablets four times per day for sore throat. If you have a

Continued ➡

fever, increase the dosage to three tablets every 2–3 hours. This remedy is for the very beginning of a cold, within twenty-four hours (optimally, within 1–2 hours) of the onset of symptoms.

- Salt-water gargle—excellent for sore throats. Salt water soothes the throat and kills bacteria and viruses. Add two teaspoons of sea salt (better than mined table salt) per glass of warm water.
- Hold Echinacea and/or Goldenseal tincture (one dropperful) at the back of the throat as long as possible, then swallow. This is only for the brave! These herbs are strong and have a local antimicrobial effect on the sore throat, as well as working internally on the cold or flu. Repeat every 3–4 hours, as needed.
- Take Hydrastis (Goldenseal) and Echinacea tincture or capsules. These herbs will boost the immune system when taken internally. Take two dropperfuls of tincture or two capsules every 2–4 hours, depending on the severity of the cold.

  —*Six years old*: half the adult dosage (one dropperful every 2–4 hours)

  —*Three years old*: one-quarter the adult dosage

  —*One year old*: one-sixth the adult dosage

  Hydrastis has a drying effect on the mucous membranes, making it ideal for any kind of upper-respiratory infection (sinus, lung, nasal). Echinacea stimulates white blood cell production and activity.

  Note: Some people are sensitive to Hydrastis (Goldenseal). If you notice a skin rash or other allergic reaction developing, stop taking Goldenseal.
- Herbal teas also can help speed the resolution of a cold.

  Combine equal parts:

yarrow	blue vervain
mint	ginger (dried or fresh)

  This is a warming tea and may cause sweating. Add one tablespoon of the above mix to one cup boiling water and steep for ten minutes. Drink one cup 3–4 times per day.

Homeopathic remedies: 30c potency. Take three pellets 2–3 times per day until improvement is noted, then stop taking the remedy.

- *Occilococcinum*—use at the very first hint of a cold, right after the first sneeze. The remedy will not be effective after the first twenty-four hours. Take six of the small pellets every 3–4 hours. You do not need to take the entire tube, as the directions on the bottle may suggest—that is a way of selling you more tubes! Remember that homeopathic remedies act according to frequency of dosage, not the amount.
- *Aconite*—take after the first sneeze, when feeling anxious or fretful; symptoms may have developed following exposure to a cold, dry wind.
- *Allium cepa*—for lots of mucus drainage, sore upper lip, excoriating discharge from the nose, bland discharge from eyes; feels worse in a warm room, better in fresh air.
- *Arsenicum*—if affected by changes in weather; thin, painful, burning discharges; patient seeks warmth.
- *Pulsatilla*—for thick, bland discharges, often green or yellow. Changing symptoms: pains move around and do not localize. Patient feels better outside, worse in stuffy room. Wants company, wants to be held (children), improves with sympathy. Best for late-stage, "ripe" colds.

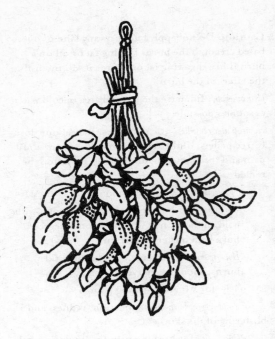

- *Gelsemium*—if slow onset, for colds that begin in warm weather or during a mild winter. Patient feels achy, the limbs heavy, as in a Southern swamp in August. No thirst.
- *Bryonia*—if feels worse with motion, better with pressure. Very hot, very dry, aches all over. Great thirst for cold drinks.
- *Nux vomica*—if very chilly, even while bundled up in bed. Worsens with slight uncovering, or the least movement. Feels chilled from drinking. Aching in limbs and back. Nose stuffed at night. May have upset stomach or other digestive symptoms.

When to consult a physician:

- If you have followed the above suggestions (especially regarding rest) and still have symptoms after seven days.
- If a child has a severe sore throat, especially if she is drooling profusely and cannot swallow.
- If a child has cold and fever symptoms accompanied by a stiff neck or arched back.
- If sore-throat symptoms persist longer than three days.
- If you have a fever above 102°F that does not respond to the suggestions in the "Fever" section of this chapter.

Colic

Be sure to rule out any possible organic causes of colic, such as bowel obstruction or lactose intolerance. Any major problems usually become apparent from a couple of days to a week after birth.

Nutritional therapy:

- Breast-feed children as long as possible. Developing infant digestive and immune systems are not able to handle solid foods until at least six months of age. Many children develop food intolerances because of early exposure to food other than human breast milk. Recent research links adult-onset diabetes with early exposure to cow's milk.
- Smaller, more frequent feedings.
- Skin-to-skin contact can soothe and calm the infant, helping the digestive system to function more smoothly.
- Breast-feeding mothers may experiment with eliminating certain foods to discover any foods that are irritating the infant. Cabbage, caffeine, onions, garlic, and highly spiced foods are common irritants. Laxatives, such as large amounts of prune juice (more than one cup per day), also may irritate the baby's digestive system.

- Feed your baby in a quiet, relaxed environment whenever possible.
- Slippery elm is a good food substitute for extreme cases of colic, acting as a demulcent to soothe the infant's digestive tract. Mix two tablespoons of slippery-elm-bark powder with a small amount of sweetener (maple syrup or molasses). Add hot water or hot milk—mother's milk, if you are still breast feeding—until the mixture is the consistency of porridge. Feed the baby slippery elm in place of other solid foods.

Botanical medicines:

- For breast-feeding mothers, drink chamomile tea to soothe the infant's digestive system.
- For children receiving formula, add 1/4 cup chamomile tea to a bottle of formula.
- Aromatic seeds have a soothing effect on the digestive system. Prepare an infusion of one of the following seeds (one teaspoon of seed per cup of water): cardamom, fennel, anise, cumin. Strain and add 1/4 cup to infant's formula, or drink a cup of this tea 10–15 minutes before breast feeding.

Physical therapy:

Gently massage the infant's abdomen with a good vegetable oil (e.g., sesame, almond, or other cold-pressed oil) in a clockwise, circular motion.

Homeopathic remedies: 30c potency

- *Magnesium phosphorica*—for cramping pain that improves with warm applications.
- *Chamomilla*—if the child is extremely irritable, wants to be carried, then demands to be put down. Inconsolable. One cheek is red, the other pale.
- *Cholocynthis*—forcramping, abdominal pain that is relieved by pressure and by drawing the knees toward the chest.
- *Bryonia*—if feels worse following the slightest motion; generally irritable.

When to consult a physician:

- If the infant is losing weight.
- If colic routinely disturbs the infant's sleep cycle.

Constipation

A healthy person with a healthy digestive tract will have one to three bowel movements per day. Normal stools are light brown with no mucus or blood, well-formed, soft, and easy to pass.

Persons suffering with constipation go two or three days without having a bowel movement. Difficulty passing stools does not necessarily mean one is constipated. The following suggestions will also benefit patients who have daily bowel movements that are difficult to pass.

- Stop taking laxatives. If laxatives are used over a long period of time, the bowel loses its ability to stimulate movement (peristalsis) in the colon. Eventually, the body grows resistant to the laxatives, and movement in the colon ceases altogether. During the bowel-restraining time, you may use herbal laxatives 2–3 times per week, before going to sleep, to replace this action of other laxatives. Decrease the herbs by half a dose per week until you no longer need laxatives to stimulate bowel activity.
- Increase water consumption to at least two quarts per day. Often constipation results from simple lack of fluid in the digestive tract.
- Eliminate coffee, black tea, and other stimulants. Coffee has the effect of increasing gut peristalsis (the contraction of smooth muscle

Continued

in the digestive tract), but also acts as a diuretic, decreasing fluid in the body. (Each cup of coffee results in the loss of two cups of fluid from the body.) Water and herbal teas are better sources of fluid.

- Increase fiber in the diet. Fiber creates bulk in the intestines, which helps stimulate elimination. The simplest way to increase fiber is to eat foods as close as possible to their natural state. Brown rice, for example, contains more fiber than white rice, which contains more than white-rice flour. Apples have more fiber than apple juice. Focus on whole grains, steamed vegetables, and fresh fruits in the diet.

- Develop a regular rhythm for elimination. Some people become constipated because they never make time to have a bowel movement. Generally, early morning is the best time to set aside for bowel training. (From a Chinese perspective, each organ has a time of day when it is most active; large intestine time is 5–7 a.m.) Drink a glass of warm water or herb tea when you get out of bed. Fifteen minutes later, sit on the toilet for at least five minutes. Do not strain or try to force a bowel movement. Get up after five minutes and go about your day. Avoid reading or doing any other activity while sitting on the toilet, to ensure that the mind and body associate the toilet with elimination only. Over time, the body will get used to the rhythm and respond with regular bowel movements.

- Never repress an urge to defecate.

- Exercise at least twenty minutes per day, three days per week (the minimum amount of exercise to maintain aerobic fitness). Exercise stimulates colon activity.

Homeopathic remedies: 30c potency

- *Nux vomica*—for "ineffectual urging to stool," never feel completely emptied. Overuse of laxatives. Chilly, irritable.

- *Sulphur*—for frequent urge with incomplete evacuation. Hard, dry, black stools expelled with great effort, pain, and burning, especially around the anus. Alternating constipation and diarrhea. 5 a.m. diarrhea.

- *Bryonia*—for dry mouth, dry lips, dry tongue. Stools dry and hard, as if burnt. Thirst for large quantities of water.

- *Calc carb*—if feels better the longer the patient doesn't have a bowel movement.

Botanical remedies:

- *Psyllium seeds*—one or two tablespoons taken with water or diluted fruit juice after each meal increases bulk in the stool. The seeds are also mucilaginous, helping to lubricate the stool. With any bulk stool softener, you must increase water intake; otherwise, the fiber will bind the stool and make the constipation even worse.

- *Aloe vera*—aloe vera gel, made from the inner part of the leaves, is a mild laxative that also helps to lubricate stools. Take one tablespoon after each meal. The skin of the aloe vera leaf is a powerful cathartic that should be used only in extreme situations, not on a regular basis.

- *Buckthorn (Cascara sagrada)*—stimulates peristalsis. Some people experience intestinal cramping with cascara. With long-term use, cascara can have the same side effects as chemical laxatives, so short-term usage (1–2 months maximum) is best during the bowel retraining program.

- *Cassia senna*, similar to cascara in its actions and effects.

- *Slippery elm (Ulmus fulva)*—helps to lubricate the stool and increase bulk.

- *Smooth Move* (made by Traditional Medicinals)—a good prepared tea that combines several of the above herbs. As noted above, some people experience intestinal cramping after taking cascara.

When to consult a physician:

- If more than a week passes without having a bowel movement.

- If you follow the above suggestions and still experience constipation. Your physician can test for other causes.

Coughs

Steam inhalation: three to five drops of peppermint oil added to a pan of boiling water. Drape a towel over your head and inhale the steam for 5–10 minutes, or until the vapor begins to cool. Peppermint oil has high concentrations of free menthol, soothing irritated mucous-membrane tissues (which constitute the lining of the entire respiratory tract). Menthol also helps to fight viral and bacterial infections. A steam inhalation at the earliest signs of a cold or flu may abort an illness before it starts.

Essential oils (applied to the chest and neck)

- Combine ten drops each of thyme, rosemary, eucalyptus, and camphorated oil. Rub ten drops of this mixture on the chest and neck 2–3 times per day. Stop if the skin develops a rash or becomes excessively irritated. Some reddening of the skin is normal, as the oils will draw circulation into the area.

- Olbas oil, a commercial preparation, also can be used following the directions given above.

Cuts

- Apply direct pressure to the wound, pressing the area with a clean cloth, bandanna, or T-shirt until bleeding stops.

- Wash the wound with water, or soap and water if available. Washing a puncture wound is especially important, as bacteria can move into a deep wound and remain after the area has healed on the skin surface. Even such virulent bacterial infections as tetanus and rabies can be aborted by carefully washing the wound. Of course, you cannot rely on soap and water alone.

- Apply *Calendula succus* (fresh plant extract of calendula). If stinging results, dilute one part *Calendula succus* in ten parts water. The mixture may be stored in a sterilized spray bottle for use as an antibacterial spray. If soap and water are unavailable, applying *Calendula succus* can take the place of washing.

- *Yunnan pai yao* is a Chinese herbal formula that was brought to the West from Vietnam, where U.S. soldiers witnessed its seemingly miraculous effects. The powder can be packed into wounds to stop bleeding, or taken internally. *Each package comes with one small red pill, which is to be used only for severe hemorrhaging.* The orange-powder capsules, however, may be taken internally, one pill 3–4 times per day, to stop bleeding. Stop taking the medicine as soon as the bleeding stops.

Homeopathic remedies: 30c potency. Take three pellets every 15–30 minutes for acute bleeding. Stop taking the remedy when the bleeding stops.

- *Arnica*—helps stop bleeding, especially bleeding associated with soft-tissue injury.

- *Phosphorous*—for arterial bleeding (bright red blood, usually cascading in spurts).

- *Belladonna*—helps infection, especially staph and strep.

- *Mag phos*—releases muscle tension associated with cuts and other physical trauma.

- *Ferrum phos*—helps stop bleeding.

When to consult a physician:

- If you are bitten by an animal (wild or domesticated).

- If you cannot completely clean a cut or wound. ("Dirty" wounds, especially puncture wounds, may develop tetanus.)

- If you cannot stop the bleeding with direct pressure.

- If infection develops during healing.

Diaper Rash

Most diaper rashes are caused by prolonged exposure to wet, soiled diapers. Keeping the infant's bottom as dry as possible decreases the chances of developing diaper rash.

General recommendations:

- Change diapers frequently, right after each bowel movement.

- Expose baby's bottom to light and air as often as possible.

- Use cotton diapers without plastic pants whenever possible; cotton breathes more than do plastic-coated diapers. Use wool "soakers" instead of plastic pants.

- For severe rashes, apply calendula ointment and/or dust with calendula powder. Calendula promotes skin healing and has antibacterial action.

- Use arrowroot powder or bentonite clay instead of commercial baby powders.

- Use olive oil instead of Vaseline or commercial ointments, which have chemical additives that may irritate the baby's skin.

- Wash diapers with soap flakes. Avoid harsh detergents. Add vinegar to the final rinse water, and dry diapers in the sunshine if possible.

For severe rashes:

- Apply comfrey-root ointment to the diaper rash. Comfrey leaf does not contain as much allantoin, the active constituent that promotes skin healing.

- Apply Calendula ointment, which also promotes skin healing.

- Avoid ointments with goldenseal, as this herb may irritate sensitive tissue in the genital area.

When to consult a physician:

- If you have tried the above suggestions and the rash has persisted for more than a week.

- If the skin is raw or bleeding.

Diarrhea

General recommendations:

- Fast or reduce food intake until the diarrhea has passed.

- Increase water intake to avoid dehydration, especially in young children. For adults, drink at least two to three liters of fluid (dilute juices—half water, half juice) each day.

- Dissolve one tablespoon of bentonite clay in a glass of water and drink the clay solution. The clay will draw irritants and toxins from the intestines.

- Eat burnt toast (one or two slices), or activated charcoal dissolved in water. Dissolve one tablespoon of the charcoal in a glass of water

Continued ➡

and drink. The carbon will absorb toxins and reduce fluid loss.

Note: Activated charcoal will turn the stool black.

- Slippery-elm-bark gruel is easy to digest and soothes the digestive tract. Combine 1/4 cup powdered slippery elm with 3/4 cup water. Bring to a boil, then simmer for approximately five minutes. You also can add one or two tablespoons of slippery elm to oatmeal or other cooked cereal. Eat several tablespoons of the slippery elm gruel every 2–3 hours.

Homeopathic remedies: 30c potency

- *Arsenicum*—for explosive diarrhea with vomiting. Patient is exhausted, restless, anxious; desires hot drinks, in small sips.
- *Bryonia*—following exposure to cold, dry wind, or after a fright.
- *Chamomilla*—for diarrhea with teething (infants); grass-green stools with undigested food. The diarrhea has mucus and blood, and smells like rotten eggs.
- *Cholocynthis*—for frequent urging, severe colicky pains, relieved by pressure and bending double.
- *Nux vomica*—for diarrhea caused by "dietary indiscretion" (eating too much or eating heavy, rich foods). Diarrhea alternating with constipation. Frequent urging, often with no passing of stool; irritable; chilly.
- *Pulsatilla*—for diarrhea from rich foods and pastries. Diarrhea at night. Diarrhea from taking cold drinks. Variable, no two stools alike.
- *Sulphur*—if diarrhea drives patient out of bed at 5 a.m. Stools are painless, variable in consistency and amount. Red anus.
- *Gelsemium*—for nervous diarrhea ("stage fright").

When to consult a physician:

- If the diarrhea persists for more than two days
- If a high fever (above 102°F) accompanies the diarrhea.
- If you see pus or blood in the diarrhea.
- If you have severe, continuous abdominal pain with the diarrhea.

Earache

Earaches are especially common in children, in large part because the developing Eustachian tubes do not effectively drain the ear. Whether young or old, the pain associated with ear infections is usually intense and requires immediate care.

The best treatment is prevention. Many children respond well to dietary changes. Eliminating dairy and sugar reduces mucus-forming foods; dairy and wheat are the two most common food allergens in North America. Sometimes removing these three foods—milk, sugar, and wheat—is enough to stop recurrent ear infections.

Most children with chronic ear infections are caught on a merry-go-round of antibiotic treatments. The antibiotics clear the infection, but another quickly follows, usually within 4–6 weeks. Antibiotics wipe out the good bacteria in the body, as well as the invading bacteria in the ear. After antibiotic treatment, the body is more susceptible to infection.

Keeping the ears warm and covered when outdoors also helps prevent ear infections, as does increasing vitamin C during the cold season. For children, 500 mg of vitamin C twice per day is an adequate dosage. Adults may supplement 2–3 grams twice per day.

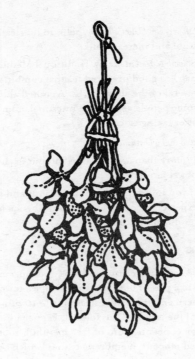

The following suggestions are for acute ear infections, when preventive measures have not succeeded.

General recommendations:

- Sit the patient near a 40-watt lightbulb, with the ear close enough to feel warmth, but not close enough to cause burning. Carefully monitor. The warmth will soothe ear pain and increase circulation in the area, which brings more immune cells to fight the infection.

Hydrotherapy:

- Alternate hot and cold applications to the ear. Wring out a washcloth in water as hot as you can stand and apply for five minutes to the ear. Follow with a cold application (a wet washcloth put in the freezer, or a bag of frozen peas) for one minute. Repeat the cycle, alternating hot and cold, at least three times. Always end with a cold application.
- Wet-socks treatment at bedtime (see "Hydrotherapy" section).
- Constitutional hydrotherapy treatment once per day (see "Hydrotherapy" section).

Botanical therapy:

- *Oil of mullein and/or garlic*—Place two or three drops of gently warmed oil in the ear. (Warm the oil by placing the bottle in a bowl of hot water for a couple of minutes.) Mullein oil reduces pain and inflammation. Both garlic and mullein have antimicrobial action.

  Caution: Use ear drops only if the tympanic membrane (eardrum) is not broken.
- *Echinazea and goldenseal tincture or capsules*—Dose according to age

  —*Twelve and older:* full dose (two dropperfuls, or two capsules every 2–4 hours)

  —*Six years old:* half the adult dosage (one dropperful, or one capsule every 2–4 hours)

  —*Three years old:* one-quarter the adult dosage

  —*One year old:* one-sixth the adult dosage

Homeopathic remedies: 30c potency

- *Aconite*—if earache begins after exposure to cold, dry wind. Bright red ears, high fever, sudden onset. Very sensitive to noise. Sharp pain. Anxious, restless. Thirst for cold drinks. Onset after shock.
- *Belladonna*—for sudden, violent onset. Dilated pupils. Throbbing blood vessels in the neck. Pain causes delirium. Child may have nightmares and call out in sleep. Throbbing,

shooting, sharp pains. No thirst with fever. Red-hot throbbing ear.

- *Chamomilla*—for irritable, intense pain. One cheek is red, the other pale. The child wants to be held and carried, yet arches her back. Inconsolable. Earaches from teething. Grass-green stool.
- *Ferrum phos*—for first stage of infection, before pus develops. Pulsating, throbbing pain. Flushed face. High fever with few symptoms. Use when Belladonna fails.
- *Hepar sulph*—for mucus, pus in ear. For later stage of infection, when pus has developed behind the eardrum. Hates drafts, wants to cover ears or head. Chilly, oversensitive, sweats easily. Feels better with hot, damp weather.
- *Pulsatilla*—for a "ripe" (second or third stage) cold and ear infection. Copious, thick, yellow-green discharge. Changing symptoms. No thirst. Feels better in fresh, cold, open air; worse in warm, stuffy room. Feels worse in the evening.

When to consult a physician:

- If ear infections occur more than once or twice in a year.
- If ear infection and pain persist for more than four days.
- If ear infection is accompanied by a high fever (above 102°F).
- If the child has a stiff neck or arches the back.
- If the ear oozes pus or blood.
- If redness or swelling develops in the bony area behind the ear.

Eye Injuries

The major causes of eye injuries include:

- sunburn
- foreign body
- bruising
- laceration

Important: Eye injuries are very serious and require emergency care for all but the simplest of irritations.

TREATMENT FOR SUNBURNED EYELIDS

Sunburn often occurs when someone falls asleep while sunbathing. This is one eye injury you may treat at home without concern about consulting a physician *unless the burn affects the eyeball.*

- Apply aloe vera or sliced cucumber to the eyelids. Be sure to keep aloe vera out of the eye itself.

Homeopathic remedies: 30c potency. Take three pellets 2–3 times per day until symptoms improve.

- *Hypericum*—for redness with extremely sensitive, burning pain; first-degree burn.
- *Ruta*—for burns to the eyeball. Administer while en route to the hospital.
- *Apis*—for swollen lids. Profuse, hot tears. Photophobia (aversion to bright light), but can't bear covering eyes.

When to consult a physician:

- When the eyeball is affected.
- If the sunburned eyelid is blistered or looks charred.

TREATMENT FOR FOREIGN BODIES IN THE EYES

These suggestions are for care en route to the hospital.

- Loosely patch both eyes, even if only one side is injured. Tight bandaging may cause the

Continued ➡

object to move deeper into the eye. Loosely bandaging both eyes reduces movement. (If only one eye is bandaged, both eyes will continue to move in response to what one eye sees.) You can use anything for a bandage, although a dry, sterile bandage is ideal. A clean T-shirt or other soft cloth will work in an emergency situation.

- If something is sticking out of the eye, cut a hole in the bottom of a paper cup and affix the lip of the cup to the facial surface (cheeks, forehead, etc.) surrounding the eye, with the object protruding through the hole in the cup. The cup will keep the object from moving and protect the eye from further damage.

- Never put ointment in the eye.

- For sand or grit, you may not need to go to the hospital if you are able to remove it by using one or more of the following suggestions:

1. Blink, up to 100 times. Blinking moves objects to the corners of the eye, where they are easy to remove.

2. Flood the eye with water.

3. Push up the lower lid, pull upper lid out and down (over the lower lid), then roll the eye. This will move the object to the center of the eye.

4. Touch the foreign body with a damp sterile cotton applicator (best), or a clean damp handkerchief or bandanna.

5. End with a Calendula wash—ten drops of *Calendula succus* in two tablespoons of water (best to use sterile water or saline solution).

Homeopathic remedies: 30c potency, three pellets 2–3 times per day until symptoms resolve.

- *Silica*—pushes out foreign objects

Herbs to soothe the eye after removing sand or grit: make a tea of euphrasia ("eyebright") by placing one tablespoon of dried herb (leaf) in a cup of boiling water. Steep for ten minutes, then strain through cheesecloth or other filtering material. Allow the tea to cool to room temperature, then flush the eye with tea using an eye cup (available at most pharmacies). Make a new batch of tea each day.

Treatment for Bruises to the Eye

Administer the following treatments en route to the hospital.

General recommendations:

- Immediately apply washcloths wrung out in cold water, replacing as they are warmed by the eye, or apply tofu that has been in the refrigerator.

- After 24 hours, alternate hot and cold applications, five minutes with a warm washcloth, one minute with a cold washcloth. Repeat the cycle at least three times, always ending with a cold washcloth for one minute.

Homeopathic remedies: 30c potency. Take one dose of the remedy 2–3 times per day until symptoms improve.

- *Ruta*—is called the "Arnica of eye." For acute trauma or for slow healing of the eyeball. After serious injury, you can take *Ruta* every 20–60 minutes as required.

- *Hypericum*—for sharp, shooting nerve pain and numbness around eye.

- *Ledum*—for black eye. Feels better with cold applications.

- *Aconite*—for sudden heat. Feels anxious. Use during the first twenty-four hours after injury.

Fever

Fever is a response to

- endogenous pyrogens (fever-causing chemicals produced in the body)
- bacteria
- exercise
- dehydration

The body produces endogenous pyrogens when bacteria or viruses overgrow in the body. These pyrogens signal the body to increase the core temperature. They also are responsible for many of the symptoms associated with a fever—achiness, fatigue, mental dullness. Again, these reactions can be seen as protective. Often the body needs rest more than anything else.

As mentioned earlier, the body knows that bacteria and viruses can survive only in a narrow temperature range. A fever creates an inhospitable environment for the pathogens. The inability to spike a fever in response to an infection is a sign of weakness and debility. Patients with serious diseases such as AIDS and cancer often do not have enough strength to generate a fever. Elderly people also may have serious infections without any signs of fever, also a sign of weakened vitality. Diagnosing infections in the elderly and in those with serious illnesses can be more difficult precisely because they cannot run a fever.

Elevated temperature in response to exercise is a normal reaction. In fact, this naturally generated "fever therapy" may help reduce infections during the cold and flu season. Fever due to dehydration, on the other hand, is never a healthy response. If you are working hard or exercising heavily outdoors in a hot climate, make sure that you are drinking plenty of fluids (at least 2–3 quarts per day).

Prolonged fever, especially in children, can produce brain damage. Serious diseases, however, may result from giving aspirin to children with high fevers. For example, Reye's syndrome, characterized by brain dysfunction (acute encephalopathy) and replacement of organs with fatty tissue (fatty degeneration of the viscera), can result from giving aspirin to feverish children suffering from viral infections. Obviously, not every child with a viral infection and fever who is given aspirin will manifest Reye's syndrome, but the risk of such side effects of aspirin is far greater than the risk associated with high fevers.

Parents often fear convulsions that may result from high fevers, but according to Dr. Alvin N. Eden, "a child who has a fever during a seizure does not have epilepsy. Furthermore, simple febrile seizures do not lead to mental retardation." In fact, reports pediatrician Uwe Stave, "Fever attacks can affect children in quite a positive way. Even though . . . physical strength is reduced, the child may disclose a wealth of new interests and skills. He may find new advanced ways to communicate, think, and handle situations, or display a refinement of his motor skills. In short, after a fever, the child reveals a spurt of development and maturation." (Both sources quoted in Rahima Baldwin, "Childhood Fevers," *Mothering*, Spring 1989, p. 36.)

Convulsions rarely occur in children when the fever runs at or below 102°F. The best approach is to work with the fever, keeping it in safe range, rather than giving aspirin or Tylenol to reduce it. Often anti-inflammatory drugs merely suppress a fever; afterward, the temperature can rebound even higher, especially with children. Choosing to use hydrotherapy or other therapeutics requires close monitoring of the child's temperature.

General recommendations:

- Drink plenty of fluids (two to four quarts per day).

- Rest. Stop your activities and go to bed ASAP.

- Stop eating. The proper translation of the old adage is "If you feed a cold, you will have to starve a fever." Digestion slows dramatically when the body spikes a fever. Food tends to ferment and putrefy, so the best treatment is to fast and drink plenty of fluids, allowing the body to use its energy to support the immune system rather than the digestive system.

- Encourage sweating (if your temperature is below 102°F to break the fever and push out what the Chinese refer to as "external pernicious influences" (EPIs), which may include wind, dampness, heat, and cold. Simmer a tablespoon of fresh ginger in two cups of water for ten minutes. Draw a hot bath. Sip the ginger tea while relaxing in the bath. Once you begin to sweat, get out of the bath, towel dry, and get into bed. Wrap up in warm blankets and allow yourself to sweat. In the morning, take a shower to rinse off the sweat and excreted toxins.

  Caution: (1) Make sure that you are not exposed to drafts or chills during this treatment. Your pores are open and, therefore, more susceptible to drafts and chills. (2) Sweating therapy can further weaken someone who is debilitated, e.g., the elderly or those with long-term chronic illnesses. Also, children usually do not require such aggressive therapy.

- Continue resting for another twenty-four hours after your temperature returns to normal. The body needs time to recover fully. If people return to their busy schedules too quickly, they are often sick again with another round of cold or flu within six weeks.

Homeopathic remedies: 30c potency. Take three pellets 2–3 times per day until improvement is noted, then stop taking the remedy.

- *Aconite*—if hot, dry, cranky. Fever often develops after exposure to cold wind. Fearful, anxious.

- *Ferrum phos*—for fever without other specific symptoms.

- *Belladonna*—for glassy-eyed, dilated pupils; hot, red, dry face; sweaty body; possible delirium. Sudden onset. No thirst. Specific for strep.

When a fever goes above 102°F:

- Place a cold washcloth on the forehead.

- Use a cold application on at least one-quarter of the body surface (see "Hydrotherapy" section).

- Take a sponge bath in cool or tepid water, every 1–2 hours if necessary (especially with children).

- Soak the feet in a basin of cool or tepid water.

- Do not reduce a fever too quickly or too far. Remember, the optimal range for a fever is 99–102°F.

- Drink a glass of fluid (water is best) every hour.

When to consult a physician:

- If the fever persists more than three days.

- If the fever stays above 102°F, despite using the methods outlined above.

- If a child has a stiff neck, or is arching the back.

- If patient has other symptoms, such as burning urination, severe low-back pain, persistent sore throat (for longer than three days), or infected skin abrasions.

Continued ➡

Headache

Headaches may be caused by a variety of conditions. The suggestions below are meant for acute care, not to substitute for a thorough physical history and examination of those suffering with chronic headaches.

General recommendations:

- Progressive relaxation exercises. Many headaches are caused by muscle constriction and tension. Practice the following exercise during an acute headache and as a daily preventive measure.

BODY SWEEP

Sit or lie down in a comfortable position. Begin at the feet and slowly move through each body part, foot, ankle, calf, knee, thigh, etc., noticing any areas of tension. When you sense a tight area, imagine the body becoming warm and heavy there. Continue moving toward the head until your entire body is warm and relaxed.

Once you have completed the "body sweep," imagine yourself relaxing in a favorite environment (by the ocean, in a shady forest, by a beautiful lake). Take a mini-vacation for at least five minutes in this favorite spot. When you are ready, return your attention to the room where you are sitting or lying, open your eyes, and take three deep breaths.

- Take a hot foot bath, or alternating hot and cold foot bath, to reduce congestion in the head area.
- Place a cold washcloth on the forehead. A cold application reduces congestion in the head. Combining a cold compress to the head with a hot foot bath will increase the effect of the treatment.
- Rub a drop of essential oil of lavender into each temple.
- Drink lots of water, a minimum of two to three quarts per day. Some headaches are caused by simple dehydration.
- Increase fiber (whole grains, fruits, and vegetables) in the diet. Constipation may cause reabsorption of toxins, leading to "sick headaches." Be sure to increase water consumption so that increased fiber does not bind the stools.
- Eliminate coffee, cola, and black tea from the diet. These are common contributors to headaches. Migraines are the exception: caffeine causes blood-vessel constriction, which reduces early migraine symptoms. (Most migraines are caused by excessive dilation of blood vessels; common headaches are caused by blood-vessel constriction.)
- Tobacco causes blood-vessel constriction. Reduce or eliminate cigarette smoking, tobacco chewing, etc.
- Acupressure stimulation of the following points:
  1. Large Intestine 4: the web between the thumb and first finger.
  2. Liver 3: the web between the first and second toe.
  3. *Yin tang:* just above the bridge of the nose.
  4. *Tai yang:* the temple area on either side of the forehead.
  5. Stomach 36: just below the knee on the lateral (outer) side, one finger breadth away from the shin bone.
- Keep the extremities (arms and legs) warm.
- Take a brisk walk in the fresh air, being sure to keep the extremities warm (mittens, hat, scarf, and boots in winter months).

- Drink red clover or catnip tea at the first sign of a headache.

Homeopathic remedies: 30c potency

- *Belladonna*—for intense, throbbing pain. Extreme sensitivity to noise, light, touch, strong smells. Pain comes on suddenly, usually in the frontal area. Pain may extend to the back of the head. Feels worse after jarring. Face may be red and hot, extremities cold. Pupils may be dilated.
- *Bryonia*—if worse with any motion, even slight movement of the head or eyes. Better with firm pressure to the painful area. Steady, aching pain may be concentrated over the left eye or over the forehead area. Irritable, wants to be left alone. Improves with warmth.
- *Nux vomica*—for headaches following excesses in eating or drinking; hangovers. Generally sick feeling, with possible digestive upset. Aversion to light and sound. Avoids company. Irritable.
- *Gelsemium*—for heavy head, as if full of molasses. Dull headache. Sensation of having a band around the head. Joints are achy, heavy. Wants to be alone.

Indigestion

Indigestion usually results from eating too much food, or eating the wrong kinds of food for our particular bodies. The best treatment is preventive, eat fresh, well-cooked foods prepared and eaten in a relaxed environment. Avoid arguments while eating. Chew each bite well (some say at least fifty times). Some days, I'm lucky if I chew each bite ten times! Eat while sitting down, preferably in a chair, and not while hurtling along the freeway in your car. Remember that the digestive system works best when we are relaxed, which is when the parasympathetic nervous system is most active (see the section on "Nutrition").

- Avoid eating when you are rushed or emotionally upset. The body shunts energy and circulation away from the digestive tract during stressful periods, whether the stress is physical, mental, or emotional.
- Avoid eating excessive amounts of cold or raw food. From a Chinese medical perspective, the stomach functions best when it is warm (but not overheated). Steamed and baked foods are easiest to digest. Raw foods, as well as cold or frozen foods, tend to be very cooling and therefore difficult to digest. In general, the body tolerates a modest amount of raw food better in the warm summer months than during the winter.
- Avoid highly spiced, fried, or greasy foods, which may overheat the digestive system and cause irritation.
- Choose water and herb teas for beverages. Avoid coffee, black tea, and alcohol, all of which are heating and irritating to the digestive tract.

Botanical therapy:

- *Peppermint oil*—one drop in a cup of hot water. Essential oils are very strong, so one drop really is enough.
- *Ginger tea*—grate one or two tablespoons of fresh ginger into two cups of water. Bring to a boil and simmer for ten minutes. Sip the warm tea as needed. Ginger is warming, which helps stimulate digestion.
- *Chamomile and/or mint tea*—add one tablespoon of dried herb to one cup of boiling water. Allow to steep for ten minutes, then drink.
- *"Pill Curing"*—a Chinese patent formula. Take

one vial of the pellets every 2–3 hours as needed.

Homeopathic remedies: 30c potency

- *Nux vomica*—classic for overeating and overdrinking. The patient tends to overwork and keep a demanding schedule, which irritates his already weak digestive system. Tendency to constipation.
- *Arsenicum*—for burning pain in the stomach, with desire to drink small sips of water, although water may cause vomiting. Food poisoning, with both diarrhea and vomiting.

When to consult a physician:

- If indigestion becomes a regular occurrence (more than once or twice per week).
- If you notice changes in the bowel movements.
- Black, tarry stools (may be an indication of stomach or duodenal ulcer).
- Excessive gas and bloating (may be an indication of parasite infection). This does not include gas caused by eating too many or poorly cooked beans!
- Regular or severe episodes of heartburn.
- If symptoms of indigestion, bloating, and burping consistently follow ingestion of fatty, greasy, or rich foods (may be a symptom of gall bladder irritation).

Insect and Other Bites

In general, clean the wound with soap and water.

Botanical therapy:

- *Calendula succus* (plant juice, preserved with a small amount of alcohol)—encourages wound healing and prevents infection. Apply after washing the bite.
- *Comfrey or mullein compresses*—also encourage healing. Comfrey contains allantoin, a plant constituent that increases cell division and thereby speeds wound healing. Mullein has soothing properties to ease the stinging and itching associated with insect bites. Make a compress by crushing the leaves or putting fresh leaves in the blender with a small amount of water. Spread the crushed leaves on muslin or cheesecloth and apply to the affected area.
- *Fresh potato*—cut in slices and apply to affected areas to draw out inflammation and swelling.
- *Bentonite clay*—reconstituted to a paste and applied to the area, this will draw out inflammation and swelling and reduce pain.

Homeopathic remedies: 30c potency

- *Ledum*—specific for bites and puncture wounds of all kinds, especially those that are cold and pale blue in color. Ledum is especially helpful for "dirty" bites, or animals bites that are susceptible to infection.
- *Cantharis*—for bites with intense itching, small red bumps, vesicles.
- *Tarantula*—for spider bites.
- *Apis*—for bee stings, or any kind of sting that causes intense, painful swelling and stinging.
- *Hypericum*—for shooting pain.
- *Lachesis*—for snake bite.

When to consult a physician:

- If the insect bite becomes infected.
- If you have an allergic reaction to the insect sting, e.g., excessive swelling in the local area or difficulty breathing.
- If you suspect you may have been bitten by a poisonous insect.

Continued ➔

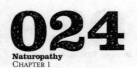

Menstrual Cramping

From the perspective of Chinese medicine, stagnation leads to pain. Stagnation may be caused by cold or, paradoxically, by a decrease in the cooling, nourishing *yin* fluids of the body. A deficiency of blood, a yin substance, causes irritation, cramping, and scanty blood flow. The deficiency is a qualitative decrease in blood, not a quantitative deficiency that would show up on a blood test.

Cold also causes constriction. Generally, cramping worsens with cold, whether the source of the cold is internal or external.

- Avoid cold foods and drinks the week before menses begins. Cold causes constriction and exacerbates cramping, whether the source of the cold is internal (food and drink) or external (cold drafts, swimming in cold water, etc.)
- Exercise is a good preventive, increasing circulation and decreasing stagnation.
- Clear your schedule as much as possible the day before you begin bleeding. If possible, have a completely quiet, unscheduled day when you begin bleeding.

Botanical therapy:

- *Yarrow*—acts as a diuretic for bloating associated with premenstrual syndrome (PMS).
- *Wild yam*—to reduce cramping and balance hormones.
- *Valerian officinalis*—to reduce cramping and relax smooth muscles. (The uterus is smooth muscle tissue.)
- *Red raspberry leaf*—uterine tonic.

Combine equal parts of the above. Drink three to four cups of tea per day, or take two dropperfuls every 1–2 hours during acute, severe cramping.

Nutritional therapy:

- Increase fiber in the diet. Slow, sluggish bowels encourage the re-uptake of hormones the body is trying to excrete through the intestines. High hormonal levels may exacerbate menstrual cramping, as well as PMS symptoms.
- Drink at least two quarts of water per day to increase elimination from the body.
- Eat magnesium-rich foods. Magnesium encourages muscle relaxation.
- Take 50–100 mg of vitamin B_6 per day for at least two months.
- Exercise aerobically at least twenty minutes, 3–4 times per week. Exercise increases circulation in the reproductive organs and decreases stress levels, both of which can decrease menstrual cramping.

Homeopathic remedies: 30c potency

- *Belladonna*—for heavy sensation in abdomen. Menses bright red, profuse. Restless. Head sensitive to drafts. Feels worse after jarring or even when touched.
- *Borax*—if fears downward motion. Membrane and tissue pass with menses. Early, profuse bleeding, with colic and nausea. Application of pressure eases discomfort. Feels better during cold weather.
- *Bryonia*—for "vicarious menses," i.e., nosebleed rather than menstrual flow. Inter-menses pains with pelvic and abdominal soreness. Avoids the least motion. Thirsty for large amounts of water.
- *Calc phos*—for violent backache. Chilly. Menses is early, excessive, bright red; occurs every two weeks.
- *Chamomilla*—dark, clotted blood with labor-like pains. Irritable, cross, quarrelsome. Thirsty.

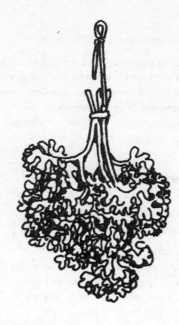

Feels worse at night, when angry, or after drinking coffee.

- *Colocynthis*—if patient bends over double; pain "bores into" ovary. Pain eases with pressure. Restless. Waves of violent, gripping pain.
- *Pulsatilla*—for sensation of band around throat just before menses. Clotted, intermittent, changeable menses.

When to consult a physician:

- If severe menstrual cramping occurs more than twice in a year.
- If menstrual cramping worsens over time (possible indication that endometriosis may be developing).
- If the cramps are severe enough to stop your daily activities.

Motion Sickness

General Recommendations:

- Relaxation exercises, before and during travel. Move through the body from head to foot, noting and releasing any areas of muscle tension. Take up to ten deep breaths and allow your body to grow heavy and relaxed.
- Drink ginger tea. Grate one or two tablespoons of fresh ginger into a saucepan with two cups of water. Bring to a boil, then simmer for ten minutes. Drink one-half cup of ginger tea every half hour, or as needed for stomach upset.
- Mint and chamomile teas also soothe the stomach. Steep one tablespoon dried herb in a cup of boiling water for ten minutes. Drink as needed.

Homeopathic remedies: 30c potency. Take the remedy one hour before travel, then every 15–30 minutes as needed once travel begins.

- *Borax*—for motion sickness during air travel. Symptoms worsen with downward motion.
- *Rhus tox*—for nausea and vomiting with complete loss of appetite. Giddiness on attempting to rise. Severe frontal headache. Unquenchable thirst.
- *Cocculus*—for car sickness. Also for morning sickness in pregnancy. Person cannot stand the sight or smell of food. Hollow, empty feeling.

When to consult a physician:

- If the above remedies do not alleviate motion sickness.
- If you have difficulties with balance that are exacerbated by travel. You may have an inner-ear problem that needs further treatment.

Physical Trauma

Most trauma is caused by stretching tissues beyond their capacity. Overstretching connective tissues (muscle, blood vessels, tendons, bones) leads to tissue damage, pain, and swelling. Swelling may serve as a natural splint, to protect and immobilize the traumatized area. Unfortunately, swelling may also lead to a dangerous decrease in circulation.

The treatments listed below apply to most physical injuries. Please see other sections of this chapter for information on specific conditions (bruising, burns, etc.).

- Give homeopathic Arnica as soon as possible after the injury. Arnica is specific for trauma, bruising, head injury, and soft-tissue injury, and can also slow bleeding and treat shock. Often someone needing Arnica will deny that she is injured. Imagine a construction worker falling two stories, landing hard, getting up, and saying she is fine, she needs Arnica!
- Continue giving Arnica as needed for 3–4 days. You may repeat the remedy as often as every thirty minutes immediately after the injury. Remember, homeopathic remedies act according to the frequency of dosage, not the amount.
- For the first twenty-four hours, use cold applications to the affected area. There is some controversy here: one school of thought says cold applications are best because they reduce circulation, and therefore swelling, in the local area; another school of thought argues that cold applications cause "stagnation" (as defined in Chinese medicine) by slowing the circulation. A compromise approach involves alternating hot and cold applications to increase circulation and decrease stagnation.
- After twenty-four hours, use alternating hot and cold applications—five minutes of hot, followed by one minute of cold. Continue for at least three cycles of alternating hot and cold applications. Always end with a cold application.

Other Homeopathic remedies: 30c potency

- *Ledum*—for bruised area that is cold and blue. Follows *Arnica* well, after three or four days.
- *Ruta*—for injury to periosteal tissue (surface of the bone). Area is red; condition worsens with motion. Also for injuries to ligaments.
- *Rhus tox*—for sore, painful joints that improve with warmth and motion (painful when first moved, better with continued movement).
- *Hypericum*—for injury to areas dense with nerve tissue (eyes, hands, genitals). Sharp, nerve-like pain.

Botanical remedies:

- *Arnica oil*—apply to the affected area every 3–4 hours. Because Arnica is a counter-irritant (increasing circulation in an area by causing mild irritation) it should not be used on broken skin.

  Caution: for external use only. Do not take Arnica internally. Use on unbroken skin only.

- *Hypericum oil*—causes blood-vessel dilation; warning to injured area, soothing to nerves. **Caution:** for external use only.
- *Symphytum (comfrey) oil or lotion*—stimulates cell production and tissue healing. Apply externally, or take as tea internally. Comfrey tea is especially healing for bone breaks.

  Caution: for skin injuries (cuts and abrasions), apply comfrey only after scab formation. Applying comfrey to a deep, open wound can cause the wound to close too quickly, trapping

Continued ➡

anaerobic bacteria in the wound and possibly causing a serious infection.

- Any plant with chlorophyll will stimulate healing. Plantain is exceptionally soothing to the skin. Crush the leaves and apply to cuts and abrasions, especially if you are outdoors and have no other first-aid supplies with you. Plantain is called "nature's Band-Aid."

Acupressure: Deeply massage points on the limb opposite the injured area. Massaging points on the left wrist will decrease pain and increase circulation to a sprained right wrist.

When to consult a physician:

- If the patient shows signs of shock (see the section on "Shock," at right).
- If the injury involves blood loss (more than minor oozing from a cut).
- If you cannot voluntarily move the injured area.
- If you can see bone protruding through the skin.
- If you begin to see red streaks developing above an injury, moving up the arm or leg, a sign of internal infection.
- If pain and swelling persist for more than 3–4 days after injury.

Poison Ivy and Poison Oak

General recommendations:

- Learn to identify these plants and keep a respectful distance away from them.
- Wash with soap and water. The rash and irritation associated with poison oak and ivy are caused by an oil in the plant's leaves and stems. Washing with soap, which emulsifies and removes oils, decreases and sometimes completely removes the irritant.
- Remove the irritant with drawing agents. Moisten bentonite clay with enough water to form a smooth paste. Add one or two drops of peppermint oil. The clay will absorb oils and oozing discharge from poison ivy rashes. A very small amount of peppermint oil will decrease itching. If you do not have clay, apply a fresh slice of potato to the area. (Potato also acts as a drawing agent.)
- Avoid touching or brushing the affected area. You may spread the irritant oil accidentally by scratching the rash, then touching another body part. This is usually how poison ivy spreads to the eyes and face. If you tend to scratch in your sleep, wear cotton gloves. Wash your hands often during the day.

Homeopathic remedies: 30c potency

- *Rhus tox*—for itchy, red vesicles. The area feels better with hot-water applications and motion.
- *Rhus lobatum*—made from poison oak, which is more common on the West Coast. Some people respond better to this remedy than to *Rhus tox*, which is made from poison ivy.
- If you are extremely sensitive to poison ivy or oak and must work in or near it (e.g., clearing poison ivy in your yard), take one 30c dose of *Rhus tox* before beginning work. This prophylactic dose can reduce and sometimes prevent a rash.

When to consult a physician:

- If the rash continues to spread despite treatment.
- If the rash persists for more than seven days.
- If the area becomes infected.

Shock

When someone goes into shock, the body suspends all but the most vital functions. If shock goes untreated, even those vital functions may shut down. Symptoms of shock include:

- confusion
- very slow or very fast pulse
- very slow or very fast breathing
- trembling or weakness of the arms and legs
- cool, moist skin
- enlarged pupils
- pale or bluish fingernails, lips, skin

Treatments for shock:

Call 911. Most shock is caused by major trauma and requires immediate medical attention. The following suggestions are meant to support the patient until emergency medical care arrives.

- Keep the patient lying down.
- Address the cause of the shock: remove any live electrical source (if you can do so without endangering yourself), stanch bleeding, remove causes of severe pain, use first-aid procedures to restore breathing.
- Keep the patient warm. Cover him or her with a blanket, and elevate the feet.
- Give "Rescue Remedy," a blend of Bach flowers available at most health food stores. Give three or four drops under the tongue every fifteen minutes, or as necessary once recovery begins.

Homeopathic remedies: 30c potency. Give every 15, 30 minutes until improvement is noted.

- *Aconite*—for fear, fright, anxiety. Sudden, violent onset. Numbness. Vomiting from fear. Face is deathly pale when patient sits up. Fear of death.
- *Carbo veg*—for icy coldness. Stagnant blood. "Air hunger" (can't catch breath). Wants windows open; wants to be fanned; wants cold drinks during chills.
- *Gelsemium*—if dull, droopy, drowsy, dazed. Dilated pupils. No thirst. Heat stroke. Heavy, drooping eyelids.
- *Arnica*—especially after head injury. Denies need for help ("I'm fine. Just leave me alone.").

When to consult a physician:

- Always consult a physician for illnesses and injuries involving shock.
- If the patient has minor injuries (e.g., a scraped leg or arm) and does not respond to the above treatment within 10–15 minutes.

Sunburn

Fair-skinned people always have been susceptible to sunburn. Now, with the increasing emissions of hydrocarbons and fluorocarbons and subsequent destruction of the ozone layer, even dark-skinned people are at risk. The long-term effects of excessive sun exposure include skin cancer. One severe sunburn during a lifetime can increase the risk of multiple myeloma, i.e., bone cancer. The best treatment is preventive:

- Stay out of the sun during the middle of the day (11 a.m.–3 p.m.), when the sun's rays are strongest.
- Wear hats that screen the face, especially the nose. Wear light clothing that covers the arms and legs.
- Apply sunscreen to areas of the skin that are not covered by clothing. Sunscreen increases

the number of minutes the skin can withstand burning rays by the factor noted on the product. For example, a fair-skinned person without protection might normally stay in the sun for ten minutes before noticing signs of burning. If that person uses a "15" sunscreen, he or she could stay in the sun for 10 x 15 minutes, or 150 minutes (i.e., two and a half hours). Reapplying the sunscreen after 150 minutes will not increase the length of protection. Washing off the sunscreen will reduce the effective time.

If you are unable to avoid overexposure, use the following treatments:

- Apply cool water as soon as possible. Take frequent cool showers (e.g., two minutes in the shower, every one or two hours). Pat dry; do not rub the skin. If the burn is localized, apply cold wet washcloths, changing the cloth as it warms.
- Apply aloe vera gel every 3–4 hours.
- Avoid applications of oil-based products or butter. Oils and fats increase the burn, just as throwing grease on a fire will feed the flames.
- Drink plenty of fluids. Often the body becomes dehydrated, especially if the burn covers a large area of the body.

Homeopathic remedies: 30c potency

- *Hypericum*—for first-degree sunburn (no blistering).
- *Cantharis*—especially if blistering is present (second-degree burn).

When to consult a physician:

- If a second-degree burn (i.e., with blistering) covers more than 10 percent of the skin surface.
- If the patient shows signs of:

a. heat stroke, collapse in the heat with hot, dry skin. Other symptoms include a rapid, strong pulse and high body temperature (105°F or higher). Heat stroke is a very serious condition requiring immediate medical attention.

b. Heat exhaustion, collapse in the heat with moist, clammy skin. Other symptoms include profuse perspiration, weakness, nausea, dizziness, headaches, and possibly cramps. Heat exhaustion is a serious condition, although not as life-threatening as heat stroke.

Teething

Many symptoms may accompany the eruption of teeth in an infant, including colds, ear infections, and diarrhea. The following suggestions are meant specifically for the gum and mouth symptoms.

- Soak a clean cloth in chamomile tea, wring out, and place in the freezer. Give to baby to chew on when he or she shows signs of discomfort.
- Water-filled plastic "teething rings" can soothe inflamed gums.
- If you are breast feeding, drink chamomile and oatstraw tea (equal parts). The herbs will pass into the breast milk.

Homeopathic remedies: 30c potency

- *Calc carb*—for late dentition (teeth slow to emerge). Fontanelles slow to close. Ear infections sometimes accompany teething.
- *Chamomilla*— a classic remedy for teething, especially for inconsolable children, or children who are extremely irritable and demand to be carried, yet arch their back away from

Continued ➡

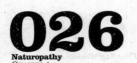

whomever is carrying them. One cheek is red, the other pale. Grass-green, runny stools may accompany teething.

· *Ignatia*—if child is distressed, but not as irritable as in previous case. The baby sobs, sighs, and cries. The whole body, or single body parts, may tremble.

—From *Pocket Guide to Naturopathic Medicine*

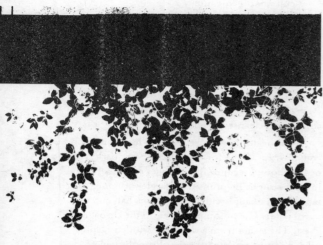

HOW TO CHOOSE A NATUROPATHIC PHYSICIAN

Judith Boice, N.D.

Choosing a physician is like choosing a car, you need someone you can trust who will take you where you need to go. As with any human relationship, "chemistry" is part of the equation. Your dream physician may be like the flashy sports car, or the car with the best gas mileage, or the one with the sensible upholstery.

In all states in which naturopathic physicians are licensed, they function as primary-care physicians, meaning they are qualified to diagnose and treat disease. The naturopathic doctor (N.D.) functions as a family doctor, the equivalent to conventional medicine's general practitioner (G.P.). A naturopathic physician employs physical exams, patient health histories, and lab tests to arrive at diagnoses, just like any other physician. An N.D. varies from conventional medical practice only in the treatments that he or she prescribes to address illness. In some states, naturopathic physicians may prescribe pharmaceutical drugs.

In states without a naturopathic licensing board, anyone may call him or herself a "naturopathic doctor," or use the initials "N.D." after his or her name, because the term is not legally defined or regulated by the state. Before making an appointment with an N.D., ask where he or she went to school. In North America, there are three accredited four-year schools of naturopathic medicine. Physicians who have graduated from one of these schools have completed a rigorous medical training, equivalent to that offered at conventional medical schools, with the addition of natural therapeutic modalities absent from most medical school curricula. Check with the schools listed at right or with the American Association of Naturopathic Physicians (AANP) to find a trained naturopathic physician in an unlicensed state.

In licensed states, naturopathic physicians must pass a national board exam (three days of written exams) before they are licensed. Most naturopathic physicians who have graduated from an accredited school pass national board exams and retain a license in a licensed state, even if they are practicing in a state that does not recognize naturopathic physicians.

States presently licensing naturopathic physicians include: Alaska, Arizona, Connecticut, Florida, Hawaii, Maine, Montana, New Hampshire, Oregon, Utah, and Washington. The following Canadian provinces license naturopathic physicians: Alberta, British Columbia, Manitoba, Ontario, Quebec, and Saskatchewan.

Keep in mind that each licensed naturopathic physician is likely to emphasize particular therapeutic approaches in his or her practice. Always ask what therapeutic methods a particular practitioner uses (e.g., nutrition, homeopathy, botanical medicine, physical medicine, hydrotherapy, etc.). I know of one patient who went to a naturopathic physician for several months, always expecting that the physician eventually would prescribe a homeopathic remedy. Finally, this extremely patient patient asked the physician when he was going to prescribe a remedy. "Oh," said the physician, arching his eyebrow in surprise, "I don't work with homeopathic remedies. I suggest you contact Dr. So-and-so!"

General guidelines for choosing a physician (of any kind):

· The physician listens well and encourages questions.
· The physician asks what *you* think is happening with your health.
· The physician takes time to explain things.
· The treatment plan includes lifestyle changes, not just pills.
· The physician outlines options and helps you make educated health-care choices.
· The physician educates patients during an office visit and, ideally, also offers lectures and trainings for patients who desire more information.
· The physician conducts physical exams and orders appropriate lab tests. This does not apply to naturopathic physicians in unlicensed states, where N.D.s must refer patients to other physicians for lab testing. In licensed states, naturopathic physicians can order lab tests, draw blood, etc.

Accredited North American naturopathic medical schools:

Bastyr University
14500 Juanita Drive NE
Bothell, WA 98011
(206) 823-1300

National College of Naturopathic Medicine
Ross Island Center
049 S.W. Porter
Portland, OR 97201
(503) 225-4860

Ontario College of Naturopathic Medicine
60 Berl Avenue
Toronto, Ontario M8Y3C7
Canada
(416) 251-5261

Currently undergoing accreditation:

Southwest College of Naturopathic Medicine
and Health Sciences
2140 East Broadway Road
Tempe, AZ 85282
(602) 990-7424

American Association of Naturopathic Physicians (AANP) referral line: (206) 323-7610.

—From *Pocket Guide to Naturopathic Medicine*

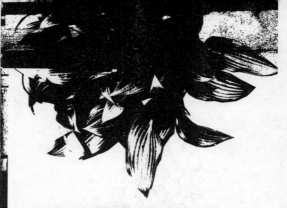

A SELECTION OF NATURAL REMEDIES

Ellen Tart-Jensen

Bedsores

A bedsore is caused by repeated friction on the skin from bedsheets when someone is confined to bed for an extended period of time. Here is a healing paste that has worked well in the treatment of bedsores.

SOOTHING HERBAL PASTE

2 parts slippery elm powder
1 part marshmallow root powder
1 part goldenseal root powder

Mix the powders with hot distilled water, enough to form a paste. Spread the paste on bedsores and cover with a bandage.

Bee Stings

If you are severely allergic to bee stings, go to the hospital immediately if you are stung. Otherwise, use raw, organic honey or bentonite clay on the sting. If it is available, use natural mud. A plaintain poultice is also great for bee stings.

Bleeding

Place cayenne pepper in the wound. Cayenne will stop external bleeding. For internal bleeding, bleeding with colitis, and vaginal bleeding that is not from menstruation, take two cayenne capsules, three times per day. Shepherd's purse, horsetail, and stinging nettle teas or capsules will also help stop the bleeding. Midwives often use it to help stop postpartum bleeding.

Boils

A boil usually begins with a painful red area on the skin due to some type of infection. After a while, a boil will swell with fluid and pus. This is caused by white blood cells that move in to fight the infection. Eventually a "head" will form on the boil. Sometimes doctors will lance a boil to surgically remove the liquid. Teenagers can get cystic acne, which is an infection that forms in a pore clogged with oil. Some boils are caused by the staphylococcus germ. These are called foruncles or carbuncles and can have one or several openings and cause chills and fever. Boils usually occur around hair follicles—on the face, neck, under the arms, pubic area, buttocks, or thighs. All boils can be quite painful. Many boils can be drained through the surface of the skin using natural methods. However, if you have a severe boil causing fever, see a competent physician. The following are some natural home remedies for boils.

DISINFECTING SOLUTION

6 drops tea tree oil or 4 drops oregano oil
1 cup hot distilled water

Mix the oil and the water. Wet a cloth with the solution, and hold it on the boil. Keep wetting the cloth with the solution until the boil breaks open. Then put a salve on the boil made from one-half

Continued ➡

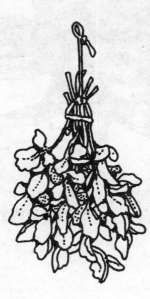

teaspoon olive oil, six drops oregano oil, and one capsule goldenseal. Open the capsule and pour goldenseal into the oil, and mix well. Apply to the affected area, and bandage well. There is also a colloidal silver herbal salve that works great as well.

Bronchitis

Bronchitis is an infection that causes inflammation in the bronchi, the pipes that carry oxygen and air into your lungs. Bronchitis is usually caused by a virus in the lining of the bronchi that causes swelling and the production of mucus. Mucus is made to help protect the bronchi from the inflammation and carry off the germs. However, the mucus causes congestion and makes it very difficult to breathe. Many times, a person will begin to cough in order to rid the body of the mucus and infection. We get viruses when the body is worn down, exhausted, and the immune system is weak. People that smoke or live in areas where there is lots of pollution are more likely to get bronchitis because the bronchi and lungs are already weak. Here is a home remedy that has helped in many cases to relieve and heal bronchitis. If the condition persists, see a physician.

OREGANO SOLUTION

> 10 drops oregano oil
> 4 ounces warm distilled water

Mix the oil and warm water, then drink it four times daily. Mix twenty drops of oregano oil or twenty drops of garlic oil with three tablespoons of olive oil and rub on the chest and feet. Cover the chest with warm onion poultices. If coughing is severe, take valerian root to relax the throat. Gargle with one tablespoon of raw apple cider vinegar in six ounces of water. Take two propolis, twice daily and one echinacea or goldenseal twice daily. Grapefruit seed extract is also very beneficial in helping break up the mucus and stop a cough. Recommended dose is two capsules, twice daily with food. If the throat is sore, spray with a colloidal silver solution of ten parts per million.

Bruising

If you tend to bruise easily, take five hundred milligrams of bioflavonoids and one hundred milligrams of rutin three times per day. If you have a severe bruise, use arnica cream or salve on it. Arnica cream can be found in any health food store and contains the arnica herb that has proven to be beneficial in healing bruises. It contains the essential oil called thymol that helps reduce inflammation and flavonoids that knit tissue back together. A comfrey poultice is also very healing for severe bruises. Or apply Complete Tissue and Bone Cream.

Burns and Sunburns

Raw organic honey mixed half and half with fresh organic wheat germ oil will heal a burn quickly. Place the honey and oil on the burn, and keep a sterile white cotton cloth over it. Aloe vera juice and gel are also wonderful for healing burns. According to Anne McIntyre in *Herbal Medicine*:

> The University of Pennsylvania Radiology Department has found that the juice of this plant [aloe vera] is more effective in treating radiation burns than any other known product. It is now one of the most popular herbs used commercially in face creams, hand and body lotions and shampoos.

In treating severe burns, be careful when changing the bandages. The bandages may stick and cause severe pain or, worse, pull off the healing skin. John W. Keim writes about this in *Comfort for the Burned and Wounded*. He discovered that placing clean, moist plantain leaves over the salve worked well. The leaves should be wrapped with gauze and a towel. This wrapping allows air to get through to the burn. In addition, the leaves are very healing. If plaintain leaves are not available, Mr. Keim found that burdock and dandelion leaves work well also. Soaked dried leaves may also be used. The bandage can be changed every twelve hours and will not tear or pull the skin or tissue. With this type of treatment, there should be no infection and little or no scarring.

Bursitis

Bursitis occurs when the bursae have become inflamed. Bursae are small sacs filled with fluid that are located between the tendons and bones throughout the body. Bursitis is treated much the same way tendonitis is. Avoid alcohol and caffeine. Soak in Epsom salts baths and apply castor oil poultices. Apply arnica cream or Complete Tissue and Bone Cream and wear an ace bandage. Take marshmallow herb, tumeric, calcium, magnesium, trace minerals, B complex, and vitamin C to reduce inflammation. Rest the injured tendon.

Calluses

Rub castor oil on calluses on the hands or feet. They will soften and come off beautifully.

Calluses are composed of several layers of skin produced to protect an area from wear and tear. Wearing shoes that are too tight, for example, can put daily pressure on a specific area on the foot. Some people stand or walk in such a way that the same area of the foot is stressed daily. Over time, calluses can become hardened and painful.

To prevent calluses, change your shoes and wear different pairs. Wear shoes that are made of leather or cloth and allow the foot to breathe. Wear shoes that are supportive but do not put extreme pressure on specific areas. Notice how you stand and walk. If you are putting undue pressure on a certain area, practice standing and walking so that you are no longer causing that pressure. If you have a severe problem with your feet, see an expert. If you are overweight, this can cause extra pressure on the feet as well. Follow the healthy eating plans presented in chapter 1, and drop those extra pounds.

Soak the affected foot each day in hot water with a half cup of baking soda for twenty minutes to an hour. Rinse your foot, then scrub the callus gently with a pumice stone. Apply castor oil and put on an old cotton sock before going to bed. Rinse your foot in the morning with warm water and baking soda. Baking soda removes castor oil from your body as well as from your clothes. If the callus is

painful, put a bit of castor oil or Complete Tissue and Bone Cream on a bandage and keep it bandaged during the day.

Colds and Coughs

Dr. Jensen had wonderful results treating coughs with the following recipe.

COUGH SYRUP

> 6 yellow onions, chopped, or 6 lemons, chopped
> 1 cup raw organic honey

Place the onions or lemons over water in a double boiler. Cover them and bring to a boil. Lower the temperature to a simmer. Cook the mixture for one hour. Remove the mixture from the heat and add the honey. Blend the mixture and then strain it. Take one teaspoon of warm syrup every hour. It will soothe your throat, help stop a cough, and cleanse the bowels.

Your health food store may also have some good cough syrups. Look for wild black cherry bark syrup or horehound syrup. Zinc lozenges or Swiss Herbal lozenges can be helpful. Also, gargle with one tablespoon of apple cider vinegar to a half cup of warm water. Use onion poultices on the throat and chest. The steam from a vaporizer with eucalyptus oil can soothe irritated throats. Propolis tablets, liquid, or tincture, elderberry tea, echinacea and goldenseal, vitamin C, and Dr. Christopher's antiplague formula can all help to heal the body.

Constipation

For occasional constipation, take cascara sagrada capsules or tea before bedtime.

CASCARA SAGRADA TEA

> $1/3$ teaspoon cascara sagrada bark powder
> $2/3$ teaspoon cardamom powder
> a pinch of ginger powder
> 1 teaspoon honey
> 1 cup boiling water

Pour the boiling water over the herbs. Add the honey and stir. Cover for five minutes, then drink slowly.

If constipation is a chronic problem, you may need to change your lifestyle. Make sure you are drinking eight glasses of distilled water daily with fifteen drops of ionic liquid trace minerals in each glass. Constipation is often related to a magnesium deficiency. Peristalsis, or movement of the colon, depends upon minerals and trace minerals in order to function properly.

The colon must have adequate fiber each day to work well. Fiber comes from fruits, vegetables, whole grains, nuts, and seeds. Have a tablespoon of ground flaxseeds each morning on a bowl of cooked millet. Flaxseed tea is mucilaginous and also beneficial in promoting healthy elimination. Eat papayas, pineapple, and apples in between meals. These fruits are high in enzymes. Apples contain pectin, a wonderful natural fiber. Chewing alfalfa tablets works wonders for some people. People who are sensitive to alfalfa tablets fare better with chlorella tablets. The fiber is finer in chlorella tablets (you must get the shattered-cell wall type of chlorella in order to utilize the storehouse of nutrients). Take five to eight chlorella tablets just before each meal with two teaspoons of flaxseed oil. This combination makes an oily bolus that lubricates and sweeps the colon clean. Raw beet juice and spinach juice promote peristalsis in the intestinal tract.

Grated raw beets and steamed beets are great for the colon. Watermelon eaten first thing in the morning helps encourage good bowel movements.

Continued ➡

Dried fruits help tremendously as well, but you must pour boiling water over all dried fruit in order to kill parasites. Remember it is best to eat fruit alone. Combining your foods properly, as well as taking digestive plant enzymes just before meals, helps improve digestion.

Make sure you have plenty of good bacteria, such as acidophilus, lactobacillus, and bifidus, in your digestive tract. Eating yogurt is a good choice for people who do not have allergies to milk. Many people with milk allergies can tolerate yogurt because it has been predigested and is high in friendly bacterial cultures. It is best to make your own yogurt with raw organic goat's or cow's milk. If this is not possible, try to find certified organic yogurt in your health food store.

Dandruff

Do a colon cleansing and kidney cleansing. Take two tablespoons of flaxseed oil, fifty milligrams of zinc, and six hundred international units of vitamin E daily. Drink two cups of oatstraw tea daily, and take horsetail herb. Rubbing a bit of eucalyptus oil mixed half and half with olive oil has also helped many get rid of dandruff.

Diarrhea

When you have diarrhea, there is usually a poison in your system that needs to be released. Taking medicine to stop it prevents the toxicity from getting out of the body. Instead, stop eating regular meals. Prepare some barley or brown rice gruel, cooking the barley or rice really well until it is almost a mush. Eat several small bowls of it throughout the day. You also may eat a very ripe banana at separate times from the gruel.

Alternate between drinking red raspberry leaf tea, thyme tea, cinnamon tea, and ginger tea. These help check diarrhea and relieve nausea.

Diarrhea also can be the result of an inflammation of the intestinal tract caused by bacteria, viruses, or parasites. Viruses are spread through close human contact. Bacteria and parasites are transmitted through contaminated water or food. A rainforest herb called Sangre de Drago has proven to be very beneficial in healing intestinal inflammation and stopping diarrhea. Colloidal silver can kill viruses and bacteria, so it's very useful in stopping diarrhea caused by any of these micro-organisms. Black walnut, wormwood, and cloves are helpful if diarrhea is caused by parasites. In all cases of diarrhea, you should take acidophilus and bifidus to reinstate friendly bacteria into the colon. If diarrhea persists more than three or four days, you can become dehydrated and need to seek medical advice. Symptoms of dehydration include dry mouth, little urination, and intense thirst. If you have a fever of 100°F, abdominal pain, or black or red blood in the stools, go to the doctor. Call your doctor if your child has diarrhea for more than twenty-four hours. Children can dehydrate much more rapidly than adults. A doctor will be able to test your blood and run a stool test to determine the cause of the diarrhea.

Ear Infections

Ear infections are common in children and swimmers. They are caused by germs, including bacteria and viruses, that get into the ear and middle ear (just inside the ear canal). These germs can also get into the Eustachian tubes, which are passages between your middle ear and throat. These tubes are important because they allow air to move in and out of your middle ear, killing germs and preventing pressure from building up. Little children have very tiny Eustachian tubes and they are less able to

keep germs out. Allergies and colds can cause mucus to become trapped in the Eustachian tubes and middle ear allowing infection to grow. Water from swimming can become trapped in the middle ear forming damp breeding grounds for germs. Ear infections are not spread from person to person. They occur when germs grow in the middle ear due to congestion. Ear infections can be extremely painful and cause fever. You might even have difficulty hearing. If you get an ear infection, the following oil has proven to be very helpful time and again for healing the ears.

Garlic-Mullein Ear Oil

1 part garlic oil
3 parts mullein oil

Combine the oils. Put the mixture in a dropper bottle, and place it in a cup of hot water. Put one to two drops of warm oil in each ear. This oil helps reduce inflammation and swelling, fight infection, and soften hardened earwax. Avoid dairy products, wheat, and sugar, and make sure the bowels are working well. Keep the immune system strong by taking two propolis tablets daily.

Swimmers should use the following: one ounce colloidal silver at 125 parts per million with ten drops of tea tree oil added. Natural Path/Silver Wings carries a great colloidal silver with herbal tincture of Swedish bitters and tea tree oil that I also highly recommend for ear infections.

Fever

To relieve a fever, soak in a hot ginger bath, then rinse in cool water. Take an enema with two quarts of cool distilled water, two tablespoons of chlorophyll, one tablespoon of white willow bark powder, and one cup of catnip tea. Aspirin was originally made from willow bark, which is like a natural aspirin without the side effects. Take two capsules of white willow bark three times daily. Children should take half that amount. A small enema can be made for children with one cup of cool distilled water, two teaspoons of chlorophyll, and one teaspoon of white willow bark powder.

Gum Disease

Gum disease, or periodontal disease, is common throughout the United States. People with gum disease have bad breath. Gum disease is caused by bacteria, plaque (mucus and bacteria), and particles of food and sugar that deteriorate on the gums. Gingivitis, or gum inflammation, is the beginning of periodontal disease. In the advanced stage, called pyorrhea, gums become infected, swollen, and red, and they bleed easily. Too much bleeding can cause anemia. Eventually, the teeth may fall out.

Avoid sugar and white flour. Use a water pick to loosen plaque. Floss your teeth gently, and brush with a soft brush. Rub clove oil or thyme oil directly on your gums to kill bacteria and relieve any pain. Rinse your mouth with food-grade peroxide (one-half teaspoon mixed with eight ounces distilled water).

Headaches

Many headaches are caused by poor circulation to the head. Rub peppermint oil mixed half and half with safflower or lavender oil on the temples, but be sure not to get it in the eyes. Peppermint oil contains menthol and promotes blood circulation as well. Lavender oil has relaxing properties that can promote rest and reduce headaches. Take fifty milligrams of niacin together with B complex to promote blood flow to the head and ease a headache. Rosemary tea is helpful in treating headaches. Feverfew is often useful in stopping migraines. Follow the

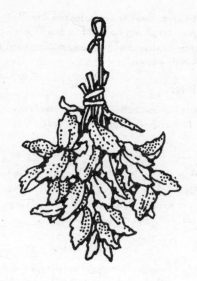

directions on the bottle. If headaches persist, consult a knowledgeable physician.

Hemorrhoids

Hemorrhoids are actually swollen veins in the anus and rectum, similar to varicose veins. The tissue of the veins has weakened, often due to prolonged constipation and straining. Grind flaxseeds and use one teaspoon daily for three days, then increase gradually to three teaspoons daily. Too much fiber at once can cause gas. Use one tablespoon of flaxseed oil three times daily to lubricate the colon and soften stools. Flaxseeds are high in fiber, which helps the colon function well. A cup of flaxseed tea, taken three times daily, can soothe the intestinal tract and promote good peristalsis. Slippery elm tea and capsules also soothe the alimentary tract and rectum.

Drink a cup of oatstraw tea daily. Oatstraw is high in silicon, which can strengthen the walls of the veins and arteries. Take two thousand milligrams of vitamin C with bioflavonoids three times daily. Bioflavonoids help to strengthen connective tissue. If hemorrhoids are persistent, take extra rutin, fifty milligrams three times daily. Rutin is one of the bioflavonoids that has proven to be very effective in reducing hemorrhoids.

Soak in a warm sitz bath of two quarts of water and one cup of calendula tea and one tablespoon of witch hazel (which can be found in liquid form at your health store). Calendula tea soothes hemorrhoids. Witch hazel acts as an astringent and can help relieve bleeding. Rinse off and apply castor oil to the anus and rectum. If hemorrhoids are bleeding, take one capsule of cayenne mixed with ginger three times daily to help stop the bleeding. Be sure to eat foods high in iron (dark green leafy vegetables, beets, figs, and blackstrap molasses) if you have been bleeding.

Infections, Topical

Antibacterial Herbal Paste

⅓ ounce tea tree oil or oregano oil
1 ounce olive oil
4 capsules of goldenseal root powder (broken open and poured into paste)
2 capsules of marshmallow root or slippery elm (broken open and poured into paste)

Mix the oils, goldenseal root powder and marshmallow root or slippery elm powder to form a paste. Apply the paste to the infected area, and cover it with a bandage.

Lice

Wear rubber gloves and apply tea tree oil or oil of oregano mixed half and half with lavender oil to a

Continued ➡

lice-infested area, three to six times per day. Wash scalp with pine tar shampoo and hands with pine tar soap. Tea tree oil shampoo and soap may be used as well. Avoid eating sugar.

Mosquito Bites

To repel mosquitoes, rub lemongrass oil on the skin or eat lots of garlic and brewer's yeast.

Nausea

Nausea can be caused by a stomach virus, vertigo, or car sickness.

To relieve nausea, drink ginger tea, red raspberry leaf tea, or peppermint leaf tea.

Ringworm

Ringworm is a fungus that occurs on the skin and looks like a rounded, slightly raised red patch. Make a paste with goldenseal root powder and tea tree oil. Place the paste on the infected area and keep it bandaged. Ringworm can be contagious!

Shingles

Shingles is caused by the varicella zoster virus, which also causes chicken pox. The virus can live in the body for years before being triggered by stress. Symptoms include a rash and severe pain. Soak in a tub of warm water and four cups of calendula tea. Use calendula cream on the sores to promote healing and reduce the pain. Echinazea, olive leaf, garlic, and colloidal silver minimize replication of the virus. Take lots of vitamin C, vitamin E, and beta-carotene, and cleanse the colon.

Skin Rashes

For skin rashes, soak in a bath of warm water and two cups of raw apple cider vinegar for twenty minutes. Raw apple cider vinegar will often help stop itching. Rinse off, then rub on a salve made of chickweed, marigold (calendula), and olive oil. If rash does not improve within two to three days, colon cleansing can be most helpful. Also, you may need to see a qualified dermatologist to tell you what type of rash you have and make suggestions for healing. If it is coming from an allergy, you may have to avoid all foods that could be causing it, wear only cotton clothing, use natural soaps with no perfumes and dyes, and make sure your home is free from mold.

Snoring

To relieve snoring, lie on your back. Place a castor oil poultice over your abdomen so it covers the top side of the areas where the adrenal glands are located, in the back above the kidneys and the liver. Losing weight and cleansing the colon and liver will often solve problems with snoring. Rubbing peppermint oil mixed half and half with lavender oil on the bridge of the nose and just beneath the nostrils will help open up air passages and reduce snoring. If snoring continues, go for a sleep apnea test.

Sore Throat

To soothe a sore throat, try the gargle below.

APPLE CIDER VINEGAR GARGLE

 1 tablespoon apple cider vinegar
 6 ounces distilled water

Mix the vinegar and water. Use it to gargle several times a day.

Get plenty of rest. Keep the colon clean. Take propolis, echinacea, grapefruit seed extract. Colloidal silver can help heal a sore throat as well. Avoid sugar, dairy products, and wheat. Take extra

B_6 unless you are taking a B complex. Fluids build up in the body when the kidneys are not releasing fluid properly as urine. Herbal teas can flush the kidneys and help improve their function. Drink juniper berry tea. Eating watermelon is also very cleansing for the kidneys. Watercress is a natural diuretic.

Tendonitis

Tendonitis is the inflammation of a tendon. Symptoms include pain, numbness, tingling, and tenderness. Avoid alcohol and caffeine. Have some spinal adjustments and massages. Soak in Epsom salts bath and apply castor oil poultices. Apply arnica cream and wear an Ace bandage. Take tumeric, calcium, magnesium, trace minerals, B complex, and vitamin C to reduce inflammation. Rest the injured tendon.

Varicose Veins

Varicose veins are quite common and affect about 60 percent of Americans. They are often raised lumpy areas, dark blue or purple and appear on the backs of the legs or calves and sometimes on the insides of the legs. Varicose veins result when the veins lose their elasticity and stretch. Valves in the legs may stop working, causing blood to flow backward away from the heart. Constipation, pregnancy, and standing jobs can all contribute to varicosities because of pressure placed on the veins. To help heal varicose veins, take a warming bath with ginger four to five times per week. Dry off well and apply a cabbage poultice to the areas with varicosities. Sleep with your legs propped up. Drink three to four cups of oatstraw tea per day. Oatstraw tea is high in silicon, which builds connective tissue. Use horse chestnut cream to help strengthen veins. Take two thousand milligrams of bioflavonoids and two hundred milligrams of rutin per day. Bioflavonoids build and repair connective tissue as well. If you are constipated, see and follow directions under "Constipation." If you have a job where you have to stand on your feet all day, do your best to change jobs to one that allows more sitting. If legs become swollen and red or painful, see your doctor right away because it may indicate a blood clot.

Warts

Warts are produced on the skin by a virus from the human papillomavirus (HPV) family. They can be passed from one person to another. Some people have very strong immune systems and do not get warts as easily as others. To heal warts, combine equal parts castor oil and oregano oil or garlic oil. Massage the mixture onto warts in a circular motion ten times, three times per day. Work to boost the immune system by eating properly, drinking purified water, exercising, and taking two propolis tablets daily. Eating garlic can also be helpful.

Yeast Infections

Yeast infections of the vaginal tract often occur when a person is under stress or consuming lots of sugar or beer. Vaginal yeast can be contracted from a sexual partner that has a yeast infection. Try taking four tablets of propolis three times per day. Use two capsules of acidophilus every two hours until well, then two capsules three times a day for one month. Use two capsules of grapefruit seed extract two times per day. Use caprylic acid as directed on the label (this comes from coconut). Take one capsule of essential fatty acids (black currant seed oil, flaxseed oil, borage oil, and pumpkin seed oil are

good sources) three times per day. Drink one cup of Pau d'Arco tea per day and one cup of clove tea per day (both teas are antifungal and antibacterial).

Your diet must be fruit-free, sugar-free, and yeast-free. Avoid aged cheeses, alcohol, chocolate, honey, maple syrup, fermented foods such as pickles and vinegar, and grains containing gluten. Eat vegetables, fish, brown rice, quinoa, and millet. Eat plain yogurt that contains live yogurt cultures. Drink distilled water only.

VAGINAL DOUCHE FOR YEAST INFECTIONS

 16 ounces distilled water
 1 teaspoon ground Pau d'Arco bark
 6 capsules goldenseal root powder
 6 capsules acidophilus
 6 drops tea tree oil or 4 drops oregano oil
 2 droppers colloidal silver at 250 parts per million

Boil the distilled water and pour it over the Pau d'Arco bark. Steep the mixture for fifteen minutes, then strain it. Break open the capsules of goldenseal root powder; pour the Pau d'Arco tea over the goldenseal. Stir the mixture well, then let it cool. Add the remaining ingredients, and stir everything together. Pour the mixture into a douche bag. Stand in the shower and gently insert the tip of the douche tube, lubricated with olive oil, into the vagina. Let the contents of the bag flow in. A large part will flow back out, but some of the ingredients will remain and work to heal the yeast infection. Douche in the morning and at night for seven days.

A vaginal implant will also help heal a yeast infection. Insert a garlic clove that has been dipped in olive oil into the vagina each night before going to sleep. It will come out easily in the morning. On the third night, cut the garlic clove once with a sharp knife before inserting it. On the fourth night, cut the garlic clove twice before inserting it. Garlic cloves may be worn during the day as well with a sanitary napkin. Discontinue when the vaginal tract is healthy.

An alternate vaginal implant requires a large two-ounce syringe. Mix the implant as follows.

VAGINAL IMPLANT FOR YEAST INFECTIONS

 2 ounces plain raw yogurt
 6 capsules acidophilus
 3 capsules goldenseal
 1 dropper colloidal silver
 1 dropper fresh-squeezed wheatgrass juice

Break the capsules open, and pour the contents into a bowl with the yogurt, wheatgrass juice, and liquid colloidal silver. Stir all the ingredients together. Draw some of the mixture up into a syringe. Insert the contents into the vaginal tract. Lie with your hips up on a pillow for at least one hour. This mixture can be inserted at night before bed.

—From *Health Is Your Birthright*

Herbalism

AN INTRODUCTION TO HERBALISM

Debra St. Claire

In order to use this herbal guide wisely, it is essential that you understand some basic principles of herbology. Hippocrates stated, "Let your food be your medicine and your medicine be your food." Most of the food plants that we currently use have medicinal properties. For instance, Celery and Parsley have diuretic effects; Apples, Prunes and the Squash family have laxative effects; certain spices such as Black Pepper and Ginger have stimulant effects; etc.

The use of plants as medicines is our oldest form of healing, and traditional botanically based medicine is still the predominant form of medical treatment in today's world. At certain periods in human history, herbalism had peaks of knowledge and usage, the last one being in the late 1800s during the reign of the eclectic physicians. After the ability to synthesize medicine from inert substances such as petroleum and minerals was developed, the therapeutic use of herbs diminished. The art of pharmacy turned to the production of drugs that could bring the quickest relief of symptoms, ignoring the reason that the symptoms appeared.

As we look back, perhaps it is time to reconsider that path. The use of these substances has spawned a myriad of unexpected problems, such as suppression of the very signals that our bodies produce to alert us to a need for change. Pain itself is a call to action—a call to remedy an imbalance in our lifestyle. From the perspective of Ayurvedic medicine (the oldest recorded healing system), the period of body imbalance which is easiest to correct is that first, often vague sense of unrest which precedes the onset of an illness. The proficient use of herbal therapy is directly connected to our ability to sense that first signal and to adjust our lifestyle accordingly. It is when these signals are continually ignored that disease has a chance to seat itself more deeply within our body.

The appropriate use of herbs is only one of many healthy alternatives to our present medical system. It is my hope that as you use this booklet, you will be inspired to explore your own lifestyle and body balance and to study this and other forms of natural healing as you take increasing responsibility for your own health.

Our government is faced with an incredible resurgence of interest in natural healing. While creating laws which were originally designed to protect people from medical fraud, it unfortunately included laws that limit our freedom to choose our own form of medical treatment. Herbs are currently tossed back and forth between "food" and "drug" classifications like a hot potato with no place to rest. With due respect for traditional cultures, and the thousands of years of clinical experience that they represent, herbalists propose that a third classification be created for medicinal plants, namely as agents of traditional medicine, with proven safety being the criteria instead of medical efficacy. Once out of the realm of food and drug, more responsibility would lie with the consumer as to personal use.

Because of the often well-founded prohibition on practicing medicine without a license, making medical claims, etc., the research presented in this booklet must be used only as a guide to the historical use of herbs. Each person's body chemistry is different, and what works for one may not work for another. Your personal responsibility is to pay attention to your own body's reaction to the herbs, and to adjust your use of them as necessary.

I believe that as people turn to natural plant-based medicine, they will rediscover their appreciation for the earth. Due to the increase of industrialization and its destructive effect on the environment, we are losing one species of plants each day, and it is estimated that if the current pattern prevails, it could soon be one species per hour. Once a genetic code is lost, it can never be regained. We are losing potential foods and medicines which could be the solutions to our most important health issues.

As herbalists, we believe that ecological stewardship is essential; therefore, we are faced with several issues as we produce our herbal products. As the use of herbal medicine increases, we could easily extin-

Continued ➜

guish our stands of wild herbs; thus our goal is to protect all plant species and to organically grow the plants we use so that we can insure their survival and continued availability on our planet.

A final note: For goodness' sake, be sensible about all this. . . if symptoms persist, pay attention to them. It is always advantageous to seek the diagnostic services of a qualified holistic physician. If you experience nausea or any other adverse reaction, stop taking the herbs! Too many people, familiar with the terms "detoxification" and "healing crisis," put up with unpleasant reactions to natural products in the belief that these reactions are part of the process of healing (penance for past improprieties?), when, in fact, the body is communicating its need for an adjustment in the choice of therapy. Your skill at interpreting your own body's language will improve with practice; in the meantime, when in doubt, stop what you're doing and study! There is a list of some of the most useful herbal and natural therapy texts at the end of this booklet. *Use them.*

Frequently Asked Questions About Herbal Medicine

Q: I hear the word "herb" pronounced two different ways. Which is correct?

ANS: In every country in the world except the United States, the word is pronounced with the "h," as in "house." Therefore, many people are ceasing to pronounce it as "erb."

Q: What is a herbal extract?

ANS: Herbal extracts are the medicinal properties of herbs extracted into fluids that act as solvents and preservatives such as grain alcohol/distilled water, vinegar or glycerin. No heat is needed in the extraction, therefore the volatile oils and healing properties are preserved.

Q: How do herbal extracts work?

ANS: Herbal extracts support the body's ability to heal itself by cleansing and strengthening the tissues. They also catalyze certain body actions, such as diuresis (urination) or diaphoresis (sweating). Extracts are quickly assimilated by the body, and are best used to support and maintain the body's own efforts to defend itself from disease. Therefore herbal extracts play an important role in preventive medicine.

Q: Why take a herbal extract instead of other forms of herbal preparations?

ANS: Extracts are the most convenient way to ingest herbal medicines. Capsules and most teas are made from dried herbs, and their potency is vulnerable. Herbal extracts can be produced from *fresh* plants, and maintain their potency for 3–5 years if stored out of direct sunlight in a cool place. They do not require refrigeration.

Q: How are herbal extracts taken?

ANS: Many people prefer diluting the dosage (usually 20–30 drops) with ½ cup water, then drinking it like an instant "tea." If there is an acute problem like a sore throat, however, it can be squirted back so that it coats the throat full strength. Hold the dropper forward so that it doesn't touch the mouth to preserve its sterility.

Q: Is it necessary to use alcohol in herbal extracts?

ANS: Yes. The medicinal constituents of plants fall into two basic categories—water soluble and alcohol soluble. Many constituents are not water soluble and will only give up their medicinal properties to an alcohol base. If only water is used, the alcohol soluble constituents will remain in the plant matter

and not be bio-available. Therefore, a specific balance of distilled water and grain alcohol is required to extract the full spectrum of medicinal properties from the plant.

Q: What if one does not want the alcohol?

ANS: If you want to remove the alcohol, put the dose in a cup, pour ½ cup hot water over it, and let it sit, uncovered, for 5 minutes. The alcohol will dissipate, leaving the herbal concentrate behind. (The amount of alcohol in an average dose [30 drops] of a herbal extract containing 50% alcohol is roughly equivalent to 1/50 of a can of beer.)

Q: What is the proper amount to take?

ANS: Always a sticky subject due to personal metabolism, dietary habits, stress levels and other vagaries of our individual bodies, dosage guidelines are nevertheless important. Well put in Felter's *Materia Medica*, vol. 1, "It is better to err on the side of insufficient dosage and trust to nature, than to overdose to the present or future harm or danger to the patient." In other words, try a little, and watch for your reaction, before you take a lot. In acute cases people have taken a dropperful every hour and usually take 1–3 droppers full per day in chronic problems. If one is sensitive enough, and listens well to one's own body, the dosage should be apparent. If you have dosage questions, consult a competent wholistic practitioner for assistance.

Q: Can herbs be taken with prescription drugs?

ANS: The key is to use herbs and a healthy diet to correct the imbalance before prescription drugs are necessary. Consult a holistic physician with botanical training for the herb's compatibility with specific prescriptions.

Q: What is the difference between Chinese, Ayurvedic and American herbal products?

ANS: Other than the locality of their production, the real difference between the three is in the diagnostic systems which are the foundation of their use. The plant itself is no more efficient just because it was grown in another country.

American herbal products are often associated with the Western medical model, which treats symptoms instead of the cause of the "dis-ease." The Chinese and Ayurvedic systems use herbs as *foods* to increase the body's systemic integrity. American herbs can be used in the same manner.

U.S. regulations require spraying of imported plant products which are not prepackaged. These fumigants and other chemicals leave a residue on the plants that I feel makes them unsuitable for medicinal purposes. It is also difficult to guarantee whether the plants were organically grown or fumigated prior to packaging.

When we utilize locally grown U.S. plants, we can closely monitor their growing and harvesting conditions to assure the highest standards of quality, while also supporting the local economy.

Q: Why do some manufacturers use fresh herbs in their extracts instead of dried ones?

ANS: Because they feel that the best extract is made by capturing the *vital potency* of the *fresh plant*. The greater the distance and time between harvest and processing, the greater chance of quality deterioration in the final product. Dried plants are exposed to the influences of moisture, atmosphere and in-storage contamination. From the time they are gathered until they are used, a constant change is occurring. Oxidation, the loss of volatile oils, and other biochemical breakdowns decrease the quality of the product. Fresh plants are also much easier to identify, thus preventing the substitution of inferior materials.

The Language of Herbal Preparation & Usage

The array of teas, capsules, extracts and tinctures displayed on the market shelves can be confusing. Questions like, "What is the difference between an extract and a tincture?" are often heard. The following section provides insight into the basic language of herbology. Once you have become acquainted with the fundamental terminology, understanding how and when to use the various preparations will easily follow.

Fluid Preparations

The chemical constituents found in plant life dissolve in different types of fluids. The following list is organized according to solvency.

WATER-BASED PREPARATIONS

Infusion
Extraction of the medicinal or flavor elements of plants by soaking in cold or hot water. Used for leaves, stems and flowers.

Decoction
Extraction of medicinal constituents by gently simmering the denser parts of plants for extended periods of time (i.e., roots, barks, seeds, etc.).

Medicinal or Beverage Tea
Prepared by placing the herbs in a vessel of water (preferably distilled) that has just been boiled, then stirring, covering, and letting steep for 10–15 min. (Can also be made as a cold infusion.)

HYDRO-ALCOHOLIC PREPARATIONS

These preparations are best made with a mixture of distilled water and pure grain alcohol (ETOH).

Weight/volume ratio *refers to the proportion of* **plant** *to the* **liquid** *it is being extracted into: i.e., water, grain alcohol, vinegar, etc. More plant matter does not necessarily increase the potency of the extract, as the point is to adequately "saturate" the plant matter in order to extract the full spectrum of available constituents (impossible if there is not enough liquid to "flush" out the active ingredients).*

USP Fluid Extract
- **Weight/volume ratio:** 1:1 (Herb weight & liquid volume are equal, producing an extract in which 1 cc = 1 gm dried herb.)
- **Extraction method:** Percolation of dried plant material according to specifications in United States or British pharmacoepias.
- **Quality control:** It is harder to identify adulterations of dried and pulverized specimens without chemical analysis. Imported herbs and those in storage are subjected to chemical sprays to prevent insect infestation and molds.
- **Note:** The advantage of drying a plant is that it concentrates some medicinal properties. Unfortunately, important constituents are lost along the way. This is particularly evident in botanicals of storage before extraction, leading to oxidation and rancidity.

Fresh Plant Fluid Extract
- **Weight/volume ratio:** By the time reliable research on *fresh* plant extraction had begun, the focus of pharmacy had shifted to isolation and synthesis of active constituents. Therefore, fresh plant or "green extractions" had limited reference in the early pharmacoepias. As a result, there is a lack of standardized definition in the industry. We are only now, in the recent rise of interest in botanical medicine,

Continued ➡

able to redefine and perfect this processing technique. Most manufacturers define them as highly concentrated extracts prepared in a range between 1:0.75 and 1:3, depending on moisture analysis and the physical nature of the fresh plant.

- **Extraction method:** Maceration (grinding up and blending with dissolving solution for specified period)
- **Quality control:** Plants should be set into the menstruum (the combination of plant matter and dissolving fluid) as soon as possible after harvesting, optimum being no later than 24 hours. All plants should be organically grown or ecologically wildcrafted in pure surroundings, away from power lines or environmental pollutants.
- **Note:** Most botanicals can and should be extracted while fresh. A few are dried to alter potentially irritating constituents, as in the case of Cascara Sagrada.

Tincture
- **Weight/volume ratio:** 1:5
- **Extraction method:** Maceration (fresh or dried plants) or percolation (dried plants) **Quality control:** Process techniques vary. Question manufacturer about plant condition at time of extraction (fresh or dry, length of time between harvest and extraction). Ask about extraction method.
- **Notes:** Less strong than the first two categories. Can be prepared with either fresh or dried plants, depending on method of extraction, although standard definition of tincture indicates the use of dried material.

Homeopathic Mother Tincture
- **Weight/volume ratio:** 1:10
- **Extraction method:** Maceration, most often prepared with fresh plants.
- **Quality control:** As above
- **Notes:** Generally used as a base for further dilutions and sucussions as per standard homeopathic pharmacy technique.

Solid Extract
- **Weight/volume ratio:** Generally 4:1
- **Extraction method:** (1) With fresh plants, maceration then concentration from a liquid down into a solid, utilizing the rotary evaporation technique. (2) Dried plants are usually percolated, then concentrated.
- **Quality control:** As above. Ask manufacturer if extraction is performed in line with advertised quality standards or performed as an out-lab service.

ELIXIRS
Elixirs are sweetened, aromatic and spirituous solutions, designed as vehicles for small amounts of active medicines. As a class they are very unsatisfactory, though pleasant preparations.

—*The Eclectic Materia Medica, Pharmacology and Therapeutics,*
H. W. Felter, M.D.

ESSENTIAL OILS
The pure, volatile, aromatic essence of the plant. Usually steam distilled, although there are other methods such as effleurage and direct expression.

GLYCERITES
Vegetable Glycerin is a hydrolized vegetable fat that is between water and alcohol in its ability to dissolve plant constituents. It has weaker preservative properties than alcohol. Very sweet taste, making it use-ful in the preparation of elixirs and syrups. Glycerites are most safely made with dried herbs to prevent spoilage, because fresh plants have higher percentages of active bacteria.

HERBAL OILS
Created by soaking or gently simmering herbs in a carrier oil such as olive or almond.

SYRUPS
Syrups are generally made by simmering fresh or dried herbs down into a concentrate. Honey, glycerin, Sucanat, Nutri-Cane, maple syrup, rice syrup, or other natural sweeteners are added, then simmered down until the mixture reaches the desired syrupy consistency. Quick syrups can also be made by adding herbal extracts to honey or other sweeteners, with the advantage of not using heat. This method best preserves the volatile constituents.

VINEGARS
Vinegar also dissolves medicinal constituents, however, it is not as effective as the hydro-alcoholic solution. Its preservative strength is more than plain water and less than alcohol. Will extract constituents from fresh or dried herbs.

Dried Herbs
Herbs are also available in dried form. They should be purchased from companies who utilize organically grown herbs. Smell them to see if the aromas are still present, one indication of proper harvesting and storage. Store in tightly closed glass containers away from direct sunlight. If properly cared for, their potency lasts approximately one year.

BULK HERBS
May be used to brew beverage or medicinal teas, make poultices, baths, steams and a number of other herbal preparations. Available in single herbs or combinations.

TEA BAGS
Should be purchased in bleach-free paper to avoid dioxin contamination. A very easy way to prepare herbal beverages. Also useful as emergency poultices.

CAPSULATED HERBS
As of this printing, the new animal-free gelatin capsules still have some problems with early disintegration, which are expected to be corrected soon. The problem with gelatin capsules is that they short circuit the digestive process by prohibiting oral "recognition" of the herb. I have seen many cases where they moved through the entire digestive tract and were eliminated as a whole capsule without ever dissolving. Although it may not taste good, it helps to open one capsule and sprinkle it over the rest of the capsules in the jar. This way the body has a greater chance of secreting the proper digestive enzymes by analyzing the "taste"—similar to the social courtesy of telephoning before you visit.

Another issue is the difficulty in swallowing capsules. They should not be given to small children. Open the capsule and mix it with a carrier such as a bit of honey. (This type of herbal preparation is known as an electuary.)

POWDERS
When a herb is broken down in small enough particles to be considered a powder, it has a much shorter shelf life, due to the fact that more surface area is exposed to oxygen and light. The volatile oils and other medicinal constituents are easily lost, decreasing the potency.

Herbs are powdered previous to the capsulation process and in the percolation process of using dried herbs to make fluid extracts. Some companies also provide them as powdered formulas.

If you must use powdered herbs, it is best to powder them immediately before use. This is most easily accomplished with a coffee grinder or mortar and pestle.

Glossary of Herbal Preparations
Balm: See *Salve.*

Baths: Water-based infusion designed to achieve herbal therapy through immersion/osmosis.

Capsules: Inclusion of dried, powdered herbs in gelatin, primarily to hide their taste.

Cerates: A fatty preparation resembling an ointment, but having a firmer consistency and a higher melting point. True cerates always contain wax.

Cold Compresses: Used to prevent swelling and reduce fevers. An infusion or decoction which is chilled, soaked into a cloth and externally applied.

Creams: Herbs captured in a fatty or oily base with a light, airy texture which is easily spread on skin for a healing or moisturizing effect.

Decoctions: Roots, barks, seeds and other dense plant parts gently simmered for extended periods to dissolve water soluble constituents.

Douches: An infusion or decoction administered vaginally to cleanse, disinfect, and soothe.

Electuaries: The medicinal or nourishing constituents of herbs in a sweet base such as honey.

Elixirs: Thin, syrupy liquid carrier used to make herbs more palatable. Very sweet.

Enemas: Infusion or decoction rectally injected to relieve constipation, cleanse, and soothe the large intestine.

Eyewashes: Infusion or decoction used to cleanse, disinfect, and soothe ocular tissue.

Fluid Extracts: The medicinal properties of herbs in a concentrated liquid form for internal consumption or external application.

Fomentation: Applied hot—an infusion or decoction of herbs soaked into a cloth for external application.

Gargle: An infusion, decoction or diluted extract used to cleanse, disinfect and soothe the throat. Normally not swallowed.

Glycerites: The medicinal or nourishing constituents of herbs extracted into this highly sweet hydrolized vegetable fat. Does not sufficiently extract full spectrum of available constituents.

Granules: Sugar pellets impregnated with medicinal matter which is applied in liquid form and absorbed by the pellets, then dried. Usually used as a carrier for homeopathic preparations.

Infusions: Leaves, flowers, and other tender parts of plants soaked in freshly boiled water to capture their water-soluble constituents. Internal and external use.

Juices: See *Succus.*

Liniments: Alcoholic or hydro-alcoholic solutions of medicinal constituents used for external application.

Lotions: Oil/water-based preparation, allowing healing benefits to be absorbed through skin.

Lozenges: Small, sweetened, candylike disks or drops (preferably with natural base ingredients) which are sucked to obtain medicinal benefit (dependent on specific formula).

Mucilages: Fresh or dried herbs which become slick and slimy when mixed with water. Used internally and externally to soothe and heal irritated tissue.

Ointments: Herbs mixed with lard, lanolin, petroleum, or wax for external application to skin afflictions. Gradually melts with skin heat and is absorbed.

Continued ➜

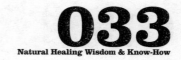

Oxymel: Neutralizes acrid or pungent taste of herbs like garlic with vinegar and honey.

Pessaries: Bullet-size, cocoa butter-based pellet which carries herbs for vaginal absorption.

Pills: Masses of medicinal matter, round or oval in shape, designed for internal consumption. Sometimes contain carrier material such as starch, gelatin, or milk sugar.

Plasters: Medicinal herbs stirred into a sticky base which is then spread on skin, silk, cotton cloth or paper. Solidifies into a hard mass which mechanically supports the injured area while the medicinal constituents are absorbed.

Poultices: Fresh or dried herbs mixed with enough liquid to make a thick, pasty consistency for external application to skin and muscular injuries.

Powders: Dried herbs comminuted (ground) into small particles for encapsulation or extraction.

Salves: Oil and beeswax preparation useful for external skin application to promote healing of injured skin. Also known as a *Balm*.

Sinus Snuff: A powdered herb mixture designed for nasal inhalation. Produces copious discharge, aiding decongestion of the sinuses.

Spray: Herbal extracts, teas or diluted essential oils in spray bottles for internal or external use.

Steams: Infusion or decoction of herbs or small amounts of essential oils in hot water which rises up and surrounds the affected area for a detoxifying or decongesting effect.

Succus: Freshly expressed herbal juice, usually preserved with grain alcohol.

Suppositories: Bullet-shaped pellets of powdered herbs in a cocoa butter base designed for rectal absorption.

Syrups: Sweet, thick carrier for herbal medicine. Base usually consists of honey, glycerin, maple syrup, rice syrup, etc.

Tablets: Dry or moistened powdered herbs compressed into a variety of swallowable shapes. Sometimes contain carrier material such as starch, gelatin, or milk sugar.

Tinctures: Herbal constituents extracted into a standard weight/volume ratio of 1 part herb to 5 parts solvent.

Vinegars: Herbal constituents dissolved into vinegar for internal ingestion. Should be raw apple cider vinegar.

Wines: Herbal constituents dissolved into wines. Adds flavor. Best made with organic wines.

Therapeutic Actions

Abortifacient: Produces abortion

Adaptogenic: Decreases the harmful effects of stress

Alterative: Promotes healthy changes in the organism

Analgesic: Relieves pain

Anaphrodisiac: Subdues sexual desire

Anesthetic: Produces insensibility to pain

Anodyne: Relieves pain

Antacid: Counteracts acidity

Antagonist: Opposes action of other medicines

Antidote: Counteracts effect of poison

Antiemetic: Prevents vomiting

Antigalactic: Diminishes secretion of milk

Anthelmintic: Destroys parasites

Antihypnotic: Prevents sleep

Anti-inflammatory: Reduces inflammation

Antilithic: Helps prevent stone or gravel

Antimicrobial: Destroys microbes

Antimycetic: Destroys fungal infections

Antiseptic: Prevents or arrests putrefaction

Antispasmodic: Reduces spasms, relaxes

Antitussive: Relieves or prevents coughs

Aperient: Gently laxative

Aphrodisiac: Stimulates sexual desire

Astringent: Contracts tissue, restrains discharges

Bactericide: Destroys bacteria

Bitter: Increases tone and activity of gastric mucosa

Calmative: Gently calms nerves

Cardiac: Heart stimulant or tonic

Carminative: Prevents or relieves flatulence

Cathartic: Hastens or increases evacuation of the bowels

Cholagogue: Stimulates flow of bile

Demulcent: Soothing to mucus membranes

Deodorant: Removes/corrects foul odors

Depuritive: Removes impurities from the body, cleansing action

Diaphoretic: Increases perspiration

Digestant: Aids digestion

Disinfectant: Destroys the cause of infection

Diuretic: Increases secretion of urine

Drastic: Acts quickly and violently, said of cathartics

Emetic: Causes vomiting

Emmenagogue: Promotes menstruation

Emollient: Softening, soothing

Expectorant: Promotes mucus discharge from respiratory passages

Febrifuge: Reduces fever

Galactagogue: Promotes flow of milk in nursing mothers

Hemostatic: Arrests flow of blood

Hepatic: Stimulates function of liver

Hypnotic: Induces sleep

Irritant: Excites inflammation

Laxative: Produces gentle action of the bowels

Narcotic: Induces sleep or unconsciousness

Nervine: Calms nerves

Nutritive: Nourishes and sustains life

Palliative: Relieves morbid conditions without curing

Parasiticide: Destroys parasites

Parturient: Hastens labor

Pectoral: Relieves diseases of the lungs

Prophylactic: Prevents disease

Pyrogenic: Produces fever

Refrigerant: Cooling, reduces heat

Relaxant: Relieves tension, relaxes

Restorative: Brings back normal function and vitality

Rubefacient: Increases superficial circulation, producing irritation or redness

Sedative: Diminishes vital functions

Sialagogue: Stimulates secretion of saliva

Stimulant: Excites or increases vital action

Stomachic: Induces healthy action of stomach

Styptic: Stops bleeding

Sudorific: Produces perspiration

Tonic: Produces permanent increase in functional tone of the system

Toxic: Poisonous

Vermifuge: Destroys or expels worms

Vulnerary: Stimulates healing of wounds

—From *Pocket Herbal Reference Guide*

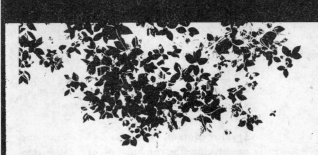

THE ACTIONS AND LANGUAGE OF HERBALISM

James Green, Herbalist

Using an Herbal

One finds information about the actions and affinities of an herb by reading an herbal. Many books are published about herbs and herbalism today, but few are written by experienced, knowledgeable herbalists. I strongly advise that readers seek out truly accurate herbals from the current glut of books about herbs that have become fashionable to publish.

While referencing an herbal, readers are confronted with a blend of information the author has selected to illustrate his or her particular herbal emphasis. As you peruse various herbals, you can note the prime bent of the authors. Some herbalists emphasize the botany and cultivation of herbs, for this is the aspect of herbalism that intrigues them most; some emphasize the more therapeutic and medicinal aspects of herbs, and others focus on the native habitat and harvesting and medicine-making details. But whatever is the author's particular experience and pleasure, the information shared is commonly organized in the general order given in the following example.

Common Name: Horse Chestnut

Botanical (binomial) name: *Aesculus hippocastanum*

Plant family: *Hippocastanaceae*

Parts used: (This section lists the parts of the plant used therapeutically.) Fruit and inner bark.

Description: (This section gives a fairly detailed macroscopical and often microscopical description of the plant to help the herbalist accurately identify it.) The trunk is very erect and columnar; bark is smooth and grayish; large leaves are divided into five or seven leaflets, spreading like fingers from the palm of the hand; flowers are mostly white with reddish tinge, growing in dense, erect spikes; fruit is a shining chestnut-brown nut having a bitter taste; the fruit has a large, green husk. It is protected with short spines that split into three valves when it falls to the ground, which dislodges the nut…

History: Horse Chestnut is indigenous to Persia and north India…was introduced into central Europe in the sixteenth century…now common in many parts of the United States…extensively cultivated for shade and ornamentation…

Flowering season: May–June

Collection season: Ripe nuts are collected in September and October as they fall to the ground; the bark is harvested in the early spring.

Cultivation and habitat: The plant is generally raised from the nuts sown in early spring…thrive in most soils and situations, but do best in a good sandy loam…

Actions and medical uses: (This section is alternatively termed "Properties," "Affinities," or

Continued ➡

"Virtues.") The fruit is a circulatory tonic and astringent. The bark is tonic, astringent, febrifuge, narcotic, and antiseptic.

Energy, taste, and organs affected: Cool, dry; mildly bitter, astringent, spicy; circulatory, particularly the venous system, genitourinary, digestive, blood.

Specific indications: (This section discusses the specific uses of the herb's actions and affinities.) The unique actions of Horse Chestnut are on the vessels of the circulatory system…increasing the strength and tone of the veins in particular…used internally to aid the body in the treatment of problems such as phlebitis, varicosity, and hemorrhoids. A remedy for congestion and engorgement, nerve pain in the viscera due to congestion, soreness of the whole body, with vascular fullness, throbbing, and general malaise, as well as rectal uneasiness with burning or aching pain.

Combinations used: (An herb often combines particularly well with certain other herbs in the treatment of specific conditions, so usually both the combination and the condition are discussed.) Combines well with Hawthorn, Yarrow, and Prickly Ash for internal use to treat varicosity. Combines with Witch Hazel for preparing a lotion to use externally on varicose veins or hemorrhoids.

Constituents: (This section lists isolated chemical constituents theorized to be most relevant to the action of the plant.) Saponins, tannins, flavones, starch, fatty oil, and the glycosides aesculin, aescin, and fraxin.

Precautions: Do not inject extracts hypodermically.

Preparation and dosage: (This section discusses common preparations of the herb and general dosage.)

Infusion: 1–2 full teaspoons of the dried fruit steeped in 1 cup of boiling water for ten to twenty minutes. Drink 1 cup three times a day.

Tincture: Take 1–4 milliliters of tincture three times a day. Externally: This plant is used as a lotion for the above conditions and is also appropriate for treating skin ulcers.

Toxicity: Eating the leaves or green outer casing of the fruit can lead to symptoms of gastroenteritis, reddening of the skin, and drowsiness.

Other uses: Shade and aesthetic ornamentation. The seeds or "conkers" are used by English children like marbles.

(An exceptional herbal usually features a drawing of each herb's pertinent parts.)

Few herbals will speak to all the attributes listed above, the format of each being custom designed according to the author's emphasis, but all these attributes are commonly used in some combination throughout the herbals in our Western culture. The one category of attributes that you will always find, however, is the actions. This is the most important empirical information given and is often also the most misunderstood and confusing to the student. Some herbals will present a long list of actions, which leaves one more befuddled than informed. It frequently appears that a particular herb is good for just about everything, which can leave one in a state of dismay due to oversaturation. Unfortunately, what has not been defined, and is often not understood, is the particular body system (for example, the digestive system, the respiratory system, or the lymphatic system) or systems that each herb has a natural affinity with. In some cases, various parts of a particular plant (leaf, root, flower, seed, and so on) provide different actions and have affinities for distinct systems of the body. But in many herbals, this information is all lumped into one amalgamated list and becomes nearly useless as a practical guide.

Seed (nut)

Green seed pod

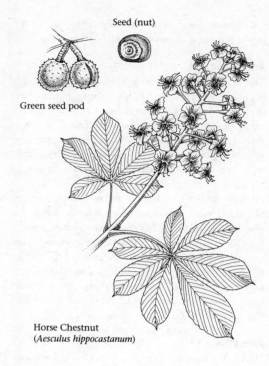

Horse Chestnut
(*Aesculus hippocastanum*)

What will help a learner most is to study and recognize the actions of an herb in relationship to its natural body-systems affinity. This affinity between an herb and a body system can also be thought of as a biochemical kinship, a natural spontaneous relationship, or a mutually attractive force. From centuries of human observation, the herb has demonstrated a consistent, predictable affinity with a particular body system, and the herb's actions cause a specific effect or action on that system. Ginkgo, for example, will move to the peripheral-vascular systems and other outlying regions and will dilate the blood vessels, and—voilà!—more blood and oxygen will ultimately reach the brain. A Horse Chestnut fruit extract, meanwhile, having a natural affinity with the circulatory system, will move to the vessels of this system and act to give them strength and tone, while an extract of its bark will readily cruise to the rectal area and supply astringent action for congested hemorrhoids (varicose rectal veins)—a true ally indeed.

Therefore, it is imperative that individuals who choose to use herbs for their personal and family health care become familiar with the action words of the language of herbalism that introduce them to the unique attributes of each herb. An herb can then be used most appropriately with the greatest efficiency. Combinations of herbs can be formulated to work synergistically in a more holistic approach, treating not only the obvious symptoms but, at the same time, supporting the health of all the other systems. Each herb has an array of actions and affinities, so a knowledgeable person can take care to combine herbs such that they enhance each other's actions to build health and tend to a range of problems. Armed with the understanding of the actions and affinities of a few herbs, one can devise a specific strategy for toning, balancing, and cleansing one's systems, thereby bolstering vital energy and simultaneously treating causes as well as symptoms.

An example formula for treating a prostate infection will illustrate this approach. Note the actions of the following herbs:

- The actions of Saw Palmetto berries are tonic, nutrient, and antiseptic, and this herb has a strong affinity for the reproductive and nervous systems. It acts to nourish the nerves and tone and strengthen the male reproductive system, particularly the prostate gland.
- Echinacea is an overall systemic (which means that it works throughout the whole body),

antimicrobial, lymphatic, alterative, and immune enhancer.

- Damiana is a nerve tonic, a prostate tonic, a urinary antiseptic, and an antidepressant, and it is mildly laxative. It, too, has an affinity for the reproductive and nervous systems.
- Yarrow is an astringent, bitter, and urinary antiseptic; is diuretic and diaphoretic, aiding the body in dealing with fever; and has an affinity for the circulatory system, directly assisting in normalizing blood pressure.

Using the combined actions of these four herbs, we can create at once a strong glandular tonic that is astringent and strengthening for a debilitated and, most likely, swollen prostate gland. In all cases of infection, the body's natural resistance is somehow compromised. This may be caused by stress, constipation, or inadequate diet, so I have included bitters in this formula to help stimulate appetite and the secretion of digestive juices. I have included immune system—enhancing herbs with genitourinary system antiseptics to support the overall immune system, especially targeting the prostate. I also have circulatory system and nervous system tonics with an alterative herb. These herbs support circulation, nerve impulses, and blood conditioning, respectively, with a mild laxative action present, if needed.

So, by taking advantage of the specific actions and system affinities of these herbs, we are attending to the major symptom, the infected prostate gland, while also enhancing the health of the nervous, circulatory, and digestive systems and firmly assisting the body's overall systemic immune action. If there is discomfort and pain, Cramp Bark and/or Black Haw can be added to the formula. These two herbs are nervine, analgesic, and antispasmodic, having an affinity with the reproductive system. If flavor is an issue, we can add Fennel seed, which is a pleasant-tasting herb having carminative, aromatic, and antispasmodic actions, to the formula. Fennel has an affinity with the entire digestive tract, stimulating appetite and digestion while relieving flatulence.

An herbal remedy specific for treating infection in the male genitourinary system that simultaneously nourishes and strengthens supportive systems combines the above herbs as follows:

2 parts	Saw Palmetto
2 parts	Echinacea
1 part	Damiana
1 part	Yarrow
1 part	Cramp Bark

I suggest including Saw Palmetto and Echinacea in 2 parts, because they possess the primary properties required to treat the prostate infection.

Prepare a pot of tea (using 1 rounded teaspoon of this formula per cup of water) and drink 1 cup three times a day. In place of taking a tea, you can take the herbs as a tincture blend, combining the individual plant tinctures in the same proportions, and using 30 to 50 drops of the blended liquid formula three times a day.

With wholesome diet, adequate water, regular exercise, and rest, a blend of herbs similar to the above formula can assist a man in ridding himself of prostate infection and reproductive-organ debility. Preventive care, including regular Kegel exercises and continued use of prostate tonics such as Saw Palmetto, Nettle Root, and Red Raspberry leaf, will then become the key to his continued experience of health.

Continued ➡

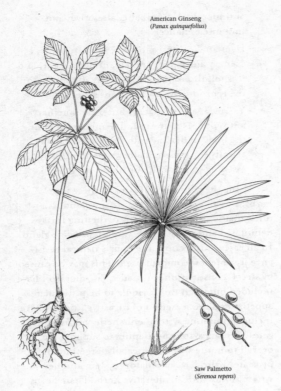

American Ginseng
(*Panax quinquefolius*)

Saw Palmetto
(*Serenoa repens*)

Herbal Actions

Now that there no longer exists even a wisp of doubt about the importance of knowing the actions and affinities of the herbs one uses, I will list and discuss some of the main actions of herbs. Reductionist science has undertaken difficult research to determine the plant constituents responsible for these actions and has classified these constituents according to their chemical groups and physiological properties or effects. Thus, for example, plant gum and mucilage constituents are said to give rise to the soothing demulcent and emollient actions; the tannins give rise to astringent and hemostatic actions, and some saponins are believed to give rise to anti-inflammatory and expectorant actions. Using this reductionist insight and technology to determine the chemical constituents of herbal medicines newly introduced to us by the regional folklore of the plant's native environment, we can gain valuable hints as to the actions of these new plants. At the same time, when experimenting with these plants therapeutically, I feel it is important to keep in mind an herbalist's perspective that the integrity and therapeutic value of a medicinal herb remains biomedically unique only when the herb's individual constituents remain in the context of the natural organization of the hundreds of synergistic biochemical constituents contained in the whole herb.

Approximately 120 actions have been identified through the ages. However, only about a third of them are commonly considered. In the specific context of male health care, we need to be most functionally cognizant of the following actions.

Tonic

Along with adaptogens, tonic action is perhaps the most profound contribution of herbal medicine to natural health care. Tonic herbs stimulate nutrition by improving the assimilation of essential nutrients by the organs and improve systemic tone, lending increased vigor, energy, and strength to the tissues of either specific organs or to the whole body. This is the central essential action to consider when devising a healing therapeutic formula. Once an individual has undertaken sufficient cleansing of his body's systems, the other herbal actions work symbiotically with toning to evolve full healing....The long list of tonic herbs includes Oats, Hawthorn, Saw Palmetto, Nettles, Garlic,

Goldenseal, Dandelion, *Ho shou wu*, *Dong Quai*, *Askwagandha*, Ginseng, Raspberry, and Yarrow.

Adaptogen

This is a timely, newly recognized action concept unique to herbal therapeutics. Adaptogenic or hormonal modulating actions increase the body's resistance to, and endurance in the face of, a wide variety of adverse influences from physical, chemical, biological, and emotional stress, assisting the body's ability to cope and adapt. Adaptogens are nontoxic and possess normalizing actions. For example, adaptogens tend to normalize high or low blood pressure, overactive or underactive adrenal glands and possibly other endocrine glands, and high or low blood sugar. Adaptogen action appears to work through hormonal regulation of the stress response, which, in turn, has a modulating effect on the human immune system. Adaptogenic herbs include Siberian Ginseng, Chinese and American Ginseng, Schisandra, and *Ashwagandha*.

Alterative

Herbs that have this property, referred to as blood cleansers, gradually restore health and vitality to the body by helping it assimilate nutrients, eliminate metabolic wastes, and restore proper function. Alterative herbs are used to help treat infection, blood toxicity, skin eruptions, impotence, and chronic degenerative conditions. Alterative herbs include Burdock, Red Clover, Nettle, Cleavers, and Oregon Grape.

Amphoteric

These herbs normalize a hyperactive or hypoactive process in the body: Garlic (which normalizes both high and low blood pressure), Chaste Tree, Lobelia, Elder, Mullein, and Schisandra.

Analgesic, Anodyne

These nonnarcotic herbs relieve pain when administered orally or externally: Skullcap, Valerian, and Passion Flower.

Antacid

These herbs neutralize excess acid in the stomach and intestinal tract: Fennel, Catnip, Dandelion, Slippery Elm, Mullein, Umeboshi (or Japanese) Plum, and Meadowsweet (which clears symptoms of hyperacidity).

Anthelmintic

These herbs destroy or expel worms from the digestive tract: Garlic, Onion, Wormwood, Rue, and Thyme.

Anticatarrhal

These herbs counteract inflammation that causes the buildup and increased flow of excess mucus from the sinuses or other upper respiratory parts: Eyebright, Echinacea, Garlic, Black Pepper, Cayenne, Sage, Hyssop, Goldenrod, Yarrow, and Yerba Santa.

Antiemetic

These herbs lessen nausea and help relieve or prevent vomiting: Balm, Peppermint, Ginger, Fennel, Dill, Gentian, and Meadowsweet.

Anti-inflammatory

Moderate inflammation is the body's appropriate reaction to infection, injury, or irritation, resulting in enhanced tissue repair and containment of invaders. One does not always want to lessen this inflammation but often finds it more efficacious to stimulate it by using rubifacients or systemic vasodilators. (See page 37.) One uses anti-inflammatory action to combat extensive or too painful

occurrences of inflammation. Anti-inflammatory herbs include those having demulcent, emollient, and vulnerary actions when applied externally: St. John's Wort, Calendula, Turmeric, Arnica, Licorice, Chamomile, and Wild Yam.

Antilithic

These herbs help prevent or dissolve and discharge urinary and biliary stones and gravel. For urinary-system kidney and bladder stones: Gravel Root, Hydrangea, Dandelion, Cleavers, Buchu, Goldenrod, Corn Silk, and Bearberry (also known as *Uva Ursi*). For gallbladder: Oregon Grape and Chaparral.

Antimicrobial

These herbs help the body's immune system destroy or resist pathogenic microorganisms: unripe Black Walnut hulls, Echinacea, Chaparral, Garlic, Goldenseal, Wormwood, and herbs high in volatile oils such as Anise, Caraway, Clove, Eucalyptus, Myrrh, Peppermint, Rosemary, and Thyme.

Antipyretic

These herbs reduce fever and inflammation: Feverfew, Boneset, Yarrow, Elder, and Catnip.

Aphrodisiac

These herbs help correct conditions of impotence mostly by strengthening sexual excitement and desire. They tend more to stimulate sexual arousal than to improve performance. A combined use with alteratives helps restore proper function. The substantial list of herbal aphrodisiacs includes Damiana, Yohimbe, Long Jack, Maca, and Muira Puama.

Aromatic

These herbs have a salient, usually pleasant aroma, which stimulates the gastrointestinal system (see Carminative) and are frequently used to improve the aroma and taste of medicines and foods: Lavender, Peppermint, Angelica, Cardamom, Cinnamon, Dill, and Citrus Peel.

Astringent

This action promotes greater density and firmness of tissue by precipitating protein and condensing the cellular structure of the tissue, contracting and firming relaxed weakened tissue such as hemorrhoids and prolapsed organs. Astringency can reduce excessive discharge of fluids such as diarrhea in the intestines, blood hemorrhaging from the lungs and kidneys, or excessive perspiration from the skin. These herbs include White Oak, Pipsissewa, Horse Chestnut, Partridgeberry, and Witch Hazel.

Bitter

These herbs stimulate the secretion of digestive juices, benefiting digestion and assimilation, and stimulate the liver and the pancreas, aiding the elimination of toxins: Gentian, Hops, Artichoke, Mugwort, and Dandelion.

Carminative

This action excites intestinal peristalsis, promotes expulsion of gas, soothes the stomach and promotes digestion, and relieves gripping (severe cramping pain) in the gastrointestinal tract. These herbs, rich in aromatic volatile oils, include Anise, Fennel, Chamomile, Peppermint, Caraway, and Ginger.

Cholagogue

This action promotes the discharge and flow of bile from the gallbladder into the small intestine. This is beneficial in treating gallbladder problems. Bile helps disinfect the bowels and can have a laxative effect, as bile normally stimulates peristalsis elimi-

Continued ➡

nation. Cholagogues include Barberry, Goldenseal, Dandelion, Oregon Grape, and Wild Yam.

Demulcent

This action relieves and soothes the tissue of the digestive tract upon direct contact, and triggers reflex mechanisms that travel through the spinal nerves, effectively reducing inflammation and irritation in the respiratory and urinary systems. These mucilaginous, gelatinous, soothing, and protective herbs include Comfrey, Marshmallow, Slippery Elm, Mullein, and Corn Silk.

Diaphoretic

Fever is a very appropriate response of the body for dealing with infection. Contrary to accepted medical technique, stimulating a fever is often highly beneficial. Just drink lots of water. Doing so increases perspiration, bringing the heat and inflammation outward to the surface of the skin, cooling the skin by evaporation, and facilitating excretion of waste matter. These herbs, taken hot, induce increased perspiration, dilate capillaries, and increase elimination through the skin: Elder, Osha, Ginger, and Peppermint.

Diuretic

These herbs increase the elimination and regulate the flow of urine. For best results, drink lots of pure water while using diuretics, which include Dandelion, Couchgrass, Bearberry, Plantain, and Horsetail.

Emetic

Emetics cause vomiting, helping the stomach empty. To produce this effect, these herbs usually need to be taken in large doses: Lobelia, Ipecac, and Boneset.

Emollient

Applied to the skin, emollients soothe, soften, and protect externally, much like demulcents do internally. They include Comfrey, Chickweed, Plantain, Slippery Elm, and Marshmallow.

Expectorant

Stimulating expectorants, including Elecampane and White Horehound, stimulate the nerves and muscles of the respiratory system to manifest a coughing

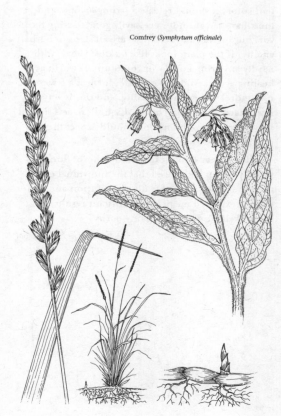

Comfrey (*Symphytum officinale*)

syndrome, causing expectoration by encouraging the loosening and expulsion of mucus. *Relaxing* expectorants, including Coltsfoot (excellent for children), Gumweed, Licorice, and Hyssop, reduce tension in lung tissue, easing tightness and allowing natural coughing and flow of mucus to occur. *Amphoteric* expectorants, including Lobelia, Mullein, Horehound, Coltsfoot, Elder, and Garlic, can stimulate or relax the respiratory system, relying on the body's intelligence to determine what is necessary.

Febrifuge

These herbs assist the body in reducing fever: Catnip, Elder Blossom, and Yarrow.

Hemostatic

These herbs are internal astringents that arrest hemorrhaging: Bayberry, Blackberry, Cayenne, Shepherd's Purse, and Goldenseal.

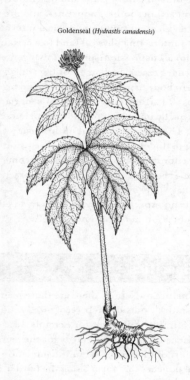

Goldenseal (*Hydrastis canadensis*)

Hepatic

These herbs strengthen and tone the liver, stimulating its secretive function and causing an increase in the flow of bile: Oregon Grape root, Dandelion, Goldenseal, and Wild Yam.

Hypnotic

These herbs have a powerful relaxant and sedative action and help induce sleep: Hops, Valerian, and Wild Lettuce.

Hypotensive

These herbs reduce elevated blood pressure: Cramp Bark, Onion, Garlic, Yarrow, and Hawthorn berries and flowers.

Laxative and Aperient

Laxative herbs stimulate bowel action, promoting evacuation: Cascara Sagrada, Yellow Dock, and Rhubarb root. Aperient herbs, which have a very mild laxative action, include Dandelion root, Boneset, and Beet root.

Lymphatic

These herbs support the health and activity of the lymphatic system: Cleavers, Calendula, and Echinacea.

Nervine

These herbs affect the nervous system, having either a tonic (Oats, Damiana), relaxing (Chamomile, Hops), or stimulating (coffee, Green Tea, Yerba Mate) effect.

Pectoral

These herbs have a general strengthening and healing effect on the entire respiratory system: Elecampane, Coltsfoot, Comfrey, Mullein, Yerba Santa, and Yerba Mansa.

Rubefacient

When applied locally to the skin, rubefacients cause gentle irritation, promoting capillary dilation and increased circulation in the skin, drawing blood from deeper areas of the body. This action relieves inflammation and congestion in these parts, often reducing pain. These herbs are useful for treating acute sprains, chronic arthritis, rheumatism, and other joint afflictions: Stinging Nettle, Mustard seed, Cayenne, Horseradish, and Black Pepper.

Sedative

These herbs calm the nervous system by decreasing the functional activity of an organ or by reducing stress and nervous irritation throughout the body: Valerian, Skullcap, Passion Flower, and Black Cohosh.

Sialagogue

These herbs promote the secretion and flow of saliva from the salivary glands: Echinacea, Spilanthes, Prickly Ash, and Black Pepper.

Stimulant

These herbs warm the body, quicken the circulation, break up obstruction and congestion, increase energy, and possess a notably intense energy: Cayenne, Ginger, Horseradish, Mustard, and Wormwood.

Styptic

These herbs arrest or reduce external bleeding by causing astringent action on blood vessels: Yarrow, Horsetail, Cayenne, Bayberry, and Plantain.

Vasodilator

These herbs expand blood vessels, allowing increased circulation: Ginkgo, Feverfew, Ginger, Cayenne, and Bayberry.

Vulnerary

These herbs, applied externally, help the body heal wounds, bruises, and cuts: Comfrey, Calendula, Chickweed, St. John's Wort, and Marshmallow.

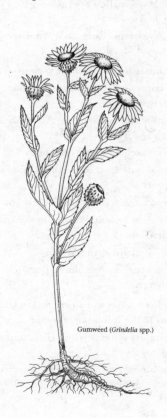

Gumweed (*Grindelia* spp.)

Continued ➡

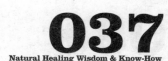

The Systems' Affinity for Herbs

Each system of the body has plants particularly suited to it, plants that have a natural affinity with it. So we find that within each of the action categories listed above are plants embodying that action that carry the action to a particular body system. To illustrate this affinity, the following lists of body systems will denote some herbs that carry anti-inflammatory, demulcent, bitter, or astringent actions to these systems.

These herbs carry anti-inflammatory action (reduced pain and discomfort) to various systems:

- Circulatory system: Hawthorn berries, Horse Chestnut, Yarrow, and Lime blossom
- Digestive system: Chamomile, Peppermint, Fennel, and Ginger
- Musculoskeletal system: Willow and Meadowsweet
- Nervous system: St. John's Wort
- Reproductive system: Lady's Mantle and Blue Cohosh
- Respiratory system: Licorice and Coltsfoot
- Skin: St. John's Wort, Calendula, Chickweed, Arnica, and Plantain
- Urinary system: Corn Silk, Goldenrod, and Marshmallow

These herbs carry demulcent action to various systems:

- Circulatory system (generally does not require demulcent action; however, Horse Chestnut and Linden blossoms, applied externally, have a soothing emollient action on the blood vessels)
- Digestive system (the anti-inflammatories will have a more direct therapeutic effect on this system than will demulcents): Slippery Elm
- Nervous system (demulcents have direct value only when applied to the skin for nervous conditions like shingles): Slippery Elm and Marshmallow
- Reproductive system: Marshmallow root, Mullein, Licorice, and Coltsfoot
- Respiratory system: Mullein, Marshmallow root, Plantain, and Licorice
- Skin: Marshmallow root, Comfrey, Plantain, and Chickweed
- Urinary system: Corn Silk, Couchgrass, Bearberry, and Marshmallow

These bitter herbs affect the various systems:

- Circulatory system: Yarrow, Gentian, and Goldenseal
- Digestive system: Gentian, Artichoke, Goldenseal, and Yarrow
- Musculoskeletal system: Bogbean
- Nervous system: Chamomile, Hops, and Mugwort
- Reproductive system: Goldenseal and Yarrow
- Respiratory system: White Horehound and Goldenseal
- Skin: Goldenseal and Myrrh
- Urinary system: Agrimony, Burdock, and Bearberry

These herbs carry astringent action (tone and strengthen) to the following systems:

- Respiratory system: White Horehound and Goldenseal
- Circulatory system: Bayberry (internally); Yarrow, Horse Chestnut, and Arnica (externally)

- Respiratory system: White Horehound and Goldenseal
- Digestive system: Agrimony and Oak Bark
- Respiratory system: White Horehound and Goldenseal
- Musculoskeletal system: Agrimony
- Nervous system: Rosemary
- Reproductive system: Red Raspberry
- Respiratory system: Sage, Goldenrod, and Yarrow
- Skin: Witch Hazel and Oak Bark
- Urinary system: Bearberry, Horsetail, and Yarrow

With these four actions, an herbalist can perform most of the therapeutic work he or she might need to accomplish (especially when dealing with the digestive system). The anti-inflammatory action helps reduce inflammation, pain, and discomfort; the demulcent action soothes, nourishes, and protects; the bitter element stimulates normal internal secretions, counteracting physical (and to a certain extent emotional) depression; and the astringent action can reduce excess discharge, toning and giving strength to body tissues. Of course, the many other actions and affinities of our herbal materia medica are equally important to understand and learn to use. The scope and intent of this male herbal is not to undertake an in-depth discussion of all these actions and system affinities. I recommend that one acquire a small collection of practical herbals that will provide a diversity of information and experience contributing to a well-rounded foundation of herbal knowledge...

Herbal Specifics

True to the nature of Nature, there are those plants that can act entirely outside their recognized actions and systems affinity. Wild Yam, for example, has been experienced as a specific remedy for the pain and discomfort of diverticulitis (an inflammation in abnormal pouches that form along the border of the colon wall). This is known not by studying its normal actions but, rather, based on folkloric knowledge; herbalists find that it has exceptionally helpful energy for this specific condition. Agrimony, when it is used in time, is specific for treating appendicitis. Red Sage, taken as a tea internally and used as mouthwash, is a specific for treating mouth ulcers. Gumweed is a respiratory antispasmodic, while Mugwort is a digestive-system and reproductive-system bitter, but the combination of these two herbs, prepared for external application, creates a traditional remedy for allergy to Poison Oak. This knowledge of the use of certain herbs as specifics is a gift of folkloric wisdom.

An Herbal Light Show

Using one's inherent ability for direct knowing is a gift of one's own intuition that must be trusted when selecting herbs for health care. The more one acquires therapeutic knowledge and experience by studying and working with herbs and people, the more frequently one's intuition brings the two together in a successful experience. The practical use of intuition in times of crisis and healing is a quality we tend to let go in face of the onslaught of authoritarian information that continuously bombards us. But let your intuition not be denied. All scientific knowledge and hypotheses are inspired by the proverbial flash of insight. Like healing, intuition is a basic human function. Trust it. Let the forest be with you....

Herb Quality

Herb quality is an important issue when it comes to picking the right herbs for herbal therapeutics and health maintenance. Discrimination is most necessary when selecting an herbal product, for the fact that it is herbal is not enough. To be effective, it must be of high quality. Many people assume that all herbs are organically grown and properly harvested, but this is not so. Many are grown for the commercial market using standard agricultural techniques and chemical fertilizers, are harvested and dried improperly, and so forth. For example, flowering tops often provide the medicinal actions in plants, but the parts harvested and sold will include a large percentage of extraneous leaf and stem, all of which may have been harvested incorrectly by machine, or overheated when oven dried in large batches and stored for long periods of time. Plants must be harvested and processed carefully to ensure the quality of their constituents, and plants gradually lose their potency when stored for too long or in unsuitable conditions.

Once you have picked and processed your own fresh herbs, you will know what high-quality herbs are like. It is always best to prepare medicine from herbs you have harvested and dried yourself, but obviously this is not always possible. When selecting an herb from a source other than yourself, use your senses to determine its quality. It must show excellent color, it should release a strong aroma, and it must have flavor—not necessarily good-tasting flavor, but intense flavor. These are all signs of herbal vitality. If the plant looks like lackluster hay, with hardly any aroma or flavor, question its worth as a healing agent. And buy organic: for just a few pennies more, you get high quality, and this is very important when using herbs. Liquid extracts should also be scrutinized; and you should expect them to pass the same sensual tests.

If you hear from someone that herbs don't work, you can be assured that the individual either used the wrong herbs for his constitution and condition, expected magic-bullet/instant results, or, most likely, used poor-quality herbs.

—From *The Male Herbal*

Continued ➤

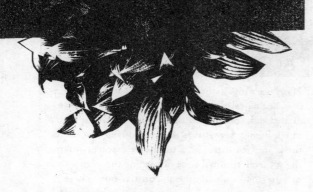

HERBAL FUNDAMENTALS

Lesley Tierra, L.Ac., Herbalist, A.H.G.

There are many aspects to learn about herbs…. Here we cover plant parts and chemistry, herbal families, safety, herb/drug interactions and herbal forms, administration, formulary, processing, harvesting, preparing and storing.

Plant Parts

Any part of an herb may potentially be used as medicine: **root**—grows into the ground; **rhizome**—grows horizontally under the ground; **root bark**—a root's outer bark; **above ground parts**—entire herb growing above the ground—leaves, stems, seed, flowers; **bark**—bark of a tree or shrub; **twigs**—the small branches of a shrub or tree; **leaf, stem, seed, flower, fruit, vine**—these are exactly as named.

Herbal Families

Taxonomy, the science of plant classification, groups plants according to their botanical classification, usually based upon the comparative study of their flower, fruit and leaf structures (botany is the study of plants). These groupings are ordered according to kingdom, division, class, subclass, order, family, genus, species and common name. Plants are generally identified by their genus and species (the two Latin words botanically naming a plant), much like the last (genus) and first (species) names of people. An example classification of **lemon balm** (*Melissa officinalis*) follows:

Kingdom: Plantae (plant kingdom)

Division: Magnoliophyta (the angiosperms, including flowering plants)

Class: Magnoliopsida (the dicots)

Subclass: Asteridae (gentian-aster subclass)

Order: Lamiales (mint order)

Family: Laminazeae (mint family)

Genus: Melissa

Species: officinalis

Common Name: lemon balm

Knowing these details enables herbalists to not only peg one exact herb, but also to identify commonalities between herbs sharing the same family and genus, giving hints at what possible uses other herbs in that family might have. For example, most herbs in the Rose Family (*Rosaceae*), such as **blackberry** and **agrimony**, have an effect on the intestinal tract, while many of those in the *Umbelliferae* family have a zesty flavor.

On the other hand, because Chinese **ginseng** and North American **spikenard** are both members of the *Araliaceae* family and both plants have saponins as major constituents, **spikenard** may have similar tonifying effects to ginseng. Further exploration in these areas could be very valuable for learning the uses of lesser-known herbs of North America.

Plant Chemistry

The science and study of plant chemistry, called pharmacognosy, covers all aspects of a plant's structure, growth, reproduction, active ingredients and nutrients. The primary compounds of a plant are the elements it needs to live: vitamins, minerals, sugars, starches, and so forth. Yet, plants also produce secondary compounds in small quantities that have various biological effects. These are the **chemical constituents** (or active parts) of a plant studied for therapeutic use.

When scientists began separating individual constituents and looking at them closely, they found out why plants affect the body. Further, they learned that these effects correspond to the way the whole plant is traditionally used. For instance, Digitoxin was created from a cardiac glycoside found in **foxglove**, an herb (though a poisonous one) known to regulate the heart.

Likewise, salicylic acid was extracted from **meadowsweet** to form aspirin, having the same analgesic effect as the herb does (salicylic acid is also found in **willow bark** and **poplar bark** and buds). Thus, active ingredients were separately extracted, then concentrated, to treat specific conditions. Later, these laboratories synthetically produced the drugs without using the herbs, usually changing one molecule to make the product stronger or "better" (and, of course, patentable and more expensive).

While learning chemical constituents can be very useful to scientifically determine how and why herbs work, it is not a holistic method for using herbs themselves. Keep the big picture in mind, for the territory is not the map: the isolated components are not responsible for the healing action of a plant—the whole plant is.

Herbs are a complex synergistic whole in which each of its chemical parts contributes to, or buffers, the other parts. In separating out and concentrating one active principle from the rest, this important balance is lost. Since an herb can actually be separated into hundreds, even thousands, of isolated constituents, it ultimately teaches us *less* about a plant, not more. Further each individual constituent may have different uses on its own than when combined within the whole plant.

Therefore, only learning about herbs through their chemical constituents limits the use of an herb to the effects of that constituent rather than using its traditional broad functions. The result is possible toxic side effects and, eventually, a drug rather than a useful herb. Further, it perpetuates the symptomatic approach to treating illness rather than treating the person and his/her unique condition! Several valuable herbs are being lost to this way of thinking, which doesn't represent herbalism as a healing system.

Interestingly, those who do experience difficulty with certain plant chemicals (like pyrrolizidine alkaloids) are generally the folks with Liver imbalances, since this Organ is responsible for processing anything foreign in the body. If the Liver is imbalanced in any way, then it can't properly process chemicals and symptoms arise.

Thus, those who have Liver congestion (stagnation), Heat, or Damp-Heat, liver diseases, or who are taking medications with liver side effects, are more susceptible to any potential issues around certain plant chemicals. Liver imbalances generally arise from long-term or excessive consumption of alcohol (including those who don't drink but are children of alcoholics), caffeine, fats, fried foods, nuts and nut berries, avocados, cheese and/or turkey, as well as taking drugs (including recreational), or having a history of hepatitis or mononucleosis.

As there are thousands of chemical constituents in plants, only the main ones are listed here. This is a brief reference and not intended to fully describe the details of plant constituents or plant chemistry (consult the *Bibliography* for further informational sources).

Carbohydrates: A carbohydrate is any form of sugar; it provides basic nutrition and energy. It appears as starch, monosaccharide, disaccharide, polysaccharide, insulin, pectin, gum, and mucilage (a slippery stringy exudate that serves as a soothing and healing gel on damaged mucus membrane linings in the lungs, digestive and urinary tracts, the tissues, and nerves). Gums are commonly used as stabilizers in cosmetics and foods. Examples: **marshmallow, comfrey, plantain, slippery elm, aloe vera.**

Glycosides: A glycoside is a sugar combined with a nonsugar (a-glycone) compound. Found in many combinations, they are soluble in water and alcohol. There are many types of glycosides.

Cardiac glycosides: These have a marked effect on the heart and increase its efficiency by increasing the force and power of the heartbeat without increasing the amount of oxygen needed by the heart muscle. These are very dangerous plants and shouldn't be used internally. Examples: **foxglove** (from which the drug, Digitoxin, is made) and **lily of the valley.**

Anthraquinone glycosides: These irritate the large intestine, creating a laxative or purgative effect. They should always be combined with a carminative, like **ginger** or **fennel**, to relieve any gripping pain they can cause. Examples: **rhubarb** and **senna.**

Flavonoids and Flavonone glycosides: These compounds are safe for people and animals, but toxic to microorganisms. Many are antiviral, antispasmodic, anti-inflammatory, antifungal, antibacterial, diuretic, heart, and circulatory stimulants and antioxidants; Vitamins C, E, and P are flavonoids. Examples: **hawthorn berries, raspberry, ginkgo.**

Phenols and Phenolic Glycosides: Phenols, always carbon-based, are basic building blocks of many plant constituents and other glycosides. Some have antiseptic, febrifuge, analgesic and anti-inflammatory activities and externally, antiseptic, and rubefacient properties. Examples: **clove, thyme.**

Coumarins: There are more than 100 kinds of coumarins and they have a sweet smell (best known for their aromatic components used in perfumery) and anti-inflammatory and antibacterial properties. They are also anticoagulants, thus thinning the blood and reducing blood clots (and therefore, shouldn't be taken by those on blood-thinning medication and vice versa). Examples: **black haw, red clover, angelica, licorice**

Saponins: These glycosides dissolve in water (water-soluble) and form lather when shaken. Saponins have a structure similar to human sex and stress hormones and so have been used in synthesizing these types of drugs. Examples: **fenu-greek, licorice, sarsaparilla, wild yam.**

Other glycosides: Others include sulfur glycosides, cyanide glycosides. and furanocoumarin glycosides.

Acids: Weak acids are found throughout the plant kingdom in many forms. Acids cleanse and detoxify, astringe tissues and stimulate pancreatic and bile secretions. **Citric** and **tartaric acids**, for example, are most concentrated in unripe fruit. They stimulate saliva flow and are mildly laxative, diuretic and antibacterial. Citric acid provides vita-

Continued ➡

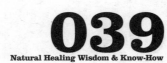

min C to the body whereas **oxalic acid**, found in spinach, chard and sorrel, binds with calcium, making it unavailable and ultimately causing kidney stone formation. **Salicylic acid**, found in **meadowsweet**, **willow bark**, **white poplar** and **wintergreen**, has recognized analgesic effects that were synthesized into the drug, aspirin. **Formic acid**, found in animals and plants to protect themselves, causes a temporary inflammation but easily breaks down with cooking.

Tannic acid, as its name suggests, tans leather. In small amounts, tannins are astringent, acting on protein to form protective skin on wounds and inflamed mucus membranes, thus promoting their rapid healing. Tannins are used externally for minor burns, cuts, inflammations and infections, swellings, hemorrhoids and varicose ulcers. Internally they treat diarrhea, peptic ulcers, colitis secretions, and bleeding. Tannins are soluble in water, glycerine and alcohol.

Example herbs with acids: **red clover**, **yarrow**, **willow bark**, **black haw**, **blackberry**.

Alkaloids: When nitrogen isn't fully utilized by plants for protein production, it accumulates in the form of alkaloids. There are around 5,000 known alkaloids that produce diverse and profound effects. Alkaloids act on particular parts of the body, such as the liver, nerves, lungs, digestive system and especially, the central nervous system.

Usually alkalinizing and having a bitter taste, some alkaloids are anti-inflammatory and antibacterial while others are irritating stimulants, narcotics or toxic. Some are in poisonous and hallucinogenic plants, including nicotine, caffeine, morphine, opium poppy and codeine (all characterized by their *-ine* ending). Plants normally contain several alkaloids in combination. Alkaloids have limited solubility in alcohol and are comparatively insoluble in water. Some better-known alkaloids include **indole**, **quinoline**, **isoquinoline**, **purine**, **tropane**, **pyridine**, **piperidine**, **quinolizidine** and **terpenoid alkaloids**.

One alkaloid group, **pyrrolizidine alkaloid**, causes liver blockage in humans and cancer in mice. Usually this occurs when the plant is taken in very high doses over a long period of time since this alkaloid slowly accumulates in the body. If you are uncertain how to use a plant containing PAs, then consider taking it only for short periods of time, and avoiding it altogether if pregnant, nursing, a young child, having liver disease or Liver stagnation, Heat or Damp Heat (**comfrey** and **coltsfoot** have PAs).

Example herbs with alkaloids: **Oregon grape root**, **goldenseal**, **barberry**.

Essential or Volatile Oils: As the name implies, volatile oils are unstable and easily separate from the plant to vaporize into air, especially when the plant is crushed or exposed to the sun. In various combinations these oils provide plants' rich smells, and because they permeate and travel through the body quickly and easily, they have a wide range of use. Essential oils are antiseptic, carminative, antispasmodic, antifungal, analgesic, febrifuge, vermifuge, sedative, diaphoretic, anti-inflammatory and/or rubefacient in action and stimulate the production and activity of white blood cells. They are also used in perfumes, aromatherapy and insect repellents. Most are soluble in alcohol and slightly soluble in water. Examples: **rosemary**, **thyme**, **mint**.

Bitter Principles: Because these substances have a very strong bitter taste, they stimulate the secretion of digestive juices and bile, thus activating digestion, bowel elimination and bile flow and increasing appetite. Bitters, as some herbal combinations

have traditionally been called, are often taken before meals for just these reasons, although they are valuable after meals for indigestion. They are also antibiotic and antifungal in action. Bitter compounds are soluble in water and alcohol. Examples: **gentian**, **wormwood**, **goldenseal**.

Resins: These transparent or translucent plant secretions or excretions are usually yellowish to brown in color and sticky or gummy. Formed from oxidized volatile oils, they are expectorant, stimulating, diaphoretic, and diuretic in action, and are soluble in alcohol, fixed oils, and volatile oils, and insoluble in water. Examples: **myrrh**, **frankincense**.

Plants have other components, such as vegetable oils, vitamins, trace elements, chlorophyll, oleoresins, alcohols, acrids, latex, gelatins, lipids, enzymes, and other proteins, balsams and coloring matter. The myriad aspects that comprise a plant's chemistry truly give it a unique character which, when combined with the plant's energy, properties and special qualities, yield the unique healing ability of that plant.

Herbal Safety

Most herbs are mild and act like special foods in the body. With some exceptions, they lack the concentration of active biochemical ingredients that cause side effects, as do Western drugs. They also possess hundreds to thousands of constituents that counterbalance each other, making most herbs quite safe. Generally, herbs regulate chemical physiological imbalances, not cause adverse reactions, and when taken together in formula, they buffer any of the strong effects of one individual herb while synergistically enhancing each other's functions and purposes.

People rarely consider foods as toxic, yet when exposed to sunlight the green tuber of potatoes create a poisonous alkaloid. Wheat rye, barley and oats contain protein gluten that can irritate the intestines. Similarly, there are toxic herbs most people know to avoid such as **oleander**, **hemlock**, and **poison oak**, **ivy**, and **sumac**. The point is that just because a few plants are poisonous doesn't mean all herbs are dangerous or unsafe. Rather, it's wise to familiarize yourself with and avoid the few toxic plants (**aconite**, **belladonna**, **fox glove**, **mandrake**, **may apple**, and **arnica** are some, though they are not commonly available, except perhaps in homeopathic remedies). Most herbs are safe to use if you heed their dosage and precaution guidelines.

Periodically, public warnings against herbs occur. These often arise either when the herb is used inappropriately, such as for the wrong intention or in excessive doses, or when the whole herb is ignored and instead only the actions of one particular constituent is investigated and condemned (and it's usually given in much higher doses than can ever be taken when consuming the whole plant). Such information can be misleading because some specimens of an herb may contain a constituent that others do not, or occur in higher amounts in one plant part versus another.

Sometimes warnings are issued before all the evidence is in, or is checked for true accuracy. For example, women with estrogen-sensitive tumors and fibroids were warned against using **dang gui** for several years because people believed it contained phytoestrogenic substances, while later studies demonstrated it doesn't after all. Another time a study pointed to the false presence of colchicines in **ginkgo**, yet it later was learned that the paper itself was flawed, as the herb doesn't contain this substance (this is actually herbal slander).

Herb Standardization: Pros and Cons

Many warnings actually arise from using standardized herbal extracts. This is because some of these extracts take one constituent and concentrate it to a much higher percentage than is naturally found in the plant (for instance, a turmeric extract containing 95% curcumin), thus displacing the herb's ratio of other naturally occurring constituents. These extracts create something different than the herb itself and thus they often have druglike actions.

Further, when one constituent is pumped up at the expense of the others, it can create actions that aren't present in the whole herb itself (for instance, **ginkgo** taken in its whole herb form doesn't cause bleeding, but in its 24% flavoglycoside extract form it does). On the other hand, all of ginkgo's circulatory and memory-enhancing properties are based on this standardized extract, and so this is the form that should be used to treat those issues.

Thus, not only are all of an herb's uses lost, but now a different product is created that has no precedent in traditional herbal practice. While a ginkgo standardized extract is valuable in certain circumstances, this general approach can be dangerous to herbalism as a whole. Not only do such products create herbal warnings, but eventually the herb may be taken away from public use, and the more druglike standardized product eventually be exclusively used by doctors (and become patentable). While this may seem far-fetched, it's exactly what's occurring in Europe today.

Interestingly, and perhaps most importantly, standardizing herbs doesn't always increase their effectiveness. In fact, according to herbalist and researcher, Roy Upton, tests of various herbs, like **St. John's wort** and **Echinacea**, determine that the whole plant extracts containing all the herbs' compounds are more effective than their standardized extracts. To avoid these problems, some standardized products use a chemical component only as a marker, presuming that if the herb meets a certain content level of that component, the other chemical constituents will meet it as well (for instance, a **feverfew** extract that contains 2.6% parthenolides, or a **goldenseal** extract that contains 5% hydrastine). Others use standard markers in their extracts and then add it back into the whole herb (called "full spectrum"), thus buffering some of the boosted constituent's side effects and making a very potent, but safe product....Overall, the majority of most readily available herbs are extremely safe for general use, particularly when consumed in their whole, rather than standardized, forms. When an herb has been used for thousands of years and we "suddenly" believe it's toxic, perhaps the investigation should turn to our stressful and toxin-laden lives and how this disables our bodies to handle such herbs, rather than labeling the herb itself as dangerous. In other cases, herbs cause problems because they are used improperly.

For instance, in most of the **kava kava** cases reported in Europe, the users also heavily drank alcohol, had hepatitis or a history of drug abuse, or took medications with known liver disease-causing side effects. Yet, kava kava was reported to be the cause for hepatotoxicity rather than the other factors, all of which are known to cause liver damage. In other cases, the herb is used inappropriately, such as **ephedra** (*ma huang*), a major Chinese herb for treating asthma, taken as a power pill to reduce weight and stimulate energy. This is inappropriate lifestyle usage and herbal substance abuse.

The real issue then isn't if an herb is safe or not, but the data given and how it's reviewed. It's

Continued ➡

important such information be discriminately checked for inaccuracies and true issues needing attention. Thus, don't throw the baby out with the bath water, assuming the current hype on an herb tells the whole story. This type of sensationalism is generally inaccurate and overemphasized, especially in relation to the acceptable daily consumption of known dangerous substances such as alcohol and tobacco. Further, people generally turn to herbs in the first place because they're safer than drugs. You do not have to be a professional herbalist to use herbs safely. Look at the whole picture, be informed and critically review all the data.

Herb/Drug Interactions

As the spotlight turns more on herbs, how they affect medications (and vice versa) is now coming into focus. In general, it's safe to take most herbs while taking medications. According to herbalist Christopher Hobbs, 20 million people take herbs and drugs together with only a handful of adverse reactions reported. Many people like to study the theoretical adverse interactions between herbs and drugs and get others excited about potential problems, but most of their study results are just that: hypothetical and not actual.

In fact, I frequently see people who are on 5-10 medications (I am not exaggerating) and, with the use of herbs and diet, I am able to help these folks eliminate most, if not all, of them. To me, this is the ideal goal, and rather than looking at which herbs you should not take while on medications, you might consider which medications you won't take while on herbs.

As some herbs do have interactions with certain medications, it's wise to know about them. There are two main red **flag categories** of drugs to watch when taking herbs: **blood thinners** and **tranquilizers/antidepressants**.

Blood thinners: If you are undergoing surgery or taking any blood-thinning medications (including anticoagulants, Warfarin, etc.), then any herb with *coumarin* should be avoided: **angelica** (*Angelica archangelica*), **prickly ash**, **red clover** and western **licorice**. Further, herbs that thin blood should be avoided, too (**garlic** and standardized **ginkgo**). However, seriously consider that if your blood needs thinning, perhaps taking a blood-thinning herb, such as red clover, might do the job without needing to use medication. If on blood thinners and you take herbs with coumarins, then have your doctor monitor your clotting time and adjust your medication appropriately.

Tranquilizers/antidepressants: Certain herbs can interact with tranquilizers and antidepressants, increasing their actions, such as **St. John's wort** or **kava**. On the other hand, these herbs can be extremely useful alternatives after eliminating these medications. Any herb with MAO inhibitors can also interfere with certain antidepressants (and anesthesia—St. John's wort has MAOs). As well, **ephedra** (*ma huang*) should never be taken while on MAO inhibitors, or it can skyrocket blood pressure.

Other: Other possible herb/drug interactions to be aware of include taking herbs that alter thyroid function (**bugleweed**, **lemon balm**, **myrrh**) if on hypothyroid medication, or herbs that interfere with interferon, such as **bupleurum**. Further, because spices, like **cayenne**, **black pepper**, and **kava** speed absorption of various chemicals, including phytochemicals (since they influence how the liver processes and eliminates these substances), taking them in frequent or high doses while on medications can make drugs more potent. As well, it is wise to avoid combining herbs and drugs that have opposite effects, such as taking **astragalus** while on an immunosuppressive medication (and vice versa).

Dosage of Herbs

The proper dosage of herbs is very important. First, it's necessary to take a sufficient quantity of herbs for them to be effective. Quite often people take the right herbs or formulas but don't realize results simply because they didn't take enough of them. Most traditional herbalists give herbs in fairly high doses, while Western herbalists tend to give lower ones. On the other hand, it's possible to take too many herbs (and supplements), for over a long period of time excessive quantities can injure digestion, eventually impairing the body's ability to metabolize food. At other times, a low dose of a formula over time can give results without any aggravating effects, especially if it contains strong-acting herbs.

How do you know which dose to use? Once you've chosen an herbal treatment plan, take the herbs for three days. If after this time you experience a positive reaction, continue your plan until your symptoms are relieved. If you don't experience any changes, increase the dose and continue for another week, then reevaluate your condition. Sometimes subtle changes occur slowly which take time to feel. Other times you have the right herbs but need to take a higher dose for better results.

If you experience a mild negative reaction, cut down to a minimal dose (1 tablet or 10 drops tincture, 2 times/day) and continue for another 3 days. If the reaction continues, or if you experience a marked negative reaction, stop the herbs until the reactions disappear, you definitely know that it's the wrong herbal approach and needs reevaluation. Don't be discouraged if this occurs. Herbal medicine is a matter of strategy and herbalists often give a test formula or treatment to see if they have the right diagnosis. If an adverse reaction occurs, this may be used diagnostically to help reveal the correct treatment plan.

The most effective form to take herbs is as teas since they assimilate easily. Yet, some herbs are too bitter to drink as teas while others are more potent in alcoholic extract form. Thus, other forms are useful, such as liquid extracts, powdered extracts, pills, and tablets. Generally, most herbs are better absorbed when taken warm, either by drinking the warm teas, or by swallowing the pills, powders, capsules, tablets, or extracts with warm water. This is because warm water assists their assimilation and protects digestion.

General dosages are calculated for a person weighing about 150 pounds. However, even if weighing this, each body responds differently to herbs and therefore, a particular dosage may be too

Herbal Safety Guidelines

- Mild herbs are specific foods, as safe as practically any vegetable.
- Examine all the evidence on an herb rather than swallowing a little carte blanche.
- Know your sources—only purchase herbs from quality sources, companies with GMP. If an herbal product company withholds information about, or won't tell you who's in charge of quality control, search for another source.
- Be cautious when purchasing herbs that are commonly adulterated, such as **chickweed**, **plantain**, and **skullcap**, and make sure you obtain the correct one. Also beware of herbs that are sometimes substituted by others, such as **true unicorn** for **false unicorn**; **barberry**, **Orego grape**, or some other berberine-containing herb for **goldenseal**; or Russian **comfrey** for *symphytum officinale* (it's more concentrated in PAs and so less desirable).

- Don't exceed given doses and heed the few herb/drug interactions.
- Read labels and doses carefully.
- Use common sense.
- Choose commonly available herbs and if you don't experience results within several weeks, stop and rethink your approach.
- Don't believe sensational claims about miraculous cures.
- Monitor yourself for reactions and discontinue use if you notice any adverse effects.
- Don't use herbs just for specific vitamin and mineral supplementation, as they have many other effects you may be unaware of.
- Only use herbs as necessary during pregnancy or lactation, or to promote those functions (such as **raspberry** for pregnancy and **fennel** for lactation).
- If you have any questions, consult a professional herbalist for guidance.

Guidelines for Taking Herbs and Medications

- Check the "red flag" categories of heart/drug interactions.
- Take herbs in formulas rather than singly.
- Begin herbs at low doses, then gradually increase.
- Take herbs and medications separately, about 3–4 hours apart.
- Monitor your body's response for any adverse reactions after taking herbs.
- Have you doctor monitor your body's response and reduce medication does as appropriate.
- If you have any questions, consult a professional herbalist for guidance.

Continued →

high or too low for your own needs and sensitivities. As a guideline, start with the given dosage, then increase or decrease according to your body's response and size.

For babies, the same dosage rule may be used. However, the best way to treat nursing babies with herbs is to treat the mother. Any herbs Mom takes go directly into her milk and then to the baby (the same is true of any foods or substances). Use the same herbs given for baby's ailment and drink as a tea. Start with teaspoon doses at first to make sure the baby doesn't have a reaction, then increase to a cup, twice a day, if needed.

For those who cannot nurse, there are several other effective ways to give herbs to babies. A plastic eyedropper is useful for administering mild herbal teas. Squeeze a dropperful of tea into baby's mouth several times throughout the day. Keep fresh tea in dropper bottle for convenient traveling and administration throughout the day. (This is especially a good method for treating colic—try a combination

For children, a convenient rule of thumb helps determine herb dosages by calculating according to the child's body weight as compared to the adult dosage:

$$\frac{\text{Child's weight in pounds}}{150 \text{ pounds}} = \frac{\text{the fraction of the adult}}{\text{dose to use}}$$

For example, if a child weighs 50 pounds:

$$\frac{50}{150} = .33 = 1/3 \text{ of the adult dose is used for this child}$$

of equal parts **chamomile**, **fennel**, and **lemon balm** for this.)

Herbal baths are also very effective for treating babies and quite safe. Baby quickly absorbs the herbs' healing properties through the skin and from there into the bloodstream. This can be done 2–3 times/day until the problem is alleviated. (Fevers respond especially well to **poplar bark** bath.)

Dosage Guidelines

Age	Fractional Adult Dosage
0 to 1 year	1/10 to 1/75 of adult dosage
2 to 6 years	1/8 to 1/10 of adult dosage
6 to 12 years	1/4 to 2/3 of adult dosage
15 to 70 years	Full adult dosage
Over 70 years	1/2 adult dosage

Administering Herbs

How herbs are taken also affects their efficiency:

- Take herbs that treat the lower part of the body (Bladder, Kidneys, Intestines, genital area, lower body conditions, and sometimes the Liver and Gallbladder) between and up to ½ hour before meals.
- Take herbs that treat the middle of the body (Stomach, Spleen, Liver, Gallbladder, and digestive disorders) with meals.
- Take herbs that treat the upper part of the body (Heart, Lungs, and upper body ailments) ½ to several hours after eating.
- If a diaphoretic or tonic effect is desired, take the herbal tea warm.
- When a diuretic effect is wanted, take the herbal tea cool.
- Take herbs on an empty stomach for detoxification (creates a stronger effect).
- Taking herbs before meals most effectively treats intestinal issues, tonifies and reduces fat.
- Herbs taken after meals treat gas, indigestion, lung conditions, sinus ailments, and prevents mucus.
- Herbs mixed with food, or taken with a meal, are best for weak individuals, or those with poor digestion or having digestive disturbances.
- Taking herbs between meals is best for urinary and nervous disorders.
- Infants and young children respond well to herbal baths and fomentations, or to teas (add **licorice** or **slippery elm** to improve taste) when put into dropper bottle and given several dropperfuls throughout the day. Children over two may be given herbs powdered and mixed with honey to form a paste.
- Herbs with strong therapeutic actions, such as strong diaphoretics, and purgatives should be used with great care in those with severe weakness.
- Blood-moving herbs, emmenagogues and purgatives with a strong downward action should not be used by pregnant women or during menses.
- Excessively cooling and bitter herbs should not be taken too frequently, or over a prolonged period, since they can damage digestion and injure Blood and Yin.

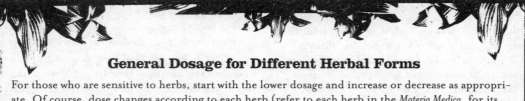

General Dosage for Different Herbal Forms

For those who are sensitive to herbs, start with the lower dosage and increase or decrease as appropriate. Of course, dose changes according to each herb (refer to each herb in the *Materia Medica*, for its specific dose). Dosage can be varied according to body weight, age and severity of condition (for instance, heavier bodies need a higher dosage while lighter bodies need a smaller dosage; the more severe the condition, the more herbs need to be taken).

Bulk herbs in formulas	3–9 gms (1/9–1/3 oz.)
Teas	1 oz. herbs/1 pint water; drink 1 cup, 3 times/day
Tinctures*	20–60 drops, 3–4 times/day (traditional herbalists tend to give 1 tsp., 3 times/day—depending on the herb)
Capsules	2–4 capsules, 3–4 times/day
Dry Concentrated and Freeze-dried extracts	3–5 gms., 3 times/day
Tablets/Caplets	2–6 tablets, 3–4 times/day
Patents	4–8 pills, 3 times/day (depending on patent)
Powdered Herbs	1 tsp, 3–4 times/day
Standardized Extracts	Follow directions on bottle
Syrups	1 Tbsp., 3–4 times/day (every 2 hr. for acute conditions)
Compress/fomentations	1–2 times/day leaving on for 20–60 minutes
Poultices	Replenish 2–3 times/day and continue generally for 3 days
Essential Oils	Add 1–2 drops to an oil and apply locally
Liniments, salves, crèmes, oils, sprays and other external ointments	As needed

To evaporate the undesirable alcohol, boil tincture in water uncovered for 20 minutes.

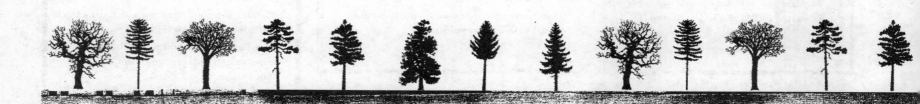

Continued ➡

- Excessively heating herbs should rarely be used in summer, while cold herbs with strong eliminative properties should rarely be used in winter.

- For a more rapid recovery from skin diseases and disorders of the throat, vagina, rectum, lungs, eyes, ears and nose, use external applications along with internal ones, such as fomentations, gargles, douches, boluses, herbal enemas, suppositories, eye and ear drops, syrups, fomentations, poultices and herbal vapor inhalations.

- If there is an acute disease occurring at the same time as a chronic one, the acute disease should be treated first by using fewer herbs in a formula. Small frequent doses should be taken every 1–2 hours, tapering off frequency as symptoms subside. If too many herbs are combined for acute conditions, their individual effects are weakened and effectiveness diluted. Acute diseases should show improvement within 13 days at most. If they don't, herbs should be reevaluated and possibly changed.

- Chronic diseases are treated more slowly and gently with a balanced formulation given over a prolonged period of time. If treated too quickly or strongly, the body's reserves may diminish, or the body itself weaken. Combine several herbs together in a formula to temper any strong effects of one individual herb. Take larger amounts of the herbs regularly, 2–3 times/day, and last the equivalent of one month to each year since the symptoms began. Chronic diseases should show benefit within two weeks or so. If they don't, reevaluate and possibly change your treatment approach.

- When treating illness naturally, it is important to take plenty of herbs and use several natural therapies to heal the condition. For example, if you have pneumonia, then it isn't effective to only drink three cups of herb tea a day. Instead, you also need to rest, use onion poultices on the chest twice a day, do a ginger foot bath, take an herbal syrup and herbal formula every 2–4 hours as well as drink 4–6 cups of strong herb tea per day. This may be why some people who try herbs don't feel they are effective: they didn't take enough herbs nor do enough therapies to overcome the disease.

- In general, Excess diseases are easier to cure while Deficiency conditions take longer and can be more difficult to heal (refer to *The Energy of Illness*, to understand Excess and Deficiency). This is because it is easier to eliminate too much of something than it is to build from a depleted physical state. Deficient conditions often involve more complex issues, such as healing emotional needs, work or relationship issues, or poor dietary habits. On the other hand, prolonged Excess conditions ultimately cause Deficiency in the body because over time they deplete the body's resources and reserves. As with Deficiencies, healing then becomes harder, taking more attention, time, and patience....

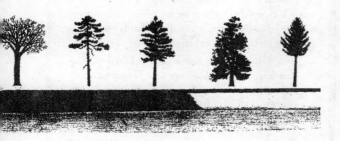

Processing Herbs

Many traditional medicines, such as Chinese, Ayurvedic and Tibetan, have developed methods of processing herbs to reduce toxicity, increase therapeutic effectiveness, alter energies or properties and remove any offending odors. For example, when **astragalus** is uncooked it is diaphoretic and diuretic, but when stir-fried with honey, it more directly tonifies the Spleen and Stomach and raises Qi, lifting prolapsed organs. Uncooked **dang gui** lubricates the intestines, acting as a laxative, while dang gui in wine form more strongly tonifies Blood. You may process your own herbs, or purchase them prepared from herb suppliers. Following are a few of the processing methods and their effects:

Steamed and Dried: When herbs are steamed with wine and then dried, the herb's energy becomes warmer. Example: cooked **rehmannia** (*Rehmannia glutinosa*).

Dry-Roasted: Herbs dry-roasted in a dry pan (in the oven or on the stove, while stirring constantly until slightly brown) creates a warmer energy and enhances flavor. Examples: **roasted dandelion** and **chicory** roots.

Stir-Fried: Stir-frying herbs in a wok or skillet with honey enhances moistening properties and tonification (particularly of the Spleen and Stomach). Examples: **licorice** and **astragalus**.

Spirits or Wine: Herbs soaked in grain spirits or wine increases Blood-moving, warming, and ascending energies. Generally the herbs are left in the alcohol and taken in teaspoon doses 3–4 times/day as a tonic, or for rheumatic or circulatory complaints. Examples: **deer antler** and **dang gui**.

Processing with Salt: Salt added to an herbal formula enhances its descending and Kidney-tonifying energies (although omit if cleansing the urinary system).

Processing with Vinegar: Processing herbs with sour substances, such as vinegar, increases their descending and contracting energies and actions on the Liver, and helps extract alkaloids found in herbs.

Charring/Carbonizing: Charring (calcining, carbonizing) herbs is cooking them until burnt. This increases their astringency so they more effectively stop bleeding, diarrhea, dysentery and other undesirable discharges. Examples: charred **agrimony**.

Harvesting Herbs

Harvesting, preparing and storing your own herbs is an enriching and satisfying experience. Directly working with herbs teaches invaluable information that can't be substituted by reading books. Pick herbs from your own garden as well as in fields, woods or mountains. Harvesting your own herbs is called *wildcrafting* and provides the purest and best source for making herbal medicines.

When wildcrafting, harvest plants in a manner that increases their number and perpetuates healthy plant populations. Indiscriminate harvesting practices in the past have endangered several herbs native to America, such as **goldenseal**, **wild American ginseng** and **lady's slipper**. Thus, it's important to follow ethical harvesting practices to protect the plants and their environment. Following are several guidelines for picking and processing your own herbs, whether they are wild-crafted or grown yourself:

1. **Bring along** gloves, cutting knives, shears, string and large bags to carry your harvest

home. Avoid wearing hard-soled shoes that damage delicate hillside ecosystems.

2. **Choose your harvesting locations wisely.** Pick herbs far from common highways to avoid pollution and car exhaust. Harvest in areas not used by other herbalists. Don't pick herbs growing near high-tension electric wires (this may cause mutation), on lawns or in public parks that are chemically fertilized, or located downstream from mining or agribusiness, around parking lots and areas sprayed with chemicals, herbicides, or pesticides. Avoid picking herbs in fragile locations and ecosystems, as one irresponsible wildcrafter can easily destroy an herbal environment.

3. **Pick herbs during their prime therapeutic state** as follows:

   Roots and rhizomes: in early spring before sap rises, after seeding, in the early morning before sunshine, or in late autumn when sap returns to ground and aerial parts have died back.

   Barks and root-barks: in spring or fall when they easily peel from wood.

   Seeds, fruits, and berries: when fully ripened and mature.

   Leaves and stems: when fully matured, usually before full development of flower.

   Flowers: when fully developed, scent is strong, oil content is evident and before fruiting and seeding stages.

   Saps and Pitches: in late winter or early spring.

   Buds: when sticky.

   All plant parts: in early morning after dew dries and before noon when life force is strongest. Avoid wilted or withered plants, as they have weaker energy.

4. **Harvest herbs in such a way as to not deplete or inhibit their future growth and development.** Take only what you immediately need. Pick where there's an abundance of herbs and only take about one-third. Don't harvest the same stand year after year. You may need to tend the area by thinning, cleaning and preserving a selection of grandparent plants to seed and guard young plants. Spread any seeds to help propagation, especially when taking roots. Fill any holes you dig and cover with leaves. When harvesting leaves, don't pull the roots. Flower pruning of certain plants increases root yields as well as foliage. Keep your picking places secret so others don't crudely plunder them.

5. **Taste, but don't swallow, a plant you don't know.** Have positive identification of the plant before harvesting. Use identification keys or a specimen when necessary.

6. **When getting barks from trees**, only take longitudinal strips—never strip a complete circumference around the tree, as this kills the tree. Only pick from smaller branches.

7. **Never gather endangered or threatened plant species**, such as goldenseal, American ginseng and lady's slipper. Harvest no more than 10% of the native and 30% of the naturalized plant species from an area. Gather only from abundant stands. The overharvesting of certain wild herbs has caused many to become endangered. Rather than harvesting any endangered or at-risk herbs, purchase cultivated ones. To learn more about this as well as to help protect endangered plants and locate seeds and cultivated plants, contact the organization, United Plant Savers. The following herbs are now endangered or at risk:

Continued ➡

Endangered Herbs

American ginseng (*Panax quincfuefolius*)

Black Cohosh (*Cimicifuga racemosa*)

Bloodroot (*Sanguinaria Canadensis*)

Blue Cohosh (*Caulophyllum thalictroides*)

Echinacea (*Echinacea spp.*)

Eyebright (*Euphrasia spp.*)

Goldenseal (*Hydrastis Canadensis*)

Helonias Root (*Chamaelirium luteum*)

Lady's Slipper (*Cypripedium spp.*)

Lomatium (*Lomatium dissectum*)

Osha (*Ligusticum porteri, L. spp*)

Slippery Elm (*Ulmus rubra*)

Sundew (*Drosera spp.*)

Trillium, Beth Root (*Trillium spp.*)

True Unicorn (*Aletris farinose*)

Venus Flytrap (*Dionaea muscipula*)

Virginia Snakeroot (*Aristolochia serpentaria*)

Wild Yam (*Dioscorea villosa, D. spp.*)

Endangered in Hawaii: **Kava Kava** (*Piper methysticum*)

At-Risk (To Watch) Herbs

Arnica (*Arnica spp.*), **Butterfly Weed** (*Aslepias tuberose*), **Cascara Sagrada** (*Rhamnus purshiana*), **Chaparro** (*Casatela emoryi*), **Elephant Tree** (*Bursera microphylla*), **Gentian** (*Gentiana spp.*), **Goldthread** (*Coptis spp.*), **Lobelia** (*Lobelia spp.*), **Maidenhair Fern** (*Adiantum pendatum*), **Mayapple** (*Podophyllum peltatum*), **Oregon Grape** (*Mahonia spp.*), **Partridgeberry** (*Mitchella repens*), **Pink Root** (*Spigelia marilaandica*), **Pipsissewa** (*Chimaphila umbellate*), **Spikenard** (*Aralia racemosa, A. californica*), **Stillingia** (*Stillingia sylvatica*), **Stone Root** (*Collinsonia Canadensis*), **Stream Orchid** (*Epipactis gigantean*), **Turkey Corn** (*Dicentra Canadensis*), **White Sage** (*Salvia apiana*), **Wild Indigo** (*Baptisia tinctoria*), **Yerba Mansa** (*Anemopsis californica*), **Yerba Santa** (*Eriodictyon californica*)

Preparing Herbs

1. First wash herbs gently, scrubbing roots well and rinsing barks (usually flowers, leaves, and seeds don't need to be washed—instead, shake to remove bugs and dust). After washing, immediately slice roots into small pieces (they are too hard to cut when dry).

2. Dry herbs in a shaded and well-ventilated area, spreading on screens or sheets (avoid wire screens and newspaper print). It's important to keep most herbs out of sunlight or else they'll scorch and lose medicinal properties (although some barks, like wild cherry, may be dried in the sun to activate their medicinal properties). If plants are too close to each other, they'll mold or turn down, losing much healing value. Don't dry too quickly. If plants contain natural oils, dry slowly to retain.

3. Herbs may also be gathered together and tied in a bundle (with a diameter no bigger than 1½") near the end of the stems. Suspend upside down from a ceiling bean or wall. This allows the plant's sap to run from the stems into the leaves and flowers while drying, making those parts more potent. Hang in a well-aired, dry and shady place for several weeks, or until completely dry. All plant parts are dry when they feel brittle. You can pinch the lowest part of hanging plants to check this, or cut a sample root in half to see if the center is dry.

4. Crush and "garble" harvested herbs for easy storage (clean by removing stems and other unwanted items). Strip leaves from stems by running your hand along the stem from the top toward its bottom.

Storing Herbs

Herb potency is destroyed by heat, bright light, exposure to air and bacteria. Therefore, store herbs in well-sealed or tightly capped and dark-colored jars and containers. Place in a cool, dry place away from windows, direct sunlight, the stove or other places of high heat. Be sure to label herbs and herbal preparations with date, name of herb(s), name of preparation, if wildcrafted, organically grown or store bought, location, and any other relevant information you think necessary.

The shelf life of dried loose herbs is 1–2 years, and some parts, like barks, last much longer and even improve with age, such as **cascara bark**. Broken or crushed herbs lose potency more rapidly than whole, uncut herbs. If herbs begin to lose smell, taste and/or color, they are best used in an herbal bath rather than as medicine. Herbs bought at the store, especially if whole, should last about one year in a well-sealed jar. Herbs you harvest and dry can last 1–2 years. Herbs with strong plant oils lose potency first, while roots and barks keep medicinal energies longer.

An herbal tea keeps about three days when tightly bottled and refrigerated (when reheating, do not boil the tea). Tinctures and wines last 7–10 years. Vinegar extracts last 3 years or more if stored in a cool, dark place. Oils last up to seven years if a small amount of vitamin E or benzoin tincture is added as preservative and they're stored in tightly covered jars in a cool, dark place. Likewise, salves last for 5 years or more when properly preserved and stored in the same way. Powders lasat from 3 months to a year or two at most, depending on how well they are stored. Powders particularly need to be well sealed to prevent exposure to air and kept in a cool, dark place. Herbal poultices, fomentations, washes, plasters, milks, gargles, gruels, and potherbs are not stored, but made as needed.

—From *Healing with the Herbs of Life*

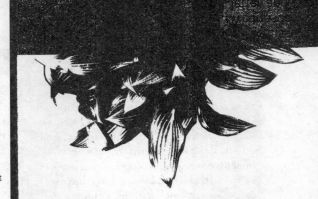

A SUCCINCT COURSE IN PREPARING TEAS, TINCTURES, AND OTHER HERBAL EXTRACTS

James Green, Herbalist

The techniques of making herbal medicine remain simple, and the materials necessary are minimal. They are:

- Measuring cups that also indicate metric measures.
- Glass, stainless-steel, or porcelain teapot and saucepans (avoid aluminum cooking vessels like you do red ants).
- Electric coffee-bean grinder (a post-Edison mortar and pestle) for powdering dried herbs.
- A mortar and pestle for ambience.
- An electric blender for mixing fresh plant preparations.
- Glass jars and other glass containers that have good, tight-fitting lids (especially save all amber glass containers for storing herbs and herbal preparations).
- Fine-mesh stainless-steel kitchen sieves and natural, undyed cotton muslin cloth for straining and filtering.
- Assorted funnels, rubber spatulas, and stirring sticks.
- A kitchen scale that indicates metric weight.
- A food and herb dehydrator; this is not essential, but it is extremely useful. (After you have owned one and used it for a while, it becomes essential to you.)

How to Prepare

Infusions (Tea)

Variances exist in the recommended dosages for individual herbs. However, in general, to prepare a medicinal tea, put 1 ounce of cut or crushed herb leaves and/or flowers (the tender, more delicate plant parts, which frequently contain aromatic volatile oils) into a quart jar, add 1 quart of boiling water for a solvent*, stir, cover, and let steep for fifteen to twenty minutes; then strain and drink. (*A solvent—water, alcohol, wine, glycerin, vinegar, fruit juice, or a combination of any or all of these—is also called a menstruum.) You have made a natural medicine or beverage that is called an herbal infusion—or call it an herbal tisane. It is best to use this infusion within forty-eight hours, and keep it refrigerated, for it deteriorates rapidly. Standard dosage is 1 cup three times a day. When preparing an herbal-beverage tea, you will probably want to use less herb to suit your taste.

Some mucilaginous herbs such as Marshmallow root and Slippery Elm bark are best prepared as cold infusions. This process extracts the most mucilage from these herbs, and this constituent

Continued ➜

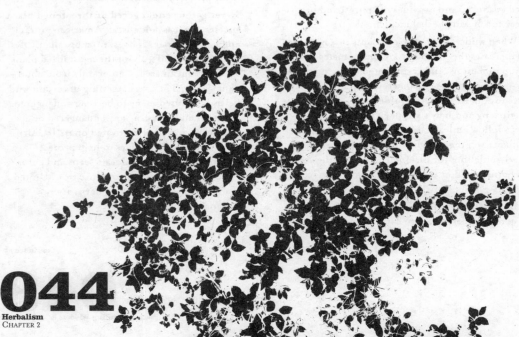

won't coagulate in a cold-water menstruum, as it might in a hot menstruum.

To make a cold infusion, simply place the cut or powdered herb into a container of cold (room-temperature) distilled water, stir it well, let it steep for five to twelve hours, until the water is slimy, and strain. Adding a little maple syrup gives it flavor.

Note: Bitter herbs do hot require as large a quantity of crude herb as other herbs do, and only a pinch of a very intense herb such as Cayenne is needed for an effective infusion. For those who have been trained to make tonic and therapeutic teas using much larger proportions of herb to water than recommended in this section—for example, an once of herb to a pint of water—note that it is my feeling that the energetics of an herb are more significant than a high dosage. Many Western herbalists today tend to make their recommended dosages smaller than traditionally administered, which is what I am doing in this book.

Decoction

Put ½ to 1 ounce of cut or crushed herb seeds, root, rhizomes, and/or bark (the tougher, woodier, more dense plant parts) into a saucepan and add 1 quart of cold water; allow this mixture to soak for a few hours if you have the time. Place on a low fire, bring to a boil, cover and simmer for fifteen minutes, and strain and drink. This is called an herbal decoction. You can keep a decoction for up to seventy-two hours if you refrigerate it. The standard dosage is 1 cup three times a day.

Combination Decoction/Infusion

First, make a decoction with the hard, woody plant parts. Then, turn off the heat and add the softer plant parts to the pot. These more delicate flowers and leaves usually contain volatile oils that would evaporate and be lost if decocted. Cover and steep the mixture until ready, then strain the tea.

Concentrate

You can continue to simmer at low heat a completed decoction that has had the spent herbs removed; this used-up herb pulp is referred to as the marc. Evaporate the tea down to one-half or one-fourth the original volume, and you make an herbal concentrate. Concentrates are considered more potent due to their condensed form, so they are often used to prepare compresses and syrups.

Syrup

To make an herbal syrup, begin with an herbal concentrate. To approximately 1 pint of this concentrate, add 2 to 4 tablespoons of raw honey and 2 to 4 tablespoons of vegetable glycerin. (Alter these amounts depending on the consistency you desire.) Tinctures can be added to syrups by adding 2 tablespoons of the tincture to 1 cup of the syrup. Store syrups in the refrigerator. The honey and glycerin will preserve them for approximately a year. Syrups are generally used to treat coughs and sore throats, because they coat the throat lining, keeping the herbs in contact with the throat tissue. (Think of a syrup as a sweet, flowing poultice.) They are also a good vehicle for administering herbs to children and fussy adults. The standard dose is approximately 1 tablespoon three to four times a day. If the condition is very irritating and acute, take 1 tablespoonful every two hours.

Tincture

Combine approximately 1 ounce of powdered dried herb (powder the dry herb by grinding it in the electric coffee grinder) with 1 pint of 80- or 100-proof alcohol (vodka, gin, brandy, high-quality moonshine—whatever you prefer) in a glass jar, stir well, and cap the jar tightly. If you choose to use a fresh, undried herb, cut it into small pieces, put it in a blender, cover it with 100-proof alcohol, and blend it all to a pulpy mash. Pour the dried-plant or fresh-plant mixture into a glass jar and shake it vigorously once or twice a day for fourteen or more days. (Shaking the tincture daily is necessary to keep the extraction process most active.) After two weeks, strain out the liquid (the extract) through muslin cloth and squeeze as much liquid out of the remaining pulp (the marc) as possible. Discard the marc and store the deeply tinted liquor in a dark, cool place in a tightly covered jar (preferably a light-retarding amber-colored jar) that has been appropriately labeled. You have made an herbal tincture. This tincture will keep for years. The standard dosage is 15 to 40 drops three times a day. Some practitioners suggest 1 to 4 milliliters three times a day depending on the herb. (A milliliter is about 25 drops.)

Solvent Exchange

Some herbs discussed in this book appear to be most efficiently extracted by using pure 190-proof ethyl alcohol for a menstruum to make a tincture. Examples of appropriate herbs are Milk Thistle seed (*Silybum marianum*), Chaparral (*Larrea tridentate*), Myrrh (*Commiphora mol-mol*)—useful for treating infections and inflammation of the mouth and throat—Valerian (*Valeriana officinalis*), and Calendula (*Calendula officinalis*).

If one—for example, an alcohol-intolerant individual wanting to heal and nourish the liver with Milk Thistle—wishes to use these extracts but does not want to ingest alcohol, the following simple technique can be used to remove the alcohol and replace it with glycerin as a preservative after having first used the alcohol to extract the plant constituents:

1. Make an extract of the desired plant using undiluted (no added water) 190-proof ethyl alcohol (basically, pure ethyl alcohol) as the menstruum. Everclear brand supplies 190-proof alcohol; however, California residents will have to go to Oregon to get it. (Please note, however, that you should never use rubbing alcohol for internal use.)

2. Make note of the exact amount of alcohol used in the menstruum. (Metric scale measurements are simplest to use.)

3. Decant and press the finished extract.

4. Measure the total amount of this extract after pressing.

5. Measure an amount of glycerin equivalent to the amount of alcohol used in the menstruum (as noted in step 2).

6. Pour the glycerin into the extract and place this entire mixture into a stainless steel or glass pot.

7. Over a low heat, gently warm the liquid extract/glycerin mixture until its volume is equivalent to the original amount of the extract in step 4. Keep the heat low, because glycerin will vaporize at 212°F. The alcohol will boil off, and you will be left with an alcohol-free glycerated extract.

8. Cool, bottle, cap tightly, and store in amber-colored bottles. The dosage is the same as that for tinctures.

Liniment

The method you use to make a tincture is the same you use to make an herbal liniment, only with the liniment, you can use rubbing alcohol in place of the liniment, you can use rubbing alcohol in place of beverage (ethyl) alcohol. If you do use rubbing alcohol, be sure to label your liniment "For external use only."

Glycerite

To make a concentrated extract similar to a tincture but with no ethyl alcohol content, make a glycerite using fresh or dried herbs.

When using a fresh, undried herb, cut it into small pieces, place them in a blender, and add enough pure vegetable glycerin to cover the herb. Blend the mixture until the herb is well blended with the glycerin. Initially, it might be difficult to position the herb in the blades of a blender, so use a blunt-ended wooden stick or a long-handled wooden spoon to assist you; persevere and be careful of the blender blades. You may need to add a small amount of distilled water to dilute the syrupy glycerin—use as little added water as possible—but this is not usually necessary when using fresh plants, for they bring their own water to the blend. After the herb and the glycerin are well blended, proceed the same as if making a tincture. (See the section titled "Tincture" at left.)

When using a dried herb, crush the herb well or powder it in your electric coffee-bean grinder, then place the powdered herb in a jar. Prepare a mixture of six parts glycerin to four parts water, and stir this mixture well to thoroughly blend the glycerin and the water. Pour this liquid onto the powdered herb, enough to saturate it, stir thoroughly, and proceed the same as if you are making a tincture.

In order for the glycerin to be an adequate preservative, your final preparation, after it has been strained, must contain at least 50 percent glycerin by volume. (Most commercial glycerin contains approximately 5 percent water; allow for this in your calculations.) This preparation will store for one to two years if it is prepared correctly. The standard dosage is 20 to 40 drops taken internally three times a day. (*Note:* In general, mucilaginous herbs such as Comfrey and Marshmallow and highly resinous plants such as Myrrh and Grindelia do not lend themselves to this form of extraction.)

Oil Infusion

Put dried powdered plant parts into high-quality cold-pressed olive oil and stir well, creating a mixture with the consistency of a mud pie, so that it will drip off a spoon but is not too runny. Keep this mixture in a warm place (approximately 100°F). Stir or shake it frequently throughout the day for ten days. While the mixture is still warm, strain out the oil through a cotton muslin cloth. Press the remaining oil from the marc. (This step can be messy, so start out in a mellow, patient mood and have sufficient cleaning materials at hand.) Store herbal-oil infusions in a tightly covered jar in a cool place. You have made a soothing medicinal-oil infusion.

Salve

Put ½ ounce (14 grams, or about 2 tablespoons) of pure beeswax shavings (do not use large, whole chunks, as this requires overheating of the herbal oil) with ½ cup vegetable oil (or a previously made herbal-oil infusion) into a small saucepan; place over low heat and gently warm until the beeswax is melted. Test for desired consistency by dipping a spoon into the mixture, removing the spoon, and letting the mixture harden on it. (Stick this in the freezer to speed the process.) If, upon cooling, the mixture is too hard, add a little more oil to the warm mixture still in the pan; if it's too soft, add a little more beeswax. Retest until the consistency is to your liking. Remove the oil-and-wax mixture

Continued ➡

from the heat and pour it into a container with a tight-fitting cap; allow the mixture to harden. You have made an herbal salve.

If you want to include aromatic essential oils in a salve, place 10 to 20 drops of the essential oil(s) into the empty glass container just before pouring in the completed salve, then pour in the salve mixture and let it all cool. When tightly capped, herbal salves can keep for a long time, but it's best to store them in a relatively cool place. Apply salves directly to your skin as needed.

Suppository

Suppositories are designed for insertion into orifices of the body. They act as carriers for any herb or herbs being used for treatment. Suppositories are normally shaped for inserting into the rectum (to treat the lower intestinal tract and as the most direct route for treating the prostate gland) or the vagina. Their form is usually cone shaped, with a rounded apex (torpedo-like), about the length and width of the first two joints of your little finger (with a volume of approximately 30 grams). Their consistency should be such that they will retain their shape at ordinary room temperature but will readily melt at body temperature, liberating the herbs contained therein. Cocoa butter is an excellent base to use, for it fulfills both of the above requirements and it is easily obtained. If you dwell in a very warm climate, it may be necessary to add a small amount of beeswax to raise the melting point of the cocoa butter (about 6 parts cocoa butter to 1 part shaved beeswax).

To prepare a suppository using powdered herbs, make a mold by forming aluminum foil into the length and shape you need for the suppositories. An easy way to shape foil is to form it around a medium-width writing pen, crimp one end of the foil, and remove the pen out the other end. This will mold a long suppository that can be cut into appropriate lengths (that can be further shaped) once it has cooled.

Grind the herb(s) to be used to a fine powder. Use an electric coffee-bean grinder to powder the herbs if necessary. Melt cocoa butter over low heat. Mix the finely powdered herb(s) with the melted cocoa butter. Herbs vary in texture and "fluff," so it is difficult to give exact proportions. Begin by mixing equal parts by volume (for example, 1 level tablespoon of herb powder to 1 tablespoon of melted cocoa butter). Hold aside some extra herb and cocoa butter in case they are needed to adjust the final consistency of this mixture.

Pour the final mixture into the aluminum foil mold. Crimp closed the open end of the filled mold and let it cool. You can now cut the pen-shaped suppository into 1-inch lengths and shape them further for use, or store them in a jar in the refrigerator for future use. Label the jar, informing others that it is not a jar of candy—or don't; they'll figure it out.

Employing a liquid extract in a suppository form requires the use of a base other than cocoa butter. To prepare a suppository using liquid herbal extracts (for example, infusions, decoctions, or tinctures), shape your aluminum mold as above and measure forty parts liquid extract, fifteen parts glycerin, and ten parts gelatin.

Soak the gelatin in the liquid extract for a half hour. Then, using a very low heat, dissolve the gelatin into the extract. Add the vegetable glycerin to the mixture and stir well. Using a water bath or a double boiler, heat the mixture to evaporate the water. The final consistency of the suppositories will depend on how much water is removed; if all is removed, you end up with a very firm consistency.

Pour the final mixture into the aluminum foil mold and let it cool. These suppositories can also be stored for a while in the refrigerator for future use.

Compress (Fomentation)

Dip a clean, freshly laundered, white cotton cloth into a warm herbal infusion, decoction, or tincture (even an oil infusion, if you can live with the unctuous experience). Wring out excess liquid and place on an injured or stressed body part. You have made a healing herb compress. Cover this compress with a recycled plastic produce bag, wrap a towel around it to hold it all in place, and then apply a blanket, a hot pad, or a hot-water bottle if warmth or added heat is appropriate. Apply the compress once or twice a day or more if appropriate. Leave it on for twenty minutes to an hour at a time.

Poultice

Crush, bruise, pummel, chop, juice, or—in an emergency—merely chew up fresh plant parts and lay them directly on injured, stung, bitten, or otherwise irritated body parts. Wrap the herbs with a clean cloth to hold them in place. Alternatively, moisten powdered dried herbs with hot tea or plain hot water and place the mixture directly on the body. You have made an herbal poultice. Apply poultices thick and wet (but not runny wet); this is when they draw and soothe most efficiently. Replenish the poultice two or three times a day and continue this procedure for about three days.

A Part of an Herbal Formula

When putting together a formula, herbalists design the formula and communicate its composition by referring to numbers of parts. For treating an irritated prostate gland, for example, mix 16 parts Saw Palmetto, 8 parts Echinacea, 8 parts Damiana, 8 parts Yarrow, and 1 part Ginger.

The question, "What is a part?" often arises. Is it a drop, a gram, an ounce, a cupful, a shovelful, or a truckload? The answer is that it can be any of these measures. You retain the proper proportions as long as each measure used to make up a part is the same measure as each of the other measured parts in the mixture. It all comes down to how much mixture you want to end up with. If you choose shovelfuls as a measure for each part in the sample formula above, however, you'll prepare enough mixture for all the prostates in the NFL. Therefore, a more reasonable measure to use is the avoirdupois ounce (there are 16 ounces in a pound) when compounding bulk herbs or the fluid ounce (there are 32 ounces in a quart) for blending liquid extracts. (Metric measures—grams and milliliters among them—are much better to use, of course, but we won't pursue that political issue here.) Referring again to the sample formula, you would blend together 2 ounces of Saw Palmetto, 1 ounce of Echinacea, 1 ounce of Damiana, 1 ounce of Yarrow, and 1/8 ounce of Ginger, ending up with 5 1/8 ounces of the formula. If you want only half that amount, make each part equal 1/2 ounce. It doesn't matter what measure you use: a household coffee scoop works fine as a (volume) part measure, but use the same scoop for each part throughout.

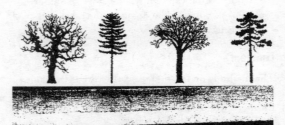

A Drop

What is a drop? This is questionable. A drop of water is supposed to be equivalent to a minim, and in pharmacy-speak is often referred to as such. But this is true only when applied to water—and then, only when the water is expelled from an international standard dropper. The shape and quality of the surface from which a drop descends influences its size. However, even when you use a standard dropper, these presumptions are seldom true when applied to liquids other than pure water. Thick, viscous liquids such as syrups produce a drop five times larger than a drop of a heavy, mobile liquid such as chloroform, and three times that of alcohol. If we use a fluid drachm as a liquid measure, we will find that it holds 250 drops of chloroform, 146 drops of alcohol, or 130 to 150 drops of an aqueous-alcohol tincture or fluid extract. It will hold 105 to 140 drops of oil but only 45 to 110 drops of syrup. So, because 8 fluid drachms are equivalent to 1 fluid ounce, for all practical posological purposes (those concerning dosages), we can assume that 1 fluid ounce of most commonly used tinctures holds approximately 960 to 1,200 drops. But none of this is any big deal, unless of course one is administering highly intense or toxic extracts or when administering medicines to infants, puppies, and kittens. In these situations, measuring doses by the metric milliliter (ml) or cubic centimeter (cc) instead of by drops is more reliable.

Calculating Dosage

If you intend to make extracts and calculate dosages, do yourself a big favor and acquire a scale, ideally one that speaks metric as well as avoirdupois.

The world has gone metric. Covered wagons and typewriters are obsolete, and so are pounds and ounces. Only the United States (and I think maybe Myanmar, formerly known as Burma) remains in the weights-and-measures dark ages, stubbornly steeping itself in feet and miles, and teaspoons and tablespoons. Therefore, we have to contend with this convoluted system of weight and measures based on the sizes of ancient European kings' feet and arms and fingers.

Regarding communicating and preparing dosages, if you deal in metric measures, it is most practical and explicit (tailored to each specific herb) to suggest a dosage of dried herb as follows: Damiana, 3 to 5 grams, taken as an infusion three times a day. This means to weigh out on a metric scale 3 to 5 grams of the herb and make a tea of it. All metric scales measure weight in grams. Prepare and drink this dose three times a day. You might use only 1 to 3 grams of a stronger herb or 4 to 6 grams of a less intense one. Regardless, it doesn't really matter how much water you use for the infusion as long as you use enough water to extract the herb's properties, which would be more or less 1 cup of water. It's only the amount of herb you're taking that matters.

You can say all this using teaspoons and tablespoons and ounces and cup measurements, too: Damiana, 1/10 to 1/6 of an ounce, taken as an infusion three times a day. However, scales that accurately measure 1/10- and 1/6-ounce increments are hard to come by and are probably unduly expensive, and any attempt to convert these fractions of ounces to teaspoons or tablespoons will drive you nuts. So, you usually see, for practical reasons and regard for sanity, simplified instructions such as those at the top of this section direct that you pour 1 quart of

Continued ➡

User-Friendly Table of Approximate Equivalencies

Liquid Measures

30 milliliters = 1 fluid ounce = 2 tablespoons

1000 milliliters = 1 liter = 1 quart = 4 cups

500 milliliters = 1 pint = 2 cups

1 teaspoon = 5 milliliters = 5 cubic centimeters = 1/6 fluid ounce

1 tablespoon = 15 milliliters = 15 cubic centimeters = 3 teaspoons = 1/2 fluid ounce

1 cup or glass = 240 milliliters = 8 fluid ounces

1 U.S. gallon = 128 fluid ounces = 3.8 liters

1 British Imperial gallon = 154 fluid ounces = 4.6 liters

Weights

30 grams = 1 ounce (avoirdupois)

454 grams = 1 pound (avoirdupois)

1 kilogram = 2.2 pounds

---

boiling water onto 1 ounce of herbs, stir, cover, and let steep for ten minutes, then strain, and drink—dosage 1 cup twice a day or 1/2 cup three to four times a day, or whatever. So, regardless of what herb you are using, you create a standardized weight-to-volume (ounce-to-quart) herbal tea and you adjust the dosage by the amount of tea you drink per dose. It's simpler that way and much easier to comply with. (The herbs discussed in this book are safe—they are not pharmaceuticals—and therefore they are not dangerous and not too dose specific.)

Meanwhile, you will see below some approximate equivalencies you might find useful. However, as far as a teaspoon measurement (or tablespoon measurement) is concerned, I'm not sure where one can buy a bona fide spoon. Can one find an accurate teaspoon? Is there a teaspoon somewhere out there in the world that is the international standard? If so, I've never heard of it; I find teaspoons sold in all different sizes and fancy configurations—some slightly smaller, some a bit larger. I think it's a fact of life that we all have to live with: some guys will just have bigger teaspoons than others.

Individuals seventy years old and older might consider taking half doses for starters to see how they feel. Actually, I suggest that everyone take previously untried herbs in smaller-than-recommended doses to check out the herbs' effects on his system.

To convert adult doses to a child's dose, use the following rule of thumb; obtain the child's body weight in pounds, and divide the number by 150 (the average weight in pounds of an adult). This calculation will give you the approximate fraction of the adult dose to give to the child. For example, if your child weighs in at an energetic though not-feeling-quite-up-to-par 50 pounds, divide 50 by 150 (50/150, or 1/3). If the recommended adult dose of the herb(s) in question is 30 drops of extract three times a day, your child's dose will be one-third of that, or 10 drops three times a day. This is known as Clark's rule.

Capsules

Unless you're a hard-core herbalist, nasty-tasting herbs (Saw Palmetto, Chaparral, Goldenseal, and so on) just have to be put into capsules so you can get them down. It's that simple. After you've gained experience tasting bitter and pungent herbs, you might choose to take them down as tinctures, which I recommend. Liquid extracts are a more easily assimilated form to use. One ounce of powdered herb (depending entirely on the density of the herb at hand) when firmly packed fills about fifty to sixty "0" capsules and about twenty-five to thirty "00" capsules. Take capsules with a drink of warm water or tea to assist their assimilation.

As you can see, making herbal medicines is a relatively simply process. Do it a couple times and you'll get it. Selecting the appropriate herbs to take as tonics or to successfully treat a condition is the rest of the art and science of herbalism, and that is what the scope of this herbal is prepared to help you learn. If you become interested in learning further techniques and insights into making herbal medicines, including how to harvest, dry, and store herbs, how to prepare herbal wines, lotions, and creams, and more detailed instructions on dosage, along with dazzling illustrations and mesmerizing wit, you may be interested in my publication *The Herbal Medicine-Maker's Handbook*, published by Crossing Press and illustrated by my daughter, Ajana.

—From *The Male Herbal*

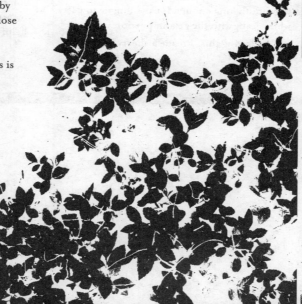

A FEW HERBS ARE ALL YOU NEED

James Green, Herbalist

It's a jungle garden out there; roots and flowers are everywhere. That's why this leafy turquoise planet is so dear to the hearts of herbalists. Here we enjoy an unending variety of plants and animals to embrace as our allies and teachers. But for an enthusiastic student herbalist, who has just entered through some unassuming personal gate into the vast forest of Herbalism, sorting out Earth's immense herbal diversity can be somewhat bewildering.

Question: How many herbs should I know to be an effectual herbalist?

Answer: 30...well, maybe 35...and probably a fungus as well.

How's that for an assertive air of authority? Someone has to act like he or she knows the answer to that question. I'll reference the source of this authority shortly.

Certainly, most herbalists I know strongly recommend that a student limit his or her studies to "a few select herbs." Get to know them well by learning to identify them, experience growing them when possible, communicate with them, discern when, where, and how best to harvest them, make medicine with them, *touch, taste, smell,* and *use them.* The energies of thirty to thirty-five herbs will enchant you and keep you sufficiently busy for the following year or two. Distinguished individuals from the remaining myriad of herbs that dwell on Earth will, one by one, as situations arise, attract your attention and attach themselves to your initial repertory.

So, the subsequent question arises: "Which few select herbs should I choose?"

Well, the most important principle to guide you in this very personal selection is to embrace any and all plants that you are intuitively attracted to: those that touch your spirit in an exceptionally deep and personal way. These are relationships that you never want to ignore. A second reliable criterion is to select herbs that grow near you and can be found thriving in the bio-region you inhabit, or in closely neighboring bio-regions. The plants you select should be fairly easy to acquire and always of excellent quality. Flirt with the currently fashionable and exotic imports, by all means, but don't become dependent on their availability.

Most herb students commence their studies by gleaning information found in popular herb books, and the number of herbs discussed in today's herbal literature can be overwhelming. At least, I have found this to be the experience of many students before they connected with a teacher or attended an herb school. So, if I may assist you with some specific suggestions, I will give you an historic and authoritative list of plants that you might consider as you orchestrate your first line of green allies, or you can at least refer to this list as a model for choosing a comparable group of plants that live in your area.

The authoritative history: In the late 1980s the California School of Herbal Studies (CSHS) was codirected by six herbalists: Tim Blakley, David Hoffmann, Amanda McQuade Crawford, Mindy Green, Gina Banghart, and myself. We decided that, in order to align our individual classes throughout the year, it would be helpful for all of us to focus on the personalities, actions, and indications of a central core of tonic and therapeutic

Continued ➡

Herb Jello

James Green, Herbalist

One afternoon, as I was manipulating the makings of glycerated-gelatin suppositories,...I discovered (actually crashed into) an interesting new(?) herbal vehicle—a medicinal herbal jello.

As a result of this impact and the events that followed, I have reason to suspect that tonic and therapeutic herbal jellos offer notable potential for assisting herbalists and parents to increase child and "ill-tempered adult" patient compliance.

This discovery stemmed from a blunder of mine that involved a particularly precious tincture of primo-wildcrafted Oregon Grape root (OGR). The simple pharmaceutical event was supposed to culminate in a manifestation of many, perfectly molded glycerated-gelatin suppositories, but instead, ended up as an unintended mass of OGR jello. Momentarily deranged by my frustration and self-pity (I was racing toward a publishing deadline at the time), I lost control. In my mindless anguish, I took a spoon to it all, slashing and scooping at it blindly as I cried out, "Why me!? Why now!? Why all that glycerin? Why my finest OGR tincture!?"

Immediately following the gelatal carnage, as I stood at the kitchen counter, bewildered, remorseful, emotionally spent, questioning the meaning of life and the purpose of man's toil on earth, gazing aimlessly at the sordid glycerated remains, the empty tincture bottle laying on its side, the soiled beakers, I ate a spoonful of the still quivering blunder...and behold...I was instantly uplifted! It was fun, like eating jello always is (even for those cranky adults who won't admit it). And it tasted....."all right!" which OGR tincture never does. Right, kids?

I discovered that jellofied herb effortlessly jiggles and diffuses ghastly flavors, distracting one's taste buds from the roots of bitterness, and the glycerin follows up smoothly with a pleasantly sweet aftertaste. I liked it! I ate another scoop. The herbalized jello played in my mouth. I slurped another scoop, then another. My face smiled big; the universe, amused by my blunderability had given me an answer to my questions...*herb jello* (*Botanica wiggleus; Gelatinaceae* family)! What an idea! (Individuals requiring a more sophisticated air of credibility in their future discussions concerning this important new clinical vehicle can use the currently more fashionable European-flavored term "phytojel." Such a joyous footnote this will be scribed in the herb section of the Akashic records and in the future archives of twenty-first century American phyto-folklore. Herbal pharmacy of the new millennium will have a wiggle.

Not long thereafter, creativity ablaze, I boarded my bike and sped to the local grocery store, where I bought myself a couple packs of lime-flavored Jell-O® (what can I say, lime is green). I flirted with the idea of getting the sugar-free type Jell-O, but its label said "aspartame" on the ingredients list, so I reconsidered and bought the ones that said "sugar" instead. In my belief system, aspartame makes white sugar the good guy. And, with all that good herb that's going to be taken, a little sugar isn't going to hurt anyone.

Upon returning home, I opened my box of lime Jell-O, immediately poured a little bit of the green powder into my palm, and proceeded to lick it, mm-*mm*! You've gotta do that; every kid does. Then I poured the rest of the powder onto a scale and weighed it. I wanted only to use ¼ of the Jell-O to experiment with. I weighed out 22 Gm (the 3 oz box said 85 Gm, but I got 86 Gm + my approximately 2 Gm compulsive lick).

HERB JELLO

¼ box	lime Jell-O (I did cherry Jell-O next) = approximately 22 Gm
¼ cup	boiling water (60 ml)
1 oz.	tincture (I used Feverfew for my first intentional herb jello) (30 ml or ⅛ cup)
1 oz.	cold water (30 ml or ⅛ cup)

1. Put the jello powder into a small rectangular shaped baking tin. (I used a small loaf tin that measured 2½ inches by 4½ inches. Using this squared-off shape makes it easy to divide the herb jello into equal-sized pieces in order to give relatively equal-sized doses.)

2. Pour the boiling water onto the jello powder and *stir well* for 2 to 3 minutes, *making sure that the gelatin is completely dissolved*.

3. Add the tincture and stir this well.

4. Then add the cold water and stir well.

5. Pour this mixture into the pan and/or into any other molds you wish to use. I bought some candy molds of various forms (shells, cars, cigars, Christmas trees, etc.) that make kid-approved shapes for eating. (The research that remains for us to discover the jello flavors that work best with each uniquely flavored herb or herbal blend. This is why I use only ¼ of the pack, or less, at a time.)

6. Once the herb jello has hardened, cut it into 6 equal portions, each one delivering about a 5 ml dose of tincture.

The Feverfew jello turned out tasting "all right." At least it is the best-tasting, most palatable dose of Feverfew I've taken so far, and taste-wise, Feverfew is one of the herbs most folks applaud the least.

This water-gelatin vehicle scoots the herbal flavors quickly past the taste buds and on down to the stomach with a minimal amount of gustative resistance; yet in passing, it makes its moves on the mouth long enough for the tongue to party whimsically with the gelatin portion.

Following this, I made a cherry St. John's Wort jello and called it "cherry up." Next, I assembled a relaxing nervine jello using Valerian and California Poppy with lemon Jell-O and called it "mellow yellow jello" (naming your herb jello is optional).

I feel a great potential here for parents, grumps, and wee ones. One can experiment with all types of flavored Jell-O® brand jellos in order to find those that cohabit harmoniously in a jelly-body with otherwise strange and frightful tasting herbal extracts, like Feverfew, Oregon Grape Yarrow, and Mugwort.....Glycerin is a non-sugar sweetener. Or one can experiment with using Stevia, which has been infused into the water that is used to dissolve an unsweetened gelatin. Stevia (*Stevia rebaudiana*) is an herb that has come to us from its native land Paraguay. It tastes sweeter than sugar, but by FDA (the Federal Denial Attendants) pronouncement, cannot be called a sweetener (this edict is probably another side effect of the aspartame industry). Use Hains® brand vegetarian jello or a flavored pectin if you prefer a vegetarian variety.

You can incorporate herbal infusions, decoctions, tinctures—any and all forms of loathsome tasting herbal liquids children and ill-tempered adults often refuse to take or complain about so incessantly it's hardly worth the effort trying to help them. Of course, all the naturally good-tasting herbal teas, glycerites, and tinctures like Lemon Balm, Mint, Chamomile, and Fennel are also garnished with fun when transformed into a phytogel.

Adults (senior kids) can take a bit of dessert before meals as a digestive aid, using an herb jello incorporating Peppermint, Chamomile, Lemon Balm, Ginger, or any of the other carminatives. Merely the name "Lemon Balm-lemon-lime jello" shimmies with vibrations of gastric approval and upliftment.

I'm planning to prepare a Meadowsweet jello which will be a consoling herbal therapeutic treat for any child who is experiencing diarrhea. The jello portion will proceed to make his or her insides feel soothed and happy, and the Meadowsweet will supply its gently efficient internal action to help balance out the child's troubled intestine. Catnip and Fennel is an herbal blend I strongly recommend having on hand in all households inhabited by babies and young children. It is an excellent compound to use for soothing children's colicky digestive systems and for allaying children's fevers, especially during childhood fever diseases such as measles, mumps, chickenpox, etc. The name "Catnip-Fennel-jello" carries an inherent giggle and just sounds like a good time. The babe will love it as a medicinal treat, and a touch of party. (If the child's fever is prolonged and quite troublesome, the insertion of a homecrafted Meadowsweet, Yarrow suppository will be quite helpful.)

—From *The Herbal Medicine-Maker's Handbook*

Continued ➤

plants. As an initial step to develop this group of medicinals, each of us agreed to provide a list of thirty favored plants that we felt could be relied upon to supply an herbalist with pretty much any and all the herbal actions and uplifting virtues required to provide good health care in a home and community. The succeeding task of grafting our lists together and then pruning the aggregation back to thirty plants proved to be an interesting journey of forbearance and compromise; the results of that saga attest to the fact that, on a rare occasion, even experts can come to an agreement, or at least cross-pollinate their opinions. The hybrid list we ultimately compiled and felt reasonably good about included the following thirty plants.

CSHS List of 30 Herbs

Blackberry (*Rubus villosus*)

***Black Cohosh** (*Cimicifuga racemosa*)

Calendula (*Calendula officinalis*)

Cayenne (*Capsicum annuum*)

Chamomile, German (*Matricaria recutita*)

Cleavers (*Galium aperine*)

Comfrey (*Symphytum officinale*)

Crampbark (*Viburnum opulus*)

Dandelion (*Taraxacum officinale*)

***Echinacea** (*Echinacea purpurea*)

Elder (*Sambucus nigra*)

Fennel (*Foeniculum vulgare*)

Ginger (*Zingiber officinale*)

***Goldenseal** (*Hydrastis canadensis*)

Gumweed (*Grindelia spp.*)

Hawthorn (*Crataegus oxyacanthus*)

Marshmallow (*Althaea officinalis*)

Mugwort (*Artemisia vulgaris*)

Mullein (*Verbascum spp.*)

Nettle (*Urtica spp.*)

Peppermint (*Mentha piperita*)

***Pipsissewa** (*Chimaphilla umbellate*)

Plantain (*Plantago lanceolata or P. major*)

St. John's Wort (*Hypericum perforatum*)

Scullcap (*Scutellaria spp.*)

Valerian (*Valeriana officinalis*)

Vitex (*Vitex agnus-castus*)

Willow (*Salix alba*)

Yarrow (*Achillea millefolium*)

Yellow Dock (*Rumex crispus*)

*I have asterisked the plants which are broadly used in commerce and which, due to overharvest, loss of habitat, or by the nature of their innate rareness or sensitivity are either at risk or have significantly declined in numbers within their current range. Use substitute plants when possible.

Yes, I know; where's Milk Thistle, where's Sage, where's Usnea, where's....Undeniably, this list screams out the names of countless time-honored herbs that have not been included, and I must say (using this opportunity to get in a "last word"), the herbs that would be at the top of the list of thirty (if anybody would have listened to me) are listed next.

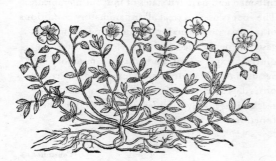

Green's Long-Awaited Embellishments

Burdock (*Arctium lappa*)

Ginkgo (*Ginkgo biloba*)

Oat (wild: *Avena fatua*, cultivated: *Avena sativa*)

Saw Palmetto (*Serenoa serrulata*)

Siberian Ginseng (*Eleuthrococcus senticosus*)

And then there's **Reishi** mushroom (*Ganoderma lucidum*), a fungus, and...Well, you can appreciate the problem we faced.

Please note that most of the thirty plants on the CSHS list grow in abundance in the northern California region where our school is located, but as you may also notice, love transcends all rules and common sense, and some of our most favored plants that made it onto the list don't normally grow here. Ginger thrives in moist tropical regions; Goldenseal and Black Cohosh live in moist and shady Eastern hardwood forests; Echinacea lives in the open plains of the Midwest; and Pipsissewa, although it lives in Pacific Northwest forests, grows very slowly, and therefore, even if harvested correctly does not recover rapidly. With the recently ballooning popularity of herbal medicine in this country, these five plants have all become highly sought-after medicinals, and while Ginger is abundantly cultivated and therefore not threatened by its popularity, the other four plants are not yet being adequately cultivated and are being plucked from their relatively small native stands at far too rapid a rate. They are simply being overharvested from their native environment in order to supply the soaring commercial demands of people living in the other bio-regions of the U.S. as well as in Canada and many countries overseas.

The survival of these four plants is currently at great risk, and therefore humans need to find substitutes whenever possible (preferably plants that grow in our own backyard bio-regions) until these plants can be cultivated adequately to supply our commercial demands. As you can see, since the time we developed our CSHS list of thirty herbs, herbalists and other plant people have become quite alert to the fact that a number of important medicinal plants (in addition to the four on our list) are currently extremely harvest-sensitive. So, with deep regard for all these plants, I offer the following suggestions and ask you to heed them:

In general, regarding the four at-risk plants that appear on the list of thirty:

- Please become familiar with United Plant Savers' (UpS) list of "at-risk" medicinal plants and avoid using them until we can escort them back to their natural state of abundance.

- Use Black Cohosh sparingly, *only* when it is specifically indicated (see indications, p. 50) and when there is no substitute available. In this regard, for those living in the Pacific Northwest region, there is our Baneberry (*Actea rubra*), a close relative of Black Cohosh, that can be harvested and prepared as a reliable substitute. The root of Baneberry offers nearly all the same actions as Black Cohosh root. Yes, the berries of Baneberry are toxic, but its root is not (that's why we don't call it Baneroot). In fact, in the early 1900s batches of Black Cohosh were often adulterated by mixing Baneberry root with the Cohosh. When taken as a tincture, Baneberry root bestows the same anti-inflammatory, sedative, and antispasmodic action for relieving the vast array of dull aching pains as does Black Cohosh. For a multitude of reasons, but specifically for invaluable insight into the use of this plant as an important substitute for the endangered Black Cohosh, I suggest and highly recommend that you consult *Medicinal Plants of the Pacific West*, researched and written by herbalist Michael Moore.

- In place of Pipsissewa when treating urinary tract inflammation, substitute Uva Ursi (*Arctostaphylos uva-ursi*) for its excellent diuretic, antiseptic, and astringent properties. Prepare it as a cold infusion to eliminate the extraction of most of its condensed tannins that can be irritating to some folks, and combine this with Marshmallow root to help soothe and protect any irritated tissue.

- When utilizing Goldenseal to employ its berberine alkaloid component, use it only when the plant's overall specific indications are absolutely required; otherwise use other berberine-containing plants such as Barberry (*Berberis vulgaris*), or Oregon Grape (*Mahonia aquifolium*), or at least dilute Goldenseal whenever using it: mixing 1 part Goldenseal to 4 parts Barberry or Oregon Grape root. When you feel you must use Goldenseal undiluted, use a reduced dosage, for, when it is truly the specific plant to use, a small dose is wholly adequate.

- Use only *organically cultivated* Echinacea. Avoid using wild Echinacea or any commercial products that use wildcrafted or wild-harvested Echinacea in their ingredients. Three species of Echinacea are used commercially: *E. purpurea, E. angustifolia*, and *E. pallida*. Echinacea purpurea is easily and presently cultivated, whereas the other two species are more difficult to grow and therefore not so widely cultivated. Due to overaggressive wildcrafting, the native stands of all three of these species of Echinacea are disappearing rapidly.

Goldenseal, Black Cohosh, Echinacea, and Pipsissewa are four plant allies that are due a collective show of human appreciation and currently require our concerted acts of tender loving care. Discontinuing the wild harvesting of these plants while using other herbs as appropriate substitutes will give these generous medicinals time to repopulate their natural habitats and will give herb growers time and resources to develop their skills in cultivating these herbs for commercial use. *Merci.*

In addition to the drama of innumerable heartbreaking revelations of personal love affairs with certain herbs, there was a rational method to the madness that was conjured up as we six herbalists compiled the above CSHS list of thirty herbs. Along with seeking plants that grow well in our climatic zone, we looked very closely at the *actions* (also referred to as therapeutic or medicinal *properties*) of these plants, and we made sure our final group of herbs embraced all the actions that we know are essential and therefore necessary in a well-endowed herbal pharmacy.

Pertaining to these actions, the science of Herbalism, like all therapeutic sciences, has its particular language. The nutritional and medicinal actions of each herb in our materia medica constitute the fundamental vocabulary of the language of Herbalism. Knowledge of the actions (the biochemical energetics) of each plant and the plant's spontaneous affinity for various systems of the body is basic to successfully employing herbs in health maintenance, disease prevention, and curative self-care.

Understanding the inherent energetics of each plant that one uses gives insight and increased autonomy in personal and family health care. It is too limiting to think or ask, "What herb do I take for..." or "What herb will cure my..." This

Continued →

approach stems from the "magic bullet" (one drug for one disease) myth conjured by pharmaceutical drug marketing. Herbs are more clever and practical than that. Each herb can do many things and have more than one effect on the human body and mind. The therapeutic actions and the unique blend of organic nutrients of each herb have a *natural affinity* for a variety of tissues, organs, and systems of the body. Supervised by the body's cellular intelligence which attracts to itself whatever is needed for toning and healing, these actions are contributed by the herb to the appropriate systems for preventing and/or curing a wide variety of conditions....

Actions and Indications for the CSHS List of 30 Herbs

Blackberry (Bramble) is astringent, especially for the gastrointestinal tract. It allays excessive fluid loss from diarrhea, and when medical intervention is not available may save lives. Hemostatic—it stops bleeding of the gastrointestinal tract.

Black Cohosh (an at-risk plant, seek organically cultivated or employ substitutes when possible) is antispasmodic, anti-inflammatory, and analgesic and is most useful for its ability to reduce dull aching pain just about anywhere in the body. Along with this generalized effect, Black Cohosh has a specific affinity for the reproductive organs. It relieves the aching pains in the reproductive tract of males, but is most often used as a regulator of female imbalances. As an emmenagogue, it is used for relief of painful menstruation, but is also very effective for relieving suppressed menstruation. This, along with the fact that its effects are often long-lasting, suggests that it has a generalized tonic effect on the uterus and most likely on the male reproductive organs as well. This plant is widely used for the treatment of rheumatism and neuralgia and all cases characterized by that kind of pain known as rheumatic, dull, tensive, and intermittent. Black Cohosh is nervine, hypotensive, having a powerful influence over the nervous system as it appears to have a sedating effect on the perception of pain.

When using Baneberry root (*Actea rubra*), which is recommended as a substitute for Black Cohosh for relieving pain, use a reduced dosage....

Calendula (Marigold) is anti-inflammatory, vulnerary, lymphatic, antimicrobia, and antifungal. It is unsurpassed for treating local skin problems that are due to infection, and for treating wounds, burns bruises, or strains due to physical damage. It is excellent for internal digestive inflammation and ulceration. Calendula is antispasmodic, lymphatic, and emmenagogue for normalizing the menstrual process, and cholagogue for aiding in the relief of a gallbladder problem and its accompanying digestive complaints; hepatic.

Cayenne (Capsicum) is a general tonic, but it's also quite specific to the circulatory and digestive systems. It is the most useful of the systemic stimulants, strengthening the heart, arteries, capillaries, blood flow, peripheral circulation, and nerves. It helps in conditions of debility, especially of the elderly, and wards off colds and catarrh. It is also carminative and sialagogue. Applied externally, it is rubefacient and is most useful for cold hands and feet (sprinkled in socks), and problems like rheumatic pains and lumbago, and for hoarseness as a gargle; antimicrobial and an ouchful! but very effective styptic (S & M variety).

Chamomile is anti-inflammatory and a pain-relieving for a wide range of conditions along the entire digestive tract; antispasmodic for easing muscle cramps; nervine. Chamomile is probably the most widely used relaxing nervine tonic. It is also used to relieve mental stress and tension. It is carminative and a mild bitter.

Cleavers is lymphatic; a lymphatic cleanser that relieves lymphatic swelling, particularly where there is an acute "hot" inflammation; it is a cooling diuretic that soothes an irritable urinary tract; tonic, and alterative.

Comfrey (Knitbone) is vulnerary and demulcent, having unparalleled wound, ulcer and fracture healing action. It is anti-inflammatory and soothing to dry inflamed digestive tract; astringent, able to allay hemorrhaging wherever it occurs; and expectorant as an age-old remedy for dry irritable coughs, especially when accompanied by blood streaked mucus.

Comfrey has been praised throughout history as a premier healing plant used extensively in folkloric Herbalism internally and externally for the repair of innumerable body wounds and illnesses. However, in the past few years reductionist science has proclaimed Comfrey (in particular, the root and the early spring leaves) to be the possessor and conveyer of certain toxic components called pyrrolizidine alkaloids that are said to cause damage to the liver of human beings. Many herbalists have accepted this as truth and a number of us have not. Therefore, in order to provide full disclosure in this printed manual concerning the use of Comfrey, I feel it prudent to inform the reader of this debate and give current standard precautions: It is recommended that pregnant women, young children, and persons with manifest liver disease avoid the consumption of Comfrey (external use is no problem). Others are advised to use Comfrey root and leaf on a short-term basis and preferably avoid the use of the spring leaf, but instead use the leaf that appears on the latter (second) growth of the year. There are available in the marketplace pyrrolizidine-free Comfrey tinctures in which the suspect alkaloids have been removed.

Crampbark is an antispasmodic that relieves voluntary and involuntary muscular spasm of the entire pelvic viscera, bladder, womb (antiabortive), ovaries, and the limbs; it allays convulsions, asthma, thigh and back pain, and it's an anti-inflammatory and nervine, helping to restore sympathetic/parasympathetic balance. Its astringent action helps allay excessive blood loss in menstruation and especially in menopause; emmenagogue.

Dandelion has many healing actions. The root a general tonic and an effective liver tonic, hepatic, which acts to "cool" (detoxify) the liver; its cholagogue action decongests the gallbladder by increasing bile flow; and its choleretic action promotes bile production. It is antirheumatic, as it stimulates cell metabolism in the body, assisting the body to dump metabolic waste into the blood to be cleansed by the liver. It is alterative, relieving skin disorders and degenerative joint disorders, lowering blood cholesterol. It is a mild laxative, bitter. The leaf is a safe, highly effective diuretic, the best natural source of potassium which avoids potassium depletion, so common with the use of other diuretics; bitter. Young leaves can be eaten raw in salads; they are best mixed with other salad greens and tossed with a favorite salad dressing.

Echinacea (an at-risk plant, use only organically cultivated) is an immune stimulant, assisting the body to resist infection more efficiently; it is antimicrobial and increases cellular resistance to virus, and activated the macrophages that destroy both cancerous cells and pathogens; it is anticatarrhal and alterative.

Elder, Black, if I recall correctly, stood at the top of each of our CSHS lists, being nearly a complete pharmacy by itself. Elder's leaves used externally are vulnerary and emollient. When used internally the leaves are purgative, expectorant, diuretic, and diaphoretic. Its flowers prepared as a cold infusion are diuretic, alterative, and cooling; as a warm infusion the flowers are diaphoretic and gently stimulating. Its berries are diaphoretic, diuretic, aperient, and when fresh they make good juice and jam. Elder is the reliable home remedy for cold, flu, fever, skin eruptions, sprains, bruises, wounds, hayfever, sinusitis, tension, constipation, rheumatic discomfort, and so on. Look this plant up in a variety of sources; probably no single herbal tells Elder's complete story.

Fennel is carminative, relieving flatulence and colic, and stimulating digestion and appetite. It is very helpful in improving the flavor of other herbs. Combined with Catnip (*Nepeta cataria*), it makes the best child's remedy for fever, colic, and general restlessness; it is antispasmodic, having a calming effect on coughs and bronchial disorders, and anti-inflammatory as a compress and eye wash for infected eyes and inflamed eyelids, and galactogogue.

Ginger is a diffusive stimulant that is warming by increasing peripheral circulation; an emergency remedy whenever immediate stimulation is needed, a master herb for relieving nausea and motion sickness; an anodyne in gastric and intestinal pain; a carminative- and anti-spasmodic in the digestive tract; diaphoretic for promoting perspiration in feverish conditions; anti-inflammatory particularly useful in rheumatic conditions that benefit from heat; anti-microbial; rubefacient; and a reliable emmenagogue.

Goldenseal (an at-risk plant; use cultivated Goldenseal or replace with other berberine-containing plants or other plants that offer similar actions) is hepatic, cholagogue, a bitter digestive stimulant, and a primary antimicrobial for acute infection. It is an invaluable tonic stimulant for overrelaxed, profusely secreting mucous membranes having a wide effect on the respiratory, digestive, and genito-urinary systems, and it has an anticatarrhal effect, especially in sinus conditions. It is astringent and emmenagogue.

Gumweed is a relaxing expectorant, which relaxes the smooth muscles. It is antispasmodic and hypotensive, useful for treatment of asthmatic and bronchial conditions, especially when accompanied by rapid heartbeat and nervous response.

Hawthorn is a heart tonic of the first order which maintains the heart in a healthy condition. It directly effects the cells of the heart muscle, enhancing both activity and nutrition. It is a specific remedy in most cardiac disease and facilitates a gentle but long-term sustained effect on degenerative, age-related, changes in the entire cardiovascular system; astringent. It is hypotensive and diuretic.

Marshmallow, due to its abundance of mucilage, is emollient when used in salves for external use. Used internally, it is a soothing demulcent indicated for inflamed and irritated states of mucous membranes. The root is used to treat all inflammatory conditions of the gastrointestinal tract, including the mouth, gastritis, peptic ulcers, colitis, etc. The leaves are diuretic, expectorant, and anti-inflammatory, and are used to relieve dryness of lungs and a burning or irritated urinary tract; its abundant mucopolysaccharides mildly stimulate the body's immune function.

Continued ➡

Mugwort is a bitter tonic and foremost digestive stimulant. It is antioxidant, which helps in the metabolism of rancid fats and protects the liver from damage from free radicals. It is cholagogue, giving a general stimulating effect on bile flow, helping to remove liver congestion, especially for those, who have eaten (rancid) oily food. As a nervine tonic, it eases tension, and is antidepressant, as it aids in depression, particularly when this is due to liver congestion, a virus, and/or a sedentary lifestyle; it is emmenagogue.

Mullein is expectorant, an extremely beneficial respiratory remedy that tones the mucous membranes, reduces inflammation, and stimulates fluid production, thus facilitating expectoration. It is also demulcent, diuretic, nervine, antispasmodic, alterative, astringent, anodyne, vulnerary, and anti-inflammatory. The oil infusion of the fresh flowers is particularly effective for soothing and healing any inflamed surface and easing ear problems (pain). As a fomentation of leaves it is excellent for local application to any inflamed parts.

Nettle leaf is a spring tonic and a general alterative detoxifying agent which clears out waste products, strengthens the mucosa of the urinary, digestive, and respiratory systems, and when taken fresh works against the allergic response to hayfever. It prevents uric acid buildup in joints and is extremely helpful in cases of gout, rheumatism, and arthritis. It is an astringent, which is useful for relieving excessive discharge and bleeding, and is diuretic and hypotensive. Nettle root is tonic for the genito-urinary system. It is a good prostate tonic and quite helpful for benign prostatic enlargement. It is an excellent potherb cooked like spinach or any other fresh greens.

Peppermint is one of humanity's favorite and most uplifting flavors. It is carminative and antispasmodic, having a relaxing effect on the muscles of the digestive system; it combats flatulence and stimulates bile and the flow of digestive juices. It is carminative, diaphoretic, and antiemetic. As a mild anesthetic to the stomach lining, it often allays feelings of nausea. It is nervine, and antimicrobial. This plant (combined with Elder and Yarrow) is a traditional treatment for fevers, colds, and influenza and thereby has saved countless lives throughout the ages.

Pipsissewa is an at-risk plant, well substituted for by using an Uva Ursi and Marshmallow combination. Therefore, Uva Ursi (Bearberry) is diuretic; it has a specific antiseptic and astringent effect upon the membranes of the urinary system, which it can be relied upon to soothe and tone. With its anti-microbial action, it is wonderfully effective for treating bladder infection, gravel, or a stone in the kidney. It is helpful to blend this plant with Marshmallow root to increase the soothing and protectant demulcent action.

Plantain is a magnificent weed that grows everywhere and is readily available throughout the year. It is vulnerary, expectorant, demulcent, anti-inflammatory, astringent, diuretic, and anti-microbial, having excellent healing properties. It is a gentle expectorant that will soothe inflamed and painful membranes, ideal for coughs and bronchitis. Its astringency aids in diarrhea, hemorrhoids, and bladder inflammation where there is bleeding. It relieves inflammation of the skin and intestinal tract. It is a valuable treatment for diseases of the blood and glandular conditions. It is a traditional cure taken internally, and as a poultice for treating the stings and bites of snakes, spiders, and insects, and as a dressing for cuts, wounds, and bruises.

St. John's Wort is nervine. Taken internally, it has a sedative and pain-relieving effect appropriate for treating neuralgia, anxiety, and tension, and any irritable and anxious effects of menopausal changes. As an antidepressant, it is highly recommended for treatment of melancholia or "the blues." As an astringent, it is used externally as an oil or salve. It is a valuable healing vulnerary and anti-inflammatory remedy for nerve injuries, muscular bruises, painful wounds, swelling, varicose veins, and mild burns.

Scullcap is a nerve tonic, having a mild sedative, anti-spasmodic edge. It is especially appropriate as a primary nervous system tonic and relaxant for stalwart individuals who have fiery emotions that promote nerve and muscle tension. This plant is also used specifically in the treatment of seizure, hysterical states, and epilepsy, as well as for general muscular and nervous irritability and tension. It is also well used where there is nervous disorder that develops twitching, tremors, restlessness, or irregular muscular action. As a cardiac relaxant, it is useful in sedating heart imbalances caused by overactive nerves; bitter.

Valerian is primarily a nervine tonic. It is helpful to know Valerian has a stimulating, warming nature which does not work well for those who tend to have too great a blood flow to the brain, and too great a nerve force already. Rather, Valerian, having a warming and stimulating effect on the body, is a remedy used better for a nervousness and irritability that comes secondarily to deficiency. It is best used in people with poor blood circulation in general, but particularly poor circulation to the brain and nervous centers. It is well used for anxiety, despondency, and nervousness in individuals whose face and skin look pale and lifeless, and the skin and body is cool. It is a particularly useful remedy when there is intestinal tension leading to gas, cramps, constipation, or irritable bowel–type conditions. For a tonic effect, it should be taken as a fresh plant extract. This plant is also hypotensive and is used as a relaxing remedy in hypertension and stress-related heart problems. As a hypnotic it is well known to improve sleep quality, especially amongst those who consider themselves to be poor sleepers. Besides its wonderful relaxing effects, Valerian is also antispasmodic and emmenagogue. It is a suitable remedy for excessive caffeine intake.

Vitex (Chasteberry) is a uterine tonic which stimulates and normalizes pituitary gland functions, especially its progesterone-stimulating function, and therefore acts to normalize the activity of female sex hormones. This is the basis for its use in everything from PMS and recovery from taking birth control pills, to dysmenorrhea and menopause. It is used to stabilize the ovulation cycle. It is well used to help reduce the undesirable symptoms of menopause and is helpful in irregular menstruation, especially if accompanied by endometriosis. It helps relieve hormonally related constipation, and can assist in the control of acne in teenagers.

Willow is an ancient analgesic remedy used for its pain-relieving, anti-inflammatory effects. In various forms, it has been employed to relieve the discomforts of headache, cold, flu, fever, gout, and the aches and pains of all description.

Yarrow is one of the best of the diaphoretic herbs, making it a standard remedy for reducing fever. It is used for treating hypertension. This action is attributed to its vaso-dilating and diuretic properties. As a tonic, this herb's main uses are as an astringent, antiseptic, anti-inflammatory, antispasmodic, and a diuretic remedy for the genito-urinary system. It is used as an astringent, anti-inflammatory, and bitter tonic in the gastrointestinal system, where it can help normalize irritated and inflamed

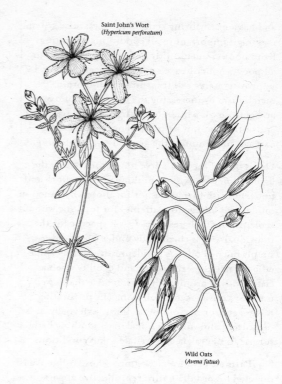

Saint John's Wort
(Hypericum perforatum)

Wild Oats
(Avena fatua)

states of the digestive tract, as its volatile oils contain similar anti-inflammatory constituents as Chamomile. Its astringent, hemostatic, and anti-inflammatory properties also make this plant useful for intestinal bleeding, hemorrhoids with bloody discharge, uterine hemorrhage, profuse, protracted menstruation, and leucorrhea. It is also quite effective in relieving menstrual cramps. Used externally, it is styptic and a wound-healing vulnerary.

Yellow Dock is a hepatic liver stimulant and laxative. As a laxative, its activity lies somewhere between the bile stimulants (Dandelion, Oregon Grape) and the more strongly laxative anthraquinone group (Bitter Aloe, Senna, Buckthorn). Its combination of liver-cleansing properties and laxative effect seems to assist the body in dealing with the metabolic wastes often associated with a low-fiber, high-fat, and meat diet. As a cholagogue, it stimulates the flow of bile and has a therapeutic effect on jaundice when this is due to congestion. Yellow Dock is a wonderful alterative for treating oily and exudative skin conditions. It seems to work through the liver and bowel to help remove metabolic wastes from the blood. By improving the liver's ability to metabolize wastes and fats it takes the burden off of secondary pathways of elimination, such as the skin.

Green's 5 Additional Herbs and the Fungus

Burdock is a "deep food" and alterative that moves the body to a state of well-nourished health, promotes the healing of wounds, and removes the indicators of system imbalance such as low energy, ulcers, skin conditions, and dandruff. As a diuretic and alterative, it works through the liver and kidneys to protect against the buildup of waste products and is considered to be one of the best tonic correctives of skin disorders. Burdock is a classic remedy for skin conditions which result in dry, scaly skin and cutaneous eruptions (eczema, psoriasis, dermatitis, boils, carbuncles, sties), as well as also being helpful in relieving rheumatism and gout. As a mild bitter that stimulates digestive juices and bile secretion, it aids appetite and digestion and is well used in anorexia. Externally, it is an exceptional fomentation or poultice to promote the healing of wounds and ulcers, especially when also taken internally on a regular basis.

Ginkgo is first and foremost a vasodilator. It improves circulation to the brain and periphery

Continued ➡

and has a normalizing action on the vascular system, making it important in all conditions stemming from poor circulation. It improves circulation to all poorly nourished areas. It enhances memory by improving nerve cell transmission and brain metabolism by increasing the utilization of oxygen and glucose. As a brain tonic, free-radical scavenger, and antioxidant, it helps prevent cardiovascular damage and counters the general effects of aging.

Oat is one of the best nerve tonics for feeding the depleted nervous system of those who overwork and undernourish themselves, or for those who function on nervous energy (or caffeine) for too long without replenishing their reserves. Oat is specific for the individual who is chronically under stress and is simply burned out. Its antidepressive activity is specific for nervous exhaustion and debility when associated with depression. It is a nutritive that is well used for convalescence following any prostrating disease and/or nervous breakdown. Externally, it is demulcent and vulnerary, making a soothing bath for use in neuralgia and irritated skin conditions.

Saw Palmetto is a nutritive tonic whose influence is directed toward the entire reproductive apparatus. It works cleverly as a remedial tonic that stimulates the nutrition of the nerve centers upon and through which it operates. For the male, this action focuses particularly on the prostate gland, which it keeps in a state of wellness. For an enlarged prostate gland and accompanying diminished sexual drive, it is remarkably therapeutic, as it reduces the size of the gland and quickly relieves the other disorders that commonly occur with this condition's symptoms (e.g., dribbling urine, slow initiation or urination, incomplete bladder evacuation). In females, this plant is beneficial for treating ovarian enlargement, weakened sexual drive, and with continual use its nourishing components can help develop small underdeveloped mammary glands. As a diuretic, antiseptic, and tonic it is a valuable remedy in treating any infection of the genitor-urinary system. As a nutritive endocrine agent, it is safely used to give a boost to the male sex hormones and has been reported to reverse sterility in women where there is no organic disease or injured tissue. This berry tastes to me like rancid soap, so I find it is most palatable when taken in capsule form. For those whose nature will do well with the actions and flavor of Licorice, this herb does a decent job of covering Saw Palmetto's controversial flavor.

Siberian Ginseng is a classic adaptogen in that when taken consistently it produces a state of nonspecific stress resistance. It helps modify the underlying imbalance caused by stressors, regardless of the specific nature of the stressor (chemical, physical, psychological, etc.). In order for an herb to be classified as an adaptogen, not only must it help one deal with "stress," but it cannot cause an imbalance in physiological functions; it must basically be harmless and should help normalize functions, regardless of whether they are underactive or overactive.

Siberian Ginseng's adaptogenic qualities have been shown to improve generalized resistance to infectious diseases, to lessen muscular fatigue, to help balance hypertension, and to reduce damage from radiation. Although its effect on the adrenal cortex gives it wide-ranging uses, it seems to have a special affinity for the circulatory system. It has been shown to balance both high and low blood pressure, reduce serum cholesterol levels, and relieve anginal pain.

The wide-ranging effects of Siberian Ginseng can be traced largely to its ability to have positive effect on the general adaptation syndrome. When confronted with long-term stress, the original response known as the "alarm reaction" is less severe; the resistance phase (i.e., when you are coping with a stress) is prolonged, and the exhaustive stage that can follow long-term stress is better handled. All in all, Siberian Ginseng allows one to better handle a tougher work load, emotional and chemical stressors, living in congested cities, and the general frazzle of living in our twenty-first-century civilization.

Reishi (*Ganoderma lucidum*) is a remarkably beneficial fungus for the human body. First of all, it is a primary supporter of the immune system, as it is believed to enhance white blood cell production, stimulate macrophage (scavenger cells of the immune system) activity, help protect against cancer, and work against viruses. It is shown to modify the body's allergic response. Reishi also provides cardiovascular protection by helping to lower excessively high blood pressure. It helps lower cholesterol while it increases the ratio of HDL (good cholesterol) to the LDL (not so good) cholesterol. At the same time, it inhibits platelet dysfunction (platelets are components of blood that promote clotting). In addition to all this, Reishi is a liver protective against damaging agents, and it seems to have a calming and strengthening effect on the nervous system, as it is mildly adaptogenic and antioxidant by protecting the body against free radicals. That's an herbal ally, my friends!

Herbs to Avoid in Pregnancy

Barberry (which I suggested using as a substitute for Goldenseal)

Black Cohosh (except for the last month of pregnancy) and its substitute Baneberry (see page 50)

Cayenne (use sparingly)

Comfrey

Ginger (use very sparingly)

Goldenseal

Mugwort

Oregon Grape (which I suggested using as a substitute for Goldenseal)

Yarrow

Parts of Plants Employed as Herbal Medicines

James Green, Herbalist

Plant Part	Example
Barks (Cortices)	Willow, Crampbark
Bulbs (Bulbi)	Garlic, Onion
Cellular	
Hairs	Cotton
Piths (Loose spongy tissue)	Sassafras pith
Spores (Primitive reproductive bodies)	*Lycopodium*
Glands	Lupulin (from the strobiles of the Hop)
Excrescences (An abnormal outgrowth)	Nutgall (highest source of tannic acid)
Corms (Cormi; a short, bulblike, underground, upright stem having a few scalelike leaves)	Trillium
Flowers (Flores)	Calendula, Chamomile, Hawthorn, Elder, Clove buds, Gumweed
Fruits (Fructi)	Cayenne, Vitex, Elder berry, Hawthorn berry, Saw Palmetto, Fennel
Fruiting bodies of fungi	Reishi, Maitake, Turkey Tail
Herbs (Herba)	St. John's Wort, Yarrow, Scullcap, Nettle, Peppermint, Mugwort
Juices (Succus; the fluid portion of a plant)	Cleavers, Plantain, Wheatgrass
Leaf and **leaflets** (Folia et Foliola)	Comfrey, Mullein, Ginkgo, Uva Ursi, Plantain
Lichen (Thallus; a composite organism consisting of a fungus living symbiotically with an algae)	Usnea
Rhizomes (Rhizomata; an underground rootlike stem)	Ginger, Wild Yam, Goldenseal, Black Cohosh, Valerian
Roots (Radices)	Echinacea, Burdock, Yellow Dock, Comfrey, Dandelion, Marshmallow, Siberian Ginseng
Seeds (Semina)	Burdock, Echinazea, Psyllium, Chia, Flax (Linseed), Nettle
Thallus (A plant body showing no differentiation into distinct members, as stem, leaves, roots, etc.)	Kelp, Dulse
Tubers (Tubera; a short, fleshy, usually underground stem or shoot)	Aconite, Devil's Claw, Western Peony
Woods (Ligna)	Quassia, Sandalwood

—From *The Herbal Medicine-Maker's Handbook*

Continued ➡

Suggested Methods of Extraction

James Green, Herbalist

	Bolus/Suppository	Decoction	Fomentation	Infusion	Lotion	Oil	Poultice	Salve	Syrup	Tincture
Blackberry		•							•	•
Black Cohosh		•							•	
Burdock (root and/or seed)		•	•				•		•	•
Calendula	•		•	•	•	•	•	•		•
Cayenne				•		•		•		•
Chamomile				•					•	•
Cleavers				•						•
Comfrey	•	•	•	•	•	•	•	•	•	•
Crampbark		•								•
Dandelion		•		•					•	•
Echinacea	•	•					•			•
Elder				•		•			•	•
Fennel				•					•	•
Ginger		•		•					•	•
Ginkgo				•						•
Goldenseal				•		•		•		•
Gumweed				•						•
Hawthorn		•		•					•	•
Marshmallow				•		•		•	•	•
Mugwort				•						•
Mullein				•		•			•	•
Nettle				•		•			•	•
Oat				•			•			•
Peppermint				•					•	•
Plantain				•		•	•	•	•	•
Reishi		•								•
Saw Palmetto		•								•
Siberian Ginseng		•								•
St. John's Wort				•		•		•	•	•
Scullcap				•						•
Uva Ursi				•						•
Valerian				•					•	•
Vitex				•						•
Willow				•						•
Yarrow			•	•			•	•		•
Yellow Dock		•					•		•	•

—From *The Herbal Medicine-Maker's Handbook*

Continued ➜

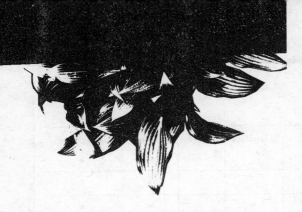

MATERIA MEDICA: HERBS AND THEIR APPLICATIONS

Debra St. Claire

A condensed, concise list of useful herbs and their therapeutic application. The...nature of this book makes it impossible to discuss everything the following herbs can be used for. The purpose is to get you started and to whet your appetite for more.

[P/C] indicates that the herb should he used with professional supervision and caution during pregnancy.

Alfalfa (Medicago sativa)

Nutritive herb with high mineral and vitamin content including Vitamin K and iron; estrogen precursor for menopause; mild diuretic.

Aloe (Aloe vera) [P/C]

Applied fresh as a burn and wound remedy, astringent. Fresh peeled leaf gel inserted as a rectal suppository for hemorrhoids. For chronic constipation with atonic bowel.

Angelica Root (Angelica spp.) [P/C]

Antispasmodic, for strong menstrual cramps with scanty flow, intestinal colic and poor digestion; stimulating expectorant for coughs.

Anise Seed (Pimpinella anisum)

Eases indigestion, flatulence and colic. Antispasmodic and expectorant.

Arnica Flower (Arnica cordifolia) [External Use Only]

Topical use for bruises, sprains, strains and other athletic injuries, including swelling. Use on unbroken skin.

Balm of Gilead (Populus balsamifera)

Soothes, disinfects and astringes mucous membranes. Specific for laryngitis, coughs and sore throat.

Barberry Root (Berberis fendleri) [P/C]

Digestive and appetite stimulant; stimulates bile flow and liver function; refrigerant; reduces fevers; antiseptic. Anticonvulsant.

Bayberry Bark (Myrica cerifera)

Astringent, used for bleeding gums and sore throat, diarrhea, gastrointestinal inflammation, postpartum hemorrhage; vasodilator of skin and mucus membranes.

Beth Root (Trillium erectum) [P/C]

Uterine tonic containing natural precursor of female sex hormones. Astringent, used for excess menstrual flow, postpartum hemorrhage.

Bilberry (Vaccinum myrtillus)

Astringent, antiseptic, absorptive, antiemetic. Used for intestinal dyspepsia and to halt diarrhea. Helps heal irritated intestina mucosa resulting from chronic constipation. Large quantities of freshly ripened berries, eaten raw, are laxative. Used as anti-inflammatory mouthwash. Used to enhance vision when taken for long periods of time.

Bistort (Polygonum bistorta)

Astringent; anti-inflammatory; used for diarrhea, dysentery mouth inflammations, laryngitis, pharyngitis.

Black Cohosh Root (Cimicifuga racemosa) [P/C]

Antispasmodic used for menstrual cramping, coughs, muscle spasms; emmenagogue; relieves hot flashes in menopausal women; mild sedative.

Black Walnut Hulls (Juglans nigra)

Antifungal (for Candida, athlete's foot, ringworm, etc,); astringent, used for skin eruptions; vermifuge in larger doses. Helps break down cystic tissue.

Bladderwrack (Fucus vesiculous)

Thyroid balancer, specific in treating obesity associated with underactive thyroid. Antirheumatic. Alleviates diarrhea and hemorrhage.

Blessed Thistle (Cnicus benedictus)

Increases lactation; emmenagogue; carminative, for indigestion and chronic headaches; astringent, for diarrhea and hemorrhage.

Bloodroot (Sanguinaria canadensis)

Expectorant. For chronic bronchitis, croup, laryngitis. Gargle for mouth sores and plaque buildup. Topical for eczema.

Blue Cohosh (Caulophyllum thalictroides) [P/C]

Uterine tonic, emmenagogue; diuretic; Antispasmodic; diaphoretic; mild expectorant. Helps prevent threatened miscarriage. *For use in last trimester only.*

Blue Flag Root (Iris versicolor)

Liver purgative; blood purifier; cathartic; sialagogue; diuretic. For constipation and biliousness, eruptive skin conditions. *Low doses only.*

Blue Vervain (Verbena spp.)

Soothes cranky children, sedative, antidepressant, diaphoretic, febrifuge, antispasmodic, mild analgesic.

Boneset (Eupatorium perfoliatum)

For flu symptoms, aches and pains; clears mucus congestion; reduces fevers; muscular rheumatism.

Borage Leaf (Borago officinalis)

Restorative for adrenal cortex, especially after cortisone or steroid treatment. Diaphoretic; expectorant; anti-inflammatory; antidepressant; galactagogue.

Buckthorn Bark (Rhamnus frangula)

Moderately strong laxative, very useful in chronic constipation. Must be dried before use to avoid intestinal cramping and nausea.

Burdock Root (Arctium lappa)

Blood cleanser, antimicrobial. Used for skin eruptions, dry/scaly skin conditions; digestive stimulant. Lowers blood sugar. Cancer preventative.

Burdock Seed (Arctium lappa)

Diuretic, kidney tonic, demulcent. Specific for chronic skin disease.

Butterbur (Petasites hybridus)

Muscle relaxant, used for intestinal colic, asthma, painful menses; mild febrifuge.

Butternut Bark (Juglans cinerea)

Mild laxative; hepatic decongestant; vermifuge. Used for dysentery.

Calendula Flower (Calendula officinalis)

Anti-inflammatory; astringent; styptic; antifungal; emmenagogue; cholagogue; topically for wounds, ulcers, burns, abscesses.

Cascara Sagrada Bark (Rhamnus purshiana) [P/C]

Laxative, mild liver stimulant, bitter tonic.

Catnip Herb (Nepeta cataria)

Carminative, diaphoretic, antispasmodic, mild febrifuge. For indigestion, flatulence and colic; mild astringent, specific for childhood fevers and diarrhea.

Cayenne Fruit (Capsicum frutescens)

Equalizes circulation, for cold hands and feet; strengthens heart; stimulant; carminative; styptic. Antiseptic, used as gargle for persistent cough.

Chamomile Flower (Matricaria recutita)

Sedative, carminative, antispasmodic, anodyne. Children's herb, especially for fever and restlessness. Mouthwash for gingivitis.

Chaparral Leaf (Larrea tridentata)

Blood cleanser, antioxidant; antibiotic; anti-viral; antiseptic; specific for infections, sluggish liver, skin problems, arthritis, tumors.

Chaparro (Castela emoryi)

Active inhibitor of intestinal protozoa. Used to prevent and alleviate amoebic dysentery and giardia.

Chaste Berry (Vitex agnus castus)

Reproductive tonic, stimulates and normalizes pituitary function. For menstrual cramps, PMS, menopause, post–birth control pill rebalancing.

Chickweed Herb (Stellaria media)

Nutritive; restorative; demulcent; diuretic; regulates thyroid; high in saponins (increases cell membrane permeability) and lecithin (emulsifies and mobilizes fat).

Cleavers (Galium spp.)

Lymphatic tonic; alterative; diuretic. For swollen glands, cystitis, ulcers and tumors, skin disorders, painful urination.

Coltsfoot (Tussilago farfara)

Soothing expectorant, demulcent, antispasmodic, astringent, anti-inflammatory. For irritating coughs, bronchitis, asthma, laryngitis, throat catarrh; externally for sores and ulcers.

Comfrey Root/Leaf (Symphytum officinalis)

Speeds healing of sprains, strains, fractures and surface wounds. Is not currently recommended for internal use.

Coriander Seed (Coriandrum sativum)

Carminative, eases intestinal griping and diarrhea (especially in children). Appetite stimulant, increases secretion of gastric juices.

Corn Silk (Zea mays)

Soothing diuretic, for renal and urinary irritation; used for bed-wetting, cystitis, urethritis, prostatitis.

Cotton Root (Gossypium herbaceum)

Works in conjunction with oxytocin to increase contractibility of uterus, seminal vesicles, and mammary tissue. Aids ability to ejaculate. Helps stimulate postpartum contractions. Useful to aid withdrawal from birth control pills.

Couchgrass Root (Agropyron repens)

Demulcent; antimicrobial; antilithic; for cystitis, urethritis, prostatitis, kidney stones and gravel.

Cow Parsnip Root/Seed (Heracleum lanatum)

Anti-nauseant; stimulant; hypotensive; emmenagogue; antispasmodic; carminative. Analgesic for sore teeth and gums.

Continued ➔

Cramp Bark (Viburnum opulus)

Relaxes muscle tension and spasms, ovarian and uterine cramps. Used to prevent threatened miscarriage.

Cranberry (Vaccinium oxycoccus)

Diuretic and urinary antiseptic; for kidney and bladder infections.

Damiana (Turnera diffusa)

Diuretic, relieves irritation of urinary mucus membranes; genitourinary stimulant effect leading to its use as an aphrodisiac; improves digestion; laxative; tonic; relieves bronchial irritation and coughs.

Dandelion Root/Leaf (Taraxacum officinale)

Blood cleanser; powerful and safe diuretic, high in potassium; cholagogue; for inflammation and congestion of the liver and gall bladder, congestive jaundice. Mild laxative, aids weight loss, lowers cholesterol and blood pressure.

Desert Willow Leaf/Bark (Chilopsis linearis)

Antifungal. Used to treat Candida albicans, specifically the symptoms of Candida suprainfections which are abundant after antibiotic therapy, e.g., indigestion, loose stools, hemorrhoids, rectal aching, foul burping, etc.

Devil's Club (Oplopanax horridus)

Pancreatic tonic, blood sugar regulator, increases endurance.

Dill Seed (Anethum graveolens)

For flatulence and colic, especially in children; stimulates lactation.

Dong Quai Root (Angelica sinensis)

Female hormone regulator, alleviates cramping and premenstrual distress.

Echinacea Root (Echinacea angustifolia)

Powerful immune stimulant; antiseptic; antimicrobial; antiviral; used for sore throats, flu, colds, infections, allergies.

Elder Flowers (Sambucus canadensis)

Diaphoretic, anticatarrhal, diuretic, expectorant. For upper respiratory infections, colds, flu, hayfever, sinusitis, fevers.

Elecampane Root (Inula helenium)

Expectorant diaphoretic; antibacterial; antitussive; stomachic; for irritating bronchial coughs, bronchitis, emphysema, asthma and bronchitic asthma.

Ephedra (Ephedra spp.) *Mormon Tea*

Vasodilator; antispasmodic; hypertensive; circulatory stimulant; used for asthma, bronchitis, whooping cough, hayfever; opens air passages.

Eyebright Herb (Euphrasia officinalis)

Anticatarrhal, astringent, anti-inflammatory. Internally for sinusitis, nasal congestion, eye inflammations. Used as an external infusion/wash for sore or inflamed eyes.

False Unicorn (Helonias) (Chamaelirium luteum)

Uterine tonic, used for delayed menses, leucorrhea, ovarian pain. Contains estrogen precursors. Eases vomiting in pregnancy (small doses). Helps prevent threatened miscarriage.

Fennel Seed (Foeniculum vulgare)

Aids digestion; relieves flatulence and colic; expels mucus; increases lactation; aids weight loss; flavoring agent; increases digestibility of other herbs.

Fenugreek Seed (Trigonella-foenum-graecum)

Soothes irritated mucus membranes, promotes lactation, mild febrifuge.

Feverfew Leaf/Flower (Tanacetum parthenium)

Anti-inflammatory, used for rheumatoid arthritis, migraine headache relief (long-term basis), asthma and bronchitis. Mild febrifuge, especially good for children. Used topically to relieve swelling from insect bites.

Figwort Herb (Scrophularia spp.)

Used internally and topically for eczema, scrofula, cradle cap, psoriasis, itching and irritated skin. *Avoid in cases of tachycardia.*

Flax Seed (Linum usitatissimum)

Excellent bulking agent that cleanses and lubricates digestive tract.

Fringetree Bark (Chionanthus virginicus)

Hepatic; cholagogue; alterative; diuretic. Used for liver problems, gall bladder inflammation and stones. Gentle, effective laxative.

Garlic Bulb/Seed (Alliumsativum)

Antibiotic; antimicrobial; antiseptic; antiviral; anthelmintic. For colds, flu, chronic bronchitis, infections, also to reduce blood pressure and cholesterol.

Gentian Root (Gentiana lutea)

Bitter, promotes production of gastric juices and bile. For sluggish digestion, dyspepsia, and flatulence. Restores appetite lost during morning sickness.

Ginger Root (Zinziber officinalis)

Used for nausea, motion sickness; diaphoretic, helps break fevers; stimulant; carminative; aids in utilization of other herbs.

Ginkgo Leaf (Ginkgo biloba)

Stimulates cerebral circulation and oxygenation, mental clarity and alertness, improves memory. Used to prevent strokes.

Ginseng Root (Panax quinquefolium)

Adaptogenic, decreases the effect of stress. Increases capillary circulation in brain; reproductive tonic; antidepressant; equalizes blood pressure. Used for general exhaustion and weakness; aids digestion. Promotes longevity.

Goldenrod (Solidago virgauria)

Anti-inflammatory; urinary antiseptic; diuretic; diaphoretic; expectorant, astringent. For cystitis, urethritis, upper respiratory catarrh, diarrhea and internal hemorrhage. Gargle for laryngitis and pharyngitis. Diaphoretic, sedative, carminative. Reduces congestion.

Goldenseal Root (Hydrastis canadensis)

Antiseptic, used for internally and topically for infection, sore throat, gastritis ulceration and colitis. Root infusion used as douche for vaginitis. Should not be taken daily for more than a week or so as overuse can stress the liver.

Gotu Kola Leaf (Centella asiatica)

Used to increase mental stamina, alleviate depression and anxiety, improve memory and promote longevity. Increases energy and endurance.

Gravel Root (Eupatorium purpureum)

For kidney and urinary infections and stones, prostatitis, pelvic inflammatory disease; painful menses; rheumatism and gout.

Grindelia Buds/Flowers (Grindelia spp.)

Expectorant; antispasmodic; for bronchitis, sinus congestion, bladder infections; topically for poison oak and ivy, insect bites.

Hawthorne Berry (Crataegus oxycantha)

Heart and circulatory tonic. Used for heart weakness, palpitations, high blood pressure, arteriosclerosis, angina pectoris.

Hops Strobile (Humulus lupulus)

Sedative; hypnotic. Used for anxiety, tension, insomnia. Reduces nervous irritability, promotes restful sleep. Astringent, used for mucous colitis.

Horehound Herb (Marrabium vulgare)

Excellent expectorant for respiratory congestion.

Horseradish Root (Armoracia rusticana)

Stimulant; for flu, fevers, sinus and respiratory congestion. Sialagogue, carminative, mild laxative, diuretic.

Horsetail Herb (Equisetum arvense)

High in silica and calcium, used to strengthen hair, skin and nails.

Hydrangea Root (Hydrangea aborescens)

Diuretic, cathartic, tonic. Helps evacuate gravelly deposits from the bladder and alleviates the pain of their passage. Styptic. Helps correct bedwetting in children.

Hyssop Leaf (Hyssopus officinalis)

Antispasmodic; nervine; expectorant; diaphoretic, sedative, carminative. For chronic congestion.

Inmortal Root (Asclephis asperula)

Bronchial dilator; stimulates lymph drainage from the lungs. Used for asthma, pleurisy, bronchitis, lung infections. Laxative, diaphoretic, mild cardiac tonic.

Jamaican Dogwood (Piscidia erythrina)

Sedative; anodyne; smooth muscle antispasmodic. For insomnia, neuralgia, menstrual cramping. Relieves coughing, reduces fevers.

Jewelweed (Impatiens aurens) External Use

Used topically to reduce the itching and inflammation of skin irritating plants such as poison ivy.

Juniper Berry (Juniperus spp.)

Urinary tract antiseptic, used for cystitis, urethritis. Should not be used in kidney inflammation or chronic kidney weakness.

Kelp (Nereocystis luetkeana)

Radiation protective properties. Reduces amount of strontium-90 absorbed by bone tissue by 50–85%.

Lemon Balm (Melissa officinalis)

Very useful in reducing fevers during colds and flu as it induces mild perspiration. Aids digestion, reduces flatulence. Wonderful herb for children. Antiviral, used externally on herpes lesions.

Licorice Root (Glycyrrhiza glabra)

Specific for adrenal gland insufficiency; demulcent; expectorant for coughs and respiratory congestion; anti-inflammatory, laxative.

Lobelia Herb (Lobelia inflata)

Respiratory stimulant; antiasthmatic; antiemetic (small dose), emetic (large dose); used for bronchitis and bronchitic asthma, whooping cough, muscular cramping and pain.

Lomatium Root (Lomatimn dissectum)

Antiviral; immune stimulant, for colds, flu, viral sore throats, respiratory infections and congestion.

Marshmallow Root (Althaea officinalis)

Soothing demulcent, used for gastrointestinal inflammation; expectorant in respiratory congestion and bronchitis. Used externally as a poultice for mastitis and skin ulcers.

Meadowsweet (Filipendula ulmaria)

Digestive herb, antacid. Used for heartburn, nausea, gastritis, hyperacidity, peptic ulcers. Mild

Continued ➡

astringent, used for diarrhea in children. Diaphoretic, anti-inflammatory, reduces fever and pain.

Milk Thistle Seed (Silybum marianum)
Powerful liver detoxifier, antidote for Amanita mushroom poisoning. Increases secretion and flow of bile. Galactagogue.

Motherwort Herb (Leonurus cardiaca) [P/C]
Sedative, useful in transition labor. Eases fake labor pains. Antispasmodic; emmenagogue; cardiac tonic; reduces tension, anxiety.

Mullen Leaf (Verbascum thapsus)
Expectorant; demulcent; reduces respiratory inflammation. Flowers steeped in olive oil used as an earache remedy.

Myrrh Gum (Commiphora myrrha)
Antiseptic; antimicrobial; astringent. Used for mouth ulcers, sore throat, gingivitis, pyorrhea, sinusitis and pharyngitis. Used externally on cuts and abrasions, forms natural bandage.

Nettle (Urtica dioica)
Nutritive herb, specific for childhood and nervous eczema. Rich in iron, silica, and potassium. For anemia. Diuretic; galactagogue; antihistamine; for hayfever and allergies.

Oatseed (Avena sariva)
Antispasmodic; soothes and supports nervous system; for depression, insomnia, hysteria, irritation, and anxiety. Helpful in breaking addictions.

Ocotillo (Fouquieria splendens)
Stimulates lymphatic drainage; improves dietary fat absorption into the lymph system. Helps drain pelvic congestion, making it useful in the treatment of hemorrhoids and varicose veins.

Onion (Allium cepa)
Diuretic, expectorant, carminative, antiseptic, antispasmodic, anthelmintic. Helps alleviate putrefaction in the gastrointestinal tract. Used to alleviate cold and flu symptoms.

Oregon Grape Root (Mahonia repens)
Liver and blood cleanser; cholagogue; antibacterial. Stimulates digestion and absorption. For sluggish liver, hangovers, acne, eczema.

Osha' Root (Ligusticum porterii)
Strong antiviral, used for herpes, sore throat, colds, flu; bronchial expectorant; immune stimulating properties.

Parsley Leaf/Root (Petroselenum crispum) [P/C]
Diuretic, carminative, antispasmodic, emmenagogue, expectorant.

Passionflower (Passiflora incarnata)
Sedative, hypnotic, antispasmodic, anodyne. Relieves nerve pain, promotes restful sleep. Has been used for seizures and hysteria.

Pau d' Arco (Tabebuia impetiginosa)
Blood cleanser; antifungal; for Candida, lymph congestion, tumors. Improves gastrointestinal utilization of nutrients.

Peppermint Leaf (Mentha piperita)
For upset stomach, heartburn, nausea, colds, flu, congestion, nervous headache, and agitation, also diarrhea and flatulence. Adds flavor to other herbs.

Pipsissewa (Chimaphila umbellata)
Diuretic, used for chronic kidney weakness, nephritis, bladder stones and rheumatism.

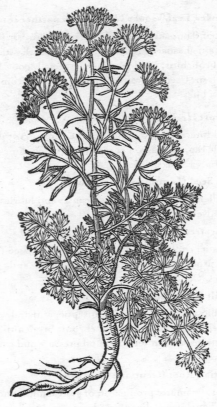

Parsley

Plantain Leaf (Plantago spp.)
Expectorant; astringent; for coughs, bronchitis, diarrhea, hemorrhoids, bleeding cystitis, chronic catarrhal problems, external wounds and sores, insect bites, hoarseness, gastritis.

Pleurisy Root (Asclepias tuberosa)
Respiratory infections, bronchitis, pleurisy, pneumonia, flu. Reduces inflammation and encourages expectoration.

Poke Root (Phytolacca americana)
Emetic, purgative. Cleanses lymph, for tonsillitis, mumps, laryngitis, swollen glands mastitis, rheumatism. Small doses only. *Physician or Herbalist supervision advised.*

Potentilla (Potentilla spp.)
Astringent mouthwash and gargle for sore throats or gum inflammation. Used for stomach ulcers, abrasions, sunburn, poison oak, fevers, diarrhea.

Propolis
Antiseptic, antibacterial. Waxy nature makes it useful for coating and isolating areas of throat inflammation to prevent spread of infection.

Psyllium Seed (Plantago ovata)
Commonly called the intestinal janitor, softly "scrubs" the sides of the intestinal wall for maximum cleansing effect.

Quassia (Pycrasma excelsa)
Bitter tonic and stomachic; antispasmodic; anthelmintic. Used to rid the body of parasites and improve digestion.

Red Clover Flowers (Trifolium pratense)
Blood cleanser, nutritive; for childhood eczema, psoriasis, coughs, bronchitis, ulcers, inflammation and infection. Galactagogue. Principal ingredient of the Hoxey cancer formula.

Red Raspberry Leaf (Rhubus idaeus)
Pregnancy herb; nutritive; relieves nausea. Uterine tonic, eases painful menses, checks hemorrhage. Remedy for childhood diarrhea, gargle for sore throat, bleeding gums.

Red Root (Ceanotlius americanus)
Stimulates lymphatic and interstitial fluid circulation, aids in the transport of nutrients and the elimination of waste products. Used for tonsillitis, sore throat, enlarged lymph nodes and spleen, fibrous cysts. Expectorant, hemostatic.

Reishi Mushroom (Ganoderma lucidum)
Adaptogenic, used to alleviate the effects of stress. Strengthens heart, protects liver, soothes nerves. Normalizes blood pressure. Inhibits the release of histamine, thus relieving the allergic inflammatory response. Supports adrenal function. Stimulates the immune system. Slows the aging process. Anti-carcinogenic.

Rhubarb Root (Rheum officinale) [P/C]
Stomachic, astringent, small doses relieve diarrhea, large doses laxative.

Rosehips (Rosa canina)
Nutrient, mild diuretic and laxative, mild astringent. Excellent source of vitamin C. Used for colds, flu, general debility and exhaustion, constipation.

Rosemary Leaf (Rosmarinus officinalis)
Circulatory and nerve stimulant, used for tension headache associated with dyspepsia, also depression. Antibacterial; antifungal. Externally for muscular pain, neuralgia and sciatica.

Sarsaparilla Root (Smilax ornata)
Antirheumatic, diuretic, diaphoretic, soothes mucous membranes, possible progesterone precursor.

Saw Palmetto (Serenoa repens)
Tones and strengthens male reproductive system, used for prostate enlargement and infection, enhances endurance. Femal fertility aid, galactagogue.

Shepherd's Purse (Capsella Bursa-pastoris)
Hemostatic; astringent; helps stop passive uterine or gastrointestinal bleeding. Diuretic; breaks up urinary stones.

Shiitake Mushroom (Lentinus edodes)
Adaptogenic. Increases the production of interferon, thus reducing the possibility of tumor development. Antiviral. Helps the body excrete excess cholesterol.

Siberian Ginseng (Eleutherococcus senticosis)
Stimulates the adrenal-pituitary axis, increasing resistance to stress. Improves cerebral circulation, increasing mental alertness.

Skullcap Herb (Scutellaria lateriflora)
Nervine; sedative; antispasmodic; used for nervous tension, hysteria, epileptic seizures, withdrawal from substance abuse and the irritability of PMS.

Slippery Elm (Ulmus rubra)
Nutrient, reduces inflammation, soothes mucus membranes, specific for ulcers.

Spikenard (Aralia racemosa)
Stimulant, diaphoretic, expectorant, alterative. Used for coughs and asthma.

Spilanthes (Spilanthes oleracea)
Anti-fungal, anti-bacterial; used for Candidiasis. Anodyne, anesthetic, relieves toothache.

Squawvine/Partridge Berry (Mitchella repens)
Uterine tonic, promotes easy labor, eases menstrual cramping, mild nervine, improves digestion.

Stillingia Root (Stillingia sylvarica)
Stimulating expectorant for bronchitis; blood

Continued ➡

cleanser, used for skin disorders. Small dose laxative and diuretic, large dose cathartic and emetic.

St. John's Wort (Hypericum perforatum)

Extract and oil used externally for bruises, strains, sprains, contusions, wounds. Extract used internally as an immune system stimulant; for retroviral infections; expectorant; antibacterial, speeds wound and burn healing; antidepressant; used to treat bedwetting and children's nightmares.

Stone Root (Collinsonia canadensis)

Strengthens structure and function of veins, used for varicose veins, hemorrhoids, anal fissures, and rectal spasms. Strong diuretic, helps prevent and dissolve urinary stones and gravel.

Thyme Leaf (Thymus vulgaris)

Anti-bacterial; anti-fungal; anti-microbial; antispasmodic; expectorant; astringent, anthelmintic; diaphoretic. Used as throat gargle for laryngitis, tonsillitis, sore throats, coughs. Reduces fevers, expels worms.

Toadflax (Linaria vulgaris)

Liver cleanser; stimulates bile production; used in hepatitis, jaundice, sluggish liver. Potent—best used in small amounts in formulas.

Tronadora (Tecoma stans)

Antiviral, particularly helpful for herpes simplex, use internally.

Usnea Lichen (Usnea spp.)

Strong antibiotic; antiviral; antifungal; for internal infections, strep, staph, trichomonas, etc., infected wounds. Also used for pneumonia, TB, and lupus.

Uva Ursi (Arcostaphylos uva-ursi)

Urinary antiseptic; antimicrobial; for cystitis, urethritis, prostatitis, nephritis. Antilithic, used for kidney and bladder stones.

Valerian Root (Valeriana officinalis)

Powerful nervine, used for tension, anxiety, insomnia, emotional stress, intestinal colic, menstrual cramps, migraine headache and rheumatic pain.

Wahoo (Euonymus atropurpureus)

Primary liver decongestant, bile stimulant; used for jaundice, gall-bladder pain and inflammation, constipation.

Watercress (Nasturtium officinalis)

Expectorant, diuretic, appetite stimulant, aids digestion.

White Oak Bark (Quercus alba)

Astringent, used for diarrhea, hemorrhage, leucorrhea, bleeding or ulcerated gums. Topically for sores, hemorrhoids. Strengthens capillaries.

White Willow Bark (Salix alba)

Astringent, contains salicin, reduces inflammation. Used for headache, neuralgia, fevers, hayfever, arthritis and rheumatism.

Wild Cherry Bark (Prunus serotina)

Expectorant, antitussive, astringent, sedative, digestive bitter. Used for irritating coughs, bronchitis and asthma.

Wild Geranium (Geranium maculatum)

Astringent, used for diarrhea and hemorrhage, bleeding gums, hemorrhoids.

Wild Ginger (Asarum canadense)

Diaphoretic, expectorant, carminative. Relieves flatulence, colic and upset stomach. Expels mucus. Helps reduce fevers by causing mild sweating, thus dropping the body temperature. Not as hot as the cultivated Ginger (Zinziber officinalis).

Wild Indigo Root (Baptisia tinctoria)

Emetic; purgative; lymph cleanser; for focused local infection such as sore throat, laryngitis, tonsillitis, pharyngitis, gingivitis, mouth ulcers and pyorrhea. Also inflamed lymph nodes. Best used in small amounts in a formula. *Caution: Large doses may be toxic.*

Wild Lettuce Herb (Lactuca spp.)

Sedative, calms restlessness and anxiety, subdues irritating coughs.

Wild Yam Root (Dioscorea spp.)

Antispasmodic; carminative; anti-inflammatory; hepatic; cholagogue; diaphoretic. Used for intestinal colic, diverticulitis, painful menses, ovarian and uterine pain, rheumatoid arthritis, flatulence.

Wormwood Leaf (Artemisia absinthium)

Brings down fevers; will inhibit roundworm and pinworm infestation when used consistently for a week or two. Stimulates sweating in dry fevers. Aids uterine circulation. *Use small amounts, preferably with herbalist or physician supervision.*

Yarrow Flowers (Achillea millefolium)

Diaphoretic, helps release toxic waste and reduce fevers. Lowers blood pressure; specific for thrombotic conditions associated with high blood pressure.

Yellow Dock Root (Rumex crispus)

Blood cleanser, used for anemia, hepatitis, chronic skin disorders. Mild laxative, aids fat digestion.

Yerba Mansa Root (Anemopsis californica)

Soothing to mucus membranes, used for diarrhea, dysentery, malarial fevers, gonorrhea, catarrh, digestive weakness.

Yerba Santa Leaf (Eriodycton spp.)

Expectorant; bronchial dilator; mild decongestant, for chest colds, asthma, hayfever, bronchitis.

Yucca Root (Yucca spp.)

Anti-inflammatory, used for arthritic pain, rheumatism, gout, asthma, urethral and prostate inflammation.

—From *Pocket Herbal Reference Guide*

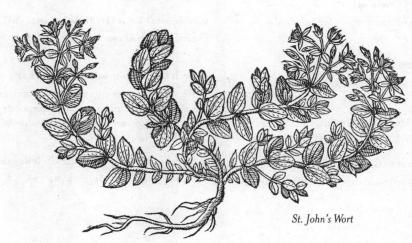

St. John's Wort

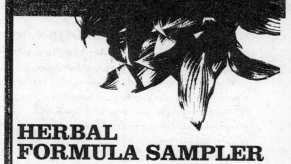

HERBAL FORMULA SAMPLER
Debra St. Claire

Again I must emphasize that the following information is for suggested use only and that no claims are made for its medicinal efficacy. The herbs listed may be used singly or combined into formulas. The therapeutic value of the herb as related to the specific condition is noted. A non-specific overview of the herb's therapeutic effect can be found in the Materia Medica section. Instructions and ideas for using these sample formulas are found here, in the Common Problems/Natural Remedies section and in the Natural Therapies section. The herbs in these formulas have been traditionally and historically used in the manner described in each listing.

NOTE: Except in the case of oils which should be used in smaller quantities, ingredients are listed in alphabetical order—not in the order of proportional quantity. For more information on creating herbal formulas, see my video/workbook series, *Herbal Preparation and Natural Therapies—Creating and Using a Home Herbal Medicine Chest.*

[P/C] indicates that some sources have listed this herb with a pregnancy caution. It should only be used after you have educated yourself about the possible side effects or if you are under the supervision of a herbalist or holistic practitioner.

Herbal Formulation Tips

- First, look up the condition you wish to alter. You can use all the herbs listed as one complete formula, or you can custom-create your own formula by selecting only the ones you want.

- Choose the ingredients for your custom formula according to the primary effect you wish to achieve. Then add smaller quantities of the circulatory stimulants (e.g., Ginger and Cayenne) or buffers (e.g., Licorice and Marshmallow root) to round out the formula. Generally, spicy herbs are stimulating and increase circulation. These would be added to help carry the medicinal benefits of the other herbs deeper into the body. Mucilaginous herbs (those which have a viscous texture when mixed with water) are soothing. You would use these to alleviate irritation in the body, as when treating inflammation.

- When mixing your own formulas, it is helpful to add a little vegetable glycerin to prevent the ingredients from separating and to sweeten it a bit.

- 99% of the herbs listed grow in North America. I have utilized the local plants for four reasons:

  1. Plants grown in other countries are generally fumigated before being allowed entry into the US.

  2. It is easier to assure that the medicinal plants in this country have been organically grown.

  3. The plants which grow in your own bioregion are most naturally effective in healing your body.

Continued ➡

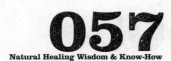

4. Local plants are more readily available.
- The very best medicine is made when you correctly grow, harvest, and prepare the plants yourself. For most people, however, this is not a possibility. Herbs can be purchased in natural food markets in the form of dried herbs, tinctures, dried plant extracts, or better yet, fresh plant extracts.

Formulas

Adrenal Formula

A supportive formula for overworked, under appreciated adrenals. Use during high-stress periods.

Borage Leaf (Borago officinalis)

Restorative for adrenal cortex, especially after cortisone or steroid treatment. Helps the body cope with intense and prolonged stress. Anti-inflammatory.

Cayenne Fruit (Capsicum frutescens)

Helps remedy the physiological effects of stress by equalizing circulation and strengthening the heart. Stimulant, increases assimilation and distribution of the other herbs throughout the system.

Ginseng Root (Panax quinquefolium)

Adaptogenic—decreases the effect of stress. Improves adrenal gland function and counteracts shrinkage of the adrenal gland due to continued stress or corticosteroid drugs. Increases capillary circulation in brain, thereby increasing mental alertness and improving quality of performance. Antidepressant. Equalizes blood pressure. Used for general exhaustion and weakness; aids digestion. Promotes longevity.

Gotu Kola Leaf (Centella asiatica)

Used to increase mental stamina, alleviate depression and anxiety, improve memory, and promote longevity. Increases energy and endurance.

Licorice Root (Glycyrrhiza glabra)

Specific for adrenal gland insufficiency. Anti-inflammatory, contains constituents that are similar to cortisone. Soothing demulcent, helps to meld and balance the rest of the formula.

Allergy Formula

This formula addresses the Type I common histamine reaction which is produced by the body when it is exposed to an allergen (a substance that provokes an allergic reaction in sensitive individuals). It is useful for early onset of nasal congestion, sneezing, drippy nose, and tearing eyes.

Ephedra (Ephedra spp.) *Mormon Tea*

Vasodilator, relieves congested sinuses; reduces spasms; stimulates circulation. Specific for asthma, bronchitis, whooping cough, hayfever. Not as intensely drying as the Chinese Ephedra.

Goldenrod (Solidago canadensis)

Helps alleviate upper respiratory congestion by reducing inflammation, producing sweating, and encouraging the elimination of excess mucus.

Nettle (Urtica dioica)

Nutritive herb with antihistamine properties, used for childhood and nervous eczema. Rich in iron, silica, and potassium. Specific remedy for hayfever and allergies.

Yerba Santa Leaf (Eriodictyon spp.)

Used for all forms of bronchial congestion. It stimulates the salivary and other digestive secretions, thus correcting the congestion resulting from inadequate digestion. Excellent remedy for both acute and chronic chest conditions, including asthma. Expectorant, stimulates the discharge of mucus. Opens air passages; mild decongestant.

Aloe Burn Spray Formula

Used for sunburn, windburn and common household burns. Can also be used as an antiseptic spray.

Aloe (Aloe vera) [P/C, internally]

Applied fresh or as a prepared juice to alleviate the pain and inflammation of burns and wounds; astringent. Known as "Nature's Band-Aid." Speeds healing.

Calendula Flower (Calendula officinalis)

Anti-inflammatory; astringent; styptic; used topically for wounds, ulcers, burns, abscesses.

Comfrey Root/Leaf (Symphytum officinalis) [external]

Demulcent, soothes irritation, promotes healing.

Lavender Oil

Antiseptic, soothing, healing.

Antifungal Formula

For internal or external fungal infections such as Candidiasis.

Angelica Root (Angelica spp.)

Antifungal.

Black Walnut Hulls (Juglans nigra)

Antifungal, (for Candida, athlete's foot, ringworm, etc.); astringent, used for skin eruptions.

Calendula Flower (Calendula officinalis)

Anti-inflammatory; astringent; antifungal.

Coltsfoot (Tussilago farfara)

Astringent, anti-inflammatory. Externally for sores, ulcers, and fungal infections.

Desert Willow Leaf/Bark (Chilopsis linearis)

Anti-fungal. Used to treat Candida albicans, specifically the symptoms of candida supra-infections which are abundant after antibiotic therapy, e.g., indigestion, loose stools, hemorrhoids, rectal aching, foul burping, etc.

Garlic Bulb/Seed (Allium sativum)

Antifungal; antibiotic; antimicrobial; antiseptic.

Goldenrod (Solidago virgauria)

Anti-inflammatory; antifungal.

Pau d'Arco (Tabebuia impetiginosa)

Blood cleanser; antifungal; used for Candida.

Rosemary Leaf (Rosmarinus officinalis)

Anti-bacterial; antifungal.

Spilanthes (Spilanthes oleracea)

Anti-fungal, antibacterial; used specifically for Candidiasis.

Usnea Lichen (Usnea spp.)

Strong antibiotic; antifungal; for internal infections, infected wounds.

Antifungal External Spray Formula

For external fungal infections such as athlete's foot, ringworm, and jock itch.

Black Walnut Hulls (Juglans nigra)

Antifungal, astringent, used for skin eruptions.

Calendula Flower (Calendula officinalis)

Anti-inflammatory; astringent; styptic; antifungal.

Garlic Bulb/Seed (Allium sativum)

Anti-fungal; antibiotic; anti-microbial; antiseptic; antiviral; anthelmintic.

Pau d'Arco (Tabebuia impetiginosa)

Blood cleanser; antifungal; used for candida.

Spilanthes (Spilanthes oleracea)

Anti-fungal; antibacterial; used for Candidiasis. Relieves pain.

Usnea Lichen (Usnea spp.)

Strong antibiotic; antiviral; antifungal.

Clary Sage Essential Oil (Salvia sclarea)

Antifungal.

Tea Tree Oil (Melaleuca alternifolia)

Antifungal; antiseptic; vulnerary; speeds healing.

Antiseptic Spray Formula

For prevention of infection in minor cuts and scrapes or as a spray for sprains and strains.

Calendula Flower (Calendula officinalis)

Anti-inflammatory; astringent; styptic; antifungal; topically for wounds, ulcers, burns, abcesses.

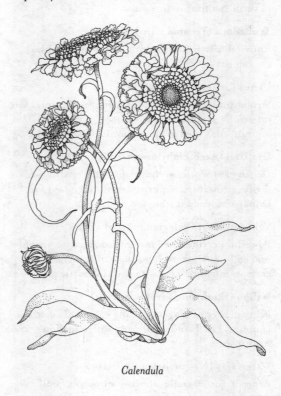

Calendula

Cayenne Fruit (Capsicum frutescens)

Antiseptic. Styptic. (Yes, it stings.)

Chaparrel Leaf (Larrea tridentate)

Antibiotic; antiviral; antiseptic; specific for infections.

Echinacea Root (Echinacea augustifolia)

Antiseptic; antimicrobial; antiviral; stimulates immune response.

Goldenseal Root (Hydrastis Canadensis)

Antiseptic, used topically for infection, sore throat, ulceration.

Myrrh Gum (Commiphore myrrha)

Used externally on cuts and abrasions, forms natural Band-Aid. Antiseptic, antimicrobial; astringent. Used for mouth ulcers, sore throat, gingivitis, pyorrhea.

Eucalyptus Oil (Eucalyptus citriodora)

Antiseptic, bactericide, disinfectant.

Continued ➡

Antiviral Formula

For herpes, shingles, flu, warts, and other viruses. Can be taken internally or applied externally.

Boneset (Eupatorium perfoliatum)

For flu symptoms, aches and pains; clears mucus congestion; reduces fevers and muscular rheumatism.

Chaparrel Leaf (Larrea tridentata)

Blood cleanser; antibiotic; anti-viral; antiseptic; specific for infections, sluggish liver, skin problems.

Echinacea Root (Echinacea angustifolia)

Immune stimulant; antiseptic; antimicrobial; antiviral; used for sore throats, flu, colds, infections, allergies.

Ginger Root (Asarum canadense)

Helps break fevers by causing the body to sweat; stimulant; aids in utilization of other herbs.

Lomatium Root (Lomatium directum)

Antiviral; immune stimulant; for colds, flu, viral sore throats, respiratory infections and congestion.

Osha' Root (Ligusticum porterii)

Strong antiviral, used for herpes, sore throat, colds, flu; bronchial expectorant; immune stimulating properties.

St. John's Wort (Hypericum perforatum)

Immune system stimulant; for retro-viral infections; expectorant; antibacterial.

Tronadora (Tecoma stans)

Antiviral, particularly helpful for herpes simplex.

Usnea Lichen (Usnea spp.)

Strong antibiotic; antiviral; for internal infections, strep, staph, trichomonas, etc., infected wounds. Also used for pneumonia, TB, and lupus.

Asthma Formula

Relaxing, decongestant formula.

Butterbur (Petasites hybridus)

Muscle relaxant, mild febrifuge.

Coltsfoot (Tussilago ferfara)

Soothing expectorant, demulcent, antispasmodic, astringent, anti-inflammatory. For irritating coughs, bronchitis, asthma, laryngitis, throat catarrh.

Elecampane Root (Inula helenium)

Expectorant; diaphoretic; antibacterial; antitussive; stomachic; for irritating bronchial coughs, bronchitis, emphysema, asthma and bronchitic asthma.

Ephedra (Ephedra spp.) *Mormon Tea*

Vasodilator; antispasmodic; hypertensive; circulatory stimulant; used for asthma, bronchitis, whooping cough, hayfever; opens air passages.

Inmortal Root (Asclepius asperula)

Bronchial dilator; stimulates lymph drainage from the lungs. Used for asthma, pleurisy, bronchitis, lung infections. Laxative, diaphoretic, mild cardiac tonic.

Lobelia Herb (Lobelia inflata)

Respiratory stimulant; anti-asthmatic; antiemetic (small dose), emetic (large dose). Used for bronchitis and bronchitic asthma, whooping cough, muscular cramping and pain.

Peppermint Leaf (Mentha piperita)

For upset stomach, heartburn, nausea, colds, flu,

congestion, nervous headache, and agitation. Adds flavor to other herbs.

Wild Cherry Bark (Prunus serotina)

Expectorant, antitussive, astringent, sedative, digestive bitter. Used for irritating coughs, bronchitis and asthma.

Yerba Santa Leaf (Eriodycton spp.)

Expectorant; bronchial dilator; mild decongestant, for chest colds, asthma, hayfever, bronchitis.

Bronchial Formula

For bronchitis, deep chest inflammation and congestion.

Coltsfoot (Tussilago farfara)

Soothing expectorant, demulcent, antispasmodic, astringent, anti-inflammatory. Helps alleviate irritating coughs, bronchitis, laryngitis throat catarrh.

Elecampane Root (Inula helenium)

Expectorant; diaphoretic; antibacterial; antitussive; for irritating bronchial coughs, bronchitis, and bronchitic asthma.

Licorice Root (Glycyrrhiza glabra)

Demulcent; expectorant for coughs and respiratory congestion; anti-inflammatory; laxative.

Peppermint Leaf (Mentha piperita)

Decongestant. Mild diaphoretic. Digestive herb.

Pleurisy Root (Asclepias tuberosa)

Reduces inflammation and encourages expectoration.

Stillingia Root (Stillingia sylvatica)

Stimulating expectorant. Small dose laxative and diuretic; large dose cathartic and emetic.

Wild Cherry Bark (Prunus serotina)

Expectorant, anti-tussive, astringent, sedative, digestive bitter. Used for irritating coughs, bronchitis and asthma.

Yerba Santa Leaf (Eriodictyon spp.)

Expectorant; bronchial dilator; mild decongestant, for chest colds, asthma, hayfever, bronchitis.

Bug Spray Formula

To discourage insects from trespassing on your body. The following essential oils are all known for their insect repellant properties.

Citronella (Ceylonese or Javanese)

Eucalyptus (Eucalyptus citriodora)

Lavender (Lavendula officinalis)

Pennyroyal (Mentha pelugium)

Children's Calming Glycerite Formula

Glycerites are made by extracting the herbs in vegetable glycerin and distilled water. They do not contain the full range of medicinal constituents, but still have mild therapeutic effects. Makes bitter-tasting extracts more palatable for children when used as a base. This formula is particularly useful to soothe children on airplanes and in other stressful situations. It is also very helpful to alleviate crankiness during the teething period.

Alfalfa (Medicago sativa)

Nutritive herb with high mineral and vitamin content, including vitamin K and iron.

Catnip Herb (Nepeta cataria)

For indigestion, flatulence, and colic; mild astringent, specific for childhood fevers and diarrhea.

Chamomile Flower (Matricaria recutita)

Reduces fever and calms restlessness. Mild pain reliever, helps relieve colic, dispels gas.

Fennel Seed (Foeniculum vulgare)

Aids digestion; relieves flatulence and colic; expels mucous; flavoring agent; increases digestibility of other herbs.

Lemon Balm (Melissa officinalis)

Very useful in reducing fevers during colds and flu since it induces mild perspiration. Aids digestion, reduces flatulence.

Licorice Root (Glycyrrhiza glabra)

Soothing demulcent; mild laxative.

Red Raspberry Leaf (Rhubus idaeus)

Nutritive, relieves nausea. Remedy for childhood diarrhea.

Rosehips (Rosa canina)

Nutritive, mild diuretic and laxative, mild astringent. Good source of vitamin C. Used for colds, flu, general debility and exhaustion, constipation.

Clear Eyes Formula

An internal formula for eye strain and infections. Do not place in eyes.

Bilberry (Vaccinum myrtillus)

Astringent, antiseptic, absorptive. Used to enhance vision when taken for long periods of time.

Echinacea Root (Echinacea angustifolia)

Powerful immune stimulant; antiseptic; antimicrobial; antiviral. Helps the body combat infections.

Eyebright Herb (Euphrasia officinalis)

Anticatarrhal, astringent, anti-inflammatory. Internally for sinusitis, nasal congestion, eye inflammations.

Goldenseal Root (Hydrastis canadensis)

Antiseptic, used for infections. Should not be taken daily for more than a week or so as overuse can stress the liver.

Red Raspberry Leaf (Rhubus idaeus)

Nutritive; astringent; helps strengthen eyes.

Red Root (Ceanothus americana)

Stimulates lymphatic function, helping to carry toxins out of the body.

Usnea Lichen (Usnea spp.)

Strong antibiotic; antiviral; antifungal; for internal infections, staph, etc., infected wounds.

Clear Thought Formula

To increase mental clarity; also helpful when adjusting to higher altitudes.

Cayenne Fruit (Capsicum frutescens)

Equalizes circulation; for cold hands and feet; strengthens heart; stimulant.

Ginkgo Leaf (Ginkgo biloba)

Stimulates cerebral circulation and oxygenation, mental clarity and alertness, improves memory.

Ginseng Root (Panax quinquefolium)

Adaptogenic, decreases the essect of stress. Increases capillary circulation in brain; reproductive tonic; antidepressant; equalizes blood pressure. Used for general exhaustion and weakness; aids digestion. Promotes longevity.

Gotu Kola Leaf (Centella asiatica)

Used to increase mental stamina, alleviate depression and anxiety, improve memory and promote longevity. Increases energy and endurance.

Licorice Root (Glycyrrhiza glabra)

Supports adrenal glands.

Continued →

Computer Stress Formula

To alleviate the effects of computer radiation exposure, metabolic depression, eyestrain, nervous tension, lack of libido, and mental fatigue.

Bladderwrack (Fucus vesiculosus)

Thyroid balancer, specific in treating obesity associated with underactive thyroid.

Dandelion Root/Leaf (Taraxacum officinale)

Blood cleanser; powerful and safe diuretic, high in potassium. Mild laxative, aids weight loss, lowers cholesterol and blood pressure.

Echinacea Root (Echinacea angustifolia)

Powerful immune stimulant; antiseptic; antimicrobial; antiviral.

Eyebright Herb (Euphrasia officinalis)

Helps strengthen eyes, decreases eyestrain.

Ginkgo Leaf (Ginkgo biloba)

Stimulates cerebral circulation and oxygenation, mental clarity and alertness, improves memory.

Gotu Kola Leaf (Centella asiatica)

Used to increase mental stamina, alleviate depression and anxiety, improve memory and promote longevity. Increases energy and endurance.

Kelp (Nereocystis luetkeana)

Radiation protective properties. Reduces amount of strontium-90 absorbed by bone tissue by 50–85%.

Licorice Root (Glycyrrhiza glabra)

Supports adrenal gland; anti-inflammatory; laxative.

Oat Seed (Avena sativa)

Antispasmodic; soothes and supports nervous system; for depression, hysteria, irritation and anxiety.

Cough Calm Formula

An antispasmodic, mildly expectorant formula for the dry, annoying, unproductive cough that prevents restful sleep.

Blue Vervain (Verbena spp.)

Soothes cranky children; sedative; diaphoretic; febrifuge; antispasmodic mild analgesic.

Cayenne Fruit (Capsicum frutescens)

Stimulant; antiseptic, used as gargle for persistent cough.

Coltsfoot (Tussilago farfara)

Soothing expectorant; demulcent; antispasmodic; astringent; anti-inflammatory. For irritating coughs, bronchitis, asthma, laryngitis, throat catarrh.

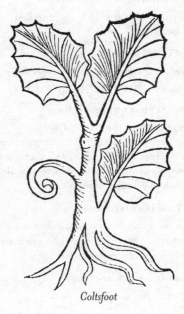

Coltsfoot

Elecampane Root (Inula helenium)

Expectorant; diaphoretic; antibacterial; anti-tussive; stomachic. Used for irritating bronchial coughs, bronchitis, emphysema, asthma and bronchitic asthma.

Jamaican Dogwood (Piscidia erythrina)

Sedative; anodyne; smooth muscle antispasmodic. For insomnia, neuralgia. Relieves coughing, reduces fevers.

Licorice Root (Glycyrrhiza glabra)

Demulcent; expectorant for coughs and respiratory congestion; antiinflammatory; laxative.

Lobelia Herb (Lobelia inflate)

Respiratory stimulant; antispasmodic.

Cramp Relief Formula

To relieve menstrual and muscular cramping.

Black Cohosh Root (Cimicifuga racemosa) [P/C]

Antispasmodic, used for menstrual cramping, coughs, muscle spasms; emmenagogue; relieves hot flashes in menopausal women; mild sedative.

Cramp Bark (Viburnum opulus)

Relaxes muscle tension and spasms, ovarian and uterine cramps. Used to prevent threatened miscarriage.

Lobelia Herb (Lobelia inflata)

Anti-emetic (small dose), emetic (large dose); Used for muscular cramping and pain.

Valerian Root (Valeriana officinalis)

Powerful nervine, used for tension, anxiety, insomnia, emotional stress, intestinal colic, menstrual cramps, migraine headache, and rheumatic pain.

Detox Formula

A cleansing formula which gently encourages the elimination of excess waste.

Anise Seed (Pimpinella anisum)

Eases indigestion, flatulence and colic. Antispasmodic and expectorant.

Buckthorn Bark (Rhamnus frangula)

Moderately strong laxative, very useful in chronic constipation. Must be dried before use to avoid intestinal cramping and nausea.

Burdock Root (Arctium lappa)

Blood cleanser, used for skin eruptions, dry/scaly skin conditions, digestive stimulant.

Dandelion Root/Leaf (Taraxacum officinale)

Blood cleanser; powerful and safe diuretic; high in potassium; cholagogue for inflammation and congestion of the liver and gall bladder, congestive jaundice. Mild laxative, aids weight loss, lowers cholesterol and blood pressure.

Echinacea Root (Echinacea angustifolia)

Powerful immune stimulant; antiseptic; antimicrobial; antiviral; used for sore throats, flu, colds, infections, allergies.

Oregon Grape Root (Mahonia repens)

Liver and blood cleanser; cholagogue; antibacterial. Stimulates digestion and absorption. Used for sluggish liver, hangovers, acne, eczema.

Stillingia Root (Stillingia sylvatica)

Blood cleanser, used for skin disorders. Small dose laxative and diuretic, large dose cathartic and emetic.

Stone Root (Collinsonia canadensis)

Strong diuretic, helps prevent and dissolve urinary stones and gravel.

Wahoo (Euonymus atropurpureus)

Primary liver decongestant, bile stimulant; used for jaundice, gallbladder pain and inflammation, constipation.

Yarrow Flowers (Achillea millefolium)

Diaphoretic, helps release toxic waste and reduce fevers.

Digestive Formula

Carminative and bitter herbs to stimulate digestion and reduce flatulence. Best taken with meals.

Alfalfa (Medicago sativa)

Nutritive herb with high mineral and vitamin content including Vitamin K and iron.

Anise Seed (Pimpinella anisum)

Aids digestion, reduces flatulence and colic. Antispasmodic.

Cayenne Fruit (Capsicum frutescens)

Equalizes circulation; stimulant; carminative.

Dill Seed (Anethum graveolens)

Carminative, used to prevent flatulence and colic, especially in children.

Fennel Seed (Foeniculum vulgare)

Aids digestion; relieves flatulence and colic; expels mucous; aids weight loss; flavoring agent; increases digestibility of other herbs.

Gentian Root (Gentiana lutea)

Bitter, promotes production of gastric juices and bile. For sluggish digestion, dyspepsia and flatulence. Restores appetite lost during morning sickness.

Ginger Root (Asariun canadense)

Carminative; aids in utilization of other herbs. Stimulant.

Meadowsweet (Filipendula ulmaria)

Digestive herb, antacid. Used for heartburn, nausea, gastritis, hyperacidity, peptic ulcers. Mild astringent, used for diarrhea in children. Anti-inflammatory.

Peppermint Leaf (Mentha piperita)

For upset stomach, heartburn, nausea, colds, flu, congestion, nervous headache and agitation, also diarrhea and flatulence. Adds flavor to other herbs.

Diuretic Formula

To decrease water retention by increasing the flow of urine.

Burdock Seed (Arctium lappa)

Diuretic, kidney tonic, demulcent.

Chickweed Herb (Stellaria media)

Nutritive; restorative; demulcent; diuretic.

Corn Silk (Zea mays)

Soothing diuretic, for renal and urinary irritation; used for bedwetting, cystitis, urethritis, prostatitis.

Cranberry (Vaccinium oxycoccus)

Diuretic and urinary antiseptic; for kidney and bladder infections.

Dandelion Root/Leaf (Taraxacum officinale)

Powerful and safe diuretic, high in potassium. Mild laxative, aids weight loss.

Continued ➤

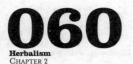

Goldenrod (Solidago virgauria)

Anti-inflammatory; urinary antiseptic; diuretic; diaphoretic; astringent.

Parsley Leaf/Root (Petroselemim crispum) [P/C]

Diuretic, antispasmodic.

Stone Root (Collinsonia canadensis)

Strong diuretic, helps prevent and dissolve urinary stones and gravel.

Uva Ursi (Arcostaphylos uva-ursi)

Urinary antiseptic; antimicrobial; for cystitis, urethritis, prostatitis, nephritis. Anrilithic, used for kidney and bladder stones.

Eczema Formula

For dry, scaly, itchy skin.

Alfalfa (Medicago sativa)

Nutritive herb with high mineral and vitamin content including Vitamin K and iron; mild diuretic.

Burdock Root (Arctium lappa)

Blood cleanser, used for skin eruptions, dry/scaly skin conditions; digestive stimulant.

Chaparrel Leaf (Larrea tridentata)

Blood cleanser, antioxidant; antibiotic; antiviral; antiseptic; specific for infections, sluggish liver, skin problems.

Figwort Herb (Scrophularia spp.)

Used internally and topically for eczema, scrofula, cradle cap, psoriasis, itching and irritated skin. *Avoid in cases of tachycardia.*

Horsetail Herb (Equisetum arvense)

High in silica and calcium, used to strengthen hair, skin and nails.

Nettle (Urtica dioica)

Nutritive herb, specific for childhood and nervous eczema. Rich in iron, silica, and potassium. Diuretic.

Expectorant Formula

To help move excess mucus out of the body, while soothing irritated membranes.

Bloodroot (Sanguinaria canadensis)

Expectorant. For chronic bronchitis, croup, laryngitis.

Boneset (Eupatorium perfoliatum)

For flu symptoms, aches and pains; clears mucus congestion; reduce fevers.

Coltsfoot (Tussilago farfara)

Soothing expectorant, demulcent, antispasmodic, astringent, anti-inflammatory. For irritating coughs, bronchitis, asthma laryngitis, throat catarrh.

Ginger Root (Asaram canadense)

Used for nausea. Diaphoretic, helps break fevers; stimulant; aids in utilization of other herbs.

Grindelia Buds/Flowers (Grindelia spp.)

Expectorant; antispasmodic; for bronchitis, sinus congestion,

Inmortal Root (Asclepius asperula)

Bronchial dilator; stimulates lymph drainage from the lungs. Used for asthma, pleurisy, bronchitis, lung infections. Laxative, diaphoretic.

Licorice Root (Glycyrrhiza glabra)

Demulcent; expectorant. For coughs and respiratory congestion; anti-inflammatory; laxative.

Mullein Leaf (Verbascum thapsus)

Expectorant; demulcent; reduces respiratory inflammation.

Osha' Root (Ligusticum porterii)

Strong antiviral, used for herpes, sore throat, colds, flu; bronchial expectorant; immune stimulating properties.

Pleurisy Root (Asclepias tuberosa)

Respiratory infections, bronchitis, pleurisy, pneumonia, flu. Reduces inflammation and encourages expectoration.

Female Glandular Formula

Formulated to gently balance female glandular function. Warning—has been known to increase libido.

Black Cohosh Root (Cimicifuga racemosa) [P/C]

Antispasmodic, used for menstrual cramping; emmenagogue; relieves hot flashes in menopausal women; mild sedative.

Chaste Berry (Vitex agnus castus)

Reproductive tonic, stimulates and normalizes pituitary function. For menstrual cramps, PMS, menopause, post–birth control pill rebalancing.

Dandelion Root/Leaf (Taraxacum officinale)

Blood cleanser; powerful and safe diuretic, high in potassium. Mild laxative, aids weight loss, lowers cholesterol and blood pressure.

Dong Quai Root (Angelica sinensis)

Female hormone regulator, alleviates cramping and premenstrual distress.

Hops Strobile (Humulus lupus)

Sedative; hypnotic. Used for anxiety, tension, insomnia. Reduces nervous irritability, promotes restful sleep.

Rhubarb (Rheum palmatum)

Stomachic, astringent, small doses to relieve diarrhea, larger doses laxative.

Squawvine/Partridge Berry (Mitchella repens)

Uterine tonic; promotes easy labor, eases menstrual cramping, mild nervine, improves digestion.

Fresh Breath Gum Tonic

Drop this antiseptic, astringent formula on your toothbrush and brush up under your gums to cleanse and strengthen the tissue. Freshens breath.

Bloodroot (Sanguinaria canadensis)

Alleviates mouth sores and reduces dental plaque.

Calendula Flower (Calendula officinalis)

Anti-inflammatory; astringent; styptic; antifungal. Use topically for wounds, ulcerations, abscesses.

Myrrh Gum (Commiphora myrrha)

Antiseptic; antimicrobial; astringent. Used for mouth ulcers, sore throat, gingivitis, pyorrhea.

Peppermint and Cinnamon Oils

For flavor, and to freshen breath.

Peppermint Leaf (Mentha piperita)

Cooling, astringent. Adds flavor to other herbs.

Potentilla (Potentilla spp.)

Astringent mouthwash and gargle for sore throats or gum inflammation.

White Oak Bark (Quercus alba)

Astringent, used for bleeding or ulcerated gums. Strengthens capillaries. Helps tighten teeth.

Wild Yam Root (Dioscorea spp.)

Anti-inflammatory.

Healthy Skin Formula

A cleansing and supportive formula for internal or external use in acne, eczema, and easily irritated skin.

Alfalfa (Medicago sativa)

Nutritive herb with high mineral and vitamin content including Vitamin K and iron; mild diuretic.

Blue Flag Root (Iris versicolor)

Liver purgative; blood purifier; cathartic; sialagogue; diuretic. For constipation and biliousness, eruptive skin conditions. *Low doses only.*

Burdock Root (Arctium lappa)

Blood cleanser, used for skin eruptions, dry/scaly skin conditions; digestive stimulant.

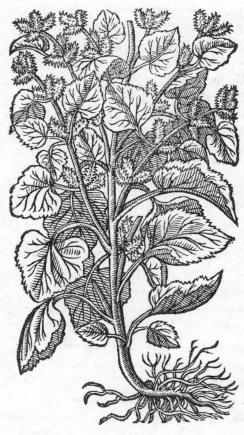

Burdock Root

Horsetail Herb (Equisetum arvense)

High in silica and calcium, used to strengthen hair, skin and nails.

Nettle (Urtica dioica)

Nutritive herb, specific for childhood and nervous eczema. Rich in iron, silica, and potassium. For anemia. Diuretic; antihistamine.

Oat Seed (Avena sativa)

Antispasmodic; soothes and supports nervous system. Calms irritation and anxiety.

Oregon Grape Root (Mahonia repens)

Liver and blood cleanser; chologogue; antibacterial. Stimulates digestion and absorption. Used for sluggish liver, acne, eczema.

Red Clover Flowers (Trifolium pretense)

Blood cleanser; nutritive; used for childhood eczema, psoriasis, ulcers, inflammation and infection. Principal ingredient of the Hoxey cancer formula.

Continued ➡

Immune-Strengthening Formula

An immune stimulant formula to help prevent susceptibility to disease. Best taken when you know you've been exposed to the latest grunge that's been going around, before it has developed into full-blown symptoms. Echinacea seems to work best when it is not over-utilized.

Echinacea Root (Echinacea angustifolia)

Powerful immune stimulant; antiseptic; anti-microbial; antiviral; used for sore throats, flu, colds, infections, allergies.

Ginseng Root (Panax quinquefolium)

Adaptogenic, decreases the effect of stress. Increases capillary circulation in brain; reproductive tonic; antidepressant; equalizes blood pressure. Used for general exhaustion and weakness; aids digestion. Promotes longevity.

Lomatium Root (Lomatium dissectum)

Antiviral; immune stimulant; for colds, flu, viral sore throats, respiratory infections and congestion.

Osha' Root (Ligusticum porterii)

Strong antiviral, used for herpes, sore throat, colds, flu; bronchial expectorant with immune stimulating properties,

St. John's Wort (Hypericun perforatum)

Extract used internally as an immune system stimulant; for retro-viral infections; expectorant; anti-bacterial, speeds wound and burn healing; antidepressant.

Infection Formula

This is the formula to use when you know you've definitely "got the bug" that's been flying around. The sooner you take care of it, the easier it will be to get rid of. The first sniffle is the most appropriate time to nip it in the bud.

Boneset (Eupatorium perfoliatum)

For flu symptoms, aches and pains; clears mucus congestion; reduces fevers; muscular rheumatism.

Cayenne Fruit (Capsicum frutescens)

Equalizes circulation; stimulant; styptic. Antiseptic, used as a gargle for persistent cough and laryngitis.

Chamomile Flower (Matricaria recutita)

Sedative, antispasmodic, anodyne. Children's herb, especially for fever and restlessness. Mouthwash for gingivitis.

Echinacea Root (Echinacea angustfolis)

Powerful immune stimulant; antiseptic; anti-microbial; antiviral; used for sore throats, flu, colds, infections, allergies.

Oregon Grape Root (Mahonia repens)

Liver and blood cleanser; cholagogue; antibacterial. Stimulates digestion and absorption.

Osha' Root (Ligusticum porterii)

Strong antiviral, used for herpes, sore throat, colds, flu; bronchial expectorant with immune stimulating properties.

Red Root (Ceanothus Americana)

Stimulates lymphatic system. Used for tonsillitis, sore throat, enlarged lymph nodes and spleen, fibrous cysts.

Usnea Lichen (Usnea spp.)

Strong antibiotic; antiviral; antifungal; for internal infections, strep, staph, trichomonas, etc., infected wounds. Also used for pneumonia, TB, and lupus.

Intestinal Fiber Maintenance Formula

Healthy intestines are vital to health in the rest of the body. Proper digestion, assimilation and elimination are essential for balanced metabolism and a strong immune system. This formula is best made with freshly ground seeds and should be refrigerated so the oils in the seeds do not go rancid. Keep it tightly closed when not in use. All the ingredients must be organically grown and cold processed. To use this formula, it is best to keep a small covered container handy to mix it in. Add one rounded teaspoon to 8 ounces of water or juice, shake well and drink immediately, because it thickens quickly. Follow with another glass of water and drink water throughout the day. This formula should be an integral part of any detoxification or weight loss program as well as daily maintenance. Different dietary fibers produce specific metabolic effects in the body. This formula provides a full spectrum of these fibers with herbal catalysts for maximum benefit.

Alfalfa Leaf (Medicago sativa)

Antibacterial. High fiber, binds and neutralizes substances that are carcinogenic to the colon.

Apple Pectin

Soft bulking agent which binds with bile acids. Used to reduce blood pressure and cholesterol.

Bentonite Clay

Highly absorbent. Helps draw impacted matter from the sides of the intestinal wall, further enhancing the detoxifying effect of the rest of the formula.

Buckthorn Bark (Rhamnus frangula)

Moderately strong laxative, very useful in chronic constipation.

Butternut Bark (Juglans cinerea)

Mild laxative; hepatic decongestant; vermifuge. Used to treat dysentery.

Cascara Sagrada Bark (Rhamnus purshiana) [P/C]

Laxative, mild liver stimulant, bitter tonic.

Cayenne Fruit (Capsicum frutescens)

Equalizes circulation; stimulant; carminative; styptic, antiseptic.

Dandelion Root/Leaf (Taraxacum officinale)

Mild laxative, liver/gall bladder decongestant, aids weight loss, lowers cholesterol and blood pressure. High in potassium.

Flax Seed (Linum usitatissimum)

Excellent bulking agent that cleanses and lubricates digestive tract.

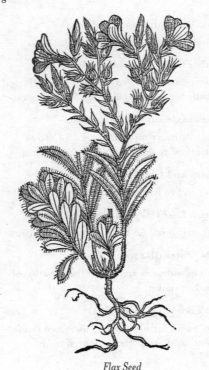

Flax Seed

Garlic Bulb/Seed (Allium sativum)

Antibiotic; antimicrobial; antiseptic; antiviral; anthelmintic. Help reduce blood pressure and cholesterol.

Gotu Kola (Centella asiatica)

Tonic, blood purifier, antispasmodic. Increases circulation, decrease fatigue. Helps heal ulcerated tissue.

Jerusalem Artichoke (Helianthus annus)

Helps stimulate the growth of healthy intestinal flora.

Kelp (Nereocystis luetkeana)

Used for radiation detoxification and to balance metabolism. Reduces amount of strontium-90 absorbed by bone tissue by 50–85%.

Lactobacillis Acidophilus and B. Bifidum/Longum

Restores the balance of healthy intestinal flora, thus inhibiting the growth of putrefactive bacteria.

Oat Bran Fiber (Avena sativa)

Bulking agent, helps reduce cholesterol. Calming.

Psyllium Seed (Plantago ovata)

Commonly called the intestinal janitor, softly "scrubs" the sides of the intestinal wall for maximum cleansing effect.

Remember to keep this formula refrigerated for maximum benefit!

Iron-Rich Formula

Increases the body's ability to utilize oxygen, thus increasing energy. Iron is essential for growth in children and resistance to disease. Iron is reduced in the body during infections, stress and the menstrual flow, and by the dietary consumption of carbonated soft drinks, alcohol, aspirin, coffee, and black tea. Iron deficiency is common in people who have either chronic herpes infection or candidiasis. It is recognized as one of the most prevalent mineral deficiencies in humans. Iron deficiency is indicated in chronic fatigue, lethargy, listlessness, depression, sleeplessness, brittle hair and fingernails. It also decreases the ability to tolerate cold weather.

Burdock Root (Arctium lappa)

Helps detoxify the bloodstream. Abundance of iron and insulin makes it of special value to the blood. Clears the kidneys of excess wastes and uric acid by increasing the flow of urine. Used for skin eruptions, dry/scaly skin conditions; increases digestion.

Chickweed Herb (Stellaria media)

A medicinal food which is high in B-complex vitamins, ascorbic acid, iron, calcium, sodium, zinc, lecithin and molybdenum. Used to build the blood and restore nutritional balance. Chickweed also assists in regulating the thyroid and has been used in weight loss programs. Increases cell membrane permeability, thus increasing the absorption of nutrients.

Mullein Leaf (Verbascum thapsus)

One of the highest herbal sources of bio-available iron. Demulcent, soothing to the gastrointestinal tract.

Nettle (Urtica dioica)

Nutritive herb, specific for childhood and nervous eczema. Rich in iron, silica, and potassium. Used to correct anemia.

Yellow Dock Root (Rumex crispus)

Nutritive tonic, aids in the assimilation of iron. Mild laxative, stimulates the flow of bile and aids fat digestion.

Continued ➡

Itch-Ease Spray Formula

Relieves itching of insect bites, poison ivy, poison oak, etc.

Echinacea Root (Echinacea angustifolia)

Antiseptic; antimicrobial.

Grindelia Buds/Flowers (Grindelia spp.)

Relieves swelling, itching, and pain of poison oak/ivy and insect bites.

Jewel Weed (Impatiens aureus)

External Use. Used topically to reduce the itching and inflammation of skin irritating plants such as poison ivy.

Nettle (Urtica dioica)

Nutritive herb, specific for childhood and nervous eczema. Rich in iron, silica, and potassium. Antihistamine, reduces inflammation and itching.

Plantain Leaf (Plantago spp.)

Astringent; used for external wounds and sores, insect bites.

Potentilla (Potentilla spp.)

Astringent, used for abrasions, sunburn, poison oak.

Joint Formula

For the stiffness and soreness associated with arthritis. Increases lymphatic drainage.

Echinacea Root (Echinacea angustifolia)

Powerful immune stimulant; aids lymphatic drainage; used for sore throats, flu, colds, infections, allergies.

Meadowsweet (Filipendula ulmaria)

Digestive herb, antacid. Used for heartburn, nausea, gastritis, hyperacidity, peptic ulcers. Mild astringent. Diaphoretic, anti-inflammatory, reduces fever and pain.

Red Root (Ceanothus americana)

Stimulates lymphatic and interstitial fluid circulation. Aids in the transport of nutrients and the elimination of waste products.

Wild Yam Root (Dioscorea spp.)

Antispasmodic; anti-inflammatory; helps alleviate the pain and swelling of rheumatoid arthritis.

Yerba Mansa Root (Anemopsis californica)

Soothing to mucus membranes, used for catarrh, aids digestion.

Kidney/Bladder Formula

Antiseptic and demulcent herbs to help alleviate urinary irritation and promote healing. Mild diuretic.

Burdock Root (Arctium lappa)

Blood cleanser, digestive stimulant.

Corn Silk (Zea mays)

Soothing diuretic, for renal & urinary irritation; used for bedwetting, cystitis, urethritis, prostatitis.

Couchgrass Root (Agropyron repens)

Demulcent; antimicrobial; antilithic; for cystitis, urethritis, prostatitis, kidney stones and gravel.

Cranberry (Vaccinium oxycoccus)

Diuretic and urinary antiseptic; for kidney and bladder infections.

Goldenrod (Solidago virgauria)

Anti-inflammatory; urinary antiseptic; diuretic; diaphoretic; expectorant, astringent. For cystitis, urethritis, upper respiratory catarrh, diarrhea, and internal hemorrhage.

Gravel Root (Eupatorium purpureum)

For kidney and urinary infections and stones; prostatitis; pelvic inflammatory disease; painful menses; rheumatism and gout.

Marshmallow Root (Althaea officinalis)

Demulcent, soothes inflamed membranes.

Pipsissewa (Chimaphila umbellata)

Diuretic, used for chronic kidney weakness, nephritis, bladder stones, and rheumatism.

Uva Ursi (Arcostaphylos uva-ursi)

Urinary antiseptic; antimicrobial; for cystitis, urethritis, prostatitis, nephritis. Antilithic, used for kidney and bladder stones.

Laxative Formula

A balance of cleansing and soothing herbs to tone the lower intestine and promote effective elimination.

Anise Seed (Pimpinella anisum)

Eases indigestion, flatulence and colic. Antispasmodic.

Barberry Root (Berberis fendleri) [P/C]

Digestive and appetite stimulant; stimulates bile flow and liver function; refrigerant, reduces fevers; antiseptic.

Buckthorn Bark (Rhamnus frangula)

Moderately strong laxative, very useful in chronic constipation. Must be dried before use to avoid intestinal cramping and nausea.

Dandelion Root/Leaf (Taraxacum officinale)

Blood cleanser; powerful and safe diuretic, high in potassium; stimulates flow of bile, for inflammation and congestion of the liver and gall bladder. Mild laxative, aids weight loss, lowers cholesterol and blood pressure.

Echinacea Root (Echinacea angustifolia)

Immune stimulant; antiseptic; antimicrobial; antiviral.

Licorice Root (Glycyrrhiza glabra)

Demulcent; anti-inflammatory; laxative.

Marshmallow Root (Althaea officinalis)

Soothing demulcent, reduces gastrointestinal inflammation.

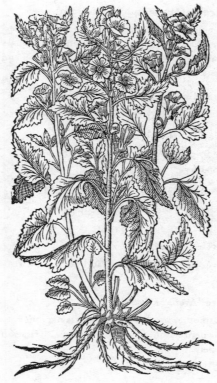

Marshmallow Root

Potentilla (Potentilla spp.)

Astringent. Used for gastrointestinal ulcers.

Rhybarb Root (Rheum palmatum) [P/C]

Stomachic, astringent, small doses to relieve diarrhea, larger doses laxative.

Wild Yam Root (Dioscorea spp.)

Antispasmodic; carminative; anti-inflammatory; hepatic; cholagogue; diaphoretic. Used for intestinal colic, diverticulitis, flatulence.

Liver Formula

Cleansing and stimulating herbs to support effective liver function.

Burdock Root (Arctium lappa)

Blood cleanser, used for skin eruptions, dry/scaly skin conditions; digestive stimulant.

Chaparrel Leaf (Larrea tridentata)

Stimulates sluggish liver.

Dandelion Root/Leaf (Taraxacum officinale)

Blood cleanser; for inflammation and congestion of the liver and gall bladder, congestive jaundice, stimulates the flow of bile. Mild laxative, aids weight loss, lowers cholesterol and blood pressure.

Fennel Seed (Foeniculum vulgare)

Aids digestion; relieves flatulence and colic.

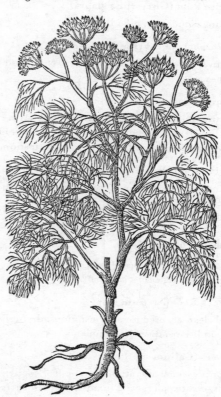

Fennel Seed

Milk Thistle Seed (Silybum marianum)

Powerful liver detoxifier, antidote for Amanita mushroom poisoning. Increases secretion and flow of bile.

Oregon Grape Root (Mahonia repens)

Liver and blood cleanser; stimulates flow of bile; antibacterial. Stimulates digestion and absorption. Used for sluggish liver and help alleviate hangovers.

Red Clover Flowers (Trifolium pratense)

Blood cleanser; nutritive; principal ingredient of the Hoxey cancer formula.

Toadflax (Linaria vulgaris)

Liver cleanser; stimulates bile production; used in hepatitis, jaundice, sluggish liver. Potent—best used in small amounts in formulas.

Continued ➡

Wild Yam Root (Dioscorea spp.)

Antispasmodic; carminative; anti-inflammatory; hepatic; cholagogue; diaphoretic. Used for intestinal colic, diverticulitis, painful menses, ovarian and uterine pain, rheumatoid arthritis, flatulence.

Lullaby Glycerite Formula

Children's aid to restful sleep.

Alfalfa (Medicago sativa)

Nutritive herb with high mineral and vitamin content, including Vitamin K and iron.

Catnip Herb (Nepeta cataria)

Mild sedative, soothes crankiness.

Chamomile Flower (Matricaria recutita)

For fever and restlessness. Mild pain reliever, helps relieve colic, dispel gas. Calming.

Fennel Seed (Foeniculum vulgare)

Aids digestion; relieves flatulence and colic; expels mucous; flavoring agent; increases digestibility of other herbs.

Lemon Balm (Melissa officinalis)

Very useful in reducing fevers during colds and flu since it induces mild perspiration. Aids digestion, reduces flatulence.

Licorice Root (Glycyrrhiza glabra)

Soothing demulcent; mild laxative.

Red Raspberry Leaf (Rhubus idaeus)

Nutritive, relieves nausea. Remedy for childhood diarrhea.

Rosehips (Rosa canina)

Nutritive, mild diuretic and laxative, mild astringent. Excellent source of vitamin C. Used for colds, flu, general debility and exhaustion, constipation.

Valerian Root (Valeriana officinalis)

Nervine, used for tension, anxiety, insomnia, emotional stress, intestinal colic, migraine headache and rheumatic pain, breaking addictions.

Lymphatic Formula

Promotes cleansing and draining of lymphatic tissue. Helps the body excrete toxic waste during infections.

Burdock Root (Arctium lappa)

Blood cleanser, used for skin eruptions, dry/scaly skin conditions; digestive stimulant.

Cleavers (Galium spp.)

Lymphatic tonic; alterative; diuretic. For swollen glands, cystitis, ulcers and tumors, skin disorders, painful urination.

Echinacea Root (Echinacea angustifolia)

Antiseptic; antimicrobial; anti-viral; used for sore throats, flu, colds, infections, allergies.

Ocotillo (Fouquieria splendens)

Stimulates lymphatic drainage; improves dietary fat absorption into the lymph system. Helps drain pelvic congestion, making it useful in the treatment of hemorrhoids and varicose veins.

Red Root (Ceanothus americana)

Stimulates lymphatic and interstitial fluid circulation. Aids in the transport of nutrients and the elimination of waste products. Used for tonsillitis, sore throat, enlarged lymph nodes and spleen, fibrous cysts. Mild expectorant, hemostatic.

Wild Indigo Root (Baptisia tinctoria)

Emetic; purgative; lymph cleanser; for focused local infection such as sore throat, laryngitis, tonsillitis, pharyngitis, gingivitis, mouth ulcers and pyorrhea, also inflamed lymph nodes. Best used in small amounts in a formula.

Male Glandular Formula

Formulated to gently balance male glandular function. Warning—has been known to increase libido.

Damiana (Turnera diffusa)

Diuretic, relieves irritation of urinary mucus membranes; genitourinary stimulant effect leading to its use as an aphrodisiac; improves digestion; laxative; tonic.

Ginseng Root (Panax quinquefolium)

Adaptogenic, decreases the effect of stress. Increases capillary circulation in brain; reproductive tonic; antidepressant; equalizes blood pressure. Used for general exhaustion and weakness; aids digestion. Promotes longevity.

Licorice Root (Glycyrrhiza glabra)

Specific for adrenal gland insufficiency; hormonal balance.

Saw Palmetto (Seronoa repens)

Tones and strengthens male reproductive system, used for prostate enlargement and infection, enhances endurance.

Menopause Formula

Balancing and supportive herbs to ease transition symptoms such as mood swings, hot flashes and irregular menses associated with menopause.

Alfalfa (Medicago sativa)

Nutritive herb with high mineral and vitamin content including Vitamin K and iron; estrogen precursor for menopause; mild diuretic.

Black Cohosh Root (Cimicifuga racemosa) [P/C]

Antispasmodic, relieves hot flashes in menopausal women; mild sedative.

Dandelion Root/Leaf (Taraxacum officinale)

Blood cleanser; powerful and safe diuretic, high in potassium. Mild laxative, aids weight loss, lowers cholesterol and blood pressure.

Dong Quai Root (Angelica sinensis)

Female hormone regulator, alleviates cramping and premenstrual distress.

Ginseng Root (Panax quinquefolium)

Adaptogenic, decreases the effect of stress. Increases capillary circulation in brain; antidepressant; equalizes blood pressure. Used for general exhaustion and weakness; aids digestion. Promotes longevity.

Hawthorn Berry (Crataegus oxycantha)

Heart and circulatory tonic.

Licorice Root (Glycyrrhiza glabra)

Specific for adrenal gland insufficiency; anti-inflammatory.

Motherwort Herb (Leonurus cardiaca) [P/C]

Antispasmodic; cardiac tonic; reduces tension, anxiety.

Nettle (Urtica dioica)

Nutritive, rich in iron, silica, and potassium. For anemia.

Oat Seed (Avena sativa)

Antispasmodic; soothes and supports nervous system; for depression, insomnia, hysteria, irritation and anxiety.

Muscle/Bruise Spray

For muscular sprains, strains and bruises. External Use Only.

Arnica Flower (Arnica cordifolia)

Topical use for bruises, sprains, strains, and other athletic injuries, including swelling. Use on unbroken skin.

Calendula Flower (Calendula officinalis)

Anti-inflammatory; astringent. Use topically. Helps reabsorb blood from bruised tissue, relieves sprains and strains.

St. John's Wort (Hypericum perforatum)

Extract and oil used externally for bruises, strains, sprains, contusions, wounds.

Nausea Formula

For motion sickness, indigestion, nausea.

Cow Parsnip Root/Seed (Heracleum lanatum)

Antinauseant; stimulant; hypotensive; emmenagogue; antispasmodic; carminative.

Ginger Root (Asarum canadense)

Used for nausea, motion sickness. Diaphoretic, helps break fevers; stimulant; carminative; aids in utilization of other herbs.

Peppermint Leaf (Mentha piperita)

For upset stomach, heartburn, nausea, colds, flu, congestion, nervous headache and agitation, also diarrhea and flatulence. Adds flavor to other herbs.

Pain Formula

Inodyne and antispasmodic herbs which have traditionally been used for headaches and muscular pain.

Blue Vervain (Verbena spp.)

Sedative, antidepressant, causes sweating, reduces fevers, antispasmodic, mild analgesic.

Chamomile Flower (Matricaria recutita)

Sedative, carminative, antispasmodic, anodyne.

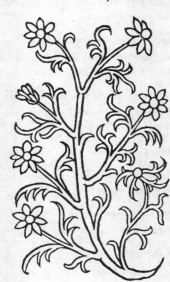

Chamomile Flower

Feverfew Leaf/Flower (Tanacetum parthenium)

Anti-inflammatory, used for rheumatoid arthritis, migraine headache relief (long-term basis). Mild febrifuge.

Ginger Root (Asarum canadense)

Diaphoretic, stimulant; carminative; aids in utilization of other herbs, reduces nausea.

Jamaican Dogwood (Piscidia erythrina)

Sedative; anodyne; smooth muscle antispasmodic. For insomnia, neuralgia, menstrual cramping. Relieves coughing, reduces fevers.

Continued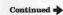

Passionflower (Passiflora incarnata)

Sedative, hypnotic, antispasmodic, anodyne. Relieves nerve pain, promotes restful sleep. Calms hysteria.

Rosemary Leaf (Rosmarinus officinalis)

Circulatory and nerve stimulant, used for tension headache associated with dyspepsia, also depression. Antibacterial; antifungal.

Valerian Root (Valeriana officinalis)

Powerful nervine, used for tension, anxiety, insomnia, emotional stress, intestinal colic, menstrual cramps, migraine headache, and rheumatic pain.

White Willow Bark (Salix alba)

Astringent, contains salicin, reduces inflammation. For headache, neuralgia, fevers, hayfever, arthritis, and rheumatism.

Wild Lettuce Herb (Lactuca spp.)

Sedative, calms restlessness and anxiety, reduces spasms.

Parasite Formula

A broad spectrum formula for intestinal parasites.

Black Walnut Hulls (Juglans nigra)

Vermifuge; antifungal, for Candida, athlete's foot, ringworm, etc., astringent, used for skin eruptions. Helps break down cystic tissue.

Butternut Bark (Juglans cineraria)

Gentle tonic, vermifuge.

Chaparro (Castela emoryi)

Active inhibitor of intestinal protozoa. Used to prevent and alleviate amoebic dysentery and giardia.

Echinacea Root (Echinacea angustifolia)

Stimulates immune response; antiseptic; antimicrobial; antiviral.

Garlic Bulb/Seed (Allium sativum)

Anthelmintic, antibiotic; antimicrobial; antiseptic; antiviral. Has long, successful history in treatment of tapeworm, round worm, pinworm and other parasites. Makes internal environment totally unfavorable to their survival.

Goldenseal Root (Hydrastis canadensis)

Antiseptic, used internally and topically for infection, sore throat, gastritis, ulceration, and colitis.

Marshmallow Root (Althaea officinalis)

Soothing demulcent, used for gastrointestinal inflammation, buffers the other herbs in the formula.

Quassia (Pycrasma excelsa)

Bitter tonic and stomachic; antispasmodic; anthelmintic. Used to rid the body of parasites and improve digestion.

Wormwood Leaf (Artemisia absinthium)

Reduces fevers, will inhibit roundworm and pinworm infestation when used consistently for a week or two. Stimulates sweating in dry fevers. *Use small amounts in the formula, preferably with herbalist or physician supervision.*

PMS Formula

For mood swings, cramping, and general misery experienced immediately prior to the female menstrual cycle.

Alfalfa (Medicago sativa)

Nutritive herb with high mineral and vitamin content including Vitamin K and iron; estrogen precursor for menopause; mild diuretic.

Black Cohosh Root (Cimicifuga racemosa) [P/C]

Antispasmodic used for menstrual cramping, coughs, muscle spasms; emmenagogue; relieves hot flashes in menopausal women; mild sedative.

Blue Vervain (Verbena spp.)

Soothes cranky children, sedative, antidepressant, diaphoretic, febrifuge, antispasmodic, mild analgesic.

Chaste Berry (Vitex agnus castus)

Reproductive tonic, stimulates and normalizes pituitary function. For menstrual cramps, PMS, menopause, post–birth control pill rebalancing.

Dong Quai Root (Angelica sinensis)

Female hormone regulator, alleviates cramping and premenstrual distress.

Oat Seed (Avena sativa)

Antispasmodic; soothes and supports nervous system; for depression, insomnia, hysteria, irritation and anxiety. Helpful in breaking addictions.

Passionflower (Passiflora incarnata)

Sedative, antispasmodic, anodyne. Relieves nerve pain, promotes restful sleep. Has been used for seizures and hysteria.

Professor Cayenne's "TNT" Formula

This formula is different, being extracted in raw, organic apple cider vinegar instead of grain alcohol and distilled water. It is used for the early onset of colds and flu. It also makes a great medicinal salad dressing!

Cayenne Fruit (Capsicum frutescens)

Equalizes circulation; for cold hands and feet; strengthens heart; stimulant; carminative; styptic. Antiseptic, used as a gargle for persistent cough.

Garlic Blub/Seed (Allium sativum)

Antibiotic; antimicrobial; antiseptic; antiviral; anthelmintic. For colds, flu, chronic bronchitis, infections, also to reduce blood pressure and cholesterol.

Ginger Root (Asarum canadense)

Used for nausea, motion sickness; diaphoretic, helps break fevers; stimulant; carminative; aids in utilization of other herbs.

Horseradish Root (Armoracia rusticana)

Stimulant; for flu, fevers, sinus and respiratory congestion. Sialagogue, carminative, mild laxative, diuretic.

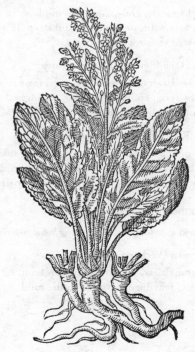

Horseradish Root

Onion (Allium cepa)

Diuretic, expectorant, carminative, antiseptic, antispasmodic, anthelmintic. Helps alleviate putrefaction in the gastrointestinal tract. Used to alleviate cold and flu symptoms.

Parsley Leaf and Root (Petroselemim crispum) [P/C]

Diuretic, carminative, antispasmodic, emmenagogue, expectorant.

Prostate Formula

Herbal allies to strengthen and support the prostate gland.

Cleavers (Galium spp.)

Lymphatic tonic; alterative; diuretic. For swollen glands, cystitis, ulcers and tumors, painful urination.

Cotton Root (Gossypium herbaceum)

Increases tone and contractibility of seminal vesicles.

Couchgrass Root (Agropyron repens)

Demulcent; antimicrobial; antilithic; for cystitis, urethritis, prostatitis, kidney stones and gravel.

Echinacea Root (Echinacea angustifolia)

Stimulates immune response; antiseptic; antimicrobial; antiviral; used for sore throats, flu, colds, infections, allergies.

Gravel Root (Eupatorium purpuremn)

For kidney and urinary infections and stones, prostatitis, pelvic inflammatory disease; rheumatism and gout.

Marshmallow Root (Althaea officinalis)

Soothes irritated tissue, buffers other herbs in formula.

Saw Palmetto (Serenoa repens)

Tones and strengthens male reproductive system, used for prostate enlargement and infection, enhances endurance.

Quit Smoking Formula

Formulated to alleviate the nervousness associated with nicotine withdrawal while stimulating detoxification and expectoration.

Anise Seed (Pimpinella anisum)

Antispasmodic and expectorant.

Chamomile Flower (Matricaria recutita)

Sedative, carminative, antispasmodic, anodyne.

Dandelion Root/Leaf (Taraxacum officinale)

Blood cleanser; powerful and safe diuretic, high in potassium: cholagogue, for inflammation and congestion of the liver and gall bladder, congestive jaundice. Mild laxative, aids weight loss, lowers cholesterol and blood pressure.

Grindelia Buds/Flowers (Grindelia spp.)

Expectorant; antispasmodic; for bronchitis, sinus congestion, bladder infections; topically for poison oak and ivy, insect bites.

Licorice Root (Glycyrrhiza glabra)

Specific for adrenal gland insufficiency; demulcent; expectorant for coughs and respiratory congestion; anti-inflammatory; laxative.

Lobelia Herb (Lobelia inflata)

Respiratory stimulant; antiasthmatic; antiemetic (small dose), emetic (large dose). Used for bronchitis and bronchitic asthma, whooping cough, muscular cramping and pain.

Continued ➡

Oat Seed (Avena sativa)

Antispasmodic; soothes and supports nervous system; for depression, insomnia, hysteria, irritation and anxiety. Helpful in decreasing the irritability associated with nicotine withdrawal.

Valerian Root (Valeriana officinalis)

Powerful nervine, used for tension, anxiety, insomnia, emotional stress, intestinal colic, menstrual cramps, migraine headache, and rheumatic pain, breaking addictions.

Reishi/Shiitake Formula

Adaptogenic, immune stimulating formula. Supports nerve and metabolic function during high-stress periods. Especially good for people who constantly out-flow energy without enough in-flow (also known as Type A personalities).

Reishi Mushroom (Ganoderma lucidum)

Adaptogenic, used to alleviate the effects of stress. Strengthens heart, protects liver, soothes nerves. Normalizes blood pressure. Inhibits the release of histamine, thus relieving the allergic inflammatory response. Supports adrenal function. Stimulates the immune system. Slows the aging process. Anti-carcinogenic. Antibacterial.

Shiitake Mushroom (Lentinus edodes)

Adaptogenic. Increases the production of interferon, thus reducing the possibility of tumor development. Antiviral. Helps the body excrete excess cholesterol.

Rejuvenation Formula

A true tonic formula for physical and mental longevity.

Alfalfa (Medicago sativa)

Nutritive herb with high mineral and vitamin content including Vitamin K, and iron; mild diuretic.

Ginkgo Leaf (Ginkgo biloba)

Stimulates cerebral circulation and oxygenation, mental clarity and alertness, improves memory. Used to prevent strokes.

Ginseng Root (Panax quinquefolium)

Adaptogenic, decreases the effect of stress. Increases capillary circulation in brain; reproductive tonic; antidepressant; equalizes blood pressure. Used for general exhaustion and weakness; aids digestion. Promotes longevity.

Gotu Kola Leaf (Centella asiatica)

Used to increase mental stamina, alleviate depression and anxiety, improve memory, and promote longevity. Increases energy and endurance.

Licorice Root (Glycyrrhiza glabra)

Specific for adrenal gland insufficiency; demulcent; expectorant for coughs and respiratory congestion; anti-inflammatory; laxative.

Oat Seed (Avena sativa)

Antispasmodic; soothes and supports nervous system; for depression, insomnia, hysteria, irritation, and anxiety. Helpful in breaking addictions.

Restful Sleep Formula

For those whose brains will not shut off at night. For the agitation generated by too much mental activity and too little physical activity. Insomnia and nervous tension. Helps promote sleep when changing time zones while traveling.

Catnip Herb (Nepeta cataria)

Calming, soothing, gently tranquilizing. Carminative, diaphoretic antispasmodic, mild febrifuge. For indigestion, flatulence and colic, mild astringent, specific for childhood fevers and diarrhea.

The Herbal First Aid Kit

The following items are useful in the first aid kit and home medicine chest.
- Aloe Burn Spray Formula
- Antiseptic Spray Formula
- Bug Spray Formula
- Cramp Formula
- Dental Poultices
- Digestive Formula
- Dr. Christopher's Burn Ointment
- Herbal Eyewash kit (herbs, filter, eyecup)
- Infection Formula
- Itch Spray Formula
- Laxative Formula
- Mullein/Garlic Ear Oil Formula
- Muscle/Bruise Salve or Liniment Spray Formula
- Pain Formula
- Restful Sleep Formula
- Skin Soothing Salve Formula
- Slippery Elm lozenges
- Tea Tree Oil
- Throat Extract/Spray Formula
- Adhesive tape; bandages; cotton gauze, roll and pads (nonstick); eyecup; mirror; Q-Tips; scissors; thermometer (Oral and Rectal); tweezers

Other useful items: Castor Oil and wool flannel, cotton diapers, enema/douche bag, handkerchiefs, hot water bottle, large enamel or glass pot, First Aid Booklet or chart describing CPR and the Heimlich maneuver.

Chamomile Flower (Matricaria recutita)

Sedative, carminative, antispasmodic, anodyne. Children's herb, especially for fever and restlessness.

Hops Strobile (Humulus lupus)

Sedative; hypnotic. Used for anxiety, tension, insomnia. Reduces nervous irritability, promotes restful sleep.

Passionflower (Passiflora incarnate)

Sedative, hypnotic, antispasmodic, anodyne. Relieves nerve pain, promotes restful sleep. Has been used for seizures and hysteria.

Skullcap Herb (Scutellaria lateriflora)

Nervine; sedative; antispasmodic; used for nervous tension, hysteria, epileptic seizures, withdrawal from substance abuse, and the irritability of PMS.

Valerian Root (Valeriana officinalis)

Powerful nervine, used for tension, anxiety, insomnia, emotional stress, intestinal colic, menstrual cramps, migraine headache, and rheumatic pain.

Stress Formula

A gently balancing, nerve supportive formula for high stress periods.

Blue Vervain (Verbena spp.)

Soothes crankiness, sedative, antidepressant, diaphoretic, febrifuge, antispasmodic, mild analgesic.

Chamomile Flower (Matricaria recutita)

Sedative, carminative, antispasmodic, anodyne. Used for fever and restlessness.

Ginseng Root (Panax quinquefolium)

Adaptogenic, decreases the effect of stress. Increases capillary circulation in brain; reproductive tonic; antidepressant; equalizes blood pressure. Used for general exhaustion, hysteria, irritation and anxiety. Helpful in breaking addictions. Alleviates exhaustion and weakness; aids digestion. Promotes longevity.

Oat Seed (Avena sativa)

Antispasmodic; soothes and supports nervous system; for depression, insomnia, hysteria, irritation and anxiety. Helpful in breaking addictions.

Passionflower (Passiflora incarnata)

Sedative, hypnotic, antispasmodic, anodyne. Relieves nerve pain, promotes restful sleep. Calms hysteria.

Prodigiosa (Brickellia grandiflora)

Helps regulate overuse of fight or flight response by moderating epinephrine's stimulation of liver to break down stored glycogen into blood sugar.

Skullcap Herb (Scutellaria lateriflora)

Nervine; sedative; antispasmodic; used for nervous tension, hysteria, epileptic seizures, withdrawal from substance abuse, and the irritability of PMS.

St. John's Wort (Hypericum perforatum)

Used internally as an immune system stimulant; for retro-viral infections; expectorant; anti-bacterial, speeds wound and burn healing; antidepressant; used to treat bedwetting and children's nightmares.

Throat Extract/Spray Formula

For sore, scratchy, irritated and inflamed throats. Works very well in conjunction with vitamin C supplementation. Can be sprayed directly into the throat, taken internally, or used as a gargle.

Cayenne Fruit (Capsicum frutescens)

Circulatory stimulant. Antiseptic, used as gargle for sore throat, persistent cough, laryngitis.

Echinacea Root (Echinacea angustifolia)

Stimulates immune system; facilitates lymphatic drainage, antiseptic; antimicrobial; antiviral; used for sore throats, flu, colds, infections, allergies.

Goldenseal Root (Hydrastis canadensis)

Antiseptic, used internally and topically for infection, sore throat.

Licorice Root (Glycyrrhiza glabra)

Soothing demulcent; expectorant for coughs and respiratory congestion; anti-inflammatory; laxative.

Myrrh Gum (Commiphora myrrha)

Antiseptic; antimicrobial; astringent. Used for mouth ulcers, sore throat, gingivitis, pyorrhea, sinusitis and pharyngitis.

Osha' Root (Ligusticum porterii)

Strong antiviral, used for herpes, sore throat, colds, flu; bronchial expectorant; immune stimulating properties.

Propolis

Antiseptic, antibacterial. Waxy nature makes it useful for coating and isolating areas of throat inflammation to prevent spread of infection, and to bind the other herbs to the throat for longer lasting effect.

Continued ➡

Usnea Lichen (Usnea spp.)

Strong antibiotic, very effective for strep throat; antiviral; for internal infections, staph, trichomonas, etc., infected wounds.

Vaginitis Formula

An antiseptic, antibiotic formula which assists the body in healing vaginal infections and irritations. Bitter taste, best mixed with juice or tea.

Echinacea Root (Echinacea angustifolia)

Immune stimulant; antiseptic; antimicrobial; antiviral; used for sore throats, flu, colds, infections.

Garlic Bulb/Seed (Allium sativum)

Antibiotic; antimicrobial; antiseptic; antiviral. Drives infection from the body.

Goldenseal Root (Hydrastis canadensis)

Antiseptic, used internally and topically for infection, sore throat, gastritis, ulceration, and colitis. Infusion of the fresh or dried root used as douche for vaginitis.

Osha' Root (Ligusticum porterii)

Strong antiviral, used for herpes, sore throat, colds, flu; bronchial expectorant; immune stimulating properties.

Peppermint Leaf (Mentha piperita)

For upset stomach, heartburn, nausea, colds, flu, congestion, nervous headache, and agitation, also diarrhea and flatulence. Adds flavor to the formula.

Red Root (Ceanothus americana)

Lymphatic stimulant, facilitating the excretion of metabolic toxins from the body. Used for infections, enlarged lymph nodes and spleen, fibrous cysts.

Usnea Lichen (Usnea spp.)

Strong antibiotic; antiviral; antifungal; for internal infections, strep, staph, trichomonas, etc., infected wounds. Also used for pneumonia, TB, and lupus.

Vein-Toning Formula

Supports and strengthens vascular integrity.

Blue Vervain (Verbena spp.)

Tonic, diaphoretic, mild analgesic.

Dandelion Root/Leaf (Taraxacum officinale)

Blood cleanser; powerful and safe diuretic, high in potassium; cholagogue, for inflammation and congestion of the liver and gall bladder, congestive jaundice. Mild laxative, aids weight loss, lowers cholesterol and blood pressure.

Hawthorn Berry (Crataegus oxycantha)

Heart and circulatory tonic.

Melilot (Melilotus officinalis)

Spasmolytic. Reduces blood stagnation.

Milk Thistle Seed (Silybum marianum)

Powerful liver detoxifier.

Ocotillo (Fouquieria splendens)

Reduces pelvic congestion and pressure on the pelvic veins.

Shepherd's Purse (Capsella Bursa-pastoris)

Hemostatic; astringent; diuretic.

Stone Root (Collinsonia canadensis)

Strengthens structural integrity of veins, used for varicose veins, hemorrhoids, anal fissures, and rectal spasms.

Syrups

Syrups are a tasty, soothing way to ingest herbs. They are traditionally made with a sweet tasting base such as honey or glycerin. Honey has antiseptic properties. The following syrups are wonderful allies to have around during the cold season.

Cough Formula Syrup

Soothing, antispasmodic herbs in a honey glycerin base to calm coughing.

Blue Vervain (Verbena spp.)

Sedative; antispasmodic; diaphoretic, promotes mild sweating to excrete toxins and decrease fever; mild pain reliever.

Cayenne Fruit (Capsicum frutescens)

Antiseptic, stimulates circulation to help metabolize nutrients and excrete toxins.

Coltsfoot (Tussilago Farfara)

Soothing expectorant, demulcent, antispasmodic, astringent, anti-inflammatory. For irritating coughs, bronchitis, asthma, laryngitis, throat catarrh.

Elecampane Root (Inula helenium)

Expectorant; diaphoretic; antibacterial; antitussive; stomachic; for irritating bronchial coughs, bronchitis, emphysema, asthma and bronchitic asthma.

Jamaican Dogwood (Piscidia erythrina)

Sedative; pain reliever; smooth muscle antispasmodic. Relieves coughing, reduces fevers.

Licorice Root (Glycyrrhiza glabra)

Soothing demulcent; expectorant for coughs and respiratory congestion; anti-inflammatory; laxative.

Lobelia Herb (Lobelia inflata)

Respiratory stimulant; antiasthmatic. Used for bronchitis and bronchitic asthma, whooping cough, muscular cramping and pain.

Expectorant Formula Syrup

Herbs which promote the expectoration of excess mucus from the respiratory system. Honey/glycerin base.

Boneset (Eupatorium perfoliatum)

For flu symptoms, aches and pains; clears mucus congestion; reduce fevers; muscular rheumatism.

Coltsfoot (Tussilago farfara)

Soothing expectorant, demulcent, antispasmodic, astringent, anti-inflammatory. For irritating coughs, bronchitis, asthma, laryngitis, throat catarrh.

Grindelia Buds/Flowers (Grindelia spp.)

Expectorant; antispasmodic; for bronchitis, mucus congestion.

Horehound Herb (Marrubium vulgare)

Effective decongestant, expectorant.

Hyssop Leaf (Hyssopus officinalis)

Antispasmodic; nervine; expectorant; diaphoretic, sedative, carminative. For chronic congestion.

Licorice Root (Glycyrrhiza glabra)

Soothing demulcent; expectorant for coughs and respiratory congestion; anti-inflammatory; laxative.

Mullein Leaf (Verbascum thapsus)

Expectorant; demulcent; reduces respiratory inflammation.

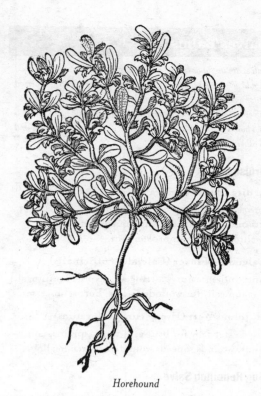

Horehound

Osha' Root (Ligusticum porterii)

Bronchial expectorant, strong antiviral, used for sore throat, colds, flu; stimulates immune system.

Garlic Formula Syrup

Garlic Syrup?!? Believe it or not, it's really tasty. Also known as an oxymel, this formula is made with fresh garlic bulbs, raw organic apple cider vinegar and raw honey. The vinegar neutralizes the odor and taste of the garlic. Once you experience how well this works, you'll make it a part of your standard home herbal remedy chest.

Garlic Bulb/Seed (Allium sativum)

Used primarily for its antibiotic effect.

Throat Soothing Syrup

In a base of honey and glycerin, this syrup is wonderful for sore throats and is also useful for laryngitis.

Balm of Gilead (Populus gileadensis)

Soothes, disinfects and astringes mucous membranes. Specific for laryngitis, coughs, and sore throat.

Coltsfoot (Tussilago farfara)

Soothing expectorant, demulcent, antispasmodic, astringent, anti-inflammatory. For irritating coughs, bronchitis, asthma laryngitis, throat catarrh.

Echinacea Root (Echinacea angustifolia)

Powerful immune stimulant; antiseptic, antimicrobial; antiviral; used for sore throats, flu, colds, infections.

Propolis

Antiseptic, antibacterial. Waxy nature makes it useful for coating and isolating areas of throat inflammation to prevent spread of infection and to bind the other ingredients to the throat for longer lasting effect.

Slippery Elm (Ulmus rhubra)

Nutritive, reduces inflammation, soothes mucus membranes.

Continued ➜

Salves/Balms

Salves are useful as topical healing agents. For wounds, they should generally be used as a skin dressing after a scab has formed. Otherwise, the body might retain bacteria underneath, leading to infection. Wash the wound and apply an antiseptic first. Salves and balms work particularly well on bruises, sprains, strains, and to otherwise decongest tissue.

Bruise Salve

Arnica Flower (Arnica Cordifolia)

External Use Only. Topical use for bruises, sprains, strains, and other athletic injuries, including swelling. Use on unbroken skin.

Calendula Flower (Calendula officinalis)

Anti-inflammatory; astringent; styptic; antifungal. Use topically for wounds, ulcers, burns, abscesses.

St. John's Wort (Hypericum perforatum)

Used externally for bruises, strains, sprains, contusions, wounds. Speeds wound and burn healing.

Bug Repelling Salve

To discourage insects from trespassing on your body. The following essential oils are all known for their insect-repellent properties. Carried in a base of olive oil and beeswax.

Citronella (Ceylonese or Javanese)

Eucalyptus (Eucalyptus citriodora)

Lavender (Lavandula officinalis)

Pennyroyal (Mentha pelugium)

Muscle-Easing Salve

In a base of olive oil and beeswax. A deep heating rub for muscle tension, soreness, sprains, and strains.

Arnica Flower (Arnica cordifolia)

External Use Only. Topical use for bruises, sprains, strains and other athletic injuries, including swelling. Use on unbroken skin.

Cajeput (Melaleuca leucadendron)

Analgesic (pain relieving).

Camphor (Cinnamomum camphora)

Analgesic, antispasmodic, antineuralgic, anti-rheumatic.

Cayenne Fruit (Capsicum frutescens)

Stimulates circulation, reduces tissue congestion. Creates heat.

Menthol (Mentha arvensis) Isolate

Cooling, anti-inflammatory, analgesic.

St. John's Wort (Hypericum perforatum)

Oil used externally for bruises, strains, sprains, contusions, wounds.

Wintergreen (Methyl salycilate) Derivative

Analgesic.

Skin-Soothing Salve

A soothing blend of skin-healing herbs in an olive oil and beeswax base.

Calendula Flower (Calendula officinalis)

Anti-inflammatory; astringent; styptic; antifungal; topically for wounds, ulcers, burns, abcesses.

Cayenne Fruit (Capsicum frutescens)

Stimulates circulation, reduces tissue congestion. Creates heat.

Chickweed Herb (Stellaria media)

Restorative; soothing demulcent.

Comfrey Root/Leaf (Symphytum officinalis)

External Use. Speeds healing of sprains, strains, fractures and surface wounds.

Goldenseal Root (Hydrastis Canadensis)

Antiseptic, used topically for infection.

Mallow (Malva rotundifolia)

Speeds healing. Astringent, demulcent, emollient, anti-inflammatory.

Plantain Leaf (Plantago spp.)

Astringent; used for external wounds and sores, insect bites.

St. John's Wort (Hypericum perforatum)

Used externally for bruises, strains, sprains, contusions, wounds. Antibacterial, speeds wound and burn healing.

Vapor Decongestant Salve

Herbal sister to Vick's VaporRub, using olive oil and beeswax instead of petroleum. Use as a decongestant rub, in steam vaporizers or smear on a tissue and inhale to decongest sinuses.

Camphor (Cinnamomum camphora)

Analgesic, antispasmodic, antineuralgia, antirheumatic.

Clove (Eugenia caryophyllata)

Stimulating antiseptic.

Lavender (Lavandula officinalis)

Antiseptic, decongestant, calming, antispasmodic.

Menthol (Mentha arvensis) Isolate

Cooling, anti-inflammatory, analgesic.

Peppermint (Mentha piperita)

Cooling, decongesting, pain relieving.

St. John's Wort (Hypericum perforatum)

Oil used externally for bruises, strains, sprains, contusions, wounds.

Wintergreen (Methyl salycilate) Derivative

Cooling, fragrant analgesic.

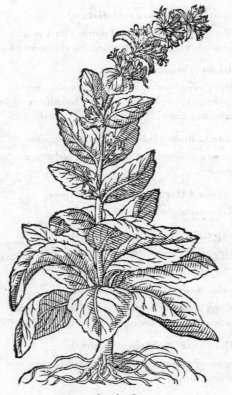

Comfrey Root

Ear Oil Formula

A soothing, antiseptic, antibiotic oil which is phenomenally effective in the treatment of both acute and chronic ear infections. Contra-indicated in cases of eardrum perforation.

Calendula Flower (Calendula officinalis)

Anti-inflammatory; astringent; antifungal.

Garlic Bulb/Seed (Allium sativum)

Antibiotic; antimicrobial; antiseptic; antiviral.

Mullein Leaf (Verbascum thapsus)

Anti-inflammatory, soothing.

St. John's Wort (Hypericum perforatum)

Soothing, healing, activates immune response.

Common Problems/Natural Remedies

This list is compiled for educational purposes. The remedies are suggestions only and are not intended as a substitute for professional assistance when needed.

Abrasions: Wash well, then apply an antiseptic spray or skin soothing salve. Bandage if necessary.

Abscesses: Infection Formula, Lymph Formula, Detox Formula, vitamin C. Eat plenty of Garlic and drink distilled water.

Acne: Healthy Skin Formula (internally and externally), Detox Formula, Liver Formula. External—vapor steam of Lemon, Lavender, Geranium and Chamomile essential oils; fresh application of Aloe vera.

Air Sickness: See *Motion Sickness*.

Anemia: Iron Formula, eat plenty of dark leafy greens.

Anxiety: Stress Formula, Adrenal Formula, Children's Calming Glycerite Formula, Essential Tranquility, or Balance aromatherapy inhalers. Dietary calcium, and B complex.

Arthritis: Joint Formula.

Asthma: Asthma Formula, Bronchial Formula, Stress Formula. (Please dissipate alcohol before using.)

Athlete's Foot: See *Fungal Infections*.

Bee Sting: Infection Formula, Antiseptic Spray Formula, Plantain, Comfrey or Clay Poultices; Papain powder, Honey.

Bladder Infections: Kidney Formula, Infection Formula, Cranberry juice or extract; plenty of vitamin C.

Bloody Nose: Apply pressure on either side of the nose. Apply cold compresses to the sinuses. Dampen a piece of gauze with water, dip it into powdered Yarrow or Horsetail, and insert into nostril. Apply strong pressure with your fingernail to the outside corner of the base of the little "pinkie" fingernail which is on the same side as the nostril which is bleeding.

Bronchitis: Onion Poultice, Infection Formula, Bronchial Formula, Expectorant Formula, Expectorant Syrup, Ginger Fomentation, Vapor Steam; plenty of vitamin C.

Bruises: Muscle/Bruise Liniment Formula, Bruise Salve, fresh Comfrey Leaf Poultice.

Burns (minor): FIRST immerse the burned area in ice cold water or apply ice, then treat with one of

Continued →

the following: fresh Aloe Vera leaf, Burn Spray Formula, Dr. Christopher's Burn Ointment (see Natural Therapies section), or vitamin E.

Chapped Lips and Skin: Skin-Soothing Salve.

Chiggers: Bug Salve or Spray, Echinacea extract, Infection Formula.

Cold Sores: Osha' Root extract or Infection Formula applied externally; Antiviral Formula internally. Supplement with nonacidic vitamin C, Acidophilus and Garlic (antibiotic).

Colds/Flu: Onion Horseradish Vinegar Formula, Infection Formula, Antiviral Formula, Immune Formula, Echinacea extract, Immune Formula, Miso soup, Peppermint tea, distilled water, Laxative Formula if constipated, Pain Formula for aches and pain, and plenty of REST!

Colic: Children's Calming Glycerite Formula, Digestive Formula; Peppermint or mild Ginger tea.

Computer Stress Syndrome: Computer Stress Formula, Stress Formula, Rejuvenation Formula, Adrenal Formula; supplement with B vitamins, sea vegetables in diet. Grow Spider plants in your office to decrease ambient radiation.

Constipation: Laxative formula; drink more water! Eat more fresh fruits and vegetables and more dietary fiber in the form of whole grains, psyllium, and flax seed. Eat less meat. Drink 2 tsp. sea salt in 1 qt. warm water on an empty stomach upon arising in the morning. Do not eat until the bowel has evacuated. Warm water enema.

Coughing: You can make a cough syrup from the Infection Formula (or any appropriate herbal extract for that matter), simply by adding honey or glycerin. Try Expectorant Formula, Cough Formula, Bronchial Formula, Cough Syrup, Garlic Syrup.

Cradle Cap; Brush the scalp gently in a circular motion with a wet baby brush dipped in shampoo. Rinse out the scales as you loosen them. Supplement the diet with Oatstraw, Nettle, Chamomile, Alfalfa, or Horsetail tea.

Cramps: Menstrual or muscular, try Cramp Formula, Ginger Fomentation, and/or Castor Oil pack. Add dietary calcium.

Cuts: See *Wounds*.

Dandruff: Healthy Skin Formula, supplement with essential fatty acids, B vitamins, Acidophilus, Sea vegetables.

Depression: Essential Joy aromatherapy inhaler, St. John's Wort extract, Stress Formula, PMS Formula, Menopause Formula, Rejuvenation Formula; supplement with B complex vitamins.

Diarrhea: As with vomiting, let the body do its work first, and only if the person becomes weak or dehydrated should you stop the process. *Do* supplement with fluids and electrolytes. Potassium rich, potato-peeling broth is helpful—wash an organic potato and cut thickly into the skin, forming peels 1/2" thick. Put into distilled water if available, simmer for 20 minutes covered, and drink. Miso soup is also good. Try Digestive Formula to increase digestion. Black Cherry juice (high in iron) is helpful, also Red Raspberry leaf tea.

Dysentery: Parasite Formula, Detox Formula, Liver Formula; Get professional diagnosis and assistance.

Earaches: Mullein-Garlic Oil. Warm oil, put 4–5 drops in ear, stuff with cotton. Onion Poultice, or Castor Oil pack. (Caution: Not to be used in cases of eardrum perforation!)

Emergency First Aid

Breathing, bleeding, and shock are the first priorities in emergency first-aid situations. Stay calm and analyze the situation, then assist. (You can take a homeopathic flower remedy here.)

Breathing: Take a class in CPR (cardiopulmonary resuscitation) at your local Red Cross. It's worth it!

Bleeding: Direct pressure on the wound helps stop the blood flow, as do styptic herbs such as Yarrow and Horsetail. Make sure the wound has been thoroughly flushed with blood, soap and water or an antiseptic solution before you encourage it to close and heal, otherwise, you will seal the bacteria inside and risk infection.

Shock: Keep the patient warm and elevate their legs. Flower essence remedies such as Rescue Remedy or Flowers formula are helpful to keep the person (and you) calm and level headed. The Essential Rescue aromatherapy inhaler is also useful. Do not give fluids to someone who is in shock.

Eczema: Eczema Formula, Healthy Skin Formula; essential fatty acid supplementation.

Eye Infections: Clear Eyes Formula, Eyewash Kit (see instructions in Therapies section). Infection Formula.

Fatigue: Iron Formula, Rejuvenation Formula, Adrenal Formula, Computer Stress Formula; supplement with B complex. Rest!

Fevers: First give the fever a chance to do its work. Give plenty of fluids such as Peppermint tea and distilled water. Each fever is different; pay attention and watch its pattern. Over 102° indicates need for professional consultation. Try Pain Formula, Infection Formula, Elder/Peppermint/Yarrow tea (equal parts), Ginger baths.

Fingernail Problems: Healthy Skin Formula; Horsetail extract. Supplement with B complex.

Flatulence: Use Digestive Formula immediately after meals. Better food combining. Better preparation procedure in cooking beans (soak overnight, add Apple Cider Vinegar, Savory). Digestive enzymes.

Fleas: Bug Formula Spray or Salve; supplement with Garlic, B complex.

Fluid Retention: Diuretic Formula, PMS Formula. Dandelion extract.

Foreign Particle in Eye: Place a Q-Tip on top of the eyelid. Hold it there while you gently grasp the eyelashes and roll the eyelid inside out over the Q-Tip. This should allow you to see and retrieve any foreign particles with another Q-Tip. Put a chia or flax seed in corner of eye. Mucilage formed by the moistened seed will carry out foreign particle. Use Eyewash kit.

Fungal Infections: For athlete's foot, jock itch, ringworm, etc. Use Antifungal Spray Formula on affected area. (Be careful, it will stain clothing.) For ringworm, soak a small piece of cotton with the formula and tape on. Reapply fresh solution at least twice daily. Internal fungal infections such as candidiasis, use 1 dropperful Antifungal Formula 3 times daily. Get a good book on Candida and incorporate its dietary guidelines.

Gas: See *Flatulence*.

Giardia: Parasite Formula (Get professional diagnostic assistance); eat plenty of Garlic.

Gum Problems: Dental poultice packs, Tooth-care kit, Fresh Breath Gum Tonic; supplement with vitamin C.

Halitosis: Fresh Breath Gum Tonic; Digestive Formula; supplement with Chlorophyll. Have dental examination for tooth decay. Colon cleansing program.

Headaches: They appear for different reasons and need to be treated differently. Try Pain Formula, Ginger Fomentation to abdomen, Digestive Formula, Laxative Formula, or chiropractic adjustment. Document when they happen and what your lifestyle was like immediately preceding the onset. Check diet, constipation, fluid intake, exposure to environmental toxins, stress level, etc. For chronic headaches, half the battle is identifying what triggers it and avoiding that stimulus.

Hemorrhoids: Fresh Aloe suppositories (see *Aloe* in Natural Therapies section). There are many other natural remedies.

Herpes: Add dietary lysine (blue corn is rich in lysine and will help strengthen the body's ability to fight the virus); apply Infection Formula internally and directly to lesion, several of the herbs in it are antiviral.

Hiccups: Take a deep breath and drink water until you burp. Try Digestive Formula or a small amount of Pain Formula for their antispasmodic and carminative herbs.

Hives: Stress Formula; Allergy Formula, Nettle extract (Make sure to dissipate alcohol); supplement with B complex, Calcium, vitamin A.

Hot Flashes: Female Glandular Formula, Black Cohosh root extract.

Hyper/Hypo Thyroid: Sea Vegetables, Computer Stress Formula.

Indigestion: Digestive Formula, Peppermint tea or extract.

Infections, swollen glands: Infection Formula, Immune Formula, Lymph Formula, Echinacea extract, Horseradish Onion Formula, Eat raw Garlic or Garlic chives. Onion Poultice, Ginger Fomentation, Castor Oil pack. Rest!

Insect Bites: Infection Formula, Antiseptic Spray Formula, Plantain, Comfrey or Clay poultices; Papain powder; Vinegar; a dab of Muscle or Bruise salve.

Insomnia: Sleep Formula; Calcium supplements 1/2 hour before bedtime (also useful to help prevent nighttime leg cramps in pregnant women).

Itching: Itch-Ease Spray Formula, Allergy Formula.

Jet Lag: Essential Rescue or Essential Balance aromatherapy inhaler; Rejuvenation Formula (Sleep Formula helps when normal sleep time is altered).

Laryngitis: Infection Formula, Throat Extract/Spray Formula, Vapor steam, Castor Oil Pack on neck.

Libido, Lack of: Female or Male Glandular Formulas, Rejuvenation Formula, Chaste Berry extract, Essential Aphrodisiac aromatherapy inhaler.

Liver Congestion: Liver Formula, Detox Formula.

Continued ➡

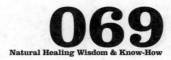

Lung Congestion: Expectorant Extract and Syrup Formulas, Bronchial Formula. Drink plenty of water, avoid dairy products. Vapor steam with vapor salve or essential oil of Eucalyptus or Sage in hot water.

Lymphatic Congestion: Lymph Formula.

Mastitis: Infection Formula, Lymph Formula; poultice of moistened, powdered or freshly ground Marshmallow root. Drink plenty of fluid; if lactating, continue nursing.

Memory, Poor: Clear Thought Formula, Essential Memory or Basil aromatherapy inhalers.

Menopause: Menopause Formula.

Menstrual Cramps: See *Cramps.*

Migraine: See *Headache.*

Morning Sickness: See *Nausea.* A chiropractic therapy is to close the ileocecal valve through external pressure manipulation. Ginger tea (sometimes contraindicated in pregnancy, although it saved me during my two!)

Motion Sickness: Nausea Formula, Ginger extract or plain Peppermint tea. Essential Rescue or Clary Sage aromatherapy inhaler.

Mumps: Antiviral Formula, Lymph Formula, Immune Formula; plenty of liquid, and vitamin C.

Muscle Aches: Muscle Liniment Spray Formula, Muscle salve Arnica or St. John's Wort extract.

Muscle Cramps: See *Cramps.*

Nausea: Nausea Formula, Digestive Formula, Ginger extract, or Peppermint tea.

Nervousness: Stress Formula, Calming Children's Glycerite Formula, Valerian Root extract; Essential Tranquility or Balance aromatherapy inhaler; supplement with B complex, essential fatty acids, calcium.

Nipples, cracked: Skin-Soothing Salve; supplement diet with essential fatty acids.

Pain: As obtuse as "headache." Try Pain Formula; supplement with calcium.

Parasites: Parasite Formula. Eat lots of Garlic and Pumpkin seeds. Giardia and amoebic infestation require special help. See a holistic practitioner.

PMS: PMS Formula.

Poison Ivy: Itch-EaseSpray Formula. See *Dermatitis.*

Ringworm: See *Fungal Infections.*

Scabies: Try Tea Tree oil soap. Bug Spray Formula. Ayurvedic medicine has some promising therapies; study.

Sinus Congestion: Professor Cayenne's Formula; Decongestant Heat Lamp Therapy (see Therapies); Vapor steam, inhale Vapor salve, salt water flush; sniff fresh Horseradish (deeply!), Essential Breath aromatherapy inhaler. Increase fluids, avoid dairy products.

Skin Rashes/Diaper Rash: Clay Poultice, Skin-Soothing Salve, Chamomile or Calendula tea wash.

Smashed Fingers/Toes: Muscle Liniment Spray, Muscle-Bruise Salve, Arnica or St. John's Wort extract.

Smoking Addiction: Smoking Formula; Stress Formula, Detox Formula, Expectorant Formula. Essential Freedom aromatherapy inhaler. Supplement with B Complex and vitamin C.

Sore Throat: Squirt Throat Extract/Spray back into the throat; Slippery Elm Lozenges; Onion Poultice, Ginger Fomentation.

Splinters and other small foreign objects (e.g., glass): If you can't get it out with tweezers, try a Plantain or Clay Poultice. Pine tar is helpful in cases where lots of small splinters are clustered in the skin. Smear it on. Splinters will pull out as you pull it off. Make sure you put some Antiseptic Formula on after you are finished.

Sprains/Swelling: Ice; Muscle/Bruise Salve or Liniment Spray; fresh Comfrey leaf Poultice, Arnica or St. John's Wort extract.

Stings: From ocean critters such as Portuguese Man-ofwar and jellyfish—First, urinate on the affected area; the ammonia in the urine will immediately relieve the sting. Then use a soothing mucilaginous herb like Comfrey Root or Slippery Elm to soothe and heal the area. (You can crush a Slippery Elm lozenge in an emergency.)

Stress: Stress Formula, Computer Stress Formula, Adrenal Formula, Reishi/Shiitake Formula; Essential Tranquility or Essential Rescue aromatherapy inhalers.

Styes: Herbal eyewash kit, Clear Eyes Formula, Infection Formula; vitamin C.

Sunburn: Aloe Burn Spray Formula, Dr. Christopher's Burn Ointment (see Therapies section), fresh Aloe vera.

Tapeworms: See *Parasites.*

Teething Pain: Pain Formula, Osha' extract rubbed on the gum. Children's Calming Glycerite Formula.

Tension: See *Stress.*

Thrush: Swab mouth with Antifungal Formula or use Antifungal Spray (stronger, contains Tea Tree oil).

Ticks: Hold incense near back of its body; tick will usually back out to get away from heat. Use Antiseptic Spray afterwards.

Toothache: Dental Poultice Pack, follow directions on pack; Cotton soaked with Osha' Root or Clove Oil.

Ulcers: Slippery Elm (make a paste with Slippery Elm powder and eat it; it will help coat the stomach and relieve pain). Cayenne (one or two capsules, twice per day). There are many other natural therapies; consult the reference section and study.

Urinary Tract Infections: See *Bladder infections.*

Vaginal infections: Goldenseal (antiseptic), Slippery Elm (to soothe), Tea Tree oil (in a pessary form to disinfect and slow fungal infections. Goldenseal powder can be used alone to make a douche). Buy some *plain* yogurt or use acidophilus capsules. A total program for vaginal infections is as follows: First use a Goldenseal douche, then insert a pessary (herbs in a cocoa butter base molded into a bullet shape—best to use are Goldenseal and Marshmallow). Be sure to wear a pad to prevent staining; leave it in overnight. Douche again with Goldenseal in the morning, and if the infection is advanced, insert another pessary for the balance of the day. In the evening, douche with Goldenseal, then insert *plain* yogurt or acidophilus capsule and leave in through the night. Alternate the douche and yogurt implant in this manner until the infection is gone. In the meantime, increase vitamin C, use a balanced vitamin supplement. Also try Vaginitis Formula.

Varicose Veins: Vein Formula; relieve pelvic congestion with Laxative Formula, PMS Formula, Diuretic Formula, Ocotillo extract. Supplement with vitamin C.

Viral Infections: Antiviral Formula, Osha' Root extract; supplement with vitamin C.

Vomiting: To induce: Lobelia extract (10–60 drops, depending entirely on the person's reaction to it and the amount of food in the stomach; rest assured, the body will tell you when it has had enough); Syrup of Ipecac.

Vomiting: To stop: 1–3 drops of Lobelia extract. (Keep in mind that the body is trying to rid itself of something it doesn't want, and respect its innate intelligence in purging itself.) Raspberry or Ginger extracts will soothe the digestive system, Nettle extract will help replenish lost nutrients. Potato peeling-broth and electrolyte replacement is a good idea if the patient can keep them down.

Warts: Topical: Banana Peel Poultice, Therapies section, Cedar oil; apply Apple Cider Vinegar then follow with fresh Milkweed juice. Antiviral Formula internally and externally.

Worms: See *Parasites.*

Wounds: Encourage initial bleeding, cleanse well, then spray with antiseptic formula. Use salves only after the wound has scabbed over, otherwise you could seal over the wound before it has had time to discharge all the harmful bacteria.

Yeast Infections: See *Vaginal infections, Fungal infections.*

Natural Therapies

The value of the skills learned in this section will be apparent in lower medical bills as well as a greater sense of personal power in your own health care. A stuffy nose or a fever is manageable without a trip to the pharmacy, and athlete's foot is controllable without harsh chemicals. If you are a visually oriented learner, these therapies are shown step by step in my video, *Herbal Preparations and Natural Therapies—Creating and Using a Home Herbal Medicine Chest.*

Simple Plantain Poultice

Plantain is one of many wayside plants that is an invaluable first aid for cuts, scrapes, bee stings and burns. It is called Nature's Band-Aid with good reason, having also the distinct advantage of being found nearly everywhere. It is well known for its ability to draw out glass and other objects that get deeply imbedded in the skin as well as simple splinters. Just make sure you gather it in a clean area where there is no traffic or animal pollution.

Fresh Comfrey Poultice

Comfrey is one of the most important plants to grow indoors as a first aid source. There are many stories which attest to the healing power of this plant, the principal ingredient of which, allantoin, is a cell proliferative. It is most useful as an external poultice to heal burns, stings, wounds and muscular sprains. Comfrey has traditionally been used to heal bone fractures.

Because it contains some potentially toxic alkaloids, it is best to take it internally only under the guidance of a competent herbalist or wholistic practitioner.

Ingredients: Fresh Comfrey leaves
Distilled water

Equipment: Blender or mortar and pestle
Gauze diaper (the thin birds'-eye kind)
Roll of gauze

Continued ➡

Poultices

A poultice is the application of plant materials (or clay) to the skin. It can be made from either fresh or dried herbs. Poultices are used to soothe, heal, regenerate tissue, stimulate circulation and organ function, warm and relax muscles, and draw out toxins or foreign particles.

Procedure: Pick the Comfrey leaves, rinse and shake them dry, then blend with enough distilled water to create a thick mash. Place in a gauze diaper, and apply to the treatment area, wrapping it with the gauze to hold it in place. Occasionally you will see a skin rash developing due to small hairs that are found on the leaves. I have seen this in instances where the comfrey was applied directly to the skin. The gauze diaper should prevent this, however if the irritation persists, discontinue use, or, if it is not an open wound, smear a little olive oil on the area to be treated first. (If you need to, a poultice can also be made from the Comfrey root powder in the burn kit; see Dr. Christopher's Burn Ointment.)

Clay Poultice

Clay has been used to draw out toxins and foreign substances, heal burns and repair damaged tissue. Its virtues are endless and deserve study. In the beginning, start out with a simple green clay and observe the effects of the poultice.

Ingredients: 1 lb. pure green clay (Cattier is a good brand)
Distilled water (set ½ cup of clay powder aside for the face mask)

Equipment: Deep nonmetal bowl
Wooden spoon
Diaper or handkerchief
Cotton gauze

Procedure: Mix the clay with enough water to make a thick paste, spread with the spoon onto center of a thin gauze diaper or handkerchief in an area approximately 6" x 8" and 1" thick. Apply the clay directly to the part of the body to be treated, pressing it into the flesh so that it adheres. Cover with gauze and leave it on until the clay pulls away on its own accord, indicating that the therapy is completed. For more information on clays, please read *The Healing Clay* by Michel Abehsera.

Onion Poultice

This poultice is used in cases of deep lung congestion and bronchial inflammation. It brings penetrating relief to that annoying itch of the lungs when it hurts too much to cough. It is also used over the ear and lymph glands to treat ear infections.

Ingredients: 3 large fresh onions (organically grown if possible)
Distilled water

Equipment: Large glass or cast-iron skillet
2 diapers or small towels
2 large towels
Rubber gloves
Wooden spoon or tongs

Procedure: Slice onions thinly and sauté them, covered, in a small amount of distilled water until transparent. Fold half of onions into a diaper so the finished pack is approximately 8" x 8". Apply to the chest as hot as the patient can stand it and immediately cover it with the towels to retain the heat. Begin preparing the next poultice. When the first one is cool, immediately replace it with the

2nd. After the therapy, gently dry the chest and tuck the patient into bed to rest. Use the same procedure for the ear, except make the poultice smaller.

Aloe Vera

This is one of the most useful first-aid plants to grow indoors Simply peel the outer structure of the leaf away to expose the inner gel, and wipe on minor burns, sunburns, cuts, scrapes, etc. You can also cut the inner gel into a suppository-size pellet and insert into the rectum as a hemorrhoid suppository.

Dr. Christopher's Burn Ointment

This formula has healed thousands of burns, and is unique in that it is not removed from the site of the injury, but is left on until the skin is completely healed. The Wheat Germ oil, Comfrey root, and Honey literally "feed" the tissue, soothing and promoting cell regeneration. It must be made fresh at the time it is needed, as it does not store well (turns into a blob of hard black goo). I highly recommend that you keep this in your medicine kit—just store the Wheat Germ oil and Honey in one container, and the Comfrey powder in another, then mix as needed.

Procedure: Stir equal parts Comfrey root powder, Wheat Germ oil, and Honey together and apply liberally to the burn. Wrap in gauze to hold it on, replenish as necessary. Carry on with the treatment until the burn is completely healed and it will prevent scarring. If you get tired of wearing a bandage, you can start putting Wheat Germ or vitamin E alone on the burn after most of the healing work has been accomplished by the ointment. This period is identified by absence of pain and general tissue healing to the point that the skin has reformed and closed with a scab or pinkish-red skin. Keep applying the oil on a daily basis until you cannot identify where the burn was.

Banana Peel Poultice for Warts

This therapy is easy. Look for brown-black bananas, the kind the grocer sells for 25 cents a pound. Take a section of the peel and place the inside part on the wart. Bind with roll gauze and leave on overnight, removing in the morning and replacing each night until the wart is gone.

Removing Moles

This therapy is not herbal, but it works so well I had to include it. I learned this method of removing moles from a macrobiotic cook, and have had 100% success with it. You first must be working with a mole that is protruding far enough to tie a hair around. Human hair works best, but fine unwaxed dental floss will also work. Simply tie the hair or floss into a circle and loop the end around an extra couple of times as if you are tying shoes. This causes it to hold its position when you tighten it. Loop it carefully around the mole and pull it snugly, but not too tightly at first. Tighten each day until the mole drops off for lack of circulation.

Caution: If the mole is black or there is any other indication of abnormality, consult a qualified practitioner before commencing this therapy.

Ginger Fomentation

This fomentation is especially good for cramps.

Ingredients: 1 cup fresh, grated Ginger root
2 quarts distilled water

Equipment: 4-quart saucepan
Cheesecloth
Rubber band
Thick diaper or cloth towels
Large bath towels

Fomentations

Fomentations are either infusions or decoctions (depending on which part of the plant is used), in which a cloth is soaked to be applied to parts of the body needing therapy. Fomentations stimulate circulation, aid in decongestion, and can be soothing to external tissue.

Procedure: Place Ginger root into cheesecloth, gather into a loose pouch, and secure with a rubber band. Put the bag into the water and bring mixture to a boil, then reduce to a simmer. Simmer for 15 minutes (covered), remove from heat, and strain. Carry the hot strained tea in a covered vessel to the patient's side. Dip a thick cloth such as a diaper into the tea. (Wearing plastic gloves will help.) Wring the cloth out and fan it in the air until it can be tested on the inside of your arm without scalding. It should be applied as hot as the patient can stand it, then covered with two towels to retain the heat as long as possible. After the cloth has cooled, remove and resoak, then reapply as before. Remember to keep the vessel covered between dippings to keep the liquid hot.

Decongesting Heat-Lamp Therapy

This simple therapy is incredibly effective for sinuses that are so stuffed that you can't breathe through your nose at all and can't sleep. Just get an ordinary aluminum mechanic's light with a spring clip that is commonly available in most department stores. Install a heat-lamp bulb in it. Clip it above you so that it can shine down on your sinuses. Cover your eyes, turn it on, and let the heat penetrate and decongest the area. Ahhhhh.

Cold Compress

This preparation is useful in preventing swelling and reducing fevers. It stimulates the production of both white and red blood cells and reduces the pulse rate. A decoction or infusion is prepared, allowed to cool and applied with a cloth as in the fomentation above.

Peppermint Cooling Compress

Ingredients: ½ cup Peppermint leaves
1 quart distilled water
Ice cubes

Equipment: 1-quart saucepan
Measuring cup
Thick diaper or cloth
Towel

Procedure: Pour boiling water over Peppermint leaves, cover, and let steep for 10 minutes, strain and cool. When tea is lukewarm put it in the freezer or add ice cubes to make it really cold, then take to the patient. Soak a cloth in the tea and apply to the patient. The cloth should be wrung out so that it does not drip yet still retains enough liquid to stay cold. If the cloth warms up resoak and reapply. Repeat this procedure three to five times, adding ice cubes if necessary, then dry the area thoroughly.

Decongestant Vapors

Ingredients: Muscle Ease salve formula or Eucalyptus oil
1 quart distilled water

Equipment: 4-quart glass or enameled pot
Towels
Headband

Continued ➜

Procedure: Boil water, remove from heat, take a toothpick and scrape out a bit of Muscle salve (try a little at first, you can always add more), stir into the pan of water. Breathe in vapor while covering head with a towel to trap steam. (Caution: Steam burns are exceedingly unpleasant, so test the heat of the steam carefully with your hand before exposing your face.)

Cleansing Facial Steam

Ingredients: Lavender, Rosebud, and Chamomile flowers (½ cup of mixture)
I quart distilled water

Equipment: 4-quart glass or enameled pot
Towels
Headband

Procedure: Boil water, remove from heat, add herbs, stir into the pan of water. Let your face bathe in the vapor while covering head with a towel to trap steam. (See caution above.)

```
Vapors and Steams
```

These preparations are useful for decongesting the lungs and detoxifying the skin. A vapor is prepared by dropping essential oils into freshly boiled distilled water, and a steam is essentially an infusion with the herbs left in it.

Herbal Eyewash

This eyewash is for tired, strained, or infected eyes. It cleanses the tear ducts and stimulates circulation, which contributes to its fame as a vision restorative.

Ingredients: I tablespoon herb mixture: Eyebright, Red Raspberry, Fennel, Goldenseal, Bayberry
I cup distilled water

Equipment: I-quart saucepan
Eyecup
Filter
White paper towels or straining cloth
2 bowls
Ladle

Procedure: Boil water, take vessel from stove, add one tablespoon herb mix, let steep (covered), for 10 minutes. While the eyewash is steeping, sterilize the eyecup by boiling. Strain tea through a filter, cool till lukewarm. At this time the strained tea should be poured into a cup measure with a pour spout so that you can keep the batch sterile as you fill the eyecup (as opposed to dipping the eyecup in the solution to fill it). Fill the eye cup with the cooled solution, look down as you place it on your eye, then tip your head back, letting the solution wash the eye as you blink several times. It is helpful to hold a folded paper towel under the eye as you do this, to catch drips. Pour used solution into separate container and refill eyecup. Apply to same eye three separate times, then resterilize eyecup (this will prevent contamination of second eye) and repeat procedure on other eye. Eyewash should be made fresh each treatment as it does not store well in the refrigerator.

Castor Oil Pack

This is a remedy popularized by the late Edgar Cayce, and has proved very useful in stimulating deep tissue and organ healing. It has drawing power up to 4" deep in the tissue, and is used for deep infection, congestion and old, hard-to-heal injuries.

Ingredients: 6 ounces castor oil
I teaspoon baking soda dissolved into:
I pint cool water

Equipment: Wool flannel cloth
Plastic sheet (a trash bag will do)
Hot-water bottle or electric heating pad
Large bath towel

Procedure: Warm the castor oil by placing the bottle in a pan of hot water. Fold the flannel so that it is 4 layers thick with a surface area of approximately 10" x 14". Lay it on the plastic sheet and pour oil the warmed oil so that it is thoroughly saturated but not dripping. Apply flannel to the area to be treated and cover with the plastic sheet, then place the heating source on top. If using the heating pad, turn it to medium, then increase it to high if the patient can tolerate it. Leave it on for 1–8 hours. If using the hot water bottle, fill it ¾ full (not totally full or it won't curve around the body), place over sheet, and cover with a towel. Change water periodically to keep hot

When the therapy is complete, remove the pack and cleanse the skin with the mixture of baking soda and water. Store the wool flannel in a plastic bag or glass jar in the refrigerator for further use. If it is not stored in the refrigerator it can go rancid.

Dosages, Weights, and Measures

Dosages

Always a sticky subject due to personal metabolism, dietary habits, stress levels, and other vagaries of our individual bodies, dosage guidelines are nevertheless important. Well put in Felter's *Materia Medica*, vol. 1, "It is better to err on the side of insufficient dosage and trust to nature, than to overdose to the present or future harm or danger to the patient." In other words, try a little and watch for the patient's reaction before you give a lot. In my own body (and truly, this is my best teacher), I take a dropperful every hour if I am fighting off an acute infection, and usually take a dropperful per day in chronic problems. The dose also depends on the potency of the preparation, so the variables are endless. If one is sensitive enough, and listens well to one's own body, the dosage should be apparent.

If you have any questions after researching the excellent sources in the book list, by all means see a competent holistic practitioner who can help you figure it out. The following is a list of comparative children's dosages.

Cowling's rule: Divide the age at the next birthday by 24. (Example: A five-year-old child—six being the age at the next birthday—divide 6 by 24 which gives you $^6/_{24}$ or ¼ the adult dose.)

Clark's rule: Divide the weight (in lbs.) of the child by 150 to give the approximate fraction of the adult dose. (Example: A 50 lb. child will require $^{50}/_{150}$ or ⅓ the adult dose.)

Young's rule: Computed by dividing the child's age by 12 plus the age. (Thus for a child of 4 years, it would be 4 divided by 12 +4 = $^4/_{16}$ = ¼ of the adult dosage.)

Weights and Measures

Liquid Equivalents (Volume)

I oz. = 29.57 ml.

I pt. = 16 oz. = 473.3 ml.

I qt. = 2 pt. = 4 cups = 32 oz. = 946.6 ml.

I gal. = 4 qts. = 8 pts. = 16 cups = 128 oz. = 3,784.95 ml.

Solid Equivalents (Weight)

I oz. = 28.4 gr.

I lb. = 16 oz. = 453.6 gr.

I kg. = 2.2 lb. = 35.2 oz. = 1,000 gr.

Herbal Extract Measurements

The following information will be useful in dispensing herbal extracts and determining how long a bottle will last, depending on the dosage specified.

Rubber stoppers sometimes give the extract a rubbery taste, and some people prefer to use extracts that are not stored with the dropper. Therefore I am including the dosage measurements by the teaspoon as well as by drops or droppers full.

Accuracy of measurement is difficult when prescribing drops (minims). Twenty drops of one extract may not equal the volume of a different extract due to glycerin content, sediment, manufacturer's design, etc. Water forms a larger droplet, while a droplet of single herbal extract is smaller. A combination extract that contains vegetable glycerin also changes the volume, as noted on the next page.

10 ml water = 265–291 drops, depending on speed of expulsion.
10 ml. single extract of Osha' Rt = 440 drops.
10 ml. combination extract = 447 drops.

Two-ounce bottles have longer droppers and contain more fluid per filling than the one-ounce dropper.

1 oz. size = approximately 30 drops per dropper.
2 oz. size = approximately 40 drops per dropper.

One-Ounce Bottle (Single or combination extract):

· Holds *approximately* 29.57 ml. of fluid.

· 4 ml. = I teaspoonful

· I dropperful = *approximately* I ml. = approx. ¼ teaspoon

· I oz. bottle holds *approximately* 7.4 teaspoons

· Average 30–40 drops (minims) per glass dropper (I oz. size)

· *Approximately* 29.5 droppersful per bottle

· *Approximately* 1,000–1,200 drops per bottle, depending on formula constituents.

· At a quantity of "one dropperful, three times daily," a one-ounce bottle would last approximately 10 days.

· At a quantity of "twenty drops, three times daily," a one-ounce bottle would last approximately 18 days.

—From *Pocket Herbal Reference Guide*

Continued ➡

HERBAL FIRST AID

Nancy Evelyn
Illustrations by Alice Muhlback

Ointments

Ointments are always used externally as dressings for skin irritations, bruises, abrasions, cuts, blisters, and the like. The benefit of using an ointment is that the base of the ointment is soothing and adds to the comfort of healing.

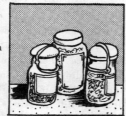

When buying an ointment, there are two things to look for. First, make sure the ingredients are on the label. Second, make sure the ointment is made up of at least 10 percent herbal extract. An ointment just won't do the job if it contains less than 10 percent of the herbal ingredient. The ointments mentioned in this book should all be readily available from health food stores.

Ointments should be bought or stored in brown glass jars and kept in a cool place. If a preservative is added, ointments stored in this manner will keep for several years.

How to Make Your Own Ointments

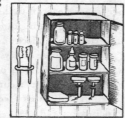

Many people enjoy making their own ointments. The ingredients are readily available from health food stores, herbal pharmacies, and old-fashioned drugstores. Ointments made with herbal extracts should last as long as the ointments you buy ready-made, but those made with an herbal infusion will last only about a year.

The basic recipe for a good ointment is to combine

2 parts herbal extract

7 parts base

1 part natural preservative

You will have to buy the herbal extract. The base can be purchased or made (see below). The best natural preservative is glycerin, which is available at most drugstores.

The procedure is simple: Mix all the ingredients thoroughly. Store in a brown glass jar and keep in a cool place.

Ointment Bases

RAW PETROLEUM JELLY

Raw petroleum jelly is vegetable in origin, made from coal before it is processed. Vaseline is petroleum jelly that has been refined three times. Using either raw or refined petroleum jelly as an ointment base requires a lot of mixing, or making the ointment in a blender—it's generally a messy affair.

LANOLIN

Lanolin is pure cholesterol extracted from the fleece of sheep. Although it is an animal product, it comes from the sheep's wool. It is much easier to mix and is far less messy than petroleum jelly. You must remember to use *pure* lanolin only.

AGAR OR IRISH MOSS

These are fine vegetable ointment bases. They gel nicely and have a soothing emollient action. They can be expensive, however. Here's the recipe for preparing the ointment base. The boric acid is optional; it adds an antiseptic action to the Agar.

> 30 grams Agar or Irish moss
>
> 300 milliliters distilled water
>
> 60 milliliters glycerin
>
> 1 teaspoon boric acid (optional)

In a large saucepan, mix the agar or Irish moss with the distilled water and bring to a gentle boil. Cover and boil gently for a few minutes. Then strain through a cheesecloth and cool.

When the jelly mixture is nearly cool, mix in the glycerin and boric acid. When the mixture is completely cool, add 2 parts herbal extract to 8 parts base.

Creams Instead of Ointments

Creams are sometimes preferred to ointments as they are absorbed more readily into the skin. In the cases of dermatitis or sunburn where large areas of skin are treated, creams are decidedly more convenient. To make a **Jiffy Herbal Cream**, use any natural product skin cream, such as Vitamin E Cream, as a base and mix 2 parts herbal extract to 8 parts cream.

Ointments for First Aid

Arnica Ointment (*Arnica Montana*)

Calendula or Marigold Ointment (*Calendula officinalis*)

Comfrey Ointment (*Symphytum officinale*)

Golden Seal Ointment (*Hydrastis canadensis*)

Hypericum or St. John's Wort Ointment (*Hypericum perforatum*)

Thuja Ointment (*Thuja occidentalis*)

ARNICA OINTMENT

As its botanical name implies, Arnica grows high on the mountains just below the snow line. This member of the daisy family, with its orange-yellow flower, is native to Siberia and northern Europe. Most of the herb we use is imported.

Part Used: The flower

Uses: Treatment for bruises

Arnica is one of the best vulneraries, which means it is used for bruises. Minor or major bruises respond very quickly to Arnica Ointment. When we bruise, it is because the blood vessels beneath the skin have broken and clotted. Arnica breaks down the bruise, or blood clot, into tiny pieces. It sends the dead cells out of the tissues where the body will take over, finally sending them out through the urine.

For those times when you've smashed your thumb under a hammer and you know it will be black and blue, applying Arnica Ointment immediately will take away much of the pain and even prevent the bruise from appearing.

One warning is necessary: *Never use Arnica on broken skin or a bleeding wound.* Arnica, because it prevents blood from clotting, will make the wound bleed more. When you treat a wound that is partly bruised and partly cut, dress it with Calendula (see below) for a few days until the skin is healed, and only then treat the bruising with Arnica Ointment.

If your household has its fair share of black eyes, fingers smashed in car doors, people who ricochet off edges of furniture, or martial artists in training, you'll become aware of the importance of Arnica Ointment in the house.

CALENDULA OR MARIGOLD OINTMENT

Calendula is a hardy annual of the daisy family, well worth growing in your garden or window box. The one to grow is the common pot marigold with the golden orange flowers. The jumbos and hybrids are not medicinal. Calendula will flower throughout the growing season if you pick the dying flowers regularly.

Part Used: The flower

Uses: As an antiseptic

Calendula is *the* household antiseptic. It is thorough and strong in its antiseptic action. Whenever you need an antiseptic, you can use Calendula in one of its many forms: ointment, poultice, or infusion.

Calendula will ease any swelling, cool down the heat of inflammation, and relieve the pain of a wound. It will heal a wound from the deepest levels through to the surface damaged skin tissue, and it prevents scars from forming.

Calendula is also a mild styptic, which means it will stop the bleeding of a wound if the bleeding is not profuse. Bloody noses stop bleeding within seconds when you put a bit of Calendula Ointment up the nose.

Calendula Ointment is a first-rate treatment for all minor wounds with broken skin—from scrapes, grazes, and gravel rash to deep cuts. The best way to treat a septic or infected wound is to wash it with Calendula Infusion (see Teas and Infusions), then dress it with Calendula Ointment or a simple Calendula poultice.

To make a simple poultice, thoroughly bruise a marigold flower in a mortar and pestle and dress the wound with it. Only use flowers that have been grown organically. Putting commercial sprays on a septic wound is *not* a good idea. Insecticides are a very good reason *not* to gather the flowers from public parks.

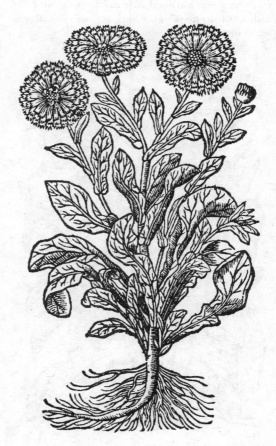

Marigold (Calendula)

Continued ➡

COMFREY OINTMENT

Comfrey, a member of the borage family, is native to Europe and temperate Asia and will grow anywhere. Even under the worst conditions, Comfrey will thrive; it fed the Irish during the potato famine. Once you have Comfrey in your garden, you'll have it forever! Its leaves are large, green, and hairy. The bottom leaves grow as large as ten to sixteen inches long. It is propagated by root division in autumn.

Parts Used: The leaf and root

Uses: To prevent and treat scar tissue and promote rapid healing

Comfrey leaf and Comfrey root are occasionally used in different circumstances. The leaf contains more enzymes than the root and is best used on festering wounds, such as skin ulcers and bedsores, where putrid tissue must be cleaned up. In my experience, the best skin ulcer treatment is an ointment mixture of Calendula, Comfrey leaf, and Comfrey root. Comfrey root is rich in vitamin B_{12} and contains a cell proliferant. The most convenient ointment to have in the medicine chest is the brown Comfrey Ointment, which is a mixture of leaf and root.

Burns and Blisters

Comfrey Ointment is the basic herbal treatment for all sorts of burns, from minor burns and blistered sunburns to third-degree burns. When we burn ourselves, we break or destroy the cell walls, and the plasma, containing the basic cell nutrients, leaks out of the cells to form a blister. Unless the blister breaks, a burn is considered a sterile wound, so there is no need to use an antiseptic.

Comfrey seals the wound and heals the burn so quickly that if you dress a burn immediately with Comfrey Ointment, the blister you would have expected does not even appear. Comfrey also takes the pain and the heat away very quickly.

The very first thing to do with any burn is to cool it to prevent the burn from reaching deeper into the tissue. Soak the affected area in ice water for several minutes. Then seal it by dressing with Comfrey Ointment.

With severe burns, change the dressing twice daily until any mark of the burn is gone—Comfrey leaves no scars.

Scar Prevention

Comfrey root prevents scarring by its cell proliferant action. Comfrey root contains allantoin, which is found in the urine of pregnant women and babies. Its presence is an indication that the cells are dividing and reproducing quickly and normally. Allantoin grows normal healthy cells at 3 times the standard rate and replaces dead cells at the same speed. Comfrey root also contains vitamin B_{12}, the master vitamin, which controls the cell replacement rate and insures that only normal and healthy cells are being reproduced. Comfrey is a cell normalizes as well as a cell proliferant, eating up the dead cells with its enzyme action and replacing them with normal cells at a very fast rate. It is this action that prevents scar tissue from forming. Any wound that you think might leave a scar will not do so if you continue to dress it with Comfrey Ointment until it is thoroughly healed.

It is safe to use Comfrey Ointment on postoperative scars only if there is no risk of infection. As Comfrey is not an antiseptic, it is best to dress postoperative wounds with Calendula, until you are sure they are free of infection. Then switch to Comfrey Ointment dressings.

Old Scars

Whether it is pock marks left over from teenage acne, stretch marks from the last pregnancy, the old appendix scar, or even those premature wrinkles, all will respond to Comfrey root. Comfrey Root Cream is the most convenient treatment. Massage it into the scarred area nightly.

A more intensive treatment is Dorothy Hall's recipe for Comfrey Root Goo: Put a handful of fresh Comfrey root in a saucepan with water to cover. Bring it to a boil and then simmer. Slowly a cream will form. Mash the root as best you can after it has cooked for a while. When the "goo" has formed, strain out any bits of root. Use the Comfrey Root Goo as an overnight mask, washing it off the next morning. Do this twice a week and the scars or wrinkles will disappear. The older the scar, the longer the treatment is necessary, but you will be able to see the changes.

Skin Irritations

Allergic reactions, rough hands from too harsh a dishwashing liquid, itching eczema, and diaper rash are all soothed with Comfrey Cream. It is not always a complete treatment, but it is soothing and heals any breaks in the skin.

Cuts and Abrasions

The one thing to remember about Comfrey is that it is not an antiseptic. If you treat an infected cut with Comfrey it can heal too fast, actually sealing the infection in, and you will have to draw it out later. It is best to use Calendula first if there are any worries of infection. If you are treating a clean cut, it is safe to use Comfrey Ointment immediately. It will heal rapidly and scarlessly.

GOLDEN SEAL OINTMENT

Golden Seal, a member of the buttercup family, grows best in its native North America, in the rich soil of shady woods. It is a small perennial herb with a horizontal, golden yellow rootstock. Golden Seal is one of the most healing of herbs, and, unfortunately, one of the most expensive, due to overcollection and urban expansion.

Part Used: The root

Uses: Skin softening and normalizing

Used as an ointment, Golden Seal has a softening, soothing, and normalizing action on calloused skin, corns, and bunions. Any corroded skin condition, such as pock marks, or any chronic peeling skin also responds to the soothing and normalizing action of Golden Seal.

Massage the ointment thoroughly into the hardened or corroded area until it is completely absorbed. You can see the skin soften and stop peeling within a matter of days.

As Golden Seal is also a dye, any excess ointment will stain your clothes or bedclothes.

HYPERICUM OINTMENT

Hypericum Ointment is made from St. John's Wort, a common pasture weed found in uncultivated open meadows and by roadsides. Growing up to 3 feet tall, this shrubby herb has bright yellow flowers.

Part Used: The flowers

Uses: Treatment for nerve ending damage or irritation

Hypericum Ointment calms down any overreaction of the nerve endings in the skin. It is good for hypersensitive allergic skin reactions, stings of insects, or nettle rashes. It soothes the sharp stinging needle pains by calming and normalizing the nerve endings.

After any major skin damage, as with burns, accidents, or operations, healing can be a painful experience. When the numbness leaves and the nerve endings begin to heal, we feel a severe pins-and-needles pain. Using Hypericum Ointment as a dressing while the skin is still numb will restore the sense of feeling and prevent the acute nerve ending pain during the healing process. I have also known Hypericum Ointment to mend severed nerve endings and ease the ghost pains that people suffer after a limb has been amputated.

If your household runs on the do-it-yourself concept, Hypericum Ointment is definitely one to have on hand. Many a finger chopped off by a power saw and many great chunks of flesh that have met the mincer have regained their function thanks to Hypericum.

One of my patients chopped the whole tip of her finger clean off in the nut grinder. Fortunately she stopped grinding quickly enough to recover the fingertip in one piece and had it stitched on. When I saw her a couple of days later, the tip of the finger was turning blue and promising not to take. Within one day, using Hypericum Ointment as a dressing, the color and sense of feeling were well on the way to being restored.

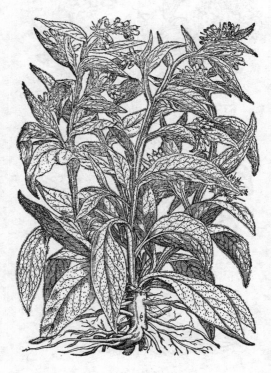

Common Comfrey

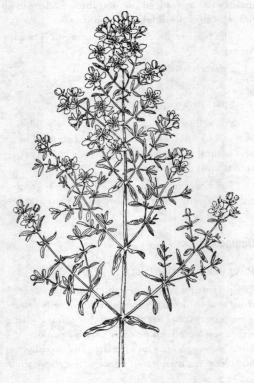

St. John's Wort (Hypericum)

Continued ➡

THUJA OINTMENT

Thuja is the North American yellow cedar. It is the arbor vitae or tree of life to many American Indian tribes because its internal uses are extensive and very powerful.

Part Used: The leaves and twigs

Uses: A fungicide

Thuja is the household fungicide. For topical ulcers, tinea (ringworm), coin spot fungus, athlete's foot, plantar's warts, or any fungus-looking infection that is making a mess of your skin, use Thuja Ointment. Yon can use Thuja Ointment on its own, or mix up an ointment of Thuja, Calendula, and Comfrey leaf and root.

At first the fungus or topical ulcer will appear to be larger but drier. Thuja is simply exposing the extent of the infection. It will soon shrink away. Change the dressing twice daily. Using Comfrey in the same ointment will insure against scarring.

If you are suffering more than one type of fungal infection, you may need Thuja internally. In this case, see a herbalist for a complete treatment, as external remedies just won't be strong enough.

Use a Thuja Infusion (See Teas and Infusions) as a fungicide wash for cleaning the shower to stop athlete's foot from spreading, or wherever you suspect a fungus lurking.

Oils

It is the essential oil of the plant that is used for medicinal purposes. The essential oil possesses the characteristic perfume as well as the healing qualities of the plant. Essential oils are also known as volatile oils as they evaporate rapidly. Extracting a high-quality medicinal oil requires a distilling process to insure against this evaporation. Unless you are skilled in extracting oils, it is wiser and definitely more convenient to buy them.

A general rule is that the purest and best-quality oils are the most expensive. Aromatherapy as a healing art was largely developed in France, and the imported French brands are by far the best of the essential oils. Some of the essential oils readily available at health food stores are also very good quality. Buying a good-quality oil may be more expensive, but it is worth it.

Fixed oils, which do not evaporate easily, also have medicinal properties. They are extracted by pressing the oils out of the plant. Castor oil, linseed oil, and olive oil fall into this category.

Heat will destroy the goodness of all oils. For this reason never buy an oil that has been standing in a shop window. Keep all oils in brown glass jars or bottles with the lid firmly in place. When an oil has lost its perfume, it is an indication that is has lost its medicinal strength as well.

Oils are generally used externally in massage or the bath. When using medicinal oils internally follow the instructions exactly as they have a very strong action.

Oils for First Aid

Castor Oil (*Ricinus communis*)

Eucalyptus Oil (*Eucalyptus globules*)

Lavender Oil (*Lavendula officinalis*)

Linseed Oil (*Linum usitatissimum*)

Olive Oil (*Olea europaca*)

Rosemary Oil (*Rosmarinus officinalis*)

Sandalwood Oil (*Santalum album*)

CASTOR OIL

Castor Oil comes from the seed of the common Castor Oil plant, with its large umbrella leaves.

Uses: Drawing poultice

Castor Oil should never be used internally. It is too strong and may be unpredictable; it often causes griping pains. There are a thousand gentler ways to cleanse the bowel, such as with senna, licorice, dried fruits, and roughage in the diet.

Used externally Castor Oil is one of the best of the emergency remedies. Remember the time you stepped on a rusty nail or walked through cow manure just after cutting your foot, and you worried about tetanus because you were so far away from the hospital? Those are the times when having Castor Oil on hand saves the day.

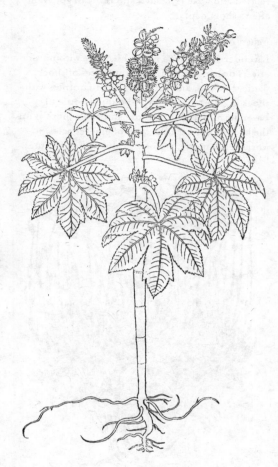

Castor Oil Plant

Castor Oil has drawing power up to 4 inches deep, and it draws thoroughly. All bits of rust or any other nasties are drawn out, preventing all kinds of infection. Pour the Castor Oil onto a wad of cotton wool, when it will sit in a small puddle. Apply it to the wound and wrap it up. Change the dressing every two hours for the rest of the day, and twice daily for the next three days. Yon can safely forget about tetanus or any other kind of infection.

Castor Oil will draw abscesses. It will draw out the irritation of tick bites, as well as any tick heads that were left behind in the tug-of-war. It will draw out splinters, and it will draw out infection from any part of the body you can put a poultice or pack on.

Castor Oil Pack

In the case of a major infection of the chest or abdominal regions, when you can feel congestion in the glands and tissues, it is wise to get rid of the infected matter as quickly as possible. This is most quickly done using a combination of internal treatments, such as garlic or slippery elm, which will break up the congestion and send it out of the body through the eliminatory organs; and external drawing treatments, such as a Castor Oil Pack, which will break up the congestion and draw it out through the skin.

To make a Castor Oil Pack, you will need an old towel large enough to wrap around the torso and be secured at the back with a safety pin. You will also need a plastic bag large enough to cover the infected area. Small garbage bags are excellent for this purpose. Lastly, you will need a double thickness of an old sheet, the same size as the plastic bag.

Lay the towel on a flat surface. Place the plastic bag in the middle of the towel and place the double sheeting on top of the plastic. Now you need to warm the Castor Oil. Put the bottle in a pan of hot water and let it stand for about 5 minutes. The oil should pour easily when it is warm. Pour the warm Castor Oil all over the top piece of double-layer sheeting, spreading it as evenly as possible.

Place the entire pack, the oil side directly on the skin, to cover the infected area. Wrap the outer towel around the body and pin it securely in place. The pack should be kept in place overnight for three nights in a row.

The drawing action of Castor Oil is quite visible. When you remove the pack in the morning, the inner sheeting will be discolored with the infected matter that has been drawn out. Never recycle the inner sheeting. Throw it away.

Eyes

The drawing action of Castor Oil is very useful with the rather serious emergency of having a s plinter in the eye, or any matter deeply buried in the eye tissue that does not respond to the Golden Seal eye wash (see Golden Seal Extract). The thick oiliness of Castor Oil oozes the splinter, or foreign matter, out slowly and will not tear or damage the sensitive eye tissue.

For splinters in the eye, metal or otherwise, put 3 drops of Castor Oil directly into the eye, place an eye pad of cotton wool soaked in Calendula Infusion (see Teas and Infusions) over the eyelid, wrapping it up for 12 hours. It does sting the eye initially, but it is a soothing treatment and the splinter should appear on the surface of the eye ready to be carefully picked up. If it is not, repeat the treatment. When the splinter has been removed, pack the closed eye with cotton wool soaked in Castor Oil and wrap it up for another 12 hours. This is to insure that the eye is free of infection.

Serious Eye Infections

Any eye infection that does not rapidly respond to the cleansing Golden Seal eye wash (see Golden Seal Extract) will certainly respond to Castor Oil. Pack the closed eye with cotton wool soaked in Castor Oil and wrap it up. Eye masks are perfect for keeping an eye pack in place. The relief is almost immediate, but keep the eye pack on overnight. In the morning when you remove the pack, you will not be able to open your eyes because they will be gummed up with matter drawn by the Castor Oil. Wash the eyes with either Golden Seal wash (see Golden Seal Extract) or Calendula Infusion (see Teas and Infusions). Repeat this overnight treatment until you can freely open your eyes in the morning.

EUCALYPTUS OIL

Eucalyptus Oil comes mostly from the blue gum tree, but many other species also have a high oil content in their fresh leaves, and all species are medicinal.

Uses: Antiseptic and expectorant

Eucalyptus is the most powerfully antiseptic of the oils, and it grows more strongly antiseptic when it is old. A substance called ozone is formed in the bottle once the oil is exposed to air, and this aids the disinfectant action. Eucalyptus works primarily in the respiratory system.

Continued →

Inhalant

One way to relieve all congestion of a cold or flu from the sinuses to the chest is to inhale Eucalyptus. Boil some water, turn off the heat, and put a few drops of Eucalyptus Oil in it. You could also use mashed fresh leaves and new shoots instead of the oil. With your head over the pot of water, drape a towel to make a tent over your head and the water and inhale. Never inhale over boiling water. Using Eucalyptus as an inhalant gets to the heart of the infection because of its antiseptic action. It is also useful for laryngitis and other throat problems as well as dry sinuses or aching raw sinuses.

Chest Rub

As a chest rub, Eucalyptus Oil has a very penetrating action, opening up the air passages and fighting infection. If your skin is at all sensitive, it may be best to dilute Eucalyptus Oil with a bland healing oil, such as wheat germ oil, before applying it to the chest.

Internally

For severe bronchial or lung infections you can use Eucalyptus Oil internally, but watch the dose. Small doses are all you need and large doses are dangerous, so don't overdo it. For chronic chest conditions or for a cold that has been hanging around for months, taking 2 drops of Eucalyptus Oil in 1 teaspoon of honey once a day for a week will shake it.

Eucalyptus has been used internally to treat tuberculosis and other microbic lung diseases quite successfully in European TB sanatoriums, where it was found that Eucalyptus Oil actually kills the TB organism outright.

Bath Oil

Putting a few drops of Eucalyptus Oil in the bath stimulates the circulation and relaxes the muscular aches and pains that often accompany a cold or flu. It also has the effect of taking a bath in an inhaler. A Eucalyptus Oil bath is a complete and relaxing cold and flu treatment.

Eucalyptus Oil baths also work wonders for muscular aches and pains after too strenuous a workout. When you have proved to yourself that you are as fit as ever and played your first game of squash in five years, a good soak in a Eucalyptus Oil bath will mean no stiff muscles the next day. It's a good treatment for the ego as well as the muscles.

Skin Parasites

For any skin parasites, such as ringworm or scabies, soak a cloth in Eucalyptus Oil and rub it on the infected area twice daily until it is gone. If the skin is too sensitive, it may be better to make a strong infusion of the leaves for this purpose (see Teas and Infusions).

Stain Remover

Here is one household use we could not possibly overlook. All sorts of stains on clothing come out when you dab a bit of Eucalyptus Oil on them. The sooner you treat a stain, the easier it will be to remove. Even with old stains, however, if you soak a bit of cotton wool in Eucalyptus Oil and rub it on the stain, letting it dry before you wash it, it usually comes clean.

LAVENDER OIL

Lavender is native to the mountainous Mediterranean regions and spread with the Romans wherever they traveled. Today it is a common garden plant. If you want your picked Lavender to last with its distinctive aroma, harvest it in full flower as midsummer approaches. The oil will then be concentrated in the flower.

Uses: Toning and calming the nerves

Headaches

Lavender Oil is good for a specific type of headache that starts with tension at the neck and base of the skull. It is the sort of headache that can be the cause of insomnia—no matter how you rest your head on the pillow, it will not relax. Lavender Oil rubbed on the back of the neck and worked into the base of the skull will ease all the tension very quickly. It is also a good idea to brush your hair thoroughly from the underside to draw out some of the tension you have accumulated in your head. You should sleep relaxed and wake refreshed and ready to go, even after a short nap.

Natural Sedative

Lavender Oil acts as a natural sedative with no side effects or hangovers. In circumstances of shock, panic, hysteria, and for a feeling of faintness with shock or sunstrokes, simply hold the bottle of Lavender Oil under the nose and rub a bit of it on the back of the neck. In cases of emergencies, it works very quickly, restoring calm within minutes.

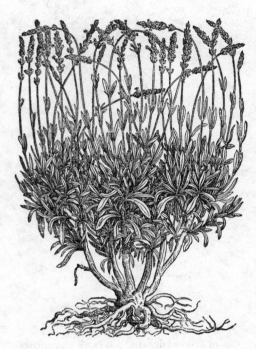

Lavender

LINSEED OIL

Linseed Oil comes from the common flax plant that grows the world over and has done so for so many centuries that its native land is unknown. We get linen from the stems and oil from the seed. Linseed Oil is best bought from a health food store.

Uses: Massage for ligaments

Linseed Oil used as a massage oil is perfect treatment for strained, sprained, stretched, twisted, and torn ligaments. It works just as well for the tight ligaments as it does for the loose ones because it tones the ligaments as well as restores their elasticity.

Linseed Oil is as essential in sports medicine as it is in home first aid for the sprained ankles and twisted knees that are an inherent part of the human experience. Massage the sprained area every few hours when the pain is acute, and follow up with a daily massage of the area until the joint has totally recovered.

OLIVE OIL

Olive Oil comes from the olive. The olive tree is native to Asia Minor and is cultivated in most warm climates. For first aid, it is best to buy a small bottle of the virgin oil, which comes from the first pressing of the olive.

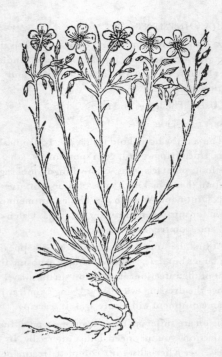

Wild Flax

Uses: Lubrication and calming of sensitive skin and ears

Olive Oil plays an important role in the diet, with its prevention of gallstone patterns and its strong lubricating ability. Most dry skin and dry scalp conditions improve with the simple addition of more oil to the diet, Olive Oil also contains natural sodium chloride, which gets the gastric juices working and ensures a good appetite as well as better digestion.

Ears

Olive Oil is the basic ingredient of herbal ear drops which are useful for treating ears that tend to waxy buildups, ears that discharge, ears that catch cold winds or ears that ache. If there is an infection deep in the ear you can mix a bit of Castor Oil with the Olive Oil to add to its drawing power.

Warm up a bit of Olive Oil by putting a small jar of it in a bowl of warm water. Put 3 drops in each ear and rub in the ear. Leave it overnight and clean the ears with a bit of cotton wool the next morning. It gives pain relief and a good general cleaning of the ears.

Skin Rashes

In all cases of skin rash, and allergic rash in particular, Olive Oil rubbed on the affected area will calm down the reaction with its soothing action. Olive Oil is bland, soothing, and lubricating to the skin and scalp, which is why it is one of the ingredients in so many good-quality soaps and shampoos.

Dry Scalp

For dry scalp dandruff, Grandma's old Olive Oil treatment is one of the best. Warm some Olive Oil, adding any scent you like, and massage it well into the scalp. Keep it on as long as you can before washing it out. Wrap your head in a towel if it is a cool day or, if you want to bring out the highlights in your hair, sit in the sun.

ROSEMARY OIL

Rosemary, the shrub that gives us our kitchen herb, is native to the Mediterranean and will grow wherever the sun shines. It prefers sandy and rocky soil.

Tension Headaches

Rosemary is treatment for the tension headache, that throbbing in the temples that usually comes with the gritting of teeth or the squinting and

Continued ➤

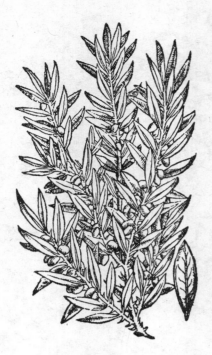

Wild Olive

straining of eyes. Massage a bit of Rosemary Oil on the temples and across the forehead. If you clench your jaw when you are tense, lightly massage Rosemary Oil along your jaw line as well. The nerves of the face will relax smartly and the headache will ease.

If tension headaches are a fact of your lifestyle, you should see how you can change your lifestyle to make it less stressful. Remember, pain is a barometer of health.

Muscles

Tight muscles, muscles in spasm, painfully strained muscles, or those weak, floppy, untoned muscles all respond to a massage of Rosemary Oil. Rosemary Oil will tone up and relax the muscles, which is why it is often an ingredient of massage oils. If your household is on the sporting side, you may want to make up a mixture of half-and-half Rosemary and Linseed Oils. With this combination oil on your shelf, you will be ready to treat strained muscles and strained ligaments in the same massage.

Hair Conditioner

If you have dark hair, Rosemary will keep your hair healthy, shiny, and dark. After you have washed your hair, put a few drops of Rosemary Oil on your hairbrush and brush it through. It won't make your hair greasy. It will keep your hair looking and smelling nice. You can get a similar effect by using Rosemary Infusion for the final rinse after shampooing your hair (see Teas and Infusions).

Sandalwood Oil

Sandalwood Oil comes from the wood of the sandalwood tree. It is native to India and has straw-colored flowers that turn deep reddish purple when they open.

Uses: Protection of the aura

Sandalwood is a necessity for sensitive, intuitive, and psychic types of people. It is for the people who listen to other people's problems—the counselors, the healers, and the neighborhood ear to whom everyone comes for guidance and nurturing. You know when you need it. It is for the times when, though you were feeling fresh and alive before your friend or client came, they left you suffering with the headache they complained of, their rheumatic pains, or their heart-breaking sadness. They feel much better, of course, and are bound to call again, so you had better be ready for the next visit!

It may be because of love or compassion for these people that you actually take their sadness or pain inside yourself in order to make them feel better. You are blending their life force, or aura, with your own. Our aura, or electrical force field, is our first line of defense. It acts very much like a permeable membrane, filtering out certain influences that may be harmful, yet allowing unharmful influences in. It can become a big problem if, because of compassion, someone has left their aura wide open. The greater problem arises when compassionate, intuitive persons think they are going around the bend because they are suffering one set of symptoms or another each time they have a visitor.

There is a solution: Sandalwood Oil, of course! Put a drop of Sandalwood Oil on your third eye, in the middle of your brow just above your nose. Put another drop on the seventh cervical vertebra (C7) of your neck. You will find the vertebra is prominent in the neck when you hang your head forward. You should be able to feel that vertebra just above your shoulder line. Within minutes after using Sandalwood Oil in this way, you will find the aches, pains, and sadness you picked up from your friend or client begin to fade. Sandalwood Oil is sealing your aura.

Using Sandalwood Oil as a preventative can enhance or even develop your psychic ability, intuition, or compassion, because you won't feel drained every time you listen to someone's problems. Some people need to use Sandalwood Oil daily.

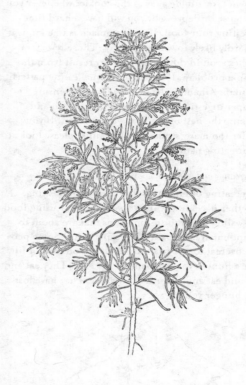

Teas and Infusions

Herbs are used as medicines in the home primarily in the form of teas and infusions. They are the nutritional part of herbal medicine, used to supplement the diet and ease the side effects of bad habits.

When you need to relieve pains or acute symptoms of ill health, drinking a cup of herbal tea or a glass of infusion will certainly help. Infusions generally are used when the symptoms are more acute because the infusions are twice as strong as teas. The beauty of herbal teas, however, is in preventing illness. It takes time to correct a pattern of ill health, so taking the right herbal tea as a regular part of your diet will prevent the illness, and therefore the symptoms, from recurring.

Teas and infusions can also be used externally as a wash for any part of the body. Simply let the tea or infusion cool down so that it can be applied externally. They can also be used as a final rinse after washing your hair. One or two cups of a tea or infusion can be added to the bath for a total body treatment. Dressings for wounds or sprains can be prepared by soaking the dressing in the tea of infusion and applying it to the affected area. Strong infusions can be used in making creams and ointments.

Teas and infusions are made easily in the kitchen using either dried herbs or herbs fresh from the garden. Dried herbs can last for several years if they are properly dried and stored in airtight containers. You can buy dried herbs in supermarkets, health food stores, herbal pharmacies, and by the mail. A packet of 3½ ounces of a dried herb is a good amount to buy when you are starting out. It will give you a chance to find out which herbs you use more frequently before you buy in bulk. Some of the more popular herbal teas are available in tea bags, making it very convenient if you want only one cup. When using fresh herbs, it is best to bruise the herb with a mortar and pestle before adding it to the teapot.

Making an Herbal Tea

Making an herbal tea is much the same as making black tea. Use 1 teaspoon of dried herb for each person and 1 for the pot. Fresh herbs are, of course, harder to measure because of varying sizes of leaf and sprig. A small handful of the fresh herb will generally make a nice cup of tea. Add boiling water, let it steep a few minutes (the longer the steeping, the stronger the brew), strain with an ordinary tea strainer, and drink. You generally do not add milk to herbal tea, though adding a spoon of honey will make it very palatable.

Making an Infusion

Making an infusion is much the same as making a strong tea. Use about 1 ounce of dried herb, or 4 small handfuls of fresh herb, to a small, 3-cup teapot. Pour boiling water over the herb, let it steep until it is cool, and strain with an ordinary tea strainer. Infusions will keep in the refrigerator for a few days. A standard dose of infusion for internal uses is a full wineglass 3 times daily.

Never use aluminum teapots for herbal teas. Porcelain or pottery teapots are best, as the herb will not be affected by the clay. This applies mainly to the brewing stage of preparation and does not necessarily apply to the tea strainer. Some people use a special teapot for herbal teas because the flavor of black tea is changed when made in the same pot. It is a matter of taste.

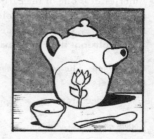

Dried Herbs for Teas and Infusions for First Aid

Calendula (*Calendula officinalis*)

Coltsfoot (*Tussilago farfara*)

Chamomile (*Matricaria chamomilla*; *Anthemis nobilis*)

Rosehip (*Rosa canina*)

Senna (*Cassia acutifolia*)

Calendula Tea & Infusion

Calendula, the household antiseptic, is worth using as an infusion any time you need an antiseptic wash.

Part Used: The flowers

Uses: Antiseptic

Continued →

For cleaning up a wound or as a facial wash for infected skin conditions, such as acne, Calendula Infusions work wonders. You can also dress a wound by soaking the dressing in a strong infusion.

Swellings

Swellings of all sorts calm down when washed or dressed with Calendula Infusion. It is lovely as a footbath for infected or swollen feet. To make a proper footbath, add a quart of boiling water to a handful of Calendula flowers and when it is cool enough, soak you feet.

Eyes

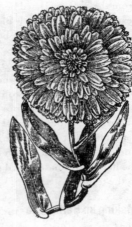

Calendula has a special affinity for the eyes. For infected eyes, conjunctivitis, inflamed eyes, sties, or tired eyes, use a cool Calendula Infusion as an eye wash. If it is an acute eye condition, wash the eyes 3 or 4 times daily. If it is not, washing the eyes morning and night will fight any infection, ease inflammation, and refresh them. If you are going to take a nap, make some Calendula eye pads by soaking some cotton wool in Calendula Infusion, Place them on your eyes during your nap. When you awake, your eye will sparkle and your vision will be very clear.

Vaginal Douche

With any bacterial type of vaginal or genital infection and irritation, using Calendula Infusion as a douche, or even patting it on the genitals, will calm down the itch, heat, and inflammation. It will generally bring comfort. In some instances of genital inflammation, it is a complete treatment. If you have a chronic problem with vaginal infections, see your herbalist—stronger treatments may be necessary.

Mild Depression

Whenever you are down in the dumps and feel like singin' the blues, Calendula Tea does a good deal to lift the spirits and warm the heart.

COLTSFOOT TEA & INFUSION

Coltsfoot is a member of the daisy family and is native to Europe, North Africa, and Asia. In North America, it is one of the earliest spring flowers, resembling dandelions in color and form. Its hoof-shaped leaves, covered in fine downy hairs, have given Coltsfoot its country name.

Parts Used: The root and leaves, and occasionally the flowers

Uses: Expectorant

Coughs and Chest Conditions

Coltsfoot is an expectorant. It removes mucus and phlegm from the pleural cavity, lungs, and bronchial tree. It eases wheezing and shortness of breath by opening the air passages and toning the nerve supply to the chest area. This also has the effect of easing any spasmodic coughing. If someone in your home is prone to chest conditions or asthma, Coltsfoot Tea as a common beverage is first-rate preventative medicine.

As an infusion, Coltsfoot is a stronger treatment and useful for bronchitis, flu, pneumonia, and even whooping cough and asthma. Coltsfoot is very useful to the frail or the aged when a cough sets in. The expectorant action of Coltsfoot helps to get behind the mucus and almost does the coughing for you, leaving you less exhausted.

In more severe chest conditions, such as emphysema, pleurisy, pneumonia, whooping cough, and asthma, you will need stronger doses of Coltsfoot and other herbs, so it is best to see an herbalist. In the meantime, Coltsfoot Infusion taken 3 times a day will bring comfort.

CHAMOMILE TEA

Chamomile, one of the favorites of the herb garden, is very useful in first aid. Both the creeping variety (*Anthemis nobilis*) and the taller variety (*Matricaria chamomilla*) are medicinal, though the latter is stronger.

Part Used: The flowers

Uses: Digestive tonic and soporific

Digestion

Poor digestion is probably the most common complaint of the western world. It is likely that someone in your home could benefit by drinking Chamomile Tea. Chamomile Tea neutralizes excess stomach acid. It both prevents and treats indigestion. It tones underactive stomachs, insuring complete digestion. It calms stomach aches, spasm, and tension; dispels nausea; releases painful, trapped wind and colic; and soothes stomach ulcers. Drinking Chamomile Tea regularly will change your digestive patterns.

Tension Eating

When you grab a bite to eat on the run in between your frantic chores, have too many working lunches, or nibble away at the cookies whenever you are tense or depressed, you will have a hard time digesting your food. If your stomach is in a knot, it is hardly likely to work properly. Those few extra inches around the waistline often result from this simple problem. If this is your usual eating pattern, drinking Chamomile Tea regularly will ensure proper digestion by relaxing your stomach and making the best of the food you've eaten. If you suffer too many stomach complaints, please look at your eating patterns.

Overeating and Anorexia

Overeating often comes down to tension eating, whether it's eating while you are tense or using food to swallow down those emotions that are about to erupt but are too painful to experience. Some people overeat to satisfy a hunger that food cannot fill, like a hunger for company or for love. They eat and eat and eat and never feel satisfied. They have lost the hunger reflex.

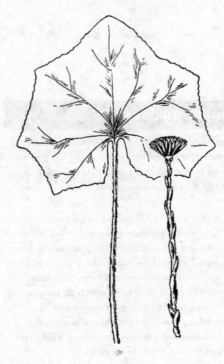

Coltsfoot

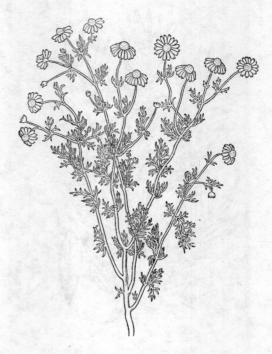

Chamomile

Anorexia is the refusal to eat. Anorexia and overeating are opposite sides of the same coin. Some people refuse nourishment for emotional reasons, and others eat to fill the emotional emptiness. Effective treatment lies in the emotional sphere. Confronting your feelings is the cure. Chamomile Tea will, however, calm down that overworked stomach. It will digest the food of the overeater and neutralize the intense acidity of the anorexic.

Headaches

Chamomile Tea is correct treatment for sick headaches where your stomach and head are both swimming. This headache usually starts with swallowing (gulp) tension, and the ache then bounces from the stomach to the head. Many migraine patterns have their beginning stages in this type of headache. Chamomile Tea for a youngster with sick headaches could prevent a life of migraines.

Sleep

Chamomile Tea is the perfect evening drink if you have a problem getting to sleep or waking in the night. Chamomile is a soporific and lulls you to a restful sleep. Certain types of insomnia are linked to indigestion. In these instances, Chamomile Tea in the evenings is just about complete treatment.

Menstrual Pain

Drinking a cup of Chamomile Tea alleviates menstrual spasms.

Babies and Toddlers

Chamomile is one of baby's best all-around remedies. As well as preventing and treating bowel and stomach pains, colic, and diarrhea, it has a number of other uses. The daily bottle of Chamomile Tea with a bit of honey (the honey increases the calcium absorption rate) gives the baby calcium phosphate for growing healthy bones and teeth, minimizes the trauma of teething by calming the pain and nausea, and helps the baby to sleep soundly. For the pain of teething, you can also put a small handful of Chamomile flowers in a handkerchief, warm it on a hot kettle, and hold it to the jaw.

Internally, and externally as a wash, Chamomile Tea does wonders for all sorts of infant skin rashes and cradle cap. It is also a lovely eye wash for gummed-up eyes.

Continued ➤

Pregnancy

During pregnancy, Chamomile is one of the herbs that ensures enough calcium phosphate for Mom's hair, teeth, and nails, as well as the baby's growing bones. It will also ease morning sickness.

ROSEHIP TEA & INFUSION

Rosehip comes from the pink wild rose that grows on land that has been tilled then left to grow wild. It is common in temperate regions the world over.

Uses: Circulatory tonic; complete source of vitamin C

If you have any circulatory problems, from varicose veins to a heart condition, Rosehip Tea should be one of your regular beverages. It is a safe circulatory tonic in all circumstances.

With its combination of vitamin C and its action as a circulatory tonic, Rosehip is the perfect drink for times of too much physical stress or anxiety. Whenever you feel that you just cannot cope or that you are falling to pieces, Rosehip Tea is a safe and sure pick-me-up. It will give you the energy to deal with your situation effectively.

Resistance to Infection

If you are run down, or have been living on adrenaline for too many days in a row, your resistance to any infection will be low. Rosehip Tea taken whenever you feel run down will restore your natural resistance and help prevent colds and flu.

If you already have a cold, flu, or any infection, have a teacup of Rosehip Infusion 3 times daily. It will help localize infection as well as help you to fight it.

Operations

In the case of any minor surgery or dental work involving a local anesthetic, drink Rosehip Tea regularly for a few days before and after the operation. Drinking Rosehip Tea before the operation will prepare the body for the trauma ahead and insure as little cell damage as possible. Drinking Rosehip Tea after minor surgery will help repair any cell damage, aid recovery, and prevent any postoperative infection.

SENNA INFUSION

Senna is a legume, indigenous to Egypt, and very well known for its laxative action. It is one of the herbs that has been continually in use through the last few generations.

Part Used: The leaf and pods
Uses: Laxative

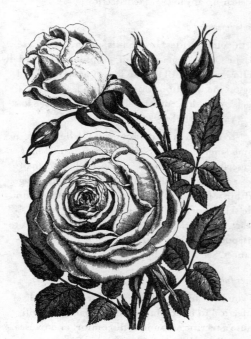

Queen's Scarlet Garden Rose

Senna is one of the safest and most thorough laxatives. It is safe for babies, children, pregnant women, and old people. Senna not only cleanses the bowel thoroughly, it also tones it. It brings no griping, no pains, and no sudden races to the toilet.

Senna pods are more effective than the leaves, as they act on the whole intestine, whereas the leaves tend to work only in the lower bowel. Make an infusion in the following doses:

Adults: 6–10 pods

Children: 3–5 pods

Infants: 2 pods

Drink a teacup of the infusion at night after a few hours without food, and the bowels will move in the morning. They will return to their normal pattern the next day.

If you are mildly constipated as a general pattern, you can use the Senna Pod Infusion regularly, with no side effects except improvement in the tone of your bowel. If you suffer a severe constipation pattern and have come to rely on a laxative to make your bowels move at all, see your herbalist. Stronger herbal treatment will be necessary as your bowels have forgotten how to work on their own.

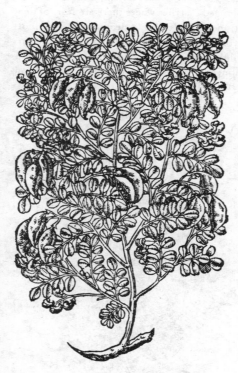

Bladder Senna

Tinctures and Extracts

Tinctures and extracts are the strongest forms of herbal medicine. In these forms, the essence of the herb is concentrated in an alcohol base. Most herbs give their characters and qualities to alcohol more efficiently than they do to water, and because alcohol is so rapidly absorbed into the bloodstream, herbs taken in a tincture or extract form are fast-acting and even dramatic in their effect. An added benefit of the alcohol base is the extended shelf life it affords. Extracts will last up to 7 years, and tinctures up to 10 years; and they will still be as effective as when they were first made—provided they are kept in brown bottles and in a cool place.

The major difference between tinctures and extracts is in their effect. Tinctures are a more vibrational treatment and will affect the whole person. Herbalists skilled at dosages can treat imbalances on mental, emotional, and spiritual levels, as well as the physical level, using tinctures. Extracts, on the other hand, have a very strong physical

effect; and depending on the herb, extracts can sometimes be too strong to be taken internally. For home use, it is a general rule to use tinctures internally, taken in a mouth full of water, and to use extracts externally in the form of washes, creams, and ointments.

All tinctures and extracts used in a medicinal practice must, by law, conform to laboratory measures. Beginning herbalists may find it far more convenient and safer to buy the tinctures and extracts for first aid. For household use, 1-ounce bottles of the tinctures and extracts listed below will probably keep you in stock for a year. They are available from herbal pharmacies and health food stores, and through the mail.

Tinctures and Extracts for First Aid

Black Cohosh Tincture (*Cimicifuga racemosa*)

Golden Seal Extract (*Hydrastis Canadensis*)

Yarrow Tincture (*Achillea millefolium*)

BLACK COHOSH TINCTURE

A member of the ranuncula family, Black Cohosh, with its white candlelike flowers, is native to eastern North America. When you put this little bottle on the shelf of your medicine chest, label it "Emergency Only."

Part Used: The root
Uses: For severe and observable spasms

Black Cohosh is a very powerful antispasmodic. All types of fits and convulsions respond to Black Cohosh, as do the severe spasms of croup and whooping cough. You can use Black Cohosh with certain menstrual cramps, but only for the violent uterine cramps complete with migraine and nausea.

Black Cohosh doesn't remedy the cause of the spasm, it simply relaxes it. It is used only while there is spasm and will cause a spasm if there is none for it to counteract. For these reasons it is a 1-dose or 2-dose treatment.

Put 7 drops of Black Cohosh Tincture directly on the tongue each 15 minutes. For children, use 4 drops each 15 minutes. It will be absorbed immediately. If someone's jaw is locked during a fit, either rub the tincture on the lips or on the pulse.

Croup and Whooping Cough

It is safe to use Black Cohosh each time there is an attack of spasmodic coughing. There is an added bonus in that Black Cohosh also has an expectorant action and will help you to cough up anything that should be coughed up. You will need other herbs to complete the treatment, so it is best to see an herbalist in these situations.

Birthing

Many a midwife in the practice of natural childbirth will know the benefit of Black Cohosh during labor. Seven drops of Black Cohosh every hour during labor will ease the spasms, relax the woman, and shorten labor. For this specific use, one of the country names for Black Cohosh is Squaw Root.

GOLDEN SEAL EXTRACT

Golden Seal Extract is useful in first aid for some of its external uses. Golden Seal is rich in vitamin A.

Uses: For the eyes and mucus membrane

Eyes

With minor eye complaints, such as conjunctivitis, sties, tired red eyes, or the scratchy, sandy feeling of a foreign particle in the eye, a Golden Seal bath brings immediate relief that lasts all day. It has an antiseptic and cleansing action for any infection, a drawing power to clean out any foreign particle, and soothing resins to calm any irritation.

Continued ➡

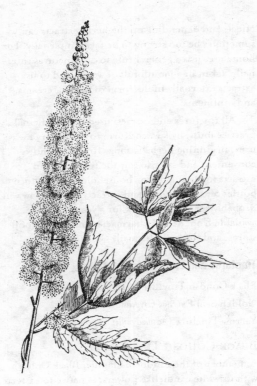

Black Cohosh

For serious eye conditions, Golden Seal has a deep action in the eyeball and will get well into the structure and fluid of the eye with its soothing detergent and antiseptic action. It is an important part of herbal treatment in serious eye conditions, such as glaucoma, but it is not complete.

To make an eye wash, put 2 drops of Golden Seal Extract into an eye cup of warm water and bathe the eyes morning and night.

Genital Infections

Whenever there is genital inflammation, pain, or irritation due to any cause, Golden Seal will soothe it. Make a mixture of 15 drops of Golden Seal Extract to a cup of warm water and pat it on the genitals or use it as a douche. The irritation and pain of vaginitis, herpes, and even STDs will respond to Golden Seal.

With most forms of vaginitis, the combination of Golden Seal as a douche and a course of Garlic Oil Capsules is complete treatment. In cases of major sexual infections, see a practitioner immediately. The major problem of genital infections is reinfection, and both parties need to be treated.

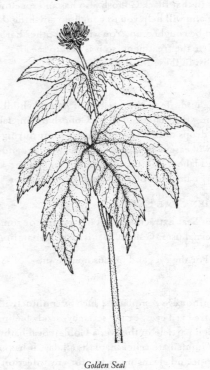

Golden Seal

YARROW TINCTURE

Yarrow, with its white to mauve flowers and feathery leaves, is a member of the daisy family. It is a common plant in herb gardens and is known as the plant's physician as it helps liven up any ailing plants around it.

Part Used: The whole plant
Uses: Astringent and styptic

Hemorrhage

In its tincture form, Yarrow will stop a hemorrhage, from a bleeding ulcer to a major hemorrhage from any organ. Even in cases of hemophilia, Yarrow will stop the bleeding.

Whenever there is a profuse, steady flow of blood, take 10 drops of Yarrow Tincture on the tongue each 10 minutes until the bleeding stops. A few doses is all that is usually necessary. Yarrow is not a complete treatment, but it is very useful while you are waiting for an ambulance. Yarrow also helps to boost the vitality that is usually fading fast in times of hemorrhage and severe fluid loss.

Fluid Loss

In cases of severe fluid loss, as with dysentery or prolonged diarrhea where there are fears of dehydration, take 10 drops (5 drops for children) of Yarrow Tincture in a bit of water every few hours until the pattern eases. Again, it is not complete treatment, though it will calm the symptoms and boost the vitality.

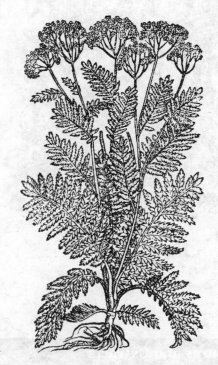

Yarrow, Milfoil

GARLIC OIL CAPSULES

Garlic Oil comes from the common garlic (*Allium sativum*) found in most kitchens. Those who regularly cook with garlic will not need medicinal doses as frequently as those who do not.

The benefit of capsules is, of course, their convenience. It is more convenient, and less socially dangerous in some circles, to take capsules rather than to chew a clove or two. It is remarkable, though, how many children will chew the capsules. Children are generally more instinctual in their eating than adults, and often less concerned with social standards. With these children, 2 cloves of crushed garlic on a slice of bread and butter will give the same results as 6 garlic capsules.

You can prepare a garlic honey for medicinal use. Thoroughly crush all the cloves of 1 corm of garlic and put it in a small sterilized jar. Pour pure honey over the garlic to cover and stir well. Add a bit more honey to approximately ½ inch above the garlic mixture and stir again. Leave it for 6 weeks to candy. Honey is a natural preservative and the mixture will keep indefinitely. Take it by the teaspoon. One teaspoon is equivalent to 2 garlic capsules. Garlic honey is not as bad as it sounds because in 6 weeks the garlic taste and smell disappears, and all you can taste is honey.

Garlic Oil Capsules are readily available from health food stores. Often they can be found in regular drugstores. There is one word of advice regarding the quality of capsules, however. A gelatin capsule should begin to melt as soon as it touches the tongue. If you do not taste the gelatin melting, it is most likely a poor-quality capsule. Some capsules that don't dissolve easily are made with plastic and should be avoided.

I can hear you asking, "What about the smell?" You can rest assured. Unless you actually chew the garlic, whenever Garlic Oil is working on an infection, you will not smell it on the breath or skin. It is when you start to recover that you begin to smell the garlic, and this is an indication that it is time to cut down the doses as you are taking more than you need.

Part Used: The oil found in the clove
Uses: A natural antibiotic

Whenever you are advised to take a course of antibiotics, you could confidently use Garlic Oil Capsules as an alternative. Garlic Oil is pure natural sulfur and will clean up any infection anywhere in the body. It is the natural sulfur drug with no nasty side effects. Even viral infections respond to Garlic Oil. It will kill a virus without harming the host cell, a great advantage over modern antibiotics.

Since it is the oil in garlic that is desirable, when you cook with it be sure to crush the clove thoroughly to get its full goodness. For the same reason, it is best to use Garlic Oil Capsules rather than tablets, which are made from dried garlic.

Chronic Infections

If you have been suffering any infection for a long time or have a recurring infection, you have a chronic condition. Chronic infected acne, cystitis, vaginal infections, and recurring boils are some of the classic conditions. Take 2 or 3 Garlic Oil Capsules daily one before each meal, until the infection is gone. You will feel much better within a week. It is good insurance, however, to take it a week longer to clear up any low-grade infection.

Acute Infections

With colds, viruses, bronchitis, or any "iris," use Garlic Oil in larger doses of 3 capsules 3 times daily before meals, until it is no longer acute. Depending on the infection, this can take a few days or a week. After the acute stage, reduce the dosage to 2 or 3 capsules daily.

To explain just how powerful Garlic Oil is, in some emergency cases of blood poisoning I have prescribed up to 5 Garlic Oil Capsules each half hour for 2 days with a follow-up infection dosage. Within a few hours, the dark line that appears on the skin, moving along the bloodstream to the heart, an indication of blood poisoning, begins to disappear. In these extremely dangerous circumstances, see a practitioner immediately.

Liver Infections

If you have any liver conditions, from a mild liver infection to infectious hepatitis, Garlic Oil will cause a terrific amount of discomfort and nausea. You will need other herbs, notably Dandelion, and will need to see a practitioner.

Continued ➡

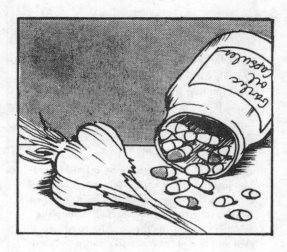

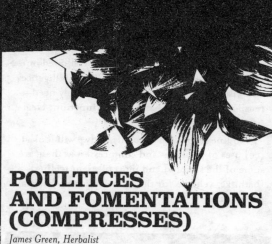

SLIPPERY ELM POWDER

Slippery Elm Powder comes from the dried inner bark of the Slippery Elm Tree (*Ulmus fulfa*). It is a native of Central and North American and has been a food source to several American Indian tribes.

Health food stores and herbal pharmacies can readily supply Slippery Elm Powder as well as the tablets and the dried bark. The powder, however, is the form most readily absorbed by the body and, therefore, offers the quickest relief. One 3½-ounce packet of Slippery Elm Powder should meet the demand of most households for several months, unless there is a need to take it daily. It should be stored in an airtight glass jar and will keep for several years, like any properly dried herb. When buying Slippery Elm Powder, you want 100 percent Slippery Elm. Make sure it is not adulterated. Mixed with hot water, it should form a jelly consistency. If it does not do this, the Slippery Elm bark either has not been ground finely enough, or it has been cut with something else. In either case, try another brand next time.

Part Used: The inner bark

Uses: Soother and healer of the digestive tract

Slippery Elm Powder is complete treatment for the entire digestive tract. Over acidic stomachs, nausea, ulcers, diarrhea, constipation, bowel pockets, hemorrhoids, colitis, colic, appendicitis, and even intestinal viruses all respond to Slippery Elm Powder. If your problem is anywhere in the digestive tract, Slippery Elm Powder is your answer.

One dose of Slippery Elm Powder coats the whole digestive tract, from the mouth to the rectum, with its soothing mucilage for 30 hours. It protects the lining of the digestive tract from any irritants: swallowed poisons, digestive acids, or viral infections. At the same time it coats, its rich calcium phosphates are working underneath, healing any ulcers, calming any spasms and generally toning the digestive tract.

Dosage: One dose of Slippery Elm Powder lasts for 30 hours. No matter what the problem is, because of its last quality, the dosage is standard: 1 tablespoon of Slippery Elm Powder daily. It is best to take it at the same time each day to insure around-the-clock coverage. Though the dosage is the same for any complaint, the duration of the treatment varies.

Slippery Elm should not be used for morning sickness in pregnancy if you are prone to miscarriage. Slippery Elm has been known to bring on a miscarriage, but only when there is already a tendency or risk of one.

How to take Slippery Elm Powder: The craziest food combinations have been invented to help people swallow Slippery Elm Powder. As a general rule, when you need Slippery Elm you usually like the taste and don't mind the thickness, but rules always have their exceptions.

The easiest and quickest way to get it down is to mix 1 tablespoon of Slippery Elm Powder with a bit of water that has just boiled and mix it into a paste. Add a spoonful of honey for a sweet woody flavor. This way it is down the hatch with one or two swallows. If you like the flavor and don't mind the thickness, sprinkle it on your breakfast cereal or mix it with yogurt.

Though Slippery Elm Tablets are available, they take a long time to break down and do not offer the immediate relief that the powder does. Since the tablets won't start working until they reach your small intestine, your stomach will not get the benefit. So whether you like the taste or not, you will get the full benefit of Slippery Elm only from the powder.

Ulcers

Slippery Elm Powder heals both peptic and duodenal ulcers, as it works in the entire digestive tract. The ulcer is protected from the irritating digestive acids and is healed at the same time. From the first dose, the relief is immediate. In cases of an ulcer, take Slippery Elm Powder daily for 6 weeks. Even major ulcers are healed in that time.

Once the ulcer is healed and you stop taking the Slippery Elm Powder, unless you learn to live in a less frantic manner, there is nothing to insure against creating another ulcer. Changing a tense lifestyle to a more relaxed one is the only permanent ulcer treatment.

Appendicitis

Chronic or acute appendicitis is soothed very quickly with Slippery Elm Powder. The thick mucilage in Slippery Elm slides into the appendix, cleans it out, and soothes the inflammation. I have seen many an appendix saved because of Slippery Elm Powder. In the case of appendicitis, take Slippery Elm Powder daily for 6 weeks.

Gastric and Intestinal Viruses

In these cases, with their sudden and severe pain, Slippery Elm Powder is emergency treatment. Even with gastroenteritis, the pain and diarrhea ease within seconds after taking Slippery Elm Powder. Have a tablespoon as soon as you are aware of the pain, and follow up the daily dosage for a week.

Swallowed Poisons

As soon as something harmful has been swallowed, whether poison mushrooms or lye, Slippery Elm Powder, with its heavy mucilage, will immediately protect the digestive lining from the irritant and begin to heal any damage that has been done. Though the relief is immediate, take it daily for 1 week.

—From *Pocket Guide to Herbal First Aid*

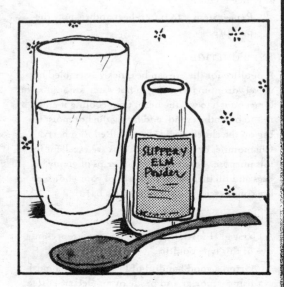

POULTICES AND FOMENTATIONS (COMPRESSES)

James Green, Herbalist

There has been an inspired reawakening of Western herb lore in the minds and hearts of the citizenry in North America. Individuals within nearly every society of our diverse culture are seeking knowledge about the utilization of self-medicating materials that were once commonly used in the homes and communities of our ancestors. One by one, we are rediscovering the simple vehicles that efficiently deliver the healing virtues residing in our garden's herbs and weeds. We are restocking our home pharmacies with herbal preparations and reviving the personal and family dignity of taking care of ourselves. This is the era of our reconnection with plant spirit; we are about to harvest the health-promoting independence of our greenselves.

Continuing the progress of this reconnection, we will review in this chapter the laying of simple herbal waters and succulent pulps upon our skin. This time-honored process is well used in concert with the vehicles discussed in the accompanying chapters.

At this point, I trust you are comfortable with the terms "self-medication" and "self-medicating." I realize we lay folk, over the last ninety years, have conditioned ourselves to believe and feel that "therapeutics," "medicine," and "medicating" are professional mysteries that are the sole domain of licensed medical doctors, and only a doctor by using medical pharmaceutical products can competently and safely medicate us. The medical/pharmaceutical licensing and marketing lobbies have successfully conjured this collective illusion. Yet I believe the current search for therapeutic "alternatives" and disease-preventive measures by ever-increasing numbers of individuals, along with the obvious swell of self-education in personal health care, illustrates our grassroots disenchantment with this tenet.

If you feel uncomfortable with the ideas of self-medicating, I respectfully suggest that it is time to root out and possibly reconsider the beliefs that underlie these feelings. Boundless numbers of us in this society are extremely intelligent human beings, fully capable of making excellent decisions about our lives, particularly when given access to valid information as a base on which to work. And in response to this collective calling there is an ever-increasing number of knowledgeably responsible books, seminars, hands-on workshops, and intensive school programs supplied by highly competent herbalists, teaching people how to use herbs safely, responsibly, and effectively for individual and family health care. We have every right to medicate our own persons, and the freedom to do so. (I believe the ninth amendment to the constitution focuses attention on this inalienable right.) And unless the state, in fact, does own our children, we have the same right and responsibility to find out what is best for them. The knowledgeable use of herbs administered in the home in place of pharmaceutical drugs is frequently a far more pragmatic, benign, and responsible choice for an ailing child's (and adult's) well-being. In the face of media blitz

Continued ➡

with its perennial promise of medical miracle cures waiting around every corner, we have allowed ourselves to lose sight of the true healing intelligence and wisdom each of us possess. We merely need to recall and revive this basic human function. Healing is inspired, not ordained.

In line with these thoughts, ...[we will look at the] uses of poultices and compresses, as these are some of the simplest and most pleasant feeling (bathlike) vehicles for the home delivery of herbal health care.

Poultices

Classically, a poultice (a.k.a. cataplasm) is a soft, mushy preparation composed usually of some pulpy or mealy substance that is capable of absorbing a large amount of liquid and of such consistency that it can be applied to any flat or irregular surface. This herbal material is made into a paste, using hot liquids, and is spread thickly upon cloths and applied directly to the body while hot. Poultices owe their primary virtues to the moist heat which they contain and therefore must be renewed every few minutes, or somehow kept warm by other means. An exception to these mechanics is the Mustard (*Brassica nigra*) poultice, which supplies its warming action through a volatile component produced when its crushed seed is mixed with water. In herb land, however, the scope of the term *poultice* has broadened and now covers a wide range of preparations, some of which are applied hot, some cold.

Poultices and fomentations in their most simple form are merely local baths that utilize *warmth* and *moisture* to relax tissue and relieve pain. Beyond this, herbal preparations can be incorporated in these soothing hot waters to add further assistance with their unique therapeutic properties. Therefore, herbal poultices can be any of the following:

Emollient, which by supplying warmth and moisture are useful for reducing pain and inflammation and assisting the ripening and suppurative (pus-generating) process. Emollient poultices can be made of Flaxseed meal (powdered Flaxseed), Oat meal, bran, bread, and milk, Plantain, Marshmallow root, or mashed vegetable materials such as Cabbage, Turnip, Potato, or Carrot.

Medicated, which are intended to exercise a specific influence on a part of the body, independent of warmth and moisture. These are made of any or a combination of a wide variety of medicinal plants, such as astringents, styptics and vulneraries, anodynes, disinfectants, etc. They are used to penetrate and reduce enlarged or inflamed glands, eruptions, abscesses, lacerations, boils, etc.

Counterirritant or *revulsive*, which, by inducing a local irritation or inflammation as they stimulate capillary dilation and action, cause skin redness.

This counter-irritation draws stagnant blood and other materials from deeper tissues and organs to the surface, thereby relieving deeper congestion and inflammation. These poultices also act as derivatives that draw pustular materials from the body through the skin. These poultices are made using stimulating herbs such as Mustard, Ginger, Cayenne, Garlic, Rosemary, etc.

Optimally, medicated herbal poultices are prepared from fresh herbs which have been chewed, chopped, mashed, bruised, or blended in an electric blender and mixed with hot water, apple cider vinegar, or some other hot liquid. A blender suits us well for these preparations, for it is important to break up the cell walls in order to gain access to the properties contained in the plant juices.

Dry (dehydrated) herb that has been rehydrated also can be used to make poultices. You can rehydrate a dehydrated herb by gently heating it in a little water, apple cider vinegar, milk, or other liquid that seems appropriate. Once the herb has absorbed the liquid and softened, it is ready to use for preparing a poultice in the same way that you would use a fresh plant.

A poultice can be used again and again during each session. However, it needs to be reheated each time before reapplying. A hot poultice should be applied as hot as can be borne. To test its temperature apply it to the back of your hand—it should feel hot, but comfortable. To prevent the rapid loss of heat, it is helpful to cover the poultice with a thick insulating cloth while it's on your body.

First clean the area of the body by using a solution of 1 part apple cider vinegar to 1 part warm water, or simply soap and water; then a thin layer of vegetable oil is rubbed on the skin to protect it, and to prevent the poultice from sticking to the skin.

The vinegar-water mixture is also an especially good solution to use for washing and conditioning the area after the poultice has been removed.

Making a Poultice

A VERY SIMPLE POULTICE

1. Put powdered or chopped fresh herbal materials into a clean white cotton sock. Use two socks and alternate them.

2. Tie it at the top (tie it in a knot, or use string, or elastic).

3. Place this into a shallow bowl.

4. Pour enough hot water over the prefilled sock to soak the dry herb or heat the fresh herb.

5. With your hands, knead the wet sock until it is quite hot, yet bearable.

6. Apply this to the affected area until the poultice is cool.

7. Repeat steps 3 to 6 to reheat and reapply the poultice.

EYE POULTICE

A poultice for the eye can be quickly assembled by merely dropping a tea bag in hot water for an instant, long enough to wet the herb, then cooling it enough not to burn the eyelid, and laying the hot moist tea bag on the closed eyelid. Fennel, Red Raspberry, Chamomile, or disinfectant herbs are excellent for this purpose. You can purchase strips of empty tea bags and fill them with the herbs of your choice or use commercial brand prefilled tea bags.

EMOLLIENT POULTICE

A Flaxseed (Linseed) poultice is a good representative of this type poultice.

1. Grind a good handful of Flaxseed into a meal using a mortar and pestle or an electric coffee bean grinder.

2. Add some boiling water [approximate proportions of 300 ml (10 fl. oz.) of water to 120 gm (4 oz.) of Flaxmeal].

3. Quickly stir the Flaxseed and water together until you have made a thick paste.

4. Spread this hot paste (at least ½-inch thick) onto a clean white cloth, leaving the edges of the cloth free from the paste and avoiding the formation of lumps in the paste.

5. Apply the poultice to the body as hot as possible, making sure it completely covers and even extends a little beyond the area being soothed. It helps to spread a little vegetable oil on the skin before applying the poultice to protect the skin and to make it easier to remove the poultice. Otherwise, it can stick to the skin.

6. When the poultice is lukewarm, another poultice should be ready to take its place, and the treatment should be continued as long as necessary.

7. Of course, you can help retain the heat by insulating the poultice. First lay a plastic bag directly over the poultice, then wrap a towel around it, and if appropriate lay a hot water bottle or heating pad on top of all this to supply prolonged heat.

Another convenient method to prepare a Flaxseed or similar poultice is to make several bags of various sizes out of cheesecloth. Fill the bags half full with Flaxseed or whatever agent you select, then sew up the open end (store these in the refrigerator or freezer to prevent the Flaxseed from going rancid over time). When needed, the appropriate size bag is submerged in boiling water for a few minutes. When the bag is taken out of the water, you will see that the Flaxseed has swelled and filled the bag. Squeeze out any superfluous water, lay the bag on the body, and cover it with insulating and or heating materials.

As a poultice, Flaxseed can be used for treating carbuncles, shingles, and psoriasis, it can be combined with Marshmallow root powder to use for reducing swellings and inflammations, and for drawing out the pus in boils.

Flaxseed poultices mixed with Onion are commonly used to provide relief in lung conditions, especially with pleurisy, which calls out for a warm poultice (pleurisy can be a symptom of serious disease—get it checked out). After removing a poultice from the chest area, a second one can then be placed onto the upper back, which will cover and treat the back regions of the lungs.

OTHER HERBAL MATERIALS USED TO MEDICATE A POULTICE

The herbs Calendula, Comfrey, and Plantain are the reigning matriarchs in the clan of herbal poultices, with Echinacea giving service as their cardinal aide when further wound healing and enhanced immune-stimulating action is needed.

Calendula (*Calendula officinalis*) promotes the healing and regeneration of bruised tissue, burns, eruptions, abrasions, and so forth. Overall, this herb is one of the most efficient of all herbs to use as a poultice or a fomentation (fomentations are discussed later in the chapter). A Calendula poultice reduces soreness and inflammation, while its antimicrobial properties assist in the cleansing of a wound, fostering rapid healing.

Comfrey (*Symphytum officinale*) is our most valuable plant ally for repairing wounds, while at the same time it soothes and softens tissue. It is probably the most healing mucilaginous remedy in our herbal materia medica, having been used for centuries to treat external ulceration and all types of lesions and injuries ranging from small cuts and

Continued →

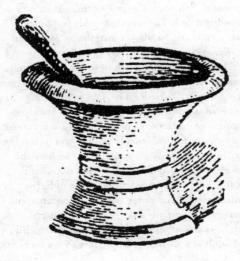

abrasions to large wounds and broken bones. A Comfrey poultice quickens the repair of the normally slow healing process of torn cartilage, tendons, and ligaments. A common name "Knitbone" refers to Comfrey's historic use as a poultice for treating skeletal fractures in humans and animals. It heals bone tissue. Its mucilage and tannins produce an astringent and contracting effect. By drawing a wound together at the surface, it reduces the need for stitching; and its generous allantoin content stimulates the regeneration of skin tissue, making the formation of scar tissue less likely.

Of all the herbs, **Plantain** (*Plantago lanceolata, P. major*) is probably the most accessible and abundant. In league with Dandelion, it is one of an herbalists two most loyal and reliable travel companions. They can be found growing nearly everywhere on our planet. Plantain is used by herbalists to remove the ouch! from wounds, especially the venomous ouch prompted by stinging and biting insects and other skin-penetrating animals. Plantain (both the narrow-leaf and broad-leaf types) helps stop bleeding, neutralizes venom and toxins, soothes inflammation, and heals wounds. This plant applied as a poultice is also helpful in withdrawing deeply lodged splinters.

Echinacea (*Echinacea spp.*) is a highly effective wound-healing plant, generously stimulating the immune system. It is especially useful in treating sluggardly, long-standing wounds that are slow to heal. The addition of this plant to any of the above plant poultices complements and amplifies their qualities.

A FIELD POULTICE

This poultice is useful if you are the recipient of an insect bite. It can be a fresh one or an old one that just doesn't seem to get better, or any kind of benign, welting, itching, insect bite including tick, wasp, yellow jacket, or a bee sting. In case of a bee sting, remove the stinger by sliding the edge of a credit card along the skin up to the stinger and gently nudging it sideways out of the skin. Don't squeeze the stinger by trying to pull it out with your fingers; you will inject more venom doing that. In case of a tick bite, pull the tick straight out first.

1. Pick a handful of Plantain.

2. Wad it up by rolling it firmly between your palms, bruising and crushing it well, or put it in your mouth and chew it (which is actually better—dogs aren't the only ones having therapeutic saliva).

3. If you chew it, don't swallow the juice. It's okay to swallow the juice, but the Plantain-infused saliva is what contacts the skin as a poultice and "makes you better."

4. Make the poultice thick and slap it on the skin.

5. Then hold the palm of your hand on top of the poultice to supply some warmth and some caring touch to the injury.

6. (*Optional*) When you can, brew a pot of Plantain tea and drink it freely. Change the poultice a couple times a day and keep one on the wound overnight with some form of a bandage. Repeat this daily until all is well again; and it will be, soon.

ONION POULTICE FOR EARACHES

To make and apply an Onion poultice for relieving the pain of an earache:

1. Cut a medium-size Onion in half and bake it at a low temperature until it is soft.

2. Place the warm flat surface of the baked Onion directly on the ear.

3. Secure it with a cloth bandage wrapped around the head, Van Gogh fashion. Unlike Vincent's

technique, however, the application of a baked Onion will soothe the ear and relieve the pain and suffering.

ONION POULTICE FOR THE BODY

While the aroma of Onion is in the air, I should explain how to make an Onion poultice for the rest of the body. (The notable refinement of detail and characteristic finesse in the preparation of the following poultice I obtained from a conversation with my friend "Herbal" Ed Smith, herbalist and president of Herb Pharm in Williams, Oregon. And although he is more than likely responsible for a lot of other things, he should not be held responsible for the wording used here.) This is what you can do at home to relieve the acute condition of cough, croup, bronchitis, strep throat kidney infection, eye infection, and whatever else hurts:

1. Chop 3 or 4 Onions finely.

2. Saute them in oil (it doesn't matter what kind of oil). Make it a little on the greasy side.

3. Cook the Onions until they become translucent, but don't cook them too much. You want them to be hot and flexible, not mushy.

4. Now, slowly pour on some apple cider vinegar (just enough to almost, but not quite, float the hot and flexible Onions).

5. Turn the flame down for the next steps to prevent the Onions from sticking to the pan.

6. Add Cornmeal or Flaxseed meal. Both of these are high in fat, so they absorb, and later, radiate the heat. You can use flour in place of the Corn or Flaxseed meals, but poultice gourmets tend to frown on this substitution.

7. Using a spatula, mix together and knead the Onions, the oil, and the meal into a wet plastic mass (not too wet, not too dry, but peanut butter-like).

8. When this is done to your satisfaction, put it on a piece of cheesecloth, or muslin, or flannel cloth, fold it over like a fat omelet, and stick the edges of the cloth together.

9. Apply the hot Onion poultice to the body.

This poultice is rich in sulfurated volatile oils and therapeutic mucilaginous substances. You will want to create a complete seal between the poultice and the skin by making sure there are no air pockets that will interfere with the "osmotic transfer" of energy between the poultice and the body.

When treating the lungs, following a chest poultice, turn the person over and apply another Onion poultice on the upper half of the back.

HONEY POULTICE

Honey is one of the best poultices to apply directly to a burn. First, cool the burned tissue with cold water, if possible, then merely spread honey on the burn or wound and leave it there for about a half hour. Reapply if necessary. Honey immediately seals off the damaged tissue from the air, reducing the pain while it works to rehydrate the wounded tissue; all the other magical bee-formulated components of honey proceed to do what they do to embellish the repair. Honey is antiseptic and helps to avoid infection.

MUSTARD POULTICE (*Brassica nigra, Sinapis nigra*)

A Mustard poultice, also known as a *sinapism*, differs from most other poultices in both its preparation and its action. Note that you shouldn't use pure, undiluted Mustard, for it is very likely to blister the skin. Mustard is ordinarily diluted with about an equal weight of Cornmeal, Flaxseed meal, or some other form of flour (sometimes these are called a *diluent*).

Prior to mixing the powdered Mustard seed

with the diluent, it is moistened with tepid or lukewarm water (140-ish°F.), never with boiling water. When water is added to the crushed seed, its ultimate warming action is aroused as an enzyme acts upon a glycoside. A volatile "isothiocyanate" is generated, which is called "volatile mustard oil" (not to be confused with an aromatic volatile "essential" oil). The formation of the warming volatile Mustard oil is greatly inhibited if too high heat is applied, so never use boiling water for this preparation. This tends to diminish the crucial enzymatic action. It is also recommended not to use vinegar as a wetting agent, for it too inhibits the formation of the heat-producing Mustard oil. To assemble and apply the Mustard poultice:

1. Mix the dry Mustard with the warm water.

2. Mix the diluent with hot water.

3. Stir these two mixtures together.

4. Place a thin cloth on the skin to protect it and to avoid adhesion to the skin.

5. Spread the poultice thickly onto the cloth.

6. The poultice is allowed to remain on the skin from 10 minutes to a half hour in order to gain its rubefacient activity.

The action is usually at its height in about 15 to 20 minutes, even though redness is usually produced in a shorter time. If an individual's skin is quite tender or there is a weakened system, a short action may be more effective overall than a prolonged one.

On delicate, sensitive skin, the Mustard poultice need not remain on the body for more than 6 to 8 minutes, for its effect continues some time after its removal. Please keep in mind that if a Mustard plaster is applied too hot and kept on too long, the skin can become inflamed, blister, and become otherwise injured.

The constituents of Mustard applied as a poultice or bath produce a lively stimulation and arouse the nervous system. This acts to disperse any pain that is due to congestion. Employ the wonderfully deep-penetrating, rubefacient, decongesting, and pain-relieving benefits of this herbal poultice, but be very attentive to the proper dilution of the Mustard with the diluent, and closely monitor the reaction of the individual's skin.

CAYENNE POULTICE

As a milder substitute for the deeper-penetrating Mustard poultice, the Cayenne red pepper or Capsicum poultice will serve well, and it will not cause blistering. Cayenne can be used as a poultice by mixing the powder with bread and moistened with a little hot milk, or mix the Cayenne powder with some form of powdered grain and moisten with hot milk or hot water.

WHITE CABBAGE POULTICE

This (vegetable) herb is good as a poultice for drawing out pus and other gloomy body exudates. Merely take the inner leaves of a common White Cabbage, wash them well, and dry them (the large middle rib is best removed and discarded for easier processing of the leaves). Bruise the leaves using a rolling pin or some other like instrument to soften them and place them on the affected area. Hold the leaves in place by wrapping a loose bandage or small towel around them. Leave the Cabbage poultice on for ½ to 1 hour, then replace it with a fresh one. You can add some powdered Myrrh gum or powdered Echinacea to this if there is any infection.

Applying raw Cabbage leaves as a poultice affords a slightly stimulating poultice, which is best used in conditions where one is treating a sluggish, ill-conditioned, offensive skin ulcer.

Continued →

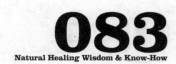

ROOT POULTICE

These emollient poultices can be prepared from any of the tender culinary roots (and tubers) like Carrot, Turnip, Potato, or Burdock. Simply boil the tender roots, remove the skin, and mash them into a soft pulp. These make a mild, nutritive, emollient poultice. Like the Cabbage poultice, when needed, a raw version of these root poultices renders increased stimulating action. Peel and shred the fresh raw roots, mash them into pulp, and apply them to the skin.

CLAY POULTICE

Clay poultices are made using bentonite clay, water, and appropriate herbal tinctures. Pharmaceutical grade bentonite can be purchased in health food stores and pharmacies.

1. Dilute an herbal tincture with about half as much water (2 parts tincture to 1 part water). Use this mixture to add to the clay.

2. Slowly add the liquid to the clay, stirring until you have made a paste. (Start out with the proportions of about a tablespoon of clay to each tablespoon of liquid.)

3. At this point you can add a few drops of Lavender or Tea Tree essential oil (5 to 10 drops) and stir them in.

4. Apply this herbal clay paste to the body.

5. Apply it thick (at least ½ inch). This helps keep the poultice warm and moist. Clay poultices that dry out too quickly are not as effectual. You want them to remain wet (when they are most active) as long as possible.

To prepare a bentonite clay poultice for the mouth, teeth, and gums for reducing the inflammation and agony of an abscessed tooth, or to help reach down and disperse the stagnating energy of swollen throat glands, you simply prepare a medicated clay roll as follows:

1. Add enough water to some pharmaceutical-grade bentonite clay to make it into a malleable peanut butter consistency.

2. Using an appropriate amount of sterile gauze, roll the clay into a joint (a controversial cigarette-like contrivance) about the size of the pain rider's small finger.

3. Rid the clay roll of any air bubbles and squeeze its ends closed to seal them.

4. Pack the cylindrical poultice between the gum and cheek and leave it there for ½ to 1 hour, 2 times a day.

5. Rest, holding the poultice in place.

6. The effect of the clay can be enhanced by mixing some finely powdered Echinacea root or Goldenseal root with the clay powder before adding the water.

When treating swollen glands, one can add a couple drops of Poke root (*Phytolacca americana*) tincture to this poultice. It is quite helpful to use hand baths also to help pump the nodes in the neck. Administer the baths by placing both hands in a hot bath for 3 minutes immediately followed by a cold hand bath for 1 minute. Repeat this several consecutive times.

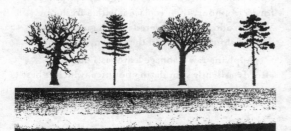

Fomentations

A fomentation (a.k.a. compress) is a form of poultice that is comprised of liquids or lotions, absorbed in woolen or cotton cloths and usually applied hot. (Cold compresses are prepared for treating some headaches and sprains, and to stop bleeding.) Basically, a fomentation is yet another species of a bath employed to convey heat, combined with moisture, to the part of the body being fomented. A fomentation, like all therapeutic and tonic baths, is administered with the intent to soothe, nurse, and/or excite one back to ebullient, healthy activity.

Material to Use for Making a Fomentation

Flannel cloths wrung out of hot liquid form the best fomentation material. In every process of fomentation there should be two cloths, one flannel ready while the other is applied. After the water has been wrung from the flannel, it should be *shaken up* and *laid lightly* over the body part. This involves a considerable amount of air which, being a poor conductor for heat transfer, retains the heat in the flannel cloth for a substantial amount of time.

When selecting a material to use for applying a fomentation, the fineness or the coarseness of the flannel is important to note. The coarser the material, the less readily it conducts heat, but it retains its warmth longer. It is therefore more efficient for fomenting. White flannel appears to retain heat longer than colored flannel. Of course, any absorbent material can be employed to apply a fomentation. Depending on the body part requiring the assistance, you can use gauze patches, stocking caps, menstrual pads, cotton gloves, jock straps, cotton bras cotton socks, and so on.

For ease of wringing out boiling hot flannel cloths, one can employ the following technique:

Purchase two pieces of white flannel each three yards long. (This is for use in large area fomenting; shorter pieces are appropriate for smaller jobs.) Sew the ends together making a very large headband-like device. This can now be wrung out of boiling liquid by means of two sticks inserted through the loop and turned in opposite directions. After the hot flannel has been wrung out, shake it up and lay the double-layered fomentation lightly on the body.

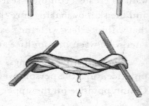

Making a Fomentation

To aid digestion in an individual whose stomach appears to be deficient in producing adequate hydrochloric acid, a simple hot-water fomentation placed over the stomach for an hour or two after eating increases the amount of hydrochloric acid secreted by the peptic glands. A hot water bottle might be more convenient to employ for this purpose, but then where is the hot-water bottle when you need it? And applications of heat over the abdomen can increase the activity of the digestive processes in the intestines and the functional activity of the pancreas and spleen. (In contrast, generally, whole-body hot baths tend to diminish the secretion of HCL.) Hot applications placed over the liver region increase the flow of bile and stimulate all the other activities of the liver.

Simple hot water fomentations are remarkably soothing and revitalizing, but the use of herbal infusions and decoctions as the hot liquid further enhances their therapeutic action. Also, tinctures diluted with water can be used to medicate a fomentation.

ARNICA FOMENTATION

A cold fomentation of Arnica (*Arnica spp.*) is well used to enhance peripheral circulation, helping to eliminate the pain of bruises, sprains, torn muscles, and tendons during the acute stage of an injury. A tablespoon of Arnica tincture to a half quart of cold water is used as the liquid in which a fomentation is soaked and laid on the injury. The injury is to be immobilized immediately and the fomentations are to be renewed frequently. Once the acute stage has run its course, one can apply warm poultices made of Comfrey root and Onion to give deeper action to assist the healing. Sprains can continue to trouble the individual long after the acute stages of the injury have passed. This is a good time to administer hot foot and leg baths or hot hand and arm bath, depending on the nature and location of the injury. These baths should be enjoyed for 20 to 30 minutes at a time.

FOXGLOVE FOMENTATION

Foxglove (*Digitalis*) is a common garden plant that is toxic when taken internally, but is quite safe and useful when used externally as a moist compress. Dr. Rudolf Weiss, in his excellent book *Herbal Medicine*, introduces this technique, which has been found to be of great value in promoting the healing of wounds that tend to persist for long periods of time. Foxglove leaves applied as a hot compress enhance the peripheral circulation of the skin and promote wound healing, especially those wounds that appear to be healing very slowly or not at all, such as chronic skin ulcers. I have found that a daily cup of herb tea made up of 1 part Comfrey root, 2 parts Burdock root, sweetened to taste, is a powerful adjunct for this task. Never drink a tea of Foxglove, however!

POPPY FOMENTATION

To help diminish pain, there is nothing as congenial than a hot fomentation made of dried Oriental Poppy (*Papaver somnifera*) heads. Drop 10 or 15 of them in water and heat the water. When it is quite warm, but not to hot to touch, pick out and tear the soggy Poppy heads in half and drop them back into the pot. When you finish doing this, bring the water to a boil, and simmer the Poppy heads for 10 to 15 minutes. The solution will turn a rich honey brown color. Dip your flannel into the hot decoction, wring it out, shake up the wet flannel, and lay it lightly on the painful area. When the flannel has cooled to warm, replace it immediately with a second fomentation. Repeat this 4 or 5 times. Leave the last fomentation on and cover it with plastic. Lay a towel over it, place a hot water bottle on this, and cover everything with a warm blanket. Let the individual lie quietly for about half an hour or so. While he or she is lying there fomenting, massage his or her feet and scalp.

CASTOR OIL FOMENTATION (HOT PACK)

It has been said and I must concur that the Castor oil hot pack (hot fomentation) is, without doubt, the high monarch of all herbal compresses; it is the Mohammed Ali, the Florence Nightingale, the '32 Ford Coup, the sensual Sultan of Swat of all poultices. I suggest that whenever you don't know what else to do for an ailing acquaintance, treat them to a Castor oil hot pack.

Mind you, a Castor oil fomentation can be a bit messy to administer. It's nothing a little attention to

Continued ➡

detail can't handle, though. It can take a while to produce noticeable, long-range results, but acute experiences of deep relaxation and central nervous system bliss are always noticed immediately. These are perfect experiences to initiate any healing journey.

A Castor oil fomentation can relieve muscular and skeletal pain, but more importantly, it can relieve the deep pain stemming from fibroids, internal scar tissue, congested lymph nodes, ovarian cysts, and infections. A series of Castor oil fomentations can restore health by invigorating scarred tissue and any deficient and sluggish glands or visceral organs.

Castor oil, which is derived from the Castor bean (*Ricinus communis*), is so similar to the natural oils of the human body it is easily received by human tissues and it is able to assist in their rejuvenation. Following is an abbreviated list of therapeutic chores expected by the judicious application of Castor oil fomentations: calming of nervous irritability and aiding sleep, detoxification of tissues including the liver when needed; reduction and healing of cysts, warts, and other unwanted growths; alleviation of uterine disorders and chronic infections; soothing the discomfort of bladder infection while promoting healing; and stimulation of the body's deep circulation, including lymphatic circulation. Castor oil fomentations promote general detoxification and deep relaxation, which in turn rejuvenates all systems of the body.

To prepare and administer a hot Castor oil fomentation:

1. Cut several pieces of laundered white cotton flannel, cotton felt, or cheesecloth large enough to more than completely cover the area to be treated. (When fomenting the liver, it is best to use pieces of material large enough to extend from the navel, over the liver, and around to the spine, and from the right hip bone up to the breast/pecs.) I suggest you cut several pieces of material because it is best for this fomentation to be several layers thick.

2. Place the cotton material into a clean glass or stainless steel pan.

3. Pour 1 to 2 cups of Castor oil onto the pieces of material, soaking them through with the oil.

4. Place the pan of oiled cotton into an oven and heat it until the oiled material is very warm but still touchable. One can put a few drops of Lavender, Chamomile, Lemon, and/or Rose essential oil onto the pack at this point if this floral oil bouquet will be appreciated.

5. Wash the area of the body to be treated with a mixture of warm water and apple cider vinegar.

6. Take the fomentation from the pan and remove any excess oil so there is no dripping.

7. Place the hot fomentation over the area to be fomented. (If this is a liver pack, the person should be lying on his or her left side. Otherwise it will be a spleen pack, and that would be okay, too.)

8. Cover the fomentation with a plastic wrap.

9. Over this lay a heating pad or a hot water bottle.

10. Wrap a large towel around all the above and tuck it comfortably under the body to hold everything in place.

11. Place a warm blanket over the individual and let him or her receive the fomentation for at least an hour up to several hours.

12. A gentle foot massage and head massage supplies a delicious touch to this healthful ritual.

13. When completed, remove the oil from the skin by using a gentle soap and then a wash of

warm water and baking soda. (This mixture will soothe the area, especially if any minor skin irritation or rash has developed from the drawing action of the Castor oil.)

When all is finished, wrap the oiled material in a plastic bag and store it in the refrigerator. It can be reheated and reused several times, *but only on the same person*. Replace it with fresh material after six to eight applications.

Repeated fomentations over a period of time are often required to heal the above conditions. These can be given in a pattern of three days in a row, then four days off. Repeat this pattern for several weeks or until the ailing condition is history. Each time you receive the effects of this poultice you will feel like you've just taken a six-week vacation, one in which you never had to look for parking places or endure airport fiascoes.

Remember, the tricks for using poultices and fomentations successfully (although there are always some exceptions) are:

· Make poultices thick.

· Keep poultices and fomentation warm and moist.

· Allow them adequate time to do their work.

Incorporating time in any therapeutic formula is valuable; you asked for the help, so give yourself the space to receive it. Enjoy post-trauma time by relaxing and being patient. More than likely, stress and impatience had major roles in creating the wounds in the first place.

—From *The Herbal Medicine Maker's Handbook*

MALE-SPECIFIC HERBALISM

James Green, Herbalist

Prostate Health

It is said that men push their worries into their prostate gland, our uniquely male chamber of silence where we store our most private concerns. What is a prostate—often called the male gland? Where is it, and why is it there? How can it be taken care of? Few people can answer these questions. Few men ever ask them until they become painful questions. And yet it appears a majority of men have trouble with their prostate gland sometime in their life.

The prostate gland is a chestnut-shaped organ, partly muscular and partly glandular, having outer and inner masses of prostatic tissue. The normal prostate is a little over 1 1/2 inches (4 centimeters) wide and about as long, approximately the size of a walnut. It is attached to the seminal vesicles, sits just below the bladder, next to the rectum, and surrounds the urethra (the urinary exit tube) in the male genitourinary system. It is undeniably a most mysterious gland. The prostate is an endocrine-dependent organ; however, knowledge of its endocrine relationship remains a blur to science. Castration (shudder) or the withdrawal of androgens, or male sex hormones, produces atrophy of the gland. The administration of androgens following castration (I promise not to use that word again) delays the development of atrophy, but

administration of estrogen, the female sex hormone, does so as well. No satisfactory explanations have come forth to explain this phenomenon of opposing hormonal influences exerting a similar effect on the male gland.

The most obvious function of the prostate gland is to secrete a milky protein fluid discharged into the urethra at the time of the emission of semen. This prostatic fluid mixes with the semen during ejaculation, helping transport sperm out of the body. Prior to puberty, the prostate gland does not secrete any fluid, but when sexual maturity occurs, prostate secretion is continuous, and even during periods of sexual inactivity a small amount of prostatic fluid is deposited into the urethra daily and passes with the urine. Some folks suspect that the prostate gland contracts during ejaculation so semen will not backflow into the seminal vesicles. If, for whatever reason, the prostate enlarges or inflames and swells, the urethra running through a hole in the prostate is pinched off, as when a drinking straw is crushed, which obstructs the flow of urine, causing the urine to stagnate, back up, and distend the bladder. Renal complications can occur if the urine backs up into the kidneys. These are potential problems perpetrated by an organ responsible for performing what appears to be such a relatively minor physical function. It must have a subtle covert function that our sciences haven't yet detected—and there must be more compassionate therapies than the common allopathic procedure of surgically reaming it out with steel devices.

Benign Prostate Enlargement

A common problem that affects men later in life is an enlargement of the prostate gland that causes discomfort and dysuria, or difficulty in urinating. This enlargement occurs very slowly and gradually, and most men are not aware they have the condition until the prostate has grown large enough to cause symptoms. Prostatic enlargement, occurring in approximately 50 to 60 percent of men ages forty to fifty-nine, is often referred to as benign prostatic hyperplasia (BPH); the last word means "excessive formation." This condition tends to be progressive; however, this is not always so. In some men, it can progress very slowly and stop at any point. Further clinical befuddlement arises from the observation that in some cases, a greatly enlarged prostate causes hardly any trouble, and in other cases, a slight enlargement causes great discomfort and difficulty in urination.

An enlarged prostate may be discovered during a routine medical checkup, or when a man complains to a doctor about symptoms. In addition to asking for details about the symptoms, the doctor will usually perform a digital rectal examination (*digital* as in "finger"). To do this, a well-lubricated, gloved finger is inserted into the rectum to feel the size and shape of the prostate. Many doctors perform this examination as part of a routine checkup for any man over the age of fifty, or sometimes starting at an earlier age. Remember, though: you can always "just say no."

Three stages of prostate enlargement seem to take place. The first stage is characterized by the stream of urine growing thinner and the urge to urinate increasing. Some men will notice that it takes more time for the sphincter muscle to relax, enabling urine to pass. Many men remain at this stage for the rest of their lives, and this stage is very responsive to herbal treatment. In the second stage, the retention of urine increases, and the bladder never fully empties. The urine that remains in the bladder is referred to as residual urine. This stage is also responsive to herbal treatment. In stage three, the residual urine increases, stagnates, and distends

Continued ➡

the bladder, creating back pressure, and eventually causes kidney damage and uremia. At this stage, surgical intervention is commonly recommended.

The medical profession uses the term *prostatism* to describe the syndrome of common uncomfortable symptoms that BPH can cause. These symptoms include:

- Urgency (feeling an extremely strong desire to urinate as soon as possible)
- Hesitancy (having a hard time getting the flow of urine started—sort of like standing at a public urinal trying to go, while a bunch of guys are standing in line behind you, waiting for you to finish)
- Decreased size and strength of stream of urine (you're no longer the contender you once were in distance-peeing contests)
- Intermittency (an on-again, off-again flow of urine)
- Dribbling that continues after urination
- Incomplete urination (the unsatisfied feeling that your bladder is still not quite empty after you urinate)
- Urinary retention (being completely unable to urinate)
- Frequency (having to urinate much more often than you used to)
- Nocturia (the need to get up and urinate during the night)
- Urinary incontinence (being unable to hold back urine until you reach the bathroom; often accompanied by feelings of urgency)

It is recommend that men experiencing mild symptoms of BPH avoid certain drugs, including antihistamines, decongestants, and alcohol, which can aggravate the condition.

Prominent medical theory suggests that BPH is caused by an accumulation of testosterone, a hormone that helps keep healthy aggression intact, in the prostate. Within the prostate, this testosterone is converted into a compound called dihydrotestosterone (DHT), which in turn causes cells to multiply excessively and eventually causes the prostate to enlarge.

When a male retires from his professional work, he often loses an arena for his normal, constructive, active aggression, so he needs to keep his lifestyle active to keep from being too retired. This may help him avoid accumulating excessive testosterone in the prostate gland.

Prostatitis

Prostatitis is inflammation or infection of the prostate gland. This condition can in turn inflame the prostatic urethra and ultimately the bladder. This completed scenario is referred to in the university-trained doctor's language as prostatocystitis. (Medical terms are undeniably impressive, literally commanding authority. Laymen should create words for prostate health symptoms such as *prostatocool* or *prostatosvelte*.)

The common symptoms of an inflamed, infected, and/or enlarged prostate gland are similar: There is an aching pain in the area of the prostate, pain when sitting, and frequent dribbling. Urination can be a challenge, with difficulty starting the stream and emptying the bladder; sometimes blood will appear in the urine, and chills and fever often accompany the condition. Causes often boil down to stress (usually, but not only, sexual stress), excesses in diet (especially excess consumption of alcohol and caffeine products), and lack of

regular physical exercise, and this condition may occur as a secondary infection caused by another infection such as a tooth abscess or a sexually transmitted disease. In this case, of course, the primary infection must be attended to concurrently and the immune system must be bolstered.

In addition to using appropriate herbal and nutritional therapy, which will be discussed below, congestion of an enlarged prostate can be relieved by the use of a firm seat on chairs; sitting in the lotus position; avoiding sitting on cold, damp surfaces or hard bicycle seats; and avoiding long rides in automobiles, trains, and so on. Men suffering from the condition should also avoid drinking alcohol (especially heavy beer drinking, because sheer volume and any festivity-induced delays in urinating can exacerbate the problem), caffeine, cooked hot spices (which appear to irritate the prostatic urethra), and sexual excesses (in many male minds, this term is handily discarded as a foolish oxymoron).

The call to urinate should be acted on immediately, and urination should be attempted every couple hours, for it's best not to overdistend the bladder. Extreme difficulty in urination may be relieved by sitting down in a tub of warm water to urinate. Also, drinking water several times a day produces dilute urine that helps flush the bladder outlet.

Nonmedical and nonsurgical treatment of these prostate problems requires focus and perseverance. Natural healing takes longer, but it is well worth the time and self-commitment. Keep in mind that as you treat these symptoms systemically using herbs, diet, and exercise, you are at the same time nourishing and normalizing your entire physical body, and you're taking care of yourself—a very good thing to do. Modern allopathic chemical therapy and surgery tend to the symptom, not to the deficiencies or excesses that caused the problem. Each man experiencing a prostate problem must make his own decision as to how he wants to treat and care for the condition.

Suggested herbal/nutritional treatments of prostate conditions are as follows:

1. First, relax. Dr. Ira Sharlip, professor of urology at the University of California at San Francisco, has acquired relevant evidence demonstrating that relaxing the body's muscles is the core of a successful method of treatment for chronic nonbacterial prostatitis. Sharlip points out that an abnormal increase in the tone of the urethral sphincter muscles due to stress (we store our worries in our prostate) is one cause of prostate difficulties. (We use the urethral sphincter muscles to close off the flow of urine.) Learning stress-management techniques, engaging in enjoyable exercise, pulling worry back out of the prostate zone, and, if necessary, using herbs—such as Valerian, Kava, Cramp Bark, and Skullcap—that help relax muscles, assist successful employment of this technique.

2. Drink lots of pure water daily, and avoid drinking cold beer.

3. Eat lightly. Adhere to a diet substantial in whole grains, fresh and steamed vegetables, fresh fruits, miso-based soups, and sea vegetables such as kelp, nori, and hijiki. This diet provides your body with a variety of foods relatively easy to digest so it can tap into a wide range of vitamins, minerals, and other essential nutrients to revitalize and heal the prostate.

4. Seeds, well chewed, are a most valuable food for developing prostate ; health. Throughout the day, chew up to 1/2 cup of Pumpkin seeds (*Cucurbita pepo*), which are a natural mucilaginous source of zinc and linoleic acid. This step is important for respiration of internal organs and to help decongest the prostate gland and lessen residual urine. Other important seed foods for males are Poppy seeds (best eaten as whole-grain poppy-seed cake), Sunflower seeds, and Sesame seeds. These are easily added to your diet in the form of sunflower-seed butter or sesame-seed butter. Be sure these seeds and seed butters are fresh when you buy them, keep them refrigerated, and, when they're not in use, keep the container lid closed so their oils do not oxidize and turn rancid.

5. Supplement your daily diet with vitamin and mineral supplements: 800 IU (international units) of vitamin E (mixed tocopherols), 400 to 600 milligrams of a calcium/magnesium supplement, and 20 to 50 milligrams of zinc picolinate or amino-chelated zinc.

6. Apply hot and cold packs to the prostate area, the area between the scrotum and the anus. Crushed ice wrapped in a face towel makes a simple ice pack. Apply the hot and cold packs in a ratio of 4:1 (for example, apply the hot pack for four to eight minutes, then follow this immediately with the cold pack for one to two minutes). Follow this routine two to three times a session, two sessions a day, or as often as you wish. This technique does a remarkable job of reducing inflammation (not just on the prostate, but anywhere on the body where inflammation is experienced), and it gives blessed relief. Make the time and effort to do it for yourself.

7. Herb teas and tinctures can provide soothing demulcent action to an inflamed and/or swollen prostate. At the same time, they can be highly nourishing and toning to the entire male system, bringing circulation to the genital area and providing effective cleansing and antimicrobial action. As exemplified by the following formulas, the strategy to consider when tending to the symptoms of an enlarged prostate should include these herbal actions:

- Male reproductive system and prostate tonics: Saw Palmetto, Stinging Nettle root, and Suma
- Genitourinary system tonics and astringents to strengthen and heal the overall system. Use the tonic/astringent herbs that also give antimicrobial and vulnerary actions: Yarrow, Horsetail, Buchu, and Dandelion
- Diuretics to prevent excess buildup of urine in the bladder due to an enlarged prostate, to prevent potential backup of urine into the kidneys, and to support preventive measures: Hydrangea, Couchgrass, Cleavers, Corn Silk, and Watermelon seed
- Immune system enhancers that help the body's defense system build resistance: Echinacea, Astragalus, and Siberian Ginseng
- Urinary system antimicrobials used even when no obvious symptoms of infection appear—these help ensure that no infection stresses the urinary tract: Oregon Grape, Echinacea, and Bearberry
- Demulcents to soothe and protect the urinary system: Couchgrass, Corn Silk, Marshmallow, and Comfrey

Each day, brew and drink alternately a total of 1 to 2 cups of each of the following herb tea formulas:

Continued ➡

An **infusion** (steeped tea) of

1 part	Corn Silk (diuretic/demulcent)
1 part	Couchgrass (very soothing demulcent/astringent/diuretic)
1 part	organic Watermelon seeds (soothing anti-inflammatory diuretic

A **decoction** (simmered tea) of

3 parts	Echinacea (immune enhancer/antimicrobial)
2 parts	Saw Palmetto (prostate tonic/nutrient)
1 part	Marshmallow root (promotes tissue healing)
1 part	Bearberry (urinary antiseptic/astringent)
1 part	Horsetail (astringent/specific for benign prostate enlargement)
1 part	Hydrangea root (gravel solvent-antilithic/astringent)

Often, during times of prostatic complaints, a man's vital energy is also depressed due to accompanying digestive and/or circulatory deficiencies. If these problems are apparent, include Hawthorn berries and flowers and Yarrow in the above formulas (1 part of each). These plants have therapeutic actions and affinities for both the circulatory and the digestive systems.

If the individual can't seem to get on top of the prostate and urinary-tract symptoms, he most likely requires some deep immune system nourishment and some adaptogenic stress-handling assistance. In this case, use immune system–enhancing herbs such as Astragalus, Siberian Ginseng, Echinacea, and Suma with reproductive-organ tonic herbs such as Sarsaparilla and Damiana.

If infection is suspected in the prostate gland or in the genitourinary system (characterized by a burning pain when urinating as well as pain in the groin area before, during, and after), combine Saw Palmetto with Oregon Grape root and Echinacea. (Add Fennel to improve the flavor.) Take 2 to 3 cups of this combination as a tea or take 25 to 40 drops of the combined tinctures three to four times a day.

German phytotherapists recommend inserting, before going to bed, rectal suppositories consisting of equal parts of Saw Palmetto berry and Echinacea root to treat irritated or inflamed prostates, and they are observing excellent results. Take care of yourself by using these herbal preparations...you'll find them very helpful.

8. Last, but definitely not least, exercise your pubococcygeal (PC) muscle regularly. This is best done by learning the Kegel exercises....

Malignant Prostatic Enlargement

Volumes of authoritative medical statistics relating to cancer, its cause, its progression, its remission, the consequence of therapies, and so forth have been published. The images and implications ingrained in our Western cultural mind-set by these comparative numbers profoundly effect our collective belief system, and each individual is left wading through his emotional preconditioning whenever he is exposed to these commanding statistics. The publication of medical statistics inform each of us at what age we will become vulnerable to various cancers (or any other disease in question) and how progressively more threatening it will become as we proceed through succeeding decades (for example, more than 41,000 men will develop this cancer annually, or one out of three men ages this to that will contract that disease).

What is a man to do with that information, except worry about it and feel bad? That's not healthy, and it's certainly not conducive to prevention. Continuing on, statistical authorities inform us which race or ethnic group is more likely to succumb to whatever and which geographic locations and occupations are most threatening, and they even predict our future: how many of us will get something, and how many will die from it. And, it looks like soon we will be supplied with statistics that inform us of gene-based risk factors that could possibly blow us away, as if we incarnated into our body with a fully designed self-destruct mechanism, and genetic science (through the medium of statistics) will tell us where we've hidden our triggers (this feels a bit like a progressed phase of the medically spent and passé germ theory). Again, I ask, what can we do with this information as the years progress?

So, what's my point? Don't be influenced by (don't even bother to read) medical statistics or mainstream beliefs concerning prostate cancer, or any other cancer, or any other disease. Ignore them. Instead, focus your attention on appreciating and enjoying your health. Spend your time taking care of yourself by making yourself feel as good as possible each and every day with every thought and decision about your life. Be acutely aware of the "nocebo" effect, the placebo's negative twin.

A placebo (the word is Latin for "I shall please") is a pretend medicine (a special sugar pill), or, by extension, a trusted authority's assurance or a feigned surgery. It contains no physical active ingredients of a medicine or consists of no actual surgical intervention but nonetheless promotes obvious healing. A nocebo ("I will harm") likewise contains no physical active ingredients and has equal power (generated in the same way by one's mind). The nocebo effect is the impact of negative expectations that can cause everything from nausea to death (perpetrated by ritual curses uttered by "witch doctors" and reported by anthropologists to sometimes occur within days).

The nocebo effect works routinely in our culture during annual flu epidemics and can be seen in those who expect they will have heart disease because they eat foods they believe raises their cholesterol, and by those individuals allergic to roses who start sneezing in a room that contains plastic roses. (Remove the artificial roses, and they quit sneezing.) A classic experiment reported in *Psychosomatic Medicine* revealed that out of forty asthmatic individuals who had inhaled pure water vapor, which they were later told contained allergens, nearly half experienced tightness in the chest, and twelve participants had an asthma attack. Soon thereafter, these folks felt their symptoms improve when they were told to inhale something that would help. It was again simple water vapor, and it worked to calm them down and ease their symptoms. The nocebo had proven to be equally effective as the placebo, depending on what the individual was told and believed.

No matter what medical science decrees or what other people believe about these pronouncements, prostate cancer is not inevitable at any age, for any race, in any place, regardless of one's genetic demeanor. It is preventable; it is curable. Medical statistics can convey powerful nocebo effects. I suggest you discount these statistics. They have no inherent bearding on your future reality. No matter how foreboding they are and how credibly they are presented, they have nothing to do with you—unless, of course, you buy into them and identify with their inferred inevitabilities. Health is our

natural most resilient state. That is what's important to understand. Hold that thought.

It is taught that there are basically two biological forms of prostatic cancer: a localized form, which is the most common form and consists of a small incidental lesion, and an advanced form, which is a much less frequent form that may metastasize and cause further (potentially fatal) harm. It has been assumed by the allopathic medical profession, without significant proof, that the localized form will inevitably become a clinically significant lesion. Like responsible lawyers, it's their job to inform you of the worst possible scenario. The problem is that, for most folks, it's nearly impossible to unwrap their mind from around an implanted, fear-goaded, negative idea. This iatrogenic factor alone negatively skews a medical prognosis, a disease-augmenting nocebo. Choose wisely which doctor you listen to.

If prostate cancer is diagnosed, keep in mind that this is a slow-growing cancer. Acquiring experienced help is prudent, and the coordinated support of a variety of healers may be needed (depending on one's temperament) to help manifest remission as the initial step of continued self-healing. With the wide variation in the inherent growth potential of tumors, many of the small localized lesions may have persisted for some time and may continue to persist as such for years.

Treatment by radical prostate surgery is often as ineffective as mastectomy is in breast cancer surgery. Each person is unique and must be dealt with individually. Consider treating a malignant prostate condition holistically with diet, herbs, attention to psychological factors, strong emphasis on building and maintaining overall health, and enhancing the immune system. Make use of alternative health care sciences and lifestyle changes rather than resorting hastily to extreme techniques such as chemotherapy, surgery, and radiation therapy. To my knowledge, the medical profession has no studies to refer to about treating this form of cancer systemically by employing intimate lifestyle change, adjusted nutrition, and herbal and other complementary therapies. Their studies merely compare radiation treatment with chemotherapy and surgical treatment.

Locate a clinical herbalist, an Oriental-medicine practitioner, a naturopath, or another natural-therapy practitioner and get a second, third, and fourth opinion on treatment. Use your time wisely and positively. Calmly choose your path. You have time, you have intelligent, knowledgeable help available, and you have your creative mind and powerful healing ability to remedy this condition. It's a call to readjust your life patterns to better comply with your true nature. Something in your life was askew that progressed into a physical symptom (which you can heal). The mark of this current condition might be the harbinger of your evolving experience of health, compelling you to make yourself happier and more deeply nourished, rather than the mark of the statistically predestined. Your life is an ever-changing experience, yours in every respect to direct and do with as you will.

Prostate cancer in men has some similarities to breast cancer in women, and both of these conditions are best prevented, controlled, and remitted with the assistance of complex-carbohydrate, low-fat, high-fiber diets. Adopting such a high-quality diet is important for complementing any form of specific treatment, and it is most effective when red meat is also eliminated from the diet. Fat does not cause disease, but may help trigger development or speed the growth of lesions and tumors. Countries with low-fat diets appear to have lower incidences of prostate cancer, leading some researchers to

Continued ➡

believe that diets employing tofu, soy flour, and soy milk, along with those emphasizing high-fiber foods such as lentils, tomatoes, carrots, peas, and oatmeal, may inhibit prostate cancer growth.

Soy is being looked at as possibly the most protective dietary factor against prostate cancer on a per calorie basis. This protective role may be associated with two components in soy, called daidzein and genistein, that may act as weak estrogens that inhibit prostate cancer. (The estrogen/prostate connection resurfaces.) It is also suggested that Asians' high intake of Green Tea can partially explain the worldwide difference in incidences of prostate cancer.

Lycopene is a red carotenoid present in tomatoes, watermelon, pink grapefruit, guavas, and rose hips. It is strongly antioxidant, proving to be an excellent protective agent for preventing cardiovascular disease and cancer, particularly prostate cancer, and also has a notably positive effect on male fertility. Heat has no effect on lycopene, so cooked tomatoes and tomato products (tomato sauce, tomato soup, ketchup, and so on) supply a concentrated amount of bio-available lycopene. Vitamin D has also been shown to be very promising to aid the control and prevention of this malady; eating low-fat dairy products and fatty fish such as salmon and tuna is also recommended. Zinc is an essential mineral for maintaining an efficient immune system and a healthy prostate: oysters, pumpkin seeds, poultry, low-fat yogurt, and baked beans are excellent foods for obtaining dietary zinc.

Exercise, as you well know, is essential for overall health maintenance. Apparently, men who exercise regularly are at far less risk of developing prostate cancer than men leading sedentary lifestyles. (I support positive statistics.) A Harvard study of 17,719 men showed that prostate cancer risk was 47 to 88 percent less in those who burned 4,000 calories a week (accomplished in about one hour of exercise daily) compared to those burning less than 1,000 calories a week. (I support uplifting health-enhancing statistics.)

Doctors recommend that men over fifty have an annual checkup that includes a prostate-specific antigen blood test. (Prostate-specific antigens are proteins produced by the cells of the prostate gland.) The PSA test (also referred to as a prostate test) measures the level of PSA in a blood sample. It is normal for men to have low levels of PSA in their blood, but prostate cancer or benign conditions (such as BPH) can increase PSA levels. This test came into use in 1986, but the pros and cons of widespread PSA screening are continually debated within the medical community. The website of the British Columbia Cancer Foundation has an excellent discussion of the pros and cons of PSA screening for prostate cancer at www.bccancer.bc.ca/ppi/screening/prostate.htm, and I recommend you check it out if you have questions about your prostate health.

Detecting cancer while it's still within the prostate allows treatment to be more successful. Once it gets outside the prostate, it becomes a greater problem. No part of a system is separate from the whole. One should also look to other urinary tract functions aside from the prostate that might need to be addressed. Use herbs that will modify, nourish, and decongest the entire genitourinary system. Herbs appropriate for this approach are Thuja, Collinsonia, Ocotilla, and Red Clover tea. For those individuals treating malignancy who have an excess-type constitution (those who are outgoing, determined, and hot-tempered, who have elevated blood pressure, whose heart and arteries are innately strong, who when stressed react with an aggressive physical response,

often giving too strong a reaction, and who manifest inflamed, red, irritated tissues), include the Hoxsey formula in your herbal therapy. This is a tonic, alterative, antitumor blend composed basically of Red Clover, Buckthorn bark, Barberry, Poke root, Burdock, Stillingia, Cascara Sagrada, Licorice root, and Prickly Ash. Men with deficient-type constitutions (those who are introverted and sensitive, who have a hyperactive and fluctuating nervous system, who have lower physical reserves and less ability to buffer themselves from the stresses of life) will do better to include Astragalus and *Reishi* mushrooms instead.

And get out into the sun, says your guynecologist. In spite of what your dermatologist tells you, sunlight is still health food. Some researchers have turned to looking at vitamin D's effect on prostate health. In the process, they have found evidence that ultraviolet radiation (the primary source for vitamin D production in the skin) has an inverse relationship with prostate cancer risk. It is possible that the higher rate of prostate cancer in the elderly is partly due to spending less time outdoors letting sunlight touch their skin. Older men can also help reduce the risk of prostate problems by simply going to the toilet as soon as the urge to urinate signals, avoiding excess alcohol and caffeine, avoiding decongestants and antihistamines (these are known to aggravate BPH symptoms), exercising their Kegel muscles regularly, reducing stress, and using adaptogenic herbs.

And now—I saved the dessert for last—for the most exciting news of all. Doctors worldwide recognize as medical fact that the most effective means for maintaining a healthy prostate gland and improving an ailing one is regular sexual intercourse. I know: as a medicine, this is a hard pill to keep down, but in fact, making love keeps the prostate working, working well, and working with pleasure. Sexual intercourse increases circulation and has a health-promoting effect on the prostate gland. No other activity seems to help as much. So much for the theory that men are less inclined toward preventive medicine than women.

Aromatherapy Treatment for an Inflamed Prostate

It is helpful to apply herbs and essential oils directly on the inflamed prostate area. One way to get herbs to the prostate is by means of an herbal rectal implant or enema. This remedy is simply to prepare and is an excellent remedy for an inflamed prostate and/or piles.

To prepare this herbal implant, mix the following:

2 ounces	ground flaxseed
1 quart	distilled water

Simmer this mixture for ten minutes, then strain it and cool it to the degree that you can comfortably leave your finger in it for ten seconds. Squeeze out all the mucilage and oil into a container.

To this mucilaginous, oily liquid, add 1/4 teaspoon of pure, steam distilled, aromatherapy-grade Lavender essential oil. (Never use synthetic essential oils, for you will not get the medicinal actions you want.) Place this mixture in a tightly closed glass container and shake it vigorously. (Always shake this mixture well before using.) Employing the use of a baby syringe (a small rubber bulb available at many stores), lie down on your side and inject anywhere from a teacup to a pint of this decoction into the rectum. Retain the herbal implant as long as possible. Repeat two to three times a day. Refrigerate and keep the remaining unused mixture tightly capped to prevent evaporation of the Lavender essential (volatile) oil, but warm the mixture before using, and use it all within seventy-two hours.

The following . . . aromatherapy-grade essential oils can give pleasant relief from the stress of prostate inflammation (and the inflammation and swelling of hernias). Use a 5 percent dilution of aromatherapy-grade essential oils of Blue Chamomile, Lavender, and/or Blue Mallee (*Eucalyptus polybractea*).

Mix the following ingredients:

50 drops	total of any one or a blend of Blue Chamomile, Lavender, and Blue Mallee essential oils
2 ounces	hazelnut, almond, wheat germ, or olive oil, or any other fixed oil

Rub this oil on the perineum (the area between the anus and the scrotum) as well as on the lower back and lower abdomen. Repeat three to four times a day. (I know, I know, but it beats a urologist's finger any day.) These essential oils provide soothing, anti-inflammatory, nervine, and antimicrobial actions to the lower body. Essential oils penetrate the skin within minutes and are an excellent medium for getting plant nutrients to inflamed internal organs.

The frequent use of alcohol, nicotine, caffeine, and white sugar retards the action of these medicines and can further irritate the organs....

Herbal Viagras: The Safe Aphrodisiacs

Impotence: The Absence of Arousal in a Man's Life

What is impotence? The concept communicated by the term *impotent* is often a rash judgment. In most cases, the absence of arousal is the more accurate issue at hand. "Erectile dysfunction" has become the politically correct new-speak for impotence. In regard to impotence or low sexual energy, I see individuals living lifestyles highly conducive to the onset of low blood sugar and sluggish adrenal function. They exist day to day in routine jobs and sedentary domestic lifestyles that neither stimulate their creative capacity nor arouse their life force.

Eventually, along with the chronic experience of this daily unmotivating, depressing occupational and/or domestic environment, come the physical symptoms of low blood sugar: diminished circulation, low immune system strength, and low adrenal and sexual procreative force. When a male individual's life does not stimulate and arouse his male spirit, how can he expect a sexual partner to wade through the emotional and physical barriers to stimulate sexual arousal? The body's central control organ of sexual response is the brain. An individual needs to be self-aroused by the joy power, and creative stimulation of his own life first; physical arousal will follow, spontaneously enhancing performance in all other arenas.

I don't think that, in most sexual relationships, it is either the man or his sexual partner who is the cause if all isn't going well. The mutual relationship is expressing impotence. Each sexual relationship develops its own sexual and emotional patterns, and both partners contribute to and are responsible for this evolution. If either or both partners don't enjoy the experiences of this mutually generated sexual energy, dissatisfaction needs to be communicated, suggestions must be made, and the pattern should be changed to once again arouse the participants.

Sometimes, however, a man can become sexually impotent (his erectile tissues becoming dysfunctional) because he has made sexuality and sexual activity too important in his life. Impotence,

Continued ➡

in this instance, may be a plea for balance, an expression of one's wise inner being providing equal time for development of other aspects.

Many herbs and exercises can assist a couple in stoking the fires of expressive love, reducing impotence to an ash....

Regaining Virility with Herbal Viagras

Following is a list of male-potency herbs, prepared for the edification and emancipation of our country's finest. Bear in mind as you prepare your shopping list amid blissful anticipatory visions of—well, that's your business—that these herbs are not Viagra clones. (They're far safer than that.) Herbalists will not recommend these herbs with the suggestion that they are magic bullet plants promising instant studliness. Some herbal-product marketers might (and do), but credible herbalists won't. Anyway, Viagra and its band of similar pharmaceutical swashbucklers target only the physical aspects of sexual dysfunction by enhancing circulation (and that works), but we're aiming for more than this one-night-stand gang can deliver. (Actually, Cialis will give you a couple nights.)

The Green Citizens for Erectile Function are looking to bestow aphrodisiacal blessings on humankind, which address desire (a.k.a. libido) and feelings of sexual response (and that works even better!). Herbs help build strong reproductive systems and maintain sexual health, but they don't do this immediately, and they work best with exercise and good nutrition setting the stage. Realize that sexual health develops over time; very few herbs give an immediate effect. Some do, but these are very stimulating and need to be taken with prudence.

And be aware that dosage is an important factor to consider. The effective amount varies to some extent with each individual, depending on one's constitutional nature. Most herbal aphrodisiacs are quite safe, and taking too much is normally not the issue, it's more a matter of taking enough. The person using them must monitor the correct amount. Always start with a modest recommended amount, see how you respond, and modify the dosage in small degrees as you proceed. Continue to eat good foods, exercise regularly, manage your stress, drink scads of pure water daily, and make love to your partner as often as ye both shall lust.

One more thing regarding male potency, function, and performance: inevitably, the question, "Is bigger better?" comes up. Personally, I'm sure most women don't really care how big your tongue is. And the beauty of a tongue is that it's propelled solely by fervent desire and depends not the least on erectile tissue for demonstrating its skill and functionality. There are no reports to my knowledge of male lingual dysfunction (MLD); it's usually more an issue of a man's foreplay naiveté contributing to his limited lingual performance (LLP) that occupies female conversation.

The tongue is always wet, notably supple, and highly trainable, and merely needs to be animated by one's lively affectionate gusto. And—have no doubt about this—when asked, every woman is eager to train her lover and, her secrets bared, encourage his exploratory lingual prowess. A wise adage, which I believe dates back to Mr. Adam and Ms. Eve, says, "Ask and you shall receive." All in all, a talented, loving tongue is probably "better than bigger" and a most satisfying surrogate to help pass the time, as time and sexual tonic herbs "abilitate" the other player.

Without further ado, I introduce to you the following herbs...

Ashwagandha (*Withania somnifera*)

This herb been used in the East as an aphrodisiac for three thousand years and is impressively effective. One translation of the name is "sweat of a horse," alluding to the idea that, if the powdered root is taken with milk or ghee (clarified butter) as a tonic, over time it will give a man the strength and sexual vitality of a horse (without having similar effects on the personality). It contains withanolides, molecules that resemble steroids in action and appearance. *Ashwagandha* is classified by some as an adaptogen and is often referred to as Indian or East Indian Ginseng, for the traditional uses of it and Ginseng were similar. Like Ginseng, it was thought to be an energy tonic capable of generally strengthening the body, enhancing libido, and restoring fertility and sexual potency. *Ashwagandha* root is safe and nonirritating and will not overstimulate sexual energy.

Catuaba (*Erythroxylum catuaba* and *Trichilia catigua*)

These trees are native to the Brazilian forests. Brazilians prefer these two species, but other varieties that are entirely different trees have been harvested and imported to the United States. An infusion of the bark is used in traditional Brazilian medicine as an aphrodisiac and as a stimulant for the central nervous system, primarily for treating erectile dysfunction and disorders of the central nervous system. It is commonly used in combination with Muira Puama (see right) for its aphrodisiac properties. Other uses include aiding memory, insomnia, pain associated with the central nervous system, fatigue, hypertension, and anxiety.

Damiana (*Turnera diffusa; var. T. aphrodisiaca*)

A mood-elevating aromatic herb that helps calm anxiety and induce a relaxed state of mind, Damiana is one of the more notorious herbal aphrodisiacs and has the reputation of being a superlative sexual tonic. It is considered especially useful when anxiety and depression are discouraging sexual arousal. It lends a delightful energy and flavor to wines and sundry other erotic potions.

Garlic (*Allium sativum*)

According to Oriental science, seven to eight cloves a day will balance systemic yin and yang. However, you may find it difficult to get a date with the quality of breath this dosage will bring forth. Garlic enhances the nervous system's ability to react to nitric oxide, an essential step in the erection process. Garlic is well known to assist in preventing and helping cure several medical conditions that are often the cause of erectile dysfunction, including hypertension, heart disease, and atherosclerosis. Garlic is an effective agent for treating nervous-problems such as headache, the prime anaphrodisiacal prompter of "Not tonight, dear..."

Ginkgo (*Ginkgo biloba*)

As a reliable peripheral vasodilator, Ginkgo is an excellent supportive agent to help remedy erectile dysfunction. It increases blood circulation and flow of oxygen to the brain, helping counter the negative effects of antidepressants (Prozac, Fluoxetine, and so on) on sexual function. It has a direct effect on endothelial cells that enhance blood flow of both penile arteries and veins without any change in systemic blood pressure. Ginkgo supports sexual function by enhancing blood circulation while concurrently improving the nitric oxide pathways. Ginkgo works best when combined with more specific carrier herbs that target the genitourinary system. The first sign of improved circulation and blood supply can be seen in about six to eight weeks, but continue this herbal supplementation for up to six months.

Ginseng (*Panax, Ginseng, Chinese Ginseng,* and *Panax quinquefolium, American Ginseng*)

Both Chinese and American Ginseng promote energy, stamina, and endurance. Ginseng supplies ginsenosides, compounds that affect hormonal balance, and its overall chemistry supports strong sexual function by nourishing the kidneys. Chinese medicine contends that Ginseng's potent ability to enhance sexual activity lies in its ability to nourish the kidneys, major players in the vital nurturing cycle of the body. Strong kidneys affect the other major organs of the body, which feed and nurture each other, ultimately supporting healthy sexual function. Ginseng enhances blood circulation by increasing blood levels of nitric oxide. This effect allows arterial walls to relax, allowing blood to flow freely when and where needed.

Gokshura (*Tribulus terrestris*)

A rejuvenating Ayurvedic herb, *Gokshura* is used to support proper function of the urinary tract and the prostate and is an excellent circulatory system tonic that can help build muscle and strength. This fruit contains a steroidal saponin shown to improve libido in men experiencing impotence. Men taking it have experienced an increase in sexual desire and fantasies and, most important, the feeling of sexual self-confidence. Some men experienced prolonged duration of intercourse before ejaculation, and most experienced improved erection and enhanced joy, pleasure, and satisfaction with their sexual experiences. This saponin also shows an ability to stimulate sperm production and increase the quality, motility, and survival time of sperm. Research indicates that *Gokshura* increases the endogenous production of luteinizing hormone; some researchers believe LH in turn stimulates endogenous testosterone, elevating sexual performance and desire in both men and women.

Horny Goat Weed (*Epimedium sagittatum, E. grandiflorum*)

This Chinese herb, named *yin yang huo*, also translates as "licentious Goat Weed," suggesting desired lusty effects. Traditionally, it has been used to increase libido and improve sexual performance by correcting erectile dysfunction and premature ejaculation. Horny Goat Weed elicits a moderate androgenlike effect on the testes and the prostate, increasing sperm production while stimulating the sensory nerves by which it indirectly increases sexual desire. It contains a notable flavonoid (icariin) that, like Viagra, Cialis, and Levitra, is a cGMP-specific PDE-5 inhibitor.

Kapi kacchu (*Mucuna pruriens*)

An Ayurvedic herb used to balance kidneys and the nervous system, this is one of the premier rejuvenating herbs for men and women, having a highly esteemed reputation as a powerful aphrodisiac. It is used to enhance sexual potency and as a tonic herb to reverse the aging process. *Kapi kacchu* seed also shows fertility promoting and spermatogenic effects in men, improving sperm count and motility. This powdered seed is reported to increase testosterone, and, due to its natural ability to generate L-dopa, it ultimately, stimulates the production of human growth hormone (HGH), which acts as a prolactin inhibitor in the pituitary gland. (Increased prolactin is said to be responsible for up to 70 percent of erection failure in males.) In a study involving fifty-six men, each was treated with *Kapi kacchu* for merely four weeks. The results showed stronger erections, longer duration of coitus, and enhanced postcoital satisfaction. (It's reported that hundreds of males and a number of female volunteers lining up for the subsequent study had to be dowsed with buckets of cold water and turned away by force. Just kidding. No force was used.)

Continued ➡

Long Jack (*Eurycoma longifolia*)

This small tree, found throughout the jungles of Malaysia and Southeast Asia, goes by many names, but is commonly known as *tongkat ali* and Malaysian Ginseng. Natives consider every part of the tree as medicine; however, the extract known as Long Jack—or *Eurycoma longifolia* Jack (ELJ)—is taken from the roots. Long Jack has many healing properties, but in the United States, it is especially prized as an aphrodisiac and a libido booster with the ability to improve male potency and drive. Long Jack is believed to stimulate production of endogenous testosterone and to reduce the levels of bound and metabolically inactive testosterone. It is said to achieve this action through the leutinizing-hormone pathway. Therefore, men who use this herb report increased feeling of well-being, increased sex drive, improved joint health, greater recovery from exercise, improved mental focus, and improved immune system function. Side effects are rare; however, some individuals, who probably took too much at once, report experiencing insomnia, restlessness, and impatience. It is probably best to take small amounts over a two- to four-day period.

Maca (*Lepidium meyenii, L. Peruvianum*)

A hearty root vegetable grown high in the mountains of Peru, Maca is a nutritive tonic for men and women that optimizes physical stamina and endurance, sexual health, potency, and fertility and enhances sexual appetite by increasing libido. Couples native to the Peruvian mountains prize Maca's fertility powers; men and women having difficulty conceiving eat Maca continually until conception occurs. Peruvian physicians and researchers claim it has a positive effect on ovarian function in women and erectile function in men. As a restorative tonic, it optimizes erectile function, increases quantity of semen and sperm motility in men, and stimulates ovarian, or Graafian, follicles, which release the ovum in female ovulation.

Muira puama (*Ptychopetalum olacoides*)

This Brazilian herb, known as "potency wood," is used as an aphrodisiac by Brazilian natives; the root and bark are taken internally for libido effect and increased circulation in both men and women. Muira puama is a nervous system tonic that enhances sexual libido and increases circulation, having a positive effect on the erectile tissues of both men and women. It is used to remedy sexual weakness, erectile dysfunction, and performance anxiety in men and diminished sexual desire in women. This herb is quite safe to use regularly; however, excessive quantities may have a stimulating effect.

Oats (*Avena sativa, cultivated, A. fatua, wild*)

This is an indirect sexual enhancer, as it is one of the best herbs for nourishing the nervous system, particularly where there is exhaustion, depression, and nervous debility. Oat seed has beneficial application in all forms of sexual dysfunction, particularly where a depleted nervous system is playing a role.

Sarsaparilla (*Smilax ornate*)

Empirical observation suggests that Sarsaparilla possesses mild androgen-like effects and can serve as a reasonable sexual tonic and anabolic toner. It combines with Saw Palmetto and Echinacea for nourishing and toning the reproductive organs.

Saw Palmetto (*Serenoa repens*)

Saw Palmetto berries are sexual tonics famous for keeping a man's prostate healthy and treating the problems of prostate enlargement thought to be caused by an accumulation of dihydrotestosterone (DHT), a biologically active metabolite of the hormone testosterone. It is said to be about thirty times more potent than testosterone because of its increased affinity to the androgen receptors. The buildup of DHT in the prostate can decrease sex drive and performance. Saw Palmetto stops the conversion of testosterone to DHT, aiding the shrinking and relaxing of the prostate when it enlarges. A healthy prostate is an important element of male health and is essential for male sexual health, so the harmonizing tonic energy of this herb produces the background music to which aphrodisiacs can more easily dance with male sexual potency.

Shilajit

This Ayurvedic herb (of sorts) is actually an exudates. *Shilajit* (also spelled *Shilajeet*) has powerful rejuvenative properties. For centuries, Ayurvedic physicians have relied on it with confidence to successfully treat debility or weaknesses caused by injury, dysfunction, and aging. Its rejuvenative effect increases the core energy responsible for sexual power and health. As an aphrodisiac, *Shilajit* increases vitality and stamina while toning the reproductive organs and enhancing their function. It has been shown to enhance nitric oxide's effect and facilitate multiple sexual-health functions.

Yohimbe (*Pausinystalia yohimba*)

This sexual stimulant comes from the bark of an African tree. It was used traditionally to stimulate erections, which it does. There have been several clinical studies on the use of this agent to treat erectile dysfunction (mostly using the isolated yohimbe alkaloid, not the whole herb). The results are promising, though they demonstrate the wide range of effects Yohimbe has on different individuals. Yohimbe is said to work mentally as well as physically, making orgasms more powerful by postponing ejaculation. (Strong Kegel muscles allow a man to do the same thing). Yohimbe, being a mild monoamine oxidase (MAO) inhibitor, has an uplifting effect on depression, and it dilates blood vessels, which is why it has been used for erectile dysfunction. Like Viagra and other similar prescription drugs, Yohimbe is used primarily to stimulate a physical reaction rather than promote the amorous mood of sex, as a true aphrodisiac would. (Consider taking it along with Damiana.) This is a highly stimulating herb, affecting individuals with varying constitutions in equally varied ways, so there are definite precautions for its use.

As everything in Nature is connected in some way, everything in the body and the mind is connected. Nourish and care for one part, and the other parts are cared for, too. Neglect a part, and the healthy function of the others is diminished. Combine these herbal sexual tonics and aphrodisiacs with other tonics that effect mutually supportive systems (for example, nervous system tonics such as Wild Oat and Skullcap, adaptogens and adrenal gland tonics such as Ginseng, Licorice, and Siberian Ginseng to enhance vital energy and buffer stress, and Ginkgo with Hawthorn to enhance peripheral penile circulation). This approach works holistically to promote full health and vitality, which your sexuality can celebrate with ardent frequency....

Fertility

Clinically, the most obvious contributors to male spermatogenic deficiency are:

- Low sperm count or deficiencies in maturation of germ cells in the semen, which may be a secondary effect caused by hypogonadism (deficient activity of the testis) or hypopituitarism (diminished activity of the pituitary gland).

- Low percentage of motile sperm (sperm capable of spontaneous movement).

- Short duration of sperm motility.

- Low percentage of normally formed sperm.

Other contributors to male infertility, though rare, are obstruction of the conduction system and hypothyroidism (a state produced by deficient secretion of the thyroid gland).

The cause of the above conditions is not usually so obvious. Stress, nervous anxiety, and/or an underlying low state of health are three major possibilities. Survival stress due to burnout can result in a man having no interest in anything other than personal survival issues; his body will express this trauma in multiple ways, including infertility.

Creating appropriate combinations of herbs based on the specific needs of the individual man will build a strong nutritional base for a program to help reverse male infertility. For example, system tonics that build underlying vitality to help reverse infertility and low adrenal energy include Maca, *Gokshura*, Horny Goat Weed, Saw Palmetto, and Ginseng. Discussion of these and other applicable herbs follows:

- Maca, used for centuries in the Peruvian highlands for its notable fertility-enhancing as well as adaptogenic effects, has been shown to significantly increase seminal volume, increased sperm count and quality, and sperm with improved motility. Taken over time and in adequate amounts, Maca appears to significantly increase endometrial characteristics, indicating higher fertility levels in women.

- *Gokshura* contains a steroidal saponin shown to stimulate sperm production and increase quality, motility, and survival time of sperm in male fertility.

- Horny Goat Weed is traditionally used to treat impotence and spermatorrhea and is reputed to increase the production of sperm, heighten the level of testosterone, and stimulate sensory nerves.

- Saw Palmetto is highly regarded as a general tonic with therapeutic applications for functional impotence, physical and mental debility, and male senility. Its tonic effect nurtures the entire reproductive system in both men and women, and it is used to treat atrophy conditions of the testes and ovaries.

- Ginseng is a remarkable adaptogen and sexual rejuvenator. Its ginsenoside components affect the central nervous system and gonadal tissue and help improve energy metabolism, which play a significant role in the treatment of male sexual and infertility problems.

- *Ho shou wu* helps normalize the action of the kidneys and the liver and is noted to increase sperm count and improve sperm motility. It helps retain a man's essence and stop leakage due to nocturnal emission and other forms of involuntary emission of semen. *Ho shou wu* is a renowned rejuvenating tonic that can be taken over a long time and is best used this way to help retain youthfulness, build healthy blood and sperm, and alleviate impotence.

- *Ashwagandha* is an adaptogen and energy tonic having stamina enhancing properties probably equal to those of Ginseng. This herb retards various aspects to the aging process, improves sexual performance and fertility, and is a paramount tonic in the process of recuperation from exhaustive burned out stages of stress.

Continued ➜

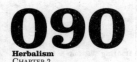

- Schisandra is one of the most highly regarded herbal tonics for enhancing sperm production and increasing RNA, as well as glycogen and enzymes to the kidneys and gonad glands.

- Astragalus is a revered herb for enhancing the immune system and has likewise shown itself to be an exceptional agent for increasing the quantity and motility of sperm.

- *Shilajit* is a peculiar exudate that increases the core energy responsible for sexual health and power. It improves the function of the entire genitourinary system in men and women and supplies high quality bioavailable trace minerals, as well as iron and calcium, that help prevent anemia and flagging sexual energy. *Shilajit* accelerates the body's recuperative process resulting from injury or strenuous exercise as well as the recovery of youthful vitality.

- The adaptogenic herbs Siberian Ginseng, American and Chinese Ginseng, Suma, and Roseroot (*Rhodiola rosea*) greatly assist a man in dealing with all forms of stress and anxiety. They are excellent tonic herbs to help build the state of health and adaptation to stress necessary to produce adequate sperm count and the joy and libido to deliver it.

- Hawthorn and Ginkgo work to increase cardiovascular power and improve circulation.

- Oat is considered one of the best herbs for nourishing and toning the entire nervous system, particularly in conditions of depression and nervous exhaustion. Likewise, it is tonifying to the genitourinary system, resulting in a positive effect on reproductive health.

- Gentian, Mugwort, and Yarrow are bitter herbs that have a secondary affinity for the reproductive organs. They stimulate appetite, digestion, and assimilation necessary for improving health and increasing energy.

- Sarsaparilla, Licorice, Wild Yam, and Ginseng provide hormone precursors to help enhance hormonal health.

- Sarsaparilla, Red Raspberry leaves, Burdock root, and Saw Palmetto berries have alterative action that improves the condition of the blood and facilitates overall improvement of health. These herbs are also specific for the reproductive system and supply primary nourishment for enhancing fertility....

Longevity

In one's quest for a long and healthy life, some well-substantiated axioms of gerontology can be relied on:

- Sustained exercise and training inhibits the decline of physique that normally comes as a person ages.

- Sustained exercise and training inhibits the decline of physical fitness that normally comes as a person ages.

- Sustained exercise and training inhibits the decline of mental function that normally comes as a person ages.

Many older athletes up to age eighty have shown themselves to be as fit or fitter than nonathletes half their age. You don't have to be a full-time athlete to remain fit, but you do have to exercise regularly to remain youthful and healthy. You have no control over your chronological aging, but you can control your biological aging. It is known for sure that what we used to call natural and inevitable aging is neither natural nor inevitable. It is simply the usual pattern we see, because the majority of people exhibit similar degenerative disorders.

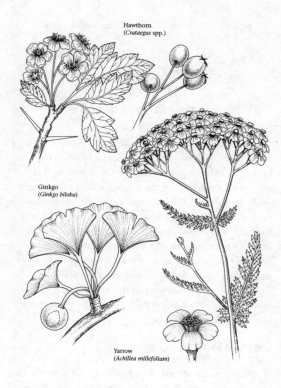

Hawthorn
(*Crataegus* spp.)

Ginkgo
(*Ginkgo biloba*)

Yarrow
(*Achillea millefolium*)

The body is a marvelously adaptive organism. If one performs regular aerobic activities, cardiovascular capacity increases; lift weights, and the muscles, bones, and connective tissues get stronger; stretch regularly, and flexibility improves; manage stress, eat a sensible nutritious diet, and get sufficient rest, and vital energy magnifies; drink sufficient water, and one's overall health will abound; and protect the skin and hair from harsh elements, and they age more slowly.

All these activities are well within each person's power to pursue. Each individual can expand his own longevity by adopting a longevity lifestyle. Cultivate a positive attitude, laugh, play in an occupation that you love, and cultivate warm friendships, and, when these factors that are in your control are in place, getting older will be a stimulating, non-enfeebling process of remaining healthy, enjoying life on this beautiful planet, and realizing more wisdom. I believe this is what longevity is all about.

As a man ages, he experiences a natural polarity reversal. His testosterone hormone production decreases, and the estrogenic side of his being becomes subtly more expressive. The male being becomes less aggressive and gentler, and his interests turn more inward for the continuation of his spiritual evolution. He becomes more a lover than a pursuer. A woman experiences a similar reversal, though estrogen decline is more confronting land firm. These are normally smooth transitions, and they facilitate the continual development of subtle, maturing awareness. It is important for boys and men of all ages to be aware of natural male-energy changes and to understand and honor this phenomenon.

Tied in with all the issues we modern folks are concerned with, such as cardiovascular health, joint health, sexual health, weight management, memory loss, blood sugar stability, obesity, and physical attractiveness, is the overshadowing concern about aging. And, though chronological aging is incessant and irreversible, physical aging is highly manageable. The experts on doing this are the healthy octogenarians, nonagenarians, and centenarians dwelling in our midst. As it has always been, wisdom resides in the life experiences of our vibrant elders. What has changed in our culture, what has shifted, is that youth has stopped revering them. But these elders have lived what we want to know most: how to remain youthful throughout our lives.

Reflected in the life stories of creatively functional elders and according to the findings of current medical research, stress can make you ill and make you old. What needs to be clearly understood is that it isn't the amount of stress you are exposed to that matters; it is how you manage the stress—you either internalize it, or you let it go. Letting it go is as pleasurable and refreshing as a sauna and a daily shower, but internalizing it accumulates emotional debris that soils your mind and clogs your vital systems. Based on ongoing studies, researchers theorize that constant unrelieved ("unshowered") stress causes one's telomeres—biological markers of aging—to get smaller at a quickened pace. They are tiny caps on the ends of cells' chromosomes that act somewhat like the protective plastic tips that keep shoelace ends from fraying. When these telomeres get too short, the cell stops dividing and eventually expires....

For herbal support, the most obvious combination is regular intake of Ginkgo and Hawthorn flowers and berries. These two tonics work exceptionally well together to tone and strengthen the heart and brain. Include a few more herbs that are well known to improve memory and central nervous system function and that neutralize free radicals (high-energy molecular fragments that can run amok in the body, contributing to the aging process), and you have an excellent longevity plant ally at hand. I suggest the following combination as a basic herbal formula for high-quality life extension:

4 parts	Ginkgo
4 parts	Hawthorn
3 parts	Siberian Ginseng
2 parts	*Gotu kola*
2 parts	*Ho shou wu*
1 part	Rosemary
1 part	Skullcap and/or Oat

Note: Whenever you boil water for herbal preparations, or for any other eating purpose, avoid aluminum pots and cookware. Health sciences strongly suspect a dietary link between Alzheimer's disease and unnatural aluminum deposits found in the cerebral cortex of the brain.

Alzheimer's disease disrupts the cognitive functions of aging people. This disease places a tremendous burden on longevity, to say the least. The use of aluminum is also suspected of greatly irritating arthritic conditions. (The aluminum industry criticizes these suspicions as flawed research; I criticize their products as flawed marketing.) If you inspect the inside surface of any well-used aluminum pot, you will find it extensively pitted. Aluminum particles have left the cooking utensil and mixed with the liquid solvents (especially the acidic and salty ones), which, unfortunately, were most likely the breakfasts, lunches, dinners, snacks, and hot beverages of the pot users.

Aluminum also enters the body through impure drinking water, commercial baking powder, aluminum cans, aluminum-containing antiperspirants, analgesic and antacid over-the-counter medicines, and many if not most current medical vaccines in which alum and aluminum phosphate are included as preservatives.

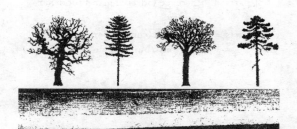

Continued ➡

I want to credit my friend and companion herbalist, Rosemary Gladstar, with the following four exotic herbal recipes. Rosemary gives these formulas freely to all who attend her classes, but I suspect that only those individuals who embody the soul of a connoisseur actually prepare them. These herbal preparations make excellent gifts for the man who has everything and intends to use it.

Power Balls

The following recipe manifests a collection of ingredients that help provide a man with a continual store of energy. It contains nutrients that are supportive for the male yang energy and is formulated to nourish and tone the male reproductive system over time.

Combine the following powders in a bowl:

2 tablespoons	Siberian Ginseng powder
2 tablespoons	Ginseng powder
1 tablespoon	Ginger powder
4 tablespoons	bee pollen
6 tablespoons	pumpkin seeds (ground)
1 tablespoon	sesame seeds (ground)
1 to 2 tablespoons	spirulina (a freshwater alga)

Combine in another bowl:

3/4 cup	sesame seed, almond, or peanut butter
1/4 cup	honey

Gradually add the first mixture to the second and knead the resulting mixture into a paste. Add roasted carob powder and, if you like, lightly roasted shredded coconut to sweeten and flavor. Roll into walnut-size balls and each day eat one before and one after your daily exercises.

Rosemary's Long-Life Elixir

The flavor and culinary presence of this male system tonic brings to mind terms such as "exquisite" and "for the gods." It is an herbal tonic that builds strength and vitality and is formulated to be taken over a long period of time.

Ingredients:

2–6 whole roots	Ginseng root (restorative tonic/adaptogen)
1 part	Saw Palmetto (reproductive system tonic)
2 parts	Sarsaparilla (anabolic agent/blood purifier)
4 parts	Wild Yam (hormone precursors/tonic)
2 parts	Sassafras root bark (alterative/tonic)
2 parts	Siberian Ginseng (general tonic/adaptogen)
4 parts	Ginger (circulatory stimulant)
2 parts	Damiana (prostate tonic/sexual vitality)
4 parts	Licorice (adrenal gland food/harmonizer)
4 parts	*Ho shou wu* (central nervous system nutrients/builds male chi)

4 parts	Astragalus (deep immune system support)
1 part	Star Anise (warming stimulator)
Brandy	(sufficient amount to cover the herbs)
1/2 cup	black cherry or other fruit concentrate

Place all the herbs in a quart-size glass jar and cover them with the brandy. Select a high-quality brandy that has not had fruit flavor added to it. Put the lid on tight and let the extract sit for six to eight weeks in a warm, shaded area. After the period has passed, strain the ingredients and discard the spent herbs (but save the whole Ginseng roots). To each cup of herbal extract add the fruit concentrate, available at natural food stores. (Important: Do not use a fruit juice; doing so will spoil the elixir.) Return the Ginseng roots to the elixir. Sip 1 to 2 tablespoons of the elixir daily; store the remaining elixir in the refrigerator.

Long-Life Wine

If this aromatic served as an herbal tonic doesn't, in fact, lengthen one's life, it will certainly help make it more romantic.

Ingredients:

1 root	Ginseng
1/4 ounce	Damiana
1/4 ounce	Astragalus
1/4 ounce	Coriander seed or pods
1/4 ounce	Star Anise
1 bottle	red or white wine

Place the herbs in a jar, warm the wine, and pour it over the herbs. (Save the wine bottle.) Cap the herbed wine and let it sit for one to two weeks. Strain the wine, pour it back into its original bottle, and add back the Ginseng root. Drink this herbal wine daily in moderate 1 tablespoon doses or drink a full wineglass once or twice a week.

Pan's Potion

This formula is designed to help increase sexual potency and vitality.

Ingredients for group 1:

1 root	Ginseng root
1/2 ounce	Saw Palmetto berries
1 ounce	Yellow Dock root
1/2 ounce	Wild Yam root
1 ounce	Damiana leaf

Ingredients for group 2:

1/4 ounce	Strawberry leaves
1/4 ounce	Raspberry leaves
1/4 ounce	Nettle leaves
1/4 ounce	Comfrey leaves
1 cup	honey
1/2 cup	brandy (optional, but highly recommended)

Simmer the herbs of group 1 in 1 quart of water over a low heat for forty-five minutes. Remove this decoction from the heat and add to it the leaves of group 2, stir, cover, and let sit overnight. The next day, strain all herbs from the tea. Place this tea on a very low fire and slowly reduce the herbal liquid to 1/2 quart (1 pint). Add the honey and brandy. Store this liquid in the refrigerator. Take 1 to 4 tablespoons daily over a period of three to six months.

Thank you, Rosemary.

Female Potency Herbs

James Green, Herbalist

In my experience, a fully functional male heterosexual is sublimely happy and fulfilled with an equally fabulous woman to love and cavort with. To this union, I submit the following list for you to share with female friends, if you feel they will appreciate it (sexual dysfunction is not at all gender specific):

Shatavari (*Asparagus racemosus*)

This herb is a reproductive system tonic having considerable nutritive, rejuvenating properties. It has an esteemed tradition in Ayirvedic medicine as a primary tonic and medicine for female sexual health (also used for male reproductive health). It is the female counterpart of *Ashwagandha* and, like that herb, is referred to as Indian Ginseng. *Shatavari* is used in Ayurvedic medicine to nourish female organs, help balance estrogen levels, improve fertility, and treat vaginal dryness and painful intercourse. One translation of the name is "she who can have a hundred husbands." A second translation is "having a hundred roots"; the former name speaks to its reputation as an aphrodisiac, and the latter bespeaks its fertility-enhancing properties. This herb has been proven an extraordinary woman's herb. *Shatavari* combines well with *Kapi kacchu* and *Shilajit* for a powerful rejuvenating tonic blend.

Kava (*Piper methysticum*)

Kava is not an aphrodisiac per se, but it's certainly a mood elevator, stress reliever, and phyto body massage. Kava relaxes the mind and clarifies thought. It releases muscle tension, reducing anxiety, nervous tension, and stress. All in all, Kava can help create a mental and physical environment more tailored to romance.

Ginger and Cinnamon

These are warming, aromatic, pleasant-tasting herbs that produce heat in the body and increase circulation in the lower abdominal and pelvic region measured to boost one's appetites both physical and sexual. Increased blood flow to the pelvic region increases vaginal moisture, which heightens vaginal response and intensifies sexual pleasure.

Damiana*, Horny Goat Weed, Maca, Oat, Muira puama, and Shilajit

These highly effective tonic and therapeutic herbs have been used for eons to help a woman who has sexual concerns such as low sexual desire, problems with arousal and attaining climax, lack of orgasm, vaginal dryness, pain with vaginal penetration, or lack of pleasure in sexual contact.

Jasmine and Rose

The aromas of these flowers, the essential oils, the aromatic hydrosols, the massage oils—these are the most transcendent of olfactory aphrodisiacs for both women and men.

—From *The Male Herbal*

Continued ➡

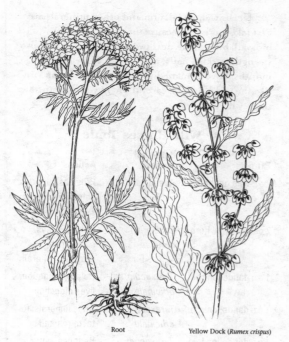

Root   Yellow Dock (*Rumex crispus*)

I want to credit one of my other herbalist colleagues, Amanda McQuade Crawford, with the next two life-inflaming herbal recipes, introducing them in Amanda's words: "'Aphrodisiacs are named for Aphrodite, Goddess of Love. Here are recipes for wild potions, tonics for women and for men. Remember that love cannot be forced, but it can be created.

Tried-and-True Tonic for Men

Ingredients:

1 ounce	Prickly Ash
1/2 ounce	Licorice
1/2 ounce	Orange peel
1/2 ounce	Thyme
1 ounce	Sarsaparilla
1 ounce	Saw Palmetto
1/2 ounce	Cinnamon
1/2 ounce	Yohimbe or Horny Goat Weed (optional)
1/2 ounce	Valerian
1/2 ounce (or more)	whole Ginseng root(s) or rootlets
to cover herbs	brandy, vodka, etc.
to taste	barley malt or honey

Cover the herbs with the brandy, vodka, or other 80-proof alcohol and store in a cool, dark place for two weeks. Shake the mixture daily. Then strain and add barley malt or honey. Pour this mixture into an aesthetically intriguing bottle, place the Ginseng roots in the bottle, and leave them indefinitely. Take 1 to 2 tablespoonfuls daily.

Red-to-Orange Chakra Express

Ingredients:

1/2 ounce	Allspice
1 ounce	Ginger
1/8 ounce	Cloves
1/2 ounce	Fennel
1/2 ounce	Cinnamon
1/2 ounce	Star Anise
1 ounce	Astragalus
1/2 ounce	Bay leaves
1/2 ounce	Nutmeg
1/8 ounce	Guarana (optional; contains caffeine)
1 to 2 bottles	Beaujolais or burgundy wine

Use leaves, seeds, barks, and roots as whole as possible. Put into a large, see-through bottle, tightly stoppered. Cover liberally with wine. Allow two weeks before straining. Warm to room temperature or over low heat before sipping slowly. Will keep in the refrigerator for two to three years.

Thank you, Amanda.

And here's one more:

Green's Male Song Tea

This tea is designed to fill the male spirit with even more pizzazz.

Ingredients:

2 parts	Sassafras-root bark
1 part	Licorice root
2 parts	Ginger root
1 part	Orange peel
2 parts	Marshmallow root
1 part	Sarsaparilla root
1 part	Ginseng root (or rootlets)
2 parts	Cinnamon bark

Combine all ingredients with water (1 teaspoon of herb mixture per cup of water). Let sit for a couple of hours, then simmer over low heat. This mixture decocts into a deliciously yang male brew. Alter the parts and add whatever to suit your taste.

—From *The Male Herbal*

- -
Endnotes

1. Thomas Luparello et al., "Influences of Suggestion on Airway Reactivity in Asthmatic Subjects," *Psychosomatic Medicine* 30 (1968): 819–25.
2. I-Min Lee et al., "Physical Activity and Risk of Prostate Cancer Among College Alumni," *American Journal of Epidemiology*, 135, no. 2 (1992): 169–79.

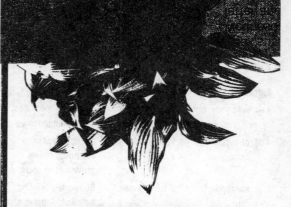

FEMALE-SPECIFIC HERBALISM
Amanda McQuaide Crawford

Fibroids

Fibroids are benign growths. The term usually refers to fibrous growths of the uterus. They commonly occur in three places: in the wall of the uterine muscle, inside the uterus, or protruding from the uterine wall into the abdomen. Uterine tissue is estrogen sensitive; that is, the surfaces of its cells have receptors that are stimulated by circulating estrogen. An excess of estrogen stimulates the overgrowth and thickening of uterine tissue, eventually producing a fibroid. High levels of human growth hormone (HGH) can also trigger the growth of fibroids, so they may increase in late pregnancy.

Fibroids may remain small and unnoticed. Most will shrink or disappear after menopause when estrogen levels naturally go down. They can, however, grow large enough before menopause to cause damage, especially if they obstruct other structures or rupture and hemorrhage (causing internal bleeding). These serious conditions mainly happen if fibroids go untreated by natural therapies or conventional medical treatment....

Fibroids respond well to changes in nutrition as well as other therapies. If they are causing you discomfort, the first step is to decrease the common foods in your diet that worsen pain and create excess estrogen. For instance, eating less protein, especially animal products with high fat content, is a good way to start decreasing excess hormones. Using less salt provides other health benefits to the bones and heart. Second, gaining physical fitness improves pelvic circulation and uterine muscle tone. Third, you may wish to try herbal remedies that are known to speed the natural processes that shrink fibroids. These are just three of the numerous alternative methods available that may help you balance your health before you consider surgery.

Herbal Medicine

The following hormone-balancing tonics assist the menopausal process in decreasing estrogen-dependent fibroids. Combined with alternatives (cleansing herbs for altering chronic conditions), these tonics promote the body's own methods of lowering excess estrogen. Some of the herbs they contain also have an observed effect of helping with inflammation, sluggish pelvic circulation, and lymphatic drainage. The astringent or toning herbs here shrink the fibrous lumps and seal the muscle walls against infection or inflammation to promote a healthy womb. The herbs combine several overlapping actions that help return overgrowths of fibrous tissue to a healthier state, perhaps even to a perfect form.

Continued ➡

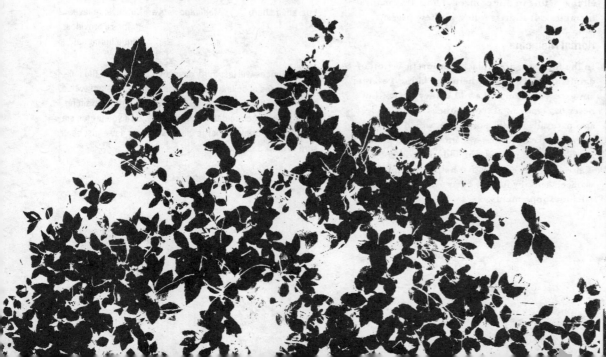

❧ Reweave Elixir ❧

Extracts	Botanical Names	Actions
4 oz. wild yam root	*Dioscorea villosa*	Balances hormones; anti-inflammatory
4 oz. chasteberry seed	*Vitez agnus-castus*	Lowers excess estrogen; slows growth of fibroids
2 oz. sarsaparilla root	*Smilax ornate*	Supports hormone balance; improves lymphatic flow
2 oz. calendula flower	*Calendula officinalis*	Stimulates liver, immune, and lymph functions
2 oz. yarrow flower	*Achillea millefolium*	Tones tissue; lessons excessive bleeding

Fourteen ounces will last thirty to forty-five days depending on need. Combine these extracts. The dose is 1/2 teaspoon to 1 tablespoon (3 teaspoons) of the combination, diluted in an 8-ounce cup of liquid, three times a day.

❧ Reweave Tea ❧

Dried Herbs	Botanical Names	Actions
4 oz. wild yam root	*Dioscorea villosa*	Balances hormones; anti-inflammatory
4 oz. chasteberry seed	*Vitex agnus-castus*	Lowers excess estrogen; slows growth of fibroids
2 oz. sarsaparilla root	*Smilax ornate*	Supports hormone balance; improves lymphatic flow
2 oz. calendula flower	*Calendula officinalis*	Stimulates liver, immune, and lymph functions
2 oz. yarrow flower	*Achillea millefolium*	Tones tissue; lessens excessive bleeding

Fourteen ounces will last two weeks. Steep 1 ounce of this tea mixture in 4 cups of boiling water for twenty minutes, covered. Strain and drink 1 cup four times daily. The volume of water is itself cleansing and moisturizing. Be sure to empty the bladder before bed, however; drinking liquid late at night may interrupt sleep for a trip to the bathroom. The herbs will not aggravate night sweats if a woman with fibroids is already experiencing this other symptom of decreased estrogen. If night sweats are a problem, especially if they aggravate loss of sleep and fatigue, add 3 ounces motherwort. The bitter flavor is worth the benefits.

❦

Whether you use tea or extract, continue for a minimum of one month before reducing the daily amount to 2 cups tea or two doses of extract. To safely double the dosage and avoid taking too much alcohol, which can occur if you are using the extract, drink both tea and extract. You can take one or both versions of this formula for another month or longer, until your body has reached a satisfying response to the herbs....

In Addition

- Exercise brings improved circulation to the pelvis, delivering nutrients to the uterus as it heals itself. Also, activity decreases tension and helps the whole body (liver metabolism, especially) to balance hormones.
- External herbal therapies. There are several excellent options, three of which are listed here. Try *just one at a time*, choosing the one that appeals most. You can alternate their use if you wish, and you don't have to do all three.

- Castor oil packs. This external remedy is effective for some women but not for others, depending on the size of the fibroids, how slowly or quickly they are growing, and how consistently a woman applies them.
- Ginger compress. Place a handful of grated fresh ginger root in a cheesecloth and squeeze out the juice into 1 gallon of very hot water. Do not boil the water or you will lose the volatile power of the ginger. Dip a cotton hand towel into the ginger water, wring it out tightly, and apply it to the whole abdominal or lower back area. It should be very hot but not uncomfortably so. A second dry towel can be placed on top to reduce heat loss. Apply a fresh, hot ginger towel every two or three minutes until the skin becomes red but not uncomfortably hot. You can use a ginger compress daily for as long as a month before you reevaluate your progress.
- Poke root compress. You can apply 1/4 to 1/2 ounce of heated poke root tincture in a wash cloth as a hot compress to the area for four hours to overnight. To keep it hot that long, cover the compress with a heating pad or hot-water bottle. As an alternative, a strong decoction (2 ounces dried poke root to 8 ounces simmering water for fifteen minutes) makes a fine poultice; use the warmed pulp and tea together. If fresh grated poke root is available (check with an herb gardener; we're always trying to get rid of some), use 1/2 to 1 ounce with sufficient hot water to make a poultice. Use this nightly up to one month before reevaluation.

Osteoporosis

Osteoporosis, the depletion of calcium in our bones, is a big concern for women throughout menopause. Bones affected by this disease are porous and weakened and may lead to fractures, back pain, loss of height, and stooped posture. The condition is quite common; according to conventional medical publications severe osteoporosis is said to affect about 25 percent of postmenopausal women.

As women go through menopause, the drop in estrogen affects the bones' ability to retain calcium. Up until menopause, estrogen has a stimulating effect on our body's bone-building activity throughout life. Around puberty, sudden increases of estrogen provide extra stimulation for growth spurts. Later, through our reproductive years, estrogen stimulates the continued formation of strong bones to pick up our growing children or to handle the mineral loss of menstruation. After our reproductive years, the decreased stimulation of bones by estrogen can be compensated for by continuing exercise and optimizing bone strength with all the factors in our control. Those that natural therapies can address follow in these pages....

Herbal Medicine

In the following formulas, the diuretic action of dandelion leaf and root helps the kidneys excrete any excess calcium and avoid kidney stones, but never by removing it from bone. Dandelion leaf is also naturally rich in potassium, which we need when we take diuretics—yet another example of nature's inherent wisdom. This multipurpose herb is also a digestive bitter that helps rebalance normal stomach acid if you have been using an excess of calcium supplements.

Herbs rich in calcium and other minerals are best taken as a tea because the water assists in bioavailability. The next two combinations can also strengthen skin, nails, and hair in three or more months. If your mane becomes glossy and you run like the wind, just be careful where you start to sow those wild oats.

❧ Wild Horses Tonic ❧

Extracts	Botanical Names	Actions
2 oz. wild oat herb	*Avena sativa*	Provides minerals; nourishes nerves, skin, hair
2 oz. horsetail herb	*Equisetum arvense*	Helps kidneys, elimination; provides minerals
1 oz. dandelion root, raw	*Taraxacum officinale*	Helps elimination, liver, digestion
1 oz. dandelion root,	*Taraxacum officinale*	Adds minerals; for taste roasted
1 oz. dandelion leaf	*Taraxacum officinale*	Reduces water retention, adds minerals
1 oz. nettle leaf	*Urtica dioica*	Nutritive; supports immune resistance
1 oz. yellow dock root	*Rumex crispus*	Stimulates liver; aids fat metabolism; adds iron
1 oz. alfalfa herb	*Medicago sativa*	Nutritive; relieves stiffness; provides gentle hormonal effects

Ten ounces will last thirty days. Combine these herbal extracts. Take 1 teaspoon twice a day (in the morning and evening) in 1 cup water, juice, or any herb tea.

❧ Wild Horses Tea ❧

Dried Herbs	Botanical Names	Actions
3 oz. wild oat herb	*Avena sativa*	Provides minerals; nourishes nerves, skin, hair
2 oz. horsetail herb	*Equisetum arvense*	Helps kidneys, elimination; provides minerals
2 oz. dandelion root, raw	*Taraxacum officinale*	Helps elimination, liver, digestion
2 oz. dandelion root,	*Taraxacum officinale*	Adds minerals; for taste roasted
2 oz. dandelion leaf	*Taraxacum officinale*	Reduces water retention, adds minerals
2 oz. nettle leaf	*Urtica dioica*	Nutritive; supports immune resistance
1 oz. yellow dock root	*Rumex crispus*	Stimulates liver; aids fat metabolism; adds iron
1 oz. alfalfa herb	*Medicago sativa*	Nutritive; relieves stiffness; provides gentle hormonal effects

Fifteen ounces will last thirty days. Add 1/2 ounce of the mixture to 4 cups of boiling water in a teapot or container with a well-fitting lid. Let stand for twenty minutes before straining. Drink 1 cup hot or cold three times a day. Or if you prefer, sip tea all day or drink two large glasses twice a day—just be sure to drink 3 cups a day.

❦

Continued ➤

Dysmenorrhea and Other Common Causes of Reproductive System Pain

Dysmenorrhea is a catch-all word meaning "painful or difficult menstrual bleeding." It can include cramps, painful arthritic inflammation, migraines, and pelvic pressure, perhaps with bloating or alternating diarrhea and constipation. Women in menopause often describe the pain as a dragging sensation. This achiness may come with a feeling that the contents of the pelvis are being pulled downward. These symptoms involve the reproductive and the nervous systems, so the herbs you use must help both. Used in conjunction with moderate exercise, a good diet, and abundant rest, the herbal remedies suggested below promote circulation, strengthen nerves, eliminate congestion, and bring better tone to the ligaments.

Sometimes a woman's pain threshold shifts around this time of the month and during the perimenopausal period. Because pain of any kind is an important message, the combinations in this section are designed so they will not suppress symptoms, but they are strong enough to take the edge off pain and provide some emergency relief. They can be used once or twice as needed for minor symptoms or for one to three months for more longstanding conditions. It takes at least ninety days for natural remedies to make significant improvements in chronic conditions. If symptoms don't feel "minor" to you, always know that a caring licensed health-care practitioner can rule out problems requiring more immediate attention.

❖ Herbal 911 ❖

Extracts	Botanical Names	Actions
4 oz. passion flower herb	*Passiflora incarnate*	Pain relieving, emotionally calming
4 oz. cramp bark	*Viburnum opulus*	Relaxes muscle spasms; relieves pain from tension
2 oz. valerian root	*Valeriana officinalis*	Sedates; relieves spasms; induces sleepiness

Ten ounces will last thirty days. Combine these herbal extracts. For pain relief right now, start with 10 drops every five minutes for twenty minutes. If that doesn't help, take ¹/₂ ounce diluted in ¹/₂ cup water, and sip over the next twenty minutes. Repeat as needed.

If you experience chronic dull or aching pain before, after, or during bleeding, take ¹/₂ teaspoon in water three times every day for three weeks before the next period and during bleeding if needed. If your cycle is erratic, so that "three weeks before" is impossible to predict, you can safely use the mixture all through the month and during bleeding.

If pain is caused by a diagnosed condition of uterine prolapse or blockage, add 2 ounces of the tissue tonic, blue cohosh (*Caulophyllum thalictroides*). This can help you heal, but you may need to do more than take the tissue tonics and connective tissue remedies. Exercise, chiropractic or osteopathic adjustments, and acupuncture may help here. If severe pain isn't lessened at all within two hours, call for more specific advice from your nearest health-care provider. For chronic lower back pain during or after menopause, try this tonic tea.

❖ I Feel Free Tea ❖

Dried Herbs	Botanical Names	Actions
4 oz. passion flower herb	*Passiflora incarnate*	Pain relieving, emotionally calming
3 oz. black haw root bark	*Viburnum prunifolium*	Relaxes ovarian, uterine muscle spasms
2 oz. sage leaf	*Salvia officinalis*	Supports hormonal balance, digestion; for taste
¹/₂ oz. ginger root	*Zingiber officinale*	Improves circulation, metabolism; for taste

Fifteen ounces will last about thirty days. Combine ¹/₃ ounce of the mixture with 3 cups of boiling water in a teapot or container with a well-fitting lid. Let stand for fifteen minutes before straining. Drink 2 cups hot or cold as needed.

Herbal Medicine

Painful intercourse caused by dysmenorrheal, fibroids, or loss of lubrication in the vaginal canal is also associated with menopause. Though sex helps all these conditions, it is hard to have good sex when it doesn't feel good. Many herbs are known to help women's enjoyment of sexuality by healing, toning, and calming inflamed vaginal tissue, lubricating thin walls, or relaxing taut muscles. For example, wound-healing herbs such as yarrow (*Achillea millefolium*) ad calendula (*Calendula officinalis*) are toning and anti-inflammatory when used directly on vaginal tissues. They are particularly beneficial if pain is caused by dryness, infection, or irritation. The following herb formulas relieve pain while healing from the inside out; also see the recommendations in "Vaginal Thinning and Dryness."

Taken internally in tea form or as extracts, many of these same herbs are also digestive bitters. This is nature's way of feeding two birds with one morsel: hormonal and digestive changes are treated together. From the inside of the body, herbs can help relieve pelvic congestion, sluggish bowels, bloating, intestinal gas, and even heavy menstrual bleeding. Other digestive herbs with helpful properties for improving the integrity of the vaginal walls and uterine muscle during menopause are sage. (*Salvia officinalis*), licorice (*Glycyrrhiza glabra*), and chamomile (*Matricaria recutita*).

Different types of pain respond to different herbs. Many common types of pain related to menopause can respond to the following two combinations. These remedies work on hormonal balance, sensory nerve endings, and adrenal stress. They also improve pelvic congestion and satisfactory elimina-

---

Herbs for Cardiovascular Disease

Amanda McQuade Crawford

The following herbal formulas help the entire cardiovascular system, especially for those women who are in higher-risk groups. While the herbs also help with hot flashes, they are specifically designed to strengthen blood vessels and heart muscle, normalize blood pressure, and improve circulation to the fingers and toes. They will not cause negative interactions with medication for high blood pressure and are safe for children or men to drink, too.

Change of Heart Cordial

Extracts	Botanical Names	Actions
4 oz. hawthorn leaf, flower, berry	*Crataegus* species	Safely relaxes blood vessels; lowers high blood pressure
2 oz. motherwort herb	*Leonurus cardiaca*	Lessens hot flashes; calms a pounding heart
2 oz. chasteberry seed	*Vitex agnus-castus*	Stabilizes hormone surges and declines
1 oz. black cohosh root	*Cimicifuga racemosa*	Hormone tonic; relaxes and nourishes nerves
¹/₂ oz. blackstrap molasses		Nutritive; provides iron without causing constipation
¹/₁₂ oz. black cherry juice concentrate		For taste; to harmonize strong herbal actions (available at natural food stores)

Twelve ounces will last thirty days. Combine these herbal extracts. Take 1 teaspoon twice a day, diluted in 1 cup of water, juice, or any herb tea, in the morning and evening.

Change of Heart Tea

Dried Herbs	Botanical Names	Actions
2 oz. linden flower	*Tilia* species	Moistens, relaxes; tones blood vessels and nerves
2 oz. hawthorn flower, leaf	*Crataegus* species	Nourishes heart; stabilizes circulation
2 oz. hawthorn berry	*Crataegus* species	Nourishes heart; stabilizes circulation
¹/₂ oz. hibiscus flower	*Hibiscus sabdariffa*	For taste, cooling; nutritive
1 oz. peppermint leaf	*Mentha piperita*	Soothes digestion; for taste

Fifteen ounces will last thirty days. Put ¹/₂ ounce of the mixture and 3¹/₂ cups of boiling water in a teapot or container with a well-fitting lid. Let stand for fifteen minutes before straining. Drink 1 cup hot or cold three times a day, either sipping the tea all day or drinking two large glasses twice a day. If you don't care for peppermint, replace it with either rosemary or raspberry leaves.

—From *The Herbal Menopause Book*

Continued ➤

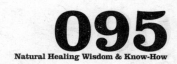

tion by activating the liver rather than stimulating the wall of the colon. This makes them milder, safer, and more comfortable to use than fast-acting herbal laxatives such as senna. *Cascara sagrada*, senna pods, and other strong anthraquinone-containing herbs are still useful in a pinch for constipation, but they only work on a symptomatic level and can be harsh on the body. The digestive bitter tonics used here are better for balancing sluggish or congested bowels in conjunction with bloating, gas, or even some alternating looseness of stools. If there's nothing wrong with the digestive tract, these herbs are mild enough not to overstimulate elimination. The combination will still offer its pain-lessening and nourishing qualities.

❧ Nepenthe's Nectar ❦

(In Greek, nepenthe means "herb that soothes away sorrow.")

Extracts	Botanical Names	Actions
4 oz. passion flowers herb	*Passiflora incarnate*	Pain relieving, emotionally calming
2 oz. licorice root	*Glycyrrhiza glabra*	Anti-inflammatory; moistening
2 oz. chamomile flower	*Matricaria recutita*	Calming to nerves, digestion; reduces bloating
1 oz. black cohosh root	*Cimicifuga racemosa*	Balances hormones; calms; anti-inflammatory
1 oz. wild yam root	*Dioscorea villosa*	Supports hormonal balance; anti-inflammatory

Ten ounces will last thirty days. Combine these herbal extracts. Take 1 teaspoon in 1 cup water, juice, or any herb tea in the morning and evening. If desired, replace licorice with skullcap (Scutellaria species).

❧ Sweet Mercy Tea ❦

Dried Herbs	Botanical Names	Actions
5 oz. passion flower herb	*Passiflora incarnate*	Pain relieving, emotionally calming
3 oz. sage leaf	*Salvia officinalis*	Supports hormonal balance, digestion; for taste
2 oz. chamomile flower	*Matricaria recutita*	Calming to nerves, digestion; reduces bloating
1 oz. dong quai root	*Amgelica sinensis*	Increases low estrogen; builds immune reserves
1 oz. cinnamon bark	*Cinnamomum species*	Warms; tones; astringent

Fifteen ounces will last thirty days. Combine ½ ounce of the mixture with 4 cups boiling water in a teapot or container with a well-fitting lid. Let stand for fifteen minutes before straining. Drink 1 cup hot or cold two to four times a day, or if you prefer, sip tea all day. If you are allergic to the daisy family, especially chrysanthemums, replace the chamomile with an extra ½ ounce of cinnamon and 1½ ounces of linden (Tilia species).

If you need to sleep to give your body a chance to escape constant or chronic pain, use the following herb as a last resort for quick symptom relief:

Extract	Botanical Name	Actions
1 oz. valerian root	*Valeriana officinalis*	Pain relieving; sedates; relaxes muscle tension

Dilute 10 to 15 drops of this pungent root in water, juice, or herb tea and take every ten to fifteen minutes until pain is gone. This usually occurs in two to three doses; don't take more than ten doses in any two-hour period. By that point, sleep will be on the horizon anyway. A tea of the root, ½ ounce to a pint of water, is also effective though it doesn't taste good and smells peculiar; drink a teacup at a time as neeed. Nonalcohol extracts with glycerin are available in many stores and taste better but are slightly less effective.

Yet another cause of pain is the menstrual migraine. This form of headache also may flare up in menopause and is aggravated by excess estrogen, caffeine, and other factors. Prevention is the best remedy for these headaches whether they are related to the menstrual cycle or changing estrogen levels in menopause. Prevention includes eating regularly to stabilize blood sugar, releasing tension before it builds up, and taking herbs to ease premenstrual or menopausal irritability. When it is too late for prevention, try one or more of the following remedies to make an immediate difference. There are three choices because each will not work for every woman, and you may need to experiment to get the relief you need.

Herbs for Depression

Amanda McQuade Crawford

The following combinations are recommended for depression, emotional vulnerability, and nervous tension. Think of them as all-natural fuel for the little engine that said, "I think I can, I think I can." Though neither extract nor tea is a delightful-tasting beverage, one or both will lighten your mood while strengthening your power. If you wish, add honey or other delicious herbs (peppermint, fennel, hibiscus) to taste. If you have blood sugar problems, don't use sugar or more than 1 teaspoon of honey per cup.

Tiger Today, Butterfly Tonight

Extracts	Botanical Names	Actions
4 oz. black cohosh root	*Cimicifuga racemosa*	Adjusts low estrogen; relaxes nerves
4 oz. St. John's wort	*Hypericum perforatum*	Repairs nerve damage; acts as antidepressant
4 oz. Siberian ginseng root	*Eleutherococcus senticosus*	Improves response to stress
2 oz. lavender flower	*Lavandula officinalis*	Lifts spirits; is cleansing and soothing
1 oz. vervain herb	*Verbena offocinalis*	Tones liver; balances mood, hormones
1 oz. licorice root	*Glycrrhiza glabra*	Moistening; anti-inflammatory

Sixteen ounces will last thirty days or more depending on need. Combine the extracts. Take 1 teaspoon in 1 cup water, juice, or any herb tea three times a day. For immediate help in coping with difficult times in the short term, take ½ teaspoon every fifteen to twenty minutes, as needed. These higher amounts can be continued for a week or two, especially if a crisis is also being handled through spot counseling or other appropriate help. If Vervain is not available, replace it with ½ ounce of mugwort (*Artemisia vulgaris*). If desired, replace licorice with wild yam (*Dioscorea villosa*).

Centered in Peace

Dried Herbs	Botanical Names	Actions
1 oz. damiana herb	*Turnera diffusa*	Stimulates nerves and sluggish digestion
3 oz. raspberry leaf	*Rubus idaeus*	Calming, nutritive; provides minerals; tones womb
3 oz. St. John's wort herb	*Hypericum perforatum*	Antidepressant; improves resistance
3 oz. lemon balm leaf	*Melissa officinalis*	For taste; improves digestion, mood
1 oz. borage flower	*Borago officinalis*	Cooling, nutritive
½ oz. motherwort herb	*Leonurus cardiaca*	Lessens hot flashes; strengthens heart
½ oz. calendula flower	*Calendula officinalis*	Tones liver, lymph, skin; anti-inflammatory
½ oz. rose petals	*Rosa species*	Tonic, astringent; for beauty

Fifteen ounces will last thirty days. Combine ½ ounce of the mixture with 3½ cups of boiling water in a teapot or container with a well-fitting lid. Let stand for fifteen minutes before straining. Drink 1 cup hot or cold three times a day. One teapot as strong as you like can be used as often as needed. Or, if you prefer, sip tea all day or drink large glasses twice a day, making sure you drink 3 cups a day. Take eight weeks or more for lasting benefits. If lemon balm or borage flowers are unavailable, replace with lemon verbena (*Lippia citriodora*).

—from *The Herbal Menopause Book*

Continued ➡

❧ Numb Skull Compound ❧

Extracts	Botanical Names	Actions
2 oz. skullcap herb	*Scutellaria laterifolis*	Relaxes tension, anxiety; nourishes nerves
2 oz. lavender flower	*Lavandula officinalis*	Cleanses; relaxes; lifts spirits
2 oz. motherwort herb	*Leonurus cardiaca*	Lowers tension, high blood pressure

Six ounces will last a long time without refrigeration; keep on hand for occasional headaches. Combine these herbal extracts. Take 1 to 3 teapoons in 1 cup water, juice, or any herb tea up to ten times a day if needed. At maximum dose, that's 30 teaspoons or just over 4 ounces in a day, so be sure to drink plain water and other fluids, eat small meals, and rest. If your headache requires that much tincture, avoid driving; instead, stay home or take a stress-relieving walk.

❧ Floral Calm Tea ❧

Extracts	Botanical Names	Actions
4 oz. skullcap herb	*Scutellaria laterifolia*	Reduces pressure, tension
2 oz. rosemary flower, leaf	*Rosmarinus officinalis*	Relaxes blood vessels
2 oz. linden flower	*Tilia species*	Reduces high blood pressure; calms; moistens
1 oz. sage leaf	*Salvia officinalis*	Supports hormonal balance; tonic, astringent
1 oz. passion flower herb	*Passiflora incarnate*	Reduces physical, emotional pain

Ten ounces stored in a closed container away from direct heat and light will last up to a year without refrigeration. Combine ½ ounce of the mixture with 3 cups of boiling water in a teapot or container with a well-fitting lid. Let stand for five to fifteen minutes before straining. Drink 2 cups hot or cold, as needed.

❧ Head for the Hills Elixir ❧

Extracts	Botanical Names	Actions
3 oz. fresh feverfew herb	*Chrysanthemum parthenium*	Stabilizes blood vessels to brain
2 oz. chasteberry seed	*Vitex agnus-castus*	Stabilizes hormones
1 oz. lavender flower	*Lavandula officinalis*	Cleanses; relaxes; uplifts
2 oz. sage leaf	*Salvia officinalis*	Tonic, astringent; supports hormonal balance

Take 1 teaspoon diluted in a cup of liquid every morning; to mask its odd taste, try it in diluted fruit juice or herb tea (try "Floral Calm," above). Take an extra dose if you feel a migraine sneaking up on you.

※

If you experience menstrual migraines, which are caused by blood vessel spasms, prevention is even more necessary than for tension headaches. The best herbal remedies for this type of headache do not get rid of a migraine once you have it; rather, they build up your resistance to future headaches. The main extract, feverfew (Chrysanthemium parthenium), must be made from the fresh flowering herb because dried tea has far less of an effect. Most companies know this; check the label of any store-bought extract to be sure it is from fresh plant material. Some women report that freeze-dried capsules work; others report they do not. When you feel like closing the door, discon-necting the phone, or heading for the hills, do that and take a cup of the following remedy.

When all is said and done, pain is sometimes not just physical or just emotional. When you know the cause of severe pain, but it has not responded to the gentle methods described above, it is not wrong or weak to suppress it. Allowing yourself escape routes in severe distress can allow your body's resources to mobilize for deep healing. A recent study shows that symptom-suppressing pain medication prescribed immediately after an operation can allow more rapid healing. The use of nature's painkillers can also contribute to healing in this way.

When physical or emotional pain is severe, take up to 1 ounce of passion flower tincture diluted in one 8-ounce cup of water or herb tea. If pain in your lower back or abdomen is causing insomnia, try massaging the affected area with the aromatherapy blend noted under "In Addition." Or take a lavender bath or even a warm shower that ends with a lukewarm or cool rinse. Then return to bed with a cup of sleep-inducing herb tea. This cam be a single herb, from mild chamomile to medium-strong motherwort (very bitter tasting) to the stronger valerian (strong tasting). Of these, only the chamomile tastes good as a tea to most women, so other useful forms are capsules (which may take up to an hour and a half to take effect) or glycerin tinctures, which have no alcohol. Alcohol-based tinctures work as well, but if you need to avoid alcohol (even a small amount of alcohol can trigger migraines in some women), do not use them.

The amount of alcohol in herbal extracts is relatively little when taken as directed, so if a small quantity of alcohol is not a problem for you, you can, of course, use alcohol-based tinctures. It is the herb, not the alcohol, that is having the effect, so you are not really using the tincture as a stiff snort, as some skeptics might scoff. If one is in great pain, it will not help to sip 1 to 3 teaspoons of Scotch diluted in a cup of water before bed. However, this dose or less of the herb extracts can work wonders. This way of using herbs is not repeated long term, but it does work well for short-term symptom management of pain or insomnia.

The purpose of using these particular pain-lessening herb formulas is not to suppress each symptom but to improve the quality of life *in the moment* while we are still working on the causes of our discomfort. Returning to sleep in itself allows deeper self-healing, even if the sleep is achieved some nights with repeated doses of valerian. Remember, we are still discussing strong plant preparations, not habit-forming pharmaceutical drugs.

Hot Flashes and Night Sweats

In Great Britain and Australia, hot flashes are known as "flushing." For the longest time, I thought it was their accent, but they really do say, "Poor dear, she's having a hot flush." For many women, hot flashes are no joke. They can be the most debilitating symptom of menopause, though they can improve or even disappear through natural means. A hot flash is a sudden sensation of heat from blood vessels near the skin, sometimes with profuse sweating and sometimes preceded by chills. A hot flash starts in the chest and rises up the neck and face, and though it happens from head to toe, it is felt most in the upper body. Hot flashes that occur at night, especially with more perspiration, are called "night sweats."…

Because women's blood vessels become more sensitive to sharp drops and floods of chemicals including hormones during the Change, the objec-tive of taking certain herbs at this time is twofold: to stabilize blood vessel sensitivity to changing hormone levels, and to slow down or smooth the overall drop in estrogen from the ovaries. Some of these herbs do this by supporting the adrenal function. Our adrenals provide a little estrogen as a hormonal cushion. Adrenal tonic herbs, called "adaptogens," help our adrenal glands help us to *adapt* to current levels of stress. Examples are Siberian ginseng (*Eleutherococcus senticosus*), borage (*Borago officinalis*), ginseng (*Panax ginseng*), and nettle (*Urtica dioica*).

Nervines are another category of herbs that do more than simply suppress hot flashes: They help the body handle stress by providing relaxation, stimulation, or pain relief. They can mitigate hot flashes because, as every women knows from experience and recent research has shown, the endocrine (hormone) and nervous systems are not two separate systems—each improves or worsens depending on the health or strain on the other. Nourishing herbs like motherwort (*Leonurus cardiaca*) that calm frazzled nerve endings can help make hot flashes disappear or at least be more comfortable (in severe cases, more tolerable).

One particular herb or another in this section may relieve hot flashes time and again for some women. But for severe or stubborn hot flashes, more women find better results from combinations of herbs that support the liver's natural function of metabolizing circulating hormones and the estrogen still made in our bodies. Wisely combined formulas also optimize the function of all types of estrogen, from ovaries, adrenal glands, and even fat cells. Hormonal tonics such as licorice (*Glycyrrhiza glabra*) can do double-duty by optimizing liver function and acting on the adrenal glands as a nourishing tonic.

Night sweats and palpitations (feeling your heart pound) can be addressed with herbal cardiovascular tonics, nervine relaxants, and hormonal balancers such as dong quai (*Angelica sinensis*), motherwort (*Leonurus cardiaca*), linden (*Tilia platyphylla/T. europea*), and yarrow (*Achillea millefolium*). These four plants, used singly or in any combination, stabilize the sensitivity of blood vessels to ebbs and flows in estrogen. Each of these has its own particular benefit, and no one needs them all, so choose the most appropriate one. The following two formulas strengthen and tone the blood vessels and, through the addition of hormone balancers such as chasteberry (*Vitex agnus-castus*), normalize your system's changing amounts of estrogen.

❧ Engine Cooler ❧

Extracts	Botanical Names	Actions
3 oz. chasteberry seed	*Vitex agnus-castus*	Stabilizes drops and surges in hormones
2 oz. motherwort herb	*Leonurus cardiaca*	Cools symptoms; calms heart palpitations
2 oz. hawthorn flower, leaf, berry	*Crataegus species*	Protects heart; strengthens blood vessels
2 oz. yarrow flower	*Achillea millefolium*	Cools temperature; stimulates liver
1 oz. dong quai root	*Angelica sinensis*	Supports estrogen balance; builds healthy blood

Ten ounces will last thirty days. Combine these herbal extracts. Every ten minutes take one dropper or ½ teaspoon diluted in ½ cup of room-temperature water. This remedy usually works in two or three doses, but the effect won't last long unless you take it consistently. For more permanent improvement, take 1

Continued ➡

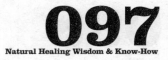

teaspoon three times a day for two weeks; then take a few days off and repeat for another two weeks. After that, repeat as needed. "Engine Cooler" combines well with the tea described below. The "cucumber" in the tea is really borage, a flowering edible plant whose peeled stalk smells and tastes a little like cucumbers. The overall effect of this tea is stabilizing, soothing, and moistening.

❧ Cool as a Cucumber Tea ❧

Dried Herbs	Botanical Names	Actions
1 oz. motherwort herb	*Leonurus cardiaca*	Cools hot flashes; lessens sweating
2 oz. linden flower	*Tilia species*	Relaxes nerves; lowers high blood pressure
1 oz. chamomile flower	*Matricaria recutita*	Soothes stomach, nerves
4 oz. skullcap herb	*Scutellaria laterifolia*	Eases tension; nourishes frazzled nerves
3 oz. borage flowers, stems, and leaves	*Borago officinalis*	Moistens; nutritive tonic
2 oz. marshmallow root	*Althaea officinalis*	Moistens; helps water balance
2 oz. hibiscus flower	*Hibiscus sabdariffa*	Cooling; for taste

Fifteen ounces will last thirty days. Combine 1 ounce of the mixtyre with 4 cups of boiling water in a teapot or container with a well-fitting lid. Let stand for fifteen minutes; then strain the tea and store it in a closed container. Allow to cool; drink at room temperature—not hot and not icy cold. During daytime hot flashes, drink 1 cup as often as needed. Or, if you prefer, sip this amount of tea all day or drink two large glasses twice a day—just be sure you drink it all sometime each day. The tea is also good for sipping while you are drying off from a cool bath or shower. Drink 1/2 to 3 cups as needed after night sweats before you return to a fresh, dry bed, but remember to empty the bladder before going to sleep.

Hops and valerian are stronger sleep-inducing herb teas or tinctures than the combinations above and taste correspondingly stronger. Either or both may replace linden and skullcap in the formula above at those times when the mind needs to turn off so the body can sleep deeply. For fewer hot flashes and sounder sleep, try 1 to 2 cups of the herbal formula earlier during the evening to help the body wind down before bedtime. Remember to empty the bladder the last thing before bed so you aren't awakened from a sound sleep for a midnight trip to the bathroom....

Single herbs make fine dietary supplements for managing the symptom of hot flashes or night sweats.

• Motherwort metabolizes fats and hormones, filters blood, and improves immunity. It is specifically helpful for heart palpitations as well as menopausal hot flashes and healthy liver function, so it may be useful in any formula taken by a woman with cardiovascular concerns. Dosage of store-bought extract ranges from 1 dropper to 1 teaspoon every ten to twenty minutes as needed and/or three times a day for prevention.

• Ginseng (*Panax ginseng*, also called Asian, Chinese, Korean, or Manchurian ginseng) taken for six weeks and longer works well too, although it may not work equally well in all women. Some traditional Chinese medical practitioners say that menopausal women should never take ginseng. Nevertheless,

numerous women have told me of the benefits it gave them, and there is research to support both view. Women who seem to react badly to ginseng are, to begin with, tired but high-strung, tense, and wound up. Women who do well with a little ginseng tend to feel, before taking the herb, emptied out, weakened in every body system, and slow to get going. The use of ginseng is certainly easier on a woman than HRT. The temporary "ginseng headache" that helps a person determine that this powerful herb may not be right for her is not as difficult a side effect to clear up as the cancer risk associated with replacement hormones.

• Licorice is a rich, affordable source of phytoestrogens. Although it should be used with some caution, moderate amounts or the conservative dosages suggested in this book are going to be helpful to most women going through the Change. An explanation of precautions is found in "Irregular Cycles," following. Formulas including this herb also indicate substitutes.

• Natural sources of phytoestrogens commonly available in herb shops or natural food stores require a different kind of caution. Sarsaparilla is often adulterated (mixed with other herb substitutes), so check with the herb seller to make sure you are buying pure Jamaican sarsaparilla, *Smilax ornate* or a related *Smilax* species. Real sarsaparilla has little fragrance; the more delicious the smell, the more likely it is to be a different plant confusingly called sarsaparilla. Because of rampant overharvesting, do not purchase the endangered wild American ginseng (*Panax quinquefolius*). Please use only cultivated roots, grown and harvested with ecological sensitivity.

Irregular Cycles

First you have a late period. Then you have two in just six weeks. You haven't bled in six months and think, "Hey, that was easy!" but the next month there's a scarlet stain on your white sheets. When your biological clock starts winding down, your cycle becomes irregular and your emotions may well become unpredictable.

The best way you can cope is to really take care of yourself. Deeply focus on stabilizing your body: Prolong your naturally occurring estrogen levels, build your health, look beyond symptoms that come and go, nourish each of the body systems affected by the Change. Focus your inner being by drawing more love to yourself in your personal, social, and spiritual relationships. Tall order? Your energy and your spirit are limitless.

And nature offers some kind assistance. One or more of the hormonal normalizers found in every habitat on Earth, such as the North American black cohosh, support a grace-filled Change, as does chasteberry (*Vitex agnus-castus*), a Mediterranean seed in human use as a hormonal tonic for more than three thousand years.

China introduced dong quai (*Angelica Sinensis*) root to the West, but my Euro-American tradition favors the use of chasteberry. In Europe, older herbal practitioners with whom I did my internship swore they could not treat menopause safely and effectively without this pungent seed. It may be that during other decades in the twentieth century, herbal alternatives such as American ginseng, red clover, and the cohoshes were not as fresh or high quality as chasteberry. Chinese herbs used for

women in menopause, such as dong quai, bupleurum (*Bupleurum Chinense*), and other companion herbs, were relatively unknown to Euro-American herbal traditions until recent years. False unicorn root (*Chamaelirium luteum*), which was a standard American remedy, is endangered in the wild, and so ethical herbal practitioners will not use it unless they personally collect it where it is locally abundant, even though it is still recommended in mass-produced herb books and formulas. Nature is generous in giving us several equally good herbs in the hormone-balancing category, so if we do not wish to destroy the plants we know and love, let us be equally generous in returning a little of our time to nature.

Herbal Medicine

...[T]he following two formulas and tea are more nourishing for women in menopause. For the quickest results, "Lunar Nectar" works with the power of the moon's pull on gravity to establish a regular menses, even if it is not twenty-eight days. If your cycles have been erratic for longer than six months, use the "Womb Rhythm" formula or tea instead.

❧ Lunar Nectar ❧

Extracts	Botanical Names	Actions
4 oz. chasteberry seed	*Vitex agnus-castus*	Regulates pituitary control of hormones
2 oz. black cohosh root	*Cimicifuga racemosa*	Reduces tension; helps balance estrogen
2 oz. nettle leaf	*Urtica dioica*	Nutritive; supports liver, kidney function
2 oz. rosehips	*Rosa canina*	Nutritive; provides bioflavonoids; cooling
1 oz. motherwort herb	*Leonurus cardiaca*	Calms, strengthens heart
1 oz. dong quai root	*Angelica sinensis*	Moistens; builds blood, low estrogen levels

Twelve ounces will last thirty days. Combine these herbal extracts. Take 1 teaspoon in 1 cup water, juice, or any herb tea three times a day morning, afternoon [3 to 5 p.m.] and after dinner. Though it may bring improvement in the first month, take for a minimum of three months for better results.

❧ Womb Rhythm Elixir ❧

Extracts	Botanical Names	Actions
2 oz. fresh shepherd's purse herb	*Capsella bursa-pastoris*	Stops or slows excess bleeding
2 oz. lady's mantle leaf	*Alchemilla vulgaris*	Protects reproductive tissue
1 oz. blue cohosh root	*Caulophyllum thalictroides*	Balances hormones; astringent
1 oz. black cohosh root	*Cimicifuga racemosa*	Balances hormones; relaxes
1 oz. chasteberry seed	*Vitex agnus-castus*	Lowers excess estrogen

Seven ounces will last approximately a week; this amount lasts three days or so if the higher dose is needed for short-term results. Combine these extracts; take 1 to 3 teaspoons every two hours until bleeding stops or slows down. For chronic problems with spotting between cycles, flooding, and fibroids, take 1 teaspoon three times a day for a minimum of three months (15 ounces per month).

Continued ➡

⚜ Womb Rhythm Tea ⚜

Dried Herbs	Botanical Names	Actions
4 oz. chasteberry seed	*Vitex agnus-castus*	Lessens excess estrogen
3 oz. sage leaf	*Salvia officinalis*	Balances hormones; astringent
3 oz. partridge berry herb	*Mitchella repens*	Lessens excess bleeding; tones
3 oz. lady's mantle herb	*Alchemilla vulgaris*	Protects reproductive tissues
1 oz. yellow dock root	*Rumex crispus*	Stimulates liver; helps iron assimilation
1 oz. cinnamon bark	*Cinnamonum zeylanicum*	For taste; soothes; lessens bleeding

Fifteen ounces will last thirty days. Add 1 ounce of the mixture to 4 cups of boiling water in a teapot or container with a well-fitting lid. Let stand for fifteen minutes before straining. Drink 1 cup hot or cold, three to four times a day. Or, if you prefer, sip tea all day or drink two large glasses twice a day, but be sure you drink 3 or 4 cups of tea in a day.

Some women find that they would like to switch to a better-tasting tea after using this mixture for a month or two. This is perfectly normal and may occur because their taste buds change as their bodies respond. Here is an alternative tea that you can switch to at any time.

⚜ In the Pink ⚜

Dried Herbs	Botanical Names	Actions
4 oz. chasteberry seed	*Vitex agnus-castus*	Tones reproductive tissues
2½ oz. wild oats herb	*Avena sativa*	Relaxes nerves; tones skin, hair
2½ oz. raspberry leaf	*Rubus idaeus*	Provides minerals; balances hormones
2 oz. St. John's wort herb	*Hypericum perforatum*	Repairs cells; anti-inflammatory
2 oz. licorice root	*Glycyrrhiza glabra*	Moistens; soothes digestion; for taste
1 oz. orange peel (organic)	*Citrus aurantium*	For taste; improves digestion
1 oz. hibiscus flower	*Hibiscus sabdariffa*	For taste; nutritive; provides bioflavonoids

Fifteen ounces will last thirty days. Add 1 ounce of the mixture to 4 cups of boiling water in a teapot or container with a well-fitting lid. Let stand for twenty minutes; then strain. Drink 1 to 3 cups daily, hot or cold. Note: This mixture uses a small amount of licorice, but if you have high blood pressure, low potassium, or a history of kidney or heart failure, replace it with Siberian ginseng (Eleutherococcus senticosus).

For irregular cycles complicated by heavy bleeding or for spotting between cycles, use one or both of the following formulas instead of those above for erratic timing....

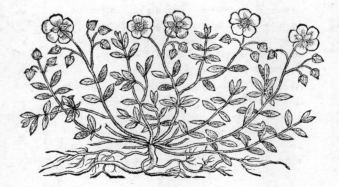

⚜ Closing the Gates ⚜

Extracts	Botanical Names	Actions
4 oz. fresh shepherd's purse herb	*Capsella bursa-pastoris*	Antihemorrhagic; fights infection
2 oz. lady's mantle herb	*Alchemilla vulgaris*	Helps reduce fibroids; protective
2 oz. blue cohosh root	*Caulophyllum thalictroides*	Balances hormones; tones tissue
1 oz. black cohosh root	*Cimicifuga racemosa*	Balances hormones; soothes nerves
1 oz. chasteberry seed	*Vitex agnus-castus*	Harmonizes; balances hormones

Ten ounces will last thirty days. Combine these herbal extracts. Take 1 tablespoon in 1 cup water, juice, or any herb tea every two hours, until bleeding slows down enough; this allows the body time to clot normally and to replace lost blood from reserves. For chronic problems with spotting between cycles, flooding (very heavy flow), and fibroids, take 1 to 2 teaspoons three times a day for a minimum of three months. Consult a health-care provider to help rule out potential dangers associated with menopausal bleeding problems.

⚜ Wise Wound Healer ⚜

Dried Herbs	Botanical Names	Actions
3 oz. chasteberry seed	*Vitex agnus-castus*	Harmonizes; balances hormones
3 oz. sage leaf	*Salvia officinalis*	Lessens excess bleeding; tones tissue
3 oz. partridge berry herb	*Mitchella repens*	Stimulates healing of uterine tissue
3 oz. lady's mantle herb	*Alchemilla vulgaris*	Protects, nourishes uterine tissue
1½ oz. yellow dock root	*Rumex cirspus*	Helps elimination; provides iron
1½ oz. cinnamon bark	*Cinnamonum zeylanicum*	Helps digestion; for taste

Fifteen ounces will last thirty days. Add 1 ounce of the mixture to 4 cups of boiling water in a teapot or container with a well-fitting lid. Let stand for fifteen minutes before straining. Drink 1 cup hot or cold three to four times a day.

Nutrition

Wise Food Choices

· In early spring, dandelion leaf in salads or mixed steamed greens

· Pomegranate fruit and seeds

· Dried apricots

· Sesame seeds, tahini (1 tablespoon plain or in prepared dishes, two to three times a week)

Supplements

· Milk thistle (1 tablespoon of seeds daily, ground into powder and sprinkled over cooked grains and salads or blended in soups). May be taken as capsules, two capsules three times a day or three capsules taken two times a day with meals. Standardized silymarin from milk thistle is also available; take as labels suggest.

· Beta-carotene obtained from yellow or orange vegetables is better than from supplements.

—From *The Herbal Menopause Book*

MORE FEMALE-SPECIFIC HERBALISM
Diane Stein

Breast Lumps

Fifty percent of women will discover a breast lump at some time, in their lives, and 50 to 70 percent of women have fibrocystic breasts. With that high a figure, it is difficult to call fibrous breasts a disease. I would consider it, rather, a condition common to women in modern American society and/or an environmental or nutritional pollution symptom. Breast lumps seem to occur under three primary factors: over–estrogen production in the body of a menstruation-age woman, overingestion of unsaturated fats in the diet, and use of high amounts of caffeine. Overproduction of estrogen and the problem with fats can possibly be traced to the hormones fed to meat and dairy animals, and also to poultry. These pollutant residues remain in the flesh and are concentrated in the fats (including milk fats) that are ingested by meat and dairy eating women. A vegetarian or organic diet, especially one free of milk products, is sometimes enough to cause breast lumps to disappear by themselves. Stopping coffee, tea, chocolate and colas—all high in caffeine—is enough to change the fibrous breast conditions of many women by itself. Decaffeinated coffee does not seem to cause this condition.

It is normal for women's breasts to feel a little lumpy, particularly around menstruation. Benign breast lumps and cystic breasts may fluctuate with the menstrual cycle but some lumps may also grow quite large. They are fluid-filled and move freely under the skin like an eye under the eyelid; they are tender and may be painful. New cysts rarely form after menopause, and 80 percent of breast lumps are benign. A malignant lump has different symptoms: it does not move freely, is not tender, and does not fluctuate in size or go away. I have had good results in helping women with breast lumps or fibrocystic breasts, using holistic methods and diet change. Begin by stopping caffeine and milk products, eating a diet low in saturated fats, and switching to either vegetarianism or organic meats and poultry. Avoid alcohol and cigarettes.

Herbs: A tea of one ounce red clover and one ounce blue violet leaf to a pint of water will cleanse the system and dissolve most breast lumps (and uterine or ovarian fibroids). Drink a pint of this daily over several months. These can be used as tinctures also and the herbs can be eaten fresh. Squaw vine or black cohosh herbs are also helpful, as well as mullein, pokeroot, or witchhazel as an external poultice. Other suggested herbs are echinacea, goldenseal, blessed thistle, ho shou wu, pau d'arco, or pokeroot. Dandelion is listed by some sources as a cancer preventive; use it internally and externally. For ovarian cysts, make a strong tea of

Continued ➡

raspberry leaf, black currant leaf, witchhazel leaf, and powdered myrrh. Strain and mix one cup of this with a cup of cooled boiled water and use as a nightly douche.

Candida Albicans

Systemic Yeast Infection

Candida can affect many parts of the body and be operant in a number of seemingly unrelated conditions. It can manifest as mouth or foot thrush, skin rashes or diseases, as vaginal infections (particularly recurrent ones), chronic fatigue, hypoglycemia, arthritis, sinusitis, digestive upsets or abdominal pain, constipation or diarrhea, joint or muscle pain, cystitis or kidney infections, PMS, depression hyperactivity, hypothyroidism, adrenal problems, environmental allergies, food sensitivities, and even diabetes. Many more women than men are affected, and women who are diabetic or pregnant, have been taking antibiotics or the contraceptive pill, are taking chemotherapy or cortisone (steroids), eat a high sugar and white flour diet, or who are under stress are particularly susceptible. Women who are deficient in the B complex vitamins or whose immune systems are lowered are also easily prone to developing systemic candida albicans. Long-term system candida has been implicated in mitral valve prolapse, a heart defect.

The cause of candida overrun is intestinal; where the natural balance of bacteria in the gut is disrupted by hormones, antibiotics, or refined carbohydrates (white sugar and flour), candida can overrun the system. Once entrenched, it can result in the wide range of symptoms and discomforts listed above and be difficult to diagnose and treat.

Herbs: Pau d'arco, black walnut, white oak bark, buchu, tea-tree tincture, or chaparral are all positive in eliminating candida albicans and rebuilding the immune system. Alternate pau d'arco and clove teas or tinctures. There are a number of herbal yeast preparations available in health food stores based on these herbs. A plant preparation called stevia can be used as a sweetener to replace sugar in the diet; it is good tasting, nontoxic, nonchemical, and won't feed the yeast. Find it from Sunrider and other companies.

Cystitis

Bladder Infections

Thirty times more women than men experience cystitis or bladder infections (urinary tract infections), and 40 percent of women will suffer it chronically at some point in their lives. Many bladder infections are caused by an imbalance in intestinal flora, the after-effect of taking antibiotics or other medical drugs. A majority of women who have chronic bladder infections seem also to have systemic Candida albicans (see above) and/or food allergies. Birth control pills can be a factor, poor-fitting diaphragms or allergy to spermicides, liver congestion, caffeine, or alcohol (they are irritants), constipation, need for spinal adjustments, stress, or frequent sexual activity (lesbian or heterosexual). A simple lack of drinking enough water can cause or aggravate this disease, and nylon underpants or pantyhose that restrict airflow to the vaginal area also make it worse. Wiping from front to back on the toilet will help to keep bacteria out of the urethra and bladder, as will urinating before and after intercourse.

Symptoms of cystitis are frequent urination, usually with burning or pain. You may have the urge to urinate again as soon as the bladder is voided, or feel an urge but nothing comes. There may be pain or cramping in the urethra, above the pubis, and/or in a line running along the pelvic bones. The urine may have a strong smell, look cloudy, or contain blood or fragments. There may be no other symptoms than frequency, and the abdomen may feel or appear to be bloated. An untreated bladder infection can spread to the kidneys, a more serious infection. If pains run along the back at about waist level, the tubes leading from bladder to kidneys are involved, or the kidneys themselves.

Herbs: Juniper berries, buchu, cornsilk, marshmallow root, nettles, parsley, dandelion, or uva ursi are used for bladder infections, as well as the herbal antibiotics goldenseal, Echinacea, or pau d'arco. Use bearberry, couchgrass, and yarrow together, or bearberry, sage, and horsetail. Use a comfrey poultice over the bladder area externally, and if there is blood in the urine use shepherd's purse.

Hair Loss

Alopecia

Hair loss is not only male heredity and vanity, but a dis-ease that affects many women. There are several cases where hair loss is expected. It is normal to lose significant amounts of hair in the last few months of pregnancy or for three or four months after childbirth. The hair usually regrows by the time the baby is six months old, and hormonal changes are the cause. It is also normal for women after menopause to experience thinning hair, particularly to the front, and graying hair with age. This is also hormone related, and much can be done to prevent and often reverse it. Radiation to the head or chemotherapy for cancer will cause hair loss, often total, which regrows after the therapy is stopped. Beyond these things, sudden falling out of women's hair in large quantities or in patches is called alopecia and can be caused by a number of factors. With holistic methods the loss can usually be stopped and very often the hair will regrow, though usually less fully than before.

Glandular imbalances are a major cause of hair loss in women, with the adrenals, thyroid (low thyroid) or pituitary glands involved. Stress, which depletes these glands, and emotional or physical trauma or shock are other causes. Hypoglycemia is another important fact. Nutritional deficiencies can cause both hair loss and graying in women. Other factors include poor scalp circulation (cranial-sacral massage work is wonderful), illness or surgery, diabetes, too-harsh shampoos, hair dyes and hot dryers, fevers, heavy metal poisoning, anemia, alcohol, and smoking. I have experienced hair loss due to adrenal exhaustion and stress, and the hair has regrown with vitamins, diet, and herbs.

Herbs: Make the following herbal preparation. Take a heaping tablespoon each of dried nettles, yarrow, and rosemary (for light hair) or black walnut (for dark) and put it into two cups of water in a nonaluminum pot on the stove. Bring to a boil, then shut off the flame and let it cool. Strain out the herbs and place the liquid in a pint plastic container, adding water to fill it. Use as a hair rinse after every shampoo; don't rinse it off. It will stimulate growth, make the hair shine and stop dandruff. Over a period of a few months it regrew my hair.

Other herbs include horsetail grass for calcium, silicon taken internally, cleavers internally, and use herbs for reducing stress. Use sage tea as a rinse for dark hair or chamomile for light hair, use comfrey rinse for dry hair, or lavender rinse for oily. Rub aloe vera gel, castor oil, or wheatgerm oil into the scalp the night before shampooing, and shampoo the next morning. Another scalp rinse infusion is rosemary, raspberry, and red sage.

Menstruation

It is only with Women's Spirituality and the honoring of women's bodies and cycles that menstruation has changed from "the curse" to the pride of modern women's Be-ing. Women bleed and do not die. Women bleed and new life is birthed. Women bleed and learn the power and beauty of being female and living with the cycles of the moon and earth. Five thousand years of patriarchy and misogynist patriarchal religions and attitudes have made women's bleeding and ability to give birth (as well as the ending of bleeding in menopause) something shameful. Women have been told that they (and their blood or because of it) are "dirty," "vessels of sin," and are not to be acknowledged in public. The verdict is changing, as women refuse the propaganda and take back their power. There would be no life without us and our ability to bleed.

Yet, menstruation for many women is not a time of joy but a time of tension and discomfort. Part of this is still from old attitudes that women have been ingrained with, and old attitudes die hard. Much of it, however, is very physical and very much caused by living in a patriarchal culture that degrades women and the earth. Few women today are able to withdraw from activity and give their bleeding time the space of quiet and peace-within that it needs. Most women live under extreme stress and tension—a byproduct of modern living and also of women's place in the patriarchy. Many women are on the contraceptive pill that wreaks havoc with normal hormones by convincing the body that it is pregnant. Most women are meat-eaters and today's meat and poultry is loaded with hormone residues that may be responsible for breast cancer, endometriosis, fibroid tumors and other diseases. Many women smoke cigarettes, which are a clear and present danger to women's lives. (Women who smoke are less fertile, have more difficult pregnancies and higher-risk babies. Women who smoke reach menopause earlier, and are at a much increased risk for osteoporosis and cancers of the lungs, breast, cervix, and uterus.) All women in industrialized America eat food that is polluted with chemicals, pesticides and drugs, and breathe air and drink water that are polluted as well. Heavy metal poisoning is a cause of PMS, along with low thyroid function, candida albicans, food allergies, high fat diets, overestrogen, hypoglycemia, poor spinal or body mechanics, poor food absorption, and vitamin deficiencies. All these things affect women's health and menstruation, and only some of them are avoidable.

Medical drugs for menstruation difficulties add more toxins and hormones to an already imbalanced mix. They worsen symptoms or have side effects that are worse than the symptoms, without touching causes. Too many women have been placed on tranquilizers for PMS, and too many hysterectomies are unnecessary. Holistic healing reaches the causes of menstrual distress while working with instead of against women's bodies. Along with the many remedy choices described below, try acupuncture or spinal manipulation instead of drugs or surgeries. They can make all the difference.

Herbs: If dong quai agrees with you, it can be the answer to PMS, cramping, bloating, vaginal dryness, fibroids, heavy bleeding, irregular cycles, and depression. Try it in tablets or tinctures and start slowly; stop if it increases the symptoms. This is the herb of choice for many women; see more about it

Continued ➡

under Menopause. Black cohosh is useful for ovarian cramps and pain, and for women who are hypoglycemic or near menopause. Try blue cohosh, or raspberry leaf with chamomile in a warm tea for PMS and cramping; raspberry also reduces flow. Motherwort is a menstrual balancer both for lack of periods (amenorrhea) and for premenopausal women, and also helps pelvic inflammation when combined with echinacea or goldenseal. Use cramp bark, wild yam, blue cohosh or squaw vine for difficult periods; squaw vine is especially good at menarche. For heavy or painful periods try cramp bark, red raspberry, strawberry leaf, white oak bark, or witchhazel (astringent and for pain). Sarsaparilla is a hormone balancer; accusations of its being a carcinogen have proved to be unfounded.

For pain or tension take a half teaspoonful of valerian tincture (or scullcap, hops, passion flower, feverfew, or cramp bark). Raspberry leaf is good for pregnancy, and use false unicorn root to prevent a threatened miscarriage. Shepherd's purse and nettles are sources of vitamin K and help heavy bleeding or hemorrhaging. They are also used after childbirth. To bring on menses, use basil, catnip, angelica, parsley, black cohosh, rosemary, ginger, or pennyroyal; do not use pennyroyal for longer than three days and do not use the oil. Siberian ginseng is used for PMS and for menopause, but is not for hypoglycemics; dong quai is more recommended. Motherwort, raspberry leaf, dong quai, wild yam, rosemary, black cohosh, and blue cohosh regulate cycles; use blue cohosh for most women under forty, black cohosh for over forty. For nausea with periods use peppermint, or peppermint with chamomile in teas. Pennyroyal increases blood flow, as does blazing star, feverfew, squaw vine, or tansy. Parsley, nettles, or blue cohosh reduce water retention.

Vaginitis

This is a vaginal irritation and inflammation with redness, odor, discharge, itching and painful sex. If trichomonas (a protozoa) is the cause, there may be a frothy, thin discharge, burning, itching and a rash; if Candida albicans (yeast, thrush, monilia) is the cause, the discharge is curdy and profuse, with odor, itching and inflammation. Leukorrhea is a watery, white vaginal discharge with the same causes as above, and hemophilus (nonspecific vaginitis) is the cause when there is a creamy white, yellowish or greyish discharge, possibly with some blood, and cramps, lower back pain, and swollen glands in the abdomen and inner thighs. Trichomonas can be stubborn to treat but will usually respond to holistic methods, and holistic methods almost always work for the other varieties. Flagyl, the antibiotic of choice for vaginitis, can cause birth defects, gene mutations and cancer. Any alternatives are more positive.

The use of antibiotics for cystitis or other infections is often the cause of Candida vaginitis, and adding more antibiotics to cure it only starts a vicious cycle, resulting in systemic Candida overrun and the triggering of multiple allergies. Other causes of vaginal infections include the contraceptive pill, cortisone or steroids, tight underwear, stress, pregnancy, diabetes, miscarriage or abortion, menstruation when the body's acid/alkaline balance is affected, postmenopausal hormone changes, immune deficiency, dry vagina during intercourse, or nutritional deficiency (B_6 and B complex). A diet high in sugar and white flour products encourages vaginitis. (See the section on Candida Albicans.) Since discovering some very simple remedies many years ago (vinegar and water douches), I have not needed to use doctors for vaginitis; the remedies work. Make sure that it is really a vaginal infection you are treating; if there is fever or lower abdominal pain, get a diagnosis. Also make sure that venereal disease is not involved. With these ruled out, the remedies below will do the trick, even for most women with trichomonas.

Herbs: A number of herbs are used as douches for vaginitis; choose among the following. For trichomonas, all vaginitis and cervicitis, use a douche of two teaspoons each of powdered myrrh and goldenseal and a half teaspoon of ginger (optional) to a pint of water. Echinacea or Echinacea and goldenseal are also positive. Boil, strain, cool, and use daily until healed; make a fresh batch each time. Take a goldenseal capsule by mouth daily, with vitamin C and yogurt, along with the douches. Three tablespoons of chickweed to a quart of boiled water is also for trichomonas, or pau d'arco, or oatstraw to drink, bathe, and douche with. For yeast infections use goldenseal and myrrh, St. John's wort, bayberry bark, comfrey, sage, yarrow, black walnut or oatstraw. Drink oatstraw tea daily for a month; use it as a douche only once a week, and lie down for half an hour after using it to saturate the tissues. For leucorrhea, use slippery elm as a douche or suppository (make it stiff with a little water), blue cohosh, lavender, white oak bark, red sage, pau d'arco, or blue flag. For nonspecific/hemophilus vaginitis use goldenseal or goldenseal with myrrh again, calendula as a douche, witchhazel, bayberry, or a combination of an ounce of uva ursi, and half an ounce each of poplar bark and marshmallow boiled for twenty minutes in a pint of water. Cool, strain, and dilute with two parts water before using as a douche.

Herbs to take internally while using the douches include blue cohosh, comfrey, or raspberry leaf, goldenseal and Echinacea together, pau d'arco, or oatstraw. For itching of the vulva dab on goldenseal with witchhazel liquid, chickweed ointment, or calendula lotion or ointment. If you don't know what type of vaginitis you have, use the goldenseal/ myrrh/Echinacea douche and take the capsules internally, or use oatstraw or pau d'arco. For chronic uterine proelems use St. John's wort. To restore the proper acid balance to the vagina, important in all forms of vaginitis, use a douche to a quart of white vinegar—this must steep for two weeks before using, so make it in advance and keep it handy.

—From *The Natural Remedy Book for Women*

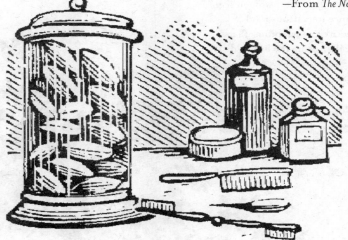

HERBS FOR MENOPAUSE
Susan M. Lark, Ph.D.

Herbs were humankind's first medicine and formed the basis of traditional healing practices for thousands of years. Their beneficial effects were discovered slowly through trial and error. By careful observation, early cultures learned to recognize the healing effects of medicinal plants for a variety of illnesses and learned to avoid the use of others because of their poisonous or harmful side effects. In modern times many research studies in the fields of botany, pharmacology, and medicine have allowed us to better understand the beneficial effects of many plant substances. Many interesting medical studies have shown that the traditional body of knowledge about herbs was correct in assigning healing properties to many plants....

Herbs can be a very useful part of your nutritional program to prevent or help balance a variety of symptoms related to menopause. They should be thought of as a form of extended nutrition, providing many nutrients that are necessary for good health in the menopause years. For example, dulse and kelp provide valuable iodine for optimal thyroid function, and red raspberry leaves are a good source of calcium and magnesium. Plants also contain natural hormones and a variety of substances that help to control bleeding, hot flashes, anxiety, insomnia, and other common menopause symptoms. In the following section I will give information on specific herbs that can help relieve menopause symptoms.

Herbs for Your Menopause Symptoms

Heavy irregular menstrual bleeding. Plants that contain flavonoids of the flavone or flavonal class (commonly called bioflavonoids) help to strengthen capillaries and prevent heavy, irregular menstrual bleeding (menorrhagia). This is a common bleeding pattern as women approach menopause. Flavonoids are found in a large variety of fruits and flowers and are responsible for their color. Excellent sources are citrus fruits, cherry, grape, and hawthorn berry. According to research studies, they have also been found in red clover and subterranean clover strains in Australia. Many medical studies of citrus bioflavonoids have demonstrated their usefulness in a variety of bleeding problems, besides those related to menopause, such as habitual spontaneous abortion and tuberculosis.

Hot flashes. Many plants are good sources of estrogen, the hormone that helps to control hot flashes. Genestine and dedzine, the isoflavones from soybeans, have weak estrogenic activity ($1/50,000$ the strength of estrogen). They are very effective in controlling such common menopause symptoms as hot flashes, anxiety, and irritability. Soy isoflavones in either powder or capsule form may be particularly useful for women who cannot take prescription hormones because of their strong side effects. Other plant sources of estrogen and progesterone used in traditional herbology include black cohosh, blue cohosh, unicorn root, false unicorn root, fennel, and licorice root. The hormonal activities of these plants have been researched in a number of studies. Black cohosh in

Continued ➤

particular has been found to help control hot flashes, mood swings, and vaginal dryness.

Plants may also form the basis for the production of medical hormones. Many common plants such as soy beans and yams contain a preformed steroidal nucleus. Estrogen and progesterone can be synthesized from plants in relatively few steps and have allowed six hormones to become available commercially at a reasonable cost.

Menopause anxiety, irritability, and insomnia. Women with menopause anxiety, irritability, and insomnia have a number of herbal remedies to choose from for relief of their symptoms. Herbs such as passionflower and valerian root have a significant calming and restful effect on the central nervous system. Passionflower has been found to elevate levels of the neurotransmitter serotonin. Serotonin is synthesized from tryptophan, an essential amino acid that has been found in numerous medical studies to initiate sleep and decrease awakening. Valerian root has been used extensively in traditional herbology as a sleep inducer. It is used widely in Europe as an effective treatment for insomnia. Research studies have confirmed both the sedative effect of valerian root and its effectiveness as a means to treat insomnia. For women with menopause insomnia, valerian root can be a real blessing. I have used it with patients for the past fourteen years and noted much symptom relief. Other effective herbal treatments include chamomile, hops, catnip, and peppermint teas. I have used all of them in my practice and many pleased patients have commented on their effectiveness.

Menopause fatigue and depression. For women with menopause fatigue and depression, herbs such as gota kola, ginger, and ginkgo biloba. Siberian ginseng (eleutherococcus), and licorice root may have a stimulatory effect, improving energy and vitality. Women who use these herbs may note an increased ability to handle stress, as well as improved physical and mental capabilities. Some of the salutary effects may be due to the high levels of the many essential vitamins and minerals contained in herbs. Siberian ginseng, ginger, and licorice root have been important traditional medicines in China and other countries for thousands of years. They have been reputed to increase longevity and decrease fatigue and weakness. These herbs have been used to boost immunity and to strengthen the cardiovascular system. In modern China, Japan, and other countries there has been much interest in the pharmacological effects of these traditional herbs. Scientific studies are corroborating the important medicinal effects of these plants. Oat straw has been found in research studies to relieve fatigue and weakness, particularly when there is an emotional component.

Menopause urinary tract symptoms. Many herbs appear to have an ability to soothe, relieve irritation, and reduce infection in the urinary tract, including goldenseal, uva ursi, blackberry root, and wintergreen. Research studies suggest that the plant coleus forskohlii also decreases urinary tract pain and discomfort. The urinary tract is a particularly vulnerable area in women during the menopause years and beyond because the lack of hormonal support causes the tissues to become more delicate and easily traumatized. Goldenseal contains berberine, an alkaloid with antibiotic activity, while uva ursi contains arbutin, a urinary diuretic and anti-infective agent. Coleus forskohlii contains forskolin, an anti-spasmodic which can relieve painful urination as well as menstrual cramps and intestinal colic.

Menopause and sexual frigidity. Herbs have also been used to treat problems of sexual frigidity and impotence. Many cultures hold certain plants in high esteem for their aphrodisiac properties. On closer inspection, some of these plants, like Spanish fly or nutmeg, have been found to be genitourinary irritants, rather than sexual stimulants. Traditional Indian medicine considers a number of plants such as saffron crocus and priya-darsa to have extraordinary aphrodisiac powers. Yohimbe, a plant aphrodisiac, is the base of several drugs currently prescribed to treat impotence.

Menopause Herbal Formulas

I have used herbs in my medical practice for years as a form of extended nutrition for menopause. They are an effective means of balancing the diet and optimizing the nutritional intake. There are three herbal formulas that I use to provide optimal nutritional support for women suffering from menopause-related complaints. Formula I can be used by women with general menopause complaints such as hot flashes and vaginal dryness due to hormonal deficiency. Formula II is very helpful for women with menopause-related fatigue, debility, and weakness. Formula III can be used by women with menopause-related anxiety, irritability, and insomnia. Formula I is the basic herbal formula for menopausal women. Formulas II and III should also be used if you have the symptoms for which are applicable.

Herbal Formula I can be put together by combining the herbs yourself. Formula I is also widely available in health food stores.

Herbal Formula I:	Black cohosh
	Fennel
	Anise
	Blessed thistle
Herbal Formula II:	Ginger
	Ginkgo biloba
	Siberian ginseng
	(eleutherococcus)
Herbal Formula III:	Valerian root
	Catnip
	Chamomile
	Hops

The herbs should be used in small amounts. You may find that specific herbs make you feel better than all of the herbs in one formula used in combination. Take herbs with your meals either in capsule form or in a tea. If you prefer to make a tea, simply empty the capsule into a cup of boiling water and let it steep for a few minutes. Do not drink more than one or two cups of the tea per day.

All foods have the potential for causing distress in some people, and herbs are no exception. They should be discontinued immediately if you notice nausea, vomiting, or diarrhea upon using. These are the most common symptoms of intolerance. The herbs in my formulas are all recommended as being safe for human consumption, but some women seem to have a specific intolerance for various foods, including herbs. If you notice any symptoms that make you uncomfortable after using the herbs, discontinue them immediately.

Herbs for Menopause and Female Health Problems

Symptoms	Herbal Treatments
Menorrhagia	Shepherd's purse
	Hawthorn berry
	Cherry
	Grape skin
	Bilberry
	Red clover
Menopause hot flashes, Vasomotor symptoms	Dong quai
	Black cohosh
	Blessed thistle
	Anise
	Fennel
	Sarsaparilla
	Red clover
	Aloe vera gel
Menopause insomnia and anxiety	Valerian root
	Passion flower
	Peppermint
	Catnip
	Chamomile
	Hops
Menopause fatigue, tiredness, and depression	Ginkgo biloba
	Ginger
	Gota kola
	Dandelion root
	Siberian ginseng
	Licorice root
Manopause bladder and lower urinary tract symptoms	Coleus forskohlii (pain)
	Goldenseal (infections)
	Uva ursi (infections)
	Blackberry root (infections)
	Wintergreen
Osteoporosis	Red raspberry leaf
	Comfrey
Hypothyroidism	Irish moss
	Kelp
	Dulse
	Sarsaparilla
Breast lumps and tenderness	Alfalfa
	Kelp
	Poke root poultices

Plants Used as Starting Materials for Commercial Hormone Synthesis

Plant Source	Performed Steroidal Nucleus
Soybean	Stigmasterol
Calabas bean	Stigmasterol
Yeast	Ergosterol
Cereal grains	B-Sitosterol
Yams	Diosgenin
Sisal	Hecogenin

—From *The Menopause Self-Help Book*

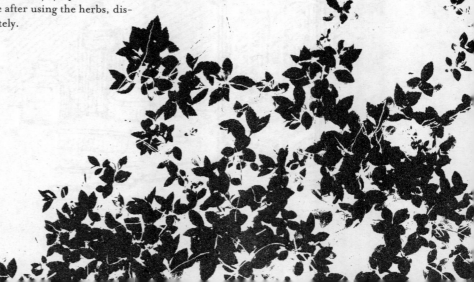

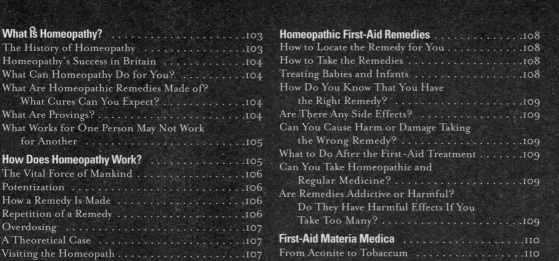

Homeo-pathy

WHAT IS HOMEOPATHY?

Ambika Wauters, R.S. Hom.

Homeopathy is a complete medicine that, when used intelligently, will heal many conditions. It can be used by anyone of any age to restore balance and well-being. It is a medicine that is both life-enhancing and revitalizing, bringing harmony to stressed bodies, frazzled nerves, and weary spirits. Homeopathy penetrates deeply into the essence of a person, relieving any emotional and mental imbalance, and correcting the effects this imbalance has on the body, mind, and spirit. It is a totally holistic medicine.

Although homeopathy has been practiced for over several hundred years and is the medicine of choice in many parts of Europe, it is just now beginning to be accepted in the United States as a reliable alternative to conventional medicine. The remedies can be administered easily at home with positive results. They are safe and can be used by the entire family at any stage of life. Babies can ingest remedies through a bottle or their mother's milk. They can be used by young people and old people. They can be used throughout pregnancy and are effective for labor, delivery, and postpartum care.

Homeopathy is practiced today as it was originally conceived nearly 250 years ago by Dr. Samuel Hahnemann in Leipzig, Germany. Nothing has changed in homeopathic philosophy since that time. Thus as a medicine, it is anchored in solid ethical principles that are taught in the international homeopathic community and enforced.

This is not to say that homeopathy is old-fashioned with rigid guidelines. Just the opposite—it has adapted to the modern industrial world which is far different from Hahnemann's own era. Because people today are psychologically more complex and physically more dysfunctional than they were 200 years ago, homeopathic research has had to become more aware of the mental and emotional causes of physical symptoms. This is where homeopathy differs fundamentally from conventional medicine.

Homeopathy has been practiced in Europe, India, and Latin America for over two hundred years. It was and is still the preferred medicine of the royal families of Europe. In Britain, the royal family takes homeopathic remedies and advocates their use. Homeopathy is currently obtainable on the National Health Service as a medicine of choice.

In America homeopathy thrived until the early 1930s, when the American Medical Association closed down the homeopathic medical schools and banned the practice of homeopathy in several states.

The History of Homeopathy

Homeopathy was developed in Germany in the early 1700s by Dr. Samuel Hahnemann, a physician who became disillusioned with the medical practices of his day—he was losing more patients than he was saving. He therefore gave up his practice and began to earn his living by translating medical reports. In the course of his work, he came upon an article written by a physician named Cullen who proposed the use of cinchona bark as a cure for malaria. Curious about what the bark would do to him—he didn't have malaria—he swallowed a gram of cinchona and immediately experienced all the symptoms of malaria. He then reasoned that if a substance could create symptoms in a healthy person, it could cure the same symptoms in a sick person. He called his practice of healing homeopathy.

The strongest opposition to Hahnemann's practice and theories came from the pharmaceutical companies who were successful in running him out of Germany. In order to continue practicing, he moved to France. There Hahnemann found other physicians who shared his beliefs, and together they continued to examine many substances and tested their effect on healthy people.

In the beginning they studied folk remedies that had been used for thousands of years and then expanded their studies when Hahnemann discovered

Continued ➡

that some substances, though toxic in their material form, were not toxic when they were diluted, and, as a matter of fact, were more effective in extreme dilution. He never hesitated to try these medicines on himself and he recorded their effects. These observations are known as provings—they form the basis for the homeopathic materia medica.

As an example of a toxic substance becoming a remedy, there is a fascinating story about a great homeopath, Constantine Herring. He traveled to South America with his wife in search of substances that could be used as remedies. He heard about the most poisonous snake known to man, the bushmaster. After obtaining a live specimen, he told his wife to record all his symptoms after he first diluted the snake's venom and then ingested the solution. After he did so, he fell into a stupor and was unconscious for three days. However, his wife did record his symptoms, and we now have one of the most widely used, most powerful remedies in the entire materia medica, which is used today to treat jealousy, grief, delirium, hallucination, menopausal symptoms, and high septic states such as diphtheria. It is known as *Lachesis*.

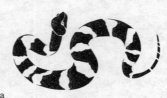

Hahnemann lived and worked during the time of the great plagues that ravaged Europe. Entire populations of towns and villages were wiped out while doctors and pharmacists stood by, helpless. Hahnemann and his colleagues were able to save thousands of lives by noting the symptoms common to each plague and administering the similimum remedy. Allopathic doctors were losing nine out of ten patients, while Hahnemann and his colleagues were saving nine out of ten. This work of treating epidemics homeopathically is not generally recognized, but probably should be, considering the ever virulent flus striking large numbers of people and with autoimmune deficiency diseases on the increase.

Hahnemann made one other observation crucial in homeopathy: he observed that people vary in their response to an illness according to their temperament. This is the reason there are few prescriptive remedies. What works for one person may not work for another, though their symptoms might be similar. Homeopaths are taught to look for what is peculiar to each case. This is where homeopathy differs fundamentally from conventional medicine.

Today Hahnemann's work is still the backbone of homeopathy and the basis upon which good homeopaths practice.

Three Principles of Homeopathy As Conceived by Hahnemann

1. A medicine which in large doses produces the symptoms of a disease will in smaller doses cure the disease.

2. Through the process of extreme dilution, the medicine's curative properties are enhanced and all the poisonous or undesirable side effects are lost.

3. Homeopathic medicines are prescribed individually by the study of the whole person, according to that person's temperament and individual responses.

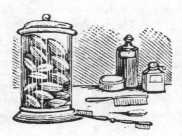

Homeopathy's Success in Britain

I was trained as a classical homeopath in Britain, where homeopathy is recognized as an important field of medicine. Today the largest growing body of alternative practitioners in Britain are homeopaths: their ranks have grown over 400 percent in the past ten years. Homeopathy is practiced in clinics run and operated by the National Health Service. Private medical insurance believes in homeopathic treatment and pays for it. Businesses investing in homeopathy for their staff have found it dramatically reduced the number of sick days. Nursing homes are investigating homeopathy for gentle, cost-efficient treatment of the elderly, and midwives are studying the ways it can relieve the trauma of childbirth. Homeopathy is also gaining credibility and acceptance by the conventional medical community in Britain who are seeking reliable alternatives to conventional drugs and their side effects.

It has been discovered that over one-third of the patients in the National Health Hospitals in Britain suffer from iatrogenic diseases, brought on by conventional medical treatment, specifically drugs. It is important to look into a form of medicine which addresses all conditions without concurrent drug toxicity. Conventional medicine could then be used for what it does best: save lives, treat the terminally ill, perform necessary surgery, and look after basic health needs. Finding a proper place for each of these medicines is worthy of consideration by both allopathic and homeopathic practitioners.

What Can Homeopathy Do For You?

In homeopathy we treat you, the individual, not the disease. We look at your physical, emotional, and mental symptoms to assess your case. We rely on the information we gather in interviews with you to help us prescribe a remedy that will address your condition and bring swift relief to your symptoms. We go over each area of your body and ask you to tell us how well you function. And if you can't express yourself, we ask those nearest you to tell us how you have been feeling and behaving. Oftentimes elderly people or very young children can't answer our questions and therefore we ask whoever takes care of them to describe their symptoms. We look for an underlying emotional cause of imbalance because we believe that your physical symptoms often mirror your emotional state.

We also look for family predisposition to conditions and diseases which may contribute to your case. We base our findings on simple facts, feelings, and experiences: how you feel and your emotional, mental, or physical response to your environment. These are all clues that will lead us to your remedy. We do not use machines to give us statistics, nor do we measure various systemic levels with tests.

What Are Homeopathic Remedies Made of? What Cures Can You Expect?

Homeopathy's cures are numerous and its supporters great in number. Case after case of clinical evidence attest to its effectiveness. There are many people who were diagnosed as hopeless and given up by the allopathic medical community, who now experience full lives.

Homeopathic remedies are made from minerals, animals, and plants. They are very effective in the treatment of pets, dairy cows, goats, and cattle.

Not only are vets using homeopathy on pets with excellent results, homeopaths are reportedly using it on wild animals who have been injured by environmental stress and pollution. Because there was evidence of an HIV-type disease decimating the dolphin population of the North Sea, several homeopaths set out in wetsuits to treat the dolphins with positive results. There is no placebo effect or psychological brainwashing possible when animals are treated with homeopathic remedies.

In order to diagnose animals, homeopaths rely on observation of their behavior. In order to diagnose people, homeopaths rely on interviews where clients report how they feel and how they respond to stress. Behavioral responses such as thirst, heat, cold, mobility, and lack of mobility must be observed. In those interviews we see what the Vital Force is doing and prescribe on that basis. We are looking for the whole range of symptoms that have upset the energetic economy so that we will understand how the remedy will work on subtle levels of the mind and emotions.

Homeopathy treats far more conditions than the medical community because it looks at the underlying emotional etiology. For example, there are no allopathic cures for bedwetting, fear, anxiety, or grief, whereas in homeopathy it is part of our practice to consider all aspects of human behavior. We also treat such conditions as asthma, heart disease, arthritis, cancer, and autoimmune deficiency diseases with success.

What Are Provings?

We gather a picture of the effect of our remedies on healthy people and register these symptoms in our homeopathic *material medica*. Each new symptom portrayed from a proving is added to our annals. This provides us with information about how a particular substance works. Our annals are based on over 250 years of experiments organized by categories. For instance, in a proving we note all the symptoms of the mind, head, face, throat, chest, respiration, heart, stomach, urination, bowels, sexual function, male and female differences, fevers, circulation, etc. This is the way a remedy portrait is developed. We want to know how a remedy works in its totality and what dimensions of the energetic economy it affects.

New provings are done annually on both old and new substances and, though our philosophy never changes, our *material medica* is constantly expanding to meet the challenge of modern times.

All well-trained homeopaths are taught to read these provings. We base our evidence on the work of generations of practitioners who went before us who were meticulous in recording their clinical and laboratory findings that describe how a substance worked. Some of our remedies are presently being made from an original source over a hundred years old. What was used in homeopathy 250 years ago is still used to this day. We value all substances found in nature, and we examine them carefully to see how they work on the entire energetic economy, whether it is the physical, emotional, or mental realm.

It becomes very important to stay current with the remedies that are needed to shift the downward spiral of illness found in the population today. We are witness to more and more autoimmune deficiency diseases, attesting to some weakening in the vital force in a significant number of people. We also see a weakening in the human organism,

Continued ➡

apparent in people's increasing allergic reactions to external stimulation such as food additives, petrochemical pollution, and sexually transmitted diseases. How this general weakening will affect future generations in terms of health no one knows. Homeopaths feel that if we were to begin treatment today, it would take four generations before we would see a rise in the general health. We feel that it is our job to fortify the immune systems of our patients to resist any further decline.

Homeopathy looks deeply within the nature of the human psyche to rebalance the conditions that destroy and immobilize the will, that part of man/woman that helps us evolve and develop, that is required for getting on with our lives. Without a viable will, there is little that can be done to get a person's life back on track. Homeopaths treat people so that they can realistically assess their lives, and their will can be reengaged through conscious, good choices. This is healing that nurtures and fosters growth at all levels.

Unfortunately, too few people understand the profound healing that homeopathic medicine can bring. It works on so many levels of our energy system that, if used correctly, it can root out fears, phobias, and neuroses, and deal with physical problems as well. By finding the right homeopathic remedy, change becomes part of the natural evolutionary cycle of a person's life, and they are better able to develop on all levels.

In effect, homeopathic healing does not separate the deeper realms from the physical reality in which healing operates. We can see that a physical condition mirrors a state of mind, that when a person is suffering physically they may be undergoing a similar internal emotional process. This is reflected by the way they respond to a situation or a condition, even when those events happened a long time ago. What happens internally is also happening externally. The body acts as a reflection of our internal state and our emotions are reflected in our body.

Classical homeopathy believes in the use of one remedy at a time. We always wait to see how the remedy affects you on all levels before considering changing a remedy or increasing the potency. Conversely, if a remedy is working we do not change it. We are taught to be patient and watch for change on all levels.

A remedy may have a stronger effect on a mental level than on a physical level and vice versa. We need to see which realm is affected as well as how the remedy is rebalancing your symptoms. This takes time and observation.

What Works for One Person May Not Work for Another

Homeopaths are taught to look for what is peculiar to each case. This is what differentiates one remedy portrait from another and one person from another. If you question ten people about their headache symptoms, you will hear ten different responses. One person will feel a sharp pain in their left eye. Another person will feel a sharp pain in the back of their neck, while a third person will feel a sharp pain on the top of their head and have a stomachache. In homeopathy each of these headache symptoms would be treated with a different remedy. This approach has been proven the most positive and refined type of treatment. It has also made it difficult to be prescriptive.

Think of the different ways individuals react emotionally to a situation. For instance, in a tragedy, one person may be hysterical and become demanding and overwrought. Another person may feel incredibly sad and weep uncontrollably, want-

ing consolation and fearful of being alone. Still another may become silent and morose, and not wish to be with other people. Each person will react differently to the same situation. Homeopathy has remedies that address each one of these different conditions, even though each one is a response to the same external stimuli.

What is required in treatment is the ability to differentiate one emotional state from another, and the way one person responds to stimuli compared to another. How we determine our choice of remedies is based on observation, and the information we gather about these particular symptoms.

There are exceptions to this rule. Homeopathy does treat specific conditions when they are common to millions of people. For instance, there are only a handful of remedies for nosebleed. These work for most people. The same is true for cold symptoms and influenza.

—From *Homeopathic Medicine Chest*

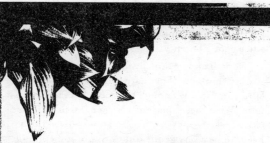

HOW DOES HOMEOPATHY WORK?

Ambika Wauters, R.S. Hom.

This medicine works differently from conventional medicine. Its philosophy that less is more may be confusing to you. Let's look at how homeopathy works.

First, homeopathy requires you to be aware of your symptoms and the aspects of your condition that are specific to you. Let us assume you have a headache that plagues you regularly. A homeopath would want to know how regularly you experience this headache. Is it periodic in its occurrence?

Whatever is unique to your condition needs to be noted. For instance, you may dislike going out in bright light when you have a headache, or you may desire cold drinks, or you may lose your appetite when you are feeling poorly. Whatever you can note that will distinguish your symptoms is important for finding the remedy that will help you.

If you take an aspirin for your headache, be assured your headache will return when a similar stress provokes it again. In homeopathy when the underlying cause is addressed, in many cases the susceptibility to the problem is completely eliminated. This is one reason it is so effective; it goes to the core of things to reestablish balance and harmony.

But before you can be given a remedy that will eliminate your headache and stop it from reoccurring, it is essential to dissect its components and analyze the manner in which it operates. Every aspect of how you feel when this headache or any other symptom occurs needs to be looked at. When this information is collated, a remedy is carefully chosen that contains the totality of your symptoms in its remedy portrait. It is then prescribed for you.

Remember, arriving at the right remedy is only as good as the information you give the homeopath. To simply say you have a headache means nothing to a homeopath. Because it is such an individual medicine, it demands that therapeutic guidelines be followed carefully for positive results. A homeopath needs to ask, What are the qualities of your condi-

tion? Where does it hurt? Is the pain in the front, side, back of your body? How would you describe the pain? Is it dull, aching, sharp, throbbing, constricting? What else is going on physically, emotionally, and mentally? Are you feeling irritable, sad, anxious, fearful? Are you thirsty or not thirsty at all? Can you think clearly, do you want fresh air, or do you want to lie down? These are the things that help determine which remedy suits your condition.

It is important to clarify symptoms when searching for a remedy. There are simple keynote symptoms that help differentiate one remedy from another. For instance, we may want to know what provoked the headache, and how you react when you have a headache. Besides the symptoms above, do you feel better or worse for eating? Do you crave milk, sweets, or some other food? Are you constipated when you have a headache? Does your stomach ache or do your legs feel weak? What makes you feel better or worse?

These concomitant symptoms will help you get the right remedy. They may seem unimportant to you, but they can make a difference to your well-being. It is important to pay attention to your temperament. Are you irritable, angry, sad, frustrated, depressed? All these symptoms are signs that will lead you to your remedy. Often a remedy will have levels of irritability, anxiety, fear, sadness, or apathy which go along with its physical symptoms. They are all noted in the *materia medica*.

When you describe your symptoms ask yourself how you feel emotionally. It will assist you in arriving at a remedy that works for you. We are too accustomed to thinking of medicine as a cure for our physicality; we do not see the accompanying emotional picture.

A recent case in point is of a woman who was moving from her home. She was surrounded by clutter and felt angry that her son was not helping her. The weather was very hot and she, a natural redhead, was very flushed. She had a headache, was not thirsty, but the top of her head was throbbing. She was given a *Belladonna* 6x and within a few minutes her color returned to normal, the headache had disappeared, and she realized how angry she was at her son for leaving her with a mess. This was quick healing. It not only brought relief, it brought self-awareness.

Whatever state you are in, the remedy that works for you will match your internal state. It will address every level of your unbalance. It not only addresses a physical symptom and leaves you in an internal state of irritability and agitation. It works at the core of your being and rebalances you at every level. It helps you to move forward in your life while eliminating the underlying factors that create the imbalance in the first place.

In homeopathy there are no biochemical statistics that will prove *how* the similimum remedy stimulates your Vital Force to respond. We do know from many trials that the remedies work when we look at the deeper mental and emotional factors that go along with the physical symptoms. We don't know how they work.

If you went to a homeopath soon after a relationship broke up, complaining of a chronic sore throat and headache, you would be asked about your grief, how you handle the expression of your feelings, and what you feel is still unresolved in that relationship. Your response would help the homeopath determine what remedy would be best suited to you right now.

You may come back to see the homeopath with the same exact sore throat a year later. But you are different now from the way you were when you saw her before. You have recovered from your grief and

Continued →

are now suffering from feelings of suppressed anger with your boss for not listening to your good ideas. It is obvious that one of your areas of susceptibility is your throat and issues of communication, but your emotional etiology is completely different this time. So the remedy that would help you with your throat symptoms and your feelings of loss would be different the second time. On your original visit your condition was caused by unexpressed grief; the second condition was caused by unexpressed anger. Though the same area is affected, the emotions are different and so are the remedies.

Homeopaths are now better able to follow scientific guidelines for how change occurs in the physical economy, and they are performing double-blind studies on the ways in which the remedies work. Homeopathy takes time to bring about healing, and it is particularly slow for long-term chronic conditions. For these we give a remedy, wait, and watch to see how you respond. However, it works miraculously for first-aid problems and acute conditions.

We measure only clinical results and evident symptom alleviation. Remedies are never repeated when the condition has cleared up. The homeopathic definition of health is not limited to the absence of disease or the relief of symptoms. Emotional stability, mental clarity, and well-functioning lives are also a part of the spectrum of health. We measure results by looking at quality of life in every case. We don't say you are healed because your ulcer is healed. We suggest that you may wish to treat other areas of susceptibility that limit your effectiveness in living the life you say you want. We suggest you explore some of the other dimensions in your life where you are not happy or fulfilled, and then treat those homeopathically. We strive for complete balance and wholeness in our patients. This is what homeopathy can offer to people. It is wonderful for people who are going through times of change and transformation.

Few people, outside of homeopaths and patients, know how deep homeopathy can go and how it can restore health and vitality. Our definition of health is broad. It includes supporting your capacity to live harmoniously. This medicine helps people adapt to change, and to undergo internal transformation that aligns them with their higher purpose in life.

The Vital Force of Mankind

Homeopathy addresses the life principle in each person. The Vital Force is that aspect of all things which is alive and vital and acts as the internal guiding principle to regulate every bodily function. It is also known as the immune system. It controls your heartbeat, reduces a fever when you are ill, and lets you know you are hungry, thirsty, irritable, sad, or happy. This part of you is shared with all things living. It does not exist in us when we die. It is that part of us that responds to life; it becomes irritated, it grieves, suffers, laughs, delights, loves, and is adaptable to change. This is the part that when it is chilled produces a fever to compensate. When it is unhappy, it creates symptoms of stress and irritability. It controls all vital functions at every level of existence and acts in all systems of the body to produce symptoms we can see and treat. In homeopathy we believe that all symptoms are there to give us a picture of the levels of health or dysfunction in a person. Symptoms are signs of how the Vital Force is functioning.

Homeopaths are taught to read, see, and hear the signs the Vital Force. We know that symptoms can be addressed with a remedy which contains similar symptoms in its portrait as your Vital Force is displaying. In response to a remedy the Vital Force once

again assumes a level of harmony and well-being.

The stronger the individual's Vital Force, the stronger their symptoms. Weak symptoms indicate a compromised Vital Force. Therefore, a healthy organism will have very strong symptoms when it is out of balance. You see this in healthy children who have high fevers and strong reactions to infection. Paradoxically, you have to be healthy to be very ill. This is a difficult concept to accept if you are not familiar with homeopathic thinking.

People with weak immunities don't have enough vitality to become ill. When a person gets a cold after taking a remedy, it is considered a sign of health, rather than weakness. It shows that the Vital Force has been stimulated and detoxification is beginning. It also means mental symptoms may move to the physical level to be expressed.

The strength and vitality of the Vital Force is apparent in new life, and when there is an imbalance it is instantly apparent. Healthy babies and young children become ill quickly. Their symptoms must also be treated promptly with a remedy that contains a similar degree of vitality in its portrait. Delicate constitutions require delicate remedies and a gentle potency.

Very ill and terminally ill patients do not have strong symptoms. They have a diminished Vital Force, not strong enough to produce vibrant symptoms. What they experience is a general malaise or lack of reactive powers. The treatment given them needs to be a very gentle dilution, not something that is going to upset their delicately balanced system. Homeopathic remedies are chosen for their similimum qualities and for the reactive force of the potency used.

Potentization

Potentization refers to the level a homeopathic remedy is diluted. Each state of dilution is called a *potency*. The higher the potency, the stronger the remedy, and the deeper its realm of action. The higher the potency, the more the remedy works at mental and emotional levels and the longer its effect is felt. Some remedies can last up to a year with one single dose.

What this means in terms of treatment is that if you have a headache you would take a dose of a 6x (or 6 dilution) of the remedy selected to match your symptoms. You may need to repeat this rem-

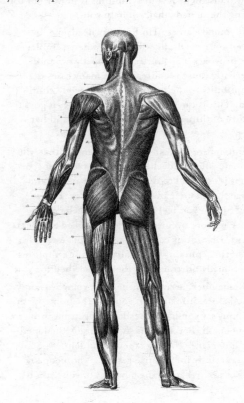

edy several times during the day. When the headache is alleviated, you stop taking the remedy. If, however, you were attempting to stop your susceptibility to headaches altogether, as in the case of chronically occurring headaches or migraine, you would take the similimum remedy in a high potency of perhaps a 200c (200 dilutions), and you would take it only once and not repeat it. In attempting to rebalance the body, this remedy could be effective for several months. It is given only one time, and the dynamic effects go on for weeks and weeks.

Potency is generally done is incremental shifts of 3, 6, 12, 30, 200, 1000, 10,000, 50,000, and 100,000. The "x" refers to dilution in decimals. This means that the substance is diluted in ten drops of water and alcohol. A "c" dilution refers to a dilution in one hundred drops of water and alcohol. They are similar in their effect with the "c" being slightly stronger in higher potency. Remedies are often potentized in "x" dilutions under 12 potencies. After that they are potentized in "c" dilutions.

The rule of thumb is that when you take a remedy of low potency of 6x and under, you treat quickly and easily. The realm of action is generally physical and does not have a deep or long-term effect on the emotions or mental attitudes.

For first-aid treatment the remedies are recommended at 6x, and occasionally 30c for serious conditions. These can be purchased at health food stores and from homeopathic pharmacies.

For higher dilution it is recommended that you see a homeopath for treatment. Once you get into higher potencies you need a well-trained homeopath because expertise is important at this level. Self-treatment with high potencies is not encouraged.

How a Remedy Is Made

A remedy is made in the following manner. A substance is taken from nature and either boiled or triturated (crushed) to produce a supply which can be made into a tincture. This is known as the *mother tincture* and is symbolized in homeopathy with this symbol (0). This means that the substance is in its most basic state before dilution.

If you were to take *Hawthorn*; for instance, which is used in the treatment of heart conditions, you would begin to make the remedy by boiling up the leaves, flowers, and bark taken from a Hawthorn tree at the time the flower was in optimal bloom in early spring. This is when the Vital Force of this plant is at its strongest, when it contains more energy than at any other time. Eventually with enough boiling you would produce a heavily concentrated serum. This serum is used in herbalism just as it is to make herbal tinctures. In homeopathic remedies the process begins by making the first dilution. This is done by taking one single drop of the serum and adding it to a mixture of ten drops of water and alcohol. You now have what is known in homeopathy as the first dilution (1x). Then if you take one drop of this mixture and add it to another ten drops of water and alcohol, you have the second dilution. This process continues of taking one drop of solution and placing it in a solution of water and alcohol until you have the number of dilutions required.

Repetition of a Remedy

Normally, higher potencies are not repeated, while low potencies of 6x are repeated often. This is because the higher the potency the more dynamic the medicine and the more powerful its realm of influence.

Continued ➡

A general rule of thumb is that if a low potency remedy is repeated three times in a short period of time and has not altered the symptoms for which it was intended, it is not the similimum and you need to choose another remedy. This applies to first aid and acute cases. Chronic treatment takes much longer to assess. It is believed that if you have the similimum remedy the potency is not as important as the remedy itself. Selecting a remedy carefully will alleviate your symptoms.

Lower potencies are very effective and quick to address symptoms. It is not normal for a patient to need more than a couple of doses of a remedy to have their first-aid symptoms alleviated.

For instance, if you had a nosebleed and you saw in the first-aid kit that *Ferrum Phos.* was the suitable remedy, you would take one dose of a 6x and wait five minutes. If the bleeding had slowed down but was not completely gone you would take one more dose. If this completely stopped the bleeding you would not take any more of the remedy. If you were to continue to do so you might create the condition you were trying to stop, in this case a nosebleed.

Remedies are taken only while the symptoms last. You do not take a remedy if there is not a symptom. This is important!

If you feel you want a higher potency for a remedy, remember that it is more important to get the similimum remedy than to worry about the potency. A low potency of a remedy (this is usually considered to be 3x, 6x, 12c) can be extremely effective, even if it is necessary to repeat over a period of time.

A middle level potency (a 30c, for instance) can be given once, even twice a day, for a short duration of up to three days and left to act. This level of potency can treat chronic symptoms very effectively, and is good for mild, chronic conditions such as sinusitis, constipation, or symptoms that are irritating but not undermining to your health.

Overdosing

Be careful. Don't overdose on a remedy. It is common in our culture to think that more is better. In homeopathy the rule is that less is more. Less can transform your energy and health to a very high degree. You do not need to pour a lot of medicine into your body for it to work. What you have to do is get the right remedy and let it stimulate your Vital Force back into balance.

When you do have the right remedy, proceed cautiously and wait to see how it affects you. If you have a headache, for instance, and you decide that the portrait of *Bryonia* suits your symptoms, you would take one 6x (not two as are prescribed by the commercial pharmaceutical companies who are trying to sell more bottles of their product) and wait for half an hour to see if your headache went away. If it did you would not need to repeat the remedy. What you are putting into your body is a frequency of vibration. If you take one small pill or a bathtub full of pills you are still only receiving that one frequency of vibration.

If your headache did not go away, but was only partially relieved, you would take a second pill and let it work. If after half an hour, you had no symptoms at all, you could take a third pill. It is not advisable to take more than five doses of a remedy in a day. If you feel that you need to do this, you most likely do not have the right remedy.

If you put a lot of different remedies into your body and none of them worked, you should give some thought to seeing a homeopath to discuss your case. A professionally trained and qualified practitioner is better able to assess your case. Moreover, they have a variety of remedies at their disposal. Also, the practitioner may be better able to access your case in terms of familial predisposition, stress-related factors, and past medical history. They are trained to evaluate your case in the light of many contributory causes, which you may not be able to see.

A Theoretical Case

Let's look at a theoretical case so that you can see how treatment works. Let's use the case of the grief-stricken patient we discussed early on in this chapter. He was upset over the loss of a relationship. He is shocked and does not cry or respond to this situation, but swallows his grief, feeling it is far too painful to feel. His temperament does not allow him to express feelings openly and he can grieve only in private. Nevertheless, he is hurt. His grief congests his energy because he holds on to his grief. After a period of time he develops symptoms which are not normal for him. He eats too many sweets that stick in his throat and he has trouble swallowing. He gets a headache that feels like a nail is being driven into his head, and he feels irritable, moody, and incommunicative. If he doesn't realize these are not normal, they will become more acute until he's forced to pay attention. This is how the Vital Force is signaling him that he is not in harmony with his deep self. It is creating a portrait of grief for him to see in the hope that healing can happen. A homeopath notes these sensations and symptoms, and matches them against the mental, emotional, and physical symptoms displayed in various remedies in the *materia medica*. In homeopathy we define disease as separation from the self. When this happens we create symptoms that tell astute observers trained to observe symptoms that something is not right. These symptoms of grief linger and somaticize in the body as pain or dysfunction and they do not improve, even with aspirin or drugs. This is more than a physical case, though many of the symptoms are on the physical plane. The person then decides to visit a homeopath. Let's look at how the procedure unfolds, and how a remedy is found to help this person feel better.

Visiting the Homeopath

After a few weeks of continuing symptoms, he calls to make an appointment. The homeopath sends a family history form to be returned before the consultation. On the first visit the homeopath has scheduled an hour and a half for the consultation which involves answering questions and talking about oneself. The homeopath wants to know all about this person, how he feels about things, his emotional response to situations, what he likes, what he dislikes, what he fears, what he loves.

Questions are asked about his general health in all the systems of the body, including sleep patterns, and other cycles such as menstruation. Questions are asked about appetite and what he likes and dislikes in food and drink. The way in which he responds is observed. It is noted if he is anxious, aggressive, closed, or open. When the consultation is completed, the homeopath may tell the person that a remedy will be sent to him with clear instructions. He will be asked to make note of how he feels after taking the remedy, and to call the homeopath with questions.

In this hypothetical case, after taking the remedy the headache completely disappears within a few days and cycles start to readjust; sleep and dreams are deeper. The craving for sweets disappears as does the lump in the throat. At some point the emotions may be engaged and the grief appropriately expressed in tears. Within a short time he feels like his old self. This treatment reflects the holistic nature of the medicine and the way in which a person is treated for his mind/body/spirit.

Can Homeopathy Work for You?

The degree of healing this medicine can provide you throughout your life is well worth investigating. You may find it worthwhile to get a consultation and find out if your condition can be treated and if you can achieve higher levels of health and vitality by taking homeopathy.

It is important to ask questions if there is something you don't understand about your treatment. Ask your homeopath about what is involved in your particular case. The more responsibility you are willing to take for your health, the better your treatment will be for you. It is important to get as much information as possible. Be sure that you fully understand the procedure and the length of time your condition needs for healing. Ask questions, keep track of how you feel, and note the changes in your body, mind, and spirit. Read books, ask questions, and take responsibility for what you want to see happen to your general well-being.

What Can and Cannot Be Treated Homeopathically?

Of course, homeopathy works best on people who are receptive to it. It can, however, be used on the elderly, infants, and animals who may have no say in their treatment. It works best in someone who is not taking conventional or herbal medicine. Each form of medicine has its unique realm of action. The only way a homeopath can observe your reaction to a remedy is to have you as drug free as possible. So it is suggested you do not mix treatments with other alternative or allopathic medicine, unless it is essential for your health.

If you are presently taking a medicine that suppresses symptoms and take a homeopathic remedy, you create confusion and conflict in your body. If you are taking cortisone or antibiotics, for instance, these powerful drugs will create a picture that may make it difficult to know what symptoms are true to your constitution and which symptoms are created by the drugs. Homeopathy can work when people are heavily medicated, though it is not ideal. Aggravation may arise and create discomfort for the patient and confusion for the practitioner. Even the birth control pill, highly suppressive of the life force, can make deep constitutional treatment slower and less effective.

Homeopathy is generally slow but effective in constitutional and chronic cases. First-aid treatment is very responsive, and because the potency is kept very low the chance of aggravating the body is minimal.

If you wish to treat a specific condition it is best to understand that homeopathic treatment is addressed to the whole person. It does not treat a disease because that is a label. It treats the totality of symptoms that create your distress and imbalance. A condition has other components that are part of an overall picture of imbalance such as feelings and thoughts.

If you have doubts about the effectiveness of homeopathy, please consult a homeopath in your area. He or she can suggest a consultation where you can talk over your case and inquire as to whether homeopathy would be an effective treatment.

Continued ➡

In terminal diseases homeopathy is a wonderful gift. As it promotes quality of life, it helps relieve symptoms that can be painful and uncomfortable. It can allow a person to end their time with dignity, minimal discomfort, and clarity of mind. Many people fear death and some of the remedies used to treat the terminally ill will help make the experience less fearful. It can ease the distress of those who are nursing the ill and dying as well.

Any time a person is in extreme conditions that stretch their emotions and nerves, homeopathy can ease his/her symptoms. It is excellent for major life changes, in childbirth, for teething infants, toddlers, youth, adults, and the elderly. It can treat asthma, eczema, and the variety of childhood diseases that make parenting a full-time job. It can help adolescents deal with this major life change, and help regulate growth, relieve acne, and other changes that accompany adolescence. It is excellent for young adults to boost job confidence and increase the possibility of success.

Homeopathy is the best ticket for aging I know. It can help regulate menopause so that it becomes a time when new options and possibilities can manifest. It can also treat bone density, ligament weakness, joint stiffness, and calcium depletion without putting dangerous drugs into the body. In fact, it is so effective in menopause that hot flashes and night sweats disappear. In short, it has been used to aid aging so that the wisdom of elders can be preserved along with a strong and viable physical body to support the spirit.

In extreme cases of mental disease where medication is necessary, homeopathy has been used to reduce episodes of violence, hysteria, and acting out. Because it addresses the mental and emotional aspects of the personality, it brings order promptly to anyone who is distressed.

Homeopathy has been used in the treatment of autistic and Asperger's disease where cognitive disorders inhibit socialization. And it has been used in mental hospitals to reduce violent outbursts without having to medicate patients heavily.

It is less effective when a person is on medications that suppress vital function, although in drug dependency of any kind this medicine works to stimulate the Vital Force again.

Homeopathy is a complete medicine. It is designed to treat the individual and not the disease. It is effective because it triggers the natural vitality of the person to respond holistically, bringing about balance and harmony over a period of time on all levels. In the case of first aid this readjustment can happen quickly. In deeper constitutional treatment the rebalancing can take a period of time.

—From *Homeopathic Medicine Chest*

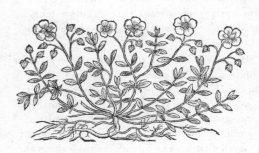

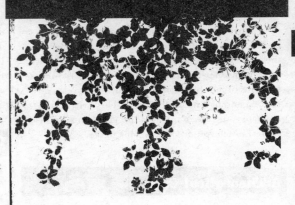

HOMEOPATHIC FIRST-AID REMEDIES

Ambika Wauters, R. S. Hom.

How to Locate the Remedy for You

You must choose the remedy which most closely matches your symptoms. Notice as many characteristics of your condition as possible and match them with the symptoms noted in the remedy. Note the location and the site affected to see if they match the location in the remedy picture. Pay attention to what makes you feel better: lying in a certain position, or if you are better or worse from such things as pressure, touch, bending, moving your head or back, in fresh air, being tightly clothed.

Other symptoms, such as your emotional state, help you to find the similimum remedy. Self-observation is crucial in treatment. It isn't enough to say you have a pain here or there. How do you feel? Are you irritable, sad, angry; do you despair of recovery, anticipate an event, or are you frightened? These emotional keynotes make a difference in determining your remedy. They go along with the specific physical questions: Where is it? What makes it feel better or worse? Which side is it on, etc.

So, in locating your first-aid remedy, pay attention to yourself or the person you are treating. Homeopathic remedies have no side effects. If you do not choose the right remedy, you will not experience any change in your symptoms. If you fail to note what goes on with your case you may fail to achieve the healing you seek. The remedy needs to be carefully chosen in order to be effective. Homeopathic first aid is gentle and very effective when you get the right remedy and you can be assured it will work for you. The remedies in this book are recommended for first aid and injuries only. They are not recommended for deeper chronic or constitutional care. When dealing with acute first-aid conditions, the remedies need to be precisely matched to the patient's symptoms. Read the symptoms over carefully and determine which remedy suits your condition.

1. Please note the *location*, which is the exact position of the symptoms.

2. Pay attention to the *sensations*, which are the feelings you experience, such as heat, cold, dizziness, pain. Note what type of pain it is, such as sharp, throbbing, aching, dull.

3. Please be aware of the *modalities*, which are whatever makes the symptoms feel better or worse.

4. If it is possible to be aware of the *cause* of the symptoms this may be very helpful in finding the remedy you need. You emotional state could be the result of a stressful or unhappy situation.

How to Take the Remedies

There are several ways to take a remedy. The easiest way is in pill form. Take one pill, place it under your tongue, and let it dissolve. Many bottles from homeopathic pharmacies require you to take two or more pills. There is no need to waste your supply of remedies when one pill does the trick.

As the remedy dissolves under your tongue, avoid water or food for ten minutes before and after you take the remedy. If you need to repeat the remedy, keep it out of the sunlight or away from strongly scented things like perfume or tobacco while you wait to repeat it. These will weaken the strength of the remedy and its effect. It is suggested that remedies be kept in cool, dark places while they are not in use. They should also be kept away from strongly scented things like camphor, lavender, eucalyptus, perfume, essential oils, detergent, or tobacco.

Another way of taking a remedy is with powder sachets. They are placed directly on the tongue. This is the way they are sold in homeopathic pharmacies in Europe, specifically in Belgium and France. You may come across a pharmacy where they are prepared in this way. Drops are sometimes used but often require that the bottle be shaken several times before each treatment. If you have a liquid remedy it can also be sniffed. This has proved effective for many people who are very responsive to remedies.

Treating Babies and Infants

For babies or small children you can do the following: if you are treating a nursing baby, have the mother take the pill and pass the remedy to the child through her milk. It is a direct way of treating and there is no time lapse once the mother has ingested the pill. For a bottle-fed baby, let the remedy dissolve in the bottle of milk, water, or juice. It is important to remember that it is not a question of quantity, it is the contact with the remedy that is important. Give the baby the amount of fluid it cares to drink. It is not a matter of how much fluid is ingested. What is important is that the fluid make contact with the baby's mouth.

In an emergency, place the remedy under the upper lip of the child and hold the lip down for at least ten seconds. Homeopathic remedies can work promptly to get into the bloodstream. The medication will be absorbed from the coated pill. The child does not need to ingest the pill, only to have contact with it for ten seconds. Remember, do not eat or drink anything for at least ten minutes prior to or after the remedy. The remedy must get into the blood without any interference as quickly as possible.

If the remedy is working and needs to be repeated, you can take it again within two minutes for an emergency, but no more than three doses more. If it is not an emergency, repeat after twenty minutes to half an hour for up to three doses. When the remedy begins to work and be effective, spread out the doses until the symptoms disappear. Once they are gone, stop giving the remedy altogether. It is meant to be used only while the symptom lasts.

Continued ➡

How Do You Know That You Have the Right Remedy?

You know that you have given the correct remedy because symptoms begin to disappear and you feel better. It is a very pragmatic form of medicine. If it is not working, you do not have the right remedy.

Check again to make sure that the symptoms match the picture of the remedy listed in the *material medica* (see page 110). Check again on the following: Are you thirsty? Do you feel better lying down or sitting up? Do you crave warmth or do you crave cold fresh air? These are the points that can make the difference in selecting the right remedy for the case. The wrong remedy has no effect. The right remedy alleviates the symptoms you are treating quickly and efficiently.

Are There Any Side Effects?

There are no side effects in homeopathy. In first aid you can expect instant results, such as an end to a hemorrhage or a headache. There are no half measures with homeopathy; either you have the similimum and it works or you have not chosen the appropriate remedy.

Chemical drugs have so-called side effects. These destabilize the body and cause the kidneys, liver, and stomach to process heavy acid that harms the delicate tissues and organs of the body. In homeopathy you can experience aggravation when taking a constitutional remedy. For instance, in order for the body to detoxify from congestion you may develop a rash, have a bout of loose bowels, or experience a headache briefly while the body readjusts itself to regain balance. This can be experienced as mild discomfort. It is not a side effect and it is not damaging in any way. It is the result of the imbalance that already exists.

Can You Cause Harm or Damage Taking the Wrong Remedy?

No. The wrong remedy is released through the urine and leaves no trace of any kind. There are stories of children getting into first-aid kits and taking a variety of remedies with absolutely no side effects. When the remedy is not the similimum, it does not act. It is not a chemical or herbal potion. It is an energetic substance that needs to match the portrait of your specific symptoms in order to restore balance.

Remember, the substance that is made into a remedy has a picture of symptoms that should match your symptoms. When you take a remedy it relieves those symptoms. It does nothing else to you.

What to Do After the First-Aid Treatment

If you feel that this form of medicine works for you, and you want to know if it can do more to help you in a general way, visit a homeopath. You can also take courses in first aid, take home study programs, and read books that will help you understand the nature of homeopathy and how it can help, balance, and bring relief to you and your family.

Can You Take Homeopathic and Regular Medicine?

Homeopathy is a complete medicine in itself. It is life enhancing and does not suppress symptoms as conventional medicine does. Taking the two together can cause disruption in your general health and is not encouraged.

In conventional medicine, symptoms are suppressed—they are pushed deeper into the body. For instance, in conventional medicine when you have a skin problem such as eczema, cortisone is given for relief of the itching and redness. Cortisone pushes the symptoms deeper into the body. The next thing you know, you experience joint aches and pains where the toxins, once on the surface of the body, are now deeper in the body. If more medicine is administered for this, systemic symptoms appear indicating weakened and debilitated organs. Eventually, after prolonged use of allopathic drugs, weakness forms in the tissues of the heart and liver. The system is so overdosed with drugs that it weakens and breaks down completely. The drugs have compromised the general immunity of the patient.

Homeopathy, because it is an energetic medicine, strives to build the energetic economy and revitalize the body. This means that it strengthens the immune system and rebalances the Vital Force. It does this by pushing symptoms up to the surface. It frees the deep organs of toxins, so that they may function properly. We want symptoms to move from the deep core out to the surface.

When you take a deep-acting constitutional homeopathic remedy it will bring symptoms out to the surface of the body. We anticipate rashes and discharges, which strengthen the core of a person and aid in the detoxification of deep tissue. We find that people generally feel better when this happens, even when they may experience external symptoms. We believe that toxins and impurities are better out of the body than congesting and weakening the system internally. So we never suppress rashes; we soothe them with homeopathic ointments, and work to detoxify the deeper organs. We want toxins out onto the surface of the body, away from the core, where they can cause severe disruption of health.

We do not encourage the mixture of allopathic, herbal, or ayurvedic medicine, or acupuncture while on a remedy. It creates confusion in the body and is not effective. In order to see how your system reacts to remedies it is best to be free of medication and off supplements. If you feel weak and debilitated, we want to see that picture and treat it. When there is a condition on the skin we know that it will eventually be relieved. We know that when you develop a skin symptom something deep within the body is discharging toxins. We would not do anything to suppress this symptom, other than see that you were comfortable. But in the case of eczema or acne, for instance, we treat the deep inner organs to establish balance so that the skin symptoms clear up.

In conventional medicine you would be given a remedy to stop any skin irritation. It is our experience in homeopathy that when this is done, symptoms internalize and disease patterns take hold from toxic congestion of the cells. When asthma develops after treating eczema or a skin rash with cortisone, you have begun the process of immuno-suppression, which eventually weakens and debilitates you.

Conventional medicine acts in the opposite way from homeopathy. However, if a person is on medicine which is life sustaining and important for the treatment of a chronic and serious condition, we would give our medicine in gentle doses that would not conflict with their medicine. For instance, in the treatment of diabetes, we would never suggest that a patient come off insulin. That would create such imbalance in the body that it could be life threatening. We would use very dilute forms of homeopathic medicine, called LM potency, and stop it immediately if the patient exhibited a stressful reaction to it. We try to stimulate the Vital Force to reactivate itself.

Medicines, such as cortisone, antibiotics, and birth control pills are suppressive. When you give homeopathic remedies along with these you can create an aggravation where the Vital Force wants to rid itself of the suppressed symptoms. Conflict develops in the physical body with one medicine trying to push symptoms down and another trying to bring them out. Also, the remedies do not work as effectively because of the level of suppression caused by these powerful drugs.

Are Remedies Addictive or Harmful? Do They Have Harmful Effects If You Take Too Many?

No. Homeopathic remedies are not addictive in any way, nor can you do any harm to the system if you take too many pills. As I mentioned, there are stories of children getting into homeopathic remedies and having no ill effects at all. A remedy needs to be the right one to have any effect, and if this is what the child needs it will work on their system. If it is not what they need it will not have any effect at all. This is what makes homeopathy such an excellent and affirming medicine.

It is important to stop taking a homeopathic remedy as soon as your symptoms cease. Otherwise your body may reproduce the symptoms it has just eliminated.

This is another way we differ from allopathic medicine. We do not give courses of remedies. We give them and take them for only the duration of the symptoms. When the symptoms cease it is time to stop the remedy.

—From *Homeopathic Medicine Chest*

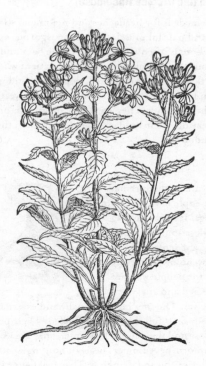

Continued ➡

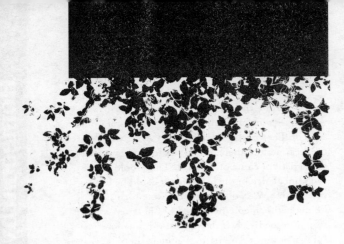

FIRST-AID MATERIA MEDICA

Ambika Wauters, R.S. Hom.

From Aconite to Tobaccum

Aconite (*Aconitum Napellus*)

Aconite is advised for the sudden onset of all symptoms that usually come on after exposure to drafts, cold wind, or icy cold weather. The symptoms appear as a dry, suffocating cough, sore throat resulting from exposure to cold, dry wind and weather. A high temperature with a great thirst and all signs of illness appear very quickly. There can be acute pain which the patient finds intolerable.

It is also good for where fear is felt. Fear is another symptom that responds to *Aconite*: fear of crowds, death, approaching events, and/or the past. The person is always anxious, fretful, and is physically and mentally restless.

Symptoms can come on from bereavement, bites, travel, or anxiety. They are always worse at midnight, while lying on affected side, in a warm room, in cold air, in tobacco smoke, or while listening to music. They are relieved in airy rooms, or when the bedding is thrown off. Use *Aconite* at the beginning of a cold, sore throat, or the flu. It can stop these illnesses if you give it immediately when symptoms appear. This remedy does not have a long-term effect and is mainly for the beginning of illness. Use for shock and injury if there is fear. The difference between *Aconite* and *Arnica* is that *Aconite* is for fear and *Arnica* is not.

Actaea Rac (Actaea Racemosa)

This remedy is for headaches and neuralgia, stiff necks and painful muscles following rigorous exercise. There is often rheumatism in the back and shooting pains along the spine. The patient who needs this remedy is confused, depressed, and despondent. They are worse in cold, damp weather and while moving. They are better in warmth or when eating; their headaches get better when they are outdoors.

Aloe

This is an excellent remedy when people have used a lot of drugs. It works for stagnant digestion, when people live a sedentary life. The psychological picture is suited for people who are dissatisfied and angry at themselves. They are hot, internally and externally. The belly feels full, heavy, and bloated. Their bowels feel loose and their limbs feel lame. They are worse in the morning, summer, heat, in hot, dry weather, and after eating and drinking. They feel better in cold, open air. The patient can have headaches

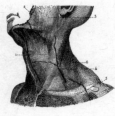

alternating with lumbago and intestinal and uterine problems. There is a disinclination to mental work. The pure juice of aloe in homeopathic potency is good for consumption and digestive problems.

Ant, Tart (Antimonium Tartarticum)

This remedy is used for rattling mucus in the chest made worse by the slightest expectoration. There is a sensation of great fatigue, weakness, and cold sweat. They are worse in the evening, lying down at night, and from warmth. They are better sitting erect, and after burping and expectoration. This is an excellent remedy for children with colds in their lungs and bronchia. The rattling noise is apparent to anyone near the patient and is the keynote symptom that calls for this remedy.

Apis Mel (Apis Mellifica)

This remedy is used for all the effects of insect stings and for symptoms where there is swelling, soreness, and intolerance to heat. The skin has a red, rosy hue. It is a remedy used for edema, congestion, and heat in any part of the body. There is always a burning, stinging sensation, whether it is with the symptoms of swollen eyes, or the burning sensation of cystitis. There is generally an absence of thirst. Apis Mel can be effective in the treatment of arthritis where joints are swollen and there is redness and burning. It is indicated where there is great irritability and depression resulting from anger, fright, and grief. Some of the symptoms that respond to this remedy are rheumatism, swollen parts, incontinence, and rash. Patients are often listless, have trouble concentrating, and can be despondent about their lives. They are worse during the late afternoon, after sleep, from heat, when touched, and in closed, heated rooms. They are better in the open air and with cold water.

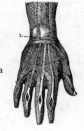

Arg, Nit (Argentum Nitricum)

This remedy works on the throat, when the mucous membranes are affected and irritated. It is also an excellent remedy for nerves, irritable stomach symptoms, and suits fearful and nervous people. It is also used when the mind is full of anxieties and fear, the memory weak, and there are errors of perception. It is a good remedy for mental exertion. It is also excellent for anticipation, when time appears to pass too slowly, stage fright, and examination nerves, or if one cannot stand heat and is worse in any form of warmth, at night, after eating, or has sweats. They are better in fresh air, when cold, and when burping. It is a good remedy when people are stressed from work and have long chronic periods of anxiety.

Arnica

This is the first remedy to be thought of for shock, trauma, accident, or injury. It takes away the shock, which is always present in accidents. It is excellent for bruising and also acts as an antihemorrhagic. It will stop bleeding instantly and should be thought of in all wounds where there is bleeding and contusion to tissue. It relieves sore, bruised feelings after injury, and childbirth. If they say they want to be left alone and always tell you that they are all right, no matter how ill or shocked they may be, Arnica is the premier homeopathic remedy. It is known to restore vitality after jet lag, and to stop bleeding, bruising, and soreness. Consider it first for any accident, injury, or shock. If you wish to apply it topically to a wound, never put it on cut skin. It will sting and cause irritation. Use it on bruised areas or where there is soreness and aching. It is excellent

for any ache or pain. Use it before and after dentistry, before and after exertion, such as workouts, long cycling trips, or running. It will save wear and tear on the body and help your metabolism respond in ways that lead to prompt regeneration.

Arsen. Alb (Arsenicum Album)

This remedy should be thought of whenever there is weakness, debility, exhaustion, and restlessness, with nightly aggravation around midnight to 2 A.M. It can revive a person during and after flu or serious illness, or with burning symptoms, and with unquenchable thirst, where the person sips drinks slowly. It is excellent for food poisoning and will bring equilibrium to the digestive system promptly. It is used with septic infections and low vitality after illness. When the patient needs this remedy, you will generally see such a restlessness around midnight that it can drive the patient from room to room. Think of this remedy for midnight to 2 A.M. asthma attacks. The patient may feel chilly, fastidious, and exacting. They are worse in cold air, with cold applications, at night, and between midnight and 2 A.M. They are better with warmth, except with a headache, and then they ask for cold applications. You may see the patient sitting wrapped in blankets by an open window. It is good for influenza, colds, and times of serious illness when pain and medication have exhausted the patient.

Belladonna

This remedy acts on the entire nervous system where there is congestion, inflammation, convulsions, and pain. It is always associated with hot, red skin, flushed face, glaring eyes, throbbing veins, and a state of excitation, violence, and anger. The sleep is restless; there can be delirium and pains that come and go suddenly and violently. This remedy works on a dry, parched throat where the patient does not wish to drink. Lack of thirst is a keynote symptom. It is a wonderful children's remedy and can stop a fever promptly. The patient is worse after 3 A.M. or after midnight, from uncovering or being in drafts, or lying down. They are better when their body is covered and their head held high. Think of this remedy for arthritic pains, fevers, and sore throats where there is sudden pain and inflammation. It can be used for throbbing, bursting headaches where patient is sensitive to light, and pain is worse on the right side, and when lying down. Remember that *Belladonna* cases are not thirsty and are hot. These are considered classic symptoms for the remedy.

Bryonia

This remedy is for a person who suffers from or dislikes movement of any kind from headaches, mastitis, colds, and flu. The patient cannot stand to get out of bed. Movement makes all symptoms worse. The patient is irritated or angered. They are thirsty and crave cold water. They are anxious about the future and often insecure, which can produce headaches, or an illness symptomatic of not having to move forward in life. They prefer to stay where they are. Even food sits in the stomach and does not move, as if a stone were in the pit of the stomach. There is often accompanying constipation. This remedy should be thought of for headaches (worse on the left side), colds and coughs, hacking and dry. It is good for fevers where the patient is sweating and chilled. The patient is worse with movement, worse in the morning, from eating, from hot weather, exertion, and touch. They feel better lying on the painful part of the body, better with pressure, rest, and cold applications. Always think of *Bryonia* for migraine. For the treatment of chronic migraine consult a homeopath.

Continued ➡

Calc. Carb (Calcarea Carbonica)

This remedy is good for over 90 percent of all children at some point in their homeopathic constitutional treatment. It is often thought of for patients who are fat, flabby, and obese. It affects nutrition, glands, skin, and bone. It is used for swellings, tickling coughs, fleeting chest pains, nausea, acidity, and a dislike of fat. The patient becomes out of breath easily. It is used when there are relapses, especially during colds with heavy mucus. The mental symptom is apprehension, which is worse toward evening. The patient is full of fears, is irrational, or fears that others will see their weakness. They can be confused, low-spirited, and forgetful. They can be obstinate and averse to work and exertion. They may be overweight, have excessive appetites, dislike dairy products, and have a tendency to feel cold and catch cold easily. They may have itching skin and profuse periods. This remedy is suited to quiet, shy, sensitive people who are subject to depression, who are worse in cold, damp weather, and when standing. They are better in dry weather, from warmth and from lying on the painful side.

Calc Fluor (Calcarea Fluorica)

This remedy is used when there is a thick, greenish discharge, excessive coughing and catarrh with tiny lumps. It is used in croup, for gumboils, toothache, and arthritis. The person is worse after rest, and from damp weather, and is better after a little movement and with warm applications.

Calc Phos (Calcarea Phosphorica)

This remedy is excellent for broken bones that are slow to knit. It is good for slow dentition in children, anemic children who are peevish, have weak digestion, and are cold to the touch. This remedy is used for headaches after weather change, severe stomach pain after eating, and for heartburn. It is useful for period pains, acne, and inflamed gums. It is helpful after grief and after injury, and for those who are worse with any change in weather, especially cold, damp, rainy weather, and from exertion and movement. They are better in warm, dry weather, with hot baths, and when resting.

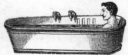

Calendula

This is the best remedy for cuts, incised wounds, and when there is injury to skin tissue in any form. It is applied topically to injuries to stop bleeding and to clean damaged tissue. It promotes quick and efficient healing to all tissue. It is suggested for cradle cap, cuts, wounds, incisions, and especially after surgery. Put ten drops of the tincture into a cup of hot water and apply to the area. Moisten bandaged wounds such as burns by dripping the solution over the wound. It can be used on eczema, rashes, and areas of the skin that are irritated. It brings soothing relief. The tincture can be applied in creams and used whenever there is irritation.

Cantharis Vesicatoria

This remedy is specific for all burns or burning pains. It is used for burns and scalds before blisters form; sunburn; burning in the bladder before, during, and after urination; in cystitis, when the urine scalds the skin; burning in the eyes, mouth, throat, and stomach. Burning is the keynote symptom made worse by touch, during urination, and after drinking cold water and coffee. The person feels better in warmth and when lying down. It will relieve the pain associated with all burning symptoms.

Carbo Veg (Carbo Vegetabilis)

This is a wonderful remedy to help people revive after they have been ill and are weak. There may be anemia and depletion of all energy. It will revive people when they have fainted, and can be useful for coma and unconsciousness. It also offers temporary relief from belching, acidity, and gas in the intestines. It is a specific remedy after food poisoning from eating contaminated fish. It is good for ailments following cold, damp weather when the person may shiver but cling to an open window for fresh air. This remedy can be used for hoarseness and voice loss. Use it also with discomfort after eating fatty food, during warm, damp weather, and in the evenings and at night. It is good for belching and passing wind.

Causticum

This remedy is used for burning, and for rawness and soreness in parts of the body, such as the throat, chest, and rectum. There may be weakness, sinking strength, and shaking in the patient who needs this remedy. It is used often for incontinence when the patient coughs, sneezes, or blows their nose, or while walking or during sleep. It is for those who are worse in dry, cold winds, in fine weather, and in cold air, and are better in damp weather, warmth, or the heat of bed. This remedy is for patients broken down from a long disease, or extended worry. Sometimes paralysis is setting in and this can reverse the symptoms.

Chamomile

This is an excellent remedy for small children, especially during teething. It is used when children are peevish, restless, and angry, with an acute sensitivity to pain and changes. They may be irritable, thirsty, hot, and their pain seems unendurable. A child may whine, be given many things and reject them all. One cheek will be red and hot, the other white and cold. This strange, rare, and peculiar symptom is always an indication for this remedy. The remedy is used for toothache and excruciating pains, such as backache, childbirth, and rheumatic pains. It is made worse by heat, anger, open air, wind, and at night. The child feels better being carried, in warmth, and in wet weather.

China

This is a remedy used for weariness and prostration. It is used as a general tonic and is especially good after malaria and asthma attacks, which occur periodically with weakness and exhaustion. It is good for fever accompanied by continuous weakness and depletion.

Coccolus Indicus

This is one of the great remedies for motion sickness with sensations of weakness or hollowness. The person suffers from lack of sleep or overwork. The head feels so heavy it can't support itself. In seasickness the patient is better in fresh air. They are worse after eating, from loss of sleep, in open air, with smoking, from riding, and in noise. It can be used in pregnancy with morning sickness and backache.

Coffea

This remedy is used for pain relief for the patient who is nervous, sensitive, and excitable. It is used as a painkiller in childbirth and extreme pain due to injury or wounding, where the patient's nerves feel on edge. They feel worse with excessive emotions, joy, narcotics, strong odors, noise, in open air, cold, and at night. They are better in warmth, lying down, and sucking on ice.

Colocynthus

This is a wonderful remedy for the treatment of painful neuralgia. *Colocynthus* is suited for angry, irritable people. When pains are so severe that the person doubles over for relief, and all pains are relieved by bending forward, doubling up, hard pressure, warmth, and lying with head bent forward.

Cuprum

This remedy is considered whenever spasms and cramps affect the body. These can be leg cramps, congestion and spasms in the lungs with asthma, or stomach cramps. Cuprum can be used for convulsions, violent contractions, and intermittent, spasmodic pain. Spasms begin with a twitching in the fingers and moving out. The patient is made worse from vomiting and nausea. They feel better perspiring and drinking cold water.

Dioscorea

This remedy is thought of primarily for colic in the belly, radiating out from the navel to all parts. The pain feels worse bending and is relieved by standing erect. Infants with colic try to stretch themselves fully to alleviate their discomfort. There may be wind and rumbling associated with stomach conditions. The patient feels worse lying down or doubled up, and is worse at night. They are better standing, stretching, in open air, and with pressure.

Drosera

This is a remedy used specifically for spasmodic coughs. Any cough which is violent, protracted, and ends in vomiting responds to *Drosera*. Symptoms are deep, hoarse, barking coughs, constant tickling coughs, laryngitis with a dry throat that makes it difficult to speak, and a sensation of a feather in the back of the throat. The patient is worse with warmth, warm drinks, while laughing, singing, talking, when lying down, after midnight, and better in open air, with activity, and getting out of bed.

Dulcamara

This remedy is used for symptoms caused by changes in weather, especially from warm to cold. The person has stiffness in the joints, especially the back, neck, and throat. They suffer from diarrhea after exposure to wet weather conditions. They may also have rheumatic pains brought on by weather changes that are worse at night and in cold, damp, rainy weather. They feel better when warm and moving about.

Euphatorium

This is one of the best remedies for flu when the bones ache, and there is a high fever and head congestion. It can take all the aches out of a bad bout of malaria or influenza, and is excellent for the aches and pains associated with any illness.

Euphrasia

This is specifically known as a remedy to treat inflammation of the eye, the conjunctiva, and when there is profuse tearing. The patient is better in open air. It is used when there is running of the eyes and nose often associated with hay fever and other irritants. It works to alleviate bursting headaches with dazzling eyes. The patient is worse indoors, in the evening, in warmth, and light. The patient feels better in the dark.

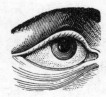

Continued →

Ferrum Phos. (Ferrum Phosphoricum)

This remedy is best used to stop a fever in its early stages. It can also be used to stop a cold that is developing. It stops hemorrhages, especially nosebleeds. It will alleviate a frontal headache that is relieved by nosebleed. The person is worse at night between 4 and 6 A.M., and with touch and movement. The right side is worse. They feel better with cold applications.

Fragaria

This is a tincture made from wild strawberries that strengthens the gums and freshens the mouth.

Gelsemium

This is an excellent flu remedy where the patient is weak, trembling, and chilly. The eyes can barely stay open, there is a dull, tired headache, and the mind is dull. The patient is unable to think clearly. It relieves sore throats, symptoms of flushing, aching, and "tight" headaches. There may be an absence of thirst even with high fever and difficulty in swallowing. It is also an excellent remedy for anticipatory anxiety, such as rehearsals, school exams, and interviews. It takes the "stage fright" away. The patient is worse at 10 A.M., in hot rooms, exposed to the sun, and on receiving bad news. They feel better in the open air and after urinating.

Glonine

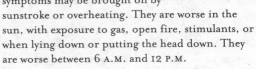

This is used for bursting headaches that start in the back of the neck and are so painful that it feels like the head will explode. The patient cannot bear anything on their head and symptoms may be brought on by sunstroke or overheating. They are worse in the sun, with exposure to gas, open fire, stimulants, or when lying down or putting the head down. They are worse between 6 A.M. and 12 P.M.

Graphites

This is used to treat unhealthy skin conditions, such as eczema, cracked fingers, or when there is a tendency for skin to suppurate. The patient is often overweight and constipated.

Gunpowder

This is used specifically as a blood cleaner for boils and carbuncles.

Hammamelis

This is used as first aid for nosebleeds, tired feeling in arms and legs, burns, bruises, and whenever the mucous membranes are inflamed.

Hepar Sulph (Hepar Sulphuris)

This remedy is used when injuries suppurate and weep, as with eczema, acne, and cracks in the lower lip. It is a wonderful remedy for croup, coughs brought on by exposure, wheezing, earaches, and tonsillitis. The patient feels worse in cold air, lying on the painful part, or when the affected part is touched. They feel better in warmth, and wrapped up in damp, cold weather.

Hypericum

This is an excellent remedy for healing lacerated wounds that involve areas of nerve endings—fingers, toes, and the coccyx. It is good for bites, abscesses, and any painful, deep wound to the body; it will promote healing rapidly. It can be used in a cream, tincture, or taken internally. The person is worse when it is cold and damp, when touched, or in a closed room. They are better bending the head backwards.

Ignatia

This is considered the first remedy for grief, when tears are shed, and when the patient wants only to be left alone. It relieves fright, prolonged grief, and helps sore throats, croup, and backaches brought on by the structure breaking down in one's life. It helps insomnia where there is much yawning but no sleep. The patient is worse with tobacco, cold air, strong odors, and alcohol, and is better in warmth, when changing positions, and when eating.

Ipecacuanha

Any time there is nausea or vomiting this remedy relieves. It is good for travel sickness, morning sickness, and asthma with nausea. It relieves rattling mucus in the bronchial area when there is nausea and vomiting. The person is worse in winter and dry weather, as well as in a warm room where they can't get enough air. They are better with open air, resting with eyes closed.

Iris Tenax

This remedy is specific for appendicitis and for headaches with vomiting.

Kali Bich (Kali Bichromicum)

This is a remedy for catarrhal conditions: sinus troubles, sore throats, and coughs with copious mucus. It is also for migraines, blurred vision, nausea, and vomiting after alcohol use. The patient is worse in the morning, when drinking, especially beer, and in hot weather. They are better with hot applications.

Kali Phos (Kali Phosphoricum)

This remedy is reserved for extreme exhaustion, when people are tired from overwork, nervous exhaustion, and from long periods of preparation for a project at school or work. It is used in stages of childbirth to keep the blood sugar up so that the mother can focus on delivering the baby. It is good for headaches with humming in the ears following long mental effort. The patient is worse with noise, excitement, and mental and physical exhaustion. They are better with nourishment, and light easy movement.

Ledum

This is a remedy used for all puncture wounds from nails, pins, and needles, especially when there is little or no bleeding. It is to be used for bites from animals, such as horses, dogs, cats, and rats. If shooting pains develop after the bite or wound use *Hypericum*. This remedy can help avoid tetanus. *Ledum* can be used in varicose ulcers that refuse to heal. The patient is worse at night, from the heat of the bed, and better in cold, when uncovered, and using cold water, especially putting their feet in cold water.

Lobelia Inflata

This remedy is used specifically for asthma attacks, when the chest feels heavy and there is nausea and vomiting. The patient is worse in motion, cold, in the afternoon, and around tobacco. They are better in warmth, and at night.

Lycopodium

This is a remedy that affects digestion and is good for acidity, hiccups, gout, and cystitis. It is used for excessive hunger, a preference to be alone, a dislike of exercise, when irritable, or when one craves sweets even though they cause indigestion. The patient is worse between 4 and 8 P.M., in stuffy rooms, in cold air, with food and liquid. They are sensitive to loud noise, and feel better with warm food and drinks, wearing loose clothes, in fresh air, and with activity.

Mag. Mur (Magnesia Muriaticum)

This is used as first aid for menstrual cramping, often when there is acne preceding the menses, and flooding during the period. The person feels worse immediately after eating, lying on the right side, and bathing in the sea. They feel better with pressure, motion, and in open air.

Magnesia Phosphoricum

This is used as an antispasmodic remedy. It is exceptionally good for muscle cramps of any nature. It is an asthma remedy, useful in dry, tickling coughs, spasmodic coughs, and whooping cough. The patient feels worse on the right side, from cold, touch, or at night. They are better in warmth, bending double, with pressure and friction.

Merc. Sol (Mercurius Sol)

This is suggested for feverish head colds with great weakness and shaking, for sore throats with overabundant saliva, mouth ulcers, thrush of the mouth, toothache, and earache. It is an excellent remedy for abscesses, and itching skin conditions. It is used if one has offensive breath, spongy, bleeding gums, or profuse, fetid sweats with no relief. The person is worse at night, in wet, damp weather, lying on their right side, and perspiring. They are better in a warm room and in a warm bed.

Nat. Mur (Naturm Muriaticum)

This is the best remedy for running noses and sinus problems. It is useful in the treatment of eczema, urticaria, and with menstrual pains when the patient is sad, irritable, and has reoccurring PMS. It is suited for people who tend to feel insecure and unsure of themselves, who worry about the future, are easily moved to tears or unable to cry at all, or are very irritable before their periods. It is used for the ill effects of prolonged grief, fright, or anger, or if they want to be left alone to experience their sadness, or feel that they will never have a good life. The person is worse in noise, with music, in a warm room, about 10 A.M., at the sea, with mental exertion, consolation, and talking. They feel better in the open air, on bright, sunny days, and washing in cold water after a sweat.

Nitric Acid

This is used for strong, splinterlike pains, or sticking pains. It is excellent for treating blisters and ulcers in the mouth, tongue, and genitals with discharges that are very offensive, or for people with chronic diseases who take cold easily and are disposed to diarrhea. It is effective when the mind is irritable, hateful, vindictive, hopeless, and in despair. The person may be sensitive to noise, touch, jarring, and often fears death. They are worse in the evening, at night, in cold climates, and in very hot weather. They feel better when driving.

Nux Vom (Nux Vomica)

This remedy can cure a multitude of modern-day problems for people stuck in offices, who do not move a lot, and eat rich food and drink regularly. The patient may be very irritable, and sensitive to all impressions. They can be violent-tempered, even malicious. They are oversensitive to odor, noise, and light, and they do not want to be touched. *Nux Vomica* is used for hangovers, indulgence in rich food, and excessive drinking. It is a good nerve remedy, especially suited for travel sickness and indigestion. This is an excellent headache

Continued ➔

remedy, one used specifically for constipation, itching hemorrhoids, stuffy colds, raw sore throats, and PMS. The patient is worse in the morning, from mental exertion, after eating and using all stimulants and narcotics, and in cold weather. They feel better with sleep, damp, wet weather, and with strong pressure.

Petroleum

This is used for many skin conditions and for asthma attacks. It is used when tissue is irritated by external stimuli. Petroleum is good for lingering gastric and lung problems and chronic diarrhea. It is suitable for lasting complaints, fright, irritability, and fears of death. The patient is worse in dampness, before and during thunderstorms, in cars, and during winter. They are better in warm air and dry weather.

Phos. Ac (Phosphoric Acid)

This is used when a patient is exhausted, weak, and nervous. It revives mental tiredness and physical exhaustion. It is useful after serious illnesses when people cannot regenerate their vitality. It is good for excesses, grief, and loss of fluids. It is also used to treat cancer pain.

Phosphorus

This is an excellent remedy for bronchitis and chest problems. It helps cure coughs, hoarseness, laryngitis, and loss of voice. It also works on stomach symptoms, such as vomiting and heartburn. The patient craves cold water, but often vomits it back up when it becomes warm in the stomach. They fear thunderstorms and lightning. The patient is also very sensitive to noise, light, and the slightest stimulation. *Phosphorus* can be used after anesthesia to clear the system of ill effects, and is considered an excellent jet lag remedy. The patient is worse with touch, exertion, at twilight, with warm food and drink, changes of weather, from getting wet in hot weather, in thunderstorms, and ascending stairs. They feel better in the dark, eating cold food and drink, in the cold, open air, and having sleep.

Plumbum

This is good for treating weakness and paralysis in the limbs, or in conditions where there is progressive paralysis. The patient may be worse at night, and with motion. They may feel better with rubbing, hard pressure, and exertion.

Pulsatilla

This is known as the weather cock remedy because pains and symptoms are always shifting to one side or the other, or from one area of the body to another. *Pulsatilla* is thought of for shy, clinging children, people who crave fresh air and always feel better outdoors, even though they may be chilly. It is used when the mucous membranes are affected, secreting copious thick yellow-green discharges. The symptoms are always changing and the patient is complaining, whining, chilly, and is not thirsty.

The emotional state is that a patient weeps easily over trifles, is timid, fears being alone, and wants consolation from others. The patient is worse in heat, after rich food, after eating, in the evening, and in warm and stuffy rooms. They are better in open air, having windows open, even in winter, after cold food and drinks, and with motion.

Rhus Tox (Rhus Roxicoderndron)

This is a wonderful remedy for sprains and muscle strain. It can relieve rheumatism, lumbago, stiff neck, and pains made worse by proximity to dampness, moisture, and cold. When a person has been sitting or lying in one position for too long and the body becomes stiff and achy, this remedy brings swift relief. The person is worse with sleep, in cold, wet, damp, rainy weather, after rain or cold bathing, with night rest, and has right-sided complaints. They are better in warm, dry weather, in motion, walking, changing positions, with rubbing, using warm applications, and from stretching out the limbs.

Ruta Grav

This remedy is for bruised bones, even old injuries where there is stiffness and bone pain. It works well where there is trouble with the wrists, and with conditions that are worse in cold, wet weather and when the person always feels better moving. It relieves eyestrain for close-up work, or when the eyes are weary and ache. The patient is worse lying down and when they are cold. It is useful for sprains, muscle strain, pulled ligaments, and backache.

Sepia

This is a predominantly female remedy, used for period pains, nausea during pregnancy, and menopause that has many symptoms. The person is sensitive to cold, sad, and fearful of being left alone, and is emotionally indifferent to those close. *Sepia* is suited for people who are depressed, and who are fearful. The person is worse in the afternoons and evenings, from cold, thunder, and from tobacco smoke. They are better in a warm bed and with hot applications.

Silica

This remedy is useful in several first aid conditions, such as colds, sore throats, hay fever, splinters, and thorns lodged under the skin. It works to alleviate constipation, migraine, chronic headaches, and sinus trouble. It is suited for people who have problems facing up to their problems and prefer not to take responsibility for themselves. They feel worse being cold, uncovered, in cold weather, and approaching winter. They are better when wrapped up, lying down, and in the summer.

Spongia

This remedy is used for coughs and croup. It is particularly good for children who continue to cough after the flu or a bad cold. There can be anxiety, difficulty breathing, and weakness after the slightest exertion. They are worse when ascending, in wind, after midnight, and are better descending and lying with head low. Children will hang their head over the bed to stop the coughing.

Sulphur

This remedy has been used since ancient times to treat skin conditions: itching skin, rashes, acne, burning and itching hemorrhoids. It is useful for treating burning pains, tinnitus, diarrhea, and a lack of energy. It is excellent for colds that go directly into the lungs. It is suited to people who are deep thinkers and have a nervous yet independent nature. The person is worse in damp, cold weather and at the sea. They are better in warmth and fresh air.

Symphytum

This is used specifically to speed up the knitting of bones.

Tarantula Cubensis

This is an effective remedy for boils, abscesses, or swelling where the tissue becomes blue and there are strong burning sensations. The patient is worse at night and is better when smoking.

Tobaccum

This is used for the treatment of sea and motion sickness.

—From *Homeopathic Medicine Chest*

FIRST-AID CONDITIONS

Ambika Wauters, R.S. Hom.

From Abdominal Pains to Wounds

Abdominal Pains

This refers to all stomach pains that arise from eating, from fear, anxiety, or for any other reason.

When food feels like a stone in the pit of the stomach and the patient feels better after resting (the discomfort is accompanied with a bilious feeling and a slight headache):
Homeopathic Remedy: **Bryonia**

When the stomach is bloated with accompanying gas after light intake of food:
Homeopathic Remedy: **Lycopodium**

When there is gas and colic after eating and drinking alcohol:
Homeopathic Remedy: **Nux Vom**

Abrasions

Clean the wound with a solution of **Calendula Tincture** using ten drops of solution in a cup of warm water. Cover the wound and moisten with a few drops of the solution. It will help heal the wound promptly.

Abscesses

This refers to skin conditions where there is redness, pus, and infection of tissue.

When irritation is accompanied by redness and throbbing pain:
Homeopathic Remedy: **Belladonna** (give every two hours, less frequently as improvement is evident)

Where there is pus and skin is sensitive to touch:
Homeopathic Remedy: **Hepar Sulph** (every two hours until pus discharges or disappears)

When the skin is very tense and painful:
Homeopathic Remedy: **Hypericum**

After discharge of pus, use three times a day for three days:
Homeopathic Remedy: **Silica**

For mouth abscesses:
Homeopathic Remedy: **Merc. Sol**

For general care, bathe affected part:
Homeopathic Remedy: **Calendula Lotion** (Put twenty drops of the tincture in a glass of hot water. Repeat three times daily to help the tissue open and heal.)

All glandular abscesses should be seen by a physician.

Continued →

Accidents

The first remedy to think of in any accident is **Arnica**. It is effective in easing shock; it also works as an anti-hemorrhagic to stop bleeding, and it will stop bruising of soft tissue, flesh, and muscle.

Homeopathic Remedy: **Arnica 30** (Needs to be given immediately after any accident and it can be repeated every fifteen minutes in serious conditions until medical help is available. If the accident is not serious, but shock or bruising are evident, give **Arnica 6** every half hour for 2–3 doses. Always remember that as symptoms disappear the remedy is needed less often. Other remedies can be administered, depending upon the type of injury. Please note any other symptoms that may accompany the accident. Check carefully for concussion, bleeding, and broken bones. Consult a physician if the condition of the patient is not better after first-aid treatment.

Acidity (Stomach)

This can come on as a result of overeating, stressful conditions, fear, anxiety, or anticipation. Pay attention to the emotional state of the patient.

Acidity which may come on from being nervous about a future event such as exams, rehearsals, etc.:
Homeopathic Remedy: **Arg. Nit**

Acidity accompanied by severe heartburn after small amounts of food, made worse from cold food and drink around 4 to 8 P.M.:
Homeopathic Remedy: **Lycopodium**

Acne

There are many types of acne. This is meant to cover general symptoms. If acne persists see a physician or consult a homeopath.

In people with red faces:
Homeopathic Remedy: **Belladonna**

With many pustules:
Homeopathic Remedy: **Hepar Suplh**

In people who have fair complexions:
Homeopathic Remedy: **Pulsatilla**

When the skin becomes scarred from pustules:
Homeopathic Remedy: **Silica**

In cases that resist treatment of any nature:
Homeopathic Remedy: **Sulphur**

Appendicitis

In any case where severe abdominal pain is present, a physician should be consulted immediately as complications can be very serious.

If a physician is not available:
Homeopathic Remedy: **Iris Tenax** (Covers intense pain in the lower right side of the abdomen and tenderness to pressure in one area. Use 3x to 30x every two hours.)

Appetite, Excessive

When there is a feeling of emptiness even after eating:
Homeopathic Remedy: **Calc. Carb**

When the appetite is excessive and then goes to complete loss of appetite:
Homeopathic Remedy: **Ferrum Phos.**

Excessive appetite, even at night, and easily satisfied:
Homeopathic Remedy: **Lycopodium**

Appetite, Loss of

Aversion to all food, hunger stops person from sleeping:
Homeopathic Remedy: **Ignatia**

A constant craving with a loss of appetite:
Homeopathic Remedy: **Arsen. Alb**

Apprehension (Anxiety)

There are many conditions and situations that can provoke apprehension. When these situations are stripping you of your vitality and energy these remedies can help considerably.

Anticipatory anxiety before an event such as an exam, a speech, or an important event which causes anxiety:
Homeopathic anxiety before an event such as an exam, a speech, or an important event which causes anxiety:
Homeopathic remedy: **Arg. Nit** (Take a single dose of 30x the day before the event or a 6x a half hour before the event.)

Apprehension accompanied with fear, diarrhea, trembling:
Homeopathic Remedy: **Gelsemium**

Arthritis

Homeopathic remedies are good for the relief of discomfort and pain associated with arthritis. For deeper treatment see a homeopath for constitutional treatment.

When the joints swell and are red and painful:
Homeopathic Remedy: **Apis Mel**

When the joints feel bruised:
Homeopathic Remedy: **Arnica**

When there appears to be no relief from pain:
Homeopathic Remedy: **Cryonia**

When pain shifts from joint to joint or extremity to extremity:
Homeopathic Remedy: **Pulsatilla**

Asthma

Chronic asthma can be treated at a constitutional level by a homeopath. For acute attacks the following may stop symptoms and bring relief. Take a pill every fifteen minutes during an attack until there is improvement and then take less frequently or as needed.

When an attack is brought on by exertion or by speaking, when there is tightness and pains in the chest, when breathing is oppressed and difficult:
Homeopathic Remedy: **Arnica**

When an attack comes in the middle of the night with anxiety, restlessness, tossing, and inability to get comfortable in one position, burning heat in the chest, cold sweats and exhaustion that accompany the attack:
Homeopathic Remedy: **Arsen. Alb** (every ten minutes until attack diminishes, then less frequently)

When there is a tight, constricted feeling in the chest and rattling in the windpipe, which may feel full of mucus; when it is difficult to expectorate; when there is gasping for air, a pale face, cold feet, and sometimes nausea:
Homeopathic Remedy: **Ipecacuanha**

For "nervous asthma" where the person experiences suffocation, dizziness, coughing, vomiting, and nausea:
Homeopathic Remedy: **Lobelia Inflata**

When an asthma attack, usually occurring in the early morning, is brought on by overeating and overdrinking, and the person feels very irritable:
Homeopathic Remedy: **Nux Vom**

Bad Breath

When there is a bitter taste in the mouth on waking:
Homeopathic Remedy: **Kali Phos**
Bach Remedy: **Holly**
Color Remedy: **Turquoise**

When there is a metallic taste in the mouth:
Homeopathic (Remedy): **Merc. Sol.**
Bach Remedy: **Star of Bethlehem**
Color Remedy: **Green**

Bereavement (Grief)

This may arise at any time one experiences loss. This can also be for losses felt acutely in the past that have not disappeared with time. Use for family members at a funeral or when a loved one is ill or in the hospital. It is better to allow the feelings to come to the surface than to suppress them.

When death comes very quickly and friends or family are in shock:
Homeopathic Remedy: **Aconite**

For grief that lingers:
Homeopathic Remedy: **Ignatia**

When grieving for an old rejection or loss:
Homeopathic Remedy: **Nat. Mur**

Bites, Animal

These should be treated immediately by a physician.

Take immediately after the bite:
Homeopathic Remedy: **Aconite**

Black Eye

Homeopathic Remedy: **Arnica** (Give every hour for up to five doses. If the bruising is relieved by cold cloths use **Ledum** for five doses. If there is pain in the eyeball use **Symphytum** every hour for three to four doses.)

Blisters

Homeopathic Remedy: **Calendula Tincture** or **Ointment** (Apply to the blister. If using tincture put ten drops of solution into a small glass of hot water and apply to the area. For intestinal use take **Causticum** 6x morning and evening. Reduce intake as symptoms disappear.)

Boils

When the skin is red, burning, and tight:
Homeopathic Remedy: **Belladonna**

To cleanse the blood when a boil is festering:
Homeopathic Remedy: **Gunpowder**

When an injury turns septic, and the boil is hot and painful:
Homeopathic Remedy: **Hepar Sulph**

When any injury festers and develops pus, and the boil is cold:
Homeopathic Remedy: **Silica**

For very acute pain, inflammation, stinging, burning, and throbbing, and the skin has gone to a purple color:
Homeopathic Remedy: **Tarantula Cubensis** (Externally bathe the boil in **Hypericum Tincture** using ten drops of tincture in warm water.)

As a preventative for recurring problems:
Homeopathic Remedy: **Arnica**

Bones

For broken bones, to aid the healing process:
Homeopathic Remedy: Symphytum

For fractured bones slow to mend:
Homeopathic Remedy: **Calc Phos**

Any bone injury mends well with:
Homeopathic Remedy: **Ruta Grav**

For bruised feeling in the bones:
Homeopathic Remedy: **Arnica**

If a bone injury was sustained and still aches:
Homeopathic Remedy: **Ruta Grav** (Use morning and night for a week. This can be repeated after a month if the treatment does not bring relief.)

Bronchitis

When there is rattling in the chest:
Homeopathic Remedy: **Ipecacuanha**

Continued ➡

When there is loss of voice or hoarseness:
Homeopathic Remedy: **Phosphorus**

When accompanied by a fever and chills:
Homeopathic Remedy: **Arsen. Alb**

With flu-like symptoms, bone ache, fever:
Homeopathic Remedy: **Euphatorium**

Burns

Serious burns should always be seen by a physician.

For shock:
Homeopathic Remedy: **Arnica** (If accompanying fear give **Aconite** in place of **Arnica**.)

To treat all burns:
Homeopathic Remedy: **Cantharis**

When the pain of a burn is accompanied by restlessness and the skin blisters:
Homeopathic Remedy: **Causticum** (Take a dose every half hour until the pain subsides.)

External application for burns:
Homeopathic Remedy: **Urtica Urens Tincture** or **Hypericum Tincture** (In both remedies use ten drops in warm water and apply to the burn by dripping it over a sterile dressing. Do not remove the covering, but keep it moist at all times.)

Carbuncles

If painful to the touch and patient finds contact from the dressing uncomfortable:
Homeopathic Remedy: **Hepar Sulph**

To expel all pus and toxins:
Homeopathic Remedy: **Silica**

If there is burning, stinging, and throbbing pain:
Homeopathic Remedy: **Tarantula Cubensis 6X**

When the skin is shiny and red, the pain is throbbing and stabbing, and when it is difficult to sleep:
Homeopathic Remedy: **Belladonna**

For external treatment:
Homeopathic Remedy: **Hypericum Tincture or Cream**
(Follow treatment recommended for boils.)

Catarrh

For the treatment of chronic catarrhal conditions it is suggested you see a homeopath. Excess mucous conditions can be treated effectively.

When the patient has a head cold with thick yellow discharge:
Homeopathic Remedy: **Calc Fluor**

With thick yellow discharge, weakness, and fretting:
Homeopathic Remedy: **Pulsatilla**

When there is stringy, glue-like discharge:
Homeopathic Remedy: **Kali Bich**

Chest Problems

Chest problems are often associated with flulike symptoms.

With a dry painful cough:
Homeopathic Remedy: **Bryonia**

With hoarseness and loss of voice:
Homeopathic Remedy: **Phosphorus**

When chest feels oppressed and person feels chilled:
Homeopathic Remedy: **Sulphur**

Chilliness

When accompanied by desire to sit next to the fire or radiator:
Homeopathic Remedy: **Arsen. Alb**

With chronically cold hands:
Homeopathic Remedy: **Calc. Carb**

When chilliness is intense with shivering:
Homeopathic Remedy: **Hepar Sulph**

When chilly at night:
Homeopathic Remedy: **Sepia**

Colds

From sudden onset of symptoms (Often made worse after exposure to dry, cold winds. Patient feels fretful, even frightened, one cheek hot, the other cold.):
Homeopathic Remedy: **Aconite**
Color Remedy: **Red**

When the symptoms are flulike:
Homeopathic Remedy: **Gelsemium**

When bones ache and flu has set in:
Homeopathic Remedy: **Euphatorium**

Colds with much sneezing and running nose:
Homeopathic Remedy: **Nat. Mur**

Colic

When there is gas, a distended belly like a drum, with tearing pains in the abdomen, gripping in the naval, and/or flatulent colic after anger, intolerance to pain, worse at night and in warmth:
Homeopathic Remedy: **Chamomilla**

When the pains are made worse by eating and the belly is distended and there is relief in bending over:
Homeopathic Remedy: **Colchicum**

When there are violent pains relieved by pressure and bending, the bowels feel as if they are being squeezed, and pain is acute:
Homeopathic Remedy: **Colocynthus**

When pains abate from lying still and are better when not moving:
Homeopathic Remedy: **Bryonia**

When pains are better when doubled up:
Homeopathic Remedy: **Belladonna**

When pains are better with stretching, standing erect, and walking about, and/or flatulence is worse with pressure and doubling up:
Homeopathic Remedy: **Dioscorea**

When pressure in the stomach feels like a stone; there is flatulence from eating "gassy" foods; frequent desire to move the bowels without effect; irritability; indicated for people who overeat and drink too much:
Homeopathic Remedy: **Nux Vom**

For violent cramps radiating to all parts of the body; stomach feels as if it is drawn into the spine by a string; belly feels hard and bowels are constipated:
Homeopathic Remedy: **Plumbum**

For sharp pains as if cut by a knife; violent nausea and vomiting; guts feel as if they are tied in knots; sweating all over, very weak and sometimes passing out or in stupor:
Homeopathic Remedy: **Veratrum Alb**

Concussion

Always see a physician after a concussion.

When the trouble is not severe:
Homeopathic Remedy: **Arnica 30** (every fifteen minutes for four doses)

Constipation

For persistent constipation seek a homeopath. For acute bouts, which may come from time to time, look at one of the following remedies:

With ineffectual urging to move bowels:
Homeopathic Remedy: **Nux Vom**

When motions recede or feces are only partially expelled:
Homeopathic Remedy: **Silica**

For large, painful motions:
Homeopathic Remedy: **Sulphur**

Coughs

Crouplike cough, in spasms:
Homeopathic Remedy: **Calc Fluor**

When crouplike cough comes after midnight:
Homeopathic Remedy: **Hepar Sulph**

When crouplike cough is accompanied by fright:
Homeopathic Remedy: **Ignatia**

Dry, painful coughing fits:
Homeopathic Remedy: **Bryonia**

Sudden and violent coughing:
Homeopathic Remedy: **Drosera**

Persistent coughing, worse at night, particularly in children:
Homeopathic Remedy: **Spongia**

With hoarseness, loss of voice, glassed-over eyes:
Homeopathic Remedy: **Phosphorus**

Spasmodic fits of coughing, tightness in chest:
Homeopathic Remedy: **Cuprum**

Cramps

When cramps are in calf and are caused by exhaustion:
Homeopathic Remedy: **Arnice**

Cramps in calf muscles:
Homeopathic Remedy: **Arsen. Alb**

Cramps in legs and feet with contracted muscles, or for cramps in fingers and/or toes:
Homeopathic Remedy: **Cuprum**

An effective remedy for any type of cramping:
Homeopathic Remedy: **Ledum**

When cramping starts at night, affects soles of the feet and person feels the need to stretch:
Homeopathic Remedy: **Nux Vom**

When cramps occur only during the day and while sitting:
Homeopathic Remedy: **Rhus Tox**

Crushed Fingers or Toes

For body parts, such as fingers or toes, that have many nerve endings and are very sensitive:
Homeopathic Remedy: **Hypericum 6x** (taken internally every five minutes)

To alleviate symptoms of shock:
Homeopathic Remedy: **Arnica** (intermittently)

Cuts

To stop bleeding:
Homeopathic Remedy: **Arnica** (can be repeated every minute until bleeding ceases)

For external application use:
Homeopathic Remedy: **Hypericum Cream or Tincture**

Cystitis

When it is painful to urinate and there is a stinging feeling:
Homeopathic Remedy: **Apis Mel**

When the above symptoms occur and there is fever:
Homeopathic Remedy: **Belladonna**

When there is frequent urination and a burning feeling:
Homeopathic Remedy: **Cantharis**

When there are pink deposits in the urine:
Homeopathic Remedy: **Lycopodium**

When symptoms shift from place to place and patient is upset:
Homeopathic Remedy: **Pulsatilla**

Dental Problems

To alleviate dental shock and to control pain and bleeding:
Homeopathic Remedy: **Arnica**

Continued ➡

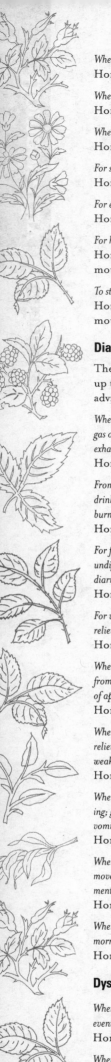

Whenever there is nerve pain:
Homeopathic Remedy: **Hypericum**

When there is great fear of visiting the dentist:
Homeopathic Remedy: **Aconite**

When there is great sensitivity to pain, especially in young people:
Homeopathic Remedy: **Chamomilla**

For sharp darting pains following drilling:
Homeopathic Remedy: **Hypericum**

For excessive bleeding following drilling or tooth pulling:
Homeopathic Remedy: **Phosphorus**

For healing a pulled tooth:
Homeopathic Remedy: **Calendula Tincture** (as a mouthwash)

To strengthen weak and bleeding gums:
Homeopathic Remedy: **Fragaria Tincture** (as a mouthwash; ten drops in water)

Diarrhea

These remedies may be taken at hourly intervals for up to four doses. If diarrhea persists seek medical advice.

When there is a constant urging to motion but uncertainty whether gas or feces will pass, or after passing a movement the patient is exhausted and sweats profusely:
Homeopathic Remedy: **Aloe**

From food poisoning, excessive amounts of fruit, ice cream, or cold drinks in hot weather; nausea, vomiting, restlessness, heat, and burning sensations; patient is very weak and body parts are chilled:
Homeopathic Remedy: **Arsen. Alb**

For frequent, watery bowel movements with gas; painless, with undigested bits of food; weakness, delicacy, associated with summer diarrhea:
Homeopathic Remedy: **China**

For watery, yellow diarrhea after eating and drinking; pains are relieved by bending over:
Homeopathic Remedy: **Colocynthus**

When diarrhea is caused by change of weather from hot to cold, or from getting wet; bowel movements are slimy green or yellow; loss of appetite and thirst:
Homeopathic Remedy: **Dulcamara**

When diarrhea is gushing, squirting, profuse, painless; cramps relieved by bending over and better with warm applications to belly; weak feeling persists:
Homeopathic Remedy: **Podophyllum**

When diarrhea is watery and profuse with cramps and colicky feeling; great thirst for ice water or acid drinks; violent nausea and vomiting; icy cold sweat:
Homeopathic Remedy: **Veratrum Alb**

When diarrhea comes on after antibiotics; smelly, offensive bowel movement; patient is irritable and exhausted after bowel movements:
Homeopathic Remedy: **Nitric Acid**

When diarrhea is offensive and drives patient out of bed in the morning:
Homeopathic Remedy: **Sulphur**

Dyspepsia (Heartburn)

When the symptoms come from nervous anticipation of future events:
Homeopathic Remedy: **Arg. Nit**

When there is gas, patient craves fresh air, and is chilly:
Homeopathic Remedy: **Carbo Veg**

When symptoms appear after small amounts of food, with pain, around 4 to 8 P.M.:
Homeopathic Remedy: **Lycopodium**

When there is an acute sensation of burning:
Homeopathic Remedy: Phosphorus

Earache

Avoid putting anything in the ear. When you select the appropriate remedy, give a dose hourly for up to three doses, and less frequently as symptoms disappear. As symptoms improve, give every two hours for a day and then three times daily for a day. If trouble persists see a physician.

When there has been exposure to cold air or wind and a fever, restlessness, and anxiety. Violent pain is better with warmth:
Homeopathic Remedy: **Aconite**

When pain develops suddenly and is severe; skin is dry and the face hot and red; the patient has no thirst and is restless:
Homeopathic Remedy: **Belladonna**

When the patient is very sensitive to pain, and it is worse with warm applications. A child is very cross and irritable. Sometimes in small children you notice one cheek is red and hot, the other white and cool:
Homeopathic Remedy: **Chamomile**

When pain begins in the early stages and there is inflammation:
Homeopathic Remedy: **Ferrum Phos.**

When the patient is worse in drafts and sensitive to touch, wants to be warm and snug:
Homeopathic Remedy: **Hepar Sulph**

When the inflammation is in the inner ear:
Homeopathic Remedy: **Merc. Sol** (Give a dose every hour, then as pain eases off give every two hours until pain is gone.)

When there is throbbing and the ear feels stopped up. The patient wants air, is worse if it is warm in the evening, is very weepy, and in want of companionship and sympathy:
Homeopathic Remedy: **Pulsatilla**

Exhaustion

When exhaustion comes after physical exertion:
Homeopathic Remedy: **Arnica**

When exhaustion comes on after a sickness:
Homeopathic Remedy: **Arsen. Alb**

When exhaustion comes after mental effort, or any time you need to keep the blood sugar up for long periods of activity, such as long-distance driving, childbirth, studying for exams:
Homeopathic Remedy: **Kali Phos**

Eyes (Inflamed, Burning, Watering, or Swollen)

When unable to bear bright light:
Homeopathic Remedy: **Euphrasia**

When eyelids are puffy and swollen:
Homeopathic Remedy: **Apis Mel**

Fainting

Select a remedy, give every ten minutes until the patient is recovered.

When there is fainting from emotional upset:
Homeopathic Remedy: **Ignatia**

When there is fainting from excitement:
Homeopathic Remedy: **Coffea**

When fainting comes from a hot, stuffy room:
Homeopathic Remedy: **Pulsatilla**

When fainting comes from pain:
Homeopathic Remedy: **Aconite or Chamomilla** (latter used in childbirth to relieve pain)

When fainting is caused by the sight of blood:
Homeopathic Remedy: **Nux Vom**

When fainting is caused by the loss of blood:
Homeopathic Remedy: **China** (If difficult to administer a pill, dissolve it in a small amount of water and wet the lips.)

Fear

When fear comes on after a frightening experience:
Homeopathic Remedy: **Aconite**

When fear becomes terror (of crowds, death, or a bad experience):
Homeopathic Remedy: **Arsen. Alb**

When there is fear of thunder or darkness:
Homeopathic Remedy: **Phosphorus**

When there is fear of appearing before groups of people:
Homeopathic Remedy: **Arg. Nit**

When there is fear of failing at something (exams, interviews):
Homeopathic Remedy: **Gelsemium**

Food Poisoning

When it is clear that sickness comes from spoiled food and the patient has diarrhea and is vomiting:
Homeopathic Remedy: **Arsen. Alb**

When the poison comes from tainted fish:
Homeopathic Remedy: **Carbo Veg**

Fractures

Always see the appropriate medical staff to set the bones properly.

For shock:
Homeopathic Remedy: **Arnica**

An old-fashioned bone-healing remedy to ensure the bones knit properly:
Homeopathic Remedy: **Symphytum** (three times daily for two weeks)

To ensure that bones are properly healed:
Homeopathic Remedy: **Calc Phos** (may be given for a further four weeks)

Grief

Grief can be the etiology for many illnesses. It affects most people at some time in their life. Remedies can be used for personal loss and for situations where disturbing news of any kind sends a person into a state of grief or loss.

When there is silent brooding, sadness, hysteria, or deep crying:
Homeopathic Remedy: **Ignatia** (three times daily for a week)

When there is deep depression from grief and the patient shuns consolation and wishes to be alone with their grief:
Homeopathic Remedy: **Nat. Mur**

When grief turns to indolence, indifference, despair, or apathy:
Homeopathic Remedy: **Phos Ac.** (Give the same dose and for the same period of time as Ignacia.)

Hay Fever

When eyes are burning and watery:
Homeopathic Remedy: **Euphrasia**

When all symptoms are better outdoors:
Homeopathic Remedy: **Pulsatilla**

In people prone to being chilly, sedentary, and weak:
Homeopathic Remedy: **Silica**

Headache

When you have selected the appropriate remedy for your type of headache, give a dose every ten minutes until symptoms are markedly reduced.

When there are sudden, violent pains with a burning sensation, as if the brain was in boiling water, the pain is intolerable, there is throbbing in the temples, the patient is restless, fearful, and thirsty.
Homeopathic Remedy: **Aconite**

When headaches reoccur periodically and the patient is weakened by them. Sometimes pain is relieved by vomiting. There is great thirst and the patient will take frequent sips of cool water. The patient is restless, fearful, and feels better when moving:

Continued ➡

Homeopathic Remedy: **Arsen. Alb**

When there is sudden pain, throbbing, bursting sensation, the pain is worse with moving, bending, and moving the eyes. The head is hot, and the face flushed. The patient can't bear light or noise. Headache often begins in the afternoon and lasts throughout the night:
Homeopathic Remedy: **Belladonna** (These headaches can come after too much exposure to sun or heat, violent emotions, or periods.)

When a headache comes on from eating rich food or too much exertion and is accompanied by great thirst or no desire for movement of any kind, is worse on the left side, and patient lingers in bed:
Homeopathic Remedy: **Bryonia**

When a headache comes on with acute sickness or great anxiety, begins in the nape of the neck and settles over the eyes. It is often worse on the right side. The patient feels heavy, sleepy, and drowsy. Sometimes the person is shivery with chills, shows no thirst, and feels better after vomiting:
Homeopathic Remedy: **Gelsemium**

When pains are violent, pulsating, throbbing, or bursting, made worse by light and bending the head backwards. These headaches are always made worse by exposure to sun or heat. The patient will actually grab their head in pain. They are flushed and hot to the touch. They cannot bear to be touched and feel better in cold air and with cold applications:
Homeopathic Remedy: **Glonine**

When the headache feels like hammers inside the head, stitching pain in the head, a sore, bruised feeling around the eyes, and movement makes the headache worse. Headache starts in the back of the neck and spreads all over the head. It can be a blinding headache, often associated with PMS or mental exertion:
Homeopathic Remedy: **Nat. Mur**

When the headache is accompanied with vomiting and nausea caused by eating rich food and drink or excessive anger. Headache feels as if a nail is being driven into the head. The patient is worse with conversation, excitement, or movement, and is very irritable and chilly. Almost always constipated as well:
Homeopathic Remedy: **Nux Vom**

When the headache is in the temples and the head is hot, better with cold applications and fresh air. This is often associated with delayed or suppressed menstrual periods. The patient is dizzy when bending over and feels worse in a stuffy room or in areas with noise and light:
Homeopathic Remedy: **Pulsatilla**

Heatstroke

When the pupils are dilated, there is a bounding pulse, burning, skin is hot and dry, patient has no thirst and is often delirious:
Homeopathic Remedy: **Belladonna**

When there is a painful headache with nausea and sometimes vomiting, and the patient is worse when moving:
Homeopathic Remedy: **Bryonia**

When there is a throbbing, bursting headache, flushed appearance, and the patient is sweating:
Homeopathic Remedy: **Glonine**

Bach Remedy: **Rescue Remedy** (taken internally and on a compress)
Color Remedy: **Indigo**

Hoarseness

When the weather is cold and damp:
Homeopathic Remedy: **Carbo Veg**

With laryngitis:
Homeopathic Remedy: **Phosphorus**

Bach Remedy: **Rescue Remedy** (Gargle with water and two drops of solution.)
Color Remedy: **Turquoise**

Horsefly Bites

To bring the swelling down:
Homeopathic Remedy: **Hypericum**

Indigestion

When accompanied with gas:
Homeopathic Remedy: **Carbo Veg**

From nervous tension:
Homeopathic Remedy: **Kali Phos**

From overeating or rich foods:
Homeopathic Remedy: **Nux Vom**

With headache and great thirst:
Homeopathic Remedy: **Bryonia**

Insect Bites

When there is numbness, sensitivity to being touched, and pain that is relieved by cold applications:
Homeopathic Remedy: **Ledum**

When there is burning, stinging pain made worse by the application of heat. There is swelling and the area is red and swollen:
Homeopathic Remedy: **Apis Mel**

When there is serious inflammation with burning, worse with touch but better with gentle massage:
Homeopathic Remedy: **Cantharis**

For insect bites:
Homeopathic Remedy: **Hypericum**

For insect stings:
Homeopathic Remedy: **Apis Mel** (Use Arnica Tincture or Calendula Tincture topically to relieve the stinging.)

Insomnia

When there is twisting and turning and person cannot settle:
Homeopathic Remedy: **Aconite**

From being overly tired, the bed feels strange and hard:
Homeopathic Remedy: **Arnica**

When there are accompanying nightmares, jerking, screaming:
Homeopathic Remedy: **Belladonna**

Much yawning but unable to sleep:
Homeopathic Remedy: **Ignatia**

When the feet and legs are hot and must be placed outside the bed:
Homeopathic Remedy: **Sulphur**

Joints

Swollen, painful:
Homeopathic Remedy: **Belladonna**

When there is rheumatism and pain:
Homeopathic Remedy: **Rhus Tox**

Menstrual Pains

When the breasts are tender and swollen:
Homeopathic Remedy: **Calc. Carb**

When period is accompanied by headaches:
Homeopathic Remedy: **Calc Phos**

When depression accompanies the period:
Homeopathic Remedy: **Lycopodium**

When sad and irritable before and during period:
Homeopathic Remedy: **Nat. Mur**

When tearful with painful breasts:
Homeopathic Remedy: **Pulsatilla**

With cramps before and during period:
Homeopathic Remedy: **Mag. Mur**

Nausea

Nausea with burning pains in the stomach and gut area:
Homeopathic Remedy: **Arsen. Alb**

Nausea and vomiting:
Homeopathic Remedy: **Ipecacuanha**

Nausea with vomiting after drinking alcohol:
Homeopathic Remedy: **Kali Bich**

Nausea and vomiting from smelling food:
Homeopathic Remedy: **Sepia**

Nausea with vomiting after eating rich food:
Homeopathic Remedy: **Nux Vom**

Neuralgia

When the pain disappears during the night and appears during the day:
Homeopathic Remedy: **Actaea Rac**

When the face is flushed, hot, and pain is throbbing:
Homeopathic Remedy: **Belladonna**

With severe pain:
Homeopathic Remedy: **Colocynthus**

Nose

Nosebleeds in children:
Homeopathic Remedy: **Ferr. Phos.**

Frequent nosebleeds:
Homeopathic Remedy: **Hammamelis**

Nosebleeds caused from a blow:
Homeopathic Remedy: **Arnica**

Nosebleeds with profuse bleeding:
Homeopathic Remedy: **Phosphorus**

Nose running during colds and flu:
Homeopathic Remedy: **Gelsemium**

Nose running constantly without stopping:
Homeopathic Remedy: **Nat. Mur**

Sciatica

When discomfort is worse in cold, damp weather and at night:
Homeopathic Remedy: **Rhus Tox**

Seasickness

When there is nausea, dizziness, feeling of faintness, and loss of direction. When traveling by sea take one every hour and also a few minutes before departure:
Homeopathic Remedy: **Cocculus Indicus**

When there is nausea with saliva in the mouth, and/or vomiting and dizziness which is better when having food in the mouth:
Homeopathic Remedy: **Petroleum**

When the patient feels icy cold, has a sinking feeling in the stomach, and is worse with the smell of tobacco smoke:
Homeopathic Remedy: **Tobaccum**

Shingles

When the scalp is affected:
Homeopathic Remedy: **Rhus Tox**

Sinus Disorders

When there is excess mucus with stringy discharge:
Homeopathic Remedy: **Kali Bich**

When there is great pain in the face and head, sometimes with nausea:
Homeopathic Remedy: **Nat. Mur**

When the pain starts at the back of the head and settles over the face:
Homeopathic Remedy: **Silica**

Skin

When the skin is blotchy:
Homeopathic Remedy: **Arg. Nit**

When the skin is cracked and there is weeping eczema:
Homeopathic Remedy: **Graphites**

Continued ➜

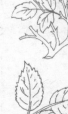

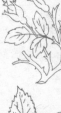
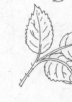

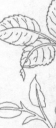
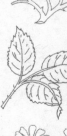

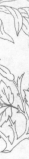

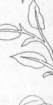

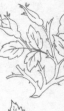
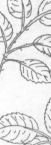

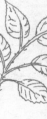

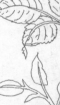
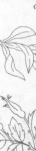

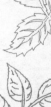

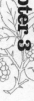

When the skin feels better when scratching:
Homeopathic Remedy: **Calc. Carb**

When the skin itches and is worse when hot:
Homeopathic Remedy: **Merc. Sol**

When the skin itches and begins to burn:
Homeopathic Remedy: **Sulphur**

Spine

When the nerve endings of the coccyx are injured:
Homeopathic Remedy: **Hypericum** (Give immediately and repeat night and day for three days or until pain subsides.)

When there is extensive bruising:
Homeopathic Remedy: **Arnica**

When the bone feels bruised:
Homeopathic Remedy: **Ruta Grav**

Bach Remedy: **Rescue Remedy**
Color Remedy: **Orange**

Splinters

To expel the splinter:
Homeopathic Remedy: **Silica** (Three times daily for a few days. If it does not expel, see a physician.)

Apply to wounded area:
Homeopathic Remedy: **Calendula Tincture** (Put ten drops of tincture in a cup of hot water. If there is deep penetration of the skin give Ledum three times in four hourly intervals.)

Sprains

When the sprain first occurs:
Homeopathic Remedy: **Arnica**

When the sprain continues to hurt:
Homeopathic Remedy: **Rhus Tox**

When the ligaments are affected:
Homeopathic Remedy: **Ruta Grav**

Sties

When there is a sticky discharge:
Homeopathic Remedy: **Graphites**

With a burning feeling in the eye:
Homeopathic Remedy: **Phosphorus**

At the beginning of the sty formation:
Homeopathic Remedy: **Pulsatilla**

If accompanied with a sore throat:
Homeopathic Remedy: **Nux Vom**

Stomach Pains

When there is burning in the stomach with a feeling of chill and sickness:
Homeopathic Remedy: **Arsen. Alb**

When food sits in the pit of the stomach like a stone:
Homeopathic Remedy: **Bryonia**

Sunburn

When the skin is red, hot, and throbbing, with no thirst:
Homeopathic Remedy: **Belladonna**

After a day in the sun when highly exposed to sun's rays:
Homeopathic Remedy: **Cantharis**

If sweating and cramping occur:
Homeopathic Remedy: **Cuprum**

Teething in Babies

To give a remedy to a baby, you can dissolve the remedy in water or milk and either give in a bottle, or in small teaspoons as a dose. For nursing infants, the mother can take the remedy and pass the remedy on through nursing. Choose the appropriate remedy and give to the baby in fifteen-minute intervals until the baby is peaceful.

When the baby awakens in a fright, jerks, and jumps in their sleep; eyes are red, pupils dilated. They are hot to the touch, restless, and feverish; may even convulse and fall asleep instantly; gums are swollen and inflamed:
Homeopathic Remedy: **Belladonna**

When the baby's head is covered in sweat during sleep. They are fretful and irritable; feet may be cool and damp; bowel movements are light colored. They vomit milk and have swollen bellies:
Homeopathic Remedy: **Calc. Carb**

When the baby is very irritable, crying, nothing will satisfy. They want to be carried all the time and will cry the minute they are put down to sleep. One cheek may be white, the other red:
Homeopathic Remedy: **Chamomilla**

When teething presents difficulties and the child is weak, delicate, and the teeth decay as soon as they appear:
Homeopathic Remedy: **Kreosotum**

Thirst (Excessive)

When there is a high temperature:
Homeopathic Remedy: **Aconite**

When there is a craving for cold drinks:
Homeopathic Remedy: **Bryonia**

When there has been an excessive use of salt:
Homeopathic Remedy: **Nat. Mur**

When the mouth and throat are dry, craving milk:
Homeopathic Remedy: **Rhus Tox**

Thirst (Lack of)

When the throat is swollen:
Homeopathic Remedy: **Apis Mel**

When there is a high temperature:
Homeopathic Remedy: **Gelsemium**

When the mouth is dry:
Homeopathic Remedy: **Pulsatilla**

Throat, Sore

When there has been exposure to cold winds:
Homeopathic Remedy: **Aconite**

For immediate relief of pain:
Homeopathic Remedy: **Kali Sulph and Nat. Phos** (Taken five minutes apart, repeat every half hour till symptoms disappear.)

When throat is sore, accompanied with constipation, irritability:
Homeopathic Remedy: **Nux Vom**

When throat is painful and there is excessive saliva in the mouth:
Homeopathic Remedy: **Merc. Sol**

Tonsillitis

When there is inflammation and pain:
Homeopathic Remedy: **Hepar Sulph**

Toothache

When there is an ache without any signs of inflammation or gum boils:
Homeopathic Remedy: **Kreosotum**

When there are no clear indications other than pain:
Homeopathic Remedy: **Merc. Sol**

When there is swelling, inflammation, and pain:
Homeopathic Remedy: **Apis Mel**

When the pain is made worse with cold drinks and air:
Homeopathic Remedy: **Calc. Carb**

When teeth are in poor condition:
Homeopathic Remedy: **Calc. Fluor**

Travel Sickness

When there is restlessness and fear:
Homeopathic Remedy: **Aconite**

When the least movement upsets:
Homeopathic Remedy: **Bryonia**

When there is irritability about movement and jarring:
Homeopathic Remedy: **Nux Vom**

When movement causes nausea and vomiting:
Homeopathic Remedy: **Ipecacuanha**

When symptoms of airsickness appear:
Homeopathic Remedy: **Belladonna**

Recovery from jet lag:
Homeopathic Remedy: **Arnica**

Vomiting

When there is nausea, vomiting with faintness, sweating, and a disgust for food; vomiting of liquid as soon as it is taken; patient has no thirst:
Homeopathic Remedy: **Ant. Tart**

When there is vomiting of solid food and patient needs to keep still as the least movement makes the vomiting start again:
Homeopathic Remedy: **Bryonia**

When there is vomiting with constant nausea; vomiting empties stomach:
Homeopathic Remedy: **Ipecacuanha**

When there has been excessive overeating and drinking, vomits are sour smelling; the stomach is worse if any pressure is applied; the patient is irritable and chilled:
Homeopathic Remedy: **Nux Vom**

When vomiting is because of suppressed period or a chill on the stomach. Stomach craves rich, fatty food like mayonnaise, butter, pastry; craves cold water and cool air:
Homeopathic Remedy: **Pulsatilla**

Wounds

To clean out wounds immediately:
Homeopathic Remedy: **Calendula Tincture**

For puncture wounds:
Homeopathic Remedy: **Calendula and Ledum** (Take internally every hour for five doses, three doses the next day. If any sign of infection occurs see a physician.)

—From *Homeopathic Medicine Chest*

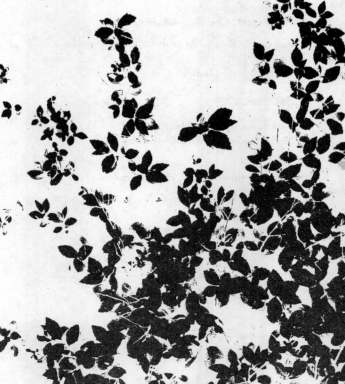

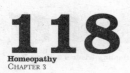

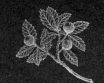

Aromatherapy & Essential Oils

WHAT IS AROMATHERAPY?

Kathi Keville

Aromatherapy describes the use of essential oils—potent aromatic substances extracted from all fragrant plants—for physical and emotional healing. Today many herbalists, body workers, cosmetologists, chiropractors, and other holistic healers are discovering how this multifaceted and versatile healing art is able to enrich their practice. Many home healers as well are using the principles and resources of aromatherapy to expand their repertoire of natural remedies.

There are many approaches to using essential oils. Applied externally, they penetrate through the skin and are deposited in the underlying tissues. They also reach the bloodstream rather quickly: compounds from lavender oil have been detected in the blood only twenty minutes after the oil was rubbed on the skin.

As a result, one can treat a wide range of physical problems with aromatherapy. For example, massaging the appropriate aromatherapy body oil directly over the abdomen will quickly banish indigestion. Rubbing an aromatic vapor balm on the chest will relieve lung congestion and fight infection in two ways—as an inhalant drawn deep into the lungs' air passages, and as a lotion that penetrates the skin. Aromatherapy cosmetics and skin preparations are also used to counter external problems such as skin infections and eczema.

Interest in the therapeutic effects of inhaling essential oils continues to grow. More and more commonly, fragrances are being pumped into offices, stores, and even some hospitals to make the atmosphere more relaxing. Large corporations are turning to other fragrances to keep their workers alert, and more content, on the job. Inhaling certain essential oils has even been shown to lower blood pressure.

The beauty of aromatherapy is that you can take advantage of its physical and emotional applications in the same treatment. For example, you can blend a combination of essential oils that will not only stop indigestion but calm you down and reduce the nervous condition that led to the indigestion. Or, you can design an aromatherapy body lotion that will not only improve your complexion but relieve depression.

In the pages that follow, I will describe all of these methods and more, providing plenty of recipes along the way to get you started. I will also be looking into the cosmetic applications of aromatherapy in skin and hair-care products. If I succeed in sparking your interest in aromatherapy, be sure to have a look at the book I wrote with Mindy Green, *Aromatherapy: The Complete Guide to the Healing Art* (from The Crossing Press), which goes into greater detail about using essential oils and making your own aromatherapy products.

Questions Most Frequently Asked About Aromatherapy

Is aromatherapy a new science?

Aromatherapy goes back to at least 4000 B.C., when Neolithic ointments combined vegetable oils with aromatic plants. Throughout the world, cultures began using aromatic steams, smoke, and water for healing. By around 3000 B.C., the uses of odoriferous herbs were being recorded on papyrus by the Egyptians, and on clay tablets in Mesopotamia and Babylonia. By 1700 B.C., trade routes had been established throughout the Middle East, mostly to permit traffic in solid aromatic unguents such as myrrh for incense, perfume and medicine, and aromatic spices for food. Eventually these routes extended into India, China, and Europe.

Essential oils were being distilled in Europe, China, and Japan by about 500 B.C., which led to the development of colognes, perfume, and facial waters. These were not only used to disguise body odor and improve the complexion, but were also ingested as medicinal tonics.

Appropriately, the birth of modern aromatherapy took place in France, the modern capital of perfume. It was Rene-Maurice Gattefosse, a French chemist descended from a long line of perfumers, who reunited the arts of perfumery and medicine. He coined the term "aromatherapy" around 1928

Continued ➜

when a laboratory explosion in his family's perfume factory severely burned his hand. After plunging his injured hand into a container of lavender essential oil, he was amazed how quickly it healed. Young Gattefosse began to look for an answer.

Eventually Gattefosse's writings inspired others to explore aromatherapy, and interest in the new science spread to Europe and, finally, to the United States. Of course, most herbalists were already using aromatic plants in their healing work.

How is aromatherapy connected to herbalism?

Aromatherapy always has been a part of herbalism. The ancient Egyptians, Arabs, Greeks, Romans, and European herbalists all referred in their writings to the use of fragrance for healing purposes.

If you have ever used herbs, the chances are you have also experienced aromatherapy. Aromatic molecules, called essential oils, occur in any fragrant plant. Whenever you make a tea of, say, peppermint or chamomile, the heat draws essential oils from the plant into the water. You receive the healing benefits of essential oils both as you drink the tea and as you inhale the aroma. It is also possible to extract essential oils directly from herbs into alcohol or warm vegetable oil. (If you have an herb garden or other good supply of fragrant herbs, you may want to experiment.)

Aromatherapy differs from herbalism inasmuch as it employs only *certain* herbs. I like to think of it as a division of herbalism—one that uses fragrant plants exclusively. While non-fragrant herbs such as comfrey or goldenseal are not used in aromatherapy, many common medicinal herbs, such as elecampane, angelica, hyssop, and myrrh, are used, as are fragrant plants that are usually not considered medicinal, but do produce therapeutic essential oils. (Examples include ylang-ylang, vanilla, and mimosa.) Because herbs often contain several different types of medicinal compounds besides essential oils, herb books describing a fragrant herb's properties may not always be referring to properties associated with the essential oil.

What are essential oils?

Essential oils consist of tiny aromatic molecules that are released from a plant when you rub it, or just from the heat of hot summer day. (This is what makes an herb garden smell so fragrant.) Each type of essential oil is composed of many different aromatic molecules—more than 30,000 have been identified and named, and it is common for a single essential oil to contain one hundred different aromatic molecules.

The vast number of possible combinations of these molecules accounts for there being so many unique plant fragrances. However, because identical or very similar molecules occur in more than one plant, some plants smell very much alike, even when the plants in question are completely unrelated. This is especially true of the variety of plants that produce a lemonlike aroma; they include lemon itself, lemon verbena, melissa (lemon balm), lemon thyme, lemon eucalyptus, citronella, and palma rosa. Even though all of these plants and their corresponding essential oils smell similar, each one possesses a slightly different combination of aromatic molecules and carries its own distinctive olfactory shading.

In a few cases, a plant's essential oil is composed chiefly of one type of molecule. For example, sandalwood may contain up to 90 percent santalol, and clove bud has between 70 percent and 80 percent eugenol.

Why do plants produce essential oils?

At first, botanists were not sure why plants contain essential oils, which they viewed as mere by-products of plant metabolism. They were at a loss to explain why some plants produce essential oils and others do not, or why the fragrances vary so much from one plant to another.

Although there is still much to learn about why plants are fragrant, modern botanical research now understands that even though plants discard essential oils as waste products, the oils do serve important functions. Fragrances attract the insects that help to fertilize their flowers. They also protect plants by repelling certain insects, along with other predators. Many essential oils contain substances called terpenes, which help to waterproof the plant and protect it from rain. (Terpenes also make it difficult for many essential oils to mix with water.) Some essential oils are highly antiseptic, preventing the growth of bacteria, mold, and fungus on a plant.

How are essential oils obtained from plants?

The pure essential oils available at the local herb shop are usually extracted from plants through a process called steam distillation. Freshly picked plants are suspended over boiling water, with the steam drawing the oils out of the plant. The next step is to rapidly cool the steam back into water. During this process, the essential oil separates from the water.

There are several other ways to produce essential oils. One method squeezes, or presses, essential oils from the plant. Another very old method, rarely used today, is enfleurage, which extracts the oils into sheets of warm fat. Although various solvents may be used to extract essential oils, aromatherapists worry about the possibility of slight traces of the solvent contaminating the oils.

New methods of obtaining essential oils are currently being developed and introduced. One of the most interesting processes, although an expensive one, extracts the oil with carbon dioxide. The resulting essential oils have an odor very much like that of the original plant.

Can I make my own essential oils?

You can indeed make essential oils at home—but don't expect to produce very much! (It isn't unusual to obtain just a small vial of essential oil from a wheelbarrow full of plants.) The process is simple enough, although even a small commercial steam distiller costs several hundred dollars. You can also have a steam distiller custom-built by someone who does laboratory-glass blowing. Check the yellow pages for a chemistry supply house.

There is, however, a much cheaper way to rig up a home steam distiller in your kitchen, although you'll end up with even less essential oil than from a laboratory distiller. At the very least, you will obtain some excellent aromatic waters and may even produce a few drops of oil. (For this reason, try distilling plants that yield a lot of oil, such as eucalyptus, rosemary, and peppermint.) Whether you purchase a distiller or rig one up at home, you will need to have a large supply of fresh plants because they release oil better and so much oil is lost when plants are dried.

To make an oil distiller at home, suspend a vegetable steamer full of fragrant herbs over a few inches of water in a pressure cooker. Place the pressure cooker on an unlit stove burner. Fasten the lid on the pressure cooker and attach the end of about six feet of plastic hose to the spout at the top. Coil the rest of the plastic tube in a bucket of ice water so that the tube's other end hangs outside the bucket. Stick this end of the tube into a quart-size glass jar. For gravity to work, the bucket needs to stand below the pressure cooker, and the end of the tube needs to reach below the bottom of the bucket. Turn on the stove and boil the water in the pressure cooker. The steam will come out the spout and travel through the tube. When it hits the cold water, the oil and water will separate and pour together into the glass jar. The essential oil, which floats on top of the water, can be skimmed off. The resulting water (or "hydrosol") will also contain some essential oil.

Why are some essential oils so much more expensive than others?

The broad price range of essential oils—they vary from about $5 to $800 per ounce—reflects the range of difficulty involved in producing various oils. It is no wonder that Bulgarian rose oil sells for $600 an ounce—it took about six hundred pounds of rose petals to produce that ounce! On the other hand, plants such as eucalyptus and rosemary yield a comparatively large amount of essential oil, placing them among the least expensive.

There are several other reasons why it may be more expensive to produce one oil than another, including difficult growing conditions and the relative scarcity of certain plants. For example, peppermint is relatively easy to cultivate and propagate, and is harvested with machinery. Compare that to roses, which must be carefully cultivated, pruned, and hand-harvested.

Another consideration is the country in which the plant is grown. Peppermint would be even less expensive than it is if most of it weren't grown in the United States, where labor and other production costs are high. Many herbs used for essential-oil production come from developing nations.

How does fragrance affect emotions?

When your olfactory sensors detect a particular aroma, this information is sent to areas of the brain that influence memory, learning, emotions, hormone balance, and even more basic survival mechanisms. Exactly how the brain processes this data is not completely understood, but we do know that certain fragrances act on the brain's primitive limbic system, also known as the "smell brain."

Researchers studying aromacology—the science of medicinal aromas—have discovered that exposure to some aromatic substances results in an alteration of brain waves. They suspect that aromas may work on the brain in still other ways. The fragrance research company International Fragrance and Flavor (IFF) has tested over two thousand subjects to better understand how certain scents relieve pain, call up deep-seated memories, and affect personality, behavior, and sleep patterns.

It is probably no surprise that many psychologists have incorporated aromatherapy into their practices. In the early 1920s, Italian psychologists Giovanni Gatti and Renato Cayola concluded that "the sense of smell has . . . an enormous influence on the function of the central nervous system." They used certain scents to sedate their patients, others as stimulants. In France, psychologist Jean Valnet uses vanilla to help his patients unlock childhood memories. Several large Tokyo corporations have followed the advice of staff psychologists and begun to circulate lemon, peppermint, and cypress through their air-conditioning systems to keep workers attentive—and reduce the urge to smoke. Aroma is also assisting truck drivers, railroad engineers, air traffic controllers, and others whose jobs require that they remain alert.

Yet another way that fragrance can affect emotion is through association. Psychologists have successfully helped people overcome anxiety and other emotional problems by first inducing a state of relaxation, often with pleasant music, then introducing a strong scent. After several exposures to the scent, the patients begin to associate it with a tranquil state.

Continued ➡

The patients are then encouraged to carry vials of that scent out into the world, and whenever they encounter a situation that makes them tense, nervous or anxious, open the bottle, sniff, and relax.

Why are so many cosmetologists working with aromatherapy?

The answer to why aromatherapy is becoming so important to so many cosmetics firms—including Revlon, Redkin, Avon, Charles of the Ritz, and the Japanese firm Shiseido—is easy: aromatherapy offers a complete health and beauty package for both skin and hair.

Actually, this is nothing new. Fragrant herbs have long been used to clear complexions and make hair silky. Certain essential oils stimulate oil production in dry skin and hair. Others slow down overactive oil glands. Still others soothe and heal irritated skin. Many cosmetics firms now add botanical derivatives in order to cash in on the popularity of natural ingredients. Be sure to read the labels carefully and thoroughly when choosing skin-care products, and remember that you, too, can make aromatherapy body-care products, for only a fraction of what you would pay at the store.

Can I learn to like scents that bother me at first?

I know several people who, consciously or unconsciously, have felt uncomfortable with, or even disliked, a person because he or she wears the same fragrance as someone with whom they once had problems. I met one man who hated the smell of lavender because the funeral parlor in his hometown had used it. Many people in his family had died when he was young, and, as a result, he had come to associate lavender with death and grief.

It takes time to change a negative reaction to a fragrance, although usually not all that much work. When you are in a good mood or in a place you enjoy, sniff a faint amount of the problematic scent combined with another scent, one that you do like. After doing this several times, you should begin to associate the once-disliked fragrance with pleasant experiences. (If this doesn't work, don't despair—aromatherapy offers so many different and appealing fragrances, you can afford to let one go.)

—From *Pocket Guide to Aromatherapy*

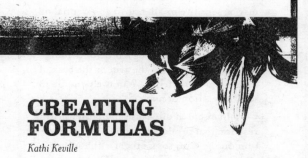

CREATING FORMULAS

Kathi Keville

Getting Started

Making and using aromatherapy products for healing or skin-care is not all that difficult. Some basic information about essential oils and a few safety tips are all you need to conduct your first experiments. Start with simple remedies and a few essential oils. As you become more familiar with the fragrances and properties of the different oils, the process will become easier and easier. For specific therapeutic and cosmetic applications, you can follow the suggestions in the five chapters following this one for your first experiments, or take inspiration from the descriptions of individual oils in the *Materia Medica*. Be sure to take careful notes so that you can duplicate a success—or avoid repeating a flop.

The most effective aromatherapy preparations have a fragrance so subtle you can barely perceive it. Use your nose as your guide, and don't be afraid to experiment. Most people prefer familiar and enjoyable fragrances. Remember, however, that not everyone likes the same fragrances. No matter how many books say that lavender is relaxing and promotes smiling, if you associate that fragrance with a bad memory, you may never learn to enjoy it.

Equipment

Unless you plan to extract your own essential oils, you will need very little equipment to make aromatherapy preparations at home. You probably have almost everything you need already in your kitchen. Vegetable oils such as almond, apricot, grape seed, and jojoba are available in most natural food stores. The glass droppers you will need to measure out small amounts of the essential oils and transfer them from bottle to bottle are sold in drugstores, and in some natural food stores. (While it is important not to contaminate your essential oils by moving the dropper directly from one vial of oil to the next, you don't need to have a separate dropper for each oil. Simply rinse the oily dropper in rubbing alcohol and wait a few minutes for the alcohol to completely evaporate before putting the dropper into another bottle.)

If you prefer, you may also use a narrow glass tube called a "pipette"—sold in chemical equipment catalogs, in some drug stores, and on the pages of aromatherapy supply catalogs—to measure out small amounts of essential oils. Place one end in the essential oil, the other in your mouth. Gently inhale to draw the essential oil slowly up the tube. Well before it reaches the top of the tube, put your finger over the end you had in your mouth and move the pipette to another bottle. Every time you raise your finger, a little bit of oil will drop out. The most useful pipettes have graduated markings along the side so you can measure out exactly the amount of oil you wish to use.

Supply Checklist

Essential oils (see below)

Carrier—vegetable oils (see right), glycerin, distilled water, vodka or grain alcohol

Pyrex measuring cup

Clean, empty glass bottles with lids

Set of measuring spoons

Glass droppers (or pipettes)

Small funnel (optional)

Notebook, pencil, labels for bottles

Cleanup supplies:

    paper towels

    rubbing alcohol

Essential Oil Starter Kit

Besides a few pieces of equipment that you probably already have in your kitchen, you will need a few essential oils. These are sold at many natural food stores and herb stores, as well as in mail-order catalogs. For a starter kit, I recommend the following oils:

Lavender—fights infection, inflammation, insomnia, pain, depression, anxiety.

Chamomile—digestive and relaxation aid; treats allergies, rashes, menstrual cramps, inflammation, anxiety, anger, and depression.

Rosemary—relieves pain, congestion, constipation, and grief; stimulates circulation and memory; helps in times of transition.

Tea tree—fights most types of infection.

Peppermint—relieves indigestion, sinus congestion, itching, panic; mental stimulant.

Lemon (or other citrus)—antidepressant: kills parasites; promotes a sense of sense of cleanliness.

Geranium—balances mind and body.

POPULAR CARRIER OILS

Almond	Coconut	Olive
Apricot	Grape seed	Rice Bran
Avocado	Hazelnut	Safflower
Canola	Jojoba	Sesame
Castor	Kukui	Squalene
Corn	Macadamia	

Media

The most technologically refined way to fragrance a room is with an electric aromatic diffuser (see Glossary). You can also scent a room by placing a few drops of essential oil into a pan of water that is gently steaming on the stove, or into a small amount of water in a potpourri cooker. You can use these methods to change the room's emotional atmosphere, or to prevent airborne bacteria from spreading infection throughout your house. Another way to scent a room is with a drop or two of essential oil on a special ring designed to rest over a hot lightbulb. Scented pillows, bed linens, clothes, and stationery are also common aromatherapy media.

Essential oils are often diluted in carrier oils (see list above). Most aromatherapy applications are 2 percent (two drops essential oil per one hundred drops carrier oil). A 1 percent dilution is better for children, pregnant women, and those with particular health concerns. Some people find it easier to measure in drops, or in teaspoons, which are more convenient for large quantities. As mentioned earlier, a drugstore dropper is usually accurate enough, although the size of drops will vary depending on the size of the dropper opening, the temperature, and the viscosity (thickness) of the essential oil. See Dilutions and Doses, page 133 for information on diluting different types of aromatherapy preparations.

Tips on Creating Custom Formulas

The many choices that go into the creation of a blend may seem intimidating at first, but they also add to the excitement. Remember to keep records of how you make your preparations; include ingredients, proportions, processing procedures, and comments. Label your finished products with the ingredients, date, and any special instructions. When combining essential oils in a therapeutic blend, it is best for a beginner to use no more than five oils at a time. That way you will avoid unpredictable results due to the complex chemistries involved. Don't worry—you can create a safe and effective remedy with even one or two oils.

You may wish to take a few hints from professional perfumers. Think of each oil as having a unique personality. In the perfume trade, the "top note," "middle note," and "low note" define an essential oil's evaporation rate. Fragrances that are light and airy, like lavender, are top notes. Those that are heavy and linger—patchouli and vetiver, for example—are low notes. The middle notes he somewhere in between. Carefully developed perfume blends that contain all three notes; beginners will especially want to avoid blends of exclusively pungent, heavy low notes.

Continued ➡

Essential oils vary in odor intensity, and you will need to add much smaller amounts of some oils to your blends than others. You can tell the oils with a high odor intensity—such as chamomile, patchouli, cinnamon, ylang-ylang, and clary sage—just by smelling them.

If all this talk about "high notes," "middle notes," "low notes," and "intensity" is beginning to make you nervous, here are a few shortcuts for beginning aromatherapists. You can start with an essential oil that has a fairly complex chemistry and already smells like a blend; try geranium, which contains hints of herbs, rose, pine, cedar, and lemon. You can then expand your formula by adding small amounts of other oils, one at a time. When in doubt, choose one of the fragrances that already exists in the complex oil. With geranium, that could be cedarwood, sandalwood, or a citrus such as bergamot or petitgrain.

Another interesting way to expand a blend is to choose oils that are similar to each other. This performs a delightful trick on the nose when the oils begin to play off one another, making your blend seem more complicated and mysterious than it actually is. Try combining peppermint and spearmint, lemon and bergamot, or cinnamon and ginger. Every choice you make will take your blend in a new and interesting direction.

Incorporating Herbs

When used together, herbs and essential oils possess a greater capacity for healing than either on its own. Oils made by soaking herbs in vegetable oil are called "infused oils" and may be used in place of plain vegetable oil in aromatherapy preparations, resulting in more potent medicines. You can also add essential oils to salves, lotions, and creams to enhance their healing properties.

Regarding Quality

To make a quality product, you will need to start with quality essential oils. Factors determining quality include purity, growing conditions, differences among species, and extraction techniques.

Purity is of concern to anyone purchasing essential oils. Rare and expensive oils are the most likely candidates for adulteration, and it is often difficult for an untrained nose to tell the difference between expensive pure essential oil of lemon verbena or melissa, and those same oils mixed with cheap lemongrass or citronella, (In fact, these oils are so often adulterated, you may never have smelled the real thing.) An essential oil that is cut with another oil will not necessarily carry the same properties, and certainly won't smell the same.

At first, it may seem difficult to judge quality, and unfortunately, store clerks do not always know a lot about aromatherapy and essential oils. Like many people, they think that anything marked "essential oil" is pure and natural. Enter the store armed with a little knowledge, and don't be shy about asking questions. You should be able to tell quickly whether the staff person is knowledgeable about essential oils. Some of the best aromatherapy companies are those run by aromatherapists, who are staking their reputations on supplying good essential oils.

Quality can vary greatly due to climate and botanical differences. A good example is lavender, available in about a dozen different grades. There is often variation even within the grades, according to where the oil comes from and the year of harvest.

Many commercial sources sell the least expensive grades of essential oil so they can offer them at a competitive price.

You don't always need to use the highest grade of essential oil, but you should at least know what you are buying. Go into a store that offers essential oils from several different companies and see if you can't smell the difference. The higher-grade essential oils generally carry more of a bouquet, a fuller-bodied fragrance.

The less expensive oils can cost more in the long run. A woman I know who makes facial creams had to use four times as much essential oil to achieve the same results when she switched to an inferior grade. Also, the fact that one essential oil smells different from another doesn't always mean that one of them is an inferior product. Sometimes variations exist in oils of comparable quality; in such cases personal preference is your only guide.

A common method of adulterating essential oils is by "extending" (i.e., diluting) them with vegetable oils, alcohol, or some other solvent. One way to tell if an oil has been diluted with vegetable oil is to put a small drop on a piece of paper. Because they are so volatile, most essential oils will evaporate rather quickly leaving no residue, and unless you are using very dark oils such as patchouli or benzoin, or a brightly colored oil such as German chamomile, no discoloration should remain. (Even with thick or colored oils, the stain should not be oily.)

While oils diluted with alcohol can be detected by a slight "boozy" odor, it is much harder to tell when the oil has been diluted with other clear, non-oily solvents. This is a potentially dangerous situation, because such solvents are readily absorbed into the body when rubbed on the skin or inhaled through the lungs. In such cases, you may have to rely on training your nose. Once you have experienced the intensity of an undiluted essential oil, oils cut with a solvent or synthetic just won't smell as good.

Problems with Synthetic Oils

When I pass around high-quality essential oils in my aromatherapy seminars, I warn my students that I am about to spoil them for life. Once you have smelled the real thing, it is difficult to use anything else. Synthetics, usually made with petroleum-based chemicals, try to duplicate natural scents; in my opinion, they never come close. They also are potentially harmful, since their tiny molecules penetrate the skin and enter the bloodstream.

Sad to say, synthetic fragrances permeate our lives. Many body-care products sold in natural food stores contain them. Most fruits and flowers do not naturally produce essential oils, so when you see "essential oil" of carnation, lily of the valley, strawberry, or gardenia, you can be sure these are synthetics. When someone says that they react adversely or are allergic to fragrances, I am always suspicious. The chances are they have encountered only synthetics.

Proper Storage

Once you've gone to the trouble of locating and purchasing quality essential oils, you will want to keep them that way. Store them in glass vials with tight lids in a cool place. The glass may be clear instead of amber, but remember to keep essential oil out of direct sunlight.

Properly stored, most essentials oil will keep for years. Citrus oils, such as orange and lemon, are the most vulnerable to oxidation and spoilage, but even they will last a couple of years if refrigerated. A few essential oils, such as patchouli, clary sage, benzoin, vetiver, and sandalwood, actually improve with age. (I have some twenty-year-old patchouli

that smells so rich, people have trouble identifying the fragrance—even those who normally hate the smell of patchouli.)

I store even diluted aromatherapy products in glass. Pure essential oils stored in plastic, or in bottles with plastic droppers, will eventually eat away the plastic. The obvious danger is that the oil will leak out of the container, but long before that occurs, the oil will have been contaminated. There are times, however, when glass can weigh you down. Say you want a lightweight first-aid kit or a toiletries case for traveling, or maybe you just want to carry a lotion or cream down to the beach or up onto the ski slopes. It is safe to temporarily store essential oils and products containing essential oils in plastic containers—just be sure that the containers are made of a durable, stiff grade of plastic.

Safety

- Overexposure to essential oils, either through the skin or by nose, can result in nausea, headache, skin irritation, emotional unease, or an overall "spaced-out" feeling. Getting some fresh air will help you to overcome these symptoms.

- To use an essential oil internally, your best bet is to take the herb as a tea or a tincture.

- Essential oils are very potent, concentrated substances, capable, if undiluted, of burning or irritating skin and other sensitive tissues. Keep all essential oils away from mucous membranes (the lining of the digestive, respiratory, and genitourinary tracts) and eyes. If you ever experience skin irritation from contact with essential oils, or accidentally get some in the eyes, flush with straight vegetable oil, not water.

POTENTIAL SKIN IRRITANTS

bay rum	citronella	thyme (except type linalool)
birch	cumin	clove
black pepper	thuja	cinnamon

- Use essential oils cautiously with anyone who is elderly, convalescing, or who has a serious health problem such as asthma, epilepsy, or heart disease. If there is any chance a person may be sensitive or allergic to an essential oil, run a patch test, placing one drop of the suspect essential oil in one-quarter teaspoon of vegetable oil and rubbing a little of the mixture into the crook of the arm or the back of the neck at the hairline. Wait twelve hours to see if a reaction occurs.

- Certain essential oils cause a photosensitizing reaction that produces an uneven pigmentation on the skin, so use them with caution—and never in a suntan lotion. The most notorious such oil is bergamot, which contains bergaptene, a powerful photosensitizer.

PHOTOSENSITIZING ESSENTIAL OILS

angelica	cumin (slightly)	lime (slightly)
bitter orange	lemon (slightly)	orange (slightly)

- Vary the essential oils you use. Uninterrupted use of some oils exposes your liver and kidneys to chemical constituents that may be harmful over time.

Potentially Toxic Essential Oils

The following oils are not included in the Materia Medica. *Never* administer these oils to children or pregnant women:

Continued ➡

bitter almond (*Prunus amygdalus*, var. *Amara*)
hyssop (*Hyssopus officinalis*)
mugwort (*Artemesia vulgaris*)
oregano (*Origanum vulgare*)
pennyroyal (*Mentha pelugium*)
sassafras (*Sassafras albidum*)
savory (*Satureja hortensis*)
thuja (*Thuja occidentalis*)

AROMATHERAPY AND EMOTIONAL HEALTH

Kathie Keville

How aroma effects the mind is not completely understood, although we do know that when you smell something, information is sent to the specific areas of the brain that influence memory, learning, emotions, hormone balance, and even basic survival mechanisms such as the fight-or-flight response. Psychologists have begun working with fragrances to enhance interaction and communication among people. Pleasant smells seem to make people more willing to negotiate, cooperate, and compromise with others.

The formulas in this section can be used as body, massage, or bath oils. If you are a health-care practitioner, one subtle way in which to practice aromatherapy with your patients is to dab a small amount of an appropriate essential oil on the back of your hand. If you would rather scent the room, use the essential oils suggested in the following formulas in a diffuser, a potpourri cooker, a pan of simmering water, or on a light-bulb ring.

Depression

Certain fragrances affect brain waves in a fashion similar to antidepressant drugs, according to research by the Olfaction Research Group at Warwick University in England. At his clinic in France, psychologist Paolo Rovesti has successfully pulled many patients out of depression with the citrus scents of orange, bergamot, lemon, and lemon verbena. One of my favorite aromatic anti-depressants, the elegant scent of neroli essential oil, is also a citrus. Sixteenth-century herbalist John Gerard said that melissa "gladdens the heart" and that clary sage counters depression, paranoia, mental fatigue, and nervous disorders. Other antidepressant essential oils include jasmine, sandalwood, and ylang-ylang.

ANTIDEPRESSIVE ESSENTIAL OILS

bergamot	lavender	orange
clary sage	lemon	petitgrain
geranium	lemon verbena	sandalwood
grapefruit	Melissa	tangerine
jasmine	neroli	ylang-ylang

Antidepressive Formula

12 drops bergamot
6 drops petitgrain
6 drops rose geranium
1 drop neroli (expensive, so optional)
4 ounces vegetable oil
Combine ingredients.

Anxiety

Aromatherapists use several fragrances to help overcome feelings of anxiety, loneliness, and rejection. I find the same oils useful for anyone undergoing a major life transition.

ANXIETY-RELIEVING ESSENTIAL OILS

basil	hyssop	orange
bergamot	lavender	rose
cedarwood	marjoram	
cypress	opopanax (similar to myrrh)	

Anxiety Formula

12 drops lavender
6 drops orange
3 drops marjoram
3 drops cedarwood
4 ounces vegetable oil
Combine ingredients.

Fatigue

A Japanese alarm clock manufacturer has designed an apparatus that uses eucalyptus and pine to awaken sleepers. Throughout the workday, lemon, cypress, and peppermint circulate through the air-conditioning systems of several large Tokyo companies to keep employees alert. The spicy aromas of clove, basil, black pepper, cinnamon, and, to a lesser degree, patchouli, lemongrass, and sage are known to reduce drowsiness, irritability, and headaches. Instead of over-amping the adrenal glands with caffeine and other stimulants, these oils actually counteract the rush of adrenaline. They also prevent the sharp drop in attention typical after thirty minutes of work. In Italy, doctors Giovanni Gatti and Renato Cayola use clove, cinnamon, lemon, ylang-ylang, cardamom, fennel, and angelica to stimulate patients.

STIMULATING ESSENTIAL OILS

angelica	cinnamon	lemon
basil	clove	peppermint
benzoin	cypress	pine
black pepper	eucalyptus	camphor
fennel		

Stimulant Formula

15 drops lemon
4 drops eucalyptus
3 drops peppermint
1 drops cinnamon
1 drop benzoin (optional)
4 ounces vegetable oil
Combine ingredients.

Memory

Researchers have learned that mental recall improves dramatically when a past event is associated with smell. That's why a whiff of a perfume or other fragrance can send you back in time, evoking long-forgotten images and feelings. Next to my computer, I keep a sprig of rosemary, whose ability to increase memory, concentration, and even cre-

ativity is legendary. Modern Japanese research confirms that rosemary is a brain stimulant. Other mental stimulants include sage, basil, and bay leaf.

MEMORY-STIMULATING ESSENTIAL OILS

bay	lavender	rosemary
jasmine	lemon	

Memory Formula

10 drops lavender
8 drops lemon
5 drops rosemary
1 drop cinnamon
4 ounces vegetable oil
Combine ingredients.

Grief

In the sixteenth century, herbalist John Gerard wrote that basil "taketh away sorrowfulness . . . and maketh a man merry and glad" and suggested a whiff of marjoram "for those given to much sighing" from grief, loneliness, or rejection. Ancient Egyptians, Greeks, and Romans also sniffed marjoram to "strengthen emotions" and mitigate grief. The Greeks used cypress and hyssop to comfort mourners; several ancient cultures burned sandalwood at death ceremonies to accomplish the same purpose. In Europe, sage, clary sage, and rosemary were used to overcome grief. These essential oils can also be used during a transition in one's life, such as a job change or the end of a romantic relationship. Other good companions include the gentle, relaxing scents of lavender and marjoram, both used traditionally to comfort the sick, the dying, and their families.

ESSENTIAL OILS TO EASE GRIEF

basil	fir	myrrh
clary sage	hyssop	rosemary
cypress	marjoram	sandalwood

Grief Formula

8 drops marjoram
6 drops melissa or lemon
4 drops clary sage
4 drops cypress or rosemary
1 drop hyssop essential oil (expensive, so optional)
4 ounces vegetable oil
Combine ingredients.

Insomnia

Lack of sleep is a problem for millions of Americans, often leading to agitation, depression, dizziness, and headaches.

ESSENTIAL OILS FOR INSOMNIA

bergamot	lavender	nutmeg
chamomile	lemon	patchouli
clary sage	marjoram	rose
frankincense	melissa	sandalwood
jasmine	myrrh	valerian
geranium	neroli	ylang-ylang

Insomnia Formula

12 drops bergamot
6 drops chamomile
5 drops geranium
1 drop frankincense
1 drop rose
4 ounces vegetable oil
Combine ingredients.

Continued ➡

Stress

Fragrances can lower your pulse and breathing rate. Place people in a room scented with lavender, bergamot, marjoram, sandalwood, lemon, or chamomile, and notice the reduction in avoidance and competition. In his seventeenth-century *Herbal*, Nicholas Culpepper agreed that chamomile "comforts" the head and brain. In more modern times, doctors Giovanni Gatti and Renato Cayola have found that the most sedating oils for their patients are neroli, petitgrain, chamomile, valerian, and opopanax.

International Flavors and Fragrance researchers have patented a blend of neroli, valerian, and nutmeg to ease stress in the workplace. Aromatherapists class ylang-ylang among the most potent of all aromatherapy relaxants.

Essential Oils to Reduce Stress

basil	jasmine	petitgrain
bergamot	lavender	rose
cardamom	marjoram	sandalwood
clove	melissa	valerian
chamomile	myrrh	vanilla
clary sage	neroli	ylang-ylang
frankincense	nutmeg	helicrysum
orange		

Sedative Formula

8 drops lavender

4 drops sandalwood

4 drops bergamot

4 drops chamomile

3 drops ylang-ylang

2 drops petitgrain

4 ounces vegetable oil

Combine ingredients.

Aphrodisiacs

Research tells us that many of the fragrances known traditionally as aphrodisiacs both stimulate and relax brain waves. Examples are ylang-ylang, rose, patchouli, sandalwood, and jasmine. Aphrodisiacs that are primarily stimulants include cinnamon and coriander (named as an aphrodisiac in *The Arabian Nights*). Both of these essential oils may also be used to relieve stress.

Aphrodisiac Oils

cinnamon	patchouli	vanilla
coriander	rose	ylang-ylang
jasmine	sandalwood	

Aphrodisiac Formula

12 drops sandalwood

5 drops ylang-ylang

5 drops vanilla

1 drop cinnamon

1 drop jasmine

4 ounces vegetable oil

Combine ingredients.

Spiritual

Throughout the world, ancient cultures have regarded incense as a mediator between the worshippers and deity, a creator of ethereal roads along which prayers travel. Aromas that smell "heavenly" were acknowledged to have powers of purification; less pleasant odors were thought to bring on disease or death, or to cleanse the impure. A special reverence was given trees, for they seemed to join earth and sky (again, the mundane with the divine); their smoke, therefore, was used to communicate between these worlds. Sandalwood, the famous "cedars of Lebanon," Tibetan cedar, American cedar, juniper, cypress, and camphor were just a few of these holy trees whose sap was correlated with blood and took its place in ritual practices. Rosemary and marjoram were included because they represented both birth and death, and were used at both weddings and funerals. Lavender is still burned with heavier resins such as myrrh in some Greek Orthodox churches.

Spiritual Essential Oils

camphor	juniper	rosemary
cedar	lavender	sandalwood
cypress	marjoram	
Frankincense	myrrh	

Spiritual Formula

8 drops sandalwood

8 drops cedarwood

6 drops lavender

2 drops frankincense

2 drops myrrh

Combine ingredients.

—From *Pocket Guide to Aromatherapy*

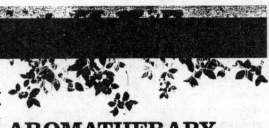

AROMATHERAPY AND SKIN CARE

Kathi Keville

The techniques and the essential oils you choose for your overall skin care should be based on your complexion type. There are several different types of complexions, the most distinctive being dry and oily. There is also a "mature" complexion (generally dry) and a "problem" complexion, associated with the kinds of conditions—such as blackheads and acne. A "couperose" complexion is sensitive skin that has fine red lines on the nose or cheeks; treat it according to whether it is oily or dry. (Essential oils that decrease inflammation will help to reduce the redness.) Many people fall into more than one skin-type category, and as a result need to be treated as though they possess two or more different complexions.

Facial Techniques Suitable for Most Complexion Types

A facial is one of the kindest things you can give your complexion. The complete treatment includes cleansing, steaming, exfoliation, and a mask, topped off with a facial toner or cream. All of these techniques increase circulation, giving your face a healthful and radiant glow. Exfoliation and steaming may be done once a week on complexions other than extremely dry or delicate skin (such as couperose). Delicate and dry complexions can use masks once a week, but stick to the gentler ones. Toners may be used as an all-over body treatment, as a facial, or as an after-shave.

Cleansing: Clean your face gently with cold cream or vegetable oil after removing any makeup.

Steaming: Besides cleansing and leaving your face looking youthful and vibrant, steaming moisturizes skin and unclogs pores.

Exfoliation: A gentle scrubbing that removes dead skin cells from the skin's surface, brings young, fresh skin to the surface, stimulates growth of underlying cells, and even gives the impression of diminishing wrinkles. Avoid the chemical exfoliants used in some beauty salons.

Mask: A facial mask absorbs, moisturizes, and may (depending upon the ingredients) remineralize the skin. Astringent masks of oats, cream of wheat, and clay also exfoliate the skin. Gentler masks include honey, avocado, egg whites, and fresh fruits such as papaya and yogurt. Adding the appropriate ground herbs will increase the skin-healing properties.
Toning: Astringent toners draw water from underlying skin levels to the surface, temporarily plumping it up and diminishing enlarged pores and wrinkles. They offer oily and "problem" skins a good alternative to oil-based moisturizers, and can double as a men's aftershave.

Facial Steam

5 drops lavender

5 drops rosemary

5 drops geranium

One quart boiling water

Bring water to a simmer, remove from heat, and add essential oils. Holding your face about twelve inches above the pan, place the towel over the back of your head and tuck the ends around the pan to enclose your face in a miniature sauna. Be sure to keep your eyes closed so they won't be irritated by the essential oils. Steam for a few minutes, then remove your head and take a few breaths of fresh air. Go back under the towel and repeat a few times. (Steam for no longer than five or ten minutes per session, or less if you have sensitive skin.)

Facial Scrub

3 tablespoons oatmeal

1 tablespoon cornmeal

water, tea, or hydrosol to moisten

Grind ingredients in an electric coffee grinder. Store powder in a closed container. To use the scrub, moisten one teaspoon with enough water, tea, or hydrosol to make a paste. Apply to a dampened face. Gently scrub and rinse with warm water.

Exfoliating Mask

1 tablespoon finely ground oats, or clay

1 teaspoon honey, slightly heated

1 drop carrot seed oil

1–2 teaspoons aloe vera juice (or herb tea)

Mash oats or clay into a thin paste with honey and aloe. Stir in essential oil. Apply to the face in an even layer, avoiding sensitive areas around eyes and mouth. Leave on 5–30 minutes, or as long as comfortable. (Don't allow the mask to dry or pull so much that it becomes irritating.) Finally, wash the mask off with warm water and gently pat the face dry.

Dry Skin

Cleanser: Instead of soap, which is drying, use a water-soluble cleansing cream that won't remove natural skin oils. Do this no more than once per day. Gently pat skin dry.

Steaming: Restrict steaming to five minutes every other week.

Exfoliation: Gently massage face for two minutes with a gentle oatmeal scrub to stimulate oil production and exfoliate flaky, dry surface skin.

Mask: Moisturize with an emollient mask of honey,

Continued ➡

yogurt, avocados, or egg yolks. Avoid drying clay masks.

Toning: Moisturize with a cream, a toner made with aloe vera, or a hydrosol to increase water content. Diluted apple-cider vinegar relieves the itching and flakiness of dry skin. Avoid alcohol, which is too drying.

Moisturizing: Use rich facial creams, and makeups that contain moisturizers.

ESSENTIAL OILS FOR DRY SKIN

The following oils balance skin-oil production, and most reduce puffiness and rejuvenate skin by encouraging new cell growth. If your dry skin is also mature skin, use the classic "anti-aging" ingredients: lavender, geranium, neroli, rosemary, and rose.

carrot seed	jasmine	peppermint
chamomile	lavender	frankincense
cistus	myrrh	palmarosa
neroli	geranium	rosewood
helichrysum	sandalwood	
rosemary (especially the chemo type verbenone)		

Dry-complexion Cleanser

8 drops sandalwood

4 drops rosemary

½ teaspoon grapefruit-seed extract

2 ounces aloe gel

1 teaspoon glycerin

1 teaspoon vegetable oil

Blend ingredients. Shake well before each use. Apply with cotton pads, then rinse off. I like to use an infused herb oil of calendula for the vegetable oil.

Dry-complexion Toner

6 drops geranium

4 drops sandalwood

1 drop chamomile

1 drop jasmine (optional)

800 IUs vitamin E oil

2 ounces aloe vera gel

2 ounces orange blossom water

1 teaspoon vinegar

Combine ingredients. Shake before using. To obtain liquid vitamin E oil, you may pop open a couple of 400 IU vitamin E gel capsules. Jasmine is "optional" only because it is so expensive.

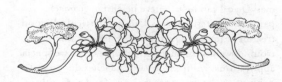

Oily Skin

Cleanser: Clean at least twice a day with a neutral pH soap, or with cleansing gel and water.

Steaming: Steam weekly to unclog pores and release excess oil.

Exfoliation: Use a mild abrasive such as corn meal mixed with oatmeal, but don't scrub vigorously, which will stimulate oil production.

Mask: Both oats and clay draw excess skin oils, but be sure to rinse before skin begins to feel tight or itchy.

Toning: Aloe vera, hydrosols, and witch hazel improve the complexion without adding oil. Grain alcohol in a tincture such as witch hazel dries the skin, although too much will cause the skin to compensate by producing even more oil.

Moisturizing: Use a light lotion instead of a cream. Just a little oil will encourage the skin to cut down on its own oil production.

ESSENTIAL OILS FOR OILY SKIN

The following oils normalize overactive sebaceous glands, slowing oil production.

basil	cypress	sage
cedarwood	eucalyptus	spike lavender
citruses	lemongrass	ylang-ylang

Oily-skin Cleanser

1 teaspoon vinegar

1 teaspoon glycerin

½ teaspoon grapefruit seed extract

6 drops lemon

2 drops cypress

2 drops grapefruit (optional)

2 ounces witch hazel

Follow the instructions given at left for dry-skin cleanser. If available, you can use an herbal vinegar. I make my own yarrow vinegar for this formula, but a basil or sage vinegar from the grocery store is fine.

Toner for Oily or "Problem" Complexion

5 drops cedarwood

3 drops lemon

1 drop ylang-ylang

1 tablespoon aloe vera

2 ounces witch hazel

Combine ingredients. Shake well before using. Without the ylang-ylang, which is too sweet-smelling for most men, this makes an excellent aftershave for men.

"Problem" Skin

Cleanser: Treat affected skin up to three times per day with a pH-balanced cleanser.

Steaming: Steam once or twice per week. Scrubbing and exfoliants only aggravate acne.

Mask: An astringent mask of clay mixed with anti-bacterial essential oils promotes peeling and reduces enlarged pores. A papaya mask will gently exfoliate.

Toning: Diluted cider vinegar is antiseptic and helps maintain the skin's acid balance. Antiseptic hydrosols or aloe vera (with its skin-healing properties and pH of 4,3) are excellent toners.

Moisturizing: Use light lotions containing mostly aloe vera.

ESSENTIAL OILS FOR "PROBLEM" SKIN

The following oils are antiseptic and drying.

clary sage	tea tree	eucalyptus
juniper	lavender	neroli
sage		
thyme (especially chemotype linalol)		
rosemary (especially chemotype verbenone)		

Zit Remover

4 drops lavender

1 teaspoon Epsom salts

¼ cup water

Bring water to a boil and pour over salts. When the salts have dissolved, add the essential oil. Soak a small absorbent cloth in the solution and press this compress onto the pimple. In a minute or two, as it starts to cool, place the cloth back in hot water, then reapply. Repeat several times. The lavender is antiseptic and anti-inflammatory.

Intensive Treatment for Acne

12 drops tea tree

½ teaspoon goldenseal root, powdered

water

Combine ingredients, adding water to create a paste. Apply directly onto acne spots. Let dry and remain on the skin for at least twenty minutes. Rinse.

Fungal and Viral Skin Infections

Aromatherapy offers many treatments against fungal and viral infections such as warts, herpes, and the related shingles virus, which causes the skin to break out in blisters along nerve endings. Treat these conditions externally by diluting an essential oil of tea tree, or with the closely related eucalyptus (especially lemon eucalyptus) in an equal amount of vegetable oil or alcohol and applying it directly to the blisters. Other excellent antiviral and anti-fungal oils are lavender, myrrh, and geranium. If applied to herpes as soon as the blisters begin to appear, these oils will often prevent a breakout. Small amounts of peppermint relieve the itching of a fungal infection, and sometimes diminish the nerve-tingling pain of herpes and shingles.

Research shows that creams made from capsaicin, a compound found in cayenne, deadens the pain of herpes and shingles. Essential oils of cayenne will work if added to a cream or oil base, but be sure to go easy with it, since too much can burn the skin.

Use the same essential oils on skin warts, which are yet another type of virus. Tea tree and thuja are two of the most effective essential oils, even in cases of skin or genital warts. However, if genital warts don't begin to disappear in a few weeks or so, have a doctor remove them. The virus that causes them is passed onto sexual partners and can eventually lead to cervical dysplasia in women.

Many different types of fungal infections appear on the skin, but athlete's foot is the most common. A fungal powder (such as that described below) or plain vinegar provide the best base for a remedy to treat fungal infections. Both the powder and vinegar are drying.

Anti-fungal Powder

12 drops tea tree (or eucalyptus)

6 drops geranium

2 tablespoons bentonite clay

Drop essential oils into clay and mix well. Apply to the problem area. If you prefer a liquid formula, add these same ingredients to ½ cup apple-cider vinegar. A soft cloth soaked in the solution makes an excellent compress.

Wart Oil

12 drops tea tree

5 drops thuja

¼ ounce castor oil

800 IU vitamin E oil

Combine ingredients. Apply two to four times per day with a glass rod or cotton swab to the warts only, since these essential oils can burn sensitive skin. If necessary, protect surrounding skin with a coating of herbal salve.

Continued ➡

Herpes Formula

10 drops tea tree (especially chemotype niaouli)

10 drops myrrh

4 drops geranium

1 ounce vodka

Apply to affected area at least two to three times per day.

Bathing

Bathing with essential oils is the ultimate aromatherapy treatment. The essential and vegetable oils float on the surface of the water and make your bath smell heavenly. When you emerge, the oils cling to your skin, scenting you for hours. Bath salts are another luxurious addition to your bath water, making the water feel silky, removing body oils and perspiration, softening the skin, relaxing the muscles, and soaking away the stresses of the day.

Floating Aromatic Bath Oil

1/2 teaspoon essential oil (your choice)

1 ounce vegetable oil

Combine ingredients. Use one teaspoon per bath. For babies, use only a few drops in the basin.

Aromatic Bath Salts

1/2 teaspoon essential oil (your choice)

1 cup sea salt

1/2 cup borax

1/2 cup baking soda

Mix salts together and add essential oils, mixing well to combine. Use 1/4 to 1/2 cup of the bath salts per bath. For muscular aches and pains, add 1/2 cup Epsom salts to this recipe. (All of the salts mentioned are sold in grocery stores.)

Hair Care

Whether you have dry, normal, or oily hair, essential oils have something to offer you. Besides making shampoos and hair rinses, you can run a couple drops of essential oil directly through the hair, which holds fragrance even better than skin, so you will remain fragrant for hours.

OILS FOR DRY HAIR

cedarwood   rosewood   sandalwood

OILS FOR OILY HAIR

cypress   lemongrass   patchouli

OILS FOR ALL HAIR TYPES

chamomile   lavender   rosemary

OILS FOR DANDRUFF

cedarwood   sage   tea tree
geranium

OILS TO COUNTERACT HAIR LOSS

basil   peppermint   ylang-ylang
cedarwood

Herbal Shampoo

1/4 teaspoon essential oil (your choice)

2 ounces unscented shampoo

2 ounces strong herb tea (your choice)

After straining and cooling, add tea to the shampoo base, then add the essential oils. Shake well before using. Use a mild and pH-balanced shampoo as the base for this recipe. Baby shampoos, which are generally made from olive and soy oils, are a good choice.

Herbal Hair Rinse

3–5 drops essential oil (your choice)

1 pint of water or herb tea

4 tablespoons vinegar or lemon juice (optional)

Shake well and pour over the scalp and hair after shampooing. Leave on for several minutes, then rinse. This formula balances the pH after shampooing, reversing the electrical charge so your hair doesn't have a flyaway look, and removes shampoo residues, leaving hair shiny and soft.

—From *Pocket Guide to Aromatherapy*

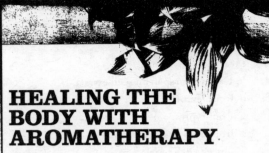

HEALING THE BODY WITH AROMATHERAPY

Kathi Keville

Most essential oils are germ-fighters, but their beneficial properties do not stop there. Essential oils can be digestive tonics, circulatory stimulants, or hormone precursors. Some oils even stimulate production of phagocytes, white blood cells that rid the body of pathogens. Fortunately, many essential oils perform more than one function, so you need only become familiar with a dozen or so to be able to tend to a wide range of common ailments.

When using aromatherapy to treat physical ailments, stick to simple disorders that you would self-diagnose and treat at home anyway, such as a minor sore throat or a bout of indigestion. Think of the remedies in this section as "over-the-counter" preparations. For more serious problems, be sure to seek the advice of a health professional, preferably one skilled in holistic healing and aromatherapy.

Although this section deals mostly with treating internal problems, essential oils are usually applied externally in a vegetable oil or alcohol base. Since the tiny molecules in essential oils are easily absorbed through the skin and into the bloodstream, external application concentrates them where they are needed. A massage oil blend designed to ease a stomach ache, for example, may be rubbed directly over the abdomen. It's also a good idea to also investigate complementary methods of healing—especially herbs, body work, diet, and lifestyle changes.

Increasing Immunity

Some of the same essential oils that are powerful antiseptic, also encourage the immune system and increase the rate of healing. Many such oils fight infection by stimulating the production of white corpuscles, part of the body's immune defense. Still others encourage new cell growth to promote faster healing. All these oils can be used in conjunction with herbal remedies designed to increase immunity.

One important way to assist your immune system is with a lymphatic massage using essential oils in massage oil. The lymphatic system is responsible for moving cellular fluid through the system, cleansing the body of waste produced through the body's simple metabolic functions. Lymph nodes in the throat, groin, breasts, under the arms, and elsewhere are filtering centers for the blood. Among the best essential oils for the lymphatic system are true bay (*Laurus nobilis*), lemon, rosemary, and grapefruit. A lymphatic massage involves deep strokes that work from the extremities toward the heart. You can even massage yourself, rubbing the oil up your arms toward the lymph nodes in your armpits, and down your neck toward the chest.

Essential Oils for Immunity

cinnamon	lemon	tea tree
eucalyptus	oregano	thyme
lavender	sage	

Oils That Stimulate Production of White Corpuscles

bergamot	lemon	sandalwood
chamomile	myrrh	thyme
lavender	pine	vetiver

OILS THAT ENCOURAGE NEW CELL GROWTH

garlic	lavender	sandalwood
geranium	rose	

Basic Immune Stimulant Blend

12 drops lavender

12 drops bergamot

5 drops tea tree

5 drops ravensare

5 drops caulophyllum inophyllum (if available)

4 ounces vegetable oil

Combine ingredients. Use as a general massage oil over areas of the body that tend to develop physical problems. For example, if you get a lot of chest colds and flus, rub this blend over your chest.

Lymph Massage Oil

12 drops lemon

12 drops rosemary

12 drops grapefruit

6 drops true bay (*Laurus nobilis*)

4 ounces vegetable oil

Combine ingredients.

Indigestion

The same essential oils that make food tasty help you digest the meals they flavor. Simply inhale the aromas of these herbs (see list below) and a signal is sent to the brain that begins a chain reaction. Your stomach starts grumbling in anticipation as digestive fluids are pumped into the digestive tract to help you assimilate the approaching meal. (Note: Smelling the essential oils of dill and of fennel may *decrease* the appetite.)

Putting essential oils that help digestion in a massage oil can help relieve belching, stomach pains, and intestinal gas. This is a particularly good treatment for young children or anyone who has trouble swallowing medicine. Some oils have special applications: cumin relieves headaches due to indigestion; rosemary improves poor food absorption; lemongrass relieves nervous indigestion; peppermint treats irritable-bowel syndrome. To overcome nausea, even from chemotherapy, try basil. Peppermint and ginger ease nausea and motion sickness. Chamomile, fennel, and melissa relax the stomach and soothe burning irritation and inflammation. Black pepper and juniper berries increase stomach acid; you can even sprinkle pepper on your meals, or chew a couple of juniper berries before eating, to obtain enough essential oil to do the trick.

GENERAL DIGESTIVE AIDS

anise	cumin	oregano
basil	ginger	peppermint
chamomile	lemongrass	rosemary
cinnamon	melissa	thyme
coriander		

Continued ➡

Digestive Massage Oil

12 drops orange

8 drops ginger

5 drops peppermint

3 drops fennel

4 ounces vegetable oil

Combine ingredients. Rub into abdomen. This all-purpose formula will help improve the appetite and digestion, and prevent nausea. (This formula can also be converted into a tea blend—see Dilutions and Doses, page 133 for proportions.)

Children's Bath for Indigestion

2 drops lemongrass

1 drop orange

1 drop chamomile

Add directly to bath water. Stir to distribute on the water's surface before getting into the tub.

Infections

Almost all essential oils are more or less antiseptic, destroying bacteria, fungi, yeast, parasites, and/or viruses. One way to use these essential oils for preventive medicine—even for internal infections—is in your bath. Another method is to rub a massage oil that contains them over the afflicted area. To treat a vaginal infection, douching brings the essential oils in direct contact with the yeast or bacteria that is causing the discomfort.

Bladder Infection Relief

8 drops tea tree

3 drops ravensare (if available)

3 drops fennel

1 ounce vegetable oil

Use as a massage oil applied over the kidney and bladder area two to three times per day. For a preventive treatment if you tend to get bladder infections, add a tablespoon of this oil to your bath.

Douche

3 drops lavender

3 drops tea tree

3 cups warm water

2 heaping tablespoons yogurt (optional)

3 cups water

Combine ingredients in a douche bag. Mix well. Use this douche once a day during an active infection. The yogurt helps establish the natural flora of the vagina and keeps the essential oils evenly distributed throughout the water. You can use these same essential oils, diluted in vegetable oil, as massage oil to rub on the abdomen, or add a few drops to a bath or a sitz bath.

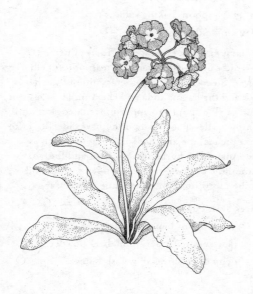

Menopause

Several essential oils that contain hormonelike substances related to estrogen are advantageous during menopause. These include clary sage, anise, fennel, angelica, coriander, and sage. Geranium and lavender are reported to be hormonal balancers. They modify menopause symptoms and relieve hot flashes. One of the easiest ways to employ them is as a bath or body oil.

Menopause symptoms can also include a dry, less-elastic vagina. An excellent essential oil to relieve this is neroli. A few drops can be added to a commercial cream—just stir it in with a toothpick—or you can blend the Rejuvenation Oil suggested below. If you buy a cream, choose one that is made with all-natural products.

In addition to these aromatherapy suggestions, seek out information on dietary and herbal treatments that may make menopause smoother.

Hormone Essential Oils

angelica	coriander	sage
anise	fennel	
clary sage	lavender and geranium (balancing)	

Menopause Body Oil

12 drops lemon

6 drops clary sage

6 drops peppermint (optional)

5 drops angelica

5 drops fennel

4 ounces vegetable oil

Combine ingredients. Use daily as a body oil. If this formula is too oily for you, add these same essential oils to four ounces of a commercial body lotion instead. The best type to use is an unscented, basic lotion with all-natural ingredients.

Rejuvenation Oil

6 drops rose geranium

6 drops lavender

1 drop neroli (expensive, and therefore optional)

1500 units vitamin E oil

1 ounces vegetable oil

Combine ingredients. (To obtain the vitamin E, either buy the liquid vitamin or open vitamin capsules and empty the contents.) Apply around and in the vagina as needed.

Nerve and Joint Pain

Essential oils of lavender, helichrysum, chamomile, and marjoram are all specific for nerve pain. I know several people with serious problems related to the nervous system, such as multiple sclerosis and chronic fatigue syndrome, who get pain relief from the Nerve Pain Oil presented below. While it may not offer a cure, it can certainly improve the quality of life. For carpal tunnel syndrome, rub this oil into the wrists. Use it on the back or hip for a pinched nerve or sciatica, and on shingles (a painful skin eruption related to herpes) to reduce pain. For arthritis, rheumatism, and other inflammatory conditions, use chamomile, marjoram, birch, and ginger.

Nerve conditions can be difficult to heal, so talk to someone skilled in natural medicine for more ideas on how to treat them.

Nerve Pain Relief

4 drops lavender

3 drops marjoram

3 drops helichrysum (if available)

2 drops chamomile

1 ounce vegetable oil

Combine ingredients. Apply as needed for relief.

Arthritic Pain Formula

4 drops birch

3 drops marjoram

3 drops lavender

2 drops ginger

1 ounce vegetable oil

Combine ingredients. Apply as needed for relief.

PMS and Menstrual Cramps

Any woman who has experienced menstrual cramps or symptoms of premenstrual syndrome (PMS) knows how uncomfortable both conditions can be. Fortunately, there are essential oils that reduce painful cramping and most of the problems accompanying PMS. Research shows some oils lower prostaglandin 2, a hormonal substance that causes blood-sugar imbalances, headaches, bowel changes, nausea, breast tenderness and cysts, joint pain, and water retention, while contributing to moodiness, irritability, and alcohol cravings—all common PMS symptoms. Among the essential oils that help reduce menstrual cramps are muscle relaxants such as chamomile, lavender, marjoram, and melissa. The best way to use them? I suggest a long, relaxing bath or massage.

Essential Oils for Cramps and PMS

chamomile	garlic	marjoram
cinnamon	ginger	melissa
cloves	lavender	thyme

Menstrual Cramp and PMS Oil

12 drops lavender

6 drops marjoram

4 drops chamomile

4 drops ginger

2 ounces vegetable oil

Combine ingredients and apply as often as needed over cramping area. This formula is also excellent for the low-back pain that sometimes accompanies menstrual cramps.

Sinus and Respiratory Congestion

Ninety percent of respiratory ailments are caused by viruses. Fortunately, several essential oils inhibit viruses, including most of the viruses responsible for flus and colds. Some oils contribute to loosening and eliminating lung and sinus congestion, making them excellent cold, flu, and hay fever remedies. Along with essential oil of peppermint and eucalyptus, anise reduces coughing and also relaxes muscle spasms around the lungs.

Anyone who has ever sniffed black pepper, eucalyptus, peppermint, or pine knows how just smelling these essential oils helps clear the sinuses. Cypress will dry up a persistent runny nose. As an extra benefit, all these oils fight the bacterial infections that so often accompany a cold or flu.

A throat spray or gargle brings the essential oils into direct contact with a sore throat or laryngitis. Vapor balms, in addition to carrying the oils, increase circulation and warmth in the chest, important factors in fighting infection. Warm, moist steam opens nasal and bronchial passages,

Continued →

making it easier to breathe, and brings the essential oils to infected sinuses and lungs. Essential oils can be used in a humidifier, or on low heat in a pan of water, to disinfect the air. *Caution:* black pepper, cinnamon, and thyme are fine in a vapor balm or gargle, but steaming with them can irritate the respiratory tract.

When steaming is impractical, use a natural nasal inhaler. You can buy one in natural-food stores, or make your own with the formula below.

Antiviral Essential Oils

bergamot	cinnamon	hyssop
black pepper	eucalyptus	melissa
peppermint	rosemary	thyme
ravensara	tea tree	

ESSENTIAL OILS FOR CONGESTION

anise	eucalyptus	pine
benzoin	frankincense	sandalwood
black pepper	myrrh	tea tree
cypress	peppermint	thyme

Steam

3–6 drops essential oils

3 cups water

Bring water to a simmer in a pan. Place a towel over the back of your head and tuck the ends around the pot so the steam is captured inside the improvised "tent." Take deep breaths of the steam for as long as is comfortable.

Homemade Nasal Inhaler

5 drops eucalyptus

1/4 teaspoon coarse salt

Place the salt in a small vial (glass is best) with a tight lid, and add oil. The salt will absorb the oil and provide a convenient way of carrying the oil without spilling it. When needed, open the vial and inhale deeply. This same technique can be used with any essential oil.

Throat Spray/Gargler

5 drops thyme or sage

1/2 cup water

1/2 teaspoon salt

Shake well to disperse the oils before gargling. Gargle a small amount throughout the day.

Vapor Rub

12 drops eucalyptus

5 drops peppermint

5 drops thyme

1 ounce olive oil

Combine ingredients in a glass bottle. Shake well to mix oils evenly. Gently massage into chest and throat.

Varicose Veins and Hemorrhoids

Medical doctors offer patients with varicose veins or hemorrhoids little hope of recovery except through surgery. I have seen essential oils of chamomile, palmarosa, myrtle, frankincense, and cypress (best

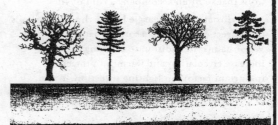

when added to an infused oil of St. John's wort) reduce the size of blood vessels associated with these problems, and also ease the inflammation and pain they cause. If the skin is ulcerated and broken, apply a compress of carrot seed essential oil. With either condition, be sure to work on ways to improve your circulation with increased exercise, improved diet, and a good herbal program.

Varicose Vein and Hemorrhoid Formula

6 drops cypress

3 drops myrtle

3 drops German chamomile

2 drops frankincense (optional)

1 ounce St. John's wort herb oil (or vegetable oil)

Combine ingredients. Apply externally. You can buy St John's wort infused oil in natural food stores.

Carrot Seed Compress

8 drops carrot seed

1/2 cup water

Add essential oil to water. Slosh a soft cloth in water, wring out, fold, and place over ulcerated veins.

—From *Pocket Guide to Aromatherapy*

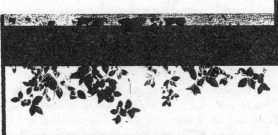

MOTHER AND BABY CARE

Kathi Keville

The gentlest oils are your best choices for use on babies and young children, and also during pregnancy. For pregnant women and children, use only one-third the amount of essential oils required in similar formulas for adults. Be cautious about using essential oils at all during the first trimester of pregnancy; even oils that are generally considered safe may be too stimulating for a woman who is prone to miscarriage.

Essential Oils for Mother and Child

chamomile	jasmine	sandalwood
citruses	lavender	spearmint
frankincense	neroli	ylang-ylang
geranium	rose	

Pregnancy

Massage and aromatherapy can help prevent stretch marks from forming as a pregnant woman's belly expands. If possible, apply the belly oil at least twice per day. Lavender is one of the gentlest essential oils, and excellent for keeping skin supple. It is also an old companion in the birthing room, and many women still appreciate being massaged with this oil during labor to help them relax. After birth, add a couple drops of clary sage to the belly oil to help counter postpartum depression.

Belly Oil

1/2 ounce cocoa butter

4 ounces vegetable oil

25 drops (1/4 teaspoon) lavender

5 drops neroli

1600 IU vitamin E

Put oil and cocoa butter in a pan over low heat. Melt the cocoa butter (sold in drug stores), then remove from heat. Stir in essential oils and vitamin E, and bottle. (Obtain vitamin E by popping open a few capsules or buying it as a liquid.) Massage your belly with the oil—or get someone to do it for you—at least once per day.

Diaper Rash

Aromatherapy baby oil and powder are good ways to protect your baby from diaper rash. The oil forms a barrier on the skin to repel moisture; the powder absorbs moisture and prevents chafing. Use one or the other with every diaper change, or more often if needed.

Baby oil also makes an excellent massage oil for babies. However, commercial baby oils and ointments are typically made from petroleum-based mineral oil, a good machinery lubricant but questionable for use on the skin. By the same token, commercial baby powders often contain talc, which may be contaminated with asbestos or other harmful substances. A good alternative is to make your own baby oils and powders.

Herbal Baby Oil

12 drops lavender

4 drops chamomile

4 ounces vegetable oil

Combine ingredients.

Fragrant Baby Powder

25 drops (1/4 teaspoon) lavender

1/2 pound cornstarch

Put the cornstarch in a plastic zippered bag and drop in the essential oils. Tightly close the bag and toss back and forth to distribute the oil, breaking up any clumps by pressing them with your fingers through the bag. Let stand at least four days, continuing to break up the clumps. Spice or salt shakers with large perforations in the lid make good powder dispensers.

Hives

Hives—rashlike skin bumps that can drive kids (as well as their parents) crazy with itching—are a symptom of food allergy. Of course, it is a good idea to address the dietary causes of the problem, but the immediate need is to stop the itching. Wash off the child's skin with the following herbal wash. If this does not provide enough relief, apply the herbal poultice. You may find that even a child who normally objects to having a poultice smeared on his or her skin will accept whatever will stop the itching of hives.

Hives Skin Wash

10 drops chamomile

3 tablespoons baking soda

2 cups elderflower tea

First make an extra strong tea by pouring 2½ cups of boiling water over four teaspoons of elderflower. Steep 15 minutes, then strain out the herbs. Now add the baking soda and chamomile. Use a soft cloth or skin sponge to apply on irritated skin until itching is alleviated. If you don't have elderflower to make the tea, use another soothing herb such as calendula. If no herbs are available, add the chamomile to plain water. Lavender essential oil can be substituted for chamomile if necessary.

Hives Skin Poultice

3 tablespoons bentonite clay

1 tablespoon slippery-elm-bark powder

1/4 cup of the hives skin wash (above)

Continued →

Stir all the ingredients into a paste and wait about five minutes for it to thicken. Apply to irritated skin with your fingers or a tongue depressor. Let dry on skin; leave at least 45 minutes before washing.

Restlessness

One of the most relaxing treatments for children before bedtime—or anytime—is a warm lavender and chamomile essential-oil bath. To completely relax the child, follow the bath with an aromatherapy massage. You can also send children off to dreamland with a "dilly pillow" filled with the herbs lavender, hops, chamomile, and dill.

Relaxing Bath

2 drops lavender

1 drop orange

1 drop chamomile

Add oils directly to bath and stir to distribute.

Relaxing Children's Massage Oil

3 drops lavender

2 drops orange

1 drop chamomile

1 drop ylang-ylang (optional)

2 ounces vegetable oil

Combine ingredients. Use for massage as needed.

Dilly Pillow

Equal parts:

Lavender flowers

Hops strobilus

Chamomile flowers

Dill seeds

5-by 10-inch piece of cloth.

Fold the cloth in half (so it measures 5 by 5 inches) and sew the edges, leaving a few inches open for stuffing. Combine the herbs and stuff them into the pillow, then sew closed. Slip this pillow inside the child's pillowcase. Add thyme to prevent nightmares.

Teething

To relieve teething pain, rub the child's gums with a little clove-bud essential oil on your finger. This can be hot stuff, so make sure the oil is diluted enough by trying it in your own mouth first.

Teething Oil

1 drop orange

4 drops clove bud

1 tablespoon vegetable oil

Combine ingredients. Rub a few drops on painful gums. Repeat every half hour or so. If your child refuses the clove teething oil, try replacing the clove with chamomile, which is a less effective pain reliever but isn't hot like the clove.

—From *Pocket Guide to Aromatherapy*

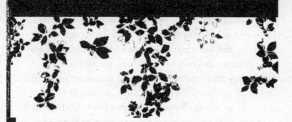

MATERIA MEDICA: SIXTY COMMON ESSENTIAL OILS

Kathi Keville

From Angelica to Ylang-Ylang

Angelica *(Angelica archangelica)*

Magical powers have been attributed to this "root of the Holy Ghost," once a common flavoring and apothecary drug. The oil distilled from the seed of this herb is spicy and peppery. The root oil, which is stronger and slightly more expensive than the seed, smells earthier and more herbal. The fragrance of angelica gives depressed people a new outlook on life. Both seed and root oils regulate menstruation and digestion, and also stop coughing. However, use angelica very carefully because it can overstimulate the nervous system. The root oil also contains the photosensitive agent bergapten.

Anise *(Pimpinella anisum)*

The delightful licorice-like scent and taste of this herb flavors pharmaceuticals, confections, toothpaste, "licorice" candy (in the U.S.), and alcoholic beverages such as French anisette and Greek ouzo. Anise reduces muscle spasms, indigestion, and coughing. It is also mildly estrogenic, and an aphrodisiac. It increases breast milk, balances emotions, induces sleep, and helps overcome nervousness and workaholic stress. Anise is even said to improve your sense of humor and overcome heartache. Large quantities, however, may be narcotic, slow down circulation, and cause skin rashes in sensitive people.

Basil *(Ocimum basilicum)*

Distilled from the leaves and flowering tops, this familiar sweet-and-spicy kitchen herb relieves headaches, sinus congestion, temporary loss of smell, nausea (even from chemotherapy), indigestion, sore muscles, and the herpes and shingles viruses. Basil gently stimulates adrenal glands, menstruation, childbirth, and production of breast milk. Basil reduces stress, rattled nerves, hysteria, and mental fatigue while increasing confidence, decisiveness, positive thoughts, and awareness of one's surroundings. Large doses can be overstimulating and may stupefy.

Bay *(Laurus nobilis)*

A pungent, spicy aroma is distilled from the leaf and, occasionally, the berry of the bay tree (also called bay laurel), which stimulants lymph and circulation while relieving sinus and lung congestion. It improves the memory; hence, the Ancient Greeks placed bay wreaths on the heads of scholars—and headache sufferers! The priestesses at Delphi sat over burning bay fumes to induce prophetic visions. If you purchase "bay," it is most likely bay rum *(Pimenta racemosa)*, which is cooler and sweeter and is used to scent colognes, soaps, and cosmetics. Unlike true bay, bay rum can irritate delicate skin and mucous membranes.

Benzoin *(Styrax benzoin)*

The sweet, vanilla-like absolute is solvent-extracted from the tree's gum resin. In India, benzoin is sacred to the Brahma-Shiva-Vishnu triad of deities. Malays use it to fend off evil during rice-harvesting ceremonies. It is antiseptic and antifungal, protects chapped skin, and increases skin elasticity. It is helpful for those who feel anxious, emotionally blocked, lonely, or exhausted, especially after a life crisis. Balsam of tolu *(Myroxylon balsamum)* and balsam of Peru *(M. balsamum, var. Pereirae)* are gum resins with similar aromas and properties. Avoid benzoin oils thinned with ethyl glycol.

Bergamot *(Citrus bergamia)*

This fresh, clean scent is cold-pressed from the almost-ripe rind of a small, green citrus fruit. Named after Bergamo, Italy, where the oil originated, it scents colognes, and flavors Earl Grey tea and some candies. It is also used as a deodorizer. Bergamot aids digestion, and reduces inflammation and infection in the genitorurinary system, mouth, throat, and skin. It kills several viruses, including those responsible for flu, herpes, shingles, and chickenpox, and is a traditional Italian folk medicine to treat fever and intestinal worms. It counters depression, anxiety, insomnia, and compulsive behavior cycles, including eating disorders. Bergamot contains photosensitizing bergapten, although a bergapten-free essential oil is available. Don't confuse *Citrus bergamia* with common garden bergamot *(Monarda didyma)*, also known as "bee balm."

Birch *(Betula lenta)*

The bark of this tree is the source of commercial "wintergreen" oil, since the chemistry, properties, and fragrance of both oils is the same. Birch relieves muscular and arthritic pain, softens skin, soothes irritation and psoriasis, and eliminates dandruff. While people tend to associate birch's scent with medicine or candy, it can be toxic in large amounts, so use carefully.

Camphor *(C. camphora)*

Unlike harsh, synthetic mothballs, the leaves and bark of this tree produce a pleasant oil, woodsy with a hint of cardamom. Camphor counters shock and depression, and helps to focus your attention. Arab cultures use it to reduce sexual desire. White camphor is a heart stimulant and potentially toxic, so use it cautiously—and don't use the even more toxic brown or yellow camphor produced from heavier parts of the oil.

Carrot Seed *(Daucus carota)*

A fruity, sharp, pungent fragrance distilled from the seeds of Queen Anne's lace, ancestor of the common carrot, carrot seed stimulates circulation and treats some genitourinary and digestive disorders. It is also gaining popularity for its ability to

Continued ➡

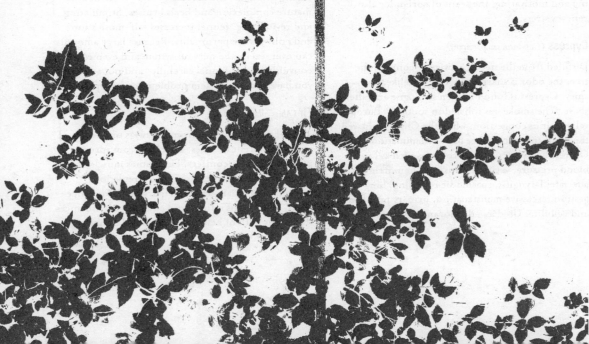

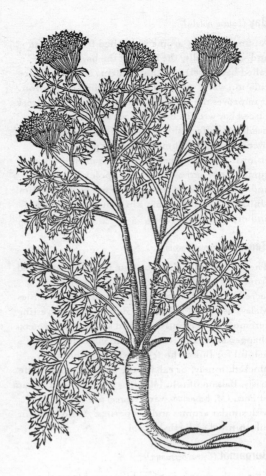

enhance skin tone and elasticity, and decrease dryness, wrinkles, dermatitis, eczema, rashes, and even certain precancerous skin conditions.

Cedarwood (*Cedrus species*)

This soft, woodsy fragrance scents soap and cologne, serving as an astringent for oily skin, acne, dandruff, dermatitis, bites, and itching. Cedar also helps in cases of respiratory and urinary infections. Emotionally, it increases self-respect, integrity, stability, meditation, and intuition, while relieving stress, aggression, and dependency. It repels wool moths and other insects. Moroccan cedar (*C. Ibani*) is the legendary "cedar of Lebanon" prized by ancient cultures. The pinelike Atlantic cedar (*C. atlantica*) is from Morocco. Himalayan cedarwood (*C. deodara*) is warm and spicy, and the least toxic cedar oil. Juniper (*Juniperus virginiana*) is actually the source of most commercial "cedar" oil—and of wood pencils. *Caution:* Avoid all cedars during pregnancy.

Chamomile, German (*Matricaria recutita*, formerly *M. chamomilla*)

A sweet, herbaceous, and applelike aroma is distilled from chamomile's flowers. Chamomile reduces inflammation due to sensitive skin; rashes; boils; sore muscles, tendons, and joints; headaches; asthma; allergies; hemorrhoids; and enlarged veins. It also treats indigestion, light constipation, PMS, menstrual pain, ulcers, and liver damage. A strong antidepressant, chamomile helps overcome oversensitivity, stress, anxiety, hysteria, insomnia, suppressed anger, and hyperactivity. The more expensive German chamomile oil is blue, while the closely related Roman chamomile (*Chamaemelum nobile*, formerly *Anthemis nobilis*) is pale yellow. Also sold as "blue chamomile" are *Ormenis multicaulis*, *Tanacetum annum*, and *Artemisia arborescens*. The last two are potentially toxic, so use them very carefully.

Cinnamon (*Cinnamomum zeylanicum*)

Distilled from the tree's leaf or bark, cinnamon is a sweet, spicy-hot fragrance. The bark is hotter smelling, hotter tasting (it can irritate skin and

especially mucous membranes), and more expensive. Cinnamon stops menstrual cramps, diarrhea, and genito-urinary infections, while increasing sweating and providing heat for liniments. It is an aphrodisiac that relieves tension, steadies nerves, and invigorates the senses. Small amounts spice up Oriental perfume blends. Cassia, or *kuei pi* (*C. cassia*), is an inexpensive substitute from China used in medicine, seasoning, incense, and cola drinks.

Citronella (*Citronella nardus*)

The sharp lemon scent of this grasslike herb is used extensively in cleaning products because it is less expensive than true lemon. It treats colds, infections, and oily complexions, and is considered a physical and emotional purifier. The most popular use of citronella is to ward off insects, especially mosquitoes. It often adulterates expensive lemon verbena and melissa, although it is much harsher and more camphoric, and can irritate the skin.

Clary sage (*Salvia sclarea*)

Although clary is related to common sage, it is quite different: relaxing and euphoric, enhancing dreams and producing smiles. Distilled from the herb's flowering tops, clary's winelike scent is sweet and heady. Clary eases muscle and nervous tension, pain, menstrual cramps, PMS, and menopause problems such as hot flashes, while slightly stimulating the adrenal glands. It also has estrogenic action. In Europe, it is used as a sore throat remedy. Clary helps rejuvenate hair and mature or inflamed skin, and reduces dandruff. It helps in cases of panic, paranoia, mental fatigue, general debility, postpartum depression, and PMS. Avoid large amounts, which can stupefy, and don't combine clary with alcohol.

Clove Bud (*Syzygium aromaticum*, formerly *Eugenia caryophyllata*)

The spicy, hot scent is distilled from the immature buds, leaves, or stems of the tree. Europeans, East Indians, and Chinese still use clove bud oil to sweeten their breath and eliminate toothache. It also treats flu, sore muscles, arthritis, colds, and bronchial congestion, and is a heating liniment. The eugenol from clove is made into drugs that kill germs and pain. As a stimulant, clove helps overcome nervousness, stress, mental fatigue, and poor memory. Avoid the leaf, which can irritate skin and mucous membranes.

Coriander (*Coriandrum sativum*)

The seed of this culinary herb yields a spicy, sharp, distinct fragrance. It soothes inflammation, rheumatic pain, headaches, cystitis, flu, and diarrhea, and is generally antiseptic. Although it was used as a love potion in Medieval times, the fourteenth-century nuns of St. Just included coriander in "Carmelite water," a combined cologne and facial toner. It still scents soaps and deodorants. Uplifting and motivating, the scent of coriander also relieves stress.

Cypress (*Cupressus sempervirens*)

Distilled from the needles, twigs or cones of the tree, the odor is sharp, pungent, pinelike, and spicy. Cypress is found in men's cologne and aftershave. The smoke was inhaled in southern Europe to relieve sinus congestion, while the Chinese chewed the small cones to reduce gum inflammation. Cypress helps circulation problems such as low blood pressure, varicose veins, and hemorrhoids. It alleviates laryngitis, spasmodic coughing, lung congestion, excessive menstruation, urinary problems, and cellulite. Used as a deodorant, cypress reduces

excessive sweating. It also eases insomnia and grief, and increases emotional stamina, helping one to move on after an emotional crisis.

Dill (*Anethum graveolens*)

A sharp herbal scent is distilled from the seed of this culinary herb to treat obesity, water retention, and indigestion. Early Americans chewed the seeds to inhibit their appetite during long church services. Babies with colic were once given "gripe water"—a syrup of dill, fennel, and baking soda—and laid to sleep on fragrant "dilly pillows" of dill, lavender, and chamomile (see page 128). Dill also refines the complexion.

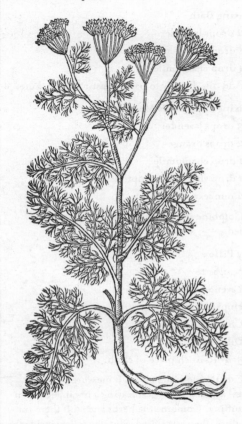

Eucalyptus (*Eucalyptus globules*)

Distilled from leaves and twigs, this essential oil is pungent, sharp, and somewhat camphoric. Eucalyptus oil (or its component eucalyptol) goes into industrial preparations, aftershaves, colognes, mouthwashes, liniments, and vapor rubs. It treats sinus and throat infection, fever, flu, chickenpox, and herpes. It is excellent on oily complexions, especially acne, boils, and insect bites, and for killing lice. The scent alone increases energy, countering physical debility and emotional imbalance.

Fennel (Foeniculum vulgare)

Distilled from the herb's seeds, the scent is herbaceous, sweet, and licorice-like. Fennel decreases obesity, water retention, urinary-tract problems, indigestion, and colic. Its hormonal properties (mostly estrogenic) increase mother's milk and slightly stimulate the adrenal glands. It refines the mature complexion and heals bruises. Stimulating and revitalizing, fennel increases self-motivation and enlivens the personality. Because large amounts can over-excite the nervous system and even cause convulsions, use fennel carefully—and not at all if you have nervous-system problems or epilepsy.

Fir (*Abies alba*)

The oil can be distilled from the twigs or needles of several different fir trees, as well as from spruces, pines, and other conifers. Fir soothes muscle and rheumatism pain, increases poor circulation, inhibits bronchial, genitorurinary, and skin infections, and lessens asthma and coughing. It enhances the senses both of being grounded and of being

Continued ➡

elevated, increases intuition, and releases energy and emotional blocks.

Frankincense (*Boswellia carteri*)

This small tree grows on the rocky hillsides of Yemen, Oman, and Somalia. When distilled, the oleo gum resin produces a soft, balsamic oil. Frankincense treats lung and genitorurinary complaints, ulcers, chronic diarrhea, breast cysts, and excessive menstruation. Use it on mature skin, acne, fungal infections, boils, hard-to-heal wounds, and scars. For centuries, frankincense has been used to increase spirituality, mental perception, meditation, prayer, and consciousness. It fortifies and soothes the spirit, slows and deepens breathing, and is relaxing. It is said to release past links and subconscious stress.

Geranium (*Pelargonium graveoloens*)

The oil is distilled from the leaves of this herb (known as "rose geranium") and smells like a combination of rose, citrus, and herb. A light adrenal-gland stimulant and hormonal normalizer, geranium treats PMS, menopause, fluid retention, breast engorgement, and sterility, and helps to regulate blood pressure. A versatile skin treatment, it reduces inflammation, infection, eczema, acne, burn injuries, bleeding, scarring, stretch marks, shingles, herpes, and ringworm. It is also said to delay wrinkling. Geranium relieves anxiety, depression, discontent, irrational behavior, and stress. It is also used to heal a passive-aggressive nature and to enhance one's perception of time and space. Some aromatherapists describe it as sedative, while others consider it stimulating, but it probably is a balancer.

Ginger (*Zingiber officinale*)

Distilled from the rhizome, the fragrance is spicy, warm, and sharp. Ginger treats colds, fevers, appetite loss, nausea, inflammation, and genito-urinary and lung infections. Studies show that ginger increases the absorption of herbs in the body, and helps to protect the liver. It is a stimulant and an aphrodisiac, and is used in warming liniments.

Grapefruit (*C. paradise*)

The oil that is pressed from the peel of this fruit encourages weight loss and gall bladder activity. Grapefruit is a favorite with children, and very useful for anyone undergoing inner-child psychological work.

Helichrysum (*Helicbrysum angustifolium*)

A pleasant spicy, sweet, almost fruity fragrance is distilled from the flowers of this everlasting, sometimes called "immortelle." It treats the infection and inflammation of chronic cough, bronchitis, fever, muscle pain, arthritis, phlebitis, and liver problems, as well as countering allergic reactions such as asthma. Use helichrysum on acne, on scar tissue, on bruises, on couperose or mature skin, and on burns to stimulate production of new cells. The scent lifts one from depression, lethargy, and nervous exhaustion, and helps alleviate stress. Some aromatherapists say it helps detoxify from drugs, including nicotine. The French oil is green, while the less-refined Yugoslavian oil has an orange hue.

Inula, sweet (*Inula graveolens* or I. *odorata*)

Distilled from the plant's root, the oil is a rich blue-green with a pungent odor that faintly resembles eucalyptus. Inula relieves muscle tension, inflammation, sinus congestion, bronchitis, and high blood pressure. A compound derived from inula is used in Europe to treat intestinal worms. It also relieves skin rashes, herpes, and itching. An essential oil is produced from the closely related medicinal herb elecampane (*Inula helenium*), but tends to cause skin reactions.

Jasmine (*Jasminum officinalis* and J. *grandiflorum*)

An enfleurage, an absolute, and a concrete are made from the plant's blossoms, whose complex fragrance is fruity, floral, and sweetly exotic, and is found in many expensive perfumes. The synthetic version is so harsh it demands a touch of the true oil to soften it. Jasmine is a nervous-system sedative that reduces menstrual cramps and is sometimes used to treat prostate problems. Good for sensitive and mature complexions, jasmine also soothes headaches, insomnia, and depression, dissolving apathy, indifference, and lack of confidence by increasing the sense of self-worth. Jasmine is an aphrodisiac and also increases receptivity. The most prized oil comes from France and Italy, although about 80 percent is Egyptian.

Juniper (*Juniperus communis*)

The berries of this North American shrub offer the highest-quality oil, although needles and branches are sometimes used. Its pungent, herbaceous, peppery odor is pine-like and camphoric. Juniper treats arteriosclerosis, rheumatic pain, general debility, varicose veins, hemorrhoids, fluid retention, cellulite, and genito-urinary tract and bronchial infections. It is suitable for treatment of acne, eczema, and greasy hair or dandruff. Juniper provides a feeling of protection when the demands of others pull too strongly, and is suggested for those who experience mental or emotional fatigue, insomnia, or anxiety. It can overstimulate the kidneys, so choose a less toxic oil when kidneys are inflamed.

Labdanum (*Cistus ladanifer*)

This is the "rock rose" grown in North American gardens. The leaves and twigs are boiled, and the resin skimmed off and aged, to produce a resinoid with a warm, spicy, balsamic odor, sometimes used as a fixative in perfumes. Oil distilled from the leaves is called "cistus," a nervous-system sedative used to treat rheumatism, colds, coughs, menstrual problems, inflamed kidneys, and hemorrhoids. Labdanum is also antiseptic on wounds, acne, dermatitis, and boils. It is both emotionally elevating and grounding, improving meditation and intuition, and raising consciousness. It calms the nerves, promotes sleep, and is an aphrodisiac. Don't confuse labdanum with laudanum, or tincture of opium poppy.

Lavender (*Lavandula angustifolia*)

Distilled from the herb's flower buds, this sweetly floral aroma is also herbal, with balsamic undertones. Lavender treats lung, sinus, and vaginal infections (including Candida), and relieves muscle pain, headaches, insect bites, cystitis, and other types of inflammation. It is also used for digestive disturbances, including colic, and boosts immunity. A skin-cell regenerator, lavender prevents scarring and stretch marks, and has a reputation for slowing wrinkles. It is suitable for all complexion types, as well as for burns, sun damage, wounds, rashes, and skin infections. Specific for central-nervous-system problems, lavender has been used to help nervousness, exhaustion, insomnia, irritability, depression, and even manic depression.

Lemon (*Citrus limonum*)

This distinctive oil, cold-pressed from the fresh peel, is antioxidant, preservative, and antiseptic, countering both viral and bacterial infections. Lemon treats hypertension and increases the rate of metabolism, relieving congested lymph, excessive stomach activity, water retention, and weight gain, and increasing mineral absorption and immunity. Lemon helps oily complexions, bruises, and skin impurities and infections. Like other citruses, it is antidepressive, increasing general well-being and the sense of humor. It also dissipates feelings of impurity or indecisiveness, and can stimulate emotional purging. The only caution is that it can be photosensitizing to some skins.

Lemongrass (*Cymbopogon citrates*)

Distilled from partly dried herb, lemongrass oil has a slightly bitter fragrance that is used in cosmetics, deodorants, and soaps (including Ivory). Lemongrass is antiseptic and treats pain resulting from indigestion, rheumatism nervous-system conditions, and headaches. It counters oily hair, acne, skin infections, scabies, and ringworm. The fragrance is sedating and soothing. Lemongrass is nontoxic, but produces skin sensitivity in some people.

Lime (*C. aurantifolia*)

The fragrance of this citrus fruit is similar to lemon, but smoother. Lime is motivating, relieving depression and increasing morale. Unlike other citruses, the peel may be distilled or pressed. Lime is slightly photosensitizing to some skins.

Marjoram (*Origanum marjorana*, formerly *Marjorana hortensis*)

Distilled from leaves of the culinary herb, the aroma is sweet-but-herbal and sharp, hinting of camphor. A sedative, marjoram eases muscle spasms, including tics and menstrual cramps, and relieves headaches (especially migraines), stiff joints, spasmodic coughs, and high blood pressure. It also counters colds, flu, and laryngitis, and is slightly laxative. Use it on the skin to tend bruises, burns, inflammation, and fungal and bacterial infections. Marjoram helps those who feel emotionally unstable, prone to hysteria, physically debilitated, or irritable—especially due to outside stimuli. Use it to ease loneliness, rejection, or a broken heart. (Old texts say that overuse may even deaden the emotions.) Note: Sometimes the much harsher oregano is commercially sold as marjoram.

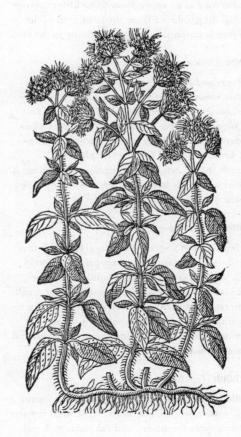

Continued ➡

Melissa (*Melissa officinalis*)

Distilled from leaves of the herb lemon balm, melissa's sweet smell is soft and lemony. Not easily distilled, this expensive oil is often adulterated with lemon or citronella. It was the main ingredient in the famous "Carmelite water," a facial toner made by nuns in the Middle Ages. Melissa treats indigestion, lung congestion, high blood pressure, menstrual problems, and infertility. It fights inflammation, and viral infections such as strep, herpes, and chickenpox. Shock, distress, depression, nervousness, and insomnia are helped by its sedative properties.

Myrrh (*Commiphora myrrha*)

The tree gum is distilled into a warm, spicy, deep, and slightly bittersweet oil. It helps with coughs, digestion, diarrhea, an overactive thyroid, scanty menstruation, and immunity. Externally, it treats wounds, gum disease, Candida, chapped, cracked, or aged skin, eczema, bruises, skin infections, varicose veins, and ringworm. Myrrh has been used since antiquity to inspire prayer and meditation, and to fortify and revitalize the spirit.

Myrtle (*Myrtus communis*)

Distilled from leaves, twigs and sometimes flowers, the spicy scent is slightly camphoric. Myrtle was the main ingredient in the sixteenth-century complexion treatment called "angel's water." It treats lung and respiratory infections, muscle spasms, and hemorrhoids. Myrtle is a treatment for oily complexions, acne, and varicose veins. The scent balances energy.

Neroli (Orange Blossom) (*Citrus aurantium*)

This sweet, spicy, and intensely heady fragrance is distilled from the blossoms of the bitter orange tree. It treats diarrhea, and circulation problems such as hemorrhoids and high blood pressure. It is used on mature and couperos skin to regenerate cells. One of the best aromatic anti-depressives, neroli counters emotional shock, mental confusion, nervous strain, anxiety, fear, and lack of confidence. It redirects one's energy in a positive direction. relieving fatigue and insomnia, and helps those who get upset without apparent reason. It is also used as an aphrodisiac. The bitter-orange essential oil produced from the fruit rind of the same tree is potentially photosensitizing to the skin.

Orange (*Citrus sinensis*)

Cold-pressed from the sweet orange peel, the familiar scent is perky and lively. Orange treats flu, colds, congested lymph, irregular heartbeat, and high blood pressure. The sedative fragrance counters depression, hysteria, shock, and nervous tension. Orange is good for oily complexions, although the oil can be slightly photosensitizing. An inferior oil comes from peel that has been pressed to make orange juice.

Palmarosa (*Cymbopogon martini*)

The lemon-rose fragrance of this grass is reminiscent of the richer and more expensive rose geranium, which it is often used to adulterate. The scent varies greatly depending on its source. A cell regenerator, palmarosa balances oil production by any complexion type, but especially with acne or otherwise infected skin. Palmarosa treats stress and nervous exhaustion.

Patchouli (*Pogostemon cablin*)

Distilled from aged, fermented leaves, the aroma is heavy, earthy, woody, and musty. Patchouli reduces appetite, water retention, and exhaustion. A cell rejuvenator and antiseptic, it treats acne, eczema, athlete's foot, inflamed, cracked or mature skin, inflammation, and dandruff. Patchouli counters nervousness and depression by putting problems into perspective and releasing pent-up emotions. It is also an aphrodisiac.

Pepper, black (*Piper nigrum*)

The oil is distilled from the same partly dried, unripe fruit we sprinkle on food. The scent is spicy, sharp, and slightly herbaceous. (A more fruity oil is produced from the fresh green fruit.) Pepper treats food poisoning, indigestion, colds, flu, urinary-tract infections, congested lungs, fevers, and poor circulation. It makes a warming liniment. The fragrance is emotionally stimulating and, some say, aphrodisiac. Though nontoxic, pepper can irritate the skin.

Peppermint (*Mentha piperita*)

Distilled from leaves of the herb, the aroma is powerful, minty, peppery, and fresh. Peppermint relieves muscle spasms, inflammation, indigestion, nausea, irritable-bowel syndrome, and sinus and lung congestion. It also destroys bacteria, viruses, and parasites in the digestive tract. Small amounts stimulate the skin's oil production and relieve itching from ringworm, herpes, scabies, and poison oak and ivy. Peppermint is used in liniments, although too much can burn the skin. As a stimulant, the scent counters insomnia shock, mental fogginess, lack of focus, and "stuck" emotions.

Petitgrain (*C. aurantium*)

Now distilled from the fragrant leaves and stems of the bitter orange, this oil originally came from the small, unripe fruit, hence the name (which means "little fruit"). Petitgrain resembles neroli, but is harsher, sharper, and less expensive. An antidepressant, petitgrain also increases perception and awareness, and reestablishes trust and self-confidence.

Pine (*Pinus species*)

The sharp fragrance from pine needles is produced from several species, but Scotch pine (*P sylvestis*) is most popular for cleansing solutions, European bath preparations (it improves poor circulation), and liniments. Pine replaces apathy and anxiety with peacefulness and invigoration. It is sometimes used to reverse male impotence.

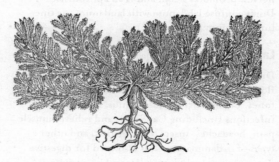

Ravensare (*Ravensara aromatica*)

Distilled from the leaves—and sometimes the fruit or bark—of this Madagascar spice tree, the scent is similar to eucalyptus, but more refined and less sharp. Ravensare is an antiseptic treatment for flu, bronchitis, viral infections (including shingles), viral hepatitis, sinus congestion, and acne. It also relieves muscle fatigue.

Rose (*Rosa damascena*, *R. gallica*, and other spices)

This costly oil is distilled, or solvent extracted, from the blossoms. It treats asthma, hay fever, liver problems, nausea, most female disorders, and impotence. A cell rejuvenator, rose soothes and heals all complexion types, and has a reputation for slowing down the skin's aging. It is also strongly antiseptic and fights infection. Rose helps alleviate depression and lack of confidence, and is useful for treating relationship conflicts, envy, and intolerance. It is comforting, supportive during a crisis, and an aphrodisiac.

Rosemary (*Rosmarinus officinalis*)

This herb's aroma, distilled from the flowering tops or leaves, is herbal, sharp, and camphoric. Possibly the first cologne, it was the main ingredient in the famous cologne "Hungary water," which doubled as a facial toner for dry or mature complexions. Rosemary gently stimulates poor circulation, low blood pressure and energy, the nervous system, the adrenal glands, and the gall bladder. It lowers cholesterol and relieves lung congestion, sore throat, and canker sores. It is used for sore muscles, rheumatism, cellulite, and parasites. Rosemary improves memory, confidence, perception, and creativity, and balances both mind and body. It prevents dizziness, dark thoughts, and nightmares, and helps in the recall of dreams. The smoke was once inhaled to counteract "brain weakness" and to stimulate spiritual awareness. There are several chemotypes with different properties.

Rosewood (*Aniba rosaeodora*)

The pleasant fragrance distilled from this tropical tree's wood is sweet, woodsy, and rosy. Rosewood eases headaches, cold, fever, infections, vaginitis, and nausea. It rejuvenates cells and benefits all types of complexions. As an antidepressive, it encourages constructive emotional work and tranquillity. Rosewood is a rainforest tree, and there is therefore concern lest it be overharvested.

Sage (*Salvia officinalis*)

Distilled from the leaves of the kitchen herb, the odor is spicy, sharp, and herbal. Sage is an antiseptic that treats throat and mouth infections. Hormonal properties help regulate both the menstrual cycle and menopause symptoms, and decrease lactation. Sage was a Medieval nervous-system tonic for tics and epilepsy. In Ancient Crete, the burning leaves were inhaled to relieve asthma. It reduces perspiration, oily skin, and acne, and is reputed to encourage hair growth. Sage helps those suffering from nervous debility, excessive sexual desire, grief, physical overexertion, and insomnia. It encourages inward focus. Sage contains the potentially neurotoxic thujone, so use it carefully and not on anyone prone to seizures.

Sandalwood (*Santalum album*)

Distilled from the tree's heartwood or roots, the scent is balsamic, soft, warm, and woody. Once a gonorrhea treatment, sandalwood is still used for genitor-urinary infections. It counters inflammation, hemorrhoids, persistent coughs, nausea, throat problems, and some nerve pain. Suitable for all complexion types, sandalwood is useful on rashes, inflammation, acne, and chapped skin. It also treats depression, anxiety, and insomnia, and helps instill peaceful relaxation, openness, and a sense of "grounding."

Spearmint (*M. spicata*)

The spearmint aroma is less peppery and sharper than the closely related peppermint. It is also slightly weaker in action, though it too is used as a stimulant. Spearmint brings back childhood joy and pleasant memories.

Continued ➡

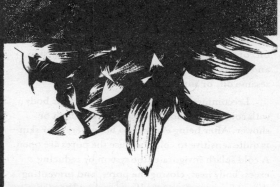

Tangerine (*C. reticulate*)

Distilled peel of tangerine produces this lively citrus scent, which counters insomnia and digestive problems, and is especially safe for children and pregnant women. The leaves are also steam-distilled for "petitgrain mandarin." The closely related mandarin orange—whose scent is very similar, but slightly richer and fuller—comes from the same species.

Tea Tree (*Melaleuca alternifolia*)

The oil distilled from the leaves of this tree is similar to the closely related eucalyptus. A good immune tonic and a strong antiseptic, tea tree fights lung, genitorurinary, vaginal, sinus, mouth, and fungal infections, as well as viral infections such as herpes, shingles, chickenpox, candida thrash, and influenza. Tea tree also treats diaper rash, acne, wounds, and insect bites, and protects the skin from radiation burns caused by cancer therapy. It is touted as one of the most nonirritating oils, but this varies with the species and the individual. It builds emotional strength, especially before an operation or during postoperative shock. "MQV" (*M. quinquenervia viridiflora*), which has a distinctively sweeter fragrance, is considered a stronger antiviral.

Dilutions and Doses

Bath: 3–15 drops in a tub

Compress: 5 drops in 1 cup of water

Cream and lotion: stir in 3–6 drops for every ounce of cream or lotion

Douche: 3–5 drops in 1 quart of warm water

Facial clay: 3 drops in 1 tablespoon prepared clay (water already added)

Foot or hand bath: 5–10 drops for every quart of water

Fragrant water: 5–10 drops in 4 ounces of water

Gargle or mouthwash: 1–2 drops in ¼ cup of water

Inhalant: 3–5 drops in bowl of hot water

Lightbulb ring: 2–3 drops on ring

Liniment: 15–18 drops essential oil for every ounce of carrier oil

Massage/body oil: 10 drops essential oil for every ounce of carrier oil

Perfume: one drop for fragrance

Potpourri: ½ teaspoon essential oils to 2 cups dried herbs

Room spray: 20 drops per 4 ounces of water (shake before using)

Salve: stir in 12–24 drops per 2 ounces of salve

Sitz bath: 5–10 drops in basin large enough to sit in

Washes: 6–12 drops in small basin of water

Thuja (*Thuja occidentalis*)

Known also as "cedar leaf or "arbor vitae," the oil is distilled from the leaves, twigs, or bark of this small tree, or sometimes from a cultivar or closely related species. The fragrance falls somewhere between the softness of cedar and the sharpness of pine. Thuja eliminates warts and treats pelvic congestion, urinary infections, and enlarged prostate. Thuja contains a skin irritant that is potentially very toxic, so use it carefully—and not at all if you are prone to seizures.

Thyme (*Thymus vulgaris*)

The scent, produced by distillation, is herbal, warm, almost sweet. Thyme is a strong antibacterial for mouth and lung infections, and destroys intestinal hookworms and roundworms. It relieves indigestion, coughs, and lung congestion, and was once a specific treatment for whooping cough. It is also a heating liniment. Thyme relieves mental instability, melancholy, and nightmares, and prevents memory loss and inefficiency. There are many chemotypes that have specific properties, including type linalol, which is not a skin irritant like the other thyme oils.

Vanilla (*Vanillaplanifolia*)

The sweet, creamy scent—obtained with a resinoid, an absolute, an oleoresin, or by CO_2 extraction—improves lack of confidence and helps dissolve pent-up anger and frustration. It is consoling, and can unleash subconscious, hidden sensuality. Some psychoanalysts use it to bring back childhood memories.

Vetiver (*Vetiveria zizanoides*)

Distilled from root, the scent is earthy and heavy. Vetiver eases muscular pain, sprains, and liver congestion, and is a circulatory stimulant. Externally it treats acne, wounds, and dry skin. Vetiver is uplifting, relaxing, and comforting, releasing deep fears and tensions. It cools the body and mind of excessive heat. In India and Indonesia, door and window screens called "tatties," woven from the roots, are sprinkled with water on hot days to scent and cool the house. An inferior oil is made from the used screens.

Ylang-ylang (*Cananga odorata*)

An intensely sweet, floral fragrance that some describe as banana-like is distilled from these tropical flowers. A strong sedative, ylang-ylang reduces muscle spasms and lowers blood pressure. As a hair tonic, it balances oil production. The fragrance makes the senses more acute and tempers depression, fear, jealousy, anger, and frustration. It is also an aphrodisiac, although high concentrations may produce headaches.

—From *Pocket Guide to Aromatherapy*

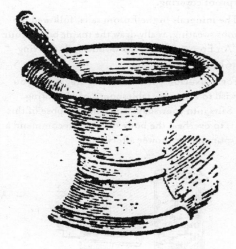

REJUVENATING BATHS
by Helen Silver

What can be more relaxing after a long, busy day than to soak in a fragrant, cleansing bath? Many people tend to cleanse themselves in a very utilitarian way—they jump in the shower, soap themselves down, rinse off, and hop out. But a bath can do so much more. It is a way to gently unwind, soothe tired muscles, open your pores, and draw wastes and toxins out through your skin. The time you take for a leisurely bath is precious personal time well invested in your health, beauty, and inner peace.

Bathing has always been a treasured ritual of personal hygiene, healing and relaxation—from the great public baths of Rome to the elegant bath ceremonies of the Orient, the sacred healing water rituals of ancient Greece, or the fashionable European spas. Your bathroom can be a sanctuary, a private retreat from the hustle and bustle of the world outside. As you luxuriate in the fragrant aromatic essences, the healing mineral salts, and the stimulating and relaxing effects of a daily water ritual, you will come to appreciate how bathing can be a way of cleansing your body of waste and your mind of stressful thought.

Different bath temperatures have different effects on the system. Hot water is very enervating. It is a great natural tranquilizer and muscle relaxant, and many people find a hot bath just before bedtime a perfect cure for insomnia. Warm baths are very pleasant, refreshing, and relaxing. Because you can stay in warm water for a long time, it helps to maximize the cleansing and healing effects of the salts or oils that you add to your bath. Cold baths are very stimulating. You may shudder at the thought of a cold bath or shower, but as your body becomes accustomed to brief exposures to cold water, you will begin to realize its benefits.

I remember when I was a girl, my mother always told me I should end my showers with cold water. Really, it was very sound folk wisdom. A cold shower might actually be considered as close to a cure-all as any other use of water I will suggest in this book. It rejuvenates the entire system, enhancing circulation, increasing muscle tone, and activating the nervous system. It stimulates the endocrine glands, improves digestion, and speeds up metabolism, and if used regularly, it can increase resistance to infections and colds.

. . . I want to encourage you to use warm, cool, and even cold baths and showers. . . . The temperature of your bath will be determined partly by the time of day. A hot bath at night can be very relaxing and help you fall asleep, while a cold shower in the morning can help to wake up your entire system.

It is not wise to use hot water too often. Hot baths tend to dry out the skin, because they draw the body's natural oils out of the skin. You may think that by adding oil to your bath you are putting oil into your skin, but bath oils simply rise to the surface of the water and do not add moisture to the skin. To protect your skin before taking a hot bath, oil your entire body before getting into the water. If

Continued ➤

you have dry skin, use almond oil, castor oil, olive oil, or peanut oil. If you have normal to oily skin and you take a lot of hot baths, use safflower oil, sesame oil, or sunflower oil.

I recommend that you always splash your body with cold water following a hot or warm bath or shower. After being exposed to hot water, your skin is quite sensitive to cold, because the pores are open. A cold splash invigorates the system by reducing excess body heat, closing the pores, and preventing the oil from seeping out. If you cannot bear the thought of standing under a cold shower, sponge yourself off with cold water. Over time, your body will get accustomed to the temperature change, and you will begin to relish a cold splash. Incidentally, you will also find that a cold sponging or a quick cold shower after a hot bath at night does not interfere with sleep, but helps you to relax even more.

One of the most invigorating kinds of showers is a contrast of alternating hot and cold. This stimulates all the body functions, especially the glandular system. It revitalizes skin function and improves circulation. Always be sure to finish a contrast shower with cold water. To prevent chilling afterward, wrap in a bath towel or do a dry skin rub to warm yourself.

Before a long, luxurious bath, it is a good idea to take a quick shower first, as is the Japanese custom, to get the day's grime off your body. When cleansing your skin, please avoid commercial deodorant soaps, because they are very drying. Many delightful moisturizing soaps are available in health food stores and body-care shops, such as those made with an olive oil or glycerin base, or with other beneficial oils. Many people use Ivory soap because it does not contain a lot of chemicals. Review the labels on soaps; remember that your skin has absorptive qualities.

While you should not expose your skin to harmful chemicals, bathing does offer an opportunity to beautify your skin and delight your senses with the aromatic essences of plants. The art and science of using natural plant essences for healing and beauty is known as aromatherapy. Although it was given that name during the present century, the use of plant essences dates back to prehistory. From the Orient to Europe and the New World, from ancient times to modern, aromatic flowers, barks, and leaves have been prized for their healing, preservative, and beautifying powers. It was not until the Middle Ages that the great Arab physician Avicenna discovered the method of distilling the pure essential oils from plants. Herbal remedies and essential oils were an important part of medicine in the Middle Ages and the Renaissance, but gradually, with the birth of modern pharmacology, these natural substances were displaced by their more powerful synthetic forms. Now, essential oils are being rediscovered by practitioners of aromatherapy and herbal medicine as we seek gentler, lasting methods of healing and rejuvenation.

Curative Properties of Essential Oils

This table will help you to customize your daily bath to benefit from the rejuvenating effects of these natural essences.

Antidepressant: Bergamot, chamomile, clary sage, geranium, jasmine, lavender, oranges, rose, sandalwood, ylang ylang

Antiseptic: Bergamot, eucalyptus, juniper, lavender, rosemary, sandalwood

Aphrodisiac: Clary sage, rose, sandalwood, ylang ylang

Detoxifying: Fennel, garlic, juniper, rose

Diuretic: Benzoin, chamomile, cedarwood, cypress, fennel, frankincense, geranium, juniper, rosemary, sandalwood

Expectorant: Benzoin, bergamot, eucalyptus, marjoram, myrrh, sandalwood

Hypnotic: Chamomile, lavender, marjoram, ylang ylang

Moisturizer: Carrot oil

Pain Relief: Bergamot, chamomile, lavender, marjoram, rosemary

Sedative: Benzoin, bergamot, clary sage, frankincense, juniper, lavender, marjoram, rose, sandalwood

Stimulant: Black pepper, eucalyptus, geranium, rosemary

Essential oils are very readily absorbed by the skin, and inhaling their fragrance in steam also has an effect on both the mind and the body. Adding the beneficial effects of essential oils to the healing properties of water offers a very wide range of possibilities for relaxation, rejuvenation, invigoration, and beautification. Today you will learn how to use essential oils to revitalize and moisturize the skin, stimulate the systems of elimination, and influence your mental and emotional states. I will be giving you recipes for baths and steams and other uses of essential oils throughout my program. You may wish to refer to the Curative Properties of Essential Oils (left) to customize the recipes to suit your own physical or emotional requirements.

Whether it is a hot soak, a fume bath, a sauna, steam room, or mud bath, the benefits of bathing are essentially the same. Bathing opens the pores and pulls the waste-laden sweat out of the system, promoting the function of your skin as an organ of elimination and restoring its youthful, glowing color and smooth, clear texture. Minerals and herbs added to your bath amplify the healing, cleansing, and beautifying properties of water. The following bath preparations will get you started in discovering the pleasures of bathing.

Epsom Salts Soak

Epsom salts, or magnesium sulfate, are an age-old favorite for hot soaks. Epsom salts are available in pharmacies, supermarkets, and health food stores. During this soak, you will be submerged in the water as deeply as possible, so your natural cooling mechanisms will not be operating. Holding the heat in the body promotes the detoxifying and drawing properties of the Epsom salts.

Pour two whole pounds of Epsom salts into a hot bath, as hot and deep as you can stand. (Cover the outflow in your bathtub if you want to raise the water to a higher level.) Soak for twenty minutes, then get out, wrap yourself in a towel or blanket, and lie down and continue to sweat. You may want to cover your bed with a plastic drop cloth or other waterproof covering.

The minerals in the Epsom salts, followed by vigorous sweating, really draw the toxins out of your skin. An Epsom salts soak is wonderfully relaxing before bedtime. . . .

For a luxurious, skin-soothing fragrance, you may wish to mix a few tablespoons of Hydrating Bath Salts into your soak. Since the purpose of this bath is to overheat the body, I do not recommend a cold sponging or shower afterward.

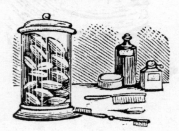

Make Your Own Hydrating Bath Salts

Enjoy the mineralizing and cleansing benefits of Epsom salts, the moisturizing effects of castor and carrot oils, and the heady aroma and complexion-enhancing properties of the floral and fruit oils.

    4-pound box of Epsom salts
    4 ounces castor oil
    1 teaspoon orange essential oil
    1 teaspoon rose essential oil
    1 teaspoon chamomile essential oil
    ½ teaspoon carrot essential oil

In a small jar, combine the castor oil with the essential oils. Pour the oil mixture over the Epsom salts. Allow the salts to stand for at least twenty-four hours so that the essences are completely absorbed. You will be using your Hydrating Bath Salts throughout the program.

You may keep the Epsom salts in the original box, but I prefer to transfer the Epsom salts to a covered glass jar, so the cardboard box will not absorb the oils. Two handfuls (about one ounce) of the Hydrating Bath Salts added to your bath will be just right.

You may vary this recipe, adding other essential oils . . . to produce your own personal combination of scents and healing and cleansing properties. You may also add a packet of concentrated seawater (available in powder form at aquarium stores) to the Epsom salts, to add the benefits of concentrated sea minerals to your bath: You may enjoy these bath salts throughout the year.

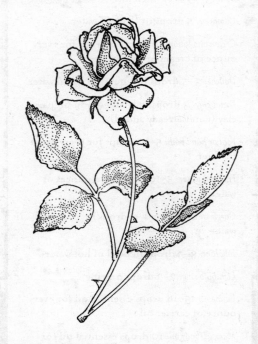

Cleopatra's Milk Bath

Milk has a well-deserved reputation for promoting a beautiful complexion when used externally. It is excellent for general skin care and will smooth dry, tired skin. . . .

Simmer half a cup of barley in one quart of water, in a covered pot, for three hours. Prepare a larger quantity if you like, storing the extra barley water in your refrigerator.

Make one-fourth cup of almond meal by grinding whole raw almonds in a coffee grinder or blender. Combine the almond meal with one-fourth cup of oatmeal. Tie the mixture securely in a washcloth or cheesecloth. Fill your bathtub with warm water and add the bag of meal. Add three cups of milk along with half a cup of the cooked liquid from the barley; warm these liquids if necessary, so they will not cool the bath water. Soak in this luxurious bath for twenty to thirty minutes, then finish off with a cold sponging or cold shower. Wrap yourself

Continued ➡

in a towel and enjoy the feeling of cleanliness and youthfulness that this bath imparts to the skin.

Optimism Bath

Draw a warm bath and add five drops each of the essential oils of rose, rose geranium, lavender, and orange. Soak for at least twenty minutes to calm and heal troubled emotions or stress.

I came across this bath late one night when I was deeply depressed over a broken romance and could not get to sleep. It was too late to call a friend, get a massage, or go to the movies, so I consulted my reference books and came up with this combination of essential oils. I even dabbed a bit of the oil on my temples and also made up the Easy Steam and let the scented fumes fill the bathroom while I soaked in my bath. My mood improved dramatically.

Rose has an age-old reputation for healing the heart, and is traditionally associated with love. There are many varieties of rose essential oils, usually blended because pure rose oil is so expensive. Lavender is also soothing for the emotions, and orange oil has an antidepressant effect, helping to lift the mood.

Tranquility Bath

Hot water is very enervating. Combined with the aromatic oils in this Tranquility Bath, it will help to calm and relax you after a busy day. Lavender and chamomile oils soothe away tension, lift the mood, and prepare you for sleep. Marjoram oil has an antispasmodic effect on tight, stressed-out muscles and deepens the relaxation provided by the other oils.

Draw a hot bath and then add each of the following essential oils:

7 drops of lavender essential oil

10 drops chamomile essential oil

5 drops of marjoram essential oil

Lie back and feel the fumes penetrate your lungs and your skin. After your bath, douse yourself with a cool-to-cold sponge to close the pores and send the heat back to the center of your body. You will find this cool sponging very relaxing. Don't worry; it will not wake you up.

Inspiration Bath

The essential oils in the inspiration bath work together to create a euphoric, self-nurturing mood that will help you affirm your resolve to take better care of yourself. Eventually, you will come to associate these scents with feelings of self-love and well-being. Essence of rose is traditionally associated with love.

Lavender essential oil

Clary sage essential oil

Rose essential oil (or blended rose oil)

To a hot bath, add six drops of each of the essential oils. Relax and inhale the fumes, allowing them to put you in a dreamy; mood. Soak for twenty minutes as the water gradually cools. Dry yourself with a coarse towel and prepare for bed.

Stress Reduction Bath

Stress puts a tremendous strain on both the nervous system and the immune system, and it can produce a state of mental and physical exhaustion. As the aromatic fumes of the essential oils in the Stress Reduction Bath envelop you, they will help to strengthen and revive your nervous system. At the same time, they will relax your body and soothe away your anxieties.

6 drops basil essential oil

6 drops rosemary essential oil

6 drops chamomile essential oil

Add the essential oils to a hot bath. Lie back in the water and inhale the wonderful fragrance. Soak for twenty minutes, allowing the water to cool and bring your body back to normal temperature. Dry off vigorously with a coarse towel, wrap yourself in a warm robe, and prepare for a good night's sleep.

Deep-Heat Bath

Draw a very hot bath, then add each of the following essential oils:

10 drops eucalyptus essential oil

8 drops rosemary essential oil

5 drops sandalwood essential oil

The hot water helps to relax your muscles, and these essential oils are all beneficial for soothing your body after exercise. Eucalyptus oil is good for aching joints and muscles, and for skin problems and chapped skin. It is also used as an antiseptic inhalant, and the vapor helps clear the respiratory passages. Rosemary oil is a nervous-system stimulant. It is used as a tonic for the heart and to enhance liver functions. Hot compresses of rosemary oil are used for the aches and pains of rheumatism. Sandalwood oil cleanses and moisturizes the skin. Its lovely aroma is used in India to induce a meditative state.

Soak in this bath for twenty minutes, inhale the fumes, and feel them clearing your mind and your breathing passages, allowing the essential oils to work their magic.

Fume Baths

Steam baths, or fume baths, use intense heat to open the pores of the skin and draw the toxins out of the system. By adding various herbal preparations to the steam, you can produce specific cleansing, healing, and beautifying effects. At the Inner Beauty Institute, my clients sit in a steam cabinet with essential oils. You may want to take advantage of the steam bath in a local health club or gym, but you can also enjoy the benefits of a fume bath by making your own at home.

Aromatic Fume Bath

Prepare a steaming unit, using an electric vaporizer, a partially covered electric frying pan, or an old electric coffeepot or tea kettle. Half-fill the container with water to make the steam, plug it in (using an extension cord if necessary), and place it in an empty, dry bathtub or shower. (Be certain the tub or shower is dry to avoid electric shock.) Place a chair or stool over the steaming apparatus, and sit down carefully. Drape a "tent" around you, made out of a large blanket or shower curtain. Leave an opening for your head, draping a bath towel around your neck to keep the steam in, or you may prefer to keep your head inside the tent. Sit inside the tent, which will fill rapidly with steam, for about twenty minutes. Be sure to wrap up in a towel afterward to prevent chilling.

For healing and beautifying benefits, there are a variety of herbal preparations that you can add to your fume bath. Witch hazel is wonderfully detoxifying and cleansing. Add tincture of witch hazel, widely available in pharmacies, to your steaming device before you turn it on. The witch hazel should constitute one-fourth of the total liquid volume. You can also use a healing essential oil . . . Some of my favorites are lavender, excellent for relieving headaches, menstrual cramps, stress, and skin eruptions; chamomile, to relax away tension and induce sleepiness; and sandalwood, a great skin moisturizer and meditation enhancer. Add six to

eight drops of essential oil on top of the water in the steaming unit.

Easy Steam

For a quick fume bath that requires little preparation, try this variation as an accompaniment to a tub bath.

Put some water in an electric frying pan or vaporizer and plug it into your bathroom outlet. If you choose to use a frying pan, place it on a dry surface near the tub. Add some almond oil to the water, as well as a few drops of essential oils that you have chosen for your bath. The almond oil adds to the moisturizing benefits of the steam, imparts a delightful fragrance, and serves as a carrier for the essential oils. Prepare a hot bath, adding the aromatic oils of your choice. Keep the bathroom door closed, sit in your bath, and let the scented steam fill the room.

While you stretch out in your tub or sit in your fume bath, relax and visualize the toxins leaving your skin. Feel your sweat glands and pores opening to expel impurities. Close your eyes and picture the dead cells gently floating off the surface of your skin. Picture the minerals or herbal aromas flowing in, cleansing and nourishing your skin, making it smooth and clear.

Breathe deeply and inhale the marvelous scent that rises in the steam around you. The relaxed, pleasant mood that this fame bath produces is an important part of my program for youthful, beautiful skin. Stress can take a toll on your complexion, and relaxation can help to smooth out the frown lines and wrinkles and promote the flow of nourishing blood and oxygen into the tissues.

Cleansing Inhalant

The regular use of this Cleansing Inhalant is a pleasant way to keep breathing passages clear. Its fragrant fumes exert a stimulating and decongesting action on the lungs and provide a healthful alternative to tobacco for smokers.

In a small wide-mouthed glass jar, preferably of dark glass, combine the following:

20 drops eucalyptus essential oil

10 drops lavender essential oil

15 drops chamomile essential oil

5 drops rosemary essential oil

15 drops tolu balsam essential oil

5 drops peppermint essential oil

15 drop tincture of benzoin

To use the Cleansing Inhalant, shake the tightly closed jar, remove the top and inhale the fumes cautiously through your mouth. Hold your breath for about twenty seconds and exhale through pursed lips. Then inhale the fumes cautiously through one nostril, hold twenty seconds, and exhale through both nostrils. Repeat for the other nostril. You will feel this fragrant inhalant open the breathing passages that have been clogged and congested.

Not only does this combination of essential oils draw the phlegm out of the lungs, but other properties of the oils also calm the emotions, stimulate the mind, and lift the mood. All the oils used in aromatherapy have multiple effects. Consult the chart on Curative Properties of Essential Oils to review some of the benefits of the oils in this Cleansing Inhalant.

Keep your Cleansing Inhalant in plain sight in your bathroom, in the kitchen, or wherever you will remember to use it several times during the day. Use it in the morning on arising, just before you go out walking, before you do your breathing exer-

Continued ➡

cises, and whenever you have a minute during the day. It is a wonderful aid in clearing your breathing passages and helping to maximize the benefits of your new practice of youthful breathing.

Foot Soaks

Foot soaks are an excellent way to stimulate lymphatic function, especially in the lower lymphatic vessels, which tend to get sluggish and clogged because of the effects of gravity. Soaking your feet helps to open the pores and draw the toxins out of the lymph system through the skin. The Romans knew the value of bathing the feet in the waters of their healing springs, and at the great French spas, footbaths were the prescribed treatment for arthritis. The effects of footbaths are aided by specific minerals or herbs added to the water and by the temperature of the water itself.

"Hot Foot" Soak

Mustard has been valued for centuries in both Eastern and Western medicine for its ability to stimulate blood and body-fluid circulation and break up stagnation. Its effects are powerful, so be careful not to use more than the recommended amount of mustard powder. This foot soak will cause you to sweat profusely, as the effects of the mustard promote the expulsion of wastes from your entire system.

In a gallon bucket or small tub, dissolve three tablespoons of mustard powder in very hot water, as hot as you can stand. Soak your feet for twenty minutes. Mustard powder is a powerful rubefacient, causing the skin to redden as it dilates the blood vessels near the surface of the skin, bringing more blood to the area. It also draws lymph to the surface, helping to flush it of toxins and waste materials. Miraculously, mustard foot soaks have been used successfully to relieve the pain of earache, tooth abscess, and sinusitis by drawing the body fluids to the surface of the feet.

Father Kneipp's Foot Bath

Father Kneipp was one of the modern pioneers in the therapeutic uses of water. This hot-and-cold contrast footbath is considered an excellent treatment for colds, sinusitis, headaches, poor circulation, neuritis, and congested abdominal organs. Try it the next time you are feeing congestion or sluggishness anywhere in your body.

Fill one small tub or gallon bucket with hot water and a second tub with cold water. The water in each tub should be eight to twelve inches deep. Place your feet in the hot tub for three to five minutes, then switch to the cold tub for thirty seconds. Repeat this procedure twice.

As with any alternating hot-and-cold bath or shower, this footbath is very invigorating. You will find it wakes up your whole body and leaves you feeling energized.

—From *Rejuvenation*

Glossary of Aromatherapy Terms

Carbon dioxide extraction: CO_2 extraction is a new process that uses high pressure and low heat to extract essential oils. The fragrance is better preserved than with high-heat methods such as distillation, and CO_2 extraction leaves no solvent residue.

Carrier: Essential oils, to be used safely, almost always require dilution. The base in which they are diluted, usually vegetable oil or alcohol, is called a "carrier."

Chemotype: A term used by aromatherapy chemists to designate a plant that has a slightly different chemistry than others of the same species. These genetic variations are reproduced by cloning or cuttings, rather than by planting seeds. Different growing conditions will often produce a greater abundance of one or another chemotype group. Aromatherapists may seek out one chemotype because it is higher in a particular medicinal constituent.

Diffuser: This handblown glass apparatus pumps a consistent fine mist of unheated fragrance into the air. Because it operates on an electric pump, try to find one that doesn't make too much noise. Do not use thick oils such as vetiver, sandalwood, vanilla, myrrh, and benzoin in a diffuser unless they are diluted with thinner essential oils, or mixed with alcohol—otherwise, they may clog your diffuser. Also don't let essential oils sit for weeks in a diffuser. If your diffuser does get clogged, or if you just want to get rid of a permeating scent, rubbing alcohol is the best cleanser.

Distillation: A common method of extracting essential oils is by steam distillation. With this method, steam passing through the plant matter lifts the essential oil out of the plant. The oil-ladened steam is then forced into an enclosed condensation tube surrounded by a cold-water bath. The cold turns the steam back into water, separating out most essential oils into beads that may be skimmed off the surface of the water.

Enfleurage: This is probably the oldest method of extracting fragrance from plants. The fragrant part of the plant is placed on thin, warm layers of animal fat, which absorb the oil. Once the fat has been saturated with fragrance, the oil is separated out. Virtually obsolete today, enfleurage is still occasionally used for plants that are unable to withstand the intense heat of distillation. This method is especially appropriate for the flowers of jasmine or tuberose, which continue to manufacture essential oils after they are picked.

Fixative: Most essential oils slowly deteriorate with age (although some actually improve as they get older). Fixative oils are used by perfumers and other fragrance-makers so the finished product will smell better and last longer. Examples of fixative essential oils are clary sage, patchouli, sandalwood, vetiver, angelica, oakmoss, and most balsams, gums, and oleo-resins, such as benzoin, balsam of Peru, balsam of tolu, frankincense, myrrh, and styrax.

Fixed oil: Vegetable oils are called "fixed" because, unlike the molecules of essential oils, their molecules are too large to escape naturally from the plant. For the same reason, vegetable oils are not easily absorbed into the skin. Most vegetable oils are extracted by a combination of heat and pressure.

Fragrant water: Fragrant waters are produced by adding essential oils to distilled water. They are less expensive, but also less effective, moisturizing agents than hydrosols (see below). Spray or splash on a fragrant water after your shower, to cool down on a hot day or just to freshen your face.

Herb infusion: This is a fancy name for herb tea. Whenever you take a fragrant herb and steep it in boiling water, the essential oils are extracted into the water. You can also make an oil infusion by extracting essential oils from plants that are submerged in warm vegetable oil.

Hydrosol: The large amount of water used during steam distillation usually picks up some of the essential oil and, along with it, its fragrance. (This is especially true of an essential oil such as rose, which is partly water-soluble.) This by-product of distillation can be used in any application for which a water carrier is desired. The most popular uses of hydrosols are as facial sprays and as room spritzers. Hydrosols are impregnated with water-soluble ("hydrophilic") compounds that are not present in essential oils.

Volatile oil: Essential oils are sometimes called "volatile" because of how quickly they evaporate into the air and dissipate.

Eastern Healing Methods

THE FOUNDATIONS OF CHINESE MEDICINE

Michael P. Milburn, Ph.D.

Chinese calligraphy by Terry Louie

The Theoretical Foundations of Oriental Medicine

By studying the organic patterns of heaven and earth a fool can become a sage. So by watching the times and seasons of natural phenomena we can become true philosophers.

—Li Quan, Yin Fu Jing (A.D. 735)[1]

The Clinical Gaze

The origins of Chinese medicine are shrouded in the mists of time. The discoveries of many of its central components—such as the flow of qi in the human body and the channels through which it circulates—date to prehistory and are the subject of legend and speculation. . . .

Much of what we "see" around us is shaped by our underlying notions of reality. . . .

One Western medical doctor, an authority on skin cancers, talked about a dilemma he faced while waiting in line at the supermarket. He could not help but notice a distinct mole on the neck of a man in the line. The mole looked suspiciously dangerous: its shape and color suggested the man should see his doctor as soon as possible and have the mole examined. It was years of training and clinical experience that caused the doctor to see something suspicious in what would appear to be a harmless mole to others.

Chinese medicine's unique "clinical gaze" can create similar experiences for its practitioners. This gaze is not fixed on specific parts of the body, but on patterns that emerge from a patient's constellation of signs and symptoms. A series of conversations with a neighbor, for example, may merge a collection of facts into a pattern of imbalance, suggesting a particular herbal treatment or acupuncture prescription.

A neighbor's complaints about acute migraine headaches, his thin appearance, agitated state, and often angry mood together with his often swollen, red eyes and his crimson tongue with a dry, yellow coating, suggest a disharmony with the liver. Too much hot and active qi coursing through the liver and meridian could cause migraine headache, problems with the eyes—a sense organ with a recognized connection to the liver—and a proclivity for anger. Of course, a careful and detailed diagnosis of the case would have to be made to confirm these suspicions.

A Contrast of East and West

The complementary clinical gazes of East and West emerge from complementary world views. In the West, the greatest effort has been applied to understanding substance by breaking things down in the search to discover what they are made of. This atomistic orientation traces back to Greek philosophers such as Democritus, who argued that the world was made of atoms, small fundamental units of matter that were quite separate from spirit. This emphasis on substance, and separation of spirit and matter, reappeared with the scientific revolution. Physical scientists such as Isaac Newton mathematically described the motion of matter and, in time, physicists discovered small, seemingly indivisible particles which they aptly called atoms. In biology, inquiry into the substance of living things began with dissection and anatomy. It then turned to smaller units of life—cells—when the discovery of the microscope opened up a world hitherto hidden by the limitations of human senses. But the cell did not turn out to be the "atom" of life, for cells were made of molecules—collections of the atoms discovered by the physicists—and soon scientists turned to the study of biologically constructed molecules. The greatest triumph came with the study of the gene, the premier molecule of life containing the blueprint for the protein molecules that lie at the heart of the structures and functions of organisms.

And so Western medicine emerged in its present form. Mental and physical disorders are dealt with by their respective experts as compartmentalized problems. Diseases are considered in terms of their

Continued ➡

molecular manifestations, and drugs—chemical substances chosen for their effects on biomolecular processes—are a mainstay of therapy. Surgery, the other foundation of therapy, is built on several centuries of anatomical exploration. Today, these therapies have evolved to an impressive level and are joined by a new frontier: the study of the genetic basis of disease. Scientists are now looking at how the blueprint of life can go awry and result in the cascade of molecular events that lie at the root of disease.

In contrast to the West's fascination with substance, the East has been enamored with form. Instead of asking what things are made of, the Chinese were intrigued by the fact that, while everything in the universe is in a constant state of flux, a wide variety of forms maintain a constant, though evolving presence. While Western natural scientists focused on specific chains of cause and effect, the Eastern naturalists noted resonances between events at drastically different scales—macrocosm and microcosm, Europeans studied things and their parts by analysis; Chinese looked at relationships, processes, and patterns from a synthetic perspective. . . .

While Western science seeks to discover the "laws" of nature—an idea that had its origins in the belief in an external lawgiver—the Chinese held to the view, described so eloquently by Joseph Needham, that "the harmonious cooperation of all beings arose, not from the orders of a superior authority external to themselves, but from the fact that they were all parts in a hierarchy of wholes forming a cosmic and organic pattern, and what they obeyed were the internal dictates of their own natures."[2] This holistic, organic view of nature implied that every system was part of a larger whole and that there was a way of nature, the Tao, ineluctably acting, not as a causal agent, but so that each actor played a peoper role in a spontaneous cosmic dance. . . .

Yin and Yang

The cosmic dance of Tao is expressed in the complementary qualities of yin and yang. Yang represents the active tendency, yin the substantive phase. While yang is hot, outward, expansive, yin is cold, inward, contracting, thus balancing yang. Yin and yang are not parts of things that can be considered in isolation, but complements that depend on each other for existence. They are innate tendencies in dynamic equilibrium.

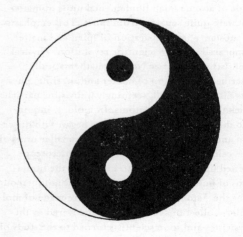

The cycle of night and day, darkness and light, for example, can be described by the interdependent dynamic equilibrium of yin and yang. While the period of darkness is yin relative to daylight which is yang, there is not an abrupt transition between two absolute qualities, but a continuous wavelike evolution. As the sun sets and a period of quiescence

begins, yin is still gaining and yang in decline. Yin does not reach its peak until the middle of the night, when yang is at its lowest point. Yet there is still yang within yin, for from midnight to sunrise yang gains strength against a waning yin. As the sun rises, yang continues to grow, reaching a peak at midday when the sun is highest in the sky. Finally, the cycle returns to its beginning as yang loses its strength and the yin within yang regains vitality.

Through yin and yang the Tao manifests itself in all things, from the daily rotation of planet Earth to the rise and fall of civilizations, from the gentle opening and closing of a lily to the economic cycle of boom and bust in industrial cultures. As an economy expands, for example, consumption increases, new factories are built, and employment rises. But this yang phase cannot last forever—yin within yang is always present, ready to contract what has expanded. Eventually the economy becomes overheated, inflation and interest rates rise, and recession looms.

Yin and yang analysis offers insight into the dynamic evolution of things. Yet the general nature of the qualities of yin and yang and their interaction, while allowing a high degree of flexibility in application, opens the way for a refinement and a description of more specific archetypal patterns of change. By representing yin with a broken line and yang with a solid line, the two lines are combined in groups of three to produce eight "trigrams." The trigrams, representing subtle sets of yin-yang interaction that appear on both cosmic and human scale, are given names and further combined in pairs to form sixty-four hexagrams. Each hexagram describes a configuration in time, and the study of these hexagrams offers insight into life circumstances.

The *I Ching* or *Book of Changes*, one of the five Confucian Classics, is a presentation of and commentary on the hexagrams. While continual change and transformation is a universal characteristic and starting point for the *I Ching*, it describes patterns and regularity within change that can be grasped. Implicit in the system of sixty-four hexagrams is the idea that the simple movement from yin to yang and from yang to yin—represented in the *I Ching* by a broken line (yin) becoming solid (yang) or solid line becoming broken—underlies the more elaborate trigrams which in turn combine to produce the hexagrams. The hexagrams are thus symbols for the subtle evolution of the universe with the dual forces of yin and yang as their root.

The Five Phases

Yin and yang and the complex, symbolic representation of the patterns of change found in the *I Ching* are not the only ways of understanding change in Chinese cosmology. The system of five phases—earth, metal, water, wood, and fire—also figure prominently in Chinese thought. Jesuit missionaries traveled to China in the seventeenth century, incorrectly interpreting these symbols as the five elements. They assumed that the Chinese were implying that earth, metal, water, wood, and fire comprised the fundamental stuff of the universe. The Jesuits' mistranslation highlights the underlying difference in Eastern and Western cosmology: the Western interest in material stuff and the Chinese emphasis on process.

The five phases (a more accurate rendering of the Chinese concept *wu xing* than "five elements") are not fundamental material substances, but five processes or activities with an interwoven set of relationships. Wood represents incipient growth, a stage of expanding activity, while fire is a symbol of an activity at its peak. Wood and fire are considered yang phases. Metal and water are yin complements,

metal connoting a decline in activity and water a fully realized period of quiescence. Earth sits as the neutral balancing point between extremes.

The phases show cycles of positive and negative feedback, known as the engendering and restraining cycles. In the engendering cycle (the cycle of creation), metal is able to "create" water, water in turn engenders .wood, wood gives rise to fire, fire fosters earth, and, in completion of the cycle, earth engenders metal. A pattern of change through the cycle of creation is found in the seasonal correspondences of metal with autumn, water with winter, wood with spring, fire with summer, and finally earth with late or Indian summer.

In the restraining cycle in contrast, metal controls wood, wood tempers earth, earth checks water, water restrains fire, and fire in turn moderates metal. The relationships between these symbolic processes do make literal sense: wood, for example, can give rise to fire and it is not hard to imagine water restraining fire. Since each phase has both yin and yang aspects, the five-phase system with its engendering and restraining cycles sets out a sophisticated set of systemic relations focused on self-regulation and organization. Such a system offers a framework for understanding the dynamic interplay between health and disease in terms of the self-regulatory organization of the complex human organism.[3]

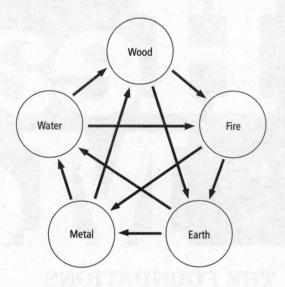

Natural Medicine

Chinese medicine is set in the cosmological milieu of yin and yang, and so it is imbued with a mystical disposition. Yet, while the Chinese had one eye to the heavens they also had two feet planted firmly on the ground. As Joseph Needham emphasized, the Chinese had an intensely practical side with an inclination to distrust theories and directly engage nature through observation and experimentation.[4] Chinese medicine combines Eastern mystical tradition with this penchant for observation and practicality.

In the realm of medicine, the Chinese discovered techniques for working with natural systems and considered health as a state of dynamic balance—a configuration of mind-body, behavior and attitude attuned to the Tao. Health in Chinese medicine is something that can be qualitatively assessed, something that requires constant vigilance to nurture, and something that can be restored when lost. Healing techniques such as acupuncture are not oriented so much toward the elimination of disease as on restoring the natural dynamic balance inherent in the human mind-body system. As balance reestablishes itself, healing will take place from within the organism. This notion of health con-

Continued ➡

trasts with the negative aspects of health by focusing on disease states and defining health as the absence of disease.

Agriculture offers a parallel to this difference between looking at health in a positive and negative sense. Conventional agriculture, like Western medicine, is disease-centered, studying the various enemies of crops—insects, fungi, weeds, etc.—and developing the (usually chemical) means to eradicate them. Organic agriculture, like Chinese medicine, is founded on a different conceptual premise, one that seeks to support the health of agricultural systems in a broader sense by working with nature. Sick plants do not mean an enemy exists to be conquered with dangerous chemicals, but that the natural balance and harmony has been lost and needs to be restored. . . .

In the East the goal and quest of the sage was to comprehend the Tao fully. Sages did not seek this understanding for personal gain or power over nature, but to be able to attune their actions with the Way. Central to this quest to live in accordance with the basic patterns of nature is the principle of *wu-wei* or "nonaction." *Wu-wei* does not literally mean nonaction as a cursory study of the characters may suggest, but rather implies a spontaneous action with the current of nature.

Wu-wei—going with the grain of things, rather than against it—is an important idea for both sage and healer. *Wei* is forcing things without accounting for their inner nature. *Wu-wei* is allowing things to follow their fate according to their inner nature. "To be able to practice *wu-wei* implied learning from nature by observations essentially scientific," claims Needham.[5]

The Chinese sages felt that good health was achieved by studying and working with nature's ways. Success in following the Tao came in the form of a long and vital life. According to the *Yellow Emperor's Classic of Internal Medicine*: "Those who follow Tao achieve the formula of perpetual youth and maintain a youthful body. Although they are old in years they are still able to produce offspring."[6]

Following the Tao means attending to balance in all things or, in Chinese terms, harmonizing yin and yang. This road to good health was described by Huang-fu Mi, a third century Taoist scholar: "It is necessary to follow the disposition of the seasons and adapt to cold and heat, to balance joy and anger and be contented with what one is, to harmonize yin and yang and adjust the unyielding and tender. Thus, no evils can arise."[7]

Imbalance between yin and yang is at the root of disease; restoration of balance is at the root of healing. Yin and yang, while metaphysical concepts, have concrete and important application to medicine. Yin and yang are not absolute categories, but a means of describing relationships in a subtle, qualitative way. The outside of the body is yang relative to the inside. The liver is yin in contrast to the gallbladder which is yang, yet the liver itself has both yin and yang aspects that are important in clinical practice. If yin has waned it can be supplemented with yin herbs, while yin symptoms such as cold limbs and low energy would call for the balancing effect of yang herbs that warm and invigorate.

The Three Treasures: Jing, Qi, and Shen

Many of the basic concepts of Chinese medicine have direct Western counterparts. After all, a liver should be a liver no matter how you look at it. Strangely, however, the idea of a liver does depend on how you look at it. In Western medicine the liver is understood anatomically, as a particular thing in a particular place. Instead of using anatomical description as the foundation of physiology, Chi-

nese reality is constructed from a study of patterns, processes, and relationships within the whole. The Chinese character *gan*, or liver, describes a set of corresponding physiological functions and mental/emotion phenomena. As American teacher, scholar, and practitioner of Chinese medicine, Ted Kaptchuk, claims: "The two paradigms embrace the body differently; there is no simple correspondence."[8, 9]

While the Eastern and Western framing of seemingly similar medical concepts needs to be carefully differentiated, there are a number of Eastern ideas without clear Western counterparts. One such concept is qi, a particularly mysterious idea central to Chinese medicine and used pervasively throughout Eastern culture. *Qi* is variously translated as "energy," sometimes as "influence," but best remains untranslated and allowed to enter the English language on its own terms as with yin and yang.

Qi represents the active organization of matter into its various forms and patterns. It is the influence that precipitates change and the quality of organization that resists it.[10] In the medical sphere qi is life itself. As a seventeenth-century text claims: "When qi gathers, so the physical body is formed; when it disperses, so the body dies."[11]

There are five major functions and over 30 specific kinds of qi distinguished in human physiology. Qi is the activity behind growth, development, and physiological processes; it acts in a defensive capacity, offering protection against pathogenic qi; it provides the foundation for metabolic warmth; it is the catalytic factor in all transformative processes; and it is responsible for keeping the blood in the vessels.

Air qi—qi absorbed from breathing—combines with qi extracted from food and essential qi stored in the kidneys to produce original qi, the basis of physiological activity. The original qi associated with the various organs is called organ qi, while channel qi flows through a network of internal and external conduits (the acupuncture channels). *Wei* qi,. or defensive qi, is a form of qi that nourishes the skin, controls the opening and closing of the pores, and resists invasion by pathogens.

Jing is another basic concept without a clear correspondence in Western science. According to Ted Kaptchuk, *jing* can be translated as "essence," and is "the substance that underlies all organic life."[12] Prenatal *jing* is inherited from one's parents: it provides the blueprint for growth and development and acts as a fundamental catalyst for digestion, thus providing a foundation for the creation of blood and acquired (or postnatal) *jing*.

In relation to each other, qi is yang, *jing* is yin, qi being active and energetic, *jing* being substantial. *Jing* helps to create qi and qi in turn plays a role in the formation of postnatal *jing*. In relation to blood—a fundamental substance, not completely equivalent to the Western conception, that circulates throughout the body providing nourishment—*jing* is yang, blood being a constant factor in regular nourishment and repair, *jing* being a guiding pattern over the scale of one's life.[13]

While qi is energetic, and *jing* substantive, *shen* or "spirit" is ethereal. *Shen* is awareness, consciousness, the foundation of self. Again Kaptchuk: "If *jing* is the source of life, and qi the ability to activate and move, then *shen* is the vitality behind *jing* and qi in the human body. While animate and inanimate movement are indicative of qi, and instinctual organic processes reflect *jing*, human consciousness indicates the presence of shen."[14]

While *shen* is linked more closely to mind than to body, it is important to appreciate that the Chi-

nese do not isolate the mind from the body, as does the West. Mind and body, *jing*, qi, and *shen*, are linked in an inseparable web of matter, energy, and spirit that etches out an evolving pattern of self in space and time.

A Landscape of Pattern and Process

A first step in organizing the landscape of human physiology is the differentiation of yin and yang organs. The yin organs, or *zang*, are interior relative to the yang organs, or *fu*, and are considered "solid" or full compared to the yang organs which are "hollow." According to the *Su Wen*, or *Essential Questions*, one of the major sections of the millennia-old *Yellow Emperor's Classic of Internal Medicine*: "The five yin organs store essential qi and do not discharge waste. They are full, but cannot be filled. The six yang organs process and convey matter, and do not store. They are filled, yet are not full."[15] The yin organs are defined by the processes they carry out in relation to fluids, blood, *jing*, qi, and *shen*, including storage, formation, and transformation. The yang organs are receptacles that process food, playing a role in the extraction of the "pure" and the elimination of the "impure."

There are five yin organs, six yang organs, and a number of "curious" organs that fall outside of the yin-yang differentiation. The five yin organs—heart, lung, spleen, kidney, and liver—are of central importance for clinical evaluation and treatment. The six yang organs are the small intestine, large intestine, stomach, urinary bladder, gallbladder, and the triple burner, an "organ" without a clear correspondence in Western biology and medicine. The curious organs are the brain, bone and bone marrow, blood vessels, uterus, and the gallbladder, which is considered "curious" since it plays a role in the processing of food like other yang organs, but produces a substance (bile) that is not a waste material.

The heart has two main functions: first, as governor of the blood vessels, and second as the abode of the spirit. Being in charge of the blood vessels emphasizes the heart's role in maintaining circulation and securing the provision of nourishment to the whole body. The heart's role in housing the spirit, or *shen*, is an example of how different aspects of mind are ascribed to various organs in Chinese medicine. (In Western thinking, mind, while classically separate from the body, is associated with the brain.) If the heart is healthy the person will have clarity in his/her thinking, but if the heart is dysfunctional the *shen* may be disturbed, resulting in insomnia and agitation or in extreme cases delirium. Heart yin and yang, heart blood and qi, are all important in the clinical practice of Chinese medicine.

The spleen is the central yin organ of digestion, governing the transformation and transportation of food and derived nutrients. The spleen is the catalyst of digestion, extracting nutrients and helping to distribute them throughout the body. It also extracts qi from food, which it sends upward to combine with air qi extracted by the lungs. As a result of its primary role in the creation of blood and qi, the spleen is referred to as the foundation of postnatal life. The spleen governs the muscles through its primary role in blood and qi production, and also "manages" the blood, by helping to create it and helping to keep the blood in the vessels.

According to the Classics, the lung governs qi, referring to its role as the organ of respiration in which fresh qi is absorbed into the body and stale qi expelled. This fresh "air qi" is a primary component, along with the grain qi extracted by the spleen and the essential qi contributed by the kidney, of the true qi that circulates throughout the body. The

Continued ➜

lung has an important down-bearing function, sending absorbed qi downward to the kidneys and helping to move fluids down to the bladder. The lung plays a role in fluid metabolism, not only in the downward movement of fluids, but also in the distribution of fluids throughout the body, particularly to the skin. There is, in fact, a close relationship between the lung and the surface of the body, including the skin. *Wei*, or protective, qi, controlled by the lung, flows on the surface of the body, helping to resist invading pathogens, and healthy lung function is manifest in healthy skin and body hair.

The kidney governs water and is the storage depot for essential qi. As the governor of water it plays an important role in water metabolism, separating the pure from the turbid, discharging the impure, and regulating the distribution of fluids. The essential qi stored in the kidneys sets the pattern for growth and development and is closely linked to reproduction. At the same time, the kidney governs the bones and produces marrow. According to the Chinese medical classics, solid and strong bones result from health of the kidney. The brain, known as the "sea of marrow," is intimately related to kidney and weak kidney qi may show itself as a lack of concentration, dizziness, or poor memory.

The liver is considered the great regulator; for it governs flowing and spreading. This function is seen in its role in maintaining the smooth and even flow of qi, indicated by smoothly coordinated physiological function. The regular and healthy expression of emotion is also related to the free-flow of qi and the liver. Excessive emotional stimulation (too much fear or too much anger, for example) can impair the free movement of qi, or, conversely, a disruption in the liver's maintenance of free-flow can give rise to an emotional disturbance, like depression. The liver is also responsible for storing the blood.

Interconnections

Oriental medicine emphasizes fundamental interconnections between the processes described in terms of the yin and yang organs. The lung, for example, has a close relationship with the heart: the lung rules qi and the heart rules blood, so that their functions are intertwined. Blood passes through the lung, where it is invigorated by lung qi. The vigor of the lung qi contributes to a smooth and vital flow of blood.

The kidney is the foundation of qi and has a close relationship with the lung, the ruler of qi. While the lung plays a pivotal role in the movement of qi throughout the body, essential qi stored in the kidney is necessary for healthy qi. The kidney plays a role in helping the lung absorb qi. The kidney is also closely linked to the liver. While the kidney stores *jing*, the liver stores blood; *jing* and blood are intimately linked. The liver's regulatory function and the kidney's storage role are interdependent and counterbalancing.

The kidney is the root of the yin and yang of the whole body. Kidney yin serves as a structural foundation for the nourishment of the other organs' yin. The kidney yang is like a pilot light for metabolism, supporting the warmth of the body and stimulating the yang aspect of the spleen, thereby engendering a robust and healthy digestion. There is also an important connection between the kidney and the heart, a link between the lower and upper parts of the body.

Each yin organ has a paired yang organ with which it forms an exterior-interior relationship, in the sense that yang organs axe considered more "external" and yin organs more "internal." These yin-yang pairs—heart and small intestine, lung and

large intestine, spleen and stomach, liver and gallbladder, kidney and urinary bladder—are closely connected. Spleen and stomach, for example, are the primary organs of digestion. The stomach receives and ripens the food, preparing it for the spleen's function of transformation and transportation. The action of the spleen moves the qi extracted from food upwards, while the stomach moves the "ripened" food downward.

Some of these connections are less obvious. The lung is paired with the large intestine, for example, without the same obvious linkage seen between the stomach and spleen. Yet in Chinese medicine the lung and large intestine are linked functionally through their roles in water metabolism. The role of the lung in transporting and transforming water in the body is described in the classics as the lung being the upper source of water. The lung helps to disperse fluids and helps water descend to the kidney. The large intestine has a complementary relationship in its role in absorbing water in the final stages of digestion. More important though, the essence of the, connection between the lung and large intestine, as with the other yin-yang pairs, lies in their energetic coupling through the meridians or channels.

The Web of Life

One of the most curious and perhaps startling facets of Chinese medicine—and one of great importance to the system—is its elaboration of a system of channels or pathways (called the *jing-luo*) for the travel of qi. There are both internal and external channels, and along the external channels are a series of points (called the *xue*). At these sites the qi can be accessed and manipulated for therapeutic effect using pressure, heat, or fine threadlike needles.

The channels provide an "energetic" linkage within the body, bringing otherwise disparate parts together into a harmonious whole. According to a modern Traditional Chinese Medicine textbook, "The organs, portals, surface skin and body hair, sinews and flesh, bones, and other tissues all rely on communication through the channels, forming an integrated, unified organism."[16] According to the two-thousand-year-old *Ling Shu*, "The twelve meridians are the place where life and death are determined, disease is generated, treated, and cared for; they are the place where beginners start and acupuncture masters end."[17]

The channels have many relationships important for the practice of acupuncture. The yin and yang organs have corresponding channels with which they connect. Also, yin-yang organ pairs are coupled by their channels. The lung channel, for example, has its origins in the middle of the body from where it travels downward to connect with the large intestine. From there it travels up to link with the lung, then courses up through the respiratory tract and throat to emerge on the surface of the body where it tracks along the edge of the arm to reach the thumb.

Fourteen channels have the greatest clinical and therapeutic value. Two of these run along the midline of the body dividing it into halves—the *ren mai* or conception vessel along the front and the *du mai* or governor vessel along the back. Twelve channels corresponding to the yin and yang organs have bilateral symmetry (they are the same on the right and left sides of the body) and are organized according to a six-fold division of yin and yang. (Yang is divided into yang ming, tai yang, and shao yang—yang brightness, greater yang, and lesser yang—and yin into tai yin, shao yin, and jue yin—greater yin, lesser yin, and terminal yin.) There are six channels, three yin and three yang, on each arm and six on each leg.

Tai yin channels move along the forward inner margin of the limb, shao yin along the back of the inner surface of the limb, and jue yin channels course the middle of the limb's inner surface. Yang ming channels move along the front outer edge of the limbs, tai yang channels along the back outer edge, and shao yang channels travel the middle of the outer surface. Hand tai yin, for example, is the lung channel, while foot tai yin is spleen. Hand yang ming is large intestine, while foot yang ming is stomach. Note that a sixth yin organ, pericardium, closely associated with the heart, pairs with the san jiao to complete the channel-organ system of correspondence.

Hand and foot channels in the same yin-yang category (tai yin, for example) are said to "communicate" with each other. Hand tai yin, lung, for example, communicates with foot tai yin, spleen, a linkage suggesting a close physiological relationship. Lung and spleen play complementary roles in the creation of qi and blood.

There are 365 classical points along the fourteen major meridians, and numerous other "extra" points. The acupoints were classically described as "the joining places and confluences, 365 in all. . . . the places where the vital qi enters in and leaves; traveling to and fro.[18] The Chinese character for acupoint, *xue*, symbolizes a cave, hole, or den and each point has an associated set of therapeutic functions.

In English, the points are assigned rather boring names, like stomach 36, the thirty-sixth point on the stomach channel. Points names in Chinese are much more poetic, rich with metaphor and multiple meaning hinting at a point's location and/or function. Stomach 36, for example, is "foot three li" (*zu san li*), which attests to the point's ability to relieve fatigue from travel by foot, so much so that one is able to manage another three li (a *li* is a Chinese "mile") after stimulating it. Points and their functions were often learned through poems and songs.

There are many groups of special points. Each of the twelve yin-yang organ meridians has five "ancient" points with five phase correspondences (see below). There are eight "influential" points that have a direct influence on qi, blood, and particular organs. Back *shu* and front *mu* points are filled with the qi of particular organs and are very useful in diagnosis and treatment. Of the over 1,000 points known today, any given practitioner makes regular use of 150 or so.

The System of Correspondence

In Chinese cosmology the link between macrocosm and microcosm is expressed through a system of correspondence based on the five phases. This has practical significance for medicine. Each organ corresponds to one of the five phases, heart to fire, spleen to earth, lung to metal, kidney to water, and liver to wood. This correspondence sets out a series of relationships via the creation and control cycles of the five phases. Kidney, for example, being water, nourishes the liver, which is wood, in what is called a mother-son relationship of the creation cycle (water creating wood). In another example, the kidney exerts a restraining influence on the heart (water restraining fire) and is itself restrained by the spleen (earth restraining water).

Other correspondences link mind and body, person and environment, and are important in diagnosis. Emotional patterns correspond directly to the Chinese organs. For example, anger is associated with the liver and wood phase, grief with the lung or metal phase. An imbalance in the liver could predispose a person to anger, while at the same time a repeated pattern of anger arising from

Continued ➡

life circumstances could precipitate a disharmony in the liver. Environmental factors show five phase correspondences and linkages to the organs. Cold, for example, corresponds to water, dampness to earth, and so the kidney is susceptible to influence by cold, the spleen can be affected by dampness.

Tastes and colors, too, are found in this system of correspondence. Sweet has an earth and salty a water correspondence, while red is a fire color and white corresponds to metal. The correspondences suggest important consequences for health, as described in the second century *Nan Jing*, or *Classic of Difficulties*: "Being upset, gloomy, sad, or thinking too much upsets and injures the heart; drinking cold fluids or being cold injures the lungs; getting angry injures the liver; overeating and drinking or tiredness from overwork injures the spleen; sitting in a damp place for a long time or bathing in cold water after working hard injures the kidneys."[19]

Zi-wu Liu-zhu

One fascinating application of the correspondence system is the theory of *zi-wu liu-zhu*. *Zi-wu* refers to the organization of space and time, with *zi* and *wu* serving as reference points of extremes. For example, *zi* can refer to midnight and *wu* to noon. The couplet *liu-zhu* symbolizes the evolution and change inherent in all things. *Zi-wu liu-zhu*, then, is a system of calculating the effect of macroscopic patterns of change on the microcosm—in this case, on the human mind-body system.

The rhythm of the human mind-body system resonates with the regular patterns of the cosmos: humans are subject to the yearly rhythm of the earth's movement around the sun, the monthly lunar cycle, the daily rotation of the earth on its axis, the regular flux of yin and yang, and the evolution of the five phases describing these cosmological cycles. This resonance can be observed as the ebb and flow of qi in various acupuncture points.

In *zi-wu liu-zhu*, calculations can determine where any particular instant of time lies in relation to the cycle of heavenly stems and earthly branches—the Chinese emblems for positions in the cosmic cycle. Five phase correspondences with the heavenly stems and earthly branches then relate to specific acupuncture channels and points through their own five phase correspondences (the "ancient" points described above).[20]

Zi-wu liu-zhu directly relates the biorhythmic movement of qi in the human mind-body system to underlying cosmological patterns. We dance to a universal beat, one that the Chinese discovered and use for practical, therapeutic purposes. Since specific acupuncture points are in resonance or "open" at specific times and the method of *zi-wu liu-zhu* allows these times to be calculated, treatments using acupuncture and other methods that influence the flow of qi in the acupuncture channels can be optimized. Patients can receive treatment during the time of peak activity of points determined to be valuable for their particular problem.

A Different Way of Thinking

The Chinese system of correspondence is the result of a distinctive thought process, a "coordinative" or "associative" type of thinking. While Western scientific thought relies on an analytical process that breaks things down into component parts, Chinese medicine's underlying thought process centers on understanding the relationship between part and whole. While the West looks for specific causes and effects, the Chinese see patterns that emerge from underlying interconnections. Joseph Needham offers a particularly clear and insightful description of the Chinese way of thinking: "The keyword in Chinese thought is *Order* and above all

Pattern. . . . The symbolic correlations or correspondence all formed part of one colossal pattern. Things behaved in particular ways not necessarily because of prior actions or impulsions of other things, but because their position in the ever-moving cyclical universe was such that they were endowed with intrinsic natures which made that behavior inevitable for them. If they did not behave in those particular ways they would lose their relational positions in the whole (which made them what they were), and turn into something other than themselves. They were thus parts in existential dependence upon the whole world-organism."[21]

Chinese medicine is founded on this different way of thinking. Instead of searching for the cause of disease, practitioners strive to identify an underlying pattern of imbalance, a configuration of the mind-body system in which illness is set. Dampness, whether internal or external or both, is not a cause of disease, but simultaneously part of a pattern's description and a potentially aggravating factor.

In the same way, emotions and mental states are not causes of disease, but important parts of the pattern identification process of Chinese medicine. Excessive and inappropriate emotional states can aggravate organ disharmony, while at the same time arising from it. As Kiiko Matsumoto and Stephen Birch, contemporary Chinese medicine practitioners and scholars put it: "There is only one energetic pattern and it manifests both internal organ problems and emotional states."[22]

The system of Chinese medicine emerges from a self-consistent and holistic conceptual framework in which the human mind-body system is viewed in relation to the cosmological whole. We are part of a great Unity, a Universal Pattern, the Tao. Our health is dependent on maintaining harmony and balance in the midst of inexorable change. By understanding the Way, the true nature of this change, the Tao manifest in each moment, our path to health becomes spontaneous and natural.

Each person is intimately linked to his or her social and physical environment. Mind and body are flip sides of the same coin and each part of the body is linked to the whole through a web of functional and energetic relationships. It is via the energetic connections forged by the meridians that a point on the ear, for example, can be used to influence the condition of the kidney.

At times we lose balance and disharmony can become disease. The clinical gaze of Chinese medicine looks for a pattern of disharmony, a configuration that describes the state of the mind-body system. It is here, in the recognition of disharmony at the system level, that resolution, the Tao of healing, lies.

Creating Balance with Needles and Herbs: The Healing Art of Chinese Medicine

Making Sense of Sickness: The Art of Diagnosis

THE FOUR EXAMINATIONS

In Chinese medicine, illness is synonymous with imbalance in the mind-body system. The overriding therapeutic goal is the restoration of balance. Over several millennia, fundamental patterns of imbalance have been catalogued and serve as the template for diagnosis, a process of bringing order to the chaos of signs and symptoms found in a particular patient. Through this pattern-identification process specific diseases are set in the broader milieu of the mind-body and parts are viewed in relation to the whole. These basic patterns serve as a guide to assessing the pattern of imbalance of an individual at

a particular time, a unique pattern that is reflected ultimately in the herbs and acupuncture points used to restore harmony and balance.

The diagnostic process of pattern identification is carried out through what are classically described as the four examinations: looking, listening-smelling, asking, and feeling. Each is a group of methods for gathering information about the state of the mind-body system. This process is logical and rational, yet not analytical, for the Chinese physician does not strive to pinpoint a specific disease location nor a precise causal agent, but works to weave the constellation of information obtained from the four examinations into a recognizable pattern.

Looking is a means of obtaining information about a patient's appearance, and can include everything from general body characteristics and facial complexion to the condition of the tongue. An obese and sluggish person with a pale, white complexion would trigger a practitioner to consider different sets of possible patterns than would a flushed, red-faced person with a nervous disposition.

Tongue observation falls into the looking category and is one of the two pillars of diagnosis. Tongues come in all shapes and sizes, colors and characteristics. There are fat, swollen tongues; red, dry tongues; furry, yellow tongues; and cracked, pale ones. These prominent differences help with pattern discrimination and (to the skilled practitioner) other subtle features help pinpoint the herbs and acupuncture points to be used for a particular case. In sticking out her tongue, the patient is presenting a mirror of the basic condition of the mind-body with characteristics matching those of the organs. Tongue diagnosis was already an important part of Chinese medicine by the time the *Yellow Emperor's Classic* was written, and was further developed during each successive era.

Tongue assessment centers on several essential features, including the color, shape, and coating, and a judgment of the deviation from the normal, healthy tongue. A healthy tongue is not too red or too pale, it is not too thin or too swollen, and it has a healthy coating or "moss" that is not too thick or moist and not too dry. Tongue signs, as with other information gleaned from the four examinations, do not have an absolute significance but must be set in the context of other signs and symptoms. A swollen tongue, for example, must be combined with tongue color, among other things, to offer meaning. A swollen, pale tongue, for example, may signify that the spleen and possibly kidneys have become deficient to the point where the movement of fluids is affected, causing the tongue to swell.

Skilled tongue observation can be compared to a walk through a vegetable field with a talented farmer who senses the close relationship between microclimate and plant health. In some areas of the field the soil might be too dry and parched, in, others it may be soggy and moist, all indications of suboptimal plant health. A broccoli crop, located in an area of full sun with exposure to the wind, might do better in a cooler, slightly moist site. The corn might be growing in depleted soil, while the rich, moist soil of the carrot bed may lack sufficient drainage. Like the farmer, the physician has an intuitive feel for the qualities that foster a healthy inner environment.

Included in the listening-smelling examination are voice quality, cough characteristics, and odors. Odors, particularly unusual ones, are a useful clue to the nature of imbalance.

From the asking examination much vital information is obtained about the history of a patient's health, details of his or her problem, and general characteristics that hint at the underlying pattern of

Continued ➜

disharmony. According to the *Essential Questions*, a major division of the *Yellow Emperor's Classic of Internal Medicine*, asking is an integral part of diagnosis: "If, in conducting the examination, the physician neither inquires as to how and when the condition arose, nor asks about the nature of the patient's complaint, about dietary irregularities, excesses of sleeping and waking, and poisoning, but instead proceeds straightaway to take the pulse, he will not succeed in identifying the disease.[23] Questions about hot and cold, perspiration, diet, sleep, and medical history are part of every exam.

The last of the four examinations, feeling, offers the opportunity for direct physical contact between patient and practitioner. There are special acupuncture points, called the back-shu and front-mu points, where the qi of the zangfu (the yin and yang organs) is "infused" and "converged," allowing the condition of the organs to be evaluated. The back-shu point of the heart, for example, is Xin Shu, the 15th point of the bladder channel beside the spine in the space between the shoulder blades. The heart's front-mu point is Ju Que, or conception vessel 14, along the midline of the abdomen below the sternum. Problems with the heart may be reflected in soreness or sensitivity at these points.

The second pillar of diagnosis, pulse taking, also falls under the category of feeling examination. While it is still an important part of the diagnostic process today, the art of the pulse was inflated to mystical heights in earlier times. The pulse is felt on the radial artery at the wrist. There are three positions at each wrist and three levels for each position, along with some thirty different qualities that can be felt, making pulse reading a complex and subtle art.[24] Each of the three positions on each wrist corresponds to particular organs and the pulse at each site reflects the health of corresponding organs.

It was Li Shi-zhen who long ago warned of overinflating the usefulness of the pulse. Li was a renowned physician of the sixteenth century and today is hailed as China's greatest naturalist. "The pulse ranks last among the four examinations," wrote Li, "and must be placed against the background of all the information gathered. All four examinations must be carried out.[25] Li wrote *The Pulse Studies of Bin Hu*, in which he set out the foundations of pulse assessment, discussing pulse states and their relationship to different diseases. According to Li, a rapid pulse is simply one that "beats six times per respiration," while the more elusive slippery pulse is one that "feels round and smooth and flows evenly. It is like a greasy round ball, which slides under the fingers. It always remains even, like a smooth stream of water."[26]

The Origin of Disease

Health is a state of balance, balance between person and environment and among the physiological and psychological components of the body-mind system—qi, blood, yin and yang, the organs and the meridians, *shen*, and emotions. Such a state of balance ensures a natural resistance against disease. Disharmony—a loss of balance—is the origin of disease. As the Yellow Emperor claimed: "If blood and qi fall into disharmony, a hundred diseases may arise."[27] When the pleasing symphony of life strikes a dissonant chord, we become susceptible to disease.

There are three general types of factors that play a role in patterns of imbalance: factors related to the external environment, factors of the internal environment, and other "independent" factors, many connected to lifestyle. These factors are much more than causes of disease: they are so intimately bound up with patterns of disharmony that they can simultaneously be considered causes and effects. In

the practical art of medicine, they are part of the descriptive landscape of a pattern, offering a clue to its true nature and the means of resolution through acupuncture or herbal therapy.

Life in modern society has largely isolated us from our environment. With our dependence on central heating and cooling we are buffered from the extremes of heat and cold. Humidifiers and dehumidifiers keep our homes from becoming too dry or too damp. It is perhaps difficult, then, to appreciate the emphasis Chinese medicine places on the meteorological factors of the external environment. Until modern times people have been under the powerful influence of wind, cold, summer-heat, dampness, dryness, and heat—the six environmental "excesses"—all of which can affect our health and, because of their constant change, to which we must continually adapt.

It is this constant need for adaptation that makes the six environmental excesses a direct factor in the development of disease. Even modern folk tradition highlights the relationship between weather and health. Exposure to a cold draft might precipitate a cold or flu, what is termed "catching a chill." A damp environment may aggravate an arthritic condition, while a sudden change in the weather might bring on a migraine headache. Other connections are obvious, like the heatstroke caused by excessive sun.

In Chinese medicine, these factors are not only catalysts for illness but the characteristics and qualities of these environmental factors are mirrored in the illnesses they generate. Wind is swift and changeable, causing movement; signs and symptoms of wind may include sudden onset, tremors, and pain that shifts location. Cold is slow, congealing, and associated with diminished activity; its signs and symptoms include lack of warmth, aversion to cold, and low energy. Heat is warm, often red and drying; it can manifest as a red face or eyes, thirst, and agitation. Dampness is wet, heavy, and lingering; its presence may be indicated by a heavy feeling in the limbs, aching joints, and lack of thirst. Similarly, dryness is indicated by signs and symptoms such as dry mouth and dry skin.[28]

These qualities and characteristics—signs and symptoms of illness in Chinese medicine—may appear without a connection to meteorological phenomena. Dampness can be generated internally by a weak spleen failing to transform and transport fluids. Weakness in the spleen and kidney yang may create a condition of cold. If the body's yin becomes deficient, the yang will no longer be held in check and heat will be generated. In this way, environmental qualities are used as descriptions of internally generated disharmonies.

These internal and external qualities—the microcosm and the macrocosm—may both play a role in a pattern of disharmony. Someone with a tendency toward an internally damp condition may be predisposed to the deleterious effects of living in a damp environment, creating a circular chain that dissolves the distinction between cause and effect. As the damp environment affects the body, the internal condition of dampness worsens, making it more susceptible to the damp environment. Damp is a description of one aspect of a pattern, a pathological process with signs and symptoms characteristic of the environmental condition that can affect it.

According to the system of correspondence, these climatic influences are linked to particular organs and to the seasons. Wind corresponds to the wood phase, the liver, and spring; heat to the fire phase, heart, and summer; damp to earth, spleen, and late summer; dryness to metal, lung, and fall; and cold to water, kidney; and winter. Various organs are thus noted as being susceptible to partic-

ular environmental excesses. The yin organ spleen, for example, has a vulnerability to damp, while its paired organ, stomach, can be affected by dryness. Environmental excesses can also combine to create a pattern of disharmony. Damp can combine with heat, for example, as part of a pattern of disharmony affecting the liver.

Emotions, the internal environmental factors, can become part of a pattern of disharmony. Joy, anger, anxiety, pensiveness, sadness, fear, and fright are healthy and natural responses to personal circumstances. Yet they can become unhealthy when extreme or recurrent. Emotions have five-phase correspondences and can be related to patterns of disharmony in particular organs. Anger, for example, may be part of a liver disharmony, while pensiveness or brooding may be a reflection of a spleen pattern. These internal factors, like the external ones, are both causes and effects. A liver disharmony may predispose a person to anger, yet the repeated expression of anger reinforces and exacerbates the liver disharmony.

The Chinese system also discusses a number of independent factors—the majority of them related to lifestyle—that play a role in patterns of disharmony. Good eating habits and proper nutrition are a foundation of qi and poor diet can create disharmony. Too much fatty food, too much sweet food, or too many raw foods can disrupt the digestive functions of the spleen and stomach, and may become part of a pattern of dampness. Too much alcohol or hot, spicy food can create or exacerbate a hot, damp condition.

Like emotions, sex is a normal, healthy part of life, but too much can weaken the body, particularly the kidney *jing*. Similarly, any kind of excessive strain can create problems. According to the *Yellow Emperor's Classic*: "Prolonged vision damages the blood; prolonged recumbency damages qi; prolonged sitting damages the flesh; prolonged standing damages the bones; and prolonged walking damages the sinews."[29, 30] From this perspective, there is always a healthy balance between extremes. Too little exercise—or sex—is not good for you, but it is also possible to get too much.

Eight Principal Patterns

In Chinese medicine, there is a structured framework with which to organize the array of signs and symptoms gathered from the four examinations into a recognizable pattern of disharmony. This framework is known as the eight principal patterns. The eight principal patterns are four pairs of complementary distinctions that assist the pattern-identification process: yin and yang, interior and exterior, deficiency and excess, cold and heat.

Exterior patterns arise when the body's exterior is assailed by external environmental pathogenic factors, especially cold and heat guided by the penetrating action of wind. As the body struggles to resist the invasion of the offending pathogen, symptoms are generated—like aversion to cold or wind, fever, and a "floating pulse." The floating pulse is a strong indicator that the pathogen is at the exterior of the body. Such exterior patterns can, if the pathogen is strong, the person's defenses weak, or the disharmony unsuccessfully treated, penetrate to the interior. Disharmony affecting the interior—an interior pattern—emerges from a variety of causes, including the inward movement of an exterior pathogen.[31]

Cold patterns are characterized by signs and symptoms reflecting cold, including a white complexion, cold limbs, desire for warm fluids, and aversion to cold. The pulse will be slow, suggesting the inhibiting influence of cold on physiological function. Heat patterns, in contrast, are indicated

Continued →

The Four Purifications

Lesley Tierra, L. Ac., Herbalist, A.H.C.

In Chinese medicine, the lungs are considered responsible in part for giving the body strength. Associated with air and its essential and vital life-giving properties, breathing exercises strengthen the lungs and body. The Four Purifications are a set of four different breathing techniques that quiet the mind, tone the lungs, blood, circulation, brain, internal organs and heart, give strength, calmness and energy to the whole body, and purify the nerve channels, stimulating digestion and strengthening the nervous system. Thus, they alleviate such ailments as nervousness, insomnia, indigestion, lung and breathing problems, poor circulation, low energy and vitality, fatigue, lethargy and poor memory. As such, they are invaluable for helping recovery from many health problems.

For those who have never done any breathing practices, these four techniques are safe to begin. For those already doing their own form of breathing practices, these are a perfect adjunct and starting exercise. Sit quietly with your back straight, either in a chair with your feet on the floor, or on the floor with your legs crossed. You may also concentrate your attention on the space between the eyebrows while doing these exercises. Do the breathing exercises in the order given. After practicing for a few months, move to the intermediate method described at the end.[1]

Alternate Nostril Breathing (Nadishodhana)

Begin by gently exhaling all air. Then close the right nostril with the thumb of the right hand and inhale slowly and deeply through the left nostril. When finished, close the left nostril with the ring finger of the right hand, releasing the thumb, and exhale slowly and fully through the right nostril. Next, immediately inhale through the right nostril in a slow and steady manner. Finally, close the right nostril with the right thumb again, releasing the ring finger, and exhale through the left nostril. This completes one round. Begin with ten rounds and gradually increase to forty.

This exercise alone is extremely beneficial to the body. It quiets the mind and strengthens the nervous system, inducing a wonderful calm state, releasing nervous tension, anxiety, agitation, anger and other disruptive emotions and inducing better sleep. It also oxygenates the system, enhancing energy and blood circulation and stimulating the proper functioning of all the internal organs. Continued practice of alternate nostril breathing strengthens the lungs and breath control.

Skull Shining (Kapala Bhati)

Skull shining is a series of forced exhalations with the breath. Begin by inhaling quickly and lightly through both nostrils. Then quickly and fully exhale all the breath through both nostrils. Emphasize the exhale, letting the inhalation come as a natural reflex. Repeat this pattern for thirty exhalations, or one round. After each round, which should last no longer than one minute, rest and breathe naturally. Then repeat the round. Begin with three rounds of thirty exhalations each and gradually increase to ten rounds of sixty exhalations each.

This technique purifies the head area, calming thoughts and enhancing breath and mind. As in alternate nostril breathing, skull shining helps release nervous tension, balances emotions and circulates Qi and blood. It also strengthens the lungs and breath control.

Cautions: Persons with high blood pressure or lung disease should not practice skull shining.

Fire Wash (Agnisara Dhauti)

Perform this exercise with all air held out of the body. Begin by taking a normal inhalation and exhalation, expelling all air. While holding the breath out, pull the diaphragm up and toward the backbone, and then release it suddenly. Repeat this in-and-out movement rapidly, as long as the breath can be held out without strain, about thirty pulls. Then inhale gently. This makes one round. Start with three rounds, gradually increasing to ten, beginning with thirty pulls per breath and working up to sixty.

This technique strengthens the "navel lock" (frequently used in breathing exercises), creating heat at the navel center (maniputa chakra) that purifies nerve channels, stimulates digestion, increases gastric fire, strengthens lungs and alleviates indigestion, abdominal diseases and menstrual disorders.

Horse Mudra (Ashvini Mudra)

This fourth exercise is an internal movement of the anal sphincter muscle. Begin by inhaling a complete and full breath and hold it in. Then contract and release the anal sphincter muscle rapidly and repeatedly. Hold the breath only so long as the following exhalation can be slow and controlled. Do not force your breath or length of holding. Begin with three rounds of thirty pulls each, and increase gradually to ten rounds of sixty contractions each. The horse mudra strengthens mula bandha, the anal lock, which increases concentration, strengthens reproductive glands and stimulates gastric fires.

Intermediate Method

When you've done the Four Purifications regularly for two to three months and feel comfortable with them, you may begin the intermediate method in this the Four Purifications are performed with no "resting breaths" in between, that is, they are done consecutively without a breath or rest in between. To perform, do 10–30 rounds of alternate nostril breathing, then after the last exhalation through the left nostril, inhale partially and immediately begin skull shining. At the end of one series of skull shining exhalations, inhale slowly and completely, then exhale all air, hold the breath out and do the fire wash. After one round of the fire wash, inhale completely, hold the breath and do the horse mudra. This entire series now completes one round.

After the horse mudra, exhale completely and immediately begin again with alternate nostril breathing, thus starting the next round. Do five rounds, gradually increasing the numbers of alternate nostril breathing and the duration of retention in each of the other three techniques.

—From *Healing With the Herbs of Life*

1. The Four Purifications are thoroughly described and illustrated, along with many other valuable breathing and yogic techniques, in *Ashtanga Yoga Primer*, by Baba Hari Dass, Sri Rama Publishing, 1981 (ox 2550, Santa Cruz, CA 95063).

---

by signs of heat, ranging from a red complexion, thirst, and restlessness to a rapid pulse indicative of the effect of heat on physiological function.

Deficiency implies weakness; excess is associated with a vigorous pathogen. Deficiency signs such as a pale face, pale tongue body, lack of energy, and a weak pulse suggest a deficit in function or substance. Any of qi, blood, yin or yang may be undersupplied, a distinction that must be made clear as the pattern recognition process proceeds. Excess is indicated by pain that is intensified by pressure, a strong pulse, and a thick tongue fur. There are several possibilities here: blocked qi and blood will form accumulations; an overenthusiastic appetite can result in digestive organ stagnation; or various environmental factors can become pathogenic.

Yin and yang, the last of the four pairs, are general qualities that shape the pattern-recognition process and can be applied to the other three pairs of complementary distinctions. Cold, deficiency, and internal are yin, while heat, excess, and external are yang. Yin and yang can also refer to specific aspects of the body-mind system, yin to the nutritious and thicker fluids of the body, and yang to the yang qi, the functional force animating physiological function and stoking the metabolic fire. . . .

Restoring Health with Herbs and Needles

From this diagnostic model the principles of therapy become apparent: heat is balanced with cold and coldness warmed; deficiencies require supplementation while excesses are cleared; yin and yang must be harmonized. To paraphrase Ted Kaptchuk, exaggerated activity must be calmed, too little activity must be tonified, a build-up of substances must be cleared, heat must be treated with cold, cold must be buffered with heat, and movement must follow its proper direction. In short, balance must be restored to the system.[32]

Over the millennia, an array of methods have been developed to accomplish these goals. Herbs can be used to cool or warm, clear or supplement, and harmonize. Through acupuncture, the qi can be manipulated to supplement deficiencies or eliminate excesses. Diet, exercise, massage, and qi gong can also help with the transition from disharmony to harmony. It is here, grounded in the perennial challenge of healing, that theory

Continued →

merges with practice, coming to life as the art of medicine.

HERBS: FROM FOLKLORE TO HIGH MEDICINE

One day while picking herbs in the mountains Master Shan noticed two young men chasing a vigorous and lithe teenager. He was told by the empty-handed and fatigued men that the girl had escaped from a foster home. Wanting to learn the girl's secret of health, the herbalist's curiosity got the best of him. Carefully placing a bowl of rice and spiced bean curd in a nearby cave, he hid in a bush by the entrance. After some hours had passed the girl appeared and began eating. Shan ran to the entrance and asked about the abundance of energy, perfect complexion, and robust health she possessed. Without hesitation the girl attributed her ability to survive the rigors of mountain life to the regular consumption of a local plant's fleshy roots. After finding the plant, Shan named the root yellow essence (huang jing).

Herbs are an important part of Chinese culture. Many herbs like huang jing are famous not for their ability to heal the sick but because they are able to build intrinsic health and prevent illness. For millennia the farmers and craftsmen of China have used herbs to strengthen and improve health. Taoists discovered and made use of herbs in their search for the elixir of immortality, while martial artists found herbs gave them strength and durability. The wealthy praised the ability of herbs to maintain youthfulness and beautify the complexion. Today, Chinese herb shops—timeless apothecaries where both abacus and calculator are used to tabulate customer accounts—throughout the world attest to the continuity of this tradition.

The use of herbs—including plants, animals, and minerals—is a key therapy in Chinese medicine. Over several thousand years Chinese herbal medicine has evolved, blending folk tradition with the learned medicine of the scholar-physicians and empirical discovery with the theory of systematic correspondence. The first book dedicated to describing the substances used in medicine was *The Divine Husbandman's Classic of the Materia Medica*, attributed to Shen Nong, the legendary Divine Husbandman, who is credited with introducing agriculture to China and honored as the patron saint of herbal medicine. From the 364 herbs recorded in *The Divine Husbandman's Classic* in A.D. 200, the materia medica grew to include 1,000 herbs by the year 1000 and close to 2,000 herbs by 1600, thanks in part to the work of Li Shi-zhen. In 1977, the Jiangsu College of New Medicine completed a massive twenty-five-year project cataloguing 5,767 medical substances.[33]

Chinese herbs are classified according to function. There are tonifying herbs to supplement blood, qi, yin and yang, herbs to expel dampness, herbs to clear heat and expel cold, and herbs to move or "regulate" stuck qi, among others.[34] All herbs have a taste—a combination of sweet, spicy, salty, bitter, sour, and bland—and temperature—a ranking on the cold to hot scale—which guide their application. Herbs are also discussed in terms of the meridians they enter, their major functions, important combinations, correct dosage, and cautions, including toxicity.

The materia medica includes many substances of plant origin, a spectrum of colorful and exotic-looking roots, berries, twigs, flowers, and fungi. Some of these, such as ginseng root and walnut, are well known in the West, while others, such as broomrape (Herba Cistanches)—a fleshy parasitic plant—are unfamiliar in the west. Minerals like gypsum and animal substances like deer antler are also widely used. In some cases, herbs are used fresh,

but often they are processed to neutralize toxicity or enhance a particular function. Many herbs, particularly those in the tonic category, are used for their nutritional, rather than medicinal, value.

Dang gui (Radix Angelica Sinensis) and *shu di huang* (Radix Rehmannia Preparatae), for example, are two of the most important blood tonic herbs. *Dang gui* is a white, hard-as-rock root that releases a unique fragrance as it is cooked. It helps invigorate and harmonize the blood and its ability to regulate menstruation makes it an important women's herb. *Dang gui* is classified as sweet, pungent, and bitter; it enters the heart, liver, and spleen meridians, and was first recorded as far back as *The Divine Husbandman's Classic*. The sticky black root *shu di huang* is prepared by steaming it with wine, a process that changes its temperature from cool to warm. It is a sweet herb that enters the kidney, liver, and heart meridians, and is used to tonify blood and nourish yin.

The earthy-colored root *dang shen* (Radix Codonopsis Pilosulae) is a sweet-flavored qi tonic with a neutral temperature. *Dang shen* strengthens qi, tonifies the lung and spleen, and nourishes fluids. *Dang shen* is similar in function to ginseng root (*ren shen* or Radix Panax Ginseng), although not as strong. North American ginseng root (Radix Panax Quinquifolium), unlike its Asian cousin, is classified as a yin tonic and has a cool temperature. It has been exported to the Orient for over 250 years, since it was first spotted by Jesuit missionaries who were familiar with ginseng through their travels to China. In addition to major areas of production in states such as Wisconsin, Canadian farmers produce close to one million pounds a year; most of this crop is exported to Asia. *Xi yang shen*, or "root from the Western seas," as it is called in Chinese, enters the lung, stomach, and kidney meridians, strengthens the qi, and supplements yin.

Wu wei zi or "five-flavored seed," a deep red pea-size berry of the magnolia vine, is predominantly sour, but contains hints of the other four flavors: sweet, spicy, salty, and bitter. Fructus Schisandra Chinensis (*wu wei zi*) is placed in the astringent category, enters both lung and kidney meridians, and has several functions related to its sour taste and astringent property. It can check excessive sweating, help stop cough in cases of lung deficiency, and is used for diarrhea with a pattern of spleen and kidney yang deficiency. *Wu wei zi* has the secondary function of calming the *shen* and is valuable for insomnia and poor memory. Modern research indicates that *wu wei zi* has an "adaptogenic" effect, normalizing various physiological functions and helping to buffer the impact of stress.

CREATING COMBINATIONS

Despite the large number of substances used in herbal medicine, the goal is not to match single herbs with particular diseases, but to create a combination of herbs that can address an individual pattern of disharmony. The first step toward this goal is recognizing effects that appear when herbs are used in combination, so that unwanted synergistic effects are avoided and the best use is made of beneficial ones. White peony root (Radix Paeonia Lactiflora), for example, can relieve pain and spasm when combined with licorice root (Radix Glycyrrhiza Uralensis), and has a special function related to the resolution of lingering wind cold patterns when combined with cinnamon twig (Ramulus Cinnamomi Cassia).[35]

Combinations of herbs are constructed according to a fourfold hierarchy of king, minister, assistant, and messenger. King refers to those herbs whose function reflects the fundamental goal of the formula, while minister herbs either support this

goal or are directed toward a secondary purpose. The assistants offer support for the king and minister or buffer their potential side effects. The messengers harmonize the actions of their superiors. The result is a combination that is more than the sum of its parts, a therapeutic agent that can address even a complex pattern of disharmony. A modern text on formulas states: "The formulas in Chinese medicine are not mere collections of medicinal substances in which the actions of one herb are simply added to those of another in a cumulative fashion. They are complex recipes of interrelated substances, each of which affects the actions of the others. . . . It is this complex interaction which makes the formulas so effective. . . ."[36]

This means that the practitioner not only has to study individual herbs and their synergistic actions, but also must be familiar with many of the hundreds of formulas that have been developed over the past two thousand years. These formulas are classified functionally in a manner similar to that of the herbs themselves. There are formulas that tonify, combinations that calm the spirit, and others that treat dryness. Such formulas serve as the starting point for developing a combination matching a patient's particular pattern of disharmony.

Rehmannia Six, used as a basis for Sue's prescription, is a skillfully crafted formula designed to tonify the kidney yin. At the core of this formula is *shu di huang*, the tarry-looking prepared root used to supplement kidney yin. *Shu di, as it is called by pharmacists, is used in the* highest dosage in the formula and its actions are supported by the astringent herb Fructus Corni (*shan zhuyu*), the purple-red fruit of the Japanese cornelian cherry, and Radix Dioscorea (*shan yao*), the tuber of a species of Chinese yam. Cornelian cherry strengthens and stabilizes the kidney, while yam is a tonic to the kidney and spleen. Support for the spleen helps to strengthen the kidney indirectly, since the spleen is the foundation of postnatal jing stored in the kidney.

These tonic actions are not without potential side effects, chief among them congestion from the sticky, hard-to-digest *shu di*. The heat that is part of a pattern of kidney yin deficiency must also be addressed. The underground stem of the water plantain (*ze xie* or Rhizoma Alismatis Orientalis) has the specific action of clearing heat, as does the "blood cooling" herb *mu dan pi* (Cortex Moutan Radicis). Together with the sixth herb completing Rehmannia Six, the subterranean mushroom *fu ling* (Sclerotium Poria Cocos), water plantain also acts to support fluid metabolism, buffering the potential congesting effect of the tonics. Together with the yam, *fu ling* bolsters spleen function, ensuring that the digestive function is not impaired by the richness of *shu di*. *Mu dan pi*, a cool herb, counterbalances the warmth of the cornelian cherry. These supporting and counterbalancing interactions make Rehmannia Six an effective way to address a pattern of kidney yin deficiency, strengthening and restoring physiological functions with a minimum of side effects.

In contrast to Sue, Dave presented a pattern of spleen qi deficiency with a complication of dampness. Dave's prescription was constructed by adding several herbs to a classic formula known as the Four Gentlemen. The king of the Four Gentlemen is *dang shen*, the spleen-supplementing herb discussed above, while its minister is *bai zhu* (Rhizoma Attractylodis Macrocephalae), a woody-looking and pungent spleen tonic with a significant drying quality. The assistant is *fu ling*, the white, chalky subterranean fungus that appeared in Rehmannia Six. *Fu ling* supports the spleen through its ability to activate the spleen's ability to transform and transport moisture, a function that is ideally suited for Dave's

Continued →

pattern. The messenger herb is *gan cao*, or Chinese licorice root, which supports the spleen qi and harmonizes the action of the other herbs. Although his underlying pattern was one of spleen qi deficiency, Dave's problem with dampness required the addition of other herbs, including dried orange peel (Pericarpium Citri Reticulatae) and *sha ren* (Frutus Amomi). Addressing a pattern of disharmony is a dynamic process set in a constantly changing landscape. During the course of his herbal treatment, Dave will change in response to the formula, and the formula will be changed to reflect his new condition.

Acupuncture: The Art of the Needle

Acupuncture and herbal medicine are the foundations of Chinese medical therapy. Many aspects of acupuncture are comparable to treatment with herbs, and its therapeutic goals, derived from the patterns of disharmony identified through the diagnostic process, are the same. Like herbs, needles can counteract excesses—relieving stagnation by circulating stuck qi, for example—or can strengthen specific meridians to overcome deficiencies. Hot conditions can be cooled; cold conditions warmed. With her fine needles the acupuncturist, like the herbalist (who are often one and the same), works to harmonize yin and yang.[37]

For the patient, acupuncture is a relatively painless procedure. It is very important that the practitioner "gets the qi"—which means obtaining a needling sensation—and when this occurs there may be a sense of pressure or fullness at the point. In the thirteenth century, Dou Han-qing noted that "a hollow, smooth, and loose sensation around the needle suggests the absence of qi, which lets you feel as if you are walking on a wild and empty ground, but a heavy, uneven, and tense feeling suggests [the practitioner has obtained the qi], which is felt as a fish biting at the hook and pulling the line downward." Over the centuries, many authors have stressed the value of "getting the qi," including Yang Ji-zhou, who wrote in the *Great Compendium of Acupuncture and Moxibustion*, published in 1601, that "[getting the qi] alone is the measure of the treatment. If the qi does not arrive, there is no treatment.[38] During treatment it is common that a patient will experience "propagated sensation along the channel," a tingling or warmth that extends along the channel being needled.

Points, like herbs, are rarely used alone and point "prescriptions" typically include from six to twelve needles. Prescriptions of points are chosen from a variety of strategies, including the king, minister, assistant, and messenger hierarchy. Needling technique is also an important part of a point prescription since various needling techniques have different effects. The two most important techniques are reinforcing and reducing; reinforcing is used to balance deficiency, reducing to balance excess. As *The Yellow Emperor's Classic* warns: "The disease will be aggravated by treatment with the wrong reinforcing or reducing method of manipulation, that is, reinforcing in excess syndromes and reducing in deficiency syndromes."[39]

In addition to using points based on the therapeutic principles required for a particular pattern of disharmony, points can be chosen based on the location of the disease, since points can affect their surrounding area. For example, large intestine 20, a point beside the lower edge of the nose, can be used to treat nose problems. Since the effect of needling is transmitted along the channel, points far from the problem can also be chosen. Large intestine 4, a point on the edge of the hand close to the vertex of the V formed by the thumb and index finger, can be used for toothache, since the large intestine channel extends from the hand along the arm, traversing the gums to end at large intestine 20 by the edge of the nose. There are also a host of points with special functions—including the front-mu and back-shu points that bear a special relation to the qi of the organs, the eight influential points which directly affect the qi, blood, and six other areas of the body, and the crossing points where two or more channels meet.

June and Heidi had both suffered for months with sleep problems, and both found that acupuncture, along with cutting out coffee and exercising regularly, virtually eliminated the problem. As they discussed their experiences over a cup of herbal tea at the office, they were surprised to learn that the treatments they received for such similar problems were different. Both recalled receiving needles at a point in the crease of the wrist, but the other needle sites appeared to be different. When they asked their acupuncturist about this strange difference, she explained that heart 7, the point on the crease of the wrist, is an important point for nourishing the heart and calming the *shen*, and this was used in both treatments. However, June, who was diagnosed with a pattern of deficiency affecting the blood, heart, and spleen, also had needles placed at spleen 6, a major point for spleen and blood tonification, bladder 15, the back-shu point of the heart, and bladder 20, the back-shu point of the spleen. Heidi, in contrast, presented a pattern of hyperactive liver and needles were placed at bladder 18, the liver back-shu point, and liver 3, a point that can settle the liver by nourishing the yin aspect of the liver. Perhaps, suggested the acupuncturist, it was their opposite traits that made them good friends—Heidi, a bundle of energy, always excited about something but often edgy and tense, and June, the calm in the center of the storm, relaxed but often unmotivated and sometimes fatigued.

The subtle power of Chinese medicine lies first in its perception of the whole and systematic organization of signs and symptoms into a pattern of disharmony. This "pattern thinking" places the clinical gaze on the milieu in which illness is set, defining the relationship between part and whole. This focus on patterns of disharmony is like a farmer who perceives a connection between the fungus on her strawberry crop and the field's poor drainage, recognizing that excessive dampness allowed the fungus to thrive. Adding sand to the soil and installing drainage pipes does not kill the fungus, but fosters the kind of environment that strawberry plants love and fungus loathes.

Intimately intertwined with Chinese medicine's "pattern thinking" is the development of therapies directed toward the restoration of balance. Patterns of disharmony are addressed using means that are subtle but persevering, flexible while precise, gentle yet effective, dynamic although directed. A contemporary practitioner can draw on an empirical body of knowledge going back thousands of years. The result is a process of healing—a realignment over space and time, rather than an event or singular solution—from which health can grow.

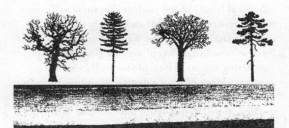

The Mind and Body in Medicine

Chinese medicine is mind-body medicine. Whether a patient's chief complaint is a mind problem or a body problem, both mental and physical signs and symptoms are included in the recognition of a pattern of disharmony. For example, a pattern of liver invading spleen, which involves both liver excess and spleen deficiency, is recognized by its combination of digestive disturbance and liver disharmony. One patient seeking treatment for a digestive problem may divulge emotional issues of irritability and frustration—typically considerd liver signs—upon questioning by the practitioner, while another seeking help for excessive anger—a sign usually associated with the liver—might reveal a minor digestive complaint during examination. Both cases could fall into the same pattern of "liver invading spleen" depending on the overall set of signs and symptoms—some of which are emotional and others physical.

Like diagnosis, treatment simultaneously addresses the mind and the body as inseparable parts of a general pattern. While the two "liver invading spleen" cases above may well share the same general description, treatments will be adjusted to match the precise manifestations of the pattern in the individual. Yet no matter what the treatment strategy taken, it will focus on adjusting the qi—the bridge between mind and body.

Acupuncture and herbs address both mental-emotional and physical disharmony. As the *Spiritual Axis* claims, the acupuncture points are the places where *shen* and qi, spirit and energy, enter and leave. Some point names reflect this connection. There is the "spirit gate"—heart 7—on the inner crease of the wrist, a useful point for treating spirit disorders such as insomnia, irritability, poor memory, and even mania. Or there are the "door of the material soul (the *po*)" and the "house of the *shen*," the 42nd and 44th points on the bladder channel, respectively. Herbs too are discussed in terms of their physiological effects and their influence on emotional and even spiritual qualities.

A modern Chinese acupuncture text illustrates the general approach in treating "depressive syndromes."[40] Such problems, the text explains, can result from overthinking or the inability to achieve an important life goal. The resulting stagnation of qi affects the "free-flow" of the liver and can impair the spleen's activity of "transformation and transportation." As fluid metabolism becomes impaired, phlegm can appear, "misting" the heart and disturbing the shen. (Phlegm, in Chinese medicine, includes discharge from the lungs and sinuses as well as congested and congealed fluids affecting other organs and body parts.)

The pattern can be resolved by restoring the liver's free flow of qi, clearing phlegm, and harmonizing the spirit, for which three "back shu" points on the bladder meridian are chosen together with heart 7, the spirit gate, to calm the mind, and stomach 40, an important point for treating phlegm. (Back shu points are special points with a direct influence on particular organ systems.) The heart-shu complements heart 7 in harmonizing the mind, the spleen-shu strengthens digestive function and supports the treatment of phlegm, while the liver-shu treats stagnant qi.

Treatments can also be more creative and less "physical." Hua Tuo, the famous surgeon, once encountered a seriously ill official, and devised a novel cure—a sort of "shock" treatment. Hua Tuo felt that if he could stimulate the patient into a rage, cure would be ensured. After collecting an

Continued ➜

exorbitant fee, he left the patient with a rather nasty and belligerent note. The official became enraged and sick to his stomach, thereafter recovering from his illness.

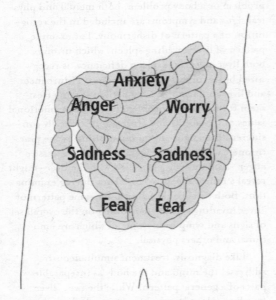

In Chinese medicine the abdominal brain stores negative emotions.

The Mystery of Qi: "Energy" in Chinese Medicine . . .

One of the most extraordinary ideas in Chinese medicine is the notion of qi and its circulation through a series of channels in the body.[42] While qi is not a material substance that can be isolated and studied, it is of fundamental importance to medicine. By adjusting the circulation of qi at an acupuncture point the physician affects physiological functions, regulating and harmonizing the organism.

Qi remains a mystery. There is little correspondence in standard Western biology to either qi, the acupoints, or the complex system of channels through which qi flows. If acupuncture has any validity say the skeptics, it may be through stimulation of the nervous system and consequent effect on various biologically active chemicals such as the endorphins, opiate-like molecules involved in pain response. Qi, according to this view, may simply be a long-held superstition or perhaps a crude metaphor for organizational and regulatory processes involving the nervous system. Yet the Western difficulty with qi may lie with the limitations of standard biology and medicine—for the new biology is offering glimpses of curious phenomena that are not without parallel to ancient Chinese ideas.

Qi in Chinese Medicine: Mystical Metaphor and Concrete Healing Tool

Cosmic Qi

Rather than using an alphabet, the Chinese language is composed of ideograms or characters built up from a set of basic symbols called radicals. The character for qi is a combination of the radical for vapor or gas and the rice or grain radical, symbolizing the fine essence drafting up from a pot of cooking grain. Qi is thus something ethereal and unseen, but known through its effects and consequences, like the saliva generated in a hungry person bending over a pot of aromatic rice.

Qi has a broad range of meanings, from simply gas and vapor to various cosmic and biological "energies." Cosmic qi, for example, played a central role in the formation of the universe. Out of

the primal nothingness emerged space and time, and from them arose original qi. This qi separated into its heavy and light components, the light rising to become heaven, the heavy coalescing to become the earth. The qi of heaven and earth in turn produced yin and yang, their qi bringing forth the seasons and differentiated things of the world.

This ancient view of the universe reached its most sophisticated level during the great Neo-Confucian synthesis of Confucian, Taoist, and Buddhist ideas during the eleventh and twelfth centuries. Chu Hsi, a Neo-Confucian who lived from 1131 to 1200 and one of China's greatest thinkers, merged the concept of qi together with *li*, the cosmic principle of organization, to set out an organic philosophy of the universe. Chu Hsi envisioned a universe oscillating eternally between order and chaos, primal unity and differentiated diversity. In the beginning, swirling cosmic qi gathered speed, coalescing to form the earth and leaving lighter qi on the outside to form the heavens. Qi was shaped over time by the innate principle of organization, *li*, creating a patterned progression from primal chaos to ever higher levels of order.

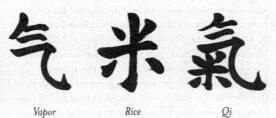

| Vapor | Rice | Qi |

QI: MATTER, ENERGY, OR VITAL FORCE?

Qi is the basic stuff of the universe, neither matter nor energy, so fine and rarefied as to fill space. Joseph Needham, who felt qi best remained untranslated as a unique cultural concept, described it as matter-energy. It is a concept that finds its way into every aspect of Chinese science and culture, from medicine to art. The acupuncture needle regulates the patient's qi, a task aided by the practitioner's own qi connecting through the needle. The space of a master's landscape painting is bursting with qi that merges seamlessly with the qi of the rocks, mountains, and trees.

Scholar Paul Unschuld warns against the common interpretation of qi as "energy," suggesting instead that qi be rendered as "finest matter influence."[44] Qi often has this connotation of a force or "influence." In medicine, for example, there is damp qi—one of the six environmental qi or influences that can affect health—and pestilential qi—a disease agent present in epidemics.

Another scholar, Manfred Porkert, in contrast, argues that while not a precisely parallel concept, qi can be considered as "energy" in a general sense. He calls qi "configurational energy," an energy with a defined direction in space, structure, or quality. There are over ten fundamental types of qi described in medicine and more than twenty secondary types. Porkert describes thirty-two of them, such as heavenly or celestial qi, denoting the effect of the ever-changing cosmic pattern, and wet qi, the body's defensive energy.[45]

In the biological realm, qi is often translated as vital energy, suggesting a connection to the mysterious "vital force" of the vitalists. Yet there are essential differences between qi and the out-of-fashion idea of a vital force. In the West, the idea of a vital force was used to differentiate living systems from non-living matter. The Chinese world view, in contrast, does not draw a demarcation line between the living and non-living. Qi is used to describe physical as well as biological phenomena. While the

physician can adjust the flow of qi in the human body, so too the practitioner of *feng shui*—literally "wind and water," an art without correspondence in the West but often translated as geomancy—works with the flow of qi in the earth to harmonize the human relationship with the environment. The Chinese universe is a living, organic one characterized by different forms and levels of organization and energy, *li* and qi.

Secondly, qi is not at heart a mysterious and unknowable philosophical concept like the vital force. As Ted Kaptchuk states: "For the Chinese, qi is not a metaphor; it is a real phenomenon that makes possible integrative descriptions of bodily changes. Diagnostic methods exist for determining its strength and motion, and there are specific treatments for supplementing its deficiency draining its excess, and regulating its flow."[46] The physician can feel the qi arrive at a point being punctured; it is like a fish grabbing the fisher's hook. The patient's sense of fullness at the point and a radiating sensation along the channel show that the qi has been activated, offering confidence in the effect of treatment. The qi gong practitioner can feel the warmth generated by concentration on the sea of qi—the center and source located just below the navel—and can, in the exercise known as "qi ball," feel the static-electricity-like ball of qi between the hands.

QI IN THE PHYSIOLOGICAL AND PSYCHOLOGICAL LANDSCAPE

As we can see in the following passage from the *Yellow Emperor's Classic of Internal Medicine*, the ancient medical book written in the form of a dialogue between the Yellow Emperor and his minister Qi Bo, qi is a central concept in medicine:

The Yellow Emperor asked, "I heard all diseases are created by qi. With anger the qi rises; with joy the qi becomes loose or moderate; with grief the qi disappears, with fear the qi descends; with cold the qi shrinks; with heat the qi leaks; with fright the qi is disordered. With tiredness, the qi wilts; with thinking the qi becomes stagnant. These nine qi are not the same. What causes these diseases?"

Qi Bo answered, "With anger the qi becomes counter flow. . . . With joy the qi becomes harmonized and the will becomes stronger. The ying and wei are able to flow through; therefore, the qi is loose or moderate. . . . With heat, the skin tissues open, the ying and wei pass through, there is a great sweating. Therefore, the qi leaks. With fright the heart cannot perform its regal tasks. The *shen* cannot return. The thoughts and consciousness are not stable; therefore, the qi becomes disordered. With tiredness there is panting and sweating; the inside and outside are overcome; therefore, the qi wilts. . . ."[47]

This exchange between the Yellow Emperor and his minister eloquently illustrates the link in Chinese medicine between the emotions, qi, and physiological processes. Qi, as this passage shows, is of pivotal importance in the theoretical foundation and explanatory framework of Chinese medicine.

Qi in the body has five functions: it plays a protective role, activates, warms, transforms, and keeps things in place. As a protective force it provides defense against pathogens. In this sense, qi is called the "correct," the mobilizing force that resists invasion by outside agents and maintains health in the face of adverse environmental conditions. Chinese medicine describes disease as a struggle between the pathogen and correct qi, which must be debilitated before a pathogen can successfully take hold.

Continued ➡

As a warming agent, qi is responsible for the maintenance of body temperature and the body's metabolic fire. Qi keeps the organs held in their proper place, prevents blood from spilling from the vessels, and checks the excessive flow of fluids such as sweat, tears, and urine from the body. Qi is also behind the transformative actions that take place in the body. Food is transformed into blood, for example, while ingested fluids are transformed into urine. As an activating agent, qi is reflected in the movement and activity inherent in everything from physiological functions to human growth and development.

VARIETIES OF QI

Manfred Porkert has discussed thirty-two distinct types of qi. Let us explore some of the most important ones, and set out a system-level model of qi in the human organism. A starting point is understanding the origins of true or genuine qi, the general designation for all the qi of the body.

Prenatal qi is inherited from one's parents. It is the root potential or basic constitution of an individual and is stored in the kidneys. The Taoists, in their great efforts to promote longevity, emphasized the importance of conserving and supporting the prenatal qi. Prenatal qi acts as the fundamental template for the functions and pattern of growth and development in the organism. When utilized and activated in this way it is known as original qi.

Original qi gushes forth from an area between the kidneys and below the navel. This is the root or source of life—the hara—so important in Eastern culture. Deep breathing combined with a relaxed concentration on the "sea of qi" below the navel is important in qi gong, the meditation-exercise used by ancient immortality-seeking adepts and modern health-seekers alike. As Qi Bo explains to the Yellow Emperor:

Each of the twelve meridians has a relationship to the source of the vital energies. The source of the vital energies is the root origin of the twelve meridians, it is the moving qi between the kidneys. This means that the source of the vital energies is fundamental to the five yin and six yang organs, the root of the twelve meridians, the gate of breathing. It is the source of the triple warmer.

"Thus" emphasize Kiiko Matsumoto and Stephen Birch, contemporary practitioners of Chinese medicine, "the abdomen is more than the physical center, the cavity in which the organs reside. It is the residence of the source of the body's energies, the energetic center from which life springs."[49] As Qi Bo describes, original qi is circulated throughout the body via the triple warmer, or sanjiao, one of the yang organ-meridian systems of Chinese medicine.

Grain qi is extracted from food by the transformative action of the spleen, while air qi is absorbed by the lungs from the air we breathe. Air qi, grain qi, and original qi combine to produce the true qi. The extraction of air qi from the respiratory processes and the circulation of qi and blood throughout the body are assisted by the ancestral qi of the chest. Ancestral qi, composed of air and grain qi, fosters the respiratory rhythm and harmonizes the heartbeat.

True qi is differentiated into its various forms according to function. True qi associated with the organs is called organ qi, the essence of each organ's physiological activity. Spleen qi, for example, is involved in the transformation and transportation of food. True qi flowing through the channels is called channel qi. The channels are the communication network of the body-mind, and channel qi the agent of information, acting to regulate and harmonize the organs.

Construction or nutritive (*ying*) qi is inseparable from the blood. As it says in the *Yellow Emperor's Classic*, "Construction qi secretes fluids, discharges them into the vessels, and turns them into blood, to nourish the limbs and supply the yin and yang organs."[50] Construction qi is involved in the transformation of food into blood, the movement of blood and the nourishment of the entire body.

Defensive (*wei*) qi, the complement of construction qi, flows outside of the vessels and offers protection against invading pathogens. Defensive qi nourishes the skin and it flows on the body exterior where it regulates sweating.

Original qi, stored in the kidneys, represents the pre-natal or inborn contribution to the qi that underlies physiological, emotional, and mental activity. Grain qi derived from eating and air qi acquired from breathing are the postnatal contribution. Proper nutrition and breathing are thus crucial components of good health, and why dietary habits and breathing exercises like qi gong are a foundation of prevention and therapy. Together, original, grain, and air qi form the true qi, which in its various forms—channel and organ qi, nutritive and defensive qi—regulates and harmonizes, nourishes and defends, allowing the mind-body in all its complexity to function in an integrated way.

OF WATER-WORKS AND CAVES

The channels (also often called meridians) through which channel qi travels are the basis of acupuncture practice. Because of the integrating, regulating, and communicating function of channel qi, its adjustment special points along the channels can harmonize and restore patterns of disharmony. As described in the *Yellow Emperor's Classic*, channels are the conduits of qi and blood, making possible the balancing of yin and yang and the moistening of the joints and sinews.[51] Channel qi circulates through the body along a network of major and minor channels (the *jing-luo*), connecting the interior with the exterior, the yin organs with the yang organs, and the organs with the various parts of the body.

The Chinese character for channel is composed of the thread or string radical and the character *jing*, signifying the underground flow of water. The top line with three arrow heads of the character *jing* depicts the flow of water beneath the ground. *Jing* also connotes the threads in a fabric that give it form and, as a verb, to pass through or to direct. The channels are thus conduits directing the flow of qi.

The character for the acupoints suggests a cave, hole, or opening. It is a picture of a roof above, with a symbol meaning to divide below, implying a shelter created by the removal of earth. The character *shu*, with an implication of transportation or movement, is also used to designate a special set of acupuncture points, hinting at the energetic transmission between point and organ.

As explained in the *Yellow Emperor's Classic*, the acupoints are places where the vital qi enters and leaves. The points, channels, and organs form an integrated, interactive, and dynamic system. When a channel connects with its organ (when the spleen channel links with the spleen, for example) it enters and saturates or belongs to that organ, implying a strong, indivisible link. When a channel connects with a coupled organ (when the spleen channel connects with the paired organ of the spleen, the stomach, for example), it "spirally wraps" the organ, implying influence and interaction but with more distinction between channel and organ.[52] The continuous circulation of qi along a sequence of channels—starting at the lung and ending at the

liver channel brings a collection of parts together into a harmonious whole.

Some scholars have pointed to the "circulation-mindedness" of the ancient Chinese, and suggest that their early conception of the circulation of blood and qi arose naturally in a society based on large-scale waterworks. Chinese civilization had it origins in a rich agricultural area prone to flooding, and waterworks were used to control water levels, irrigate crops, and provide transportation. The power and central authority of the Emperor arose from the need for a government that could organize and administer such large-scale efforts.

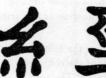

糸	坙	經
Thread	Underground Flow of Water	Acupuncture Channel

This culture of waterworks contributed many water-based descriptions and metaphors to the medical field, creating a fertile ground for the idea of blood and qi circulating through the organism. (The Chinese notion of blood circulation predated the discovery of blood circulation by William Harvey in the seventeenth century.) The characters *jing* and *luo*, for example, used to denote the main channels and the secondary connecting channels, are also found in terms for large rivers and civic drains.[53] Each of the twelve main channels has five "transporting-*shu*" points rich with water metaphor: the well, spring, stream, river, and uniting points, the latter point name suggesting a river uniting with the sea. This use of water metaphors in the East can be compared to the machine analogies used in the West and illustrates how important the cultural milieu is in shaping the understanding and interpretation of natural phenomena.

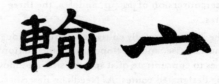

輸	亠
Shu	Roof

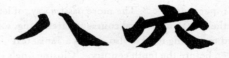

八	穴
To Divide	Acupuncture Point

ORIGINS AND REALITY

Qi, the acupoints, and the channels—unique cultural concepts whose origins are obscured in the mists of time—are without direct or obvious parallels in Western biology and medicine, making it difficult for Western biomedicine to make sense of these distinctly Eastern ideas. Modern biomedical research on acupuncture has focused on various chemical changes produced by needling. There are also electrical correspondences to the acupuncture points. Point locators based on the difference in the electrical resistance of the skin between a point and its surrounding area have emerged from this kind of inquiry.[54] So while there appears to be

Continued ➡

some objective scientific measure of the points and their ability to produce biochemical changes, the channels are on shakier ground.[55]

In describing the points as real and the channels as the result of speculation, Manfred Porkert expresses a commonly held perspective: "[The detection of the conduits] by connecting the points is analogous to the way a subterranean water course reveals itself by springs sent up through 'punctures' in the earth's crust. The sensitive points provide the positive empirical and historically primary data on which the theory is based; the conduits, on the other hand, are only the result of systematic speculations."[56] Others have suggested that acupuncture developed empirically from the systematic stimulation of the body surface, perhaps as part of ritual demon exorcism practiced by the shamanistic tribes of precivilization China.[57]

Yet early texts written before the *Yellow Emperor's Classic* suggest that the concept of the channels existed before that of the points.[58] The texts describe various channels and their zones of influence without reference to points. Matsumoto and Birch point out that it is the internal, not the external or surface, trajectories of the twelve major channels that were classically considered to be the "main" channels. While the external trajectories are important for the practice of acupuncture, they were thought of as "branches." The internal meridians are the site of "the more important energetic exchanges and interactions," the surface branches merely "superficial extensions."[59]

This suggests a completely different origin for the Chinese concepts of qi circulation, points, and channels. Out of the timeless void of prehistory arose the spiritual practice/proto-science of Taoism. Taoists were interested in spiritual development, knowledge of the natural world, and immortality, for which they practiced both outer and inner alchemy. Outer alchemy was the search for the elixir of immortality; inner or physiological alchemy was a meditative process of transforming internal "energies" for spiritual development and immortality. This process of physiological alchemy involved the cultivation and circulation of qi and the interconversion of *jing*, qi, and *shen*, the three treasures.

The Taoists carefully cultivated their qi through diet and exercise, and developed many meditation-exercises to concentrate qi at specific sites and move it along designated routes. As Needham describes: "There were two ways of making it circulate. Concentrating the will to direct it to a particular place, such as the brain, or the site of some local malady, was termed *xing* qi. Visualizing its flow in thought was 'inner vision'. . . . The more passive way, of letting the qi take its normal course in circulating, was called re-casting it." He also quotes a Taoist text written before the tenth century: "Closing one's eyes, one has an inner vision of the five yin organs, one can clearly distinguish them, one knows the place of each. . . ."[60]

The Taoists spent years practicing this kind of inner awareness, were familiar with their inner anatomy, and had some sense perception of this concentrated energy. Inner alchemy, so much a part of Taoism and Chinese civilization, likely played a key role in the discovery and elaboration of the channels and points upon which acupuncture is based. The techniques of inner alchemy were widely and continuously practiced and explain the mapping and importance of the inner trajectories of the channels. The discovery of subtle energy flows at the edge of interaction between mind and body arose in the course of systematic exploration of the inner environment by organized groups of men and women.

Endnotes

1. Quoted in Needham, *Science and Civilization in China*, Vol. 5, pretext pages.

2. Needham, *The Grand Titration: Science and Society in East and West*, p. 36.

3. The five phases play a prominent role in the history of Chinese medicine. For the interested reader, Matsumoto and Birch's Five Elements and Ten Stems offers insight into classical Chinese medical thought and the five phases, as well as their application to contemporary clinical practice. At the same time, the phases are by no means a critical facet of Chinese medicine's theoretical foundations. Indeed, TCM is commonly practiced with little practical reference to the concepts. Kaptchuk, in his *The Web That Has No Weaver*, sets out a lucid and critical discussion of the phases (pp. 343–57) and argues for the supremacy of yin-yang theory: "The Five Phases correspondence can be helpful as a guide to clinical tendencies, but the test of veracity in Chinese medicine remains the pattern. Yin-Yang theory is more applicable in the clinic because it focuses on the idea that the totality determines relationships, correspondences, and patterns."

4. Needham, *The Grand Titration*, p. 23.

5. Needham, *Science and Civilization in China*, vol. 2, p. 68, 71.

6. Veith, trans., *The Yellow Emperor's Classic of Internal Medicine*, p. 12.

7. Quoted in *The 1994 Calendar of Chinese Medicine and Astrology*, Blue Poppy Press, Boulder, CO, 1994.

8. Kaptchuk, *The Web That Has No Weaver*, p. 52.

9. As Manfred Porkert points out in his erudite book, *The Theoretical Foundations of Chinese Medicine*, "Whereas in anatomy Western medicine, causal and analytic; primarily describes the aggregate carriers (or substrata) of effects, inductive synthetic Chinese medicine is primarily interested in the fabric of functional manifestations of the different body regions." And further, "The Chinese word fei, 'lungs,' for instance, calls to mind only coincidentally and vaguely most of the ideas someone with a Western education associates with the lungs." See page 107.

10. See Bennet, "Chinese Science: Theory and Practice," Philosophy East and West, p. 445; and Porkert, *The Theoretical Foundations of Chinese Medicine*, pp. 166–96.

11. Wiseman et al., *Fundamentals of Chinese Medicine*, p. 23.

12. Kaptchuk, *The Web That Has No Weaver*, p. 43.

13. Ibid., pp. 43, 44.

14. Ibid., p. 45.

15. Wiseman et al., op. cit., p. 66.

16. Ibid., p. 37.

17. Qiu, *Chinese Acupuncture and Moxibustion*, p. 31.

18. Ibid., p. 45.

19. Matsumoto and Birch, *Five Elements and Ten Stems*, p. 48.

20. See, for example, Qiu, op. cit., pp. 393–407.

21. Needham, *Science and Civilization in China*, vol. 2, p. 281.

22. Matsumoto and Birch, *Hara Diagnosis: Reflections on the Sea*, p. 39.

23. Wiseman et al., *Fundamentals of Chinese Medicine*, p. 132.

24. The number of pulse types discussed ranges from twenty-four to thirty. Li Shi-zhen, in his *Bin Hu Mai Xue* (The Pulse Studies of Bin Hu), discusses twenty-seven pulse states.

25. Wiseman et al., op. cit., p. 149.

26. Li, *Pulse Diagnosis*, p. 68.

27. Wiseman et al., op. cit., p. 95.

28. Summer heat has been omitted for brevity. In addition to the six excesses there is "pestilential qi," a factor connected with contagious disease and not unlike the Western medical concept of viruses and bacteria.

29. Wiseman et al., op. cit., p. 103.

30. Traumas like snake bite, injury, and parasites are also listed as independent factors. There is also a class of miscellaneous factors that includes phlegm—a concept that embraces but has a broader meaning than the usual Western notion—and blood stagnation. See Wiseman et al.

31. There can be a general progression of disease from the exterior to the interior, formalized in the six stages of cold set out by Zhang Zhong-jing in the Han dynasty and the four stages of heat developed by Ye Tian-shi in the Qing. As the disease penetrates inwardly, patterns are generated that are partly exterior and partly interior.

32. Kaptchuk, *The Web That Has No Weaver*, p. 78.

33. Needham, *The Grand Titration*, p. 279; Bensky and Gamble, *Chinese Herbal Medicine: Materia Medica*, p. 6.

34. Bensky and Gamble's *Chinese Herbal Medicine: Materia Medica*, a standard English language reference, lists eighteen categories along with a number of subcategories.

35. A pattern of wind cold is an external attack by wind and cold

pathogenic factors, with symptoms that would often be considered a "cold" or "flu" by Westerners. The treatment principle is to warm and relieve the surface, using herbs that induce sweating. If the wind cold pattern is not resolved with sweating, treatment may require harmonizing the ying and the wei, the nutritive qi and the protective qi, a special function that results from the combination of cinnamon twig and white peony root.

36. Bensky and Barolet, *Chinese Herbal Medicine: Formulas and Strategies*, p. 14.

37. See, for example, Kaptchuk, *The Web That Has No Weaver*, pp. 79, 80.

38. Qiu, *Chinese Acupuncture and Moxibustion*, p. 193.

39. Ibid., p. 260.

40. Qiu, ed., *Chinese Acupuncture and Moxibustion*, pp. 292–93.

41. Porkert and Ullman, *Chinese Medicine*, p. 249.

42. Qi is pronounced chee, and sometimes spelled chi.

43. See Needham, *Science and Civilization in China*, vol. 2, pp. 455–505, and Mitukuni, "The Chinese Concept of Nature," in *Chinese Science*, Nakayama and Sivin, eds., pp. 76–89.

44. Unschuld, *Medicine in China*, p. 72.

45. Porkert, *The Theoretical Foundations of Chinese Medicine*, pp. 166–76.

46. Kaptchuk, *The Web That Has No Weaver*, p. 37.

47. Matsumoto and Birch, *Hara Diagnosis*, pp. 41, 42.

48. This is part of a passage from the Nan Jing, the *Classic of Difficulties*, a text that discusses unresolved issues found in the Huang Di Nei Jing. Matsumoto and Birch, *Hara Diagnosis*, p. 12.

49. Matsumoto and Birch, *Hara Diagnosis*, p. 12.

50. Wiseman et al., *Fundamentals of Chinese Medicine*, p. 24.

51. Ibid., p. 38.

52. For a discussion of the connection between organs and channels via the internal trajectories of the channels see Matsumoto and Birch, *Hara Diagnosis*, pp. 49–50.

53. See, for example, Unschuld, *Medicine in China*, pp. 81–82.

54. For a review of acupuncture research see G. Stux and B. Pomeranz, *Basics of Acupuncture*, Springer, Berlin, 1995, and S. Birch and R. Felt, Understanding Acupuncture, Churchill Livingstone, Edinburgh, 1999.

55. There are also electrical correspondences to the channels, but the channels do not correspond to either the nervous, lymphatic, or vascular systems. French researchers have demonstrated—using an injected radioactive tracer—pathways with a high degree of correspondence to the classically described channels. They found that the migration of the tracer did not follow the lymphatic or vascular system, and that patients with a specific organ problem showed a deviation from normal in the migration profile of the tracer. See "Etude des meridiens d'acupuncture par les traceurs radioactifs," *Bull. Acad, Natl. Med.*, 1985, 169, no. 7, pp.1071–1075.

56. Porkert, *Theoretical Foundations*, pp. 197–198.

57. See, for example, Unschuld, *Medicine in China*, pp. 95–96.

58. Kaptchuk, op. cit., p. 108.

59. Matsumoto and Birch, op. tit, p. 50.

60. Needham, *Science and Civilization in China*, vol. 5, p. 148. Needham also wonders "To what extent the later Taoist adepts pictured their qi as circulating along the tracts of the acupuncture physicians?" This question could really be inverted to ask to what extent were the acupuncture physicians concepts of the channels based on the discoveries of earlier Taoist adepts? It does seem clear from the technical details of Taoist practices described by contemporary masters that the routes of qi circulation and energy centers of inner alchemy correspond with those of the acupuncture system. See, for example, the various publications of Mantak Chia, a contemporary Taoist master.

—From *The Future of Healing*

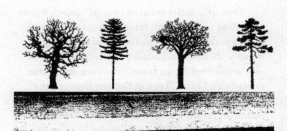

Continued →

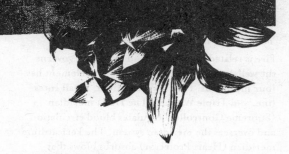

ACUPRESSURE

Cathryn Bauer

What Acupressure Can Do for You

Introduction to Acupressure

Acupressure is an age-old therapy that is easy to learn and even easier to use. You can give yourself a treatment almost anywhere. Your only tools are your fingers, your knowledge, and concentration. You can use Acupressure self-treatment for relief of symptoms such as menstrual cramps or water retention. You can also use Acupressure as a means of strengthening and balancing your body's deep energies for optimal well-being of your body, mind, and spirit.

Acupressure had its origins in ancient China. It began with the observation that when you are hurt, your hand instinctively moves to cover the injury. This generally provides a slight degree of pain relief. The Chinese sages and physicians carried this awareness further. They found that applying fingertip pressure at specific points of the body consistently helped to calm anxiety and fright, ease the pains of childbirth, and provide relief for many other symptoms of dis-ease.

Conventional treatment does not always provide workable answers for problems such as: "Why do I get colds every winter?" "How can I keep this yeast infection from coming back?" "I can't get any sleep because of these hot flashes." "I wish that I had more energy."

There are no simple answers to these broad health questions, but you'll understand more about the way your body works, if you study Acupressure self-help. Health care today is in the midst of a transformation. Women themselves are entering the health professions in increasing numbers, and, as practitioners, are paying attention to our special needs. Women as consumers of health care are making informed decisions about medical treatment.

There are differing perspectives on the reasons why the touch therapies are effective. The Asian view suggests that you are healthy when your life-energy is strong and balanced. The Western viewpoint changed in the last half of the twentieth century, and we are finally acknowledging that relaxation is the cornerstone of healthy living. Stress has been identified as the culprit in a wide variety of symptoms. This recognition has led to a new interest in Acupressure as an adjunct—not a replacement—for medical science.

How to Work with Acupressure Points

Wash your hands before you apply Acupressure. Make sure they are dry and warm before you apply pressure to a point. It is important to remember that you are doing more than pressing a button. You are relieving pain and tension. You are also balancing energy. Work with a slow and careful touch, particularly if you are not feeling well.

A good beginning is simply to hold your hand over the general area of the point. Using the tip of your index finger, approach the specific point location slowly. Move your finger around the area, probing gently until you feel a slight dip that identifies the Acupressure point. Press in lightly, holding a point until you feel the tissues underneath your fingertip soften and relax. Then, press into the point very slowly, until you sense further pressure would require force.

Pay careful attention to what is happening beneath your fingertip. Acupressure points often become warm to your touch, a sign of releasing tension. As you press into the point, note any changes in your breathing. Slower breathing is a sign that you're beginning to relax.

The point is completely released when it's neither warm nor cool in temperature and is pulsing steadily. The pulsation is similar to the pulse in your wrists and neck, but not as strong. When the point has released, ease your fingertip off slowly. An abrupt release of pressure feels uncomfortable.

Avoid two common mistakes, inaccurate point location and applying pressure for too brief a period of time. Study the charts. Accurate point location is a learned skill. Give yourself permission to be a beginner! If you feel relaxed or experience symptomatic relief after a self-treatment session, you are successfully applying the art. Keep practicing to develop sensitivity to the process. Don't be concerned if you take a while to find points. Acupressure self-care is a skill which will serve you well—for the rest of your life.

Precautions

If you are sick, tired, or weak, be sure to use a very gentle and gradual touch. Acupressure should never be applied directly to wounds, bruises, or sprains. However, you can use Acupressure points near the affected part to increase circulation and relieve muscular stiffness.

There are points which you should not press if you or a friend are pregnant, noted throughout the text. Their use can result in prenatal problems.

Acupressure is not a substitute for medical care. If you are ill or injured, consult a licensed M.D. whom you trust. You must also receive regular pelvic exams and pap smears from a doctor or nurse practitioner. In addition, check your breasts for lumps the day after your menstrual period. Your doctor or nurse practitioner will show you how.

If you ever press Acupressure points on someone else, ask their permission first and use a gentle touch.

Acupressure Self-Treatment

You have a lot to gain from taking time to care for yourself. You live in a noisy, rapidly paced society which demands a great deal from you. You are constantly being asked to produce and give of yourself, which drains energy. Make a conscious effort to replenish this energy daily. There are times when it's best to receive Acupressure from someone else. If you're feeling tired and overextended, have a professional or a friend take care of you with Acupressure. If you know a friend who shares your interest in Acupressure, take turns working with each other.

Yeshi Donden, holistic physician to the Dalai Lama of Tiber, encourages his students to develop a perception of the universe as a place where healing is possible. This outlook is your best possible supplement to Acupressure self-care or any other form of health treatment.

The Western and Asian Views of Acupressure

The Western View

The Western view suggests that Acupressure techniques stimulate the body's own resources for healing by influencing the nervous system. The Acupressure process somehow modifies the action of stress-related hormones and interferes with the transmission of pain. For example, researchers at the Harvard Medical School discovered that regular relaxation practice decreased the body's response to norepinephrine, one of the "fight or flight" hormones which elevates the blood pressure and contributes to hypertension.

When you're angry and afraid, your "fight or flight" reflex stimulates a variety of physical responses, most of them unpleasant. Your heart pounds. Your blood pressure rises. Your mouth goes dry and your muscles tighten, enabling you to run away. While these responses were essential to human survival in the past, they are inappropriate for life today. You can seldom solve job or domestic problems by fighting or running away. Yet, as long as you feel threatened, your body remains in "fight or flight mode" until the situation is resolved. You can remain in this mode for a period of less than a minute or it can continue for many years. Chronic, unmitigated stress is strongly associated with illnesses like gastric ulcer and hypertension.

Stress reduction research suggests the Acupressure is a valuable tool in a stress management program. Stress reduction techniques emphasize slow, deep breathing to induce relaxation. There are Acupressure points in the chest and upper back to reduce chest constriction and shallow breathing. You can also press points to relieve joint stiffness and other discomforts. Indirectly, Acupressure can reduce insomnia, depression, and pain.

Health professionals are reaching a better understanding of the way that touch therapies help you withstand the pressures of daily life. They also observe many situations where touch therapies ease the shock of illness or injuries.

In 1986, a ski instructor told me that ski rescue teams in the Colorado Rockies are taught "hands-on" techniques for lessening trauma at the scene of an accident. As the team reaches an injured skier, one member removes her gloves and warms her hands by rubbing them together. She makes direct skin contact with the injured skier, placing one hand on the back of the neck and gently stroking the face with her other hand. It is possible that the rescuer's touch stimulates the neural receptors (Acupressure points), activating both the inhibitory and excitatory pleasure systems that release endorphins.

The outpouring of information on stress research influences the way that people take care of themselves. Now that *stress* is an everyday word, you hear warnings on every side to reduce stress in your life or suffer the results. Yet, a life without stress is a life without challenge or personal growth. If you live a productive yet stressful lifestyle, you need a consciously planned program of stress reduction. The Western view now includes the use of Acupressure.

The Asian View

Acupressure originated from the Taoist philosophy that began centuries ago in China. Having seen how touch could relieve the pain from an injury, the Chinese physicians and philosophers discovered that life-energy flows through the body in twelve defined paths or meridians. When you are healthy, the flow proceeds unblocked, and energy is well distributed throughout the meridian pathways.

Continued ➡

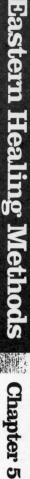

The theory was reinforced in modern times by Dr. Kim Bong-han, a professor of medicine at Korea's Pyongyang University. He found that variations in the skin's electrical resistance could be traced along the meridians as they were illustrated in ancient texts. Further research showed that skin cells along the meridians were structurally different from other skin cells. Furthermore, at certain points, there were clusters of these "meridian cells." Classic Chinese medical texts show that the clusters were located at Acupressure points.

Each point has a name and number to identify its effect or location (see Index of Pressure Points). When you apply fingertip pressure to the point, you influence the energy in its meridian in addition to relieving symptoms. You also facilitate a balance of energy among the twelve meridians which manifests itself as whole-person wellness. Disease is a sign that the energy within the meridians is out of balance.

Physicians who developed Acupressure believed that human beings are an integral part of the universe. This concept is the heart of Taoist thinking. Human beings, trees, clouds, land forms, and animals are all part of one substance, one fabric. As such, humans are subject to the laws of nature. Like the physical universe, they continually move through a yearly cycle. When they adapt to the changing cycle, living according to each system, they are healthy and productive. (An example of adaptation is wearing warm clothing during the wintertime.) When they fail to adapt, they are more susceptible to illness.

Chinese philosophers believed in a five-season year. They associated each season with one of five elements that compose the universe. Since you are a part of the natural universe, you are also composed of the elements. Each element is a part of your being, just it is a part of the world in which you live. When your Five Elements are in harmony, you are balanced and healthy.

Each element has a character of its own. It is connected with an emotion, a taste and a sound, in addition to certain meridians. When an element is out of balance, you are likely to experience one or more specific dis-eases related to that particular element. For example, you might have menstrual cramps. First-aid Acupressure can give you temporary relief from the muscular tension and pain. However, it is likely that your cramps will continue to be a monthly problem until you treat the underlying imbalance in their related element.

The Five Elements Theory

YOUR WATER ELEMENT

The Water element is your storehouse of reserve energy to be used when you're under prolonged stress or in crisis. The Water meridians are the Bladder and Kidney. The kidney meridian stores energy reserves for emergency use, and the Bladder meridian regulates fluid distribution. Your body is as much as 80 percent fluid, an amazing collection of tides and flows that must be balanced by Water. Water is also associated with your sense of hearing (taking in and remembering information), bone health, and your sexuality.

The Water emotion, fear, enables you to withdraw for self-protection. The ability to pull back in your own interest promotes your survival. However, you can go too far and be "frozen with fear," unable to move on to realize your ambitions. In this case, your voice is fear-full, sounding like a grown or a whine. Since Water governs bone health, you may refer to a frightening experience as "bone-chilling."

The colors of Water are blue and black, the "cool" colors. The Water taste is salty. Salt in excess

causes fluid retention. The Water season is Winter when the earth is at rest. Some animals hibernate for a long winter sleep and most people need more sleep during the winter months.

Symptoms and illness associated with Water imbalance include: cold hands and feet, PMS, brittle hair, fractures which are slow to heal, salt cravings, urinary and bladder infections, phobias, earache, low back pain, infertility, and pain and tension along the Water meridians.

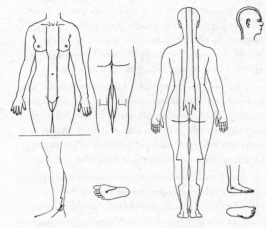

The Kidney Meridian   *The Bladder Meridian*

YOUR WOOD ELEMENT

Wood governs the health of the muscles, tendons, and ligaments. When wood is in balance, joints move easily and effortlessly. The Wood meridians are the Gall Bladder and Liver. The Liver assimilates food and purifies your blood. The Gall Bladder secretes bile to aid digestion and distributes energy (from foods you eat) throughout your meridians. Wood is related to strong, adaptable eyes and the sense of inner vision, the ability to see different sides of a situation.

Anger is the Wood emotion, an energizer that propels you into constructive action. If Wood is out of balance, you may frequently overeat with any angry response. The sound of Wood is shouting, and its taste is sour. If you frequently crave dill pickles or green olives, you may have a Wood imbalance. Wood colors are purple and green, the traditional colors of healing and transformation.

The season of Wood is spring, a time of life renewal when you grow as a person and let go of habits and ideas that no longer work for you. Wood gives you energy to reach out to get what you want from life. If Wood is healthy, you can celebrate the aging process without regret.

Symptoms and illnesses associated with Wood imbalance include: headaches, spinal problems, bursitis, muscular spasms, indecision, allergies, tendonitis, eye problems, migraine, chronic rage, and tension and pain along the Wood meridians.

The Gall Bladder Meridian   *The Liver Meridian*

YOUR FIRE ELEMENT

Fire is related to creativity and spark and governs the well-being of your heart. The Fire element has four meridians: Heart, Pericardium, Small Intestine, and Triple Warmer. The Heart meridian (Supreme Controller) regulates blood circulation and oversees the meridian system. The Pericardium meridian (Heart Protector) absorbs blows that could damage your heart. The Small Intestine processes ood, attracting nutrients and discarding wastes. The Triple Warmer protects and regulates your "Three Burning Spaces," chest, solar plexus, and abdomen. An energy presence without physical form, the Triple Warmer is the only meridian without a corresponding organ.

The emotion associated with Fire is joy. When Fire is in balance, you have a greater capacity to feel pleasure and excitement ("on fire with enthusiasm"). Laughter is the sound of Fire, and your ability to enjoy a good laugh is an indicator of health. Humor which mocks or degrades others, however, shows an imbalance.

The taste associated with Fire is bitter. Frequent cravings for unsweetened chocolate and strong, black coffee or tea indicates imbalance. Fire colors are red and pink. They can "cheer you up" or make you feel "like a neon sign." If your wardrobe contains only drab shades, or is composed entirely of red and pink, there may be a Fire imbalance. The Fire season is summer, the traditional vacation time. Like many people, you may find relief from chronic physical or emotional problems when you travel to a summery climate. However, being happy and well only in the warm months—or not being able to handle warm weather—are signs of imbalance.

Symptoms and dis-eases associated with Fire imbalance include: heart trouble, poor circulation, lack of sexual desire, depression, body temperature changes, skin changes, insensitivity to others, apathy ("losing heart", and tension or pain along Fire meridians.

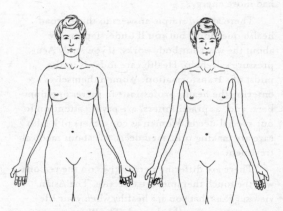

The Heart Meridian   *The Pericardium Meridian*

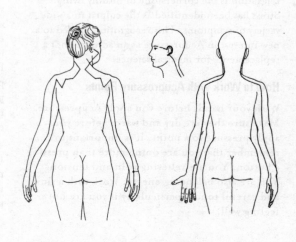

The Small Intestine Meridian   *The Triple Warmer Meridian*

Continued ➡

YOUR EARTH ELEMENT

The Earth element is your base. It gives you physical and emotional balance and, with the Water element, creates your sexuality and fertility. Spleen and Stomach are the Earth's meridians. The Spleen builds blood, and the Stomach digests food. Together, they regulate the menstrual cycle, the digestive process, and emotional reaction patterns.

Sympathy is the emotion associated with Earth. With imbalance, you can be stuck in giving too much sympathy at your own expense and excusing inappropriate behavior in yourself and others. You may also ignore your own or others' needs. A balanced Earth gives you the sense of stability, belonging whereas you are. Earth regulates your physical and emotional cycles, helping you adapt to your natural rhythms. When Earth is in balance, you understand that some days are more productive than others.

Singing is the sound of Earth. An Earth-imbalanced voice sounds like a song without a tune. Singing helps to balance your Earth meridians. The taste of Earth is sweet. With imbalance, you crave sweets, even after you've conquered a white sugar habit. The season of Earth is late summer, a period marked by weather changes. When Earth is in balance, you can enjoy any day, whatever the weather. Yellow, orange, and brown are Earth colors.

Symptoms and illnesses associated with Earth imbalance include: canker sores, stomach/abdominal pain, ulcers, nausea and vomiting, eating disorders, diabetes, yeast infections, PMS infertility, irregular ovulation, hypoglycemia, self-pity, mood swings, and tension and pain along the Earth meridians.

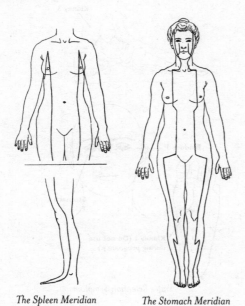

The Spleen Meridian   *The Stomach Meridian*

THE METAL ELEMENT

The Metal meridians are the Large Intestine and the Lung, and together they determine the health of your bowels, skin, and respiration. The Large Intestine which refines and filters food products is a great mover, enabling you to get rid of physical and emotional waste. When Metal is out of balance, foods may affect you badly, and you develop acne, hives, or eczema. The Lung meridian controls your breathing. When your breath is slow and regular, you're relaxed.

Grief is the emotion of Metal. If your energy is stuck in Metal, you are continually mourning the past, unable to move ahead and resolve old experiences. Your voice has a weeping sound. Metal is also related to your ability to acquire money and the material goods necessary for survival. Metal colors are white, silver, and gray, the mourning colors of several Asian societies. The taste of Metal is spicy.

With imbalance, you may overuse or avoid pepper, salsa, and other spicy condiments.

The Metal season is autumn, a time of completion and transformation. The Metal element helps you release painful experiences and replace them with hope. Metal is associated with spiritual life, inspiring you to develop a sense of justice and honor. Symptoms and dis-ease associated with Metal imbalance include: acne, eczema, frontal headache, sinus problems, colds and bronchitis, dry or chapped skin, constipation or diarrhea, delayed menstruation, asthma, pain and tension along the Metal meridians.

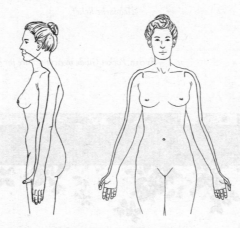

The Large Intestine Meridian   *The Lung Meridian*

THE GOVERNING VESSEL AND THE CONCEPTION VESSEL

The Governing Vessel and the Conception Vessel are extra meridians that serve as reservoirs for excess energy. They comprise a binding network that draws energy from the Kidney meridian for distribution throughout the body. Pressing points on the extra meridians calms and strengthens you, increasing the benefits derived from pressing points on the organ meridians.

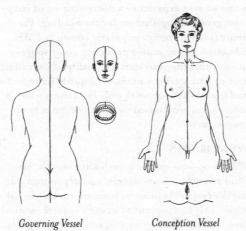

Governing Vessel   *Conception Vessel*

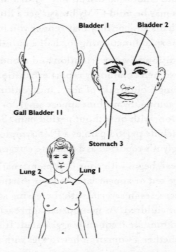

Acupressure Points for Nasal Congestion

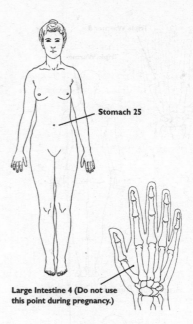

Acupressure Points for Constipation

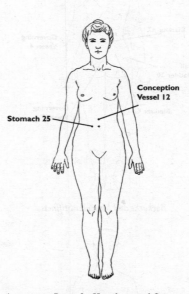

Acupressure Points for Heartburn and Constipation

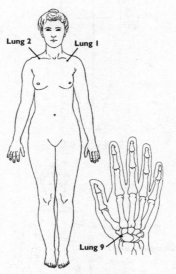

Acupressure Points to Relieve Shortness of Breath

Continued ➡

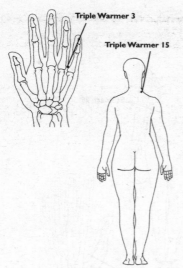

Acupressure Points for Cold Symptoms

Triple Warmer 3
Triple Warmer 15

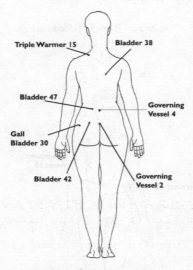

Triple Warmer 15
Bladder 38
Bladder 47
Governing Vessel 4
Gall Bladder 30
Bladder 42
Governing Vessel 2

Backache and Muscular Stiffness

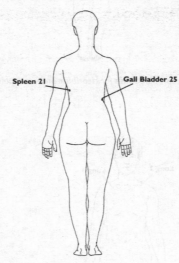

Spleen 21
Gall Bladder 25

Stitch in the Side

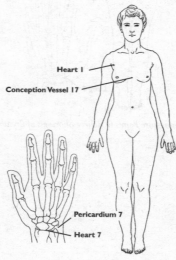

Heart 1
Conception Vessel 17
Pericardium 7
Heart 7

To Tonify the Heart*

*If you are using more than one point, proceed in the following order:
1. Heart 1, 2. Heart 7, 3. Pericardium 7, 4. Conception Vessel 17.

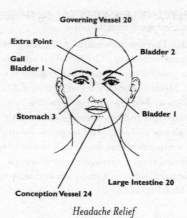

Governing Vessel 20
Extra Point
Gall Bladder 1
Bladder 2
Bladder 1
Stomach 3
Bladder 1
Large Intestine 20
Conception Vessel 24

Headache Relief

—From *Pocket Guide to Acupressure for Women*

ACUPRESSURE FOR WOMEN'S HEALTH CARE

Cathryn Bauer

Premenstrual Syndrome

PMS

Some women experience a distressing set of symptoms grouped together under the heading, Premenstrual syndrome, popularly known as PMS. Sometimes these minor problems occur so frequently that they threaten the quality of your life. You may have tried a number of quick-fix remedies and found that they work only for a short time. As soon as you are stressed or overtired, your symptoms return.

What is PMS?

PMS symptoms return month after month, causing fluid retention, nervousness, and depression during the two weeks prior to your menstrual period. While only five percent of women require medical care, countless others experience varying degrees of physical and emotional disruption. Your PMS symptoms may be mild ("My breasts get a little swollen, that's all." or they may render you incapable of normal functioning for half a month.

In addition to water retention and mood changes, women commonly report exhaustion, sweet cravings, outbreaks of acne, indigestion, and muscular aching. Symptoms appear singly or in combination, with or without period pain. Some sources include period pain as a PMS symptom, but increasingly it's reported as a separate category.

PMS can begin with your first menstruation as early as age ten or appear later in your thirties. PMS usually increases in severity with increasing age and number of children. As menopause approaches, PMS symptoms are frequently aggravated. It is still unclear whether a woman in her forties with severe premenstrual anxiety is suffering from untreated PMS or menopausal symptoms.

If you suffer regularly from PMS, there is (with minor exception) immense relief once your menstrual flow begins. However, if you also have period pain and cramping, sometimes accompanied by nausea and vomiting, distress may continue for a few days into your period.

PMS and Water Retention

When fluid accumulates in and around your cells during the luteal phase, you may gain one to three pounds. This causes abdominal bloating and breast and nipple tenderness. Less common complaints are muscular aching, wrist pain and numbness, earache, and dizziness.

While excess fluid can accumulate in any part of your body, it is drawn like a magnet to joints. Some women suffer from carpal tunnel syndrome, which causes numbness, pain, and prickly feelings in the wrist from nerve pressure. The carpal tunnel is a narrow, bony tunnel surrounding a nerve in the wrist. When the cells of the carpal tunnel are swollen with fluid, pressure on the nerve causes numbness and pain.

Your period headaches can result from buildup of water in the eyeball, in the labyrinth of the inner ear, or in your sinuses. When fluid engorges the eyeball, it causes pressure and sometimes intense pain. (If you experience these symptoms, see an ophthalmologist to rule out the possibility of glaucoma.)

Water buildup in the ear causes a similar feeling of pressure and pain. Premenstrual "sinus headaches" are due to swollen, waterlogged nasal passages. Acupressure points are effective in clearing your sinuses.

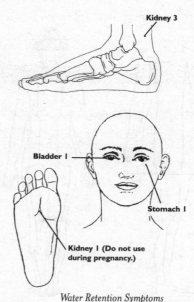

Kidney 3
Bladder 1
Stomach 1
Kidney 1 (Do not use during pregnancy.)

Water Retention Symptoms

PMS and Your Emotions

Premenstrual syndrome is usually synonymous with mood swings that make a woman suffer from low-self-esteem and seemingly inexplicable feelings of fear and anger. You may suddenly feel out of control when nothing seems to work. Your concentration is off and everything takes more of your energy. These symptoms have a way of disrupting your relationships. Gretchen says, "I used to break up with my boyfriend once every month, until I realized it was PMS picking the fights."

If PMS symptoms escalate beyond mere annoyance and become violent, you need to do something. It's unhealthy to have tantrums and/or eating or drinking binges two weeks of the month. While studies show that more antisocial acts do occur during the premenstrual period (implying that PMS makes women irrational), there is hope for PMS sufferers. Your symptoms do not make you a weak, overemotional personality.

Continued ➡

Index of Pressure Points

Cathryn Bauer

Spleen 3	Supreme White	Gall Bladder 20	Wing Pond
Spleen 4	Prince's Grandson	Gall Bladder 21	Shoulder Well
Spleen 6	Three Yin Crossing	Gall Bladder 25	Capital Gate
Spleen 12	Rushing Gate	Gall Bladder 30	Jumping Circle
Spleen 21	Great Enveloping	Gall Bladder 40	Wilderness Mound
Stomach 1	Receive Tears	Liver 3	Supreme Rushing
Stomach 3	Great Cheekbone	Liver 6	Middle Capital
Stomach 13	Energy Door	Liver 14	Gate of Hope
Stomach 16	Breast Window		
Stomach 25	Heavenly Pivot	Heart 1	Utmost Source
Stomach 36	Three More Miles	Heart 7	Spirit Gate
Stomach 41	Released Stream	Heart 9	Little Rushing In
Stomach 42	Rushing Yang		
Stomach 43	Sinking Valley	Pericardium 9	Great Mound
Lung 1	Middle Palace	Small Intestine 4	Wrist Bone
Lung 2	Cloud Gate	Small Intestine 8	Small Sea
Lung 9	Very Great Abyss	Small Intestine 17	Heavenly Appearance
		Small Intestine 19	Listening Palace
Large Intestine 4	Great Eliminator		
Large Intestine 20	Welcome Fragrance	Triple Warmer 3	Middle Islet
		Triple Warmer 4	Yang Pond
Bladder 1	Eyes Bright	Triple Warmer 15	Heavenly Bone
Bladder 2	Collect Bamboo	Triple Warmer 23	Silk Bamboo Hollow
Bladder 7	Penetrate Heaven		
Bladder 38	Rich for the Vitals	Governing Vessel 2	Loins Correspondence
Bladder 42	Spiritual Soul Gate		
Bladder 47	Ambition Room	Governing Vessel 4	Gate of Life
Bladder 64	Capital Bone	Governing Vessel 12	Body Pillar
Bladder 66	Penetrating Valley	Governing Vessel 16	Wind Palace
Bladder 67	Extremity of Yin	Governing Vessel 17	Brain Door
		Governing Vessel 19	Posterior Summit
Kidney 1	Bubbling Spring	Governing Vessel 20	One Thousand Meeting Place
Kidney 3	Greater Mountain Stream		
Kidney 11	Transverse Bone	Conception Vessel 2	Crooked Bone
Kidney 22	Walking on the Verandah	Conception Vessel 3	Utmost Middle
		Conception Vessel 4	First Gate
		Conception Vessel 12	Middle Duct
Gall Bladder 1	Orbit Bone	Conception Vessel 17	Within the Breast
Gall Bladder 11	Head Hole Yin	Conception Vessel 24	Receiving Fluid
Gall Bladder 14	Yang White		

—From *Pocket Guide to Acupressure for Women*

Do balance the amount of stress in your life and begin an Acupressure self-help program. Acupressure can calm you down when you feel upset or anxious.

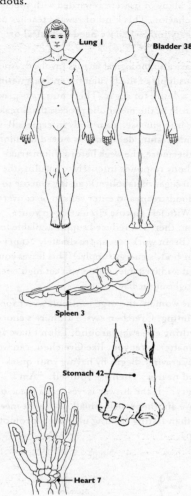

Emotional Symptoms of PMS

Premenstrual Fatigue

Just before your period, you may have little or no energy. You lack initiative and the will to carry out plans. If it weren't for coffee and sugar, you'd never make it through the day.

There are biological reasons for your fatigue. Waterlogging during the luteal phase causes a shift in mineral action. Sodium is retained while potassium is excreted, making you feel tired, weak, and irritable. Restore this mineral imbalance by limiting (or eliminating) your intake of salty foods, including hot dogs, bouillon, and potato chips. Then add potassium-rich kelp, apricots, peaches, and bananas to your diet. Acupressure provides a quick, no-caffeine pick-me-up. Instead of a coffee break, find a quiet place to relax and press one or more of the points shown.

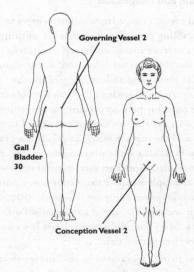

To Relieve Pelvic Tention

Continued ➡

PREMENSTRUAL SWEET CRAVING

Reaching for sugary food when you're tired or feeling negative is partially the result of childhood programming. Many of us were rewarded with sweets for good behavior. This kind of reward teaches us to crave sugary food when we need a physical or emotional lift.

There are also biological factors involved. An insufficient supply of the B vitamins and magnesium can trigger a desire for sugar. These nutrients play an important role in the metabolic process that breaks down sugar into glucose. Your body interprets B-vitamin and magnesium deficiency as a need for more sugar. Furthermore, the week before a menstrual flow, your body responds intensely to insulin (the key hormone in sugar metabolism) causing glucose to leave the bloodstream and enter cells to be converted to energy. With less glucose circulating in your bloodstream, there is a reduced supply available to the brain. (Brain work uses approximately 20 percent of your body's energy supply.) This leaves you feeling tired and irritable, unless you eat high energy foods throughout the day.

In some women, the urge to nibble sweet foods is overwhelming. Gretchen says, "If there's chocolate or anything else sweet around, I don't have any say in the matter." Yet you, like Gretchen, can work beyond this craving. Begin by having your quick energy food nearby. Then ask yourself, "Am I really hungry?" If the answer is yes, eat a piece of fruit or have another snack. Small, frequent meals are better than fasting (fasting ultimately promotes weight gain).

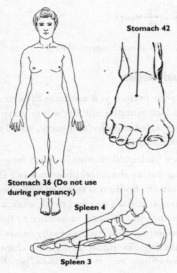

Premenstral Sweet Cravings

Period Pain and Indigestion

Menstrual cramps range from minor twinges to severe, disabling pain. Since cramps are nothing more than uterine spasms, your self-treatment program should focus on relaxation. Tense muscles in the solar plexus and abdomen aggravate the period pain and indigestion. Barbara was able to minimize monthly pain by pressing Acupressure points twice a day (before she got out of bed in the morning and during her lunch hour). If she practiced deep breathing while pressing the points, she got better results. Gretchen used natural muscle relaxants as supplements to the Acupressure points. When her cramps were intense, she took 1000 mg. of calcium and magnesium in combination with warm milk. Mary found that sex relaxed her enough to take away her period pain.

Period pain is aggravated by acid indigestion or constipation. For relief, supplement the Acupressure points by chewing a handful of ripe grapes

(grapes have a laxative effect). Do use Acupressure. You will get better results if you are familiar with points before your pain begins.

If you experience pelvic pain throughout the month, consider other causes than PMS. Pelvic pain can be the result of trauma and simple tension or it can be an indicator of a more serious problem that requires medical help. Persistent pelvic pain in a symptom of pelvic inflammatory dis-ease,

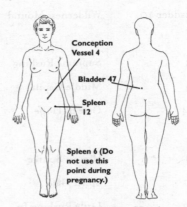

Point Series for Period Pain*

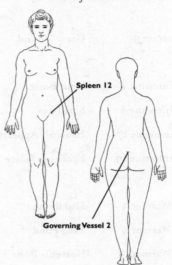

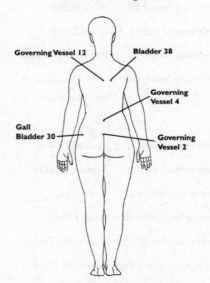

Period Pain and Indigestion

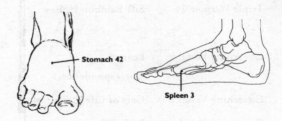

Backache and Muscular Pain

* Takes 10 minutes. Hold the points in the following order: 1. Bladder 47, 2. Conception Vessel 4, 3. Spleen 10 (do not use this point during pregnancy), 4. Spleen 13.

endometriosis, cystitis, and other illnesses. Consult a gynecologist promptly. Painful intercourse may also result from the use of a diaphragm improperly fitted or inserted incorrectly.

PMS and Acne

Acne and oily hair signal "I'm premenstrual" to many women. Curiously, this is caused by a higher level of male hormones (androgens) in your body. When your adrenal glands rev up during the luteal phase, they activate oil glands in your skin. Use a balanced diet with a minimum of sugar, fat, and chemical additives to prevent premenstrual acne. (Substitute cold chicken for the peanut butter in

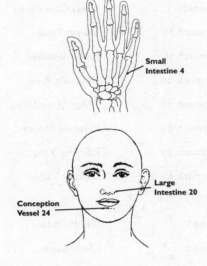

Premenstral Acne

your daily sandwich. Cut fats and oil intake by half.) Shampoo hair and wash skin frequently with nonallergenic soaps designed for oily complexions. By stimulating circulation, Acupressure points can help to prevent oil from clogging your complexion.

Pregnancy, Birth, and Nursing

Preconception

The preconception period is an optimal time to use Acupressure self-treatment. After taking stock of your health habits, including your diet and exercise program, you can start pressing Acupressure points to maximize your reproductive energies.

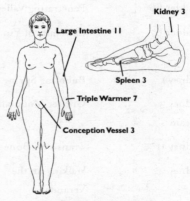

The Preconception Period

Continued ➡

Pregnancy

ACUPRESSURE POINTS TO AVOID DURING PREGNANCY

Do not use these points after your decision to become pregnant. They are traditionally forbidden for expectant mothers.

Small Intestine 7	Triple Warmer 4
Small Intestine 10	Triple Warmer 10
Kidney 1	Gall Bladder 2
Kidney 2	Gall Bladder 9
Kidney 4	Gall Bladder 34
Kidney 7	Pericardium 8
Lung 7	Pericardium 6
Lung 11	Large Intestine 2
Stomach 4	Large Intestine 4
Stomach 36	Large Intestine 10
Stomach 45	Spleen 2
Spleen 1	Spleen 6

Menopause and Aging

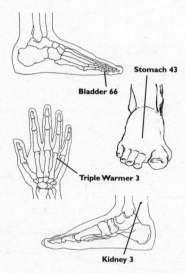

Releif of Hot Flashes

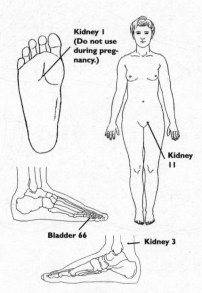

To Promote Vaginal Tone

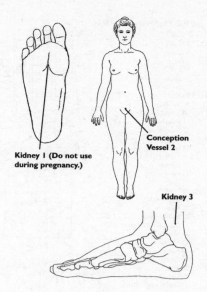

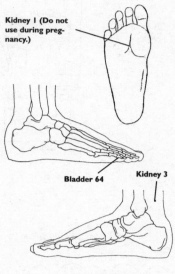

Insufficient Vaginal Lubrication

Bone Health

ACUPRESSURE/ REFLEXOLOGY

Diane Stein
Illustrations by Ken Krug

Acupressure is also known as reflexology, and consists of using finger pressure on the body, hands, ears or feet to release energy blocks. Specific points for specific organs and diseases relieve pain and symptoms. This form of healing comes from China, and is one of the most ancient healing systems. It was known in Asia by 4000 B.C.E. and in Egypt by 2330 B.C.E. It predates acupuncture, the use of needles inserted into the pressure or reflex points, by thousands of years. The Chinese Nei Jing, dated at about 300 B.C.E. is the oldest known written book of medicine, and contains information on acupressure, acupuncture and herbal healing. The system of meridians—the map of energy lines and pressure points on the body—is detailed in the Nei Jing, and is still used today. While acupuncture is done by a trained technician of Chinese doctor, acupressure is a good tool for women's self-healing.

The totality of Being, and the attainment of harmony and balance within are the central ideas in Asian healing. Health is harmony and balance; dis-ease is imbalance or the blockage of free energy flow. The physical and aura bodies are taken as a whole, and acupressure (by balancing meridian points and removing energy blocks) affects both physical and auric bodies. By applying pressure to or massaging the reflex points that are involved in a dis-ease, excess and deficiency of energy are both eliminated. With restoration of a free flow of energy, dis-ease is removed and the body returns to its natural balance and wellness.

The meridians are the energy channels of the body's organs, pathways that carry energy to and from them. There are fourteen major meridians used in pairs of yin and yang that include the five Chinese elements (water, wood, fire, earth, and metal). Yin and yang are the Chinese words for receptive and active, energy out and energy in. They are intrinsic flows that have nothing to do with gender. There are 365 classic acupuncture/acupressure points, 150 of which are standardly used. In addition there are over 2000 possible reflex massage points, used singly and multiply, that are used in acupressure to relieve dis-ease and return the body to balance. A student acupuncturist learns the meridian points and acupressure first, before using needles. Acupressure was the healing tool of laywomen and wisewomen in early China and still today.

From the meridians, energy (in China called Qi or C'hi) branches into the nadis, the multitude of tiny nerve endings in the skin. These have also been mapped in modern times by electrical means. The meridians and nadis are the electrical flows of the body. The meridian endings, where all the pathways come together, are in the ears, hands, and feet and are the basis for ear reflexology and ear acupuncture, and hand and foot reflexology. All are a part of the same system of energy flows. The skin of the ears, the palms of the hands and the soles of the feet each contain a complete energy map of the body. Every organ is represented, and pressure points on these body parts can affect healing in every part of the body and every organ. Acupressure massage of the fleshy parts of the ear, whole hand or whole foot is a powerful tool for women's overall well-being.

In this book, acupressure points are identified for each of the dis-eases in the remedy section. Use them along with other forms of healing to bring the energy flows into harmony and promote good health. Maps of the ears, hands, feet and body reflex points are included in the next few pages, as well. They provide a basis for acupressure/reflexology anatomy, and a beginning of pressure point healing for every disease. For some of the dis-eases in the remedy section, acupressure points are on the hands or feet. Remember that each reflex system has a full body map, and if points are shown for the feet, there are also hand, ear and body meridian points as well, Pressure points shown on the body are usually along the lines of the meridians, while those on hands and feet are on the seiketsu, or meridian endings. *Seiketsu* is a Japanese word.

To do this form of healing, use a finger, thumb or the whole hand to apply pressure to the designated points. Even using both hands or a blunt object like a crystal to press with is valid. Use whatever is comfortable and provides the most even pressure. Pressure is firm but without force, and may include a massaging motion. Excessive pressure that causes pain or uses undue strength is not necessary or positive. Look for the correct point to apply the pressure to. You will recognize it by the strange tingling, sometimes sharp sensation that occurs when you make contact. There is a slight depression in the skin at acupressure points which

Continued ➡

you will learn to feel in time. When you apply pressure directly to the correct reflex point, much can be accomplished with little actual pressure. In a few moments time, you will feel the tension under your fingers relax, and at that point the reflex is released. A released acupressure point pulses slightly under your fingers. One that needs releasing has a heavier, slower pulse and tighter feeling. You will soon recognize the difference.

Most points are held for about a minute, and can be massaged rather than using steady pressure. The points will be sensitive before releasing, and the sharp tingling sensation disappears from a released point. If the point is very tense and sensitive, know when to stop—years of pain may not release in one session. In acute pain, as in migraine, work the acupressure points for thirty seconds, then stop for thirty seconds before returning to them. They will be painful. Points for the abdomen and legs, and in the web between thumb and first finger, should not be pressed during a wanted pregnancy. Avoid foot reflexology in pregnancy, as well. Work more lightly and for a shorter time if you are debilitated or an elder, and work more lightly on pets, infants and children.

Full body acupressure (Jin Shin Do or shiatsu) sessions are not included in this book, as the focus here is on self-healing and they require one-on-one work with a practitioner. In using acupressure on individual points for self-healing, work for no more than five minutes twice a day in healing chronic dis-eases. In acute situations, work for a minute or two on each point, then stop and repeat a few minute later if needed; most acute dis-eases respond rapidly. In doing a full hand or foot acupressure session, do it only twice a week at first to prevent too much toxin release. Build up to twice a day but do it slowly. If you are diabetic, monitor insulin levels, as acupressure can make these change, and avoid pressure points on the legs if you have varicose veins or phlebitis (blood clots). Avoid acupressure on the legs, feet and abdomen in pregnancy unless you are knowledgeable of which points are positive. Whole hand or foot acupressure (especially feet) can be an accurate diagnostic tool for sensitive healers. Pain spots found on the body map are highly indicative, and a pain spot may appear before the dis-ease does. Be aware that every woman's body is unique and the map may vary slightly on different women's hands and feet.

In using hand or foot acupressure, the reflex points are under tougher skin and may take more probing to find than on the body. Pressure is applied in the same way, but only with the thumb or index finger. To do a complete session, rather than single points, work the thumb in a creeping motion up the sole and sides of the foot or palm. The movement of the thumb joint makes a forward motion, like a caterpillar walk. The inside edge of the thumb makes contact with the skin of the sole or palm—not fingernails or the ball of the thumb. The other fingers wrap around the foot or hand to steady it. Where less pressure is needed, as round the toes and fingers, use the index finger in the same creeping motion. Body acupressure uses a steady pressure, without the caterpillar movement.

Continue this motion until you feel a sensitive or sore spot and spend a short amount of time working the spot to release it. Then go on. Use a hooking motion of the thumb on tougher places, as where the skin on the feet is thick, and for small or hard-to-reach areas. For tender areas on the lower half of the foot or hand, use reflex rotation. This is done by holding your thumb on the pain spot and using your other hand to rotate the foot or palm gently against it until the painful point is released. Each located pain spot has its correspondence to a

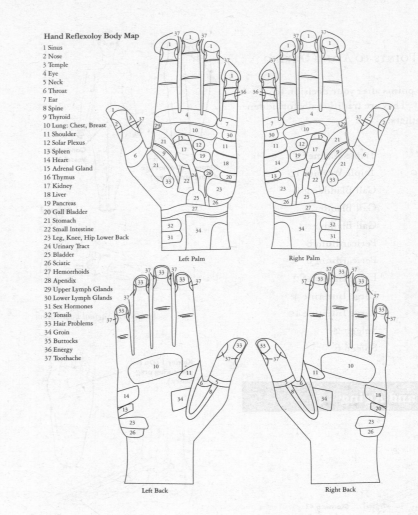

Hand Reflexoloy Body Map

1 Sinus
2 Nose
3 Temple
4 Eye
5 Neck
6 Throat
7 Ear
8 Spine
9 Thyroid
10 Lung: Chest, Breast
11 Shoulder
12 Solar Plexus
13 Spleen
14 Heart
15 Adrenal Gland
16 Thymus
17 Kidney
18 Liver
19 Pancreas
20 Gall Bladder
21 Stomach
22 Small Intestine
23 Leg, Knee, Hip Lower Back
24 Urinary Tract
25 Bladder
26 Sciatic
27 Hemorrhoids
28 Apendix
29 Upper Lymph Glands
30 Lower Lymph Glands
31 Sex Hormones
32 Tonsils
33 Hair Problems
34 Groin
35 Buttocks
36 Energy
37 Toothache

Left Palm   Right Palm

Left Back   Right Back

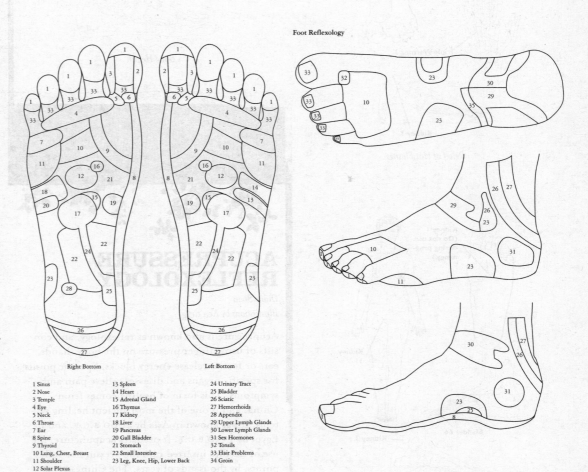

Foot Reflexology

Right Bottom   Left Bottom

1 Sinus	13 Spleen	24 Urinary Tract
2 Nose	14 Heart	25 Bladder
3 Temple	15 Adrenal Gland	26 Sciatic
4 Eye	16 Thymus	27 Hemorrhoids
5 Neck	17 Kidney	28 Appendix
6 Throat	18 Liver	29 Upper Lymph Glands
7 Ear	19 Pancreas	30 Lower Lymph Glands
8 Spine	20 Gall Bladder	31 Sex Hormones
9 Thyroid	21 Stomach	32 Tonsils
10 Lung, Chest, Breast	22 Small Intestine	33 Hair Problems
11 Shoulder	23 Leg, Knee, Hip, Lower Back	34 Groin
12 Solar Plexus		

Continued ➡

body part or organ, and will have other pain spots on the hand (or foot if working on the hand), ear and body. When doing a full foot or full hand acupressure treatment, make sure to do both feet or both hands. More accurate diagnosing and healing can probably be accomplished on the feet.

The acupressure points used in this book are single points, with often a number of points illustrated for each dis-ease. Make sure you have located the point before applying pressure, and press gradually and steadily until you feel the point release. You will feel a difference in well-being immediately. Combine acupressure with other methods of healing for dis-eases discussed in this book.

The primary acupressure references are: Cathryn Bauer, *Acupressure For Women* (The Crossing Press, 1987); three books by Mildred Carter, *Body Reflexology*, *Hand Reflexology, Key to Perfect Health*, and *Helping Yourself with Foot Reflexology* (all from Parker Publishing Co., 1983, 1975 and 1969); Iona Marsaa Teeguarden, *Acupressure Way of Health* (Japan Publications, 1978); and Moshe Olshevsky, CA, PhD., et. al., *The Manual of Natural Therapy* (Citadel Press, 1989). Also see the chapters on acupressure and reflexology in *All Women Are Healers*.

—From *The Natural Remedy Book for Women*

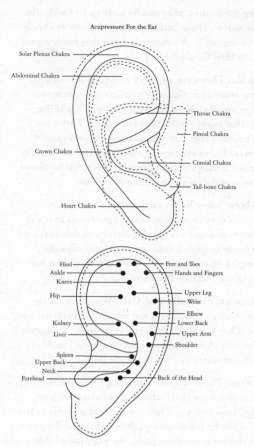

Acupressure For the Ear

Acupressure For the Ear

1 Sinus
2 Nose
3 Temple
4 Eye
5 Neck
6 Throat
7 Ear
8 Spine
9 Thyroid
10 Lung: Chest, Breast
11 Shoulder
12 Solar Plexus
13 Spleen
14 Heart
15 Adrenal Gland
16 Thymus
17 Kidney
18 Liver
19 Pancreas
20 Gall Bladder
21 Stomach
22 Small Intestine
23 Leg, Knee, Hip, Lower Back
24 Urinary Tract
25 Bladder
26 Sciatic
27 Hemorrhoids
28 Appendix
29 Upper Lymph Glands
30 Lower Lymph Glands
31 Sex Hormones
32 Tonsils
33 Hair Problems
34 Groin
35 Buttocks
36 Energy
37 General Pain, Toothache
38 Stomach Disorders
39 Mouth
40 Forehead
41 Tongue
42 Skin
43 Hypertension
44 Appetite
45 Fever
46 Stop Smoking
47 Ribs
48 Vocal Chords
49 Thirst Control
50 Wrist
51 Breathing Difficulties
52 Fingers

Body Reflexology

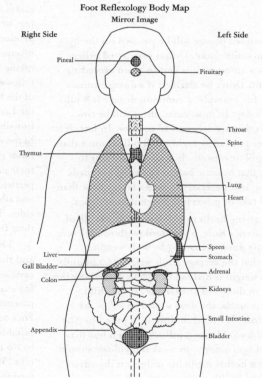

Foot Reflexology Body Map
Mirror Image

Right Side   Left Side

Right Foot   Left Foot

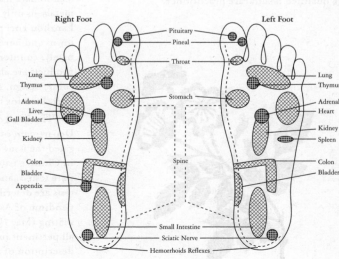

CHINESE PATENT MEDICINES

Bill Schoenbart, Lac.

Introduction to Chinese Patent Medicines

It's a familiar scenario: Seemingly out of the blue, a family member starts to feel tired and run-down. Over the next few days, she may develop a sore throat that gradually gets worse. There could be some nasal congestion that spreads into the lungs or sinuses. Over-the-counter remedies may help suppress the symptoms, but they don't affect the duration of the illness, and some can even have dangerous side effects. For example, aspirin can cause stomach ulcers, and acetaminophen can cause liver damage. Often, a sinus infection or bronchitis will develop; a visit to the family doctor may lead to a course of antibiotics. With the use of antibiotics, there is always the risk of a chronic yeast infection, gastrointestinal upset, or impaired immunity.

Is there an alternative way to deal with common colds, coughs, and minor injuries? We need only look to the other side of the planet, to the tradi-

Continued ➡

tional culture of China, where people have been using natural herbal medicines successfully for thousands of years. In China, the above scenario may begin with the same symptoms, but the response is often far different. After an injury, or at the first sign of a cold or flu, Chinese people turn not to strong pharmaceuticals to suppress their symptoms, but to a vast selection of prepackaged herbal medicines. There are hundreds of Chinese patent remedies available in convenient, easy-to-use forms like pills and liquids, typically sold in glass bottles and packaged in colorful boxes.

In the past, these prepared medicines often had secret ingredients to enable a manufacturer to distinguish their product from the competitors'. This was the Chinese version of securing a "patent" on the product. While this practice has all but disappeared due to government regulation of herbal medicines, the term "patent medicine" is still used in Western countries to describe prepackaged over-the-counter Chinese herbal formulas.

Many of these conveniently packaged herbal remedies are intended to treat easily diagnosed, acute, self-limiting conditions like the common cold, coughs, and minor injuries. For example, in the case described above, a person in China might select a remedy formulated to help the body fight off a cold, such as Gan Mao Ling ("gahn maow ling") or Yin Qiao Jie Du Pian ("yin chaow jyeh doo pyen"). If used early enough in the course of a cold or flu, these inexpensive herbal pills will often stop the illness in its tracks. If there is accompanying nasal or sinus congestion, one could also use an herbal decongestant like Bi Yan Pian ("bee yahn pyen") or Chuan Xiong Cha Tiao Wan ("chwahn shuhng chah tyow wahn"). If the cold spreads to the lungs, a cough remedy like Pinellia Root Teapills or Er Chen Wan ("uhr chen wahn") will usually clear the lungs. With the prompt application of herbal patent remedies, it is often possible to halt the progress of a simple cold or other illness before it becomes a more serious condition requiring drug therapy.

Forms of Patent Medicines

Pills: This is the most common form of patent medicines. The usual procedure is to boil an herbal formula until it becomes highly concentrated. This thickened mass is then rolled into tiny balls that are air-dried with a protective glaze. These are then typically placed in glass bottles and sealed with a cork and a plastic cap. This format has a number of advantages. The small size makes the pills easy to swallow, and the fact that they are already extracted in water makes them easy to assimilate. In Chinese, this type of pill is called wan ("wahn"), so it is common for a patent medicine's name to end with this word. For example, Six Flavor Rehmannia Pills are known as Liu Wei Di Huang Wan. Liu Wei means "six flavors," Di Huang means "Rehmannia root," and Wan means "round pill."

Tablets: This is another popular method of administering herbs. Known in Chinese as pian ("pyen"), these are either flattened discs or sugar-coated tablets (i.e., the shape of a few popular brands of coated candies). The disk-shaped tablets are a little difficult for some people to swallow, but the coated tablets are very easy to swallow. Children will have less difficulty taking this form of tablet.[1] An example of this format would be the remedy known as Bi Yan Pian ("nose inflammation tablets").

Granules or Instant Teas: Granules are an excellent way to give herbs to children. They are made by boiling down the herbs into a concentrated decoction and then crystallizing the liquid on a heated surface. They can be stirred into hot water to make a refreshing tea. For children who tend to balk at

taking medicines, they can be hidden in foods like apple sauce. These instant teas are known as chong ji ("chung jee"). An example from this book would be Luo Han Guo Chong Ji.

Liquids: There are a variety of liquid formats for patent remedies. Ginseng extracts are commonly sold in small vials mixed with honey. This is the form that many Americans have seen. There are also herbal wines, syrups, and preserved liquid extracts. These are readily absorbed and are usually pleasant tasting. Some examples from this book are Extractum Astragali and Tang Kwei Gin.

Powders: Some herbs work better in their raw form, or they contain volatile ingredients that will be destroyed by cooking. Medicines in this form are sold loose in glass bottles or in gelatin capsules. Examples of medicines in this form would be Sai Mei An or Yunnan Pai Yao.

Liniments or Medicated Oils: With rare exceptions, herbs in this form are meant for external use only. They are typically used for bruises, fractures, or sprains. An example would be Zheng Gu Shui, which translates as "setting bone liquid."

Plasters: These are self-adhering pieces of cloth or plastic that have their adhesive saturated with an herbal concentrate. They are applied directly to the skin, and the medicinal qualities of the herbs penetrate the area to relieve pain. An example of this effective type of remedy would be Die Da Zhi long Gao (Plaster for Bruise and Analgesic).

Dosage

A recommended dosage will be printed on the bottle by the manufacturer. Unless instructed otherwise by a practitioner, it is best to avoid exceeding this amount. Don't be alarmed if a dosage sounds very large; for example, a common dosage is 8 pills, 3 times per day. In most cases, these will be tiny round pills that are very easy to swallow. In fact, it is much easier to swallow eight small pills at once than one large pill or capsule. It is also important to remember that because patent remedies are made from herbs, it is necessary to take a larger dose than one would take of powerful, concentrated drugs.

When giving herbs to children, a good rule of thumb is Clark's Rule, a standard method of determining drug doses according to body weight. Assuming that the average adult weighs 150 pounds, the child's weight is divided by 150 to determine the reduction in dosage. For example, if the child weighs 50 pounds, the dose would be 50/150, or 1/3 the adult dose. If the adult dose is 15 pills, the 50-pound child would take 5 pills. Children less than one year of age, elderly, or weak individuals should not be given herbal medicine unless on the advice of a qualified health care practitioner.

Safety Issues

While Chinese patent medicines are normally a safe and convenient way to ingest healing herbs, there are some important safety issues to consider. Of greatest concern is the possible presence of heavy metals and pharmaceutical drugs in these products. These adulterants can make their way into a formula in a number of ways:

1. In China and Taiwan, herbs and drugs are intentionally mixed in certain products to achieve a synergistic action. Sometimes the drugs are listed on the label, but sometimes they are omitted.

2. Unauthorized or irresponsible factories might use polluted water containing heavy metals in the decoction process. These same factories might also skip crucial quality control procedures designed to detect the presence of pesticides in the herbs.

3. Some formulas intentionally include minerals containing heavy metals to achieve their therapeutic effect. This practice may have been acceptable in preindustrial times, when heavy metal exposure was minimal. However, in modern times people already have overly high exposures due to industrial pollution, and any further exposure is unacceptable.

Fortunately, all of these concerns can be addressed to ensure that your use of Chinese patent medicines is a safe and healing experience. The most important thing to know is that there are manufacturers in China that never use drugs, artificial coloring, or any additives or contaminants in their products. I recommend that you use medicines manufactured at facilities that adhere to Good Manufacturing Practices (G.M.P.), which are quality standards followed by Western pharmaceutical companies. One of the best examples of a G.M.P. facility in China is the Lanzhou Foci Herb Company. They have exceptionally high standards of quality control in all steps of the manufacturing process. Lanzhou Foci, like other good manufacturers, attempts to purchase all their raw herbs from farmers who avoid the use of pesticides, and will test the herbs, in their raw state and after they are extracted, for the presence of pesticides. They also filter all their water, and they test their finished products for heavy metals and molds.

There are about ten G.M.P. factories in China, and the products of other G.M.P. facilities are reviewed in this book—Qi Xing and Pangaoshou, for example, are also G.M.P. facilities. Most of the patents reviewed in this book are made by Lanzhou Foci or Plum Flower. In my experience, these are reliable lines with high standards of quality; they are by no means the only good lines of patent medicine. While Plum Flower brand—which is guaranteed to have no dyes, pharmaceuticals, or heavy metals—is only available from Mayway Corporation, Lanzhou Foci products can be found in Chinatowns and herb stores all over the world. Unfortunately, counterfeit versions of high-quality products are also very common: these use a similar color, design, or name. In the case of Lanzhou Foci, look for their *full* name on the label.

The Food and Drug branch of the California Department of Health Services has recently investigated the issue of heavy metals and pharmaceuticals in Chinese patent medicines. Over 600 products were tested, and the results of 260 of the product tests are described in a report entitled Compendium of Asian Patent Medicines. As of this writing (May 1998) the project is not complete, but all pertinent information is included in the description of any products that might be affected by contamination. In these cases, an uncontaminated product will be recommended.

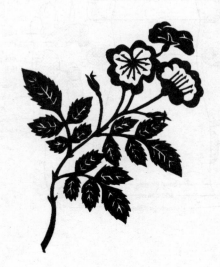

Continued →

How to Get Started

In China, people usually receive a patent medicine at a hospital or an herbal pharmacy. In either case, they are likely to have been accurately diagnosed before they select a remedy. In Western countries, licensed acupuncturists are the practitioners most likely to be thoroughly trained in the traditional Chinese diagnostic system. This is especially true in California, where all acupuncturists are required to be proficient in herbal medicine. In other states, practitioners can demonstrate their proficiency by passing an herbal exam given by the National Commission for the Certification of Acupuncturists. It is highly recommended that you consult with a qualified practitioner of Chinese herbal medicine before attempting to use patent remedies. If you are interested in becoming a practitioner of acupuncture and herbal medicine, the rigorous training takes from three to four years and involves both academic studies and clinical practice. Names of schools can be obtained from the organizations listed at the end of the book.

The remedies are organized according to organ systems and diagnostic categories. Some formulas could easily be included in several categories. In these cases the formula is listed under its most common usage. Within each category, the medicines are placed in alphabetical order. Each medicine is described in the following format:

Title: The name of the remedy, as it appears on the box. Example: Shu Gan Wan

Pronunciation and translation: To aid in pronunciation, the formulas name will be spelled phonetically. This will be followed by a literal translation of the name. Example: "shoo gahn wahn"—"soothe liver pill"

Indications: This is the range of symptoms for which the formula is indicated, though not all symptoms are necessarily present at the same time. Example: Digestive disorders that become worse under stress; abdominal distention and pain, nausea, belching, poor appetite, gas, and loose stools. Ingredients: Each ingredient in the formula is listed. Herbs are given their Latin botanical name, along with their Chinese name in parentheses. Example: Bupleurum chinense root (Chai Hu) Curcuma longa rhizome (Jiang Huang)

Description: This section will explain the action, ingredients, and Chinese and Western diagnostic categories of the formula. Lifestyle and dietary suggestions might also be included. Example: "When this pattern occurs, it is important to use a formula that soothes the Liver and also resolves the digestive difficulties. This remedy addresses both areas. While this remedy will usually resolve the imbalance, it is important to reduce the sources of stress that cause this pattern. It is helpful to avoid alcohol and high-fat foods, as well as eating on the run or while upset."

Dosage: The recommended dosage as provided by the manufacturer is given. In some cases of acute ailments, a practitioner might increase the dosage. On the other hand, dosages are decreased for children, elderly, or weak individuals. Example: 8 pills, 3 times per day

Manufacturer: Although there are often many manufacturers of a given remedy, the recommended one is listed. This is very important, since some manufacturers have very high standards of purity. They avoid using artificial coloring and pharmaceuticals, and they test for heavy metals and pesticides. Example: Lanzhou Foci

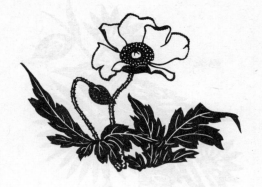

Warnings and contraindications: This will explain when the remedy is inappropriate or dangerous. Example: Do not use during pregnancy.

Traditional Chinese herbal medicine is a fascinating and intricate system of healing. While it can take a lifetime to become an expert at creating herbal formulas, studying the patent remedies provides the layperson with an excellent introduction to this ancient practice. It is my hope that this guide will kindle a lifelong interest in the healing properties of herbs. Whether they come from China or your own yard, medicinal herbs are among nature's great gifts to humanity. Used wisely and with respect, they can greatly enhance the quality of your life.

The Philosophy of Chinese Herbal Medicine

Many patent remedies are based on herbal formulas that have been in use for more than two thousand years. These formulas have gone through extensive human trials over a long period, and a skilled practitioner of herbal medicine can use them to treat extremely subtle and complex chronic conditions. To determine which formula to use, a diagnosis is made according to ancient principles that were developed by the Taoist sages, who were especially keen observers of the human body and its relationship to nature. Their worldview helped to shape the theoretical foundation for Chinese medicine as it is practiced today.

Yin and Yang in Nature and the Human Body

Through patient observation of the forces of nature, the Taoists saw the universe as a unified field, constantly moving and changing while maintaining its oneness. This constant state of change was explained by the theory of Yin and Yang, which first appeared in written form around 700 B.C. in the *I Ching* ("Book of Changes"). According to this theory, nature expresses itself in a dynamic cycle of polar opposites such as day and night, moisture and dryness, heat and cold, or activity and rest. Yin phenomena are those that exhibit the nurturing qualities of darkness, rest, moisture, cold, and structure. Yang phenomena in turn have energetic qualities such as light, activity, dryness, heat, and function. Everything in nature exhibits varying combinations of Yin and Yang. The morning fog (Yin) is dissipated by the heat of the Sun (Yang); the forest fire (Yang) is extinguished by the rainstorm (Yin); the darkness of night (Yin) is replaced by the light of day (Yang). In this way, any phenomenon in nature can be understood in relationship to another; one will always be more Yin or Yang than the other.

Since the Taoists believed that everything in the universe is essentially one, they made no distinction between the external forces of nature and the internal processes of the human body. This gave rise to the belief that "the macrocosm exists within the microcosm." In other words, any process or change that can be witnessed in nature can also be seen in the human body. For example, a person who eats cold food (Yin) on a cold, damp day (Yin) will often experience excessive mucus (Yin). Similarly, a person who performs strenuous activity (Yang) on a hot day (Yang) might experience dehydration with a fever (Yang). Some of the traditional diagnoses sound like a weather report, such as "wind and *cold* with *dampness*" (a Yin condition); or "a deficiency of *moisture* leading to *fire*" (a Yang pattern). These diagnostic descriptions illustrate the principle that the human body experiences the same fluctuations of Yin and Yang as the environment.

The internal organs also have their own balance of Yin and Yang. Yin qualities tend to be nourishing, cooling, building, relaxing, and related to the structure of the organs. Yang qualities tend to be energizing, warming, consuming, stimulating, and related to the functional activity of the organs. The organs in Chinese medicine are the Heart, Lungs, Spleen, Liver, Kidneys, Pericardium, Large Intestine, Small Intestine, Gall Bladder, Stomach, and Urinary Bladder. Each organ possesses functions that closely parallel those of its Western counterpart, but they also have additional functions that are unique to Chinese medicine. Since all the organs have Yin and Yang aspects, it is possible to monitor and adjust the levels of Yin and Yang in all parts of the body, maintaining a high level of vitality and preventing imbalances which manifest as disease. This is achieved not only with herbal medicine, but with changes in diet and lifestyle as well. In this way, the observations of the ancient Taoists have practical applications in the modern world in our quest for wellness and preventive health care.

The Vital Substances: Qi and Blood

In addition to Yin and Yang, traditional Chinese medicine also uses the concepts of two vital substances: Qi ("chee") and blood. Although Qi plays a central role in traditional Chinese medicine, it is extremely difficult to define. Existing somewhere between matter and energy, Qi has the qualities of both. It has substance without structure, and it possesses energetic qualities, but can't be measured. It is the fundamental power underlying all the activities of nature, as well as the vital life force of the human body.

It is easiest to understand Qi in terms of its functions and activities, where it is readily perceived. For example, the force of a thunderstorm can be understood in terms of its Qi; similarly, the strength of the digestive organs can be evaluated in relation to their Qi. In the storm, the power of the Qi can be observed in the fallen trees and buildings in the storm's aftermath; in the body, the strength of digestive Qi can be evaluated by the appetite and how the body assimilates nutrition.

Although there are many types of specialized Qi in the body, all varieties share some basic functions. Qi is responsible for transforming one type of substance into another. The Qi of digestion (Spleen Qi) transforms food into usable energy and blood; Kidney Qi transforms fluids into pure essence and waste water; Lung Qi transforms air into the energy to sustain life. Qi is also responsible for protecting the body from attacks by external pathogens. If the Qi is weak, a person may get frequent colds and other illnesses. Qi keeps organs in their proper place, blood within the vessels, and body fluids inside the body. Deficiency of Qi can lead to sagging organs (prolapse), bleeding disorders, and excessive sweating or urination. The Yang Qi of the Kidney is responsible for keeping the entire body warm; when it is deficient, a person can experience

Continued →

chronic cold extremities and decreased function in all activities that require warmth, such as digestion.

Blood has some parallels to its Western counterpart, such as its function of circulating through the body and nourishing the organs. However, it also has some very subtle functions in Chinese medicine, such as providing a substantial foundation for the mind and lending sensitivity to the sensory organs. It is closely aligned with Qi, having a complementary relationship with it. There is a saying, "Blood is the mother of Qi, and Qi is the leader of blood." This refers to the fact that without blood, there is no fundamental nutritional basis for Qi; without Qi, there would be no ability to form or circulate blood, and it would fail to stay within the vessels. The two are also considered to flow together through the body.

The main function of blood is to circulate throughout the body, providing nourishment and moisture to the organs, skin, muscles, and tendons. If it is deficient, there can be symptoms such as dry skin and hair, inflexible tendons, or various emotional and reproductive imbalances, depending on which organs are involved. If it is stagnant, there will be sharp pain at the site of stagnation. If there is heat in the blood, there can be irritability and skin rashes. Since Qi and blood are so closely related, a deficiency or stagnation of one of the substances will often lead to the same imbalance in the other.

Causes of Imbalance: The Six Pathogenic Factors

Another important concept that the Taoists contributed to Chinese medicine is the realization that the interior of the human body works in much the same way as the world outside the body. Through careful observation, they noted that the body could develop its own "weather patterns," often in response to the external environment. These six patterns, known as pathogenic factors, are *wind, cold, heat, dampness, dryness*, and *summer heat*.

The pathogenic factor of wind is considered to be the major cause of illness in traditional diagnosis. It readily combines with other pathogens, giving rise to syndromes like *wind cold, wind heat*, and *wind dampness*. It possesses qualities of the wind as seen in nature, appearing without warning and constantly changing. It is considered to be a Yang pathogenic factor, especially attacking the upper body, head, throat, and eyes. *Wind* causes things to move, so it is usually involved when there is twitching, spasms, and shaking. The organ most often affected by external wind is the Lung; internal *wind* is most commonly related to an imbalance in the Liver.

Cold is considered to be a Yin pathogenic factor. Its nature is to slow things down, causing tightness, stagnation, contraction, and an impairment in circulation. Externally, it can attack the skin, muscles, and Lungs. Internally, it can cause an impairment in the normal functions of the Spleen, Stomach, and Kidneys.

Heat, or *fire*, is a Yang pathogenic factor. As in nature, *heat* causes expansion and increased activity. When out of balance, it can lead to irritability, fever, and inflammatory conditions. By its nature it rises up, manifesting as a red face and eyes, dizziness, anger, and sore throat. It tends to deplete the body fluids, leading to thirst, constipation, and dark urine. Since it can produce *wind*, it can lead to spasmodic movement

In nature, dampness soaks the ground and everything that comes in contact with it, creating a stagnant situation. Once something becomes damp, especially in wet weather, it can take a long time to dry out again. The Yin pathogenic influence of *dampness* has similar qualities: it is persistent, heavy, and it can be difficult to resolve. A person who

spends a lot of time in the rain, lives in a damp environment, or sleeps on the ground can be more susceptible to an attack of external *dampness*. Similarly, a person who eats large amounts of ice cream, cold foods, cold drinks, greasy foods, and sweets is prone to imbalances of internal *dampness*. In general, symptoms of *dampness* in the body include water retention (edema), swelling, feelings of heaviness, coughing or vomiting phlegm, and wet skin eruptions. When *dampness* combines with *heat*, the condition of *damp heat* develops. This can cause a variety of symptoms such as dark, burning urine, sticky, foul-smelling stools, yellow vaginal discharges, and jaundice.

Dryness is a Yang pathogenic influence. As in nature, its influence on the body is drying and astringent. It can easily deplete the body fluids, causing constipation, concentrated urine, dryness in the throat and nose, thirst, dry skin, and dry cough. It typically enters the body through the nose and mouth, quickly affecting the Lungs.

Summer heat is a Yang pathogenic influence that usually occurs in the heat and humidity of summer. It affects the head area, causing thirst, red face, and headache; a person will tend to lie down with the limbs spread out. The excessive sweating also causes the urine to be dark and concentrated, and there can be a depletion of the body's Yin. The extreme *heat* also affects the heart, leading to restlessness or coma in severe cases like sunstroke. When it combines with *dampness* due to humidity and over-consumption of soft drinks, the Spleen is also affected. This leads to a loss of appetite, nausea, vomiting, diarrhea, and fatigue.

Diagnosis and Treatment

Before prescribing an herbal formula, a trained practitioner of Chinese medicine will look for the presence of the six pathogenic factors and assess the levels of Yin, Yang, Qi, and blood in the organs. This is done by taking an accurate history of the person's symptoms and performing a tongue and pulse diagnosis.

The condition of each of the internal organs can be determined by looking at the tongue and feeling the pulse. Different areas of the tongue represent the different organ systems. The color and shape of the tongue and its coating in each area reflects the condition of the corresponding organ. If the tongue itself is bright red this indicates *heat*, while a pale color indicates *cold*. Similarly, a yellow tongue coating is a sign of *heat*, while a white tongue coating is a sign of *cold*. For example, the back of the tongue is the area that corresponds to the Urinary Bladder. If that area has a thick and greasy yellow coating, a practitioner might suspect a bladder infection ("*damp heat* in the Urinary Bladder").

The pulses on the wrists would then be palpated. If the pulse corresponding to the Bladder is rapid and strong and has a "rolling" feeling, the physician would have further support for the diagnosis of *damp heat*. Finally, the patient's symptoms of dark, burning urine and abdominal pain would provide enough evidence to confirm the diagnosis.

Once an accurate diagnosis is made, the practitioner will select an herbal formula that has a long history of successfully treating that particular condition. Herbal formulas are organized according to traditional diagnostic categories and the organ systems that are to be treated. Each formula in a diagnostic category has a particular focus. For example, within the category of formulas that treat the common cold (*wind*), there are two subcategories: formulas that treat *cold*-type conditions (*wind cold*) and formulas that treat *heat*-type conditions (*wind heat*). Within those subcategories, some formulas might focus on symptoms that are more predominant, such as a dry cough or a sore throat, to further discriminate, certain ingredients may be added or eliminated to alter the effects of a formula.

Chinese herbal formulas are organized according to a hierarchy. The chief herb in a formula is the most important ingredient, having the most direct effect on the primary disorder. The deputy herb either augments the chief herb in treating the principal pattern, or it addresses another set of symptoms. The assistant herb can help the chief and deputy in their functions, or it can moderate their effects. Finally, the envoy herb can direct the actions of the formula to a certain area of the body, or it can act to detoxify or harmonize the other ingredients. This method of organizing formulas is quite complex, and there are differing opinions among experts over which herbs occupy various positions in the hierarchy. However, the end result is a system of diagnosis and treatment that has withstood the test of time due to its high rate of success in treating the full range of human ailments.

As you can imagine, traditional Chinese diagnosis is a very subtle and intricate process that can take an entire lifetime to master. For this reason, the beginning student of Chinese herbal medicine will have an easier time by first learning how to use the patent medicines. They often have the same ingredients as traditional formulas, but they are easier and more convenient to use. They are also less likely to cause a problem if they are used incorrectly, since they are not as strong as bulk herbs boiled in decoctions. However, it is still preferable to receive a competent diagnosis from a trained practitioner before attempting to use the patent medicines. Your learning experience will be enhanced and you are more likely to feel the full benefits of an accurately prescribed herbal formula.

Remedies for the Circulatory System

Dan Shen Yin Wan

Pronunciation and translation: "dahn shen yin wahn"—"red sage drink pill"

Indications: Pain from angina

Ingredients:

Salvia miltiorrhiza root (Dan Shen)

Santalum album wood (Tan Xiang)

Amomum villosum fruit (Sha Ren)

Description: Coronary artery disease and angina pain have become far too common in modern industrialized countries. There are a number of herbs in Chinese medicine that exert a powerful effect on the heart, clearing cholesterol deposits and increasing efficiency of the heart muscle. These herbs are a valuable supplement to Western medical treatment, and they are among the great gifts of the contemporary practice of Chinese herbal medicine.

Continued ➡

The most important herb for treating heart disease is Salvia miltiorrhiza (Dan Shen). The root of this member of the Sage genus contains constituents that have remarkable healing effects on the heart muscle and coronary arteries. In fact, it is so effective that heart attack patients in China receive an intravenous drip of a sterile Salvia extract when they arrive at the emergency room. It has multiple actions, reducing cholesterol levels, relieving pain and anxiety, and promoting a more rapid recovery. It dilates the coronary artery, adjusts the heart rate, inhibits coagulation, and increases blood flow to the heart muscle. Numerous research studies, both with the whole herb and with this patent medicine, have demonstrated the effectiveness of Salvia. In one study, 80 percent of the patients who received Dan Shen experienced a remission of angina pain and chest fullness. EKG readings showed an improvement in up to 50 percent of the patients after one month; a higher percentage showed improvement after one year.

Of course, it is essential for a person with heart disease to make radical lifestyle improvements, including diet and exercise programs supervised by their physician. No amount of medicine, whether pharmaceutical or herbal, will be successful in the long term without making these important adjustments.

Dosage: 8 pills, 3 times per day

Manufacturer: Plum Flower

Warnings and contraindications: This condition should *always* be treated by a physician; failure to receive prompt medical care increases the risk of sudden death or disability. Attempting to self-treat such a condition is extremely unwise, since even a one-hour delay in receiving medical treatment can be a fatal error if the blockage worsens and leads to a heart attack. The only appropriate use for this remedy in the event of a heart attack would be while waiting for an ambulance to arrive. For chronic heart problems, this remedy should *only* be used under the supervision of a physician.

Hawthorn Fat-Reducing Tablets

Indications: High cholesterol, angina, obesity

Ingredients: Crataegus pinnatdfida fruit (Shan Zha)

Description: Hawthorn fruit has been traditionally used in Chinese medicine for "food stagnation," the prolonged retention of food in the stomach. It is especially appropriate when the indigestion is caused by overeating fatty foods, due to its ability to break down fats. This fat-digesting action also makes Hawthorn useful in bringing down high cholesterol levels and reducing fat deposits in the body. A popular dieting tea, known as Bojenmi, is simply a mixture of tea leaves and Hawthorn.

The cardiac activity of this incredibly useful herb is not limited to its ability to break down cholesterol deposits. Hawthorn lowers blood pressure slowly and persistently, with the effect lasting for approximately three hours. It also dilates blood vessels and increases blood flow to the coronary artery. It is quite safe and can be used for extended periods of time.

Dosage: 1–2 tablets, 3 times per day

Manufacturer: Sanming Pharmaceutical Manufactory

Warnings and contraindications: Do not attempt self-treatment for heart disease. If you are taking cardiac drugs, consult your physician before using Hawthorn, as it may increase the effect of the drugs.

While this product showed no traces of contamination when tested, it does contain some sugar. Hawthorn is also commonly used in Western herbalism, so there is a wide range of high-quality solid and liquid extracts available from health food and herb stores.

Remedies for the Digestive System

Huang Lian Su

Pronunciation and translation: "hwahng lyan soo"—"coptis extract"

Indications: Diarrhea or dysentery due to bacterial infection

Ingredients: Berberine extracted from Coptis chinensis rhizome (Huang Lian)

Description: This patent medicine walks the line between herbs and drugs. The word *Su* refers to a specific constituent isolated from an herb. In this case, the constituent is berberine, a bright yellow-colored alkaloid that is also present in Western herbs like Goldenseal and Oregon Grape. Berberine is a broad spectrum antibacterial and antiparasitic, making this remedy extremely useful for the treatment of "traveler's diarrhea." On their journeys to India, China, Africa, and Central America, travelers often send postcards containing glowing references to "those little yellow pills." For best results, it is advised to combine Huang Lian Su with a remedy that normalizes intestinal function, such as Mu Xiang Shun Qi Wan.

Huang Lian (Coptis chinensis) also has strong inhibitory effects on the bacteria that cause streptococcal and staphylococcal infections, pneumonia, and dysentery. Studies have shown it to be as effective as sulfa drugs in treating dysentery, without the serious side effects. Clinical trials have also proved it to be effective in treating influenza, pertussis (whooping cough), typhoid fever, tuberculosis, scarlet fever, and diphtheria. In China herbal medicine is used with great success to treat serious disease as well as minor ailments.

Dosage: 2 pills, 3 times per day

Manufacturer: Min-Kang Drug Manufactory
Warnings and contraindications: Not appropriate for diarrhea from nonbacterial causes, such as chronic indigestion, stomach flu, or overeating.

This remedy is for acute infections only. Do not use for more than a week or two. For best results, it is advisable to replenish intestinal flora (by taking acidophilus or bifidus supplements) after using this remedy. If diarrhea persists, see your health care practitioner.

Huo Xiang Zheng Qi Wan; Lophanthus Antifebrile

Pronunciation and translation: "haw shahng jung chee warm"—"agastache Qi-normalizing pills"

Indications: Stomach flu, nausea, vomiting, diarrhea, sticky stools

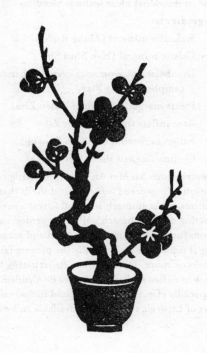

Ingredients:

Agastache rugosa plant (Huo Xiang)
Angelica dahurica root (Bai Zhi)
Areca acacia husk (Da Fu Pi)
Perilla frutescens leaf (Zi Su Ye)
Poria cocos fungus (Fu Ling)
Glycyrrhiza uralensis root (Gan Cao)
Atractylodes macrocephala root (Bai Zhu)
Magnolia officinalis bark (Hou Po)
Platycodon grandiflorum root (Jie Geng)
Citrus reticulata peel (Chen Pi)

Description: This is one of the best patent remedies for stomach flu. In traditional Chinese herbal medicine, it is indicated for a specific pattern that often occurs in the summer, with symptoms of nausea, vomiting, diarrhea, gas, headache, and sometimes fever and chills. When the symptoms are mild, it works quite well on its own, often bringing relief after just one dose. When symptoms are more severe, it is best to take it along with Gan Mao Ling (see p. 169) to enhance its ability to ward off the external pathogenic influence.

Dosage: 10 pills, 3 times per day

Manufacturer: Lanzhou Foci

Warnings and contraindications: This formula has some herbs that are drying. Do not use it when the signs of *heat* are prominent, such as a dry mouth, thirst, or high fever.

Mu Xiang Shun Qi Wan

Pronunciation and translation: "moo shahng shuhn chee wahn"—"saussurea Qi-regulating pills"

Indications: Food stagnation, indigestion, diarrhea, and intestinal gas

Ingredients:

Saussurea lappa root (Mu Xiang)
Alpinia katsumadai seed (Cao Dou Kou)
Atractylodes lancea rhizome (Cang Zhu)
Zingiberis officinalis rhizome (Sheng Jiang)
Citrus reticulata peel (Chen Pi)
Citrus reticulata green peel (Qing Pi)
Poria cocos fungus (Fu Ling)
Bupleurum chinense root (Chai Hu)
Magnolia officinalis bark (Hou Po)
Areca catechu seed (Bing Lang)
Poncirus trifoliata fruit (Zhi Shi)
Lindera strychnifolia root (Wu Yao)
Raphanus sativa seed (Lai Fu Zi)
Crataegus pinnatifida fruit (Shan Zha)
Fermentata medicinalis mass (Shen Qu)
Hordeum vulgare sprout (Mai Ya)
Glycyrrhiza uralensis root (Gan Cao)

Description: This formula relieves stagnation in the gastrointestinal tract, with symptoms such as fullness in the abdominal area, distention, gas, diarrhea, and a sensation of food sitting in the stomach without being digested. The chief herb in die remedy is Saussurea (Mu Xiang), which has the ability to reduce pain and fullness in the stomach and intestines caused by stagnation of Qi (vital energy). To enhance its effect of moving energy in the digestive tract, it is combined with other Qi-moving herbs, including Alpinia, Green Citrus, Magnolia, Areca, Poncirus, and Lindera. To alleviate the problem of food stagnating in the stomach, the following herbs are added: Raphanus (Radish seed), Crataegus (Hawthorn), Hordeum (Barley sprout), and a mixture of fermented grains and herbs (Shen Qu). The end result of this combination is a strong synergistic action that promotes

Continued ➡

peristalsis, relieves pain and fullness, and restores normal digestive function.

Mu Xiang Shun Qi Wan is especially helpful in treating traveler's diarrhea when combined with Huang Lian Su (see p.161). The latter kills the pathogens responsible for the diarrhea, while the former restores normal intestinal function. Because the combination of these two remedies is remarkably effective, it is highly recommended to include them in home first-aid or travel kits.

Dosage: 8 pills, 3 times per day

Manufacturer: Lanzhou Foci

Warnings and contraindications: If diarrhea persists, see your health care practitioner. In all cases of diarrhea, it is important to drink plenty of fluids to avoid dehydration. In severe or prolonged cases, I.V. fluids and electrolytes may need to be administered.

Peach Kernel Pills; Run Chang Wan

Pronunciation and translation: "ruhn chahng wahn"—"moisten intestines pills"

Indications: Constipation due to excess heat or dryness in the intestines

Ingredients:

Cannabis sativa seed (Huo Ma Ren)

Prunus persica seed (Tao Ren)

Cistanche salsa plant (Rou Cong Rong)

Angelica sinensis root (Dang Gui)

Rheum palmatum rhizome (Da Huang)

Description: This is a rather simple treatment for constipation. *Heat* or *dryness* lodging in the intestines can dry out the intestinal walls and the stools, preventing smooth movement of the bowels. This formula lubricates the intestines with Yin-nourishing oily seeds like Cannabis and Prunus (Peach pit). Cistanche is included for its ability to strengthen the Yang-eliminative power of the bowel, while Dang Gui nourishes the Blood and moistens the walls of the intestine. Finally, Rhubarb rhizome (Da Huang) has strong purgative qualities, effectively moving the bowels as well as clearing the *heat* that causes constipation.

Dosage: 4–8 pills, three times per day

Manufacturer: Lanzhou Foci

Warnings and contraindications: Since Rhubarb is a strong purgative herb, this remedy is for short-term use only. Constipation is usually the result of dietary indiscretions, especially insufficient fiber and fluids. It can often be rectified with a diet high in juicy vegetables, boiled whole grains, sufficient fluids, and high-quality oils like sesame, olive, and flax.

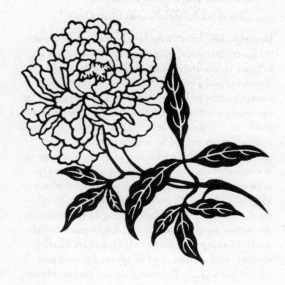

Curing Pills; Kang Ning Wan

Pronunciation and translation: "kahng ning wahn"— "healthy quiet pills

Indications: Disorders of the stomach such as nausea, vomiting, fullness, acidity, motion sickness, or acid regurgitation

Ingredients:

Gastrodia elata rhizome (Tian Ma)

Angelica dahurica root (Bai Zhi)

Chrysanthemum morifolium flower (Ju Hua)

Mentha haplocalyx plant (Bo He)

Pueraria lobata root (Ge Gen)

Trichosanthes kirilowii root (Tian Hua Fen)

Atractylodes lancea rhizome (Cang Zhu)

Coix lachryma-jobi seed (Yi Yi Ren)

Poria cocos fungus (Fu Ling)

Saussurea lappa root (Mu Xiang)

Magnolia officinalis bark (Hou Po)

Citrus erythrocarpa peel (Ju Hong)

Agastache rugosa plant (Huo Xiang)

Fermentata medicinalis mass (Shen Qu)

Oryza sativa sprout (Gu Ya)

Description: Pill Curing, also known as "Curing Pills," are extremely popular both in China and the West. They can be used for upset stomach due to overeating, weak digestion, or any other cause. For motion sickness, they should be taken 30 to 60 minutes before traveling. To enhance the effect, they can be taken with Ginger in capsules or as a tea, since Ginger has been shown in clinical trials to be more effective than Dramamine in relieving motion sickness. The combination of Ginger and Curing Pills is extremely effective. To treat nausea and vomiting that accompanies a cold or flu, this remedy can be combined with Gan Mao Ling (see p. 169).

Dosage: 1–2 vials, 3 times per day, or as needed. Each vial is filled with tiny pills, and it is quite easy to wash down a whole vial of pills with water.

Manufacturer: United Pharmaceutical Manufactory; Plum Flower

Warnings and contraindications: Many different manufacturers produce nearly identical versions of this product, and many of these contain artificial food coloring. There is now a dye-free version made by Plum Flower.

Sai Mei An

Pronunciation and translation: "sai may ahn"— "made by Sai Mei An factory"

Indications: Irritation to the stomach lining, gastric or duodenal ulcer without bleeding

Ingredients:

Stalactite mineral (Zhing Ru Shi)

Calcite mineral (Han Shui Shi)

Dryobalanops aromatica crystal [Borneol camphor] (Bing Pian)

Pteria margaritifera shell (Zhen Zhu)

Area inflata shell (Wa Leng Zi)

Fuligo herbarum (Bai Cao Shuang)

Cyclina sinensis shell (Hai Ge Ke)

Description: Sai Mei An is an interesting combination of powdered minerals and shells that neutralizes excess stomach acid and forms a protective coating on the stomach wall. This protects an ulcer from further irritation from food and acids, allowing it time to heal. Normally the process takes two weeks or more. During this time irritating foods such as coffee and spices should be avoided. An especially effective regimen could include the daily use of Licorice root. This is available in health food

stores as Deglycyrrhized Licorice (DGL); clinical studies have shown that it has a high success rate in treating ulcers.

Sai Mei An can also be used topically for mouth ulcers. Simply open a cap and sprinkle some of the powder directly on the ulcer. For damp-type skin irritations such as poison ivy/oak rashes, empty a capsule into the palm of your hand. Add a few drops of water, make into a paste with your finger, and apply it to the irritated area. The effect is soothing and cooling due to the Borneol camphor crystals, and the shell powders will help dry out the pustules. For an extra drying effect, the Sai Mei An powder can be mixed with a little French green clay powder before making it into a paste.

Dosage: 3 pills, 3 times per day, one half hour before meals

Manufacturer: Sai Mei An Medicine Factory

Warnings and contraindications: Dark, tarlike stools or vomiting blood can indicate a serious bleeding ulcer. Seek medical attention immediately.

Shen Ling Bai Zhu Pian

Pronunciation and translation: "shen ling bye zhoo pyahn"—"codonopsis, poria, and atractylodes pills"

Indications: Gastro-intestinal problems due to weak digestion, such as loose stools, bloating, and belching

Ingredients:

Codonopsis pilosula root (Dang Shen)

Poria cocos fungus (Fu Ling)

Atractylodes macrocephala rhizome (Bai Zhu)

Platycodon grandiflorum root (Jie Geng)

Dioscorea opposita root (Shan Yao)

Citrus reticulata peel (Chen Pi)

Amomum villosum seed (Sha Ren)

Nelumbo nucifera seed (Lian Zi)

Dolichoris lablab seed (Bai Bian Dou)

Coix lachryma-jobi seed (Yi Yi Ren)

Glycyrrhiza uralensis prepared root (Zhi Gan Cao)

Description: Shen Ling Bai Zhu Pian gets its name from the tonic herbs Dang Shen, Fu Ling, and Bai Zhu. These herbs strengthen the digestive Qi and remove the *damp* intestinal environment that causes diarrhea. The word *Pian* refers to a pill that is somewhat disk-shaped. In this way, a simple Chinese five-word title lists the main ingredients of the formula and describes the shape of the pill. Unlike Huang Lian Su, which treats diarrhea due to bacterial or parasitic infection, this remedy rectifies diarrhea caused by weakness in the digestive system.

In traditional Chinese diagnosis, the Qi (vital energy) of the Spleen is responsible for proper digestion and assimilation of nutrients. When the Spleen Qi is deficient, the result can be watery diarrhea or undigested food in the stools. Often this will be a chronic condition, caused by an inherited weakness or induced by poor eating habits. This situation is rectified through the use of tonic herbs that strengthen the Qi and thereby improve metabolism. In traditional formulation, some herbs will treat the cause of the problem, which is known as the root. Other herbs will address a specific symptom, known as the branch. Shen Ling Bai Zhu Pian contains herbs that treat both the root cause (Qi deficiency) and the branch symptom (diarrhea), making it effective both in the short and long term. The main herb treating the branch symptom of diarrhea is Lotus seed (Lian Zi), which has an astringent quality that helps bind

Continued ➡

the stools. Since it also has some ability to strengthen vital energy (Qi), it is an especially appropriate herb for this formula.

This is a very effective remedy that can also be used safely to treat diarrhea or excessive drooling in children, especially when they are underweight or malnourished. As always in the case of children, the dosage should be reduced in relation to the child's weight (see Clark's Rule in the dosage section of the Introduction).

Dosage: 12 pills, 3 times per day before meals

Manufacturer: Plum Flower; Sian Chinese Drug Pharmaceutical Works

Warnings and contraindications: This formula is inappropriate for acute diarrhea caused by bacteria, viruses, or parasites.

Shu Gan Wan

Pronunciation and translation: "shoo gahn wahn"—"soothe liver pill"

Indications: Digestive disorders which become worse under stress; abdominal distention and pain, nausea, belching, poor appetite, gas, and loose stools

Ingredients:

Bupleurum chinense root (Chai Hu)

Citrus aurantium fruit (Zhi Ke)

Glycyrrhiza uralensis root (Gan Cao)

Paeonia lactiflora root (Bai Shao)

Curcuma longa rhizome (Jiang Huang)

Aquilaria sinensis wood (Chen Xiang)

Corydalis yanhusuo rhizome (Yan Hu Suo)

Saussurea lappa root (Mu Xiang)

Magnolia officinalis bark (Hou Po)

Cyperus rotundus rhizome (Xiang Fu)

Paeonia suffruticosa root-bark (Mu Dan Pi)

Citrus medica fruit (Fo Shou)

Citrus reticulata peel (Chen Pi)

Citrus reticulata green peel (Qing Pi)

Amomum villosum seed (Sha Ren)

Amomum cardamomum fruit (Bai Dou Kou)

Santalum album wood (Tan Xiang)

Description: This is the standard formula for digestive difficulties due to an imbalance in the Liver. In traditional Chinese medicine, the Liver is responsible for the smooth flow of vital energy (Qi) in the body. When the Liver function becomes stagnant due to stress or environmental toxins, the effect is often felt in the digestive organs. Liver-related digestive problems will develop or get more severe under the influence of stress. There may also be a feeling of fullness and pain in the chest and abdominal area.

When this pattern occurs, it is important to use formulas that soothe the Liver in addition to herbs that resolve the digestive difficulties. This remedy addresses both areas. Bupleurum (Chai Hu), Turmeric Qiang Huang), and Peony (Bai Shao) relax the Liver and eliminate the cause of the imbalance. Digestive strength is increased with two species of Cardamom (Bai Dou Kou and Sha Ren), while the distention and pain are eliminated with Qi-regulating herbs like Saussurea (Mu Xiang), Cyperus (Xiang Fu), and Corydalis (Yan Hu Suo). While this remedy will usually resolve the imbalance, it is important to reduce the sources of stress that can cause the problem. It is helpful to avoid alcohol and high-fat foods, and not to eat when hurried or upset.

Dosage: 8 pills, 3 times per day
Manufacturer: Lanzhou Foci
Warnings and contraindications: Do not use during pregnancy.

Wei Te Ling

Pronunciation and translation: "way tuh ling"—"stomach special effective"

Indications: Heartburn, excess stomach acid

Ingredients:

Sepia esculenta bone (Hai Piao Xiao)

Corydalis yanhusuo rhizome (Yan Hu Suo)

Apis mellifera honey (Feng Mi)

Description: Wei Te Ling is the herbal version of an over-the-counter antacid. It is a very simple formula, containing Cuttlefish bone (Hai Piao Xiao) as its chief ingredient. This astringent, calcium-rich substance neutralizes excess stomach acid and helps heal stomach ulcers. Corydalis (Yan Hu Suo) is a strong analgesic to relieve pain, and Honey (Feng Mi) is nourishing to the stomach lining. The combination of the three ingredients makes this a very useful remedy for heartburn, acid stomach, or simple ulcers.

Dosage: 4–6 pills, 3 times per day before meals, or as needed

Manufacturer: Tsingtao Medicine Works

Warnings and contraindications: It is best to avoid foods and habits that cause acid stomach, especially coffee, spicy foods, and overeating.

Xiang Sha Liu Jun Wan; Aplotaxis Amomum Pills

Pronunciation and translation: "shahng shah loo juhn wahn"—"saussurea and cardamom six gentlemen pill"

Indications: Gastrointestinal symptoms due to weak digestion, with symptoms of poor appetite, nausea, vomiting, belching, chronic diarrhea, and gurgling

Ingredients:

Codonopsis pilosula root (Dang Shen)

Atractylodes macrocephala rhizome (Bai Zhu)

Poria cocos fungus (Fu Ling)

Glycyrrhiza uralensis root (Gan Cao)

Pinellia ternata rhizome (Ban Xia)

Citrus reticulata peel (Chen Pi)

Saussurea lappa root (Mu Xiang)

Amomum villosum seed (Sha Ren)

Description: This is an augmented version of the basic tonic formula to strengthen digestion, which is known as Four Gentlemen Decoction. Its combination of Codonopsis, Atractylodes, Poria, and Licorice has a synergistic effect that enhances both the immune system and the body's ability to digest and assimilate food. When Pinellia and Citrus peel

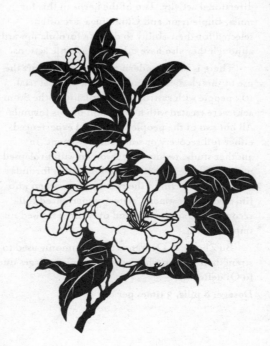

are added to further increase the digestive aspect, the formula is called Six Gentlemen Pills (Liu Jun Zi Wan). When this is further supplemented with Cardamom (Sha Ren) and Saussurea (Mu Xiang), the formula is called Xiang Sha Liu Jun Zi Wan. In this form, the remedy also has a strong ability to inhibit nausea in addition to its immune-stimulating and digestion-enhancing functions. For this reason, it is especially suitable for treating chemotherapy patients who are suffering from both nausea and depressed immunity. It is also quite useful for the symptoms of morning sickness and chronic gastritis.

Dosage: 12 pills, 3 times per day before meals

Manufacturer: Lanzhou Foci

Remedies for External Use: Plasters, Liniments, and Ointments

Ching Wan Hung; Jing Wan Hong

Pronunciation and translation: "ching wahn huhng"—"capital absolute red"

Indications: Burns of all kinds

Ingredients:

Chaenomeles lagenaria fruit (Mu Gua)

Sanguisorba officinalis root (Di Yu)

Boswellia carterii resin (Ru Xiang)

Lobelia chinensis plant (Ban Bian Lian)

Commiphora myrrh resin (Mo Yao)

Carthamus tinctorius flower (Hong Hua)

Angelica sinensis root (Dang Gui)

Dryobalanops aromatica crystal [Borneol camphor] (Bing Pian)

Description: Jing Wan Hong is one of the patent remedies that is absolutely essential in any home first aid or travel kit. In China, it is used for first, second, or third degree burns caused by hot water, steam, chemicals, radiation, or sunburn. The salve relieves pain very soon after it is applied, partly due to the analgesic action of Borneol camphor (Bing Pian). Damaged flesh is quickly regenerated, often with no scarring, since the formula also contains Myrrh (Mo Yao). Minor burns like sunburn can be healed remarkably fast, often in just a day or two.

Dosage: Apply externally as needed to cover the affected area.

Manufacturer: Tianjin Drug Manufactory

Warnings and contraindications: For external use only. This product can stain clothing.

Die Da Zhi Tong Gao; Plaster for Bruise and Analgesic

Pronunciation and translation: "dyeh dah juhr tuhng gow"—"contusion stop pain plaster"

Indications: Pain from sprains, traumatic injuries, or muscular tension

Ingredients:

Carthamus tinctorius flower (Hong Hua)

Commiphora myrrh resin (Mo Yao)

Daemonorops draco resin (Xue Jie)

Acacia catechu resin (Er Cha)

Eupolyphaga sinensis insect (Tu Bie Chong)

Dipsacus asper root (Xu Duan)

Drynaria fortunei rhizome (Gu Sui Bu)

Stegodon orientalis fossil (Long Gu)

Rheum palmatum rhizome (Da Huang)

Taraxacum mongolicum plant (Pu Gong Ying)

Mentha haplocalyx herb (Bo He)

Wintergreen oil (Dong Qing Yu)

Continued ➡

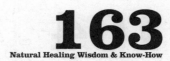

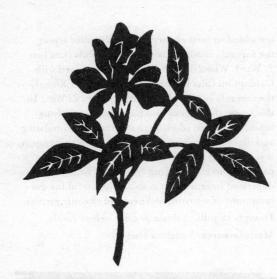

Description: Herbal plasters are still commonly used in China today. They may seem like a throwback to pioneer days, but they actually work very well. The recommended brand is good, but there are others that are very similar, such as Hua Tuo Plasters and 701 Plasters. This particular brand, Plaster for Bruise and Analgesic, made by United Pharmaceutical Manufactory, comes in a larger size than the others, but it can be trimmed to size with scissors. The plaster consists of a self-adhering patch with an herbal concentrate mixed into the adhesive. A plastic backing is peeled away, and the plaster is applied to the sore area.

Herbal plasters relieve pain from sprains, strains, fractures, sports injuries, or premenstrual back soreness. In the case of spasmodic muscles, which frequently occur on the shoulders and upper back, the plaster can be applied directly to the tight area. If this is done before bed, the tightness will often be gone in the morning. It is best to apply the plaster to both sides in this case, since the tightness may travel to the other side if only the sore side is treated.

Plasters work by promoting the circulation of blood through the injured area, and it also has ingredients that reduce swelling, stop pain, and promote healing. Typically a plaster loses its potency after 24 hours and is then removed, lb avoid irritation, it is best to let the skin air out for a few hours before putting on another plaster.

Dosage: As needed

Manufacturer: United Pharmaceutical Manufactory

Warnings and contraindications: Do not apply a plaster if the skin is broken. After 24 hours, remove the plaster and let the skin air out before applying more. Discontinue use if irritation develops. If the area to be treated has a lot of hair, it is best to use 701 brand plasters, since their adhesive is weaker.

Zheng Gu Shui

Pronunciation and translation: "juhng goo shway"—"setting bone liquid"

Indications: Traumatic injuries, bruises, fractures, sprains

Ingredients:

Panax pseudoginseng root, foliage, and flower (Tian Qi)

Angelica dahurica root (Bai Zhi)

Croton crassifolium root (Ji Gu Xiang)

Mentha haplocalyx crystal (Bo He Nao)

Cinnamomum camphora crystal (Zhang Nao)

Tiglii seed (Wu Ma Xun Cheng)

Moghania phillipinensis root (Qian Jin Ba)

Inula cappa (Da Li Wang)

Description: As its name suggests, Zheng Gu Shui ("setting bone liquid") is especially suitable for pro-

moting healing in fractured or bruised bones. In China, it is applied to the area before the bone is set in the hospital. After the bone is set, the area of the fracture is covered with cotton soaked in the liniment. The procedure is repeated twice daily until healing occurs. While this may not be practical when a plaster cast is used, it can be done when there is a removable cast or when a cast is not needed. It can also be used for sore feet, sprains, or sports injuries if the skin is not broken.

Dosage: Apply externally as needed.

Manufacturer: Tulin Drug Manufactory

Warnings and contraindications: For external use only. Wash hands thoroughly after applying. Stains clothing. Do not use on open wounds. Discontinue use immediately if a skin reaction develops. Keep tightly closed and out of reach of children. This liquid is flammable; keep away from open flame. Do not expose the treated skin to full sun when the liniment is applied.

Remedies for the Immune System and Overall Wellness (Tonics)

Central Qi Pills; Bu Zhong Yi Qi Wan

Pronunciation and translation: "boo juhng yee chee wahn"—"tonify the middle, strengthen Qi pills"

Indications: Deficiency of Qi (vital energy), weak digestion, prolapsed organs

Ingredients:

Astragalus membranaceus root (Huang Qi)

Codonopsis pilosula root (Dang Shen)

Atractylodes macrocephala rhizome (Bai Zhu)

Glycyrrhiza uralensis root (Gan Cao)

Angelica sinensis root (Dang Gui)

Citrus reticulata peel (Chen Pi)

Cimicifuga foetida rhizome (Sheng Ma)

Bupleurum chinense root (Chai Hu)

Zingiberis officinalis fresh rhizome (Sheng Jiang)

Zizyphus jujuba fruit (Da Zao)

Description: Bu Zhong Yi Qi Wan is the standard formula for organs that are prolapsed (sagging) due to a deficiency of Qi (vital energy). In addition to prolapse, other symptoms could include fatigue, poor appetite, loose stools, and a tendency to feel cold. This formula is an energetic combination of herbs that strengthen the Qi along with herbs that exert an uplifting action. In Chinese medicine, herbs are sometimes classified according to their directional activity. Two of the herbs in this formula, Bupleurum and Cimicifuga, are often selected for their ability to direct a formula upward, although they also have other therapeutic actions.

There is some modern research to support the use of this classical formula. In one clinical trial, 103 people with gastroptosis (prolapse of the Stomach) were treated with a decoction of this formula. All but two of the people in the trial experienced either full recovery or some improvement. In another study, twenty-three women with prolapsed uterus took the decoction version of this formula for two weeks. Out of the twenty-one women who finished the treatment, sixteen experienced full recovery, two improved, and only three showed no improvement.

Bu Zhong Yi Qi Wan is also commonly used to strengthen women who experience miscarriages due to Qi deficiency.

Dosage: 8 pills, 3 times per day

Manufacturer: Lanzhou Foci

Warnings and contraindications: For the above conditions, seek the help of a qualified health-care practitioner before using this remedy.

Ginseng Royal Jelly Vials; Renshen Feng Wang Jiang

Pronunciation and translation: "ren shen fuhng wahng jyahng"—"ginseng and royal jelly syrup"

Indications: Fatigue, poor appetite, feeling cold and weak

Ingredients:

Panax ginseng root (Ren Shen)

Royal jelly (Feng Wang)

Description: Ginseng is without a doubt the most well known of all Chinese herbs. What other herb from Asia can be commonly found at checkout lines of convenience stores and gas stations? This product isn't nearly as strong as an extract of Ginseng derived by boiling a root for an hour; powdered extracts of the root are also stronger. On the other hand, these little vials are very convenient, and they can provide a much-needed boost of energy during strenuous activity. Be sure to use a reputable brand that actually contains Ginseng and is free of caffeine or other adulterants.

It is important to be aware of the difference between the various types of Ginseng. There are three true species: Panax ginseng, Panax quinquifolium, and Panax notogin-seng. Panax noto-ginseng is used mostly for injuries, and it is the main ingredient in Yunnan Pai Yao (see p. 167). Panax quinquifolium is commonly known as American Ginseng. Its main distinction is that it has a cooling effect on the body. This makes it more appropriate for use in hot weather or for people with a red face, rapid pulse, irritability, and a tendency to overheat easily. A person like this will experience adverse effects from Asian Ginseng (Panax ginseng), which is very warming. Some possible side effects could be headache, stiff neck, irritability, skin rash, or a feverish feeling. Panax ginseng is the herb of choice for people who tend to look pale and feel cold, and it is indicated for low immunity, fatigue, and a host of other ailments. When it is combined with Royal jelly, as in this product, its effects are enhanced.

Ginseng has been investigated extensively, especially by the Russians and the Chinese. It is considered to be an adaptogen, meaning it helps an organism to adapt to severe stresses in the environment. Some of Ginseng's therapeutic effects include the following:

1. Reduces fatigue
2. Reduces the toxicity of certain chemicals
3. Stimulates the pituitary and adrenal cortex
4. Reduces blood sugar levels and is synergistic with insulin
5. Regulates cholesterol levels
6. Increases absorption of nutrients in the digestive system
7. Increases the body's immune response
8. Normalizes blood count
9. Stimulates production of immune globulins

After scanning this partial list of Ginseng's actions, it is easy to see why it has such an enduring reputation as a tonic for multiple purposes. When used wisely and appropriately, it can have a powerful ability to support us in our toxic and stressful modern lives.

Dosage: 1–2 vials per day.

Manufacturer: Harbin 3rd Pharmaceutical Manufactory

Continued ➜

Warnings and contraindications: Panax ginseng is very warming. It is not appropriate for a person who has *heat* signs, such as a red face, irritability, rapid pulse, restlessness, and a tendency to feel warm. Discontinue use if any of the above symptoms, or headache or stiff neck develop after taking Ginseng.

Imperial Astragali Extract; Bei Qi Jing

Pronunciation and translation: "bay chee jing"— "essence of northern astragalus"

Indications: Fatigue, weak immunity

Ingredients:

Astragalus membranaceus root (Huang Qi)

Honey (Feng Mi)

Description: The medicinal use of Astragalus root is one of the great contributions of Chinese herbal medicine. For thousands of years, it has been used to strengthen the Wei Qi ("way chee"), which is the ancients' way of describing the immune system. From a scientific perspective, Astragalus increases the production of antibodies and macrophages and improves resistance to stress. These are all important components of the body's immune response. The root slices, which look like tongue depressors, are often boiled into soup broth to be used as a daily wellness tonic. Other uses for this versatile herb include strengthening digestion, reducing edema, and regenerating flesh that is lost by injury or surgery. When combined with Ligustrurn fruit (Nu Zhen Zi), it can also normalize the blood count after chemotherapy.

While this patent medicine is a convenient way to use Astragalus, the effect is much stronger when the sliced roots are boiled into a decoction. It is also available in other forms, such as dehydrated crystals.

Dosage: 1–2 vials per day

Manufacturer: Plum Flower

Warnings and contraindications: While Astragalus can help prevent colds or infections, it is not recommended if they have already occurred. This is because Astragalus shuts down the pores, which prevents the body from expelling a pathogen. The Chinese call this "trapping the burglar," meaning it is counterproductive to lock all the doors if a burglar is already in the house. Once the pathogen has been expelled with remedies like Gan Mao Ling (see p. 169) or Yin Qiao Jie Du Pian (see p. 170), it is appropriate to use Astragalus to protect the body from future infections.

Ling Zhi Beverage

Pronunciation and translation: "ling juhr"

Indications: Frequent colds, chronic bronchitis, high cholesterol, stress

Ingredients:

Ganoderma lucidum fungus (Ling Zhi)

Description: Ganoderma (Ling Zhi), commonly known as Reishi, its Japanese name, is a beautiful, glossy black or red fungus that grows on trees in the wild. Prior to the 1970s, when researchers learned to cultivate it, Reishi was exceptionally rare and expensive. For example, in a grove of two hundred thousand plum trees, only seven wild Reishi mushrooms were found. It doesn't usually appear in the traditional herbal formulas, because it was formerly reserved for use by the emperor. Now that it can be grown in the laboratory from spores, it is widely available at a reasonable price. This particular product is an extract of the fungus, and it can be dissolved in water. A much stronger concentration can be obtained by boiling the fungus in water for an hour. Dehydrated crystals and liquid extracts are also available at retail herb and supplement stores.

Reishi has a quality that is unique among herbs that build vital energy (Qi): it is actually able to sedate and tranquilize a person while it energizes. This makes it especially appropriate for individuals who are weak and depleted but also nervous and irritable. This precious fungus has some important cardiovascular actions as well. It improves circulation to the coronary artery and heart muscles, and it decreases oxygen consumption by the heart. It also lowers blood pressure and cholesterol levels, making it exceptionally useful in maintaining cardiovascular health. Reishi is commonly included in formulas to stimulate the immune system, because it enhances immunity, increases white blood cell counts, and has antibacterial activity. It is also an antitussive and expectorant, making it an effective treatment for chronic bronchitis. Like Ginseng, it is considered a true herbal panacea.

Dosage: I cube, dissolved in water

Manufacturer: Guangxi Medicines and Health Products

Liu Wei Di Huang Wan; Rehmannia Six Teapills; Six Flavor Tea

Pronunciation and translation: "loo way dee hwahng wahn"—"six-ingredient rehmannia pills"

Indications: Thirst, irritability, night sweats, insomnia, weak lower back and knees

Ingredients:

Rehmannia ghitinosa prepared root (Shu Di Huang)

Dioscorea opposita root (Shan Yao)

Cornus officinalis fruit (Shan Zhu Yii)

Poria cocos fungus (Fu Ling)

Alisma plantago-aquatica rhizome (Ze Xie)

Paeonia suffruticosa root-bark (Mu Dan Pi)

Description: This is the classical base formula for all conditions of Yin deficiency, especially of the Liver and Kidneys. The Yin aspect of an organ refers to its structure and substance, while the Yang aspect refers to its functions and activities. Yin is cooling and moist; Yang is warming and dry. The Yin aspect of the bodyworks as a lubricant, calming and enriching the organs. It can become deficient due to a variety of factors, such as overwork, lack of sufficient rest or fluid intake, stress, an overly dry environment, or excessive sexual activity. When Yin is deficient, there can be chronic dryness and inflammation. This can be compared to running a car that is low on oil or water. The lack of lubrication or coolant will cause the engine to run hotter than normal; continued operation under these conditions can lead to long-term damage.

Symptoms of Liver and Kidney Yin deficiency include a warm sensation in the sternum, palms, and soles of the feet; red cheeks; night sweats; a feeling of heat and irritability in the afternoon and evening; sore and weak low back and knees; tinnitus (ringing in the ears); chronic dry mouth and thirst. The tongue will often be reddish with little or no coating, and the pulse typically feels thin and rapid. By focusing on nourishing the Yin and clearing the heat caused by the deficiency, this formula subtly and elegantly treats a wide range of seemingly unrelated symptoms. It contains three ingredients tjiat nourish the Yin and three that clear beat.

The chief tonifying herb in the formula is Rehrnannia glutinosa (Shu Di Huang). In its raw state, it has a cold energy and nourishes the Yin, making it useful in the treatment of high fevers and in alleviating thirst due to diabetes. In its prepared form, it is treated with wine, making it more nourishing to the Blood. In this form, it is used to treat anemia and menstrual difficulties and as an overall tonic to the Kidneys and adrenals.

Another important ingredient is Dioscorea (Shan Yao), a tonic to the Lungs, Stomach, and Kidneys. It also stimulates the immune system to produce interferon, a substance that suppresses viruses without disturbing normal body functions.

The third tonic herb is Cornus officinalis (Shan Zhu Yu), an astringent herb with a variety of actions: it is antiallergic, diuretic, anti-hypertensive, antitumor, antibacterial, and antifungal; and it increases the production of white blood cells. Being astringent, it energetically prevents further depletion of Yin through the excessive loss of semen, perspiration, urine, or uterine blood. It acts to consolidate the effect of the other tonifying herbs.

Alisma plantago (Ze Xie) is an important diuretic herb that grows wild in North America. It has a strong diuretic action, and it lowers blood pressure for prolonged periods of time. In addition to antibacterial qualities, it is an important herb for lowering blood sugar and cholesterol, another reason this formula is effective in treating diabetes. Poria cocos (Fu Ling) is another diuretic herb that also has a calming effect on the body. It is one of the important herbs for stimulating deep immunity; it induces interferon production and contains polysaccharides that stimulate macrophages to track down and destroy cells that are foreign to the body. The final herb in the formula is Mouton root bark (Mu Dan Pi), an aromatic agent that is cooling to the body on a number of different levels. It kills staphylococcus bacteria, lowers blood pressure, and decreases body temperature.

This is a highly sophisticated formula that is useful in a wide variety of conditions that manifest with the designated symptoms. There are numerous modifications to this base formula, depending on the particular focus. Some of the disorders that can be treated with Mu Wei Di Huang Wan are: diabetes, tuberculosis, hyperthyroidism, nephritis, hypertension, chronic urinary tract infection, and various degenerative diseases of the eye. In some cases, such as tuberculosis, Western pharmaceuticals would be taken along with the herbs. Obviously, many of these are serious conditions that should not be self-treated. As with most of the remedies in this book, it is essential to be under the care of a qualified physician while using these herbs. Many variations of this formula are available for specific ailments; Zhi Bai Di Huang Wa (see p. 172) and Ming Mu Di Huang Wan, discussed below, are also discussed in this book.

Dosage: 8–10 pills, 3 times per day

Manufacturer: Lanzhou Foci

Warnings and contraindications: Rehmannia can be difficult to digest, so this formula should be discontinued if excessive loose stools become a problem.

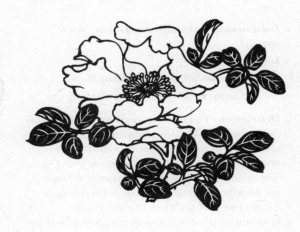

Continued ➡

Ming Mu Di Huang Wan

Pronunciation and translation: "ming moo dee hwahng wahn"—"brighten eyes rehmannia pills"

Indications: Dry eyes, blurry vision, poor eyesight

Ingredients:

Rehmannia gluti nosa prepared root (Shu Di Huang)

Dioscorea opposita root (Shan Yao)

Cornus officinalis fruit (Shan Zhu Yu)

Poria cocosi fungus (Fu Ling)

Alisma plantago-aquatica rhizome (Ze Xie)

Paeonia suffruticosa root-bark (Mu Dan Pi)

Lycium chinensis fruit (Gou Qi Zi)

Haliotis diversicolor shell (Shi Jue Ming)

Tribulus terrestris fruit (Bai Ji Li)

Description: Ming Mu Di Huang Wan is a variation of the previous formula, Liu Wei Di Huang Wan, This formula contains ingredients that focus on eye problems caused by the underlying problem of Yin deficiency, such as blurry vision, dry eyes, night blindness, and excessive tears. There may also be the general signs of Yin deficiency: dry mouth and throat, night sweats, and a sensation of heat in the palms and soles of the feet.

One of the additional herbs, Lycium fruit (Gou Qi Zi), is actually quite good to eat. It looks and tastes like raisins. These fruits are nourishing to the Liver Yin, which is the basis for healthy eyes. From a Western pharmacological perspective, Lycium fruit is hepato-protective, helping the liver eliminate toxic substances. In Chinese herbalism, it is specifically used to "brighten the eyes." The other two additions to the base formula are Abalone shell (Shi Jue Ming) and Tribulus fruit (Bai Ji Li); these are both specific for eye problems caused by heat in the Liver, making them appropriate for this remedy.

It is important to have an accurate diagnosis before using this formula. Similar eye problems can be due to a different heat pattern, and they require completely different herbs. For example, conjunctivitis due to Liver fire would require the formula Long Dan Xie Gan Wan (see p. 171), while red eyes due to Yin deficiency would be treated with this formula. This is another example of why a diagnosis from an acupuncturist is important before attempting to use this book for self-treatment.

Dosage: 10 pills, 3 times per day

Manufacturer: Lanzhou Foci

Warnings and contraindications: Not for red or swollen eyes due to conjunctivitis. Rehmannia can be difficult to digest, so this formula should be discontinued if excessive loose stools become a problem.

Shen Qi Da Bu Wan

Pronunciation and translation: "shen chee dah boo wahn"—"codonopsis astragalus great tonifying pill"

Indications: Weak immunity, fatigue, lack of appetite

Ingredients:

Codonopsis pilosula root (Dang Shen)

Astragalus membranaceus root (Huang Qi)

Description: This is a very simple formula to revive the vital energy (Qi), especially after a long illness, chemotherapy, or blood loss. This is also a good remedy to enhance the immune system (Wei Qi). The immune-stimulating properties of Astragalus are described in detail under Imperial Astragali Extract (see p. 165). When combined with Codonopsis pilosula (Dang Shen), these effects are enhanced. Codonopsis is often used as a substitute for Ginseng, since it is less warming and less expensive. It is an excellent tonic that increases red and white blood cell counts, making it very effective along with Astragalus in recovering from chemotherapy or radiation.

Both Astragalus and Codonopsis have a pleasant, mild, sweet taste. The roots are often boiled and used in soup stocks for a Chinese version of preventive medicine. They are fairly easy to grow, and seeds are available from a number of suppliers. If you live in an area with gophers, be sure to protect your plant beds with wire cages. Otherwise, after the roots get nice and juicy, they will suddenly disappear and you'll have a lot of gophers with strong immune systems!

Dosage: 8–10 pills, 3 times per day

Manufacturer: Lanzhou Foci

Remedies for Men

Kai Kit Wan

Pronunciation and translation: "keye kit wahn"—"dispel knot pills"

Indications: Benign swelling of the prostate gland

Ingredients:

Vaccaria segetalis seed (Wang Bu Liu Xing)

Patrinia scabiosaefolia plant (Bai Jiang Cao)

Paeonia lactiflora root (Bai Shao)

Astragalus membranaceus root (Huang Qi)

Paeonia suffiruticosa root-bark (Mu Dan Pi)

Akebia trifoliata stem (Mu long)

Glycyrrhiza uralensis root (Gan Cao)

Saussurea lappa root (Mu Xiang)

Corydalis yanhusuo rhizome (Yan Hu Suo)

Description: Benign prostatic hypertrophy (noncancerous swelling of the prostate gland) is very common in men over fifty years of age. Typical symptoms are difficulty in urination, frequent urination, dripping of urine, and interruption of urine flow. All of these symptoms are caused by the swelling of the prostate gland, which surrounds the urethra. Energetically, the swelling can be considered a stagnation of Qi and Blood, with a likely accumulation of heat and dampness. For this reason, treatment includes herbs that promote circulation and reduce dampness and stagnation. The chief herb in this formula is Vaccaria seed (Wang Bu Liu Xing), which has an affinity for promoting circulation in the sexual organs. Another important ingredient is Patrinia (Bai Jiang Cao), which clears stagnation and dampness. It also has an affinity for the male reproductive organs, being used with Vaccaria for testicular swelling due to mumps. Combined with the other herbs in the formula, which strengthen vital energy, promote circulation, and relieve pain, this remedy can help reduce die swelling. It is recommended to include Saw palmetto berries (Serenoa repens) in the treatment protocol, since they are a well-researched and effective treatment for this condition. Saw palmetto is available in most health food or supplement stores.

Dosage: 2–3 pills, 3 times per day

Manufacturer: Plum Flower

Warnings and contraindications: Men over age fifty should be screened for prostate cancer before attempting self-treatment for prostate problems.

Remedies for the Musculoskeletal System

Jin Gu Die Shang Wan

Pronunciation and translation: "jin goo dyeh shahng wahn"—"muscles and bones injury pill"

Indications: Traumatic injuries, bruises, sprains, and swelling

Ingredients:

Panax notoginseng root (Tian Qi)

Paeonia rubra root (Chi Shao)

Prunus persica seed (Tao Ren)

Boswellia carterii resin (Ru Xiang)

Commiphora myrrha resin (Mo Yao)

Curcuma longa rhizome (Jiang Huang)

Paeonia suffruricosa root-bark (Mu Dan Pi)

Caesalpinia sappan wood (Su Mu)

Drynaria fortunei rhizome (Gu Sui Bu)

Sparganium stoloniferum rhizome (San Leng)

Daeomonorops draco resin (Xue Jie)

Artemisia anomala plant (Liu Ji Nu)

Angelica sinensis root (Dang Gui)

Dipsacus japonicus root (Xu Duan)

Siler divaricata root (Fang Feng)

Cucumis seed (Tian Gua Zi)

Citrus aurantium fruit (Zhi Ke)

Glycyrrhiza uralensis root (Gan Cao)

Platycodon grandiflorum root (Jie Geng)

Akebia trifoliata stem (Mu Tong)

Pyritum mineral (Zi Ran Tong)

Eupolyphaga sinensis insect (Tu Bie Chong)

Description: Jin Gu Die Shang Wan is used to treat traumatic injuries. It is a combination of a large number of herbs that stimulate blood circulation, reduce swelling, stop pain, and promote healing. When combined with one of the liniments or plasters for external application, it can bring relief very quickly. Unlike Western practitioners, who use ice for traumatic injury, Chinese herbalists believe that the stagnation of Qi and Blood should be treated with warming herbs mat increase circulation to the area. While ice is very helpful in reducing swelling in the first few hours after an injury, it can actually hinder the healing process after the swelling is stabilized. When the initial swelling is under control, improved circulation to the injured area helps to carry away waste materials and bring nutrients to repair the damage.

Dosage: 8 pills, 3 times per day

Manufacturer: Plum Flower

Warnings and. contraindications: Not to be used during pregnancy. Plum Flower brand is recommended and is free of heavy metals. An alternative brand tested positive for low levels of heavy metals.

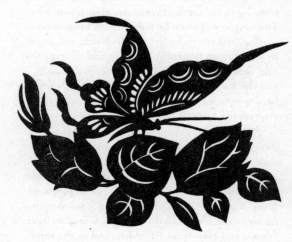

Continued ➡

Du Huo Jisheng Wan

Pronunciation and translation: "doo hwaw jee shuhng wahn"—"angelica loranthus pills"

Indications: Chronic pain and stiffness in the low back and knees; arthritis

Ingredients:

Angelica pubescens root (Du Huo)

Gentiana macrophylla root (Qin Jiao)

Siler divaricata root (Fang Feng)

Asarum sieboldi plant (Xi Xin)

Eucommia ulmoidis bark (Du Zhong)

Achyranthes bidentata root (Niu Xi)

Loranthus parasiticus stem and branch (Sang Ji Sheng)

Angelica sinensis root (Dang Gui)

Ligustdcum wallichii root (Chuan Xiong)

Rehmannia glutinosa prepared root (Shu Di Huang)

Paeonia lactiflora root (Bai Shao)

Codonopsis pilosula root (Dang Shen)

Poria cocos fungus (Fu Ling)

Glycyrrhiza uralensis root (Gan Cao)

Description: This is an excellent remedy for elderly people, since it is a well-formulated combination of herbs that tonify and strengthen the body along with herbs that improve circulation and reduce pain. It is especially helpful for pain in the low back and knees. This is due to the Achyranthes (Niu Xi), which literally means "cow's knee," and Angelica pubescens (Du Huo), an effective analgesic for pain in the lower part of the body. The formula also contains the basic combination to strengthen Qi and Blood, along with herbs that build the Yang of the Kidneys. Since pain in the low back and knees is a sign of Kidney weakness, this remedy addresses the underlying cause of the pain in addition to treating the symptoms. It is most appropriate for pain that becomes worse in cold and damp weather.

Dosage: 8 pills, 3 times per day

Manufacturer: Plum Flower

Warnings and contraindications: Contraindicated for use during pregnancy. Not to be used for inflamed joints that feel hot. Plum Flower brand contains no acetaminophen, which has been detected in another brand.

Yan Hu Suo Pian

Pronunciation and translation: "yahn hoo swaw pyen"— "corydalis tablets"

Indications: Headache, menstrual pain

Ingredients:

Corydalis yanhusuo tuber (Yan Hu Suo)

Angelica dahurica root (Bai Zhi)

Description: Corydalis rhizome (Yan Hu Suo) is one of the best pain-relieving herbs in Chinese medicine. The alcohol and acetic acid extracts are the strongest, being 40 percent as effective as morphine. It is especially useful in treating menstrual pain, but it can also be used for chest or abdominal pain or pain due to injuries or hernia. When combined with Angelica dahurica (Bai Zhi), as in this formula, it can also treat headache due to the common cold or sinus congestion.

Dosage: 4 pills, 3 times per day

Manufacturer: Plum Flower

Warnings and contraindications:

1. Not to be used during pregnancy.
2. Do not confuse this product with Yan Hu Su Zhi Long Pian, which has similar uses but contains a pharmaceutical. The word Su in the

name refers to an individual chemical constituent isolated from an herb, in this case tetrahydropalmatine, a strong analgesic drug. There is also a 100 percent herbal version known as Yan Hu Suo Zhi Tong Pian.

3. This remedy only provides symptomatic relief. It is important to treat the underlying cause, especially of chest and abdominal pain, since these can be symptoms of serious disease.

Yunnan Pai Yao

Pronunciation and translation: "yuhnahn peye yow"—"white medicine from Yunnan"

Indications: Bleeding of any kind, bruises or sports injuries, menstrual pain

Ingredients:

Panax notoginseng root (Tian Qi)

The medicine is white. A red emergency pill is included to be used in case of shock. Ingredients in the red emergency pill are a family secret.

Description: Yunnan Pai Yao is one of the essential patent medicines for the home or traveling first aid kit. Its ability to stop pain, swelling, and bleeding is legendary. The main ingredient, Panax notoginseng (Tian Qi), has a powerful ability to shorten bleeding time. In fact, during the war in Vietnam, Vietcong guerrillas were often found with a vial of this medicine around their neck, to be used in case of gunshot wounds. This formula has been a family secret for generations, and it is therefore one of the few remedies that still meets the criteria for the Chinese version of "patent medicine." While the formula itself contains mostly Tian Qi Ginseng, very little is known about the composition of the little "red emergency pill," which is taken when extensive bleeding is leading to shock.

When used for bruises and injuries, this remedy can greatly speed up the healing process. It is well known for resolving serious bruising and swelling in a matter of days. It is also used by midwives to stop any excessive bleeding after delivery. Yunnan Pai Yao is also available in powder form and as a liquid for external application.

Dosage: 2 capsules, 3 or 4 times per day

Manufacturer: Yunnan Paiyao Factory

Warnings and contraindications: Not to be used during pregnancy. Serious injuries should always be inspected by a physician to detect possible fractures or internal bleeding.

Remedies for the Nervous System

An Mien Pian

Pronunciation and translation: "ahn myehn pyen"—"peaceful sleep tablets"

Indications: Insomnia, anxiety

Ingredients:

Zizyphus spinosa seed (Suan Zao Ren)

Polygala tenuifolia root (Yuan Zhi)

Poria cocos fungus (Fu Ling)

Gardenia jasminoidis fruit (Zhi Zi)

Fermentata medicinalis mass (Shen Qu)

Glycyrrhiza uralensis root (Gan Cao)

Description: An Mien Pian is a mild sedative that can be used safely by frail or elderly people. It is useful for anxiety, insomnia, excessive dreaming, or poor memory, all signs of a deficiency of the Yin cooling system of the Heart. The chief ingredients are Zizyphus seed (Suan Zao Ren) and Polygala root (Yuan Zhi), both of which are considered to "nourish the Heart and calm the spirit." Poria fun-

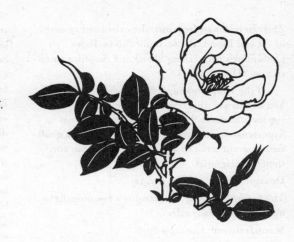

gus (Fu Ling) and Fermented mass (Shen Qu) are included to help indigestion, which can cause insomnia. Gardenia fruit (Zhi Zi) helps to eliminate internal *heat*, which can cause restlessness. This formula can be taken for a long period of time due to its mild nature.

Dosage: 4 tablets, 3 times per day

Manufacturer: Plum Flower

Emperor's Tea; Tian Wang Bu Xin Dan

Pronunciation and translation: "tyahn wahng boo shin dahn"—"emperor of heaven's pill to tonify the heart"

Indications: Insomnia, palpitations, anxiety, night sweats

Ingredients:

Rehmannia glutinosa root (Sheng Di Huang)

Angelica sinensis root (Dang Gui)

Schisandra chinensis fruit (Wu Wei Zi)

Zizyphus spinosa seed (Suan Zao Ren)

Biota orientalis seed (Bai Zi Ren)

Asparagus cochinchinensis tuber (Tian Men Dong)

Ophiopogon japonicus tuber (Mai Men Dong)

Scrophularia ningpoensis root (Xuan Shen)

Salvia miltiorrhiza root (Dan Shen)

Codonopsis pilosula root (Dang Shen)

Poria cocos fungus (Fu Ling)

Platycodon grandiflorum root (Jie Geng)

Polygala tcnuifolia root (Yuan Zhi)

Description: Emperor's Tea is the standard treatment for the pattern known as Heart Yin deficiency. This pattern may relate to the actual heart organ, but in Chinese diagnosis it is important to remember that an energetic description like Heart Yin may not always involve the heart organ itself. The Yin of the Heart gets depleted from lack of sleep, overwork, stress, or poor diet. This causes the Heart to become overheated, with symptoms such as palpitations, insomnia, restlessness, anxiety, intense dreams, and possibly thirst and night sweats. The formula goes to the root of the problem by including substances that nourish the Heart Yin and calm the spirit.

The chief ingredient in the remedy is Rehmannia root (Sheng Di Huang), which nourishes the Yin and helps clear some of the *heat* resulting from the lack of lubrication. It is combined with Scrophularia root (Xuan Shen) and Asparagus root (Tian Men Dong) to enhance the cooling effect. Salvia (Dan Shen) is incorporated to increase circulation to the coronary artery and allow the heart to work with a lower oxygen requirement. When combined with Schisandra berries (Wu Wei Zi), the palpitations can be relieved. To relieve the insomnia, nourishing herbs are used that also have a calming effect: Biota seed (Bai Zi Ren), Zizyphus seed (Suan Zao Ren), and Polygala root (Yuan

Continued →

Zhi). In order to replenish the exhausted reserves of Qi and Blood, the formula also includes Codonopsis root (Dang Shen) and Angelica sinensis root (Dang Gui).

If the symptoms support a diagnosis of Heart Yin deficiency, this remedy can be useful in treating mouth ulcers, hyperthyroidism, insomnia, hypertension, or chronic fatigue. A visit to a qualified acupuncturist or Chinese herbalist can confirm the diagnosis.

Dosage: 8 pills, 3 times per day

The formula should be taken for a few months to have a long-lasting effect.

Manufacturer: Lanzhou Foci

Warnings and contraindications: As with all formulas containing large amounts of Rehmannia, discontinue use if loose stools become a problem.

Gui Pi Wan; Angelica Longan Tea

Pronunciation and translation: "gway pee wahn"—"bring back the spleen pills"

Indications: Fatigue, palpitations, poor memory, insomnia

Ingredients:

    Codonopsis pilosula root (Dang Shen)
    Poria cocos fungus (Fu Shen)
    Zizyphus spinosa seed (Suan Zao Ren)
    Polygala tenuifolia root (Yuan Zhi)
    Angelica sinensis root (Dang Gui)
    Saussurea lappa root (Mu Xiang)
    Atractylodes macrocephala rhizome (Bai Zhu)
    Glycyrrhiza uralensis root (Gan Cao)
    Euphoria longan fruit (Long Yan Rou)
    Astragalus membranaceus root (Huang Qi)

Description: Gui Pi Wan is one of the classical ancient formulas that is available as a patent medicine. It is indicated for patterns that involve both the nervous system (Heart) and digestive system (Spleen). It is especially useful for "student's syndrome," where both of these organ systems have become depleted due to excessive studying and lack of exercise. The Heart deficiency symptoms are palpitations, insomnia, poor memory, and intense dreams; the Spleen deficiency symptoms could include fatigue, low appetite, pale face, and excessive menstrual bleeding with light-colored blood.

Since the formula treats deficiency in two different organ systems, the ingredients reflect this duality. Ingredients that tonify the Spleen include Codonopsis (Dang Shen), Poria (Fu Shen), Saussurea (Mu Xiang), Atractylodes (Bai Zhu), Licorice (Gan Cao), and Astragalus (Huang Qi). Herbs that deal with the Heart symptoms are Zizyphus (Suan Zao Ren), Polygala (Yuan Zhi), Angelica (Dang Gui), and Longan (Long Yan Rou).

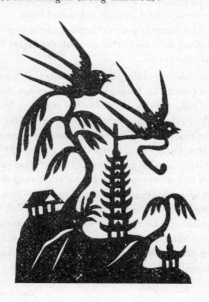

Although the Heart and Spleen symptoms may seem unrelated, there is a strong connection between them. When the digestive energy (Spleen Qi) is strong, more nutrients are assimilated from food. This enables the body to produce more Blood, which in turn nourishes the Heart. Conversely, when the Heart Blood is sufficient, the digestive organs receive the nutrients that are needed for optimal function. This symbiotic relationship is nicely explained in the ancient Chinese saying, "Blood is the mother of Qi, and Qi is the leader of blood." This refers to the fact that without blood, there is no fundamental nutritional basis for Qi; without Qi, there would be no ability to form or circulate blood, and it would fail to stay within the vessels. This formula is a practical application of this ancient principle.

Dosage: 8 pills, 3 times per day

Manufacturer: Lanzhou Foci

Remedies for the Respiratory System

Bi Yan Pian

Pronunciation and translation: "bee yahn pyen"—"nose inflammation tablets"

Indications: Nasal congestion, allergies, rhinitis, sinusitis

Ingredients:

    Xanthium sibiricum fruit (Cang Er Zi)
    Magnolia liliflora flower (Xin Yi Hua)
    Glycyrrhiza uralensis root (Gan Cao)
    Phellodendron amurense bark (Huang Bai)
    Platycodon grandiflorum root (Jie Geng)
    Schisandra chinensis firuit (Wu Wei Zi)
    Forsythia suspensa firuit (Lian Qiao)
    Angelica dahurica root (Bai Zhi)
    Anemarrhcna asphodeloides rhizome (Zhi Mu)
    Chrysanthemum indica flower (Ye Ju Hua)
    Siler divaricata root (Fang Feng)
    Schizonepeta tenuifolia herb (Jing Jie)

Description: Bi Yan Pian is a widely used and popular remedy for problems related to the nasal passages or sinuses. It can be used in both acute and chronic conditions whenever there is congestion, runny nose, or excessive mucus in these areas. It can effectively treat allergies to pollen, animal dander, mold, or any substance that causes nasal congestion and sneezing. The ingredients that make this such a useful remedy for nasal congestion are Xanthium fruit (Cang Er Zi), Magnolia flower (Xin Yi Hua), and Angelica dahurica root (Bai Zhi). The formula also contains Siler root (Fang Feng) and Schizonepeta flower (Jing Jie), which help the immune system fight off colds (external *wind*). There are also cooling ingredients, including Phellodendron bark (Huang Bai), Forsythia fruit (Lian Qiao), Anemarrhena rhizome (Zhi Mu), and Wild Chrysanthemum flower (Ye Ju Hua), that help to prevent infection. However, if a sinus infection has already developed, Bi Yan Pian should be supplemented with a formula that will help fight the infection, such as Chuan Xin Lian. When the congestion is due to the common cold, it can be taken along with Gan Mao Ling (see p. 169) or Yin Qiao Jie Du Pian (see p. 170). Many people have found this remedy to be as effective as over-the-counter decongestants with none of the uncomfortable side effects like drowsiness or over-stimulation.

Dosage: 4 pills, 3 times per day

Manufacturer: Plum Flower

Warnings and contraindications: It is preferable to use a brand such as Plum Flower, that does not contain acetaminophen or artificial coloring. Do not exceed the recommended dosage. If a sinus infection does not resolve or symptoms get worse, seek medical attention immediately. If the nasal passages, mouth, or throat get excessively dry when using this formula, decrease the dosage or discontinue its use.

Chuan Xin Lian Antiphlogistic Tablets

Pronunciation and translation: "chwahn shin lyahn"—"andrographis anti-inflammatory tablets"

Indications: Inflammation due to excess *heat*, swollen glands, severe sore throat, viral and bacterial infections

Ingredients:

    Andrographis paniculate herb (Chuan
       Xin Lian)
    Taraxacum mongolicum plant (Pu Gong Ying)
    Isatis tinctoria root (Ban Lan Gen)

Description: This remedy clears heat and inflammation from all areas of the body. It can be used for severe sore throat, coughs with yellow phlegm, urinary tract infections, or dysentery. The formula gets its name from the chief ingredient, Andrographis paniculata herb (Chuan Xin Lian). This extremely bitter herb has powerful antibacterial and antiviral properties. Clinical studies have shown it to inhibit the growth of the bacteria that cause streptococcal and staphylococcal infections, pneumonia, and dysentery It also increases phagocytosis, the ability of white blood cells to destroy bacteria. In China, it is commonly used to treat acute infections of the respiratory, digestive, and urinary tracts.

Another ingredient that has strong antibacterial activity is the common Dandelion, Taraxacum mongolicum (Pu Gong Ying). It inhibits the same bacteria as Andrographis, as well as those that cause meningitis and diphtheria. It is strange that in our culture, we spray deadly herbicides to kill a plant with such powerful healing properties! Recent studies have also shown a higher rate of cancer in children who play in areas that have been treated with these toxic chemicals. A change in our perception of wild plants, as well as our response to them, seems to be in order. While technology has brought many miracles, we still have a lot to learn from the ancient cultures.

The third ingredient in this patent medicine is Isatis tinctoria root (Ban Lan Gen). Like the other herbs, it has a cooling, antibacterial effect on infections and inflammation. Isatis is also antiviral; clinical studies have proved it to be highly effective in treating mumps and hepatitis. It has also been used along with acupuncture and Western medicine to achieve a 90 percent cure rate for encephalitis.

Dosage: 2–3 pills, 3 times per day

Manufacturer: Plum Flower

Warnings and contraindications: It is recommended to avoid brands which use artificial dyes. In any type of infection, seek the help of a health care practitioner.

Chuan Xiong Cha Tiao Wan

Pronunciation and translation: "chwahn shuhng chah tyow wahn"—"ligusticum and green tea pills"

Indications: Headache and nasal congestion due to the common cold

Ingredients:

    Mentha haplocalyx herb (Bo He)
    Ligusticum wallichii rhizome (Chuan Xiong)
    Notopterygiurn incisium rhizome (Qiang Huo)

Continued ➡

Angelica dahurica root (Bai Zhi)

Asarum sieboldi plant (Xi Xin)

Siler divaricata root (Fang Feng)

Schizonepeta tenuifolia herb (Jing Jie)

Glycyrrhiza uralensis root (Gan Cao)

Description: Chuan Xiong Cha Tiao Wan is especially indicated for headaches due to the *wind cold* type of common cold. Typical symptoms are chills, nasal congestion, stiff neck and upper back, and headache, especially in the back of the head (occiput). The chief ingredient in the formula is Ligusticum wallichii (Chuan Xiong), an aromatic herb that is indicated for a variety of headaches, especially those due to *cold*. Notopterygium rhizome (Qiang Huo) is another important ingredient, because it relaxes the upper back and neck when the muscles are contracted from the influence of *cold*. Angelica dahurica (Bai Zhi) and Wild Ginger (Xi Xin) relieve nasal congestion and have an analgesic effect on the head and sinuses. To fight off the cold, the classic combination of Schizonepeta (Jing Jie) and Siler (Fang Feng) is added. Although green tea is included in the name of the formula, it is not one of the ingredients. The traditional way to take this remedy is to wash it down with green tea. This directs the formula's effects to the head and, along with Field Mint (Bo He), adds a cooling effect to moderate the warming herbs in the formula.

Dosage: 8 pills, 3 times per day

Manufacturer: Lanzhou Foci

Warnings and contraindications: Not to be used for beat-type headaches, with fever, sore throat, or dry, burning nasal passages.

Er Chen Wan

Pronunciation and translation "uhr chen wahn"—"two old-medicine pills"

Indications: Excessive phlegm in the lungs and stomach, with symptoms of nausea and cough with abundant clear mucus

Ingredients:

Pinellia ternata rhizome (Ban Xia)

Citrus reticulata peel (Chen Pi)

Poria cocos fungus (Fu Ling)

Glycyrrhiza uralensis root (Gan Cao)

Description: The two "old medicines" referred to in the formula's name are Tangerine peel (Chen Pi) and Pinellia rhizome (Ban Xia). These herbs are highly prized when they have been aged and treated, especially Tangerine peel, which is much more expensive when its aroma is enhanced through aging. Both of these herbs have a drying effect on mucus in the Lungs and Stomach, helping to alleviate coughs or vomiting with large amounts of clear phlegm. The addition of Poria (Fu Ling) and Licorice (Gan Cao) helps to enhance digestive strength (Spleen Qi). This is essential in imbalances involving excess mucus, which is formed when digestive energy is weak. Er Chen Wan manages to treat both the cause and symptoms of this imbalance with a simple four-herb formula.

If the excess mucus is due to the common cold, it is necessary to augment this remedy with a formula that expels the pathogenic influence, such as Chuan Xiong Cha Tiao Wan (see left) or Gan Mao Ling, described at right.

Dosage: 8 pills, 3 times per day

Manufacturer: Lanzhou Foci

Warnings and contraindications: This formula has a drying effect, which is why it is indicated for excessive clear, loose phlegm. For this same reason, it should not be used when there is phlegm that is yellow or green and difficult to expectorate. For such a *heat*-type cough, Pinellia Root Tea-pills (see p. 80) is a more appropriate remedy.

Gan Mao Ling

Pronunciation and translation: "gahn maow ling"—"cold formula"

Indications: Common cold or flu, especially in the early stage

Ingredients:

Hex pubcscens root (Mao Dong Qing)

Isatis tinctoria root (Ban Lan Gen)

Chrysanthemum morifolium flower (Ju Hua)

Vitex rotundifolia fruit (Man Jing Zi)

Lonicera japonica flower (Jin Yin Hua)

Mentha haplocalyx herb (Bo He)

Description: In areas where it is well known, Gan Mao Ling is the remedy of choice when the early symptoms of the common cold arise. When it is taken in the early stage, the cold can often be completely averted. If the symptoms are full blown, it will take longer to work, but the cold will still go away faster than it would without the remedy. Although its ingredients are all cooling, Gan Mao Ling can still be used in *cold*-type illness. In this case, it should be combined with Bi Yan Pian (see p. 168) or Chuan Xiong Cha Tiao Wan (see left). If the cold is accompanied with a severe sore throat or fever, it can be combined with Chuan Xin Lian Pills (see left) or Yin Qiao Jie Du Pian (see p. 170). For stomach flu, it can be taken with Curing Pills (see p. 162) or Huo Xiang Zheng Qi Wan (see p. 161).

Dosage: 4 pills, 3 times per day

Manufacturer: Plum Flower

Warnings and contraindications: It is recommended to use Plum Flower brand, which is free of pharmaceuticals and artificial coloring.

Lo Han Kuo Infusion; Luo Han Guo Chong Ji

Pronunciation and translation: "law hahn gwaw chung jee"— "momordica fruit instant tea"

Indications: Dry, *heat*-type cough, with possible sticky phlegm

Ingredients:

Momordica grosvenori fruit (Luo Han Guo)

Description: Luo Han Guo ("smiling Buddha fruit") is the only herbal ingredient in this instant tea. This exotic fruit is round with a brittle egg-like shell; when cracked open, it reveals a clump of sweet seeds. The overall action is cooling, nourishing and moistening, making it ideal for *dryness* in the lungs with an unproductive dry cough or sticky yellow phlegm. It comes in the form of cubes that can be dissolved in water to make a pleasant-tasting tea. The cubes are 5 percent cane sugar, which contributes to the effect of moistening the lungs. The sweet taste of this remedy makes it especially popular with children.

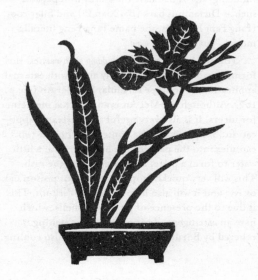

Dosage: 1 cube dissolved in 1 cup boiling water; drink 1 cup, 2 to 3 times per day

Manufacturer: Luo Han Guo Products Manufactory

Warnings and contraindications: Not for coughs with large amounts of clear phlegm that is easy to expectorate.

Ma Hsing Chih Ke Pien

Pronunciation and translation: "mah shing jih keh pyen"—"ephedra apricot stop cough tablets"

Indications: *Heat*-type cough, bronchitis, or asthma

Ingredients:

Ephedra sinica herb (Ma Huang)

Prunus armeniaca seed (Xing Ren)

Gypsum fibrosum mineral (Shi Gao)

Glycyrrhiza uralensis root (Gan Cao)

Platycodon grandiflorum root (Jie Geng)

Citrus reticulata peel (Chen Pi)

Talcum mineral (Hua Shi)

Honey (Feng Mi)

Description: This patent medicine is a variation of an ancient classic formula. It is indicated for coughs and difficulty breathing due to *heat* in the Lungs, making it useful in treating colds, flu, bronchitis, and asthma. The formula reduces fevers and clears *heat* from the Lungs due to the inclusion of two minerals: Gypsum (Shi Gao) and Talc (Hua Shi). The wheezing and difficulty breathing is resolved with Apricot seed (Xing Ren) and Ephedra (Ma Huang). Although the formula only contains 5 percent Ephedra, it is still considered the chief herb in the formula due to its great strength. Ephedra contains ephedrine, a powerful constituent that relaxes the smooth muscles of the bronchial passages and reduces mucus. This makes it ideal for treating asthma. However, care must be taken when using it, since Ephedra also can raise blood pressure and cause insomnia. For this reason, it is best to use this remedy under the care of a qualified practitioner.

Dosage: 4 pills, 2 to 3 times per day

Manufacturer: Siping Pharmaceutical Works

Warnings and contraindications: Ephedra can raise blood pressure and should not be taken by people with high blood pressure, stroke, or heart disease. Do not exceed recommended dosages. Asthma is a life-threatening condition for many people. While herbal medicine can greatly help in its treatment, it is not wise for asthma sufferers to discard their inhaler. Even if it seems like it is no longer needed, it should be kept in case of emergencies.

Pinellia Root Teapills; Pinellia Expectorant Pills; Qing Qi Hua Tan Wan

Pronunciation and translation: "ching chee hwah tahn wahn"—"clear lung, expel phlegm pills"

Indications: *Heat*-type cough, with yellow or green phlegm that is difficult to expectorate

Ingredients:

Pinellia ternata rhizome (Ban Xia)

Arisaema amurense bile-processed tuber (Dan Nan Xing)

Citrus aurantium immature fruit (Zhi Shi)

Scutellaria baicalensis root (Huang Qin)

Citrus rubrum peel (Ju Hong)

Trichosanthes kirilowii seed (Gua Lou Ren)

Prunus armeniaca seed (Xing Ren)

Poria cocos fungus (Fu Ling)

Continued ➔

Description: This is a convenient version of a classic formula with strong expectorant action. It is indicated for a *heat*-type cough, in which the phlegm is sticky, yellow or green, and difficult to expectorate. For this type of cough, the logic is to cool the Lungs, moisten and dislodge the phlegm, and clear it from the Lungs. If this is done quickly, it is possible to prevent the trapped phlegm from progressing into a serious upper respiratory infection like pneumonia.

The ingredients in the formula work together to achieve this goal. Prepared Arisaema tuber (Dan Nan Xing) and Trichosanthis seeds (Gua Lou Ren) break up sticky phlegm due to *heat*. Scutellaria root (Huang Qin) helps fight infection in the Lungs, and Apricot seed (Xing Ren) moistens the Lungs and calms the cough. Citrus peel (Ju Hong) and Poria fungus (Fu Ling) help the Lungs produce less phlegm, and PincUia rhizome (Ban Xia) eliminates phlegm and acts as an expectorant. Finally, Bitter Orange (Zhi Shi) has a descending action, relieving stagnation in the Lungs caused by the phlegm. The combination of these herbs is a very effective way to treat this uncomfortable condition.

Dosage: 6 pills, 3 times per day

Manufacturer: Lanzhou Foci

Warnings and contraindications: This formula is cooling and moistening, which is why it is indicated for phlegm that is yellow or green and difficult to expectorate. For this same reason, it should not be used when there is excessive clear, loose phlegm. For such a *damp, cold*-type cough, Er Chen Wan is a more appropriate remedy.

Yin Qiao Jie Du Pian; Yin Chiao Chieh Tu Pien

Pronunciation and translation: "yin chaow jyeh doo pyen"—"honeysuckle and forsythia clear-toxin tablets"

Indications: Acute symptoms of wind heat-type common cold with sore throat, fever, headache

Ingredients:

Lonicera japonica flower (Jin Yin Hua)
Forsythia suspensa fruit (Lian Qiao)
Arctium lappa fruit (Niu Bang Zi)
Platycodon grandiflorum root (Jie Geng)
Mentha haplocalyx herb (Bo He)
Phragmitis communis rhizome (Lu Gen)
Glycyrrhiza uralensis root (Gan Cao)
Lophatherum gracile herb (Dan Zhu Ye)
Schizonepeta tenuifolia herb (Ging Jie)

Description: Yian Qiao is probably the most commonly used Chinese patent medicine in the United States. It is indicated for the *wind heat*-type of common cold or flu, bronchitis, or tonsillitis. The symptoms are sore throat, headache, thirst, fever, and cough. While it is most effective when taken at the first appearance of symptoms, Yin Qiao can still be used to treat a cold after it has fully manifested.

The formula gets its name from the two chief herbs: Jin *Yin* Hua (Honeysuckle flower) and Lian *Qiao* (Forsythia fruit). These two herbs are often combined to treat *heat*-type flu or colds, since they can efficiently clear *heat* from the body while they fight off the external pathogens that cause the illness. Burdock seed (Niu Bang Zi) and Platy-codon root (Jie Geng) are included to relieve the sore throat, Phragmitis rhizome (Lu Gen) stops the cough, and Bamboo leaf (Dan Zhu Ye) alleviates thirst. Finally, Licorice root (Gan Cao) harmonizes all the ingredients in the formula; its anti-inflammatory action also helps soothe the sore throat.

Dosage: 4 tablets (half a vial), 3 times per day

Manufacturer: Plum Flower; Tianjin Drug Manu-

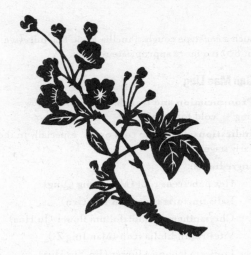

factory. There are also excellent quality American versions of this remedy, such as those made by Planetary Formulas.

Warnings and contraindications: There are numerous variations on this most popular of all patent medicines. Use caution. Some of the other Chinese blends contain over-the-counter drugs.

Remedies for the Skin

Lian Qiao Bai Du Pian; Lien Chiao Pai Tu Pien

Pronunciation and translation: "lyahn chow bye doo pyen"—"forsythia clear toxins tablets"

Indications: Inflammations and infections of the skin

Ingredients:

Lonicera japonica flower (Jin Yin Hua)
Gardenia jasminoidis fruit (Zhi Zi)
Scutellaria baicalensis root (Huang Qin)
Paeonia rubra root (Chi Shao)
Dictamnus dasycarpus bark (Bai Xian Pi)
Forsydiia suspensa fruit (Lian Qiao)
Cryptotympana atrata skin (Chan Tui)
Siler divaricata root (Fang Feng)
Rheum palmatum rhizome (Da Huang)

Description: Lian Qiao Bai Du Pian can be used for almost any type of skin condition, including infections, boils, inflammations, poison oak or ivy, and other allergic skin reactions. Skin rashes and infections are often a result of *heat* in the Blood, with accumulated *dampness* and toxicity. This is addressed by herbs that cool the Blood, such as Red Peony (Chi Shao) and Rhubarb root (Da Huang). To clear toxic *heat*, the formula incorporates Honeysuckle flower Qin Yin Hua), Forsythia fruit (Lian Qiao), Gardenia fruit (Zhi Zi), and Scutellaria root (Huang Qin). Rashes that come on suddenly or have a tendency to itch and spread are considered to be a form of *wind* in Chinese medicine. This pathogenic influence can be expelled from the body by diaphoretic (sweat-inducing) herbs that have the ability to repel *wind*, such as Dictamnus bark (Bai Xian Pi) and Siler root (Fang Feng). In fact, the name Fang Feng literally means "guard against *wind*."

For poison oak and other *damp* skin rashes, this formula can be taken internally along with external application of another formula, Sai Mei An (see p. 162). Although Sai Mei An is an internal medicine for ulcers, it is also very useful as an external application. Simply empty the contents of one or two capsules into the palm of the hand, drip in a little water to form a paste, and spread it on the rash. This will very quickly stop the itching of poison oak or ivy, and it will also help to dry the *dampness*. This is due to the presence of powdered shells, which have an astringent, drying effect. The itching is relieved by Borneol camphor, which is also cooling.

Skin problems can be eliminated much more efficiently if coffee, sweets, and spicy foods are eliminated from the diet.

Dosage: 4–6 tablets, 3 times per day

Manufacturer: Tianjin Drug Manufactory

Warnings and contraindications: Not to be used during pregnancy. This formula contains rhubarb, which acts as a laxative.

Margarite Acne Polls; Cai Feng Zhen Zhu An Choang Wan

Pronunciation and translation: "cheye fuhng jen joo ahn chwahng wahn"—"colorful phoenix pearl hide skin boil pill"

Indications: Acne, skin rashes, hives

Ingredients:

Zostera marina seaweed (Hai Dai)
Lonicera japonica flower (Jin Yin Hua)
Rehmannia glutinosa root (Sheng Di Huang)
Pteria margaritifera pearl (Zhen Zhu)
Bubalis bubalis horn (Shui Niu Jiao)
Bos taurus domesticus gallstone (Niu Huang)

Description: Margarite Acne Pills are a reliable treatment for inflammatory skin conditions such as acne, boils, rashes, and hives. Although skin problems are notoriously difficult to treat, this remedy has a good track record. The chief ingredient is Pearl, or Margarita (Zhen Zhu), a substance with a *cold* energy that clears excess *heat* from the Liver. It is combined with other herbs that have a cooling, anti-inflammatory effect. The formula also includes Water Buffalo horn (Shui Niu Jiao), a cooling agent. This is used to replace the original ingredient of Rhinoceros horn, which comes from an endangered species. Seaweed (Hai Dai) and Rehmannia root (Sheng Di Huang) are also included for their cooling, nourishing effect.

It can be very difficult to cure acne without instituting dietary changes. Coffee, greasy foods, sweets, and excessive spices can all create stagnation and *heat* which will create further skin eruptions. Plenty of fresh water, exercise, and sufficient rest are also essential.

Dosage: 6 pills, 2 times per day

Manufacturer: Plum Flower

Warnings and contraindications: Not to be used during pregnancy. Use only Plum Flower brand. Another brand of the formula contains sophoridane, which is a pharmaceutical.

Remedies for the Urinary Tract

Ba Zheng San

Pronunciation and translation: "bah juhng sahn"—"eight herbs to correct urination"

Indications: Urinary tract infection, urinary tract stones

Ingredients:

Lysimachia christinae herb (Jin Qian Cao)
Phellodendron amurense bark (Huang Bai)
Akebia trifoliata stem (Mu Tong)
Dianthus chinensis herb (Qu Mai)
Polygonum aviculare herb (Bian Xu)
Plantago asiatica seed (Che Qian Zi)
Gardenia jasminoidis fruit (Zhi Zi)
Rheum palmatum rhizome (Da Huang)
Glycyrrhiza uralensis root (Gan Cao)

Description: Ba Zheng San is a standard formula for urinary tract infections. The traditional Chi-

Continued ➡

nese diagnostic pattern is "*dampness* and *heat* in the Lower Burner" (or Urinary Bladder). The symptoms are frequent and painful urination, scanty or obstructed flow of urine, pain and distention in the lower abdominal area, and a dry mouth and throat. The tongue will often have a thick yellow coating in the back, which is the area that corresponds to the Urinary Bladder.

The formula contains Lysimachia (Jin Qian Cao), which is a diuretic. It helps eliminate stones from the urinary tract, which is another use for this formula. Other herbs that have an affinity for the urinary tract are Dianthus (Qu Mai), a common ornamental that is easy to grow, and Knotweed (Bian Xu), a weed that is common in North America. Both of these herbs are diuretic and antibacterial, as is Akebia (Mu long). Phellodendron bark (Huang Bai) and Gardenia fruit (Zhi Zi) both have the ability to eliminate dampness and heat from the Urinary Bladder.

When fighting a bladder infection, it is important to maintain an acidic urine pH. This can be done by eating protein with each meal and avoiding sweets. It is also essential to avoid coffee, since it is very irritating to the bladder and makes heat conditions worse.

Dosage: 8 pills, 3 times per day

Manufacturer: Plum Flower

Warnings and contraindications: A simple urinary tract infection can sometimes progress to become a serious kidney infection. Be sure to consult your health care practitioner whenever you attempt to self-treat any kind of infection. This remedy is for acute urinary tract infections. A chronic infection often needs to be treated with a different approach, such as nourishing Yin and clearing *heat* with Liu Wei Di Huang Wan or Zhi Bai Di Huang Wan (see p. 172).

Long Dan Xie Gan Wan

Pronunciation and translation: "luhng dahn shyeh gahn wahn"—"gentian clear the liver pills"

Indications: Urinary tract infection, conjunctivitis, prostatitis

Ingredients:

Gentiana scabra root (Long Dan Cao)
Scutellaria baicalensis root (Huang Qin)
Gardenia jasminoidis fruit (Zhi Zi)
Alisma plantago-aquatica rhizome (Ze Xie)
Plantago asiatica seed (Che Qian Zi)
Akebia trifoliata stem (Mu Tong)
Angelica sinensis root (Dang Gui)
Bupleurum chinense root (Chai Hu)
Rehmannia glutinosa root (Sheng Di Huang)
Glycyrrhiza uralensis root (Gan Cao)

Description: Long Dan Xie Gan Wan is used to treat a wide range of inflammatory conditions in addition to bladder infections. It is most easily understood when considered from an energetic perspective. Deficiency-type conditions require a strengthening or tonification of the body, but for conditions of excess, the proper treatment is clearing or draining. This formula is strictly indicated for excess-type disorders where imbalance consists of an overabundance of internal climates, such as *heat* or *dampness*. Long Dan Xie Gan Wan is specific for the patterns known as *excess heat* or *damp heat* in the Liver and Gall Bladder, with a symptom pattern that includes red eyes, headache, bitter taste in the mouth, irritability, and possible hearing loss. Other symptoms of Lower Burner *damp heat* are dark or cloudy urine, genital itching or swelling, vaginal discharge, and constipation.

Some of the numerous imbalances that can be resolved by this formula can be organized by organ system:

- Eyes: acute conjunctivitis ("pink eye"), corneal ulcers, acute glaucoma, retinitis
- Ears: acute middle ear infection, acute external ear infection
- Urinary: acute urinary tract infection (kidney, bladder, or urethra)
- Reproductive: genital herpes, pelvic inflammatory disease, vaginal discharge, testicular swelling or inflammation, acute prostatitis
- Systemic: migraine, eczema, herpes zoster
- Liver and Gall Bladder: acute hepatitis, acute cholecystitis

Although the above list of medical conditions appears to be random and unrelated, they all share the same traditional energetic diagnosis. For this reason, it is essential to treat the individual's traditional symptom complex, not the Western disease name. Just as a single Chinese diagnostic category can manifest as numerous different Western diseases, a single Western disease can also have a wide range of Chinese diagnoses, depending on the individual's symptoms and constitutional nature. For this reason, it is always wise to consult with a qualified health care practitioner before self-treating with herbal medicine.

Dosage: 8 pills, 3 times per day

Manufacturer: Lanzhou Foci

Warnings and contraindications: A simple urinary tract infection can sometimes progress to become a serious kidney infection. Be sure to consult your health care practitioner before you attempt to self-treat any kind of infection.

Remedies for Women

Chien Chin Chih Tai Wan; Qian Jin Zho Dai Wan

Pronunciation and translation: "chyen chin chih tie wahn"—"thousand-gold-piece stop leukorrhea pills"

Indications: Leukorrhea (vaginal discharge)

Ingredients:

Angelica sinensis root (Dang Gui)
Atractylodes macrocephala rhizome (Bai Zhu)
Foeniculum vulgare fruit (Xiao Hui Xiang)
Corydalis yanhusuo rhizome (Yan Hu Suo)
Saussurea lappa root (Mu Xiang)
Dipsacus asper root (Xu Duan)
Codonopsis pilosula root (Dang Shen)
Ostrea gigas shell (Mu Li)
Indigofera sufrruticosa pigment (Qing Dai)

Description: This is an effective remedy for vaginal discharges or yeast infections. The formula is appropriate for both *heat*-type discharges (dark color, strong smell) or *cold*-type discharges (light color, no smell). The *heat* symptoms can be addressed with Indigo powder (Qing Dai), which is a cooling, detoxifying antibacterial substance. The rest of the formula is tonifying in nature, since vaginal discharges are often due to a deficiency in Spleen Qi (digestive vital energy). When Spleen Qi is weak, *dampness* tends to accumulate, sometimes appearing in the form of a discharge. Chien Chin uses Codonopsis root (Dang Shen), Atractylodes rhizome (Bai Zhu), Fennel seed (Xiao Hui Xiang), and Saussurea root (Mu Xiang) to strengthen the Spleen and eliminate the *damp* environment that leads to the discharge. Oyster shell (Mu Li) is added as an astringent agent to assist in the drying effect.

Angelica root (Dang Gui) and Teasel root (Xu Duan) nourish the Blood and the Kidneys and enhance the overall nourishing the Blood and the Kidneys and enhance the overall nourishing quality of the remedy. Corydalis rhizome (Yan Hu Suo) promotes blood circulation and alleviates pain.

Dosage: 10 pills, 2 times per day

Manufacturer: Tianjin Drug Manufactory

Warnings and contraindications: If the discharge is dark-colored and has a strong smell, Yu Dai Wan is more appropriate.

Nu Ke Ba Zhen Wan; Women's Precious Pills

Pronunciation and translation: "noo keh bah jen wahn"—"gynecology eight treasure pills"

Indications: Fatigue, dizziness, anemia, scanty menses, lack of appetite

Ingredients:

Codonopsis pilosula root (Dang Shen)
Poria cocos fungus (Fu Ling)
Atractylodes macrocephala rhizome (Bai Zhu)
Glycyrrhiza uralensis root (Gan Cao)
Angelica sinensis root (Dang Gui)
Paconia lactiflora root (Bai Shao)
Rehmannia glutinosa prepared root (Shu Di Huang)
Ligusticum wallichii rhizome (Chuan Xiong)

Description: This is the classic formula for deficiency of Qi (vital energy) and blood. While this condition also occurs in men, it is especially common in women, since they lose blood on a monthly basis during their menstrual cycle. The remedy combines two formulas: one builds vital energy (Qi), and is known as "Four Gentlemen." It consists of Ginseng or Codonopsis, Atractylodes, Poria, and Licorice. The other formula nourishes blood and is known as "Four Substances." It contains Rehmannia, Peony, Dang Gui, and Ligusticum. When the two formulas are combined, as in this remedy, the result is known as "Eight Treasures" or "Women's Precious."

The reasoning behind this mixing of formulas is classic Chinese herbal logic. Blood is produced in the body through the assimilation of food by the Stomach/Spleen organ complex. When the digestive Qi is strong, more nutrition is assimilated, enabling efficient production of blood. The "Four Gentlemen" combination contains herbs that strengthen the digestive Qi of the Spleen, thereby indirectly helping the body produce more blood. At the same time, the "Four Substances" part of the formula directly builds blood. The combination of the two is an exceptionally effective way to restore normal blood counts.

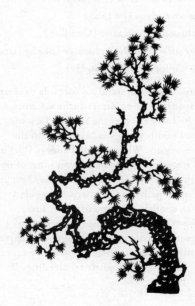

Continued ➡

Interestingly, one of the traditional uses of "Four Substances" is for poor memory induced by deficiency of blood. A recent clinical study demonstrated that this herbal combination can significantly improve working memory in rats.

Dosage: 8–10 pills, three times per day

Manufacturer: Lanzhou Foci

Tang Kwei Gin

Pronunciation and translation: "dahng gway jin"—"angelica dang gui syrup"

Indications: Fatigue, anemia, scanty menses

Ingredients:

Angelica sinensis root (Dang Gui)

Paconia lactiflora root (Bai Shao)

Rehmannia glutinosa prepared root (Shu Di Huang)

Ligusticum wallichii rhizome (Chuan Xiong)

Astragalus membranaceus root (Huang Qi)

Codonopsis pilosula root (Dang Shen)

Poria cocos fungus (Fu Ling)

Glycyrrhiza uralensis root (Gan Cao)

Description: Tang Kwei Gin is very similar to Nu Ke Ba Zhen Wan. However, it focuses more on nourishing the Blood, and it contains Astragalus root (Huang Qi), which has a synergistic action with Angelica (Dang Gui) in raising blood counts. This remedy comes in a pleasant-tasting liquid that can be mixed with water or taken by the spoonful. When used in combination with Nu Ke Ba Zhen Wan, the results can be quite dramatic. Cases of anemia and amenorrhea can often be normalized in the course of one or two months. The formula also has a beneficial effect on the immune system, since it contains many immune-enhancing herbs like Astragalus (Huang Qi), Codonopsis (Dang Shen), and Poria (Fu Ling).

Dosage: 1 tablespoon, 3 times per day

Manufacturer: Plum Flower

Warnings and contraindications: Plum Flower is made by Pangaoshou, a G.M.P. factory. It is free of sugar and preservatives.

Xiao Yao Wan

Pronunciation and translation: "shaow yaow wahn"—"free and easy wanderer pills"

Indications: Premenstrual syndrome with irritability, sore breasts and menstrual imbalances

Ingredients:

Bupleurum chinense root (Chai Hu)

Angelica sinensis root (Dang Gui)

Atractylodes macrocephala rhizome (Bai Zhu)

Paeonia lactiflora root (Bai Shao)

Poria cocos fungus (Fu Ling)

Glycyrrhiza uralensis root (Gan Cao)

Zingiber officinale fresh rhizome (Sheng Jiang)

Mentha haplocalyx herb (Bo He)

Description: This is the standard formula to clear stagnation from the Liver. In traditional Chinese medicine, the Liver ensures the smooth flow of emotions and bodily processes, especially in the reproductive organs. When the vital energy (Qi) of the Liver is stagnant, there can be symptoms of irritability, outbursts of anger, fullness in the chest and abdomen, breast pain, and menstrual irregularity. Xiao Yao Wan soothes and detoxifies the Liver, making it the treatment of choice for pre-menstrual syndrome. A course of treatment takes three to four months, using the formula every day except on the days when there is menstrual bleeding. It

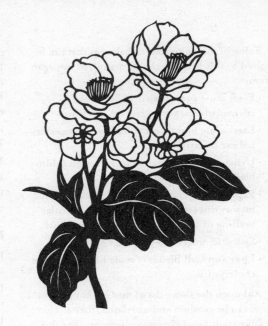

successfully treats PMS by eliminating the cause rather than merely suppressing the symptoms.

The chief herb in the formula is Bupleurum root (Chai Hu), which is the primary agent for clearing stagnation from the Liver. It is assisted by Field Mint (Bo He) and Peony root (Bai Shao), which also act to soothe and nourish the Liver. The formula also contains Atractylodes rhizome (Bai Zhu), which strengthens vital energy, and Angelica sinensis (Dang Gui), which builds Blood and has a regulatory effect on the uterus. Xiao Yao Wan, and all other remedies that treat the Liver, will work best if stress can be reduced and coffee, high-fat foods, and excessive sweets are eliminated from the diet.

Dosage: 8 pills, 3 times per day

Discontinue use during menstrual bleeding. A course of treatment is typically three to four months.

Manufactuere: Lanzhou Foci

Yu Dai Wan

Pronunciation and translation: "yoo dye wahn"—"heal leucorrhea pills"

Indications: Heat-type vaginal discharge

Ingredients:

Rehmannia glutinosa prepared root (Shu Di Huang)

Angelica sinensis root (Dang Gui)

Paeonia lactiflora root (Bai Shao)

Ligusticum wallichii rhizome (Chuan Xiong)

Phellodendron amurense bark (Huang Bai)

Ailanthus altissima root and stem bark (Chun Gen Pi)

Alpinia officinarum carbonized rhizome (Gao Liang Jiang)

Description: Yu Dai Wan is especially useful for *heat*-type vaginal discharges when there is an underlying Blood deficiency. (Chien Chin Chih Tai Wan can be used for vaginal discharges due to both heat and *cold*.) Yu Dai Wan contains a high percentage of Ailanthus bark (Chun Gen Pi), which is astringent and *cold* in nature. When combined with Phellodendron bark (Huang Bai), the two herbs powerfully clear the *heat* and *dampness* that characterize this disorder. The other herbs in the formula nourish the Blood and help alleviate the fatigue and irregular menstrual cycle associated with blood deficiency.

Dosage: 8 pills, 3 times per day

Manufacturer: Lanzhou Foci

Warnings and contraindications: For a clear-colored vaginal discharge, use Chien Chin Chih Tai Wan.

Zhi Bai Di Huang Wan; Chih Pai Ti Huang Wan

Pronunciation and translation: "jih bye dee hwahng wahn"—"anemarrhena and phellodendron with rehmannia pills"

Indications: Hot flashes, night sweats, irritability, menopausal symptoms, all due to strong *heat* arising from Yin deficiency

Ingredients:

Rehmannia glutinosa prepared root (Shu Di Huang)

Dioscorea opposita root (Shan Yao)

Cornus officinalis fruit (Shan Zhu Yu)

Poria cocos fungus (Fu Ling)

Alisma plantago-aquatica rhizome (Ze Xie)

Paeonia sufrruticosa root-bark (Mu Dan Pi)

Phellodendron amurense bark (Huang Bai)

Anemarrhena asphodeloides rhizome (Zhi Mu)

Description: This is a variation of Liu Wei Di Huang Wan or Rehmannia Six Teapills, previously described in the chapter on tonifying herbs. The name of the formula reflects the addition of two herbs, *Zhi* Mu (Anemarrhena rhizome) and Huang Bai (Phellodendron bark). These ingredients enhance the cooling effect of the formula, making it very useful in treating the hot flashes and night sweats that occur in menopause.

Zhi Bai Di Huang Wan treats both the root cause and the symptoms of menopause. The drop in estrogen levels typically reflects a deficiency of Kidney Yin essence. This is replenished with Kidney-nourishing herbs like Rehmannia root (Shu Di Huang), Chinese Yam (Shan Yao), and Dogwood fruit (Shan Zhu Yu). The rest of the ingredients address the heat symptoms that are caused by a lack of cooling, moistening Kidney Yin.

Many women have found this formula to be a welcome alternative to hormone replacement therapy, which carries an increased risk for breast cancer.

Dosage: 8 pills, 3 times per day

Manufacturer: Lanzhou Foci

Warnings and contraindications: Rehmannia can be difficult to digest, so this formula should be discontinued if excessive loose stools become a problem.

—From *Pocket Guide to Chinese Patent Medicines*

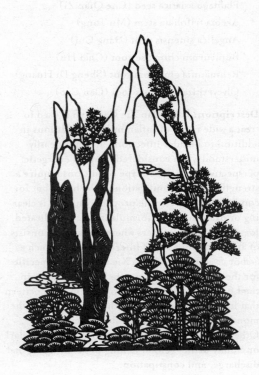

Continued ➡

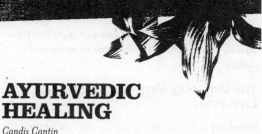

AYURVEDIC HEALING

Candis Cantin

Introduction

Ayurveda is the medicine of nature, the medicine of life. It does not give us a set of theoretical principles to impose upon our biological functioning. Rather, it seeks to present to the human mind the principles and powers of Nature herself. It teaches us to put into practice Natures great principles of health and natural living. For this reason it employs the language of nature—an energetic system of the elements and biological humors, a simple yet profound system of correspondences, not a complex scientific, materialistic or bio-chemical terminology.

—David Frawley, *The River of Life*

The system of healing known as Ayurveda—from the Sanskrit *ayur* ("life" or "longevity") and *veda* ("knowledge" or "wisdom")—helps us to harmonize our minds, bodies, and lifestyles with our spiritual purpose. The language of Ayurveda is based on that which is observable in nature. We experience things as hot or cold, sweet or sour, light or heavy, dry or damp, and so forth. As you go through this book-let, you will find out about the herbs, climates, aromas, and people that correspond to these and other qualities.

It is important, therefore, for the student of Ayurveda to develop the faculties of direct observation with all the senses, including the intuition. Through such observation, one becomes the Seer of one's life, making choices as needed from moment to moment—a skill analogous to a sailor using his knowledge of the winds and tides to steer a steady course. As directors of our own lives we need to know how to shift and regain balance, in both the inner and outer universe of our being.

Ayurveda: Cosmology as Physiology

The cosmology or creation theory of Ayurveda is complex as well as enlightening, with volume after volume dedicated to its exposition. In brief, the ancient Seers surmised that in the beginning there were two fundamental principles of existence, an absolute, unmanifested state of consciousness, called *Purusha*, and the principle of creativity or pri-mal nature, called *Prakruti*. The interplay of these two principles, of Spirit and Matter, produce the physical world and the laws that govern it.

Prakruti is said to contain three *gunas*, or attrib-utes, which are the foundation of all existence: *sattva*, the principle of light, intelligence, percep-tion, and harmony; *rajas*, the principle of energy, activity, and turbulence; and *tamas*, the principle of inertia, darkness, dullness, and resistance.

Sattva, as subjective consciousness, is responsi-ble for our perceptions, as well as for the clarity of those perceptions. In nature, sattva's balancing energy creates the seasons and other life rhythms. In the mind, sattva creates peace, virtue, and love. It also brings about the awakening of the soul and the five senses, opening us up to the experience of the physical universe.

Rajas is manifested as action and movement. In nature, we see the principle of rajas in various activities, from the wind blowing, to cars moving, to energy flowing. In the mind, rajas creates agita-tion, aggression, competition, and turbulence. From rajas are created the five motor organs of action, "the mouth for speech, the hands for

grasping, the feet for moving, the genitals for emis-sion, the anus for excretion."

Tamas gives to the world a certain steadiness and solidity—the inertia of rock, the stability of mountains—and in the body creates deep sleep or unconsciousness. Tamas in the mind, however, is responsible for periods of mental confusion and depression. From tamas come the five elements: space (sometimes called "ether"), air, fire, water, and earth.

Although all three attributes are needed to create the physical world, in the mind it is the cultivation of sattva that enables a person to feel the peace, honesty, and truth of his or her existence. Ayurveda, by emphasizing the sattvic lifestyle, moves the other gunas into a more harmonized state. The balance of the three gunas is called "pure sattva." Through healthy diet, peaceful lifestyle choices, love, faith, nonviolence, and other sattvic attrib-utes, one experiences inner peace.

The Five Elements

All things in the physical world, including our bod-ies, are made up of five elements:

Space, often translated as "ether," represents the expansion of consciousness. The "space" in our mind is the place where we experience love and compassion. Similarly, each of the body's cells con-tains "space"; without it, there would be no com-munication between cells.

Air represents the gaseous form of matter, the movement of consciousness, as well as the nerve and sensory impulses. Our breathing, sense of touch and movement are all governed by the air principle, as is the movement of our thoughts and ideas.

Fire represents the radiant form of matter. Air creates movement and friction, which in turn cre-ates heat, or "fire." In the body, "fire" is responsi-ble for digestion, absorption and assimilation. In the mind, it accounts for our ability to understand, comprehend and realize. We perceive the world around us because of the "fire" in our eyes, which digests the contents of vision. We can see the soul of a person by the light and fire in his or her eyes.

Water represents the liquid form of matter, and the "liquefaction" of consciousness. In the body, the water principle exists as plasma, saliva, mucus, sweat, urine, cerebro-spinal fluid, and other moist components. In the mind, it exists as feelings of compassion, faith, love, and devotion.

Earth represents the solid form of matter, as well as the more crystallized manifestations of con-sciousness. According to Ayurveda, the molecules of the physical world are solidified consciousness. In the body, all the solid structures—bones, carti-lage, teeth, nails, hair, and skin—are composed of the earth element. In the mind, the earth element is responsible for our feelings of groundedness and solidity.

Tri-dosha—The Three Constitutions

According to Ayurveda, there are three primary life forces, or biological humors, in the body, called "doshas." The doshas bind the five elements down into living flesh. These are called in Sanskrit *vata*, *pitta*, and *kapha*. They are the active and mobile ele-ments that determine the life processes of growth and decay. Dosha literally means "that which dark-ens, spoils, or causes things to decay," for when out of balance they are the causative forces in the dis-ease process.

Vata: the Air/Space Constitution

Associated with the elements of air and space, *vata* means "wind" or "that which moves things," and represents the force that governs biological activity. It is the prime impetus of the nervous system, con-trolling both sensory and mental balance, mental adaptability, and understanding. It is the basic life force (*prana*), and is enhanced by the consumption of pure, whole foods, the breathing of clean air, and by our connection with the Divine within, the deepest energizing force for the entire body.

Physiologically, vata governs:

- breathing
- inhalation/exhalation
- blinking of the eyelids
- movements in the muscles and tissues
- pulsations of the heart
- all contractions and expansions within the body
- movements and signals in the nerve cells
- digestion
- elimination/urine/menstruation/birthing

Mentally and emotionally, vata governs:

- mental power and movement coordination
- adaptability
- inspirations
- spiritual aspirations
- nervousness
- fear
- anxiety

Vata's main locations are:

- colon
- hips
- thighs
- ears
- bones
- organ of touch (skin)
- nerve tissues

In the mind, vata represents flexibility, ability to communicate, and creative resources. When aggravated, it can also manifest as insecurities, fears, and anxieties. In our bodies, vata is the movement of the nervous system, accumulating in the large intestines as gas, in the pelvic cavity as pains and aches, in the bones as arthritis, in the skin as neuralgia, in the ears as ringing, and in the hips and thighs as sciatic pain. If the body develops an excess of vata (air qualities), these are the first areas in which it will accumulate. When not deranged or out of balance, vata functions as nerv-ous and mental force throughout the body, and is centered in the brain and the nervous system in general.

Vata is the vital motivating force behind the other two humors, which are in themselves inca-pable of movement.

The qualities of vata (air) are:

- light
- cold
- rough
- dry
- clear
- agitated
- subtle
- hard
- dispersing
- mobile

Continued ➡

Vata rules:
- movement
- catabolism (breaking down of substances in the body)
- astringent taste (has a drying quality)
- old age (people tend to be drier and colder as they age)
- dawn and dusk (changing, transitional times)
- fall season (cold, dry, windy season)

Vata disorders:
- emaciation
- loss of warmth
- tremors
- bloating
- constipation
- insomnia
- sensory disorientation
- incoherent speech
- dizziness
- confusion
- depression
- anxiety, nervousness
- migrating pain
- arthritis

VATA CHARACTERISTICS

Just as the wind blows gently or forcefully in different directions, so the vata individual will manifest irregularity in his or her structure.

Build: Vata may be very tall (taller than the average in his or her family) or very short, with a tendency to be slender or rangy, a thin body frame, and narrow shoulders or hips. The arms may be unusually short or long. Vata people may have light, small bones, with prominent or protruding joints that tend to make cracking noises. Deviated nasal septum, bowlegs and knock-knees are also due to vata.

Weight: Vata is dry, creating a tendency to leanness in the predominantly vata constitution. Vata people may find it hard or impossible to gain weight, while some may overeat poor-quality foods and become fat; others may gain and lose weight erratically. Again, this is all part of vata's overall irregularity.

Complexion and Skin Characteristics: Vatas tend to be dark (relative to others of their race) and to tan deeply without burning. They are by nature cold, and therefore enjoy warm weather and sunlight.

Due to their high energy output, vata people tend to have dry skin that uses up lubricating dermal oils. However, due to vata's variability some areas of the skin may be dry while others are oily. Vata people may develop psoriasis, dry eczema, corns, calluses, or chapped lips. They may show wrinkles at a young age. Because they do not store up enough energy to maintain body warmth, they feel cold to the touch. Many suffer from poor circulation, with the skin showing a grayish tinge.

Hair: Hair is closely related to prana, the life force of the body. Vata hair may vary from dry to oily in different areas of the head. It is often coarse in texture, dull and lusterless, and prone to dandruff or split ends.

Nails: Vata people have hard, rough, brittle nails that may differ in size, with marked ridges or depressions. Many times the fingers will be very cold, and bluish; or grayish in color. Nail-biting is a vata attribute.

Eyes: Vata eyes may be gray, violet, slate blue, or dark chocolate. Different color eyes are also a vata characteristic. Vata eyes may be dry and scratchy, with the sclera (white part of the eye) having a grayish or bluish tinge, or dull and lusterless.

Mouth: Vata people may have crooked or uneven teeth with a mouth too large or small in proportion to the rest of the face. The teeth will tend to be brittle and oversensitive, with gums that recede early. If there is a coating on the tongue it will be thin, adherent, and grayish or pink-gray in color.

Appetite: The vata appetite is variable, with excess hunger one day and no appetite the next. If vata people do not eat regularly, they may become dizzy and weak. They do not do well with fasts, as their bodies do not store enough fat and energy to carry them through a period of food deprivation. Although vatas seem to be the people who fast the most—for purposes of cleansing, so that they can realize their spiritual aspirations more clearly—fasting may work against them, provoking the negative effects of vata.

Vatas must have breakfast; otherwise they will become anxious and tired as their blood-sugar levels drop. They may rely on caffeine to wake them up and get them going, but this will rob them of energy later in the day and will eventually exhaust them altogether by drying out their glands. (Vata tiredness is often due to adrenal exhaustion.)

Digestion/Evacuation: Vata people are usually life-long sufferers from constipation, with frequent gas and bloating, and a tendency to hard, dark-colored stools. They respond only to strong laxatives, such as cascara sagrada and castor oil. Vatas must be reminded that good eating habits are essential for easy digestion and smooth bowel movement.

Menstruation: Vata women have irregular cycles, and may miss periods if they exercise too much or if they lose too much weight. The flow is scanty, with clots due to vata dryness. Severe cramping and constipation, lasting for hours or days, may occur before bleeding begins.

Climate: Vatas feel generally cold and dry, and enjoy warm and humid climates. They tend to be weaker during the winter and must learn to bundle up if they go out in the cold. Warming tonic herbs, such as dong quai and codonopsis, may be helpful for vatas during the winter months.

Sex: Although vata types may spend much time thinking intensely about sex, their sexual appetites vary. Vata men may experience premature ejaculation. Fertility may be lower than average in the vata person.

Physical Activity: Vata types are active and restless, with low stamina. They may drive themselves to exhaustion with overactivity and excess nervous energy. Aerobics and other rigorous exercise tire them out. Gentle, slow exercises or yoga are more appropriate.

Pulse: The vata pulse is thin, fast and said to "slither like a cobra."

Sleep: Again, the variability of vatas plays a part in their sleep patterns. They may toss and turn, or wake up frequently during the night.

Emotions: Vata people in balance may be enthusiastic, idealistic, and visionary. However, a vata who is not practiced inner quiet and a peaceful lifestyle will experience fear or anxiety when confronted with difficult situations in life.

Speech/Mind: Vatas may talk very fast and breathlessly. They have original minds, and are not afraid of new ideas or sudden inspirations. They like to communicate and put ideas together. On the other hand, they may have a hard time putting ideas into action. If undisciplined, they can be spacy and chaotic.

THE VATA, AND VATA-PACIFYING, LIFESTYLES

Joe wakes up in the morning and quickly gets dressed for work. He drinks a cup of coffee, which stimulates the nervous system, and grabs a quick bite at a fast-food restaurant, which he eats while driving 65 mph through the desert outside Santa Fe—high, dry, cold, clear, windy, rough, agitated, energetic vata country. Joe rushes into work and begins to talk for hours on the phone. When lunchtime comes, he eats a salad and soft drink at his desk.

Let's see if we can pick out some of the vata elements in this story.

- First, the coffee which overstimulates the nervous system, resulting in agitation (vata), excess mobility (vata) and dryness (vata). Also, coffee is bitter and astringent (both vata qualities).
- Eating while driving is vata behavior.
- Fast foods, overcooked and lacking in nourishment, are vata.
- The salad, which is cold, light and mobile, moves through us quickly without providing deep, "building" nourishment.
- The carbonated drink, which has many gas bubbles and is cold, will increase vata qualities of lightness and coldness, and induce flatulence or burping.
- Talking all day and eating at one's desk create agitation, anxiety, indigestion, lack of inner peace, pains, tremors, twitching, and, eventually, general nervous exhaustion.

Certain lifestyle modifications will help to keep vata in balance:

Joe wakes up in the morning with a feeling of gratefulness for the day ahead. He gets out of bed and does a few gentle stretches and some deep breathing. Before his shower, he applies sesame oil to his body and allows it to stay on for a few minutes while he boils some water for spicy herbal tea and oatmeal. He takes a warm shower and puts on some comfortable natural-fiber clothing. Just before eating, he gives thanks for the nourishment and proceeds to eat his breakfast with quiet music in the background. He drives at a reasonable speed to work while listening to still more relaxing music. When lunchtime comes, Joe makes sure to get away from his desk. He orders warm vegetable soup with whole-grain bread.

This type of routine is decidedly sattvic, inducing inner peace. It will keep Joe's vata nature from getting out of hand. He feels physically better, retaining access to vata inspiration and mental acuity. Such lifestyle choices decrease the tendency to dispersion, fear, anxiety, and nervousness.

It should be mentioned that the sesame oil is warming and nourishing to the nerves, and will alleviate vata's dryness, agitation, and coldness. The warm, cooked foods are deeply nourishing and will counteract the attributes of cold, light, dryness, roughness, and hardness. In order to keep vata in its place, we must engage in practices that contrast with vata attributes: calm versus agitated, warm versus cold, soft versus hard, and so forth.

The vata person is blessed with a flexible, quick mind. There is never a lack of creative ideas and resources. Because vata is associated with motion, vata people like to be "on the move" physically, mentally, and emotionally. However, should all this nervous energy get out of hand, the vata individual may become ill with nervous exhaustion, constipation, tremors, arthritis, and so forth. The purpose of any vata-pacifying lifestyle and diet is to help regulate this motion, so that the person may continue to be inspired, but not burn out. (We will

Continued ➔

discuss vata-pacifying foods and choices in the next chapter.)

I have noticed in my practice that the biggest difficulty in working with vata people is that they often have poor follow-through with the routine suggested by the practitioner-herbalist. They get very excited about the information, but may not be grounded enough to keep the program going.

Pitta: the Fire/Water Constitution

Pitta—the biological fire humor, or "bile," means "that which digests things" or "that which heats, cooks, or transforms." It is the fire that digests the food we eat and gives our bodies warmth. Our internal fires determine our capacity to perceive reality and our power to digest life experiences.

The person with pitta predominant in her constitution is blessed with great willpower and initiative, the capacity to laugh at her troubles, great determination to reach her goals, a penetrating mind, and, usually, good "fires" for digestion.

Pitta is our enthusiasm for life, our joy and laughter. It finds negative expression in burning sensations in the body and mind, in a drive toward unhealthy competition and anger, and in the need to control.

Physiologically, pitta governs:

- hunger
- thirst
- luster
- complexion
- digestion
- body heat

Mentally and emotionally, pitta governs:

- laughter
- joy
- willpower
- enthusiasm
- anger
- competition
- judgment
- criticalness
- mental perception
- discriminating awareness
- penetrating thought
- courage

Glossary of Ayurvedic Terms

Candis Cantin

agni: "digestive fires," i.e., secretions of the digestive system that help break down undigested food (*ama*) and release energy.

ama: undigested food material that becomes lodged in the body's weakest organs and may precipitate disease conditions.

Ayurveda: the science and wisdom of life. *Ayur* means "life" or "longevity"; *veda* means "knowledge" or "wisdom."

brimhana: a tonifying therapy that uses herbs and foods to build, nourish, and strengthen tissues.

dosha: the Sanskrit word for "humor," or one of the three biological forces that bind the five elements into living flesh. They are known as vata, pitta, and kapha. Literally translated, *dosha* means "that which darkens, spoils, or causes things to decay." When out of balance, the doshas (humors) are the causative forces in the disease process. In balance, they create a healthy and harmonious body.

ghee: clarified butter. Excellent for digestion. To prepare ghee, use a medium to heavy saucepan. Melt at a very low temperature one pound of unsalted butter. (Organic and/or raw is best, if available.) The butter will make bubbling sounds as foam forms on the top. Stir in the foam and continue to cook the ghee. If you look at the bottom of the pan, you will notice milk solids forming. You will notice also that the butter no longer bubbles. (The process takes about 30 minutes or so, depending on your stove.) Take the ghee off the burner as soon as it has stopped bubbling and is clear-looking. Let it cool a bit, then pour it through a metal strainer into a glass jar. Discard the milk solids that are struck on the bottom of the pan. Ghee will store at room temperature.

gunas: the three attributes (*sattva*, *rajas* and *tamas*) that are the foundation of all existence.

kapha: one of the three *doshas* (humors) of the body; it has the qualities of water and earth.

langhana: a "lightening" therapy that focuses on effecting a decrease in weight, accumulated toxins, and excess humors.

lassi: A nourishing drink made from fresh plain yogurt, water, and spices, often served at the end of a meal as a digestive aid.

Mildly Spicy Lassi Drink

1/2 cup plain yogurt

2 cups pure water

1/4 tsp. powdered ginger

1/4 tsp. cumin powder

1/8 tsp. salt

Blend all ingredients for a few minutes. Drink at room temperature, 1/4 to 1/2 cup after meals. May be garnished with cilantro leaves.

Sweet Lassi

1/2 cup plain fresh yogurt

2 cups pure water

2 tbsp. natural sugar (Sucanat, barley malt, etc.; add less sweetener for kaphas)

1/4 tsp. powdered ginger

1/2 tsp. ground cardamom

1/4 tsp. ground cinnamon

Blend together for a few minutes. Drink at room temperature, 1/4 to 1/2 cup after meals.

ojas: the subtle essence of all the kapha, or water, in the body. Ojas is the prime energy reserve in the body, and the vitality of the immune system.

pancha karma: the five radical cleansing techniques employed in Ayurveda.

pitta: one of the three *doshas* (humors) of the body; it has the qualities of fire and water.

prana: the life force, called *chi* [Qi] in Oriental medicine.

prakruti: fixed proportions of vata, pitta, kapha established at conception; inherited nature; also, the principle of creativity or primal nature.

purva karma: various milder treatments used as a preliminary to *pancha karma*.

purusha: the absolute, unmanifested state of consciousness.

rajas: the cosmis force of action and activity; in the mind, rajas creates aggression and overactivity.

rasayana: Ayurvedic rejuvenation therapy, a special type of tonification.

sattva: the cosmic force of balance and equilibrium; helps to maintain clarity of mind.

Sucanat: a natural sugar made from organic sugar-cane juice, containing all its inherent minerals and vitamins.

tamas: the cosmic force of inactivity and inertia; in the mind, tamas creates dullness and resistance to change and growth.

tri-dosha: the three bodily humors or constitutions: vata, pitta, kapha.

trikatu: a combination of powdered ginger, black pepper, and pippali pepper. Equal amounts of these herbs are mixed together, with raw honey added to create a paste. One-quarter to one-half teaspoon may be taken with meals or after meals to facilitate digestion. The pippali pepper may be hard to find, so powdered anise seeds may be substituted. This formula is also very good for breaking up mucus.

vata: one of the three *doshas* (humors) of the body; vata has the qualities of air and space.

vikruti: the current state of your health and well-being, as opposed to the fixed state, or *prakruti*.

—From *Pocket Guide to Ayurvedic Healing*

Continued ➡

Pitta's main locations are:

- small intestine
- stomach (as digestive acids)
- blood
- eyes
- sweat
- sebaceous glands (glands that supply oil for the hair and skin)

Pitta is our inner digestive fire, acids, and bile, all of which help to combust food, providing energy and warmth. It is also the light and heat of the body and the mind.

The qualities of pitta (fire) are:

- hot
- sharp
- flowing
- light
- liquid
- oily
- smooth
- aggressive
- penetrating

Pitta rules:

- transformation
- adulthood
- metabolism (transformation of a substance)
- sour or pungent (spicy) tastes
- noon and midnight
- late spring and summer

Pitta disorders:

- yellow stool, urine, eyes, and skin
- excess hunger
- excess thirst
- burning sensations in the body
- difficult, restless sleep
- heat, fever, inflammation
- herpes
- burning eczema and rashes
- sties ("red eye")
- liver problems
- burning, bleeding ulcers

PITTA CHARACTERISTICS

Build: "Balanced" and "proportional" are the operative words for pitta. Medium-length fingers and toes, medium-width shoulders and hips, proportional frame and height.

Weight: Pittas have average weight for their height, with minor fluctuations. Fat is deposited evenly throughout the body.

Complexion: Pitta skin may be pale, pink, or copper in hue, and warm to the touch. It will tend to be delicate, irritable, and prone to rashes, pimples, and inflammations. It may have freckles, black, brown, or red moles, may sunburn easily or suffer from sun allergy, and may wrinkle early. Body hair may be light-hued and fine-textured. The lips may be deep red, showing ample blood beneath the skin. Pitta people may blush easily or turn red when angry. They may perspire very easily, even in cold weather. They may feel hot most of the time, no matter the season.

Hair: Red hair is an indication of substantial pitta in one's basic constitution. Pitta people may have light hair, or their hair may turn gray or white at an early age. Early baldness is also a pitta indicator, since it indicates high levels of testosterone, a hot, pitta-type hormone. The hair is thin, fine,

or delicate, and usually quite straight. It may be oily as well.

Nails: Pitta nails are soft, strong, rubbery and well-formed. They may be very pink in color, with a coppery tinge due to a profusion of warm blood right under the skin.

Eyes: Pitta eyes are medium in size, and may be light in color. Pitta eyes may also be hazel, green, or light blue, and may be tinged with red. The eyes look as though they are burning with an intense fire, and radiate high levels of energy. The sclera (white of the eyes) may have a reddish tinge and become fiery red when irritated.

Mouth: Pittas have medium-size teeth, prone to cavities and bleeding gums. The tongue coating may be yellow, orange, or red. The tongue itself may be irritated or bleed. Pitta-predominant people often get canker sores and experience a sour or metallic taste in the mornings.

Appetite: Pittas usually have good appetites and enjoy eating. They hate to miss meals and will grow irritable if they fail to eat when they are hungry. They do not like to fast, and if they do, may become quite agitated. In general, they like to consume and absorb new energy.

If pittas skip breakfast they will be ravenous by noon. However, if they are focused on a goal, they may skip a meal and remember later that they haven't eaten all day.

Digestion/Evacuation: Pittas are usually not constipated, enjoying frequent bowel movements. Many times the stool has a yellowish tinge and is well-formed, although it may also be loose, hot, and burning. Intense yellow or orange stool may indicate great pitta intensity (or too much salsa and chips). If a pitta person does suffer from occasional constipation, milk, figs, raisins, or dates may serve as a laxative.

Menstruation: Pittas have regular cycles, but may bleed longer and heavier than others due to their innate heat. The blood is bright red. Pitta women may have loose stools during or just before their periods. They may also experience heat and sweating before menstruation. If they have cramps, these are of medium strength.

Climate: Pittas find hot climates intolerable.

Sex: Pittas have ample sex drives and, when aroused, tend to pursue their goals. They can be quite romantic, although when thwarted they may grow angry and flare up. They are average in fertility.

Physical Activity: Pittas can endure much vigorous exercise as long as they do not grow overheated.

Pulse: The pitta pulse is full, regular, and strong, with medium speed and rhythm. In pure pitta, it is said to "jump like a frog."

Sleep: Pittas tend to go to sleep easily and sleep lightly, but if they are awakened during the night, have no trouble going to sleep again.

Emotions: Pittas can be "intense." Sometimes, because of the heat in their body, they may react with immediate anger to challenging situations. (This may or may not manifest outwardly.) However, many pittas I know are able to laugh at adversity and enjoy challenges.

Speech/Mind: Pittas are usually precise and direct in what they say. They have an acute intelligence and tend to be impatient with anyone whose intelligence is not equal to theirs. They often want to dominate. They are methodical and efficient, and love steering ideas into practical applications.

THE PITTA, AND PITTA-PACIFYING, LIFESTYLES

Jill lives in East Texas, where the summers are hot and humid, the sun so bright she has to squint her eyes to see. Jill decides to go out for a short jog, then have a bite to eat. She puts on a red running suit, laces up her sneakers and jogs to town. At the local cantina, she indulges herself with salsa and chips, followed by a spicy meat-and-bean burrito smothered in hot sauce. After her feast, she feels a little irritated about the service that she received in the restaurant and begins to tell the manager everything that is wrong with the waiter. She leaves the restaurant feeling flushed, hot and bothered.

First of all, East Texas is a predominantly pitta environment—bright, humid, aggressively hot. The red running suit is likewise hot and aggressive in nature, and jogging is a very overheating type of exercise, especially in the summer. The food too is hot, sharp, penetrating, oily—basically pitta in nature. The emotions of rash judgment and keen irritation are signs that Jill's pitta is elevated.

Now let's look at a pitta-pacifying scenario:

Jill looks outside and sees that it is another hot, sweltering day. She decides to wear a cool, light blue summer dress and anoint herself with sandalwood oil. She drives to town in her air-conditioned car, to a salad bar that has a lovely garden atmosphere with a small waterfall and pond. She orders a light meal with peppermint tea.

All the choices Jill has made are pitta-pacifying and, for her, quite sattvic, increasing coolness, calmness, and peacefulness.

I have noticed in my practice that the pitta people may want to control the Ayurvedic session. They may be contentious or aggressive, questioning the practitioner's credentials and status. It is best not to debate or argue with pittas. Try to gain their trust through discussion and presentation of facts. Once they know what they need to do, they will begin to implement the program—and may even do it to excess. (I have known pittas to carry their program with them on laminated cards so that they can follow it precisely.)

Pitta-predominant people—classic Type A's—have a tendency to do too much and burn themselves out. Chronic fatigue and liver ailments are not uncommon in the pitta person.

Kapha: the Water/Earth Constitution

Kapha, the biological force of water/earth, means both "phlegm" and "that which holds things together." It is the physical and emotional "home" in which we reside, providing the substance and support for our body, giving bulk to our tissues. Emotionally, kapha is the love and support we receive in life, governing feelings of compassion, devotion, modesty, patience, and forgiveness. Negatively expressed, kapha is greed, attachment, and self-pity.

Kapha helps to ground and control the active and consuming natures of vata and pitta. It exerts a conserving, consolidating, stabilizing, restraining force over the body and mind. Vata and pitta will squander their energy without kapha to hold them down. The subtle essence of all the kapha, or water, in the body is called ojas. Ojas is the prime energy reserve in the body and is the vitality of the immune system. If there is an excess loss of kapha due to stress, improper eating, and illness, we will suffer from a compromised immune system and will lack both physical and emotional support.

Physiologically, kapha governs:

- form and solidity
- storing of energy
- stability
- lubrication
- holding together of the joints

Continued →

- body fluids
- the sense of taste

Mentally and emotionally, kapha governs:

- patience
- forgiveness
- compassion
- love
- deep sense of satisfaction
- sense of being grounded and belonging
- attachment
- greed
- mental inertia
- dullness

Kapha's main locations are:

- stomach
- chest
- throat
- head
- pancreas
- sides
- lymph
- fat
- nose
- tongue

Its primary site is the stomach.

The qualities of kapha (water/earth) are:

- heavy
- slow
- liquid
- dense
- dull
- cold
- thick
- soft
- sticky
- cloudy
- oily
- damp

Kapha rules:

- constructing of form
- anabolism (building up of substance)
- sweet and salty tastes
- the childhood years
- morning and evening
- winter and late spring

Kapha disorders:

- depression of digestive "fire"
- nausea after eating
- lethargy
- heaviness
- paleness
- chills
- looseness of the limbs
- cough
- difficult breathing
- mucous conditions
- excessive sleeping
- accumulation of fat in the body
- congestion of the lymphatic system

Kapha in the chest or lungs produces moisture, as it does in the throat, head, sinuses, and nasal passages. In the mouth and tongue, kapha produces saliva. (The tongue is the organ of taste, the sensory quality that is said to belong to the water element.) Kapha creates fat tissue, which stores water. It is

also held along the sides of the abdominal cavity, in the form of peritoneal fluid. An excessive amount of kapha will produce an overabundance of mucus and, therefore, congestion.

KAPHA CHARACTERISTICS

Build: Kapha people are the bulkiest of the three different constitutions, with medium to broad frames, heavy bone structure and wide shoulders and/or hips. They store energy, which encourages massiveness. Kaphas are well-lubricated and normally experience none of the problems associated with dryness. Many kaphas have fingers that are squarish and short.

Weight: Kaphas can maintain moderate weight with regular exercise, but usually do not like to exert themselves. They gain weight easily, especially around fie mid-torso and the hips, and they lose weight slowly.

Complexion: Kaphas tan evenly and enjoy the sun. The skin may be cool, but not cold, to the touch. (They do not suffer from cold hands and feet to the extent that vatas do.) Many times kaphas have very beautiful skin—smooth and soft, slightly oily, with a moderate amount of body hair and very few moles. They do not have a propensity to skin disorders, but may experience stagnation of the lymphatic system due to blockages of energy. Kaphas sweat moderately, at about the same intensity in all climates.

Hair: Kaphas usually have brown or black, thick, slightly wavy hair, sometimes bordering on coarse. Oily hair may be a problem, but the hair luster is good.

Nails: Kapha nails are strong, large, and symmetrical, with very little variation.

Eyes: Kapha eyes tend to be large, liquid, calm, cool, and stable. Some people say that Kaphas have the "eyes of a deer."

Mouth: Kaphas often have large and even teeth. If there is a coating on the tongue it may be thick, white, or off-white, with a curdled look. The taste in the mouth may be sickly sweet.

Appetite: Kaphas have a stable and moderate desire for food, although they may be prone to emotional eating. Fasting is relatively easy on them due to their ability to store energy, but it rarely occurs to them to fast. Kaphas tend not to be hungry upon awakening. They may feel hungry around 10 or 11 A.M. for a light breakfast—maybe some spicy tea and a piece of fruit—but are just as likely to skip breakfast entirely. They may want coffee to stimulate them in the a.m. Two meals per day is usually sufficient for a kapha.

Digestion/Evacuation: Kapljas have regular bowel movements, with well-formed, rarely hard stools. (When constipated, they respond to medium-strength laxatives.) Kapha people may be prone to yeast conditions due to the dampness in their system, causing digestive problems. Also, they may feel heavy and lethargic after eating, due to overall slow metabolism and sluggish digestion.

Menstruation: Kaphas may have effortless, regular periods with an average quantity of blood, light in color. Cramps are usually mild and dull. Kaphas may be prone to water retention and edema, however.

Climate: Due to their stability, Kaphas are generally not disturbed by extremes of climate. They may prefer warm weather, but not humid. Cold, damp climates may be aggravating to kaphas and their physical complaints.

Sex: Kaphas have a steady desire for sex and enjoy it. They are slow to arouse, but once aroused can remain that way for a long time. Fertility is unusually high.

Physical Activity: Kaphas can endure vigorous exercise, but may not be interested in this kind of energy expenditure. When they do exercise it makes them feel strong and healthy.

Pulse: A kapha pulse is said to beat smoothly, "like a swan." It is full, slow, rhythmic, and the artery may feel cool and rubbery. Sometimes, however, a kapha pulse is hard to find due to the firmness of the flesh at the wrist area.

Sleep: Kaphas drop off quickly, sleep heavily, and wake up rested and alert. They like to oversleep to store up energy.

Emotions: Kaphas like to avoid confrontations due to their innate sweetness, which may lead to complacency. They do not like change and are stressed by unpredictable situations. They are predominantly calm, quiet, steady, and serious, and enjoy home and family. Kapha in excess may be too passive, attached, possessive, and greedy. Once they get moving and are committed to a course of action, kaphas will generally see it through.

Speech/Mind: Kaphas may speak slowly and cautiously, without volunteering much—information must be pulled out of them. They will initiate a conversation only if they have something to say. The kapha voice may be quite melodious.

THE KAPHA, AND KAPHA-PACIFYING, LIFESTYLES

On a cold, damp morning in Seattle, Pat opens her eyes, curls up in the down comforter and tries to catch a few more minutes of sleep. After a while, she lazily gets out of her waterbed and gets ready for work. She puts on some very sweet-smelling rose perfume and a pink, fluffy outfit. At work, the donut man comes around 10 A.M.—Pat purchases three donuts and a carton of cold milk. Her job at the bank keeps her sitting most of the day. At lunch, Pat orders fried chicken, french fries, cold Diet Coke, and frozen yogurt. When she goes home at night, she turns on the TV and eats nachos with extra cheese, followed by more frozen yogurt.

Cold, damp, low-elevation climates—such as that of Seattle—are kapha in nature. Sleepiness and inertia are kapha attributes. The donuts contain the sweet taste that increases kapha. The same applies to the rose perfume and pink garments; both color and aroma are sweet in nature. The sedentary job reinforces kapha's heavy, slow, thick, static, soft, dull nature. Fried chicken, french fries, cheese, frozen yogurt, and cold drinks increase the physical qualities of heaviness, slowness, coldness, oiliness, denseness, thickness, stickiness, and dullness, and will also increase mental dullness, emotional fixations, overindulgence, and greed. Waterbeds are too soft—and watery—for kapha persons.

Let us take a look at a kapha-pacifying story for Pat:

It is a cold, damp day in Seattle, so Pat keeps the house warm and dry. She sleeps on a relatively hard bed—comfortable, but not too soft or sumptuous. When she wakes up she gets out of bed immediately and does some deep-breathing and mild aerobics for a minute or two, to get the blood flowing. Before her shower, she uses a loofa sponge to dry-brush her body in order to stimulate the lymphatic system. For breakfast, she has some stewed fruit and a spicy tea. She forgoes snacks at work and has a nourishing lunch of steamed vegetables, grains, and salad, followed by a spicy warm drink and a walk before returning to work. At night she has a light meal and does not eat anything else until morning.

Kapha people have great strength and endurance. They also have faith in life, and in those close to them. They can provide the stable, nurtur-

Continued ➡

ing, grounded energy that is so rare—and so needed—these days.

I have noticed in my practice that kapha people must be treated with firmness, and aggressively enough to move them out of their complacency. You must lovingly tell them what will happen if they do not do something to overcome their inertia. They need to be motivated and put on a strict, rigorous regimen.

Prakruti/Vikruti: Constitutional Amendments

Within each of us is a place of balance and equilibrium, our basic nature or constitution, which Ayurveda calls prakruti. Prakruti is the combination of the three doshas (vata, pitta and kapha) that we received at conception, and so refers to the individual's inherent, inborn tendencies or "nature." Prakruti never changes during our lifetime. Prakruti influences activity as well as consciousness, and determines how our body-mind will respond to stress.

We also have our current state, our situation "at the moment." This is called *vikruti*. When a person is more or less free of discomfort, we can assume that his or her prakruti (inherent constitution) and vikruti (current condition) are somewhat in balance. Unfortunately, diet, lifestyle, age, emotions, environment, and so forth have a way of knocking one's constitution out of balance.

Some Ayurvedic practitioners have found it useful to attach a numerical value to the levels of vata (V), pitta (P) and kapha (K) that constitute an individual's prakruti. For the purposes of this . . . guide, the highest value level will be 4, the lowest 1.

My prakruti, for example, is:

V1, P3, K2

In other words, my prakruti is predominantly pitta, with lesser or secondary amounts of vata and kapha.

Now let's say I am lecturing, traveling extensively and therefore keeping irregular hours. Because of this, I may begin to suffer from insomnia, dry sensations in the body, gas and constipation. Because of lifestyle choices, a rough measurement of my current constitution (vikruti) shows elevated vata. I must now take remedial measures to bring vata down to its usual place of V1.

Your prakruti is the place where your health is. We are not trying to have vata, pitta, and kapha in equal proportions, which would contradict our basic natures. We are trying to honor that with which we were born, our place of balance.

Let me give another example. Again, my prakruti is:

V1, P3, K2

On a hot summer day, I decide to have a big Italian meal with lots of garlic and tomato sauce. Later that night, I begin to feel burning sensations in the intestines. My stool is very loose and burns as well. There is a slight rash on my face, and I generally feel irritated.

The foods that I ate are pitta- or fire-provoking; therefore my current situation, or vikruti, shows elevated pitta that needs to be brought down to its usual place of P3. Only then will I begin to feel well. I should take some pitta-pacifying herbs and make the appropriate lifestyle choices to bring pitta down to its proper level. (Very often a person's predominant dosha is the one that becomes unbalanced most easily.)

Because many Western treatments and medicines work with symptoms, but fail to take into account our true natures, they may throw us even more out of balance. Trying to handle a situation with more and more complicated therapies may further remove us from the simplicity and innocence of nature and our deeper selves. Health is our natural state. The aim in Ayurveda is to restore our basic nature (prakruti) and help us to live in harmony with it.

Finding Out Your Basic Constitution (Prakruti) and Current Conditions (Vikruti)

When taking the following test, keep in mind that we are trying to determine prakruti. Base your choices on what has been most constant in your life over a considerable time period. A separate test for viikruti follows.

CONSTITUTIONAL (PRAKRUTI) EVALUATION

Things to remember when taking the test:

1. Certain fixed attributes—such as body frame, weight, shape of arms and legs, and complextion—plus the state of metabolism and digestion give us a good indicator of your prakruti.

2. Lifelong habits and proclivities are also good indicators.

3. If you feel that two or three statements in some of the categories fit you, mark them all down. Mark on each line that applies to you the letter V, P, or K, then count up the total number of each letter.

4. If you do not have a clear picture of yourself in some areas, have a friend help you clarify where you stand in relation to some of the questions.

1. Body Structure:

____ Vata—taller or shorter than average; thin, wiry build

____ Pitta—medium height; moderately developed physique

____ Kapha—stout, stocky, well-developed physique; may be tall but solidly built

2. Weight:

____ Vata—low weight, or variable weight gain and loss; prominent veins and bones

____ Pitta—moderate weight; good muscle tone

____ Kapha—heavy, firm; may be obese

3. Complexion: (Take into consideration racial background):

____ Vata—dull, brown or grayish hue; dark overall

____ Pitta—red hue; ruddy, flushed, glowing

____ Kapha—white, pale; not too red or flushed

4. Skin Texture and Temperature:

____ Vata—thin, dry, cold, cracked, rough; may have prominent veins

____ Pitta—warm, moist, pink; may have moles, freckles, acne

____ Kapha—white, thick-skinned, cool, soggy, soft, smooth, oily

5. Hair:

____ Vata—dry, coarse, scanty

____ Pitta—fine, soft; may gray early; tendency to baldness

____ Kapha—oily, thick; wavy, lustrous, abundant

6. Eyes:

____ Vata—small, dry, dull, unsteady; may blink a lot; erratic eye movement

____ Pitta—medium size; may have red sclera (whites) or inflamed eyes; the eyes have a "piercing" quality and may be sensitive to light

____ Kapha—wide, prominent; white sclera

7. Face:

____ Vata—long, thin, small; may wrinkle early

____ Pitta—sharp features; moderate size

____ Kapha—round, large; soft contours

8. Shoulders:

____ Vata—thin, small, hunched; may have a caved-in chest

____ Pitta—medium size

____ Kapha—broad, well-developed

9. Arms:

____ Vata—may be too long or short for body; underdeveloped, may be bony

____ Pitta—medium arms with moderate build

____ Kapha—thick, round, well-developed

10. Joints:

____ Vata—dry, with popping or cracking sounds

____ Pitta—medium, soft, loose; may experience inflammation

____ Kapha—thick joints

11. Legs:

____ Vata—thin, often excessively long or short; bony knees

____ Pitta—medium-sized legs, medium strength

____ Kapha—large, stocky

12. Nails:

____ Vata—thin, brittle, dry, cracked; possibly bitten

____ Pitta—soft, pink, well-formed

____ Kapha—smooth, firm, large, white

13. Urine:

____ Vata—scanty, colorless

____ Pitta—profuse, dark yellow or light brown

____ Kapha—may be milky white in color

14. Stools:

____ Vata—dry, hard, difficult evacuation accompanied by gas; tendency to constipation and irregularity

____ Pitta—loose, abundant amount; sometimes yellowish in color

____ Kapha—moderate amount, solid, well-formed; may have mucus in stool

15. Appetite:

____ Vata—erratic, i.e., fine one day followed the next by gas and poor digestion; or hungry one day, not so the next

____ Pitta—strong appetite; will become irritated if he or she does not eat on time

____ Kapha—consistent appetite, slow metabolism; may eat to cope with negative emotions

16. Circulation:

____ Vata—poor, variable; cold hands, cold feet, cold body

____ Pitta—good circulation; warm

____ Kapha—slow circulation; cool hands, warm body

17. Activity:

____ Vata—fast, changeable, erratic; hyperactive

____ Pitta—motivated, goal-oriented, intense, competitive, aggressive

____ Kapha—slow, deliberate, steady

Continued ➡

18. Sensitivity:

____ Vata—sensitive to wind, cold, and dryness

____ Pitta—sensitive to heat, fire; aggravated by too much sun

____ Kapha—sensitive to cold, damp, foggy areas; likes the sun

19. Disease Tendency:

____ Vata—nervous-system diseases, arthritis, migrating aches and pains, intestinal disorders, gas, mental/emotional disorders

____ Pitta—fevers, infections, inflammations, ulcers, colitis, blood diseases, rashes, red itching skin diseases, heat

____ Kapha—mucus diseases, respiratory problems, water retention, blockages, depression

20. Resistance:

____ Vata—variable resistance; may have weak immune system

____ Pitta—medium resistance; prone to infections, heat, inflammatory conditions

____ Kapha—high resistance; generally strong immunity

21. Medications:

____ Vata—may experience rapid, unexpected reactions to medication; low doses

____ Pitta—medium reactions; medium doses

____ Kapha—slow reactions; high doses

22. Voice:

____ Vata—may be deep, weak, grating due to lack of moisture

____ Pitta—Sharp, penetrating; may be high-pitched

____ Kapha—soothing quality, deep, good tone

23. Speech:

____ Vata—quick, talkative, erratic

____ Pitta—moderate, convincing, intense, argumentative, forceful

____ Kapha—quiet, deliberate, slow

24. Sleep:

____ Vata—light sleeper; may suffer from insomnia, wakes up at night and stays up worrying

____ Pitta—moderate sleeper; goes back to sleep easily

____ Kapha—heavy sleeper; sleeps deeply, but may be groggy upon awakening

25. Pulse:

____ Vata—the pulse will be fast, feeble, "slithery," with 80–100 beats per minute

____ Pita—the pulse will feel "like a frog jumping," excited and prominent, with a moderate rate of 60–75 beats per minute

____ Kapha—the pulse will be strong, regular, broad, steady, and slow, 60–70 beats per minute, and may be hard to find due to fat and thick tissue at the wrist area

Count the number of times you selected V, P, and K, and place the totals in the appropriate boxes below.

Next, determine from the scale below the relative strength for each dosha. For example if your total for vata was 7, then the vata part of your prakruti will be 2. If the total for the pitta is 16, your pitta part will be 3. If your kapha total is 2, your kapha part will be 1.

Total Vata ____ Total Pitta ____ Total Kapha ____

1–6 = a designation of 1

7–12 = a designation of 2

13–18 = a designation of 3

18–24 = a designation of 4

My prakruti is: V ____ P ____ K ____

In all, there are seven different prakruti possibilities:

• Predominantly vata

• Predominantly pitta

• Predominantly kapha

• Equal amounts of:

   • vata/pitta

   • vata/kapha

   • pitta/kapha

   • vata/pitta/kapha

Current Condition (Vikruti) Evaluation

When you have a minor or serious imbalance, certain symptoms can be evaluated as vata, pitta, or kapha in nature. While prakruti is what we are born with, vikruti will show us what is out of balance. To determine the vikruti it is important to evaluate the dosha of the condition as it is manifesting. One easy way to do this is to list all the symptoms, then try to evaluate each one to see if it is vata, pitta, or kapha in nature. For example, if you have indigestion, try to describe to yourself the feelings associated with it, such as: "sour burps and burning sensation in the stomach and colon. I develop a rash on my face after eating." This would indicate a pitta digestive disorder. Vikruti must be dealt with until the symptoms have cleared; then we can go back to our lifestyle and diet choices for prakruti.

It should be noted that some people have been out of balance for so long that they cannot figure out what the prakruti is until some of the imbalances are taken care of. That which is manifesting now must be addressed first. With complicated conditions, more than one dosha may be out of balance. I have provided some suggestions as to how to handle this type of situation. It may be best to obtain the advice of an Ayurvedic consultant for more serious illnesses.

This test will give you an idea as to how to evaluate your current condition. You do not have to answer all the questions, as some of them may not apply to your situation. The number that is the highest will show you your vikruti. Follow the diet and lifestyle considerations until the situation is handled and you are feeling better. Then return to the diet for your prakruti.

You may find that your vikruti is an exacerbation of your prakruti. For example, if you have a pitta prakruti you may find that the vikruti is pitta in nature also. The most prominent dosha in our constitution is often the one that becomes aggravated. This test is geared toward evaluating the acute conditions of colds, flu, cough, and stomach distress.

1. Complexion:

____ Vata—dark, brown, sallow

____ Pitta—red, yellow, rashes

____ Kapha—white, pale

2. Mucus:

____ Vata—clear, light, very runny

____ Pitta—yellow, green, maybe some blood

____ Kapha—white to clear, heavy, "stuck"

3. Circulation:

____ Vata—coldness in the body; hard to keep warm

____ Pitta—generally hot; sometimes heat in different areas of the body

____ Kapha—generally cool; possibly cold hands and feet

4. Discharges:

____ Vata—gas, burping, popping joints

____ Pitta—bleeding, pus, inflammation, rashes

____ Kapha—salivation, excess moisture

5. Qualify of Pain:

____ Vata—severe, throbbing, biting, intense, variable, migratory, intermittent

____ Pitta—medium, burning

____ Kapha—heavy, dull, constant

6. Quality of Fever:

____ Vata—moderate temperature, variable or irregular; thirst, anxiety, restlessness

____ Pitta—high temperature, burning sensation; thirst, sweating, irritability, delirium

____ Kapha—low-grade fever; dullness, heaviness; constant elevated temperature

7. Unusual Tastes in the Mouth:

____ Vata—astringent, dry

____ Pitta—bitter or pungent, increased salivation

____ Kapha—sweet or salty, profuse salivation, discharge of mucus

8. Quality of Cough:

____ Vata—dry cough with little mucus; difficulty with inhalation; feeling of constriction

____ Pitta—cough feels hot; phlegm has yellow or green color, possibly with blood mixed in

____ Kapha—heavy mucous condition with much congestion

9. Throat:

____ Vata—dry, rough; painful constriction of esophagus

____ Pitta—sore throat, inflammation, burning sensation

____ Kapha—swelling, dilation, edema, puffed-up feeling

10. Stomach/Digestion:

____ Vata—decreased secretions, irregular appetite, frequent belching or hiccup, tightness in the stomach, gas, bloating

____ Pitta—good appetite, but sour burps, burning sensation or ulceration

____ Kapha—slow digestion, sweet or mucousy burps, food "just sits there"

11. Stools:

____ Vata—constipation, painful and difficult bowel movements; dry stool, small in quantity

____ Pitta—diarrhea, i.e., watery stools; quick or uncontrollable evacuation; burning sensation, increased frequency, yellowish color

____ Kapha—solid; large amount with decreased frequency of elimination; may contain mucus; anus may itch

12. Urine:

____ Vata—colorless; scanty, difficult to discharge, increased frequency or absence of urination

____ Pitta—profuse, with burning sensation; increased frequency; yellow, turbid, brown, or red in color

____ Kapha—profuse with decreased frequency; mucus in urine, white or pale in color

13. Skin:

____ Vata—dry, scaly, rough

____ Pitta—red, inflamed, itchy

____ Kapha—swollen with excess water (edema)

Continued

14. Onset of Complaint:

___ Vata—rapid, variable, irregular

___ Pitta—medium, with fever

___ Kapha—slow, constant

15. Time of the Day When the Condition Is Most Aggravated:

___ Vata—dawn, dusk

___ Pitta—noon, midnight

___ Kapha—mid-morning, mid-evening

16. Season in Which Condition Is Aggravated:

___ Vata—fall, early winter

___ Pitta—summer, late spring

___ Kapha—late winter, early spring

17. External Aggravating Factors:

___ Vata—wind, cold, dryness

___ Pitta—heat, sun, fire, humidity

___ Kapha—dampness, cold

18. Foods That Seem to Aggravate the Situation:

___ Vata—Dry foods, beans, cold foods, raw foods, stale foods, carbonated drinks, caffeine

___ Pitta—hot and spicy food, salty foods, sour foods, meats, tomatoes, caffeine, acidy foods

___ Kapha—dairy foods, salt, sweets, cold drinks, fatty fried foods, caffeine

19. Emotions You Are Experiencing Now:

___ Vata—Fear, anxiety (perhaps with hyperventilation), insecurity, tremors, palpitations, instability, insomnia

___ Pitta—irritation, impatience, anger, frustration

___ Kapha—lethargy, sadness, apathy, dullness, sleepiness, depression

20. How Have You Been Sleeping?

___ Vata—wake up at night and cannot go back to sleep; insomnia

___ Pitta—go to sleep easily, but have disturbing dreams, night sweats, or fitful rest

___ Kapha—sleep okay, but lethargic in the morning; excessively tired

Add up the totals for vata, pitta and kapha and enter these totals in the spaces below. (For this test, your number is the actual result of the addition, not—as in the first test—a range defined by the result of the addition.) Follow the pacifying diet for the dosha that is the highest or most notably out of balance relative to the prakruti (basic condition) scale.

Vata ___ Pitta ___ Kapha ___

For example: V8, P2, K3. The vata-pacifying routine would be most appropriate for now.

If two doshas are equally elevated, then follow the diet and herbs that are common to both:

• If both pitta and kapha are equally elevated, note that both of these doshas respond well to bitter herbs. However, the diet should be mild and not include any dairy, which is kapha-provoking, and the spices should not be overly hot (i.e., pitta-provoking).

• If vata and pitta are equally elevated, the diet should be mild, with sweet grains and vegetables and possibly some meat protein. The spices should be mild as well. Demulcent and sweet herbs, such as marshmallow root, may be recommended, depending on the condition (see Dietary Recommendations page 181).

• If vata and kapha are equally elevated, follow a mild, warming diet, since both kapha and vata are cold in nature. Have lots of warm, spicy tea, and foods that are easy to digest but nourishing, such as stews and soups. Avoid cold foods and congestive foods such as dairy.

• If you notice that the symptoms are changing, then retake the vikruti test and note the results.

• After the conditions have subsided, you may go back to the diet and lifestyle recommendations for your prakruti (basic constitution).

Humans frequently become habituated to foods that do not agree with them—or which moderate or exacerbate their own worst tendencies. Vata people often become hypoglycemic because they love to eat sugar, which provides instant satisfaction by temporarily leveling out vata's mental roller coaster. Workaholic pitta people may become habituated to meat, hot spices and salt, which inflame pittas and make them even more driven, intense, and goal-oriented. Kapha people may find themselves habituated to heavy, fatty foods, which reinforce their tendency to stagnation and dullness.

We need to invoke our creative intelligence and awareness to move us toward the things and qualities that will support our deepest, truest selves. When we begin to implement changes in our lives, they should be accomplished slowly, with great awareness. Do not try to change your whole life at once, or you will be setting yourself up for failure. Decide that you will *slowly* cut down on a certain activity or food choice. And be sure to thank yourself for all the little steps you have taken toward better health.

Ayurveda and Diet

The Six Tastes

In order to understand why certain diets and herbs are recommended for each of the doshas, it is important to understand the six tastes (*rasas*) that pervade our lives.

Sweet: The sweet taste is found in sugars and starches, and is composed of the elements earth and water. Examples of sweet foods include grains, sweet vegetables, and sweet fruits. The sweet taste builds and strengthens body tissue, soothes the mucous membranes, and allays burning sensations. Sweet foods increase the quality of kapha in the body and promote calmness, contentment and harmonization of the mind. The sweet taste helps the vata person and the pitta person because both these doshas are lacking some of the grounding, building, soothing qualities of kapha. Note, however, that if a person has a kapha condition of mucus or excess fat, the sweet taste will increase these qualities. "Empty" sweets such as cakes and cookies, made with refined sweetener and flours, are deranging to all constitutions.

Salty: The salty taste is found in table salt, rock salt, sea salt, and seaweeds. It is composed of the elements water and fire. The salty taste adds warmth and moisture to the body, thus increasing kapha dampness and pitta heat. In small amounts, the salty taste aids digestion, is sedating, and softens the body tissues—all useful therapies for the vata person. Pittas and kaphas must stay away from excess salt, which will cause them aggravation.

Pungent: The pungent taste is found in hot spices such as ginger and cayenne, and contains abundant amounts of the elements fire and air. The pungent taste is heating, drying and stimulating, increasing the rate of metabolism (by about 15 percent), counteracting cold sensations and aiding in digestion. Kaphas can use a generous amount of spices in their diets to counteract their general dampness, coolness, and stagnancy. Vatas can use some spice to warm them up, but they must use it with caution because it is also drying; they ought to use spices with foods that are liquid, warm, and oily, such as soups and stews. Pittas are usually warm enough and may have problems with burning sensations, so they do not need much spice. People who are suffering from pitta conditions, such as rashes or inflammation, should also avoid spices.

Sour: The sour taste contains the elements earth and fire, and is thirst-relieving and nourishing, dispels gas and stimulates growth of bodily tissues. The sour taste is found in fermented foods such as yogurt, miso, pickles, buttermilk, and sour fruits, as well as in acidic fruits. Sour is good for vatas as it will warm, moisten, and ground them. Kaphas should not eat much that is sour as it will make them damper, and pittas may become overheated or experience burning sensations in the stomach and intestines. It should be noted that although bananas taste sweet, they have a postdigestive sour quality and may create burning sensations or aggravate ulcers (a pitta condition).

Bitter: The bitter taste contains the elements air and space, and is found in herbs such as gentian and goldenseal, and in foods such as dandelion greens and chard. The bitter taste is cooling, drying, and detoxifying, reducing all bodily tissues, and creating lightness in the body and the mind. This taste will help kaphas, because it will lighten and dry up the bulk and the water in the system. It is also good for pittas, as it cools off the heat in their liver and other areas, as well as allaying inflammation such as fevers. A vata person or a person with a vata condition should not have very many bitters in the diet, however; they will be too dehydrating.

Astringent: The drying astringent taste, composed of the elements air and earth, stops excess discharges such as sweating and diarrhea, promotes the healing of tissues, and makes the cells of the body firmer. It is good for moist kaphas because it will squeeze them out like a sponge. It is also good for pittas because it will dry up excess acids and moisture. (Remember, the elements fire and water dominate the pitta institution.) Astringent herbs are good for healing wounds as well. Foods with the astringent taste include cranberries, apples, and pomegranates. Astringent herbs include oak bark, witch hazel, and raspberry leaves.

TASTE AND THE THREE DOSHAS

Vata

Aggravated by:	Balanced by:
bitter	sweet
astringent	sour
excess pungent	salty

Remember, we want to pacify vata, not aggravate it.

Pitta

Aggravated by:	Balanced by:
sour	sweet
pungent	bitter
salty	astringent

Sour, salty, and pungent are too heating for pitta.

Kapha

Aggravated by:	Balanced by:
sweet	pungent
salty	bitter
sour	astringent

The sweet, salty, and sour tastes have watery, building qualities which kapha does not need.

Continued ➔

COMPLEX AND PURE FORMS OF THE SIX TASTES

The complex forms of the tastes are less likely to aggravate vata, pitta, or kapha, as they require more assimilation and therefore do not have as strong or fast-acting effects as the pure forms.

Taste	Pure Form	Complex
sweet	sugar	complex carbohydrates, rice, grains
salty	table salt	seaweeds
pungent	cayenne pepper, garlic	mild spices such as cardamom and fennel
sour	alcohol	sour food (buttermilk)
bitter	pure bitter (gentian)	mild bitter (dandelion and aloe vera juice)
astringent	strong tannins (oak bark)	mild astringents (red raspberry)

Agni: "Digestive Fires"

Agni, named after the Hindu god of fire, is the "biological fire" that rules digestion. Agni is:

- hot
- subtle
- dry
- mobile
- light
- penetrating
- fragrant

Agni is the creative flame of transformation behind all life, as well as the acidic substance that breaks down food and stimulates digestion. Agni is increased by hot, fragrant spices such as ginger, black pepper, and cayenne, each of which has a similar nature to agni.

Agni also maintains the body's autoimmune mechanism. Strong agni destroys microorganisms, bacteria, and toxins in the stomach, as well as in the small and large intestines. It is also the protector of the good flora in the body. Skin color, the enzyme system, and metabolism all depend on agni. When agni is functioning optimally, the breakdown, absorption, and assimilation of food will be operating efficiently.

When agni becomes impaired due to an imbalance in one's constitution, the body will not receive the nutrients it needs. Eventually this will result in a breakdown of the immune system. Food material that is not digested properly becomes a foul-smelling, sticky substance that clogs the intestines and other channels, such as the blood vessels; in Ayurvedic terminology, this is called *ama*, or undigested waste. Ama accumulates, then travels through the blood to become lodged in the weakest organs. In this way, disease conditions are manifested.

Everyone, no matter what his or her constitution, should work at keeping the digestive fires strong so as not to accumulate ama, which reduces general health and clarity of mind.

Pitta types may have high agni. If it is too high due to an excess of digestive acids, the food may go through the system too quickly, resulting in burning sensations. Vatas may have irregular agni: one day they can eat anything, the next day everything bothers them. Kaphas tend to have low agni, and therefore exhibit slow metabolism and heaviness.

Agni is improved by:

- eating the foods appropriate for your constitution (prakruti) or current condition (vikruti)
- chewing well
- eating smaller portions
- taking a small amount of bitter herbs, such as dandelion extract or artichoke extract, before meals. (Bitter extracts may be purchased at health-food stores; take 20–40 drops 15 minutes before meals.)
- eating clean, natural, fresh foods
- eating fruit and vegetables in season

Agni is impaired by:

- overeating
- drinking cold or iced drinks, which put out the digestive fires
- drinking alcohol with meals
- eating too quickly
- eating poor food combinations
- watching TV, reading, or driving when eating
- eating when upset
- drinking coffee with or after meals
- eating denatured, stale, lifeless food
- eating microwaved foods, which had their "life force" destroyed

Dietary Recommendations

For predominantly vata, pitta, or kapha:

Follow the dietary recommendations for your prominent dosha throughout the year, making appropriate seasonal adjustments when necessary.

For vata-pitta:

Follow up vata-pacifying diet from fall through winter and early spring, the pitta-pacifying diet from late spring through summer.

For vata-kapha:

Follow the vata-pacifying diet from summer through fall, the kapha-pacifying diet from winter through spring.

For pitta-kapha:

Follow the pitta-pacifying diet from late spring through fall, the kapha-pacifying diet from winter through early spring.

For tri-doshic (vata-pitta-kapha):

Change diet according to the season: vata-pacifying diet during the fall, kapha-pacifying diet during winter to early spring, pitta-pacifying diet from late spring through summer.

Vata

Vata food should be:

- very nourishing
- moist
- cooked
- mildly spiced
- warm

Meals should be consumed at regular hours to alleviate the vata tendency toward hypoglycemia and nervousness. This type of food and routine will counteract vata's dry, cold, light, agitated, dispersing, mobile nature.

Grains: Well-cooked oats and rice are very healthy for vatas. Buckwheat, corn, millet, and rye are also recommended, but only when cooked with extra water; otherwise, these grains can be drying to vatas or in vata conditions.

Vegetables: Vatas do better with cooked than raw vegetables. Hard vegetables like celery are better for vatas when juiced. Tomato sauce (not whole tomatoes) with spices added is okay from time to time. Asparagus, beets, carrots, celery, garlic, okra, onions, parsnip, radish, rutabaga, turnip, sweet potato, and water chestnut are all fine. Broccoli and other vegetables of the brassica family may be added to stews and soups, or steamed well with a spice-and-oil dressing to counteract gas formation. Raw salads and vegetables may be too cooling and therefore hard for vatas to digest, so vata people are advised to stay away from them unless the digestive processes are quite healthy.

Fruits: Most fruits, excepting the astringent ones or any unripe fruit, are fine. If raw fruit causes digestive problems, take the fruit stewed with cinnamon or other mild spices. Vatas should have no dried fruit unless reconstituted; plain dried fruit dries the vata person out too much. Apricot, banana, cherry, dates, figs, grapes, grapefruit, lemon, limes, mango, papaya, peaches, pears, persimmons, pineapple, plums, oranges, and tangerines are all fine.

Meats: Meats tend to ground and nourish vatas or vata conditions, but remember that heavy meats can dull the mind. Purchase organic meat whenever possible, and choose chicken and fish over beef and pork.

Legumes: Mung beans are best for vata. Vatas may have soy products in moderation if there is no consequent discomfort.

Nuts and Seeds: Vatas may eat nuts in moderation—not big handfuls of them! Peanuts are not recommended, because they clot the blood. Nut butters are better, again in moderation. Almonds (without skins), black walnuts, cashews, Brazil nuts, coconut, pecans, pine nuts, pistachios, macadamia nuts, flax seed, halvah, psyllium, pumpkin, sesame and sunflower seed are all fine.

Oils: Sesame is the best oil for vata, while safflower oil is the worst. Olive oil, ghee (see glossary), and almond oil are also recommended.

Dairy: All dairy is good for vatas who are not allergic to it. Hard cheeses, however, should be cooked into a more liquid form. Lassi, a beverage made of yogurt blended with water and spices (see glossary), especially helps vatas.

Sweet: Vatas may use sweeteners in moderation. A healthy sweetener on the market is Sucanat(r), made from the dehydrated juice of organic sugarcane.

Spices: Spices will help with digestion and counteract gas but they are drying—so use them only in vata-pacifying foods, or as tea. Especially recommended are anise, fennel, cloves, pepper, bay, orange peel, oregano, rosemary, garlic, ginger, cumin, cinnamon, hingashtak (a combination of herbs for gas and digestion that may be purchased at East Indian markets), cardamom, and nutmeg.

Herbs: Building herbs for vata constitutions or conditions include:

codonopsis (*Codonopsis pilosula*; Chinese *Dang shen*)

American ginseng (*Panax quinquefolium*)

dong quai (*Angelica sinensis*)

angelica (*archangelica*)

marshmallow root (*althea officinalis*)

aloe vera juice or gel (*aloe barbadensis*)—mix with a pinch of ginger to counteract aloe's cold nature

shatavari (*Asparagus racemosus*)

ashwagandha or winter cherry (*withania sonnifera*)

slippery elm (*Ulmus fulva*)

licorice root (*Glycyrrhiza glabra*)

Herbs for Elimination:

triphala (*Myrobalan*)

psyllium husks (*Plantago psyllium*)

Continued ➡

Herbs for the Nerves:

basil (*Ocinum spp.*)

biota seeds (*Biota orientalis*)

valerian (*Valeriana officinalis*)

jujube dates (*ziziphus jujube*)

oatstraw (*Avena Sativa*)

The preceding herbs may be mixed with the cooling, bitter nervine herbs such as skullcap and passion flower. Combining warmer-energy herbs with cooling herbs will counteract the cooling quality.

Other Vata-Pacifying Herbs:

orange peel (*Citrus aurantium*)

fresh ginger (*zingiber officinalis*)

fennel (*foeniculum vulgare*)

hawthorn (*crataegus oxycantha*)

sassafras (*sassafras albidum*)

sarsaparilla (*smilax spp.*)

lemon grass (*cymbopogon citrates*)

rose hips (*rosa spp.*)

Vatas are prone to addiction, so all addictive substances—drugs, alcohol, cigarettes, caffeine, white sugar, et cetera—should be avoided.

Vata is calmed down by regular application of oils. I use the following blend:

2 oz. sesame oil

2 oz. almond oil

10 drops lavender essential oil

10 drops rose geranium essential oil

Mix ingredients together and use daily all over the body. The feet may be massaged at night with this formula to allow for more restful sleep.

Pitta

Pitta food should be:

- cool in nature
- very mildly spiced
- sweet in taste
- small amounts of bitter and astringent

The food should not be too spicy, hot, sour, or salty. Pittas should avoid meat and alcohol. Steamed or stir-fried vegetables are recommended, and if the pitta person has good digestion, raw vegetables may be eaten as well. Mild spices are fine, and the atmosphere for a meal should be calm. (Pittas should not eat while conducting business meetings, nor should they engage in heavy discussions over dinner.) In general, people with the pitta constitution will do best on a vegetarian diet.

Grains: barley, rice, oats, wheat, amaranth, dry cereal, couscous, tapioca.

Vegetables: All vegetables that are sweet and bitter are fine; sour vegetables such as tomatoes, as well as pungent vegetables such as radishes and garlic, should be avoided. Steamed white or yellow onions are okay occasionally; red or purple onions are too hot, as are peppers. Pittas can have asparagus, artichoke, cooked beets, broccoli, Brussels sprouts, cabbage, cauliflower, cilantro, cucumber, celery, green beans, leafy greens, lettuce, mushrooms, okra, black olives, peas, parsley, potatoes, squash, sweet potatoes, pumpkin, wheat grass, and sprouts.

Fruits: Sweet fruits are okay; avoid sour. Papaya has too great a heating quality, and bananas have a souring effect in the body. Figs and sweet grapes are especially good for pittas, as are sweet apples, avocado, berries, cherries, coconut, dates, figs, limes, melons, pears, plums, pomegranates, prunes, and raisins. Sweet oranges and pineapples are tolerated by some pittas, but others may find them irritating.

Flesh Foods: Pittas should avoid eating seafood because it is "heating" in nature and tends to cause allergies. Freshwater fish would be a better choice. Flesh foods generally encourage pitta aggression and irritability. Meats that tend to be less aggravating for pitta are white meat of chicken and turkey, rabbit, and venison.

Legumes: Pittas can have all beans, including aduki, black and white beans, chickpeas, kidney beans, lentils, lima and mung beans, mung dahl, navy beans, peas, pinto beans, soy products, split peas, and tempeh.

Nuts and Seeds: Pittas should avoid nuts for the most part because they are too oily. Peanuts are not recommended because they clot the blood. Small quantities (1 tbsp. or less) of walnuts, pecans, Brazil nuts, cashews (occasionally) are okay. Large amounts would have an unbalancing effect on pitta. Nuts that are most beneficial to pitta are almonds (soaked and peeled), coconut, pumpkin seeds (unsalted), sunflower seeds, flax, and pine nuts.

Oils: Pitta can use the following oils internally: sunflower, ghee (see glossary), canola, olive. Externally, pitta will find the use of coconut oil quite cooling.

Dairy: Pitta can have unsalted butter, soft unsalted cheese, cottage cheese, milk, the yogurt beverage lassi, and ghee (see glossary).

Sweet: The sweet taste cools off pitta. It is best to avoid large amounts of molasses and long-term use of honey, as both have a heating effect. Pittas can use fruit-juice sweetener, barley malt, maple syrup, rice syrup, Sucanat, or turbinado sugar.

Spices: fresh basil, cardamom, cilantro, cinnamon, coriander, dill, fennel, fresh ginger, mints, orange peel, saffron, turmeric, and small amounts of cumin, black pepper, and vanilla are all recommended.

Herbs: The herbs listed below are best for pitta and pitta conditions such as heat and inflammation. Herbs with a cooling, sweet, bitter, and astringent energy are best for pitta.

Herb Beverages for Pitta and Pitta Conditions:

catnip (*nepeta catarid*)

alfalfa (*medicago sativa*)

violets (*viola spp.*)

mints (*menthe spp.*)

chickweed (*stellaria media*)

nettles (*urtica urens*)

raspberry (*Rubus spp.*)

cleavers (*galium spp.*)

grain "coffee" substitutes (Pero, Cafix, Inca)

cinnamon, in moderation (*cinnamomum zeylanicum*)

cardamom, in moderation (*elettaria cardamomum*)

strawberry leaf (*fragaria spp.*)

Herbs for Calming and Relaxing:

lavender (*lavandula spp.*)

rose petals (*rosa spp.*)

skullcap (*scutellaria spp.*)

passion flower (*passiflora incarnate*)

biota seeds (*biota orientalis*)

zizyphus seeds (*zizyphus spinosa*)

chamomile (*matricaria chamomile*)

lemon balm (*melissa officinalis*)

oatstraw (*avena sativa*)

Herbs for the Liver (Pitta Organ):

barberry bark (*berberis spp.*)

dandelion leaf and root (*taraxacum vulgare*)

fennel (*foeniculum vulgare*)

gentian (*gentiana spp.*)

hops (*humulus lupulus*)

milk thistle seed (*silybum marianum*)

sarsaparilla (*smilax spp.*)

burdock root and seeds (*arctium lappa*)

red clover (*trifolium pretense*)

yellow dock (*rumex crispus*)

turmeric (*curcuma longa*)

Herbs to Strengthen and Build Energy in a Pitta Person:

aloe vera (*aloe spp.*)

licorice (*glycyrrhiza glabra*)

marshmallow root (*althea officinalis*)

peony root (*paeonia lactiflora*)

comfrey (*symphytum officinale*)

slippery elm (*ulmus fulva*)

shitavari (*asparagus racemosus*)

Herbs for Elimination:

For loose stool:

amalaki (*emblica officinalis*)

psyllium husks (*plantago psyllium*)

These two herbs work tell in combination with one another. Mix equal parts and take two "oo" capsules at bedtime.

For constipation:

prunes

cascara sagrada

Herbs for Infection and Inflammation (Pitta Conditions):

echinacea (*echinacea purpurea—angustifolia* pallida)

goldenseal (*hydrastis Canadensis*)

Oregon grape root (*mabonia repens*)

usnea or lichen (*Usnea longissima* and others)

boneset (*eupatorium peerfoliatum*)

Kapha

Kapha food should be:

- warm, dry, light in nature
- emphasize pungent, bitter, astringent tastes
- spicy
- vegetable-rich

Kaphas and those with kapha conditions need to avoid or minimize the sweet, sour, and salty tastes. Fried or greasy foods are extremely detrimental.

Grains: Hot, drying grains like buckwheat and millet are good for kapha, as are barley, rice, corn, dry cereals, couscous, crackers (unsalted), muesli, dry oats, and polenta. Breads should be avoided unless toasted.

Vegetables: Kaphas can eat most vegetables. Not recommended are sweet potatoes, pumpkin, zucchini, winter and spaghetti squash, raw tomatoes, and cucumbers.

Fruits: Avoid sweet and sour fruits. Dried fruits are okay. Cold fruit juice may be mucus-forming, so take juice warm in small amounts.

Flesh: Meats are best roasted or broiled in small amounts: white chicken, eggs, freshwater fish, shrimp, turkey (white meat), rabbit.

Legumes: Aduki, black beans, chickpeas, lentils, lima, navy, peas, pinto, soy products, tempeh, white beans.

Nuts and Seeds: Avoid nuts. Popcorn with no salt or butter is fine, as are sunflower seeds and pumpkin seeds.

Continued ➡

Oils: In general, avoid oils, but when necessary use corn, canola, sunflower, ghee (see glossary), and almond.

Dairy: Avoid for the most part, although very small amounts of unsalted butter or ghee (see glossary), cottage cheese from skimmed milk, goat's cheese (unsalted), goat's milk, the yogurt beverage lassi (see glossary), and soy milk (without added oil) are okay.

Sweeteners: Raw honey, sparingly.

Spices: All spices are good, except salt. One spice in particular is very good for kapha: trikatu (see glossary), which breaks up mucus and facilitates digestion.

Herbs: building herbs for kapha include:

aloe vera juice/gel (*aloe spp.*)

angelica archangelica

elecampane (*Inula spp.*)

Siberian ginseng (*eleutherococcus senticosus*)

dong quai (*angelica sinensis*)

ashwagandha (*withania somnifera*)

Often, kaphas do not need building as much as stimulating herbs, such as spices, to break up congestion in the body. The tonic herbs listed above—many of which have a warming energy and help move energy—are recommended for kaphas who feel weak and run-down.

Herbs for Cleansing:

barberry (*berberis spp.*)

bayberry bark (*myrica cerifera*)

cascara sagrada

hops (*humulus lupulus*)

dandelion (*taraxacum vulgare*)

burdock (*arctium lappa*)

Oregon grape root (*mabonia repens*)

milk thistle seed (*silybum marianum*)

turmeric (*curcuma longa*)

juniper berries (*juniperus spp.*)

eucalyptus (*eucalyptus globules*)

fennel (*foeniculum vulgare*)

Herbs for Mucous Conditions:

elecampane (*inula spp.*)

ginger (*zingiber officinalis*)

horehound (*marrubium vulgare*)

hyssop (*hyssopus officinalis*)

thyme (*thymus vulgaris*)

garlic (*allium sativum*)

grindelia (*grindelia robusta*)

marshmallow root (*althea officinalis*)—helps to liquify mucus; small amounts may be added to cough formulas; excess amounts may increase kapha and ama (toxins)

licorice (*glycyrrhiza glabra*)—*small amounts of licorice root may be added to help liquify mucus; excess amounts of licorice may create water retention in some people*

Other Herbs for Kapha:

alfalfa (*medicago sativa*)

chamomile (*anthemis nobilis*)

lavender (*lavandula spp.*)

lemon grass (*cymbopogon citrates*)

chicory (*cichorium intybus*)

hibiscus (*hibiscus trosa sinensis*)

lemon balm (*melissa officinalis*)

mints (*menthe*)

red clover (*trifolium pretense*)

grain beverages

FOOD QUALITY

For many thousands of years of Ayurvedic practice, there was no concern about whether food was organically grown or free of chemicals. In modern times, we should take pains to find out whether our food has been contaminated by antibiotics, growth hormones, drugs, pesticides, or herbicides. Such drugs are easily transferred to human beings through diet, creating a disruption of the beneficial flora in the digestive tract and eventually compromising the immune system.

The FDA permits milk to contain a certain concentration of 80 different antibiotics, used on dairy cows to prevent udder infections. Plant foods grown with petrochemical fertilizers are very low in mineral content; they may look pretty, but they do not contain the same level of vitality as organic produce. Such pesticide and herbicide residues also create adverse reactions in the body-mind.

White sugar is deranging to everyone—vatas, pittas, kaphas—so don't use it. Two other dangerous additives, becoming more and more prevalent in our foods, are Nutrasweet and MSG. Both of these substances can aggravate the liver and nervous system, and should be avoided whenever possible.

It is important for each of us to try our best to purchase clean produce, dairy products, and meat. For readers who do not have resources for such products close by, there are many natural-foods cooperatives around the country that will ship foods free of drugs and pesticides to different locales. I also feel that, if possible, we should all try growing some of our own food and herbs, which will enhance our sense of responsibility for what we eat, and get us in tune with the seasons and nature.

Due to the excessive consumption of antibiotics (whether prescribed by a doctor, or in milk and meats), cortisone, birth-control pills, and sugar, many people have had the favorable flora in their digestive tracts destroyed. Digestion therefore may be irregular, with excessive gas, bloating, malabsorption of nutrients, and an overgrowth of yeast. In my practice I have found it necessary to advise people to replace the good flora with acidophilus supplementation. Some people have had to stay on high doses of acidophilus—one teaspoon of the powder three times per day for six months to one year—in order to handle their yeast and digestive disruptions. As a preventative treatment, acidophilus may be taken for one month twice in a year.

Life Cycles

Times of the Day

Morning, after sunrise, is the kapha time of the day. People with a mucous condition will have more mucus flowing at this time. There may be a tendency to sluggishness, as the digestive fires may not have been awakened yet. A mild, spicy herbal tea—such as fresh ginger tea, or cinnamon blended with cardamom and orange peel—is appropriate for the morning. Stay away from cold juice and cheese, which will only create more mucus.

Evening after sunset is the other kapha time of the day. Again, one should be careful not to eat kapha-type foods, such as cheese and ice cream; otherwise, mucus may accumulate and create difficulty the following morning.

Pitta time is the afternoon, when the sun is high in the sky. The digestive fires are also high, and this is the best time for the main meal of the day. For those with pitta conditions, it is best to stay away from alcohol, spices, and other heating foods during the noon hour; otherwise, there may be some provoking of burning sensations.

Eleven P.M. until around one or two a.m. is the other pitta time of day. People with gallstones or liver problems may experience discomfort at this time because of the increased acid flow. It is therefore best to avoid acidic, spicy foods before bed; otherwise, there may be acid indigestion and other burning sensations later in the night. Try having a cup of mild, calming tea before bed for a restful sleep. A good blend is passion flower, chamomile, and spearmint.

Sunrise and sunset, and the hours just before, are the vata times of the day. Many people with vata disturbances and worries will wake up around three a.m. and start to think about their own problems or the problems of the world. This may also be a time when disturbing dreams occur. Many yogis will get up at three or four A.M. and practice meditation because this is a good time for tapping into deeper inspiration.

Sunset and sunrise are both times of great transition. Remember, vata governs our aspiration to higher consciousness. Many cultures around the world pray and meditate at these times in order to focus on the divine principles that govern life.

Seasons of the Year

Each season, with its characteristic weather conditions, expresses a certain constitution. If we become aware of the different qualities, we can moderate our activities to harmonize with the season.

Fall	Winter–Early Spring	Late Spring–Summer
(vata season)	(kapha season)	(pitta season)
windy	cold	hot
dry	damp	humid
cold	foggy	bright

Vata people and conditions will be most affected by dry, windy, cold environments; they must closely follow the vata-pacifying diet and stay out of the cold. Pitta people and conditions will be affected during hot weather; during the hot months they must stay out of the direct sun and eat cooling foods. Kapha people and conditions will be affected adversely during cold, damp times; they need to eat spicy, dry foods during those times, so as to reduce accumulation of mucus and congestion.

Seasons of Our Lives

Just as the seasons change throughout the year, human beings experience different seasons in their lives:

Kapha	Pitta	Vata
(childhood)	(adulthood)	(seniors)
development	production	detachment
building	create/transform	completions
(anabolism)	(metabolism)	(catabolism)
mucous conditions	heat conditions	bone conditions

Underlying our constitution and our imbalances are the seasons of our lives. During the kapha-building stage of life, children may experience mucous conditions and therefore need to have limits imposed on the amount of dairy they take in, or at least have their milk gently boiled with a pinch of cardamom, cinnamon, and ginger. (These spices

Continued ➔

counteract milk's mucus-producing qualities.) They will also need foods that help them to build physically and mentally.

During the adult years, people often experience inflammatory heart and blood diseases. At this phase, we require herbs and foods that help keep the digestion strong and energy moving: hawthorn berries for the heart, dandelion for the liver, marshmallow root for the kidneys.

In the senior years, bodies no longer regenerate as easily and there may be a breakdown of various systems. Seniors often experience vata conditions such as coldness, arthritis, and poor elimination. They need foods and a lifestyle that are nourishing and calming. Daily applications of oil to their bodies will help with dryness. Herbs such as ginkgo will stimulate blood circulation in the brain, which will offset any tendencies toward memory loss. Other helpful herbs are ashwagandha for building and marshmallow root for lubricating the inner organs.

Knowing that we are in a certain season of our lives, we can acknowledge and accept the changes that we are experiencing and, with greater awareness, take the appropriate steps to enhance our physical and spiritual evolution.

Simple Remedies for Common Ailments

Digestive Disturbances

Vata-type digestive disturbance:

- gas
- bloating
- variable appetite
- constipation
- insomnia
- palpitations
- nervousness

Follow the vata-pacifying diet and routine. Try to live your life rhythmically, eliminating any erratic or chaotic ways. This applies especially to mealtimes. Do not skip meals, then eat frantically because of extreme hunger. Do not eat while agitated, while working, or while running from place to place. Create an atmosphere of quiet and calm at mealtimes. Avoid sugary foods like cookies and ice cream, or dry foods like crackers or rice cakes. Have some spiced tea—e.g., ginger, fennel, cumin, cardamom or cinnamon—during the day and after meals. Cook foods with an emphasis on culinary spices. The herbal combination called *hingashtak*, which may be purchased from most Indian markets (see distributors listed in back of this guide), is recommended. One-eighth to one-quarter teaspoon may be added to vegetables as they saute to enhance digestion and absorption. A cup of ginger tea may be helpful after meals as well—or try chewing fennel seeds.

Pitta-type digestive disturbance:

- heartburn
- hyperacidity
- diarrhea or loose stool
- irritability
- gas
- burning sensation when excreting
- rash or redness of the skin

The pitta-pacifying diet should be followed, with strict avoidance of acidic and spicy foods. Try cooling carminatives (herbs that relieve intestinal gas, pain, and stomach distention), such as mints, fennel and coriander. Bitter herbs are also appropriate. Try this bitter combination:

2 parts gentian	1 part fennel
2 parts dandelion	1/8 part dried ginger
1 part Oregon grape	1/8 part licorice

This may be taken as an alcoholic extract (tincture), in capsules, or in a tea. It is best to take bitters 15 minutes before meals, or as burning sensations occur.

A tea of cumin, coriander, and fennel is also helpful. Mix equal parts of the three herbs together, put one teaspoon of the combination in a cup of boiling water and let it steep for 10 minutes. Drink after meals.

A simple tea of dandelion, mint, and licorice may be helpful as well. Aloe vera juice is also very cooling and alleviates burning.

Demulcent herbs (herbs that soothe and protect the internal membranes) may be brewed into a tea, along with some of the bitters. The following is a good combination:

marshmallow root	mint
dandelion leaf	licorice root

Mix one ounce each of these herbs together. Take one tablespoon of the combination and place it in boiling water. Let steep for 20 minutes, strain, and drink as needed.

Kapha-type digestive disturbance:

If we eat lots of foods that are mucus-forming—such as ice cream and cheese, fatty fried foods, or rancid foods—we may experience kapha digestive problems. Symptoms include:

- nausea and vomiting
- mucus in throat or chest after meals
- lethargy after meals
- general congestion

The kapha-pacifying regimen must be followed, and no cold food or drink should be taken. Do not overeat, and keep the diet simple: soups, steamed vegetables, grains. Morning and evening are the kapha times of the day. There will be a greater tendency for the body to create mucus at these times. Therefore, do not eat cold, mucus-forming foods—milk, cheese, ice cream, yogurt, et cetera—in the mornings or evenings. Hot spices are appropriate treatment for kapha disturbances. The following are kapha-pacifying spices:

- cayenne
- dried ginger
- pepper
- cinnamon
- cloves
- cardamom
- Yogi tea (available at most health stores)

Bitters may also be taken before meals when kapha is disturbed. Remember, the bitter, pungent, and astringent tastes are pacifying to kapha conditions. You may use the recipe for bitters listed under pitta digestive disturbances; however, a little extra ginger and even a pinch of cayenne will make the formula even better for the kapha condition.

Colds and Flu

Vata-type cold and flu

Symptoms include:

- dry cough
- dry nose or throat
- clear mucus, but scanty
- insomnia
- loss of voice due to dryness
- chills
- erratic fever
- fear or anxiety

The treatment for the vata-type cold and flu is basically to heat up and moisten the sufferer. This is best accomplished by using warming spices such as cinnamon, cardamom, ginger, garlic, and Yogi tea. Helpful demulcent herbs include licorice, marshmallow, comfrey, and slippery elm. A warm bath with the addition of one-quarter cup powdered ginger will help alleviate chills; a heating pad or hot-water bottle on the kidneys may also give some relief. The sufferer should stay warm and out of drafts. Generally, the vata-pacifying regimen should be adhered to, with an emphasis on simple, warming foods. Hard-to-digest food such as nuts and dairy should be avoided. If the nasal passages are dry and sore, then three or four drops sesame oil in the nostrils will help to lubricate the area.

To boost the immune system, take the herb echinacea mixed with a little licorice root, one dropperful of the tincture or two capsules every two hours during acute stages. Licorice root will help counteract the dizzy feelings some people—especially vata types—experience when taking echinacea. Cut the dose back as symptoms subside.

Pitta-type cold and flu

Symptoms include:

- high fever
- burning sensation
- heat
- yellow or green discharges
- sore throat
- agitation

Follow the pitta-pacifying diet, but avoid meat and dairy. If the sufferer has an appetite, offer mild soups and broths. Cooling herbs such as burdock, elder flowers, peppermint, yarrow, lemon balm, and mints will also be helpful. Echinacea and goldenseal may be taken every two hours until symptoms subside. These herbs are very bitter and will enhance the body's healing capacities. Bitters reduce heat in the body and are very cleansing to the system. (For a list of bitters, see the pitta food list under "Dietary Recommendations.")

To ease a sore throat, add about four or five drops tea-tree oil to one-half cup warm water and gargle. This can be done a number of times throughout the day, and it is okay to swallow after gargling. Tea tree is an excellent antiseptic and antibiotic. Echinacea and/or goldenseal extract may be used in this manner as well.

To help break a fever, make a strong tea of the following herbs:

elder flowers

peppermint

yarrow

Mix equal parts of the herbs together. Take one heaping tablespoon of the combination and let it steep in a cup of boiling water for 15 minutes. Drink up to three cups per day. To induce sweating, you may want to wrap yourself in a blanket while drinking this tea.

Kapha-type cold and flu

Symptoms include:

- low-grade fever
- loss of appetite
- excess mucus, clear or white in color
- excess salivation
- mucus in stool or urine
- lethargy or heavy feeling
- possible chilled feeling

If there is an appetite, then follow the kapha-pacifying diet. The food should be very simple,

Continued ➡

mainly soups and broths. Do not take heavy foods such as cheese, meat, or bread.

About one-quarter to one-half teaspoon trikatu paste in hot water may be taken as a tea, as needed, throughout the day. The bitter herbs listed in the section on pitta digestive disturbances may be taken as well. Strong ginger tea usually helps quite a bit: grate about three tablespoons of fresh ginger and let it gently steep in two cups of water for 15 minutes or so. Add honey and lemon to taste.

Echinacea and/or goldenseal may be taken every two hours. Echinacea helps activate the immune system; goldenseal cleanses the mucous membranes and counteracts inflammation. Continue until the symptoms subside, then cut the dose back to three times per day.

If the sufferer feels chilled, a ginger bath may be appropriate. Add one-quarter cup of ginger powder to the tub. Soak for 15 minutes or longer.

Coughs

A cough with phlegm and congestion usually indicates a kapha disorder. The kapha-pacifying diet must be accompanied by strict avoidance of iced drinks, fruit juices, soda, fried foods, cheese, milk, dairy, and white sugar. Such cold and "heavy" foods will increase mucus throughout the body. On the other hand, warm, spicy teas may be taken freely throughout the day. Ginger tea with honey will be especially therapeutic. Many times a short fast is helpful when one has a cough, cold, or flu.

A simple home remedy for relieving congestion is to chop three onions and steam them until they are soft. Place the onions between two layers of cheesecloth, then place the warm mass on the chest or upper back. Cover the area with a dry cloth and keep it warm with a hot-water bottle or heating pad for 30 minutes or longer. Onions have natural antibiotic properties and are a tremendous aid against pneumonia, lung infection, asthma, and mucous congestion due to colds.

Eucalyptus essential oil may be mixed with olive or sesame oils, 10 drops of the essential oil per ounce of base oil. Shake well, then rub directly on the chest or back to relieve lung congestion. The aroma will also help clear sinuses.

Warming expectorant herbs

The following herbs have a spicy, "warm" nature and help in the treatment of coughing, vomiting, asthma, and other mucous conditions. They help to remove energy-channel blockages in the body that may cause nerve damage, strokes, paralysis, and tremors:

- yerba santa
- platycodon
- osha root
- hyssop
- lovage
- thyme
- elecampane
- basil

Antispasmodic herbs

The following herbs, which are used mainly for conditions of cold with dampness (kapha) or heat with dampness (pitta), will help with cough spasms that leave a person exhausted or in pain, and may be combined with some of the other herbs in this section:

- wild lettuce
- mullein
- wild cherry bark
- apricot seed
- coltsfoot

- anise seeds
- lobelia

Demulcent herbs for coughs

The herbs in this category are used to help soften mucus for elimination. They also help to cool and lubricate inflamed mucous membranes:

- marshmallow root
- licorice root
- comfrey root

The following formula tastes nasty, but will also help to break up mucus:

2 parts elecampane
1 part thyme leaves
1 part grindelia
1 part Mormon tea (American ephedra)
1/2 part licorice root
1/4 part anise seeds

Gently simmer one ounce of this combination for 20 minutes in three cups of water, strain, and drink 1/2 cup of the tea four or five times per day. Add honey if desired.

Vata-Type Coughs

Coughs may be the result of imbalances in the other humors, as well. The vata-type cough will be dry with very little expectoration. When a coughing spasm occurs, there may be pain in the chest, heart, and throat. The tea adds to the vata-pacifying diet demulcent herbs such as licorice root, marshmallow root, comfrey root, and ophiopogon, which are nourishing and moistening to dry lungs. They will also lubricate, soften, and release any mucus that may have hardened and become stuck.

Mild spices such as cardamom and ginger may be added to the demulcent herbs. Spices bring warmth to the lungs and move energy. Again, strictly follow the vata-pacifying diet and lifestyle, but stay away from hard-to-digest foods such as dairy and nuts.

Try the following vata cough formula:

2 parts comfrey leaves
1 part elecampane
1 part licorice root
1/4 part anise seeds
1/4 part ginger
pinch of cloves

Let one tablespoon of the herbal combination steep in a cup of boiling water for 20–30 minutes. Strain and drink 1/4 cup four times per day. To enhance the tea's soothing properties, add honey.

Pitta-Type Coughs

With the pitta-type cough, there will be yellow, green, or blood-streaked phlegm. There may be burning sensations in the lungs, accompanied by fever, thirst, and dryness. Antibiotic herbs—goldenseal, echinacea and/or usnea—should be taken every hour or two. Demulcent herbs, such as licorice root and marshmallow root, will help cool off and soften mucus in the bronchial tubes and lungs. Other cooling expectorant herbs include:

- comfrey leaves
- horehound
- mullein
- coltsfoot

The following formula is very good for the pitta-type cough:

1 part coltsfoot
1 part comfrey
1 part mullein
1 part yarrow

1/4 part lobelia
1/4 part ginger
1/2 part licorice root

This formula does not taste very good, but it is effective. One ounce of the herb combination is gently simmered in three cups of water, keeping the lid on the pot. Strain and drink 1/2 cup four or five times a day.

The onion plaster described at the beginning of this section may also prove useful. Follow the pitta-pacifying diet, but also eliminate dairy, bread, and sweets. Do not take any cold, iced, or mucus-forming foods.

Sore Throat

Sore throats are oftentimes a complication of a flu or cold, and are of several different types.

The vata-type sore throat feels dry and scratchy. The voice may have a hoarse quality. There won't be extreme pain upon swallowing, nor will there be much of a feeling of "thickness." A simple but effective remedy is to make a paste out of slippery-elm powder mixed with raw honey. Take one-quarter teaspoon of this combination and let it melt in your mouth. Slippery elm has a demulcent quality that will help soothe the throat. The honey also will help to coat a dry throat. A tea may be made of the following herbs:

2 parts slippery elm
2 parts licorice root
1 part comfrey leaf
1 part fennel seeds
1/8 part orange peel

Take a teaspoon of this combination, place it in a muslin tea bag and let it steep in a cup of boiling water for five minutes. (Slippery elm is sold as a powder, but if this is put directly into the water, it will make the tea rather slimy.) You may prefer to make a paste out of this formula rather than take it as a tea. Powder all the herbs, then add honey until the consistency is that of a thick paste. Store the paste in a glass jar and carry it with you wherever you go for instant herbal therapy.

The Ayurvedic herb shatavari will also ease a dry throat. Add one teaspoon of the herb to raw milk or soy milk, and gently boil for fifteen minutes. Add honey to taste. Ghee (see glossary) or sesame oil also may be taken internally to soothe an irritated throat.

Painful streplike conditions of the throat usually indicate a pitta-type condition. Antibiotic herbs—such as goldenseal, echinacea and usnea (a lichen)—are appropriate for this condition. Take one dropperful every two hours. The dose is kept high until the symptoms have subsided, at which point the dose may be slowly decreased.

I have also found that gargling with lemon juice and honey mixed in water is helpful. The antiseptic quality of the lemon will help kill bacteria, and honey soothes the throat. I have also recommended a tea-tree gargle for sore throats. Add four or five drops of tea tree oil to warm water, shake well, and gargle. If sore throat is accompanied by dryness, try the demulcent formulas listed above for the vata condition. If the sufferer has an appetite, serve only broths and soups of a pitta-pacifying nature (see Dietary Recommendations).

If the sore throat is also accompanied by mucus, which indicates a complication of pitta and/or kapha, then the following warming herbs may be used in various formulas:

- sage
- bayberry
- turmeric

Continued ➡

- garlic
- cloves

Garlic stimulates the metabolism, is very warming, and is good for breaking up mucus. It is also an effective antibiotic for staphylococcus, streptococcus, salmonella, and other bacteria resistant to standard antibiotic drugs. Sage may be used as a gargle to break up mucus that is lodged in the throat and larynx. The expectorant herbs listed in the Coughs section, page 185, may be employed as well.

Nervous Debility, Insomnia and Anxiety

Nervous exhaustion and its accompanying symptoms are a sure sign of stress. There are many herbal remedies for nervous exhaustion, but the biggest consideration is lifestyle choices. Causes of nervous exhaustion, insomnia, and anxiety include:

- poor food combinations
- too much sugar
- drinking coffee and other stimulating substances
- skipping meals
- undernourishing meals
- lack of routine in life
- excess exercise, which can deplete the body of energy
- no exercise at all
- heavy use of computers and other electronic devices
- excess exposure to mass media
- overwork
- loud music and noises
- excessive sexual activity

As my teacher once said, "We are all suffering from global nervousness and anxiety." If you are suffering from nervous exhaustion, try your best to deal with some of the causes listed above. This will help to create a stronger basis for herbal healing.

Insomnia and anxiety are commonly an aggravated vata condition. Symptoms include:

- fear
- worry
- heart palpitations
- difficulty breathing
- inability to concentrate
- poor digestion
- lack of appetite
- ungroundedness
- emotional emptiness
- eating binges
- difficulty falling asleep
- disturbing dreams, especially of flying or falling

Rhythm and routine help to calm vata down. Try to eat at regular hours. The food should be nourishing and vata-pacifying. Stimulating herbs and substances, such as coffee, black tea, sugar, and Chinese ephedra (ma huang), should be avoided. Each evening before bed the feet should be massaged with almond or sesame oil. A few drops of lavender or rose essential oil may be added to the massage oil to enhance its calming properties. A time of meditation and self-reflection should be reserved for each morning and evening. Chanting a calming mantra or the repeating of a positive affirmation will help. Most people have unconscious mantras they repeat all day long, such as, "I don't have enough money," "I'm miserable," et cetera. Repeating more positive statements can change our inner as well as our outer reality.

Vata-Type Nervous Debility

For vata-type nervous exhaustion and/or insomnia, the following Western herb formula will be helpful:

2 parts valerian

1 part skullcap

1 part oatstraw

1 part hops

1 part rose petals

1 part gotu kola

1 part marshmallow

1 part licorice root

(If you can find biota seed in bulk, add it to the formula.)

Take one tablespoon of the combination and add it to a cup of boiling water. Let it steep for 10 minutes and drink three cups per day. You may also purchase the herbs in powder form and fill up "OO" sized capsules. Take two capsules three to six times per day as needed. This formula is not only calming but nourishing, which is essential for grounding high vata.

Valerian helps to clear vata from the nerve channels, and eases spasms and cramping. Because valerian contains a large amount of the earth element, it helps calm hysteria and ease vertigo. Its pungent taste also aids in digestion and alleviates gas. (The Ayurvedic herb jatamamsi is in the same family as valerian and may be used in its place. It does not create as dulling a sensation as valerian sometimes will.)

It is important to strengthen the digestive capacities of an individual when he or she is manifesting disease tendencies. If our food is not being digested and absorbed properly, then we will continue to feel run down. For example, the vata person may experience a wasting away of nerve tissue due to poor digestion and absorption, which eventually results in malnutrition. Add some mild spices to the diet to help increase agni (digestive fires). Make sure the food is chewed well and that the mealtime is peaceful.

Pitta-Type Nervous Debility

Pitta-type insomnia and nervous exhaustion is usually due to turbulent emotions such as anger, hatred, resentment, and the desire for revenge. Many times, pittas will be unable to sleep following an argument, after meeting a deadline, or during extreme heat conditions such as fevers or sunbathing. Sleep may be agitated and filled with violent dreams, which leaves pittas tired in the morning. Some of the symptoms may be the same as for vata, but they will carry more heat, more burning sensations, more agitation, and more emotional outbursts. The causes for these situations may include:

- excessive willfulness
- excessive competition
- eating hot, stimulating foods
- too much exposure to sun and heat
- high fevers
- wanting too much control over situations
- watching violent movies or TV shows

The remedy for this condition is to follow the pitta-pacifying diet, i.e., avoid excess spices, including salty and sour tastes. Meditations by a source of water or in the moonlight will help cool off heated emotions. Cooling colors and calming scents may also be helpful for pitta. Massage the feet at night with coconut oil and add a few drops of sandalwood essential oil to enhance its cooling properties. A drop of sandalwood oil on the "third eye" will cool off the mind as well.

A good Western herb formula for pitta is equal parts:

skullcap

gotu kola

passion flower

hops

spearmint

lemon balm

St. John's wort

rose petals

licorice root

Take one tablespoon of the mixture and let it steep in one cup of boiling water until the water cools to room temperature. Strain and drink three cups per day or as needed. Or powder the herbs and fill "OO" size capsules with the mixture. Take two capsules three to six times per day as needed.

For depression and hopelessness, the following formula is helpful:

2 parts oatstraw

1 part St. John's wort

2 parts lemon balm

1 part rose petals

1/4 part licorice

This can be made into a tea, one tablespoon of the herb combination to a cup of boiling water. Let steep for 20 minutes, strain, and drink three cups per day. This formula may be used for pitta and kapha constitutions. The vata person may want to add some jatamamsi and a little extra licorice root.

Kapha-Type Nervous Debililty

When we think of a kapha person, we usually get a picture of a large, contented individual who oversleeps and does not worry too much. In my practice, however, I have seen people with kapha bodies and aggravated, vata-type minds. These people are heavy and congested, but may not be able to stop talking. I usually put them on the kapha-pacifying diet to help to break down blockages and ama (toxins), but combine this with a vata-pacifying lifestyle for the mind. I recommend more routine and rhythm in their lives, and encourage them to observe more quiet time.

Try the following calming formula for herbal tea:

2 parts skullcap

1 part hops

2 parts passion flower

1 part chamomile

1 part gotu kola

1/2 part rosemary

1/2 part spearmint

1/2 part sage

pinch ginger

Saunas, massage, and exercise may also bring more balance to the kapha person.

Our modern ways are too fast and aggressive. All of us are bombarded with more information than we can possibly assimilate. No matter what our constitutional proclivities may be, everyday life in America is vata-provoking. This must always be taken into consideration.

General Fatigue

Fatigue may be due to many factors and, as with the diagnosis of nervous exhaustion, all life choices must be reviewed.

Vata Fatigue

Those who display vata imbalances should follow the vata-pacifying diet. The foods must be deeply nourishing and "building." The following herbs,

Continued ➡

which strengthen the immune system and enhance vitality, may be purchased loose, then cooked into soups, grains, and broths:

Chinese tonic herbs:

I part astragalus

I part codonopsis

I part lychee berries

I part jujube dates

Put one ounce of this blend into a muslin bag. Place the bag in the pot and cook along with the soup. Remove bag when the food is done. The tasty lychee berries may be added directly to the soup.

Another good formula for the exhausted vata person is the following:

I part American ginseng

I part dong quai

$1/2$ part marshmallow root

$1/2$ part burdock root

$1/4$ part licorice root

pinch of ginger

To make tea, simmer one ounce of this blend of herbs 45 minutes in three cups of water. Licorice root has a sweet initial taste and a bitter taste secondarily, so add the licorice root during the last five minutes of cooking. Drink two cups per day, in the morning and afternoon.

Ayurvedic tonic herbs may be blended as follows:

I tsp. ashwagandha

I tsp. shatavari

pinch of ginger

Gently simmer these herbs in one cup raw milk or soy milk for 15 minutes. If you are using the powdered herbs, do not strain them. Drink one cup in the morning and another in the afternoon.

Pitta Fatigue

A person with pitta-type fatigue must follow the pitta-pacifying diet and review the lifestyle considerations listed under "Nervous Exhaustion." Due to the burnout they are experiencing, they will also want to add "building" herbs to their foods. For example:

· astragalus

· burdock root

· jujube dates

· lychee berries

Pitta persons may also add to their herbal routine one-half cup aloe vera juice two times per day. Aloe vera juice is a cooling tonic, and is rejuvenative for the liver and spleen. It regulates metabolism of sugar and fat, and tonifies the agni (digestive enzymes). It is also excellent for the female reproductive system.

The Ayurvedic herb shatavari may be added to aloe vera juice, or it may be taken in two capsules three times per day. Shatavari is a specific rejuvenative for pitta, for the female reproductive system, and for the blood. It helps to balance women's hormones, and can be used for menopausal women and for those who have had hysterectomies.

A good Western formula for gently rebuilding and detoxifying pitta is:

Jamaican sarsaparilla

marshmallow

burdock root

nettles

red clover

licorice root

Mix together equal parts of the herbs in a jar and add one tablespoon of the combination to a cup of boiling water. Let steep 10 minutes. Drink two or three cups of this tasty tea per day. Or grind the herbs to a powder and put the mixture in "00" capsules; take two capsules three times per day. This formula will remove excess heat from the body, clear the skin of eruptions and nourish the tissues.

Kapha Fatigue

Kapha-type fatigue may be due to excess fat, water, and ama (toxins) that block the flow of prana (energy). The kapha-pacifying diet must be followed, and an effort must be made not to overeat or sleep after meals. I usually do not give a kapha person or condition strong building herbs such as the ones listed under vata and pitta, because these can increase congestion. Here are some herbal recommendations for the kapha person:

· One-quarter to one-half teaspoon of the trikatu combination (see glossary) may be mixed with honey and taken with meals two or three times per day.

· One-half cup aloe vera juice mixed with a pinch of ginger powder may be taken two times per day.

A combination of the herbs triphala and guggul may be taken in the evening. Put the mixture in "00" capsules and take two at bedtime.

The following Western herbs may be combined and placed in capsules:

2 parts elecampane

I part kelp

I part angelica archangelica

I part dandelion leaf

$1/4$ part orange peel

$1/4$ part fennel

$1/8$ part cayenne

Take two capsules between meals. This formula has many warming and bitter herbs in it, which will help to detoxify accumulated mucus and nourish the tissues. The kelp serves to normalize thyroid function.

Fatigued kaphas should not take strenuous exercise, but ought to make an effort to walk a bit after meals.

Liver Conditions

The liver is considered a "fiery" organ and is the source of most pitta disorders. The word pitta means "bile," and excessive bile or a congested bile flow can cause ulcers, heartburn, and other conditions accompanied by burning sensations. There are also many subtle enzymes (called bhuta agni) in the liver that help. They digest food particles and help build up tissue for the five sense organs.

The liver is the seat of anger, hate, resentment, jealousy, and ambition, as well as emotions associated with thwarted creativity. When stimulated and unresolved, such emotions can adversely affect the liver. An explosive temper is usually a sign of an overheated liver. The bitter taste promotes the flow of bile, cleanses the blood, detoxifies the liver and thereby relieves an exasperated pitta condition.

Herbs for cleansing and relieving liver heat

· aloe vera juice

· dandelion

· Oregon grape root

· barberry

· goldenseal

· gentian

· yellow dock

· thistle

· bhringaraj

· turmeric

· cyperus

· bupleurum

· gotu kola

· skullcap

Cyperus and bupleurum help to regulate liver energy, aiding digestion and assimilation and regulating mood swings. Gotu kola and skullcap calm the liver and help release us from addictions to substances such as sugar, cigarettes, drugs, and alcohol.

A good combination for relieving the fiery emotions is equal parts:

skullcap

passion flower

gotu kola

sandalwood

Powder the herbs and take two capsules three times per day, or as needed.

Green leafy vegetables are also good for cleansing the liver. Nettles, beet greens, chickweed, and dandelion leaves contain many vitamins and minerals, and plenty of iron and chlorophyll.

Generally, the person suffering from a liver condition should adhere to the pitta-pacifying diet, avoiding hot spices, acidic foods, fats, oils (except ghee), coffee, black tea, alcohol, and drugs. Many times I recommend that dairy products and meat products be eliminated as well.

Castor oil penetrates deeply into the tissues and gently cleanses the liver. Massage the oil over the whole liver area, just below the rib cage on the right side. If the liver should become "achy," or if you feel that the cleansing is happening too quickly and bringing you discomfort, do not continue using castor oil.

A powerful herb for the liver is seeds of milk thistle, effective against many of the deadly hepatotoxins. Studies have shown that certain milk thistle seed preparations can produce both protective and curative effects when it comes to liver damage resulting from toxic substances. It can be used for various liver diseases, including fatty degeneration of the liver, and can also be supportive treatment for chronic hepatitis and cirrhosis of the liver. I recommend milk thistle seeds in powder or tincture forms, although some herbalists with whom I have spoken sprinkle a tablespoon of the powder on various foods, such as cereals and soups. For liver conditions such as cirrhosis and hepatitis, I do not use alcoholic extracts (tinctures), because the alcohol may exasperate the condition.

Springtime is considered the "liver season," so it is a good idea to pursue a liver-cleansing regime at that time of the year to help detoxify and cleanse out all the winter sludge that may have accumulated. As always, preventative therapy is the best health insurance.

The Gallbladder and Gallstones

The gallbladder is a small gland that presses against the right lobe of the liver and serves as a storage chamber for bile. It releases its contents as needed for the digestion of various substances. When a person has gallstones, they are mainly caused by congestion and obstruction in the flow of bile. Gallstones will often manifest as acute pain in the liver and gallbladder region, and sometimes in the middle-back area. The pain may be accompanied by pronounced inflammation or fever. The herbs for cleansing the liver are appropriate for this condition, with the addition of gravel root, which helps dissolve gallstones.

I have given the following formula to clients with good results:

Continued →

3 parts gravel root

I part dandelion root

I part turmeric root

2 parts marshmallow root

¹/₂ part licorice root

¹/₄ part gingerroot

This formula is pain-relieving, detoxifying, and cooling. Take two tablets three times daily; for acute conditions take two tablets every two hours, then decrease the dose as the symptoms subside. Pregnant women should not take this formula.

Gallstones can be quite serious, so make sure that you consult a health practitioner before treating yourself for this condition.

The Woman's "Moon Cycle"

Generally speaking, the way in which a woman's menstrual cycle manifests is a good key into her health situation. In all my sessions with women I ask them about their menstruation—about regularity, discomfort, whether they are or have been on birth control pills, the number of pregnancies, births, or abortions, and so forth. If the menstruation is regular with little pain or tension, and if the emotions do not fluctuate severely each month, these are signs of good health. Most women, however, experience a degree of menstrual discomfort at different times in their lives.

If there has been some imbalance in your cycle, it may take up to four months of regular herbal treatment before you see results. The herbs work slowly to reestablish a new foundation. Be patient and continue on your healing path.

THE VATA WOMAN

The woman with a vata constitution that is out of balance may experience some of the following symptoms:

- slow start of menstruation
- brownish blood
- severe cramping and lower-back pain, sometimes lasting for days
- headaches
- chills
- nervousness, anxiety, fear
- difficulty sleeping
- gas and bloating, especially before menstruation
- irregular bowel movements
- short menstruation cycle (two or three days)
- irregular, variable cycle

The patient should follow the vata-pacifying diet, avoiding cold foods and drinks, carbonated drinks, fast foods, and ice cream. The food should be warm and nourishing. Many times excessive exercising, such as aerobics, can deplete the body of needed energy and fluids; it is best for the vata woman to practice yoga or mild exercise instead. An excessively thin person may be deficient in blood as well as energy, which will make for difficult menstruation. Excessive sexual activity can also deplete the vata person of vitality. Just before and during menstruation, observe some quiet time. This will help to calm the mind and nerves.

During menstruation, most women become introspective. Introspection helps us to before in tune with our inner voice and vision. Do not be afraid of this inner journey. Instead, learn to see it as a companion to self-realization.

Nourishing tonic herbs for the vata woman

- dong quai
- vitex
- rehmannia

- licorice root
- shatavari
- ashwagandha
- comfrey root
- wild yam root
- 8 marshmallow root
- saw palmetto

Shatavari (*asparagus racemosus*) is one of the best-known Ayurvedic herbs for the female reproductive system, nourishing, calming the heart, and demulcent for dry and inflamed membranes of the lungs, stomach, kidneys, and sexual organs. Shatavari nourishes and cleanses the blood and the reproductive organs. It can be used for menopause and for those who have had hysterectomies. It is sattvic in quality, promoting love and devotion.

Although some Ayurvedic practitioners believe that ashwagandha (*withania somnifera*) is an herb for the male system, I have used it many times, in combination with other tonic herbs, for the female system. Ashwagandha is a rejuvenative herb for the vata constitution, working in particular on the muscles, marrow, and reproductive system. It is good for all conditions of weakness and deficiency. I have had excellent results using it with pregnant women, and also with children who are weak. Try the following formula:

2 parts shatavari

2 parts ashwagandha

I part vitex

I part licorice root

¹/₄ part ginger

Take two "00" capsules three times per day with meals.

Dong quai (*angelica sinensis*) is used in the treatment of many female gynecological ailments. It regulates menstruation, tonifies the blood, promotes blood circulation, and counteracts dryness of the bowels that causes constipation. It should not be used by pregnant women or those suffering from wasting diseases, or when there is bloating, abdominal congestion, or uterine fibroids. Dong quai's phyto-estrogenic qualities make it helpful for the menopausal woman as well.

Here is another simple formula:

2 parts dong quai

I part vitex

I part wild yam

2 parts licorice root

¹/₈ part ginger

Take two "00" capsules three times per day with meals.

For cramps

I part cramp bark

I part pennyroyal

I part valerian

I part blue cohosh

¹/₂ part ginger

Put about one tablespoon each of cramp bark and blue cohosh, in a quart of boiling water. Let simmer for 20 minutes. Turn the heat off and add one tablespoon each of valerian, pennyroyal, and ¹/₂ teaspoon ginger. You do not want to boil these last three herbs, as the essential oils and active ingredients will dissipate. Let them steep for an additional 20 minutes. Drink ¹/₄ to ¹/₂ cup every 15–30 minutes until you experience some relief.

A ginger foot bath may be helpful as well, stimulating the flow of blood and warming up the system. Put one tablespoon of powdered ginger in a small tub and add warm water. Let your feet soak

for 15 or more minutes, adding hot water as needed. A hot compress of ginger tea may be placed against the uterus as well.

THE PITTA WOMAN

If the pitta woman is out of balance, then *some of* the following symptoms may occur:

- loose stool before menstruation
- feelings of irritation and anger
- heavy bleeding with some clotting
- achy breasts (due to liver congestion)
- painful cramping
- rashes, acne, or herpes outbreaks
- excess heat, night sweats, or hot flashes
- headaches
- redness of the eyes

The pitta-pacifying diet should be followed, with strict avoidance of acidic foods such as oranges and tomatoes. Hot spices, alcohol, coffee, and excess meats should be excluded from the diet. Sunbathing and saunas also may overheat the pitta woman.

Tonic herbs for the pitta woman

- aloe vera juice
- shatavari
- vitex
- sarsaparilla
- wild yam
- dong quai (high doses may aggravate pitta)
- black cohosh
- licorice root
- peony root

Cooling astringent herbs for toning the uterus

- nettles
- raspberry leaves
- motherwort
- strawberry leaves
- squaw vine

The liver herbs are important for the pitta person as well. They will keep the energy flowing and help to alleviate some of the anger, heat, and frustration that may manifest. The liver also helps to process many of the hormones in the body, thus easing menstruation.

Here's a good tonic formula for the pitta woman:

2 parts wild yam

2 parts licorice

I part burdock root

2 parts dandelion root

I part comfrey root

2 parts sarsaparilla

I part vitex

¹/₂ part dong quai

¹/₄ part ginger

Powder the herbs and take two "00" capsules three times per day.

Try out this tasty tea:

2 parts raspberry leaf

2 parts nettles

I part spearmint

I part lemongrass

Put one tablespoon of the combination in a cup of boiling water and let it steep for 10 minutes. Strain and drink two or three cups per day.

The herb motherwort may be used for night sweats and hot flashes. It is also good for heart pal-

Continued ➡

pitations. This herb is quite bitter, so I usually use it in tincture form.

For Cramping

2 parts chamomile (Note: people who are allergic to ragweed may be allergic to chamomile)

1 part yarrow

1 part cramp bark

1 part skullcap

1 part peppermint

1 part squaw vine

Gently simmer the cramp bark for 10 minutes, then add the other herbs and steep together for an additional 10 minutes. Strain and drink 1/4 cup every 15 minutes until some relief is felt. A hot ginger compress placed against the uterus may also be helpful.

THE KAPHA WOMAN

The kapha woman who is out of balance may have some of the following symptoms:

- water retention
- mucus in the blood
- mucus in the stool or urine
- feelings of heaviness and tiredness
- excess saliva and phlegm
- breasts swollen due to water retention
- teary sentimental feelings
- food feels heavy in the stomach
- nausea
- excess or emotional eating
- mild cramping with a "heavy" feeling

Follow the kapha-pacifying diet, strictly avoiding dairy, ice cream, sweets, fatty fried foods, oils, nuts, and salt. Make sure that each meal is fully digested before consuming more food. Do not drink too many liquids.

Spices such as cayenne and trikatu (see glossary) will help to stimulate the metabolism, thus relieving congestion and water retention. Another formula that works with the kidney to eliminate excess water is:

2 parts dandelion leaves

2 parts cleavers

1 part chickweed

1 part uva ursi

Take three "00" capsules three times per day, or drink three cups of tea per day. To make a tea, take one tablespoon of the herb blend and let it steep in a cup of boiling water until it cools to room temperature.

The herbs for the liver are appropriate for the kapha woman, and should be taken 15 minutes before meals.

Tonic Herbs for the Kapha Woman

- dong quai (*Angelica sinensis*)
- angelica archangelica
- black cohosh
- aloe vera juice
- false unicorn
- ashwagandha
- wild yam
- damiana

For Cramping

- blue cohosh
- black cohosh
- ginger
- "cramp bark"
- chamomile

Astringent herbs for toning the uterus

- motherwort
- raspberry leaves
- nettles
- strawberry leaves

Spices should be added to the diet, and as well as to the formulas for the kapha person. One of the actions of the spicy or pungent taste is to counteract stagnation and increase blood circulation. Many of the common spices, such as turmeric, cinnamon, ginger, cayenne, basil, cardamom, asafetida, garlic, fennel, and dill, can be used for delayed or slowed menstruation, and also to alleviate cramping.

Here is a simple but effective formula for nourishing the reproductive organs in the kapha individual:

2 parts dong quai

2 parts wild yam

1 part burdock root

2 parts dandelion root

1 part vitex

1/2 part ginger

Take two "00" capsules or one dropperful of the tincture three times per day.

Elimination, Tonification, and Rejuvenation

When we consider implementing an herbal program, we must decide whether the case calls for *eliminating* toxins or for *building* tissues, blood, or energy.

Elimination therapies focus on decreasing weight, accumulated ama (toxins), and excess humors. In Ayurveda, this type of therapy is called *langhana*, which literally means "to lighten."

When a person has an acute condition such as a cold, flu, or cough, eliminating therapies are employed. Elimination methods include:

- sweating techniques using saunas and diaphoretic herbs
- clearing the bowels with herbs that have a laxative action (purgatives)
- elimination through the urine (diuretic herbs)
- elimination through vomiting (emetic herbs)
- eliminating phlegm from the lungs (expectorants)
- discharging of gas (carminative herbs)
- destroying pathogens with blood-, lymph-, and bile-cleansing herbs (alterative herbs)

These techniques can also be used as part of a disease-prevention and internal-cleansing program to eliminate deep-seated toxins. Especially during the transitional seasons of spring and fall, it is good to undergo a light fast and cleansing program to help eliminate toxins and accumulated humors which may otherwise cause difficulties.

Tonification or supplementation therapy uses herbs and foods that build, nourish, and strengthen tissues. In Ayurveda this is call *brimhana*, meaning "to make heavy." Tonification is indicated for individuals who are elderly, malnourished, chronically ill, pregnant, emaciated, convalescent, anemic, infertile, impotent, or suffering from nervous exhaustion and emotional collapse. It is also helpful in cases of chronic insomnia.

Some tonic herbs increase the energy and vitality of the organ systems by providing deeply nourishing vitamins, minerals, and sugars. Others act to balance the energy of the organs, improving their ability to assimilate nutrients. The rule of thumb is to first eliminate toxins, then tonify. If we try to tonify while there is still accumulated ama in the

system, the tonic herbs may actually exacerbate the condition. A short fast, a series of saunas, and consumption of blood-cleansing herbs can help reduce toxins and make the tonifying therapy more effective.

A tonic is most effective taken with food. Herbs such as ginseng, astragalus, dong quai, codonopsis, and shatavari may be simmered in soups. The famous Ayurvedic formula chyavanprash combines more than 25 finely powdered herbs in a base of honey and ghee to make a delicious paste.

Other tonic herbs include:

Chinese herbs:

- panax ginseng
- Siberian ginseng
- codonopsis
- astragalus
- atractylodes
- rehmannia
- peony root
- ho shou wu

Ayurvedic herbs:

- shatavari
- triphala
- ashwagandha
- kapikacchu
- amalaki

Others:

- licorice root
- American ginseng
- marshmallow root
- comfrey root
- elecampane
- rape unicorn
- damiana
- saw palmetto
- aloe vera
- suma
- garlic
- solomon's seal
- slippery elm
- ophiopogon

Vata Tonification Therapy

Vata requires the strongest tonifying therapies, all in the context of plenty of rest, oil massage, and warm baths with mineral salts. Heavy exercising, excess sexual activity, too much talking, and the stress of travel all disperse energy and therefore should be avoided. Instead, provide a quiet environment and nourishing foods.

Tonic herbs specific for vata include:

- shatavari
- marshmallow
- comfrey root
- saw palmetto
- kapikacchu
- triphala
- astragalus
- dong quai
- Siberian ginseng
- American ginseng
- ashwagandha
- ophiopogon
- guggul (Note: guggul is not a nutritive tonic in itself, but helps to catalyze tissue regeneration, particularly of the nerve tissue, reducing toxins, increasing white-blood cell count, and

Continued ➡

helping with conditions of arthritis, gout, nervous disorders, diabetes, obesity, and skin disease. It is particularly good for vata and kapha, but will aggravate pitta if taken in large doses over a long period of time. Taken alone it may be too harsh in its action, so it is usually mixed with other herbs.)

Mild spices may be used with the formulas and in the food. These include:

- ginger
- cinnamon
- cloves
- asafoetida
- fennel
- dill
- rosemary

Pitta Tonification Therapy

The tonification therapy for pitta is moderate compared to that of vata. Mild massage is fine, but without the use of too much oil. Saunas, hot tubs, and sweat lodges should be avoided. Warm baths and showers are fine. Jogging in the middle of the day, strenuous aerobics, and heavy weight-lifting should be replaced with mild exercises and yoga. The pitta-pacifying diet should be adhered to, but with more of the building foods and herbs. Raw foods and juices should be kept to a minimum. Tonic herbs for pitta include:

- amalaki
- shatavari
- marshmallow root
- gotu kola
- rehmannia
- licorice
- aloe vera
- peony root
- ho shou wu
- Siberian ginseng

Pitta should avoid hot spices, alcohol, coffee, and other stimulants. The lifestyle should be free from competition and aggression, which will reduce vitality.

Kapha Tonification Therapy

The tonification therapy for kapha is more stimulating than building. Moderate-strength massage and mild sweating therapy are fine. Adequate rest should be taken, but do not sleep after meals or during the day. Exercise should be mild, such as walking or gently jumping on an exercise trampoline.

The kapha-pacifying diet should be followed, but with an emphasis on the more building foods. Raw foods, cold foods, dairy products, and excess oils should be avoided.

Good tonic herbs for kapha include:

- elecampane
- guggul
- aloe vera with spices
- garlic
- saffron
- angelica archangelica
- dong quai
- gotu kola
- triphala

Spices may be used in the formulas and foods to help counteract stagnation, but not in excess.

Pancha Karma and Rejuvenation

Pancha karma consists of five very intensive and radical cleansing techniques employed in Ayurveda—not just the application of the elimination methods discussed earlier, but an intensive system for guiding the toxins to specific sites for elimination. The five techniques are:

1. therapeutic vomiting
2. purgation
3. enemas
4. nasal application of herbs
5. therapeutic release of toxic blood

Prior to pancha karma, preliminary techniques called *purva karma* are employed. These consist of application of oil, followed by steam or therapeutic sweating therapy. The oils help to loosen and liquify the ama and humors in the skin and blood. They eventually drain into the gastrointestinal tract, where they are eliminated by the pancha karma techniques listed above.

Rejuvenation therapy, or *rasayana*, is a speciail type of tonification that follows pancha karma. The herbs and application are the same as for tonification therapy, but are applied in a manner calculated to bring about an energized and revitalized new person. It is beyond the capacity of this small booklet to explain these techniques in any detail. For further information, please consult one or more of the resources listed at the end of this book.

Case Studies—Ayurveda in Action

Case #1: Ken

Ken came to see me with a severe condition of ulcerated colitis, from which he had been suffering for fifteen years. He was forty-five years old, tall, medium build, dark hair, with pockmarked skin from acne, intense dark eyes, and a gentle manner. He liked to talk and was very free in describing to me his history and situation.

While a soldier in Vietnam, he had been introduced to marijuana and heroin. For five years he was a heroin addict. He had also been a heavy drinker. At one point he had kidney failure due to an overdose of heroin, and currently had a cyst on one kidney. At 28 years of age he went into a recovery house and began to eliminate drugs and alcohol from his life. He was drug- and alcohol-free when he came to see me.

His symptoms were classically those of provoked pitta (fire element). He ached in the liver and gall-bladder area, while experiencing burning sensations in the digestive tract. His stools were loose and hot. He did not sleep well and felt agitated. From time to time, he had blood in the stool and suffered from hemorrhoids. He also had chronic hepatitis with a high liver-enzyme count. He was currently on disability, and was not employed or in retraining. He never came down with acute ailments such as colds or flus.

Ken's diet was quite poor. He started the day off with two cups of coffee with Sweet 'N Low. During the day he ate just a little fruit, mostly apples and bananas, and in the evening he would eat some rice or a very light meal. I was astonished that he still had the energy to bike for 10 miles each day and still do some work around the house.

His pulse on the right wrist was strong, more a "jumping" pitta pulse. The pulse on the left hand was indiscernible due to the collapse of blood vessels that occurred during drug use.

When viewing his tongue I saw many red lines in the very back section, which indicates a heated condition of the intestines and colon. The sides of the tongue, which show the liver and gallbladder, were red, and the tongue was swollen as well.

Ken, I could see, was suffering from a condition of overall inflammation, which is pitta in nature. The stool was loose, excessively flowing, sharp (burning sensation), excessively liquid, and there was an aggressive and penetrating character to the condition.

The first obvious thing about this case was that Ken needed to stop drinking coffee, which tends to disperse energy and stimulate the nervous system, including the peristaltic action of the bowels. The seventeen alkaloids in coffee, which must be processed by the liver, strain that organ's functions. Coffee is also quite acidic, and will eat away at the mucous lining of the digestive tract.

I had Ken take amalaki, two capsules with water, each night before bed. (Amalaki is a bowel regulator for pittas and colitis. It gently cleanses the liver and kidneys, and helps regulate metabolism.) Three nights a week I had Ken rub the liver and colon area with castor oil, which penetrates deeply into the tissues, and helps cleanse the liver and heal tissue.

I also gave him a bitter formula with milk thistle seeds (two capsules 15 minutes before meals) to help detoxify the liver and protect it as well. The main formula for the ulcerated colitis was:

3 parts agrimony
2 parts wild yam
2 parts goldenseal
1 part marshmallow
1 part bayberry

Three capsules were to be taken three times per day before meals. This formula is specific for healing ulcerations of the digestive tract, calming spasms, staunching bleeding and reinstating healthy mucus in the tract lining.

Ken was already taking flaxseed oil, vitamin C, acidophilus, and psyllium. I told him to continue with these supplements.

When Ken called me a couple of weeks later, he told me that he had not stopped drinking coffee and that the colitis situation had worsened. He asked what other herbs he should take, but I insisted that the herbs would work as soon as he stopped the coffee intake. He called me again about six weeks later and thanked me for the advice. The diarrhea and bleeding had ceased about 10 days after he stopped drinking coffee. So had the symptoms of colitis. He was eating a much healthier, pitta-pacifying diet and had gained weight. He said that he felt so good that he was on a retraining program with a local college and had acquired a new girlfriend.

This example shows how important it is to address the dietary choices that the person is making. Herbs have a hard time working if the diet is counter to the treatment.

Case #2: Cheryl

Cheryl is one of my regular clients and has come to see me many times over the past six years. She is forty-eight years old, slender, small build, and has a tendency to feel cold in winter and comfortable in the summer. She has been very conscious of her food and lifestyle choices, and eats quite healthily. She has a long-term, stable relationship with her spouse and enjoys her employment as a social worker.

Her constitution is vata-pitta, with vata slightly higher than pitta. During the winter through early spring she follows the vata-pacifying diet with mostly cooked foods, extra spices, and tonifying, building herbs. In the summer she has a tendency

Continued ➡

to overheat, so she follows the pitta-pacifying diet during the very hot months.

Cheryl is in excellent health generally, but came to me complaining of headaches that occurred in the morning when she woke up, and also in the afternoon. She said she was sleeping well, with no insomnia or restlessness. We went over her diet and the herbs she was taking on a regular basis, and could not find anything that stood out as a possible cause of the headaches.

I had Cheryl describe to me the room she slept in and learned that the window was open all night and always let in a cool breeze, right at her head. At work she had a similar situation: the air vent was right over her and would cool her head all day. I told Cheryl to close the bedroom window at night and open another window that did not blow directly onto her.

The situation at work was trickier. She first tried to tilt the air vent so that it did not blow directly onto her. This proved difficult to accomplish, so I suggested she wear a hat or scarf, and that she wrap a small blanket around the kidney area and use a heating pad if her feet grew cold. I told her to report back to me after a couple of weeks.

The headaches stopped immediately upon changing the environments. She called again a few months later and said that she was still headache-free. The air vent and open window tended to create a cold, dry, mobile, agitating, and dispersing atmosphere, provoking a vata-type headache.

Looking at this example, we see that it is important to not only look at the diet and foods, but also the patient's environment.

Case #3: Susan

The next case was quite complicated. Susan, 42, had many chronic conditions that had begun to culminate in a general loss of vitality. She felt it had started three years earlier, when she had a knee operation following an injury. She had been given dozens of different anesthetics, gone into shock, and almost died. She had lost 20 pounds and felt that she had never got over that trauma.

Upon questioning her further, I found out that Susan had once suffered from colitis, which had stopped five years ago after she cut coffee out of her diet. In recent months the colitis had flared up again, but seemed to be under control now—although her stool continued to be runny.

Susan also had manifested some unusual conditions from birth. Her mother had taken different drug therapies to help with the pregnancy. The drugs created in Susan a double uterus, an appendix on the wrong side of the body, and one weak kidney. Susan also suffered from stomach bloating, arthritis of the left hand, anxiety attacks, shortness of breath, heart palpitations, allergies, eczema, and vaginal yeast. She was currently on birth control pills, Motrin for arthritis pain, and antihistamines. She had recently started on wheat grass juice and antioxidant vitamins.

Susan is medium build with light hair, skin, and eyes, a very driven person with great ambition and willpower. Her pulse was quite weak, but had a slight "jumping" quality to it. Her tongue was very red on the sides, indicating heat in the liver and gallbladder. The back of the tongue had a yellow coating, indicating heat in the lower part of her body, probably the intestines and colon.

I felt that Susan's prakruti (basic institution) was predominantly pitta, with secondary vata and kapha (i.e., V2-P3-K1) Her vikruti (current condition) was V3-P4-K1. Vata and pitta were both elevated. Among the conditions that definitely pointed

to vata were the anxiety, the palpitations, arthritis, and the shortness of breath. The pitta-provoked conditions were the colitis, the vaginal infection and the allergies.

I put Susan on the pitta-pacifying diet, but with an emphasis on the vata-pacifying lifestyle. Her meals were to be taken at regular hours and never skipped. She was to go to bed no later than 10 P.M. and was to use sesame oil on her feet, mixed with lavender essential oil for calming. She was not to watch the news or read anything that aroused turbulent emotions. I even had her make an herbal pillow stuffed with herbs for calming, such as chamomile, lemon balm, hops, lavender, and rose petals.

I had Susan cut out all alcohol from her diet, along with white sugar, all dairy, and any yeasted breads, (These foods would increase her yeast condition.) She was to take an acidophilus supplement three times per day to reinstate the good flora which had been destroyed by the drugs, antibiotics, and birth control pills.

If Susan experienced a vaginal infection, she was to do the following:

- Make a strong tea with ½ teaspoon goldenseal to one cup boiling water. Steep for 30 minutes and strain. Douche with this tea once per day for up to three days.
- Follow each douche with a second douche containing one teaspoon acidophilus powder to reinstate the good flora in the vaginal region.

The doctor had told her to ice her arthritic hand each day, but this was just stopping the flow of healing blood to the area. I instructed her in using what Chinese medicine calls "moxibustion," a method of burning herbs, such as mugwort, above the skin to warm the area and thus break down blockages. It is wonderful for sprains, injuries, and arthritis. Many times pain is due to blockage, and in Susan's case the arthritis was a definite area of congestion. I also instructed her to put some warming liniment on the area following the moxibustion.

For Susan's liver, I put together a bitter formula to help in detoxification. I did not give her any alcoholic extract, however, because I felt that the alcohol would exacerbate the situation. All the formulas were taken in capsules or teas.

In the evening before bed, Susan was to take two capsules of amalaki, and one of the herbs in the triphala compound, which is excellent for bleeding disorders, colitis, palpitations, and general debility, and is rejuvenative for pitta as well. She also was to take one-half cup of aloe vera juice two times per day.

I also gave her an arthritis formula containing:

yucca

black cohosh

white willow bark

marshmallow root

guggul (a special Ayurvedic resin for scraping toxins from the tissues)

angelica archangelica

licorice root

ginger

She took two capsules three times per day.

For a relaxing beverage tea, I mixed together the following nervines:

passion flower

lemon balm

skullcap

hops

rose petals

spearmint

lavender

chamomile

She was to drink one cup 30 minutes before bedtime.

Susan called me about a month after the session and reported that her arthritic hand was much better. She was able to work at the computer without much discomfort and was down to only one Motrin per week. She no longer suffered from anxiety attacks and was able to sleep quite well most nights. Her stools were solid and regular now, and the vaginal infection had not recurred.

She returned to work full-time, which has been a strain on her, but today she rests during her times off and believes she knows how to conduct her life in such a way that the healing process will continue.

Case #4: Bill

Bill, 48, had been suffering from a mucousy, irritating cough for about six months. It had started off as a severe cold during the winter, for which he had been prescribed antibiotics. His symptoms were worse at night and in the morning. His doctor wanted to prescribe a daily dose of antibiotics for an indefinite period of time. His digestion was poor, with a heavy feeling after meals, along with more mucus in the throat area.

After talking to Bill, I determined that his prakruti was V1-P3-K2. However, kapha was provoked at this time and stood at 3. Because he reported seeing mucus in the stool, as well as in the nasal area, I believed that the mucus had settled not only in the lungs, but throughout his system.

Some of the qualities of kapha are:

- cold
- damp
- heavy
- liquid
- thick
- slow

Bill was chilly most of the time, and his lungs and sinuses felt cool and damp. The mucus was thick and white, and tended to be heavy in texture. Bill felt heavy after eating and needed to rest more often than usual. All these symptoms pointed to a kapha condition. (Bill did not have any heat or burning symptoms, nor did he have any dryness or vata conditions, so I did not feel that the vata or pitta part of his constitution was provoked at this time.)

I put Bill on the kapha-pacifying diet with an emphasis on spices and warm foods. I told him to stop taking ice water and other cold drinks, which create mucus. He also was to eliminate all dairy, fatty foods, nuts, and oils. This was his program:

1. Bill was to start the day off with a dry body brushing with a loofa sponge or vegetable fiber brush. This would stimulate the lymphatic system and help to release congestion and toxins.

2. In the morning and evening, he was to do a nasal wash with one teaspoon of sea salt per cup of warm water.

3. He was to take a milk-free acidophilus supplement, two capsules three times per day, to reinstate the good flora that had been killed off by the antibiotic therapy.

4. He was to take bitters 15 minutes before meals; after meals, he was to take one-half teaspoon of trikatu paste (see glossary).

5. He was to take two capsules of triphala each night before bed to help regulate the bowels and cleanse the colon, liver, and kidneys.

Continued →

6. The main formula for the lungs was:

   2 parts elecampane

   I part grindelia

   I part marshmallow root

   I part horehound

   ¹/₂ part wild cherry bark

   ¹/₄ part lobelia

   ¹/₄ part ginger

   ¹/₄ part goldenseal

7. He was to drink ginger tea and other spicy beverages throughout the day, and avoid cold drinks.

Because Bill worked long hours each day, we decided that capsules would be most convenient. He took two "00" capsules three times per day on an empty stomach. I told him to take a cup of tea with the herbs listed in step number 6 at least once per day, preferably in the morning. He let one tablespoon of the herbs steep in hot water overnight so that all he had to do in the morning was strain and reheat it.

Within three weeks the coughing bouts had stopped; there was just a little residual mucus in the nasal area upon waking. We changed the formula a bit, eliminating the lobelia, goldenseal, and wild cherry bark, and added some bayberry and a little cayenne. He was soon symptom-free.

In this example we see how an illness may reflect a condition different from your basic constitution. Bill was predominantly a pitta person, but his pitta was not aggravated; it was kapha that had been provoked. In Ayurveda it is said that it is easier to cure a condition that is different than your basic constitution, because the basic constitution is not reinforcing the illness.

Appendix 1: Aromatherapy for the Three Doshas

Essential oils, used most often as perfumes or as fragrances for massage oils, may help to open the heart center and to allay negative emotions such as fear, irritation, and apathy.

For a massage oil, mix together 15 to 20 drops of essential oil (your choice) in four ounces of almond oil and shake well. For an atomizer or other spray bottle, add 15 to 20 drops of essential oil to four ounces of distilled water, and shake well.

"Candle burners," available at health food stores, are very popular as well. Place 10 drops of essential oil into the bowl of water and light the candle below it. A light fragrance will pervade into the air, creating the desired effect.

Caution: Applying essential oils directly to the skin may cause severe skin damage. Taking them internally can be extremely dangerous, and may cause death. (One ounce of essential oil is equivalent in potency to thirty two bathtubs of strong herb tea.) Unless you have studied with an aromatherapist, use the essential oils only as suggested above. And make sure that you purchase essential oils, not "fragrances," which are made from synthetic ingredients and do not carry the same health benefits.

Essential Oils for Vata

- jasmine
- sandalwood
- lavender
- rose geranium
- fennel
- pine
- camphor
- frankincense
- basil

- cinnamon
- cardamom
- orange
- angelica

These aromas are calming, warming, and grounding.

Essential Oils for Pitta

- sandalwood
- lavender
- rose geranium
- orange
- lemongrass
- fennel
- peppermint
- jasmine
- gardenia
- mints
- vetiver

These aromas are cooling, calming, and peace-inducing.

Essential Oils for Kapha

- camphor
- cedar
- cinnamon
- frankincense
- cloves
- myrrh
- musk
- pennyroyal
- thyme
- mugwort
- lemongrass
- basil
- lavender
- juniper
- rosemary
- sage

These aromas are stimulating and energizing.

Appendix 2: Color Therapy for Vata, Pitta, Kapha

Vata Colors

Warm, soft shades of:

- red
- gold
- orange
- yellow

Combining these colors with moist and calm colors, such as white or light shades of green or blue, can be very good for vata. Too-bright colors, such as flashy reds or purples, will aggravate the nervous sensitivity of vata types or vata conditions.

Under certain conditions, dark colors may be grounding for vata.

Pitta Colors

- white
- blue
- green
- pastels

Colors that are hot, sharp, or stimulating, like red, orange, and yellow, will aggravate pitta and pitta conditions. Very bright or iridescent colors will provoke pitta. Pastels of various shades are fine.

Kapha Colors

Bright shades of:

- yellow
- gold
- red
- orange

Kaphas can wear bright shades with lots of color contrasts. White, pink, or light shades of "cool" colors such as blue and green are not good for kaphas, although very bright or brilliant shades of blue and green are recommended.

—From *Pocket Guide to Ayurvedic Healing*

HATHA YOGA

Michele Picozzi

Illustrations: Iyengar Yoga Institute of San Francisco

What Is Hatha Yoga?

Yoga is skill in action.

—Bhagavad Gita

Overview

Yoga is one of India's six great ancient philosophies. A systematized body of knowledge, it represents the world's oldest method for spiritual and physical development. Modern scholars have further defined yoga as the classical Indian science that concerns itself with the search for the soul and the union between the individual, whose existence is finite, and the Divine, which is infinite.

Like any science, yoga is based on certain basic principles founded on logical conclusions and rational reasoning. The science of yoga is unique because it encompasses all the types of problems associated with the human condition. No other science can match the quality, content, methodical process, and contributions of yoga.

Noted yoga scholar, author, and historian Georg Feuegstein, Ph.D., says that yoga seeks to foster wholeness. The word *yoga* comes from the Sanskrit word *yuj* meaning "yoke" or "union." As a word, the meaning of *hatha* can best be understood by looking at its two component syllables: *ha* means "sun" and *tha* means "moon." Yoga is the union between them, suggesting that the healthy joining of opposites—in this case, the mind and body—leads to strength, vitality, and peace of mind.

Types of Yoga

While hatha yoga is the most familiar kind practiced in the West, there are five other distinct and individual practices for the purpose of unifying both body and mind.

HATHA YOGA

Called the "forceful path," this is the yoga of physical well-being. In the modern Western approach, hatha yoga is used primarily as a form of physical therapy. It consists of *asana* (postures), *pranayama* (breathing exercises), *pratyahara* (nerve control), *dharma* (mind control), *dhyana* (meditation and spiritual enlightenment). Practice is preceded by the *yama-niyama*, the ten rules of the yoga code of morality.

Continued ➨

Raja Yoga

Called the "royal path," raja yoga is commonly presented as an approach for cultivating the mind's potential for concentration and meditation or transcending the mind for the purpose of physical and mental discipline. Also known as "classical" yoga, it consists of eight "limbs":

1. moral discipline
2. self-restraint
3. posture
4. breath control
5. sensory inhibition
6. concentration
7. meditation
8. ecstasy

These components are found in many other branches of yoga as well. The practice of raja yoga typically starts with hatha yoga, which gives the body the needed health and strength to endure the hardships of more advanced stages of training.

KarmaYoga

Karma yoga is known as "enlightenment through work or action." It aims to lessen our natural tendencies to desire, which lead to actions that obscure our true identity. Karma yoga seeks to guide us to spiritual freedom through the discipline of work that is selfless and performed as a service to others.

Bhakti Yoga

Bhakti yoga seeks to cultivate an open heart and create a path for enlightenment through selfless love and devotion to the Divine, which is seen as being present in every person and thing..

Jnana Yoga

This is the path of discernment and wisdom, as taught in the *Upanishads*, the ancient Hindu mystical texts, which teach distinguishing the real from the unreal, or true happiness from fleeting pleasure.

Tantra Yoga

Tantra yoga represents the path of self-transcendence through ritual means, including consecrated sexuality. It teaches that there is no gap between the Divine and the world and the Divine can be found in ordinary existence.

What Is Hatha Yoga?

Often associated with Hinduism, yoga actually is older. It is thought to have evolved in the eleventh century as a way to prepare notices by giving them strength and equilibrium to meditate for long periods, as well as to serve as a beacon in a time the Hindus have called the kali-yuga, or the Dark Ages of spiritual decline. Despite its long and deep connections to the past, hatha yoga is tailor-made for modern Westerners, as it is a holistic form of exercise. Indra Devi, one of hatha yoga's most respected modern teachers, calls yoga a science that gives a human being the knowledge of his or her true Self.

Hatha yoga, which means "yoga for health," symbolizes the physical aspect of the practice called yoga. It aims to balance different energy flows within the human body. Over the years, yoga has been met with misunderstanding, suspicion, and sometimes ridicule. However, these attitudes have changed gradually during the past thirty years as more people take up yoga to increase flexibility and calm the mind. According to a recent Roper poll, six million Americans now practice hatha yoga. More recently, yoga's visibility and viability as an effective exercise program has been increased by the endorsements of celebrities such as Jane Fonda, Demi Moore, Woody Harrelson, and Sting.

Many people initially are attracted to hatha yoga for its ability to relieve the effects of stress, but it offers much more. Western doctors and scientists are discovering the health benefits of hatha yoga. Studies conducted abroad have shown that hatha yoga can relieve the symptoms of several common and potentially life-threatening illnesses, such as arthritis, arteriosclerosis, chronic fatigue, diabetes, AIDS, asthma, and obesity. Many believe it even fends off the ravages of old age.

A near-perfect fitness routine, hatha yoga provides the means for people of any age not only to get and stay in shape, but also to develop balance, coordination, and a sense of centeredness. It renews, invigorates, and heals the body—stretching and toning the muscles, joints, and spine and directing blood and oxygen to the internal organs (including the glands and nerves). Yoga is distinctly different from other kinds of exercise. It generates motion without causing strain and imbalances in the tiny. When practiced correctly, hatha yoga has no such negative effect on either the inner or outer body. No other form of exercise in existence today can make such a claim.

When done with dedication and purpose, hatha yoga can be a quite demanding, yet immensely rewarding type of exercise. While not inherently aerobic, it involves almost every muscle in the body and challenges the body to work in a different and often more passive way. Since the limbs function as free weights, resistance is created by moving the body's center of gravity. This strengthening gives way endurance as poses are held for longer periods of time.

Unlike conventional forms of exercise, such as weight training, walking, biking, or hiking, hatha yoga stresses quality of movement over quantity. A consistent hatha yoga practice can quiet the mind and refresh the body, bringing health, relaxation, and happiness. However, to reap the maximum benefits hatha yoga has to offer, the practice must be tailored to the needs and goals of the individual.

Yoga and Religion

Yoga does not meet the traditional definitions of a religion. Rather than broadcasting a philosophy or doctrine of its own, hatha yoga is a physical and psychological discipline that combines the learning and practice of *asana*, *pranayama*, and meditation.

Because of its roots in Eastern religion and mythology, hatha yoga has often been associated with the Hindu religion. While both Hinduism and yoga have their roots in India, yoga is an independent tradition. Its separate physical and psychological processes have no connection with religious beliefs. While yoga encourages vegetarianism and celibacy, these practices are not required to reap the many benefits hatha yoga has to offer.

There are, however, a set of ethics associated with yoga, which complements the practice of hatha yoga. While adherence to these ethics is not required, there is substantial benefit to be gained when followed. Additionally, dedicated hatha yoga practice has been found to enhance the religious practice or beliefs of practitioners, whatever their current beliefs.

Components of Hatha Yoga

Hatha yoga consists of three essential components.

Asana: derived from the Sanskrit root meaning "to stay," "to be," "to sit," or "to be established in a particular position". The word refers specifically to all yoga postures or exercises that encourage flexibility and strengthen the skeletal, muscular, glandular, and nervous systems. The spine functions as the focal point of many of the postures, and all postures require a conscious awareness, steadiness, and the ability to surrender to gravity. Patanjali, author of the bible of yoga, the *Yoga Sutras*, describes *asana* as the place on which the student sits or stands and that both the student and the posture are firm and relaxed.

Pranayama: concerns breathing practice where *prana*, vital air or energy, is contained and balanced; yama is the control and direction of that energy and is gained by conscious inhalation, breath retention, and exhalation. Regular practice regulates and harmonizes the breath and its rhythm. The compelling force behind relaxation in yoga comes from *pranayama*, or breath awareness, which increases mental and physical energy by releasing the mind from its continuous stream of random thoughts.

For thousands of years, Eastern medical practitioners have believed breathing to be the single most important factor in health, but only recently has the West caught on. Today, the combination of controlled breathing and meditation are at the core of well-known stress-reduction programs offered at the University of Massachusetts Medical Center in Worcester and the Menniger Clinic in Topeka, Kansas.

Meditation—*Pratyahara*—is withdrawal of the senses from the outer world. *Dharana* (concentration) *dhyana* (contemplation or absorption/meditatiion), and *Samadhi* (ecstatic union) are the final stages of practice and are collectively known as meditation. Like the word *yoga*, meditation refers to the goal of ecstatic union and the variety of practices used to reach this goal. Meditation could be broadly defined as a focusing of attention that results in quieting the mind, increasing intuition, and the ability to relax at will.

Specific Health Benefits

Yoga is both preventive and therapeutic. It is one of the very few exercises that invert the body, as in postures such as headstand, handstand, shoulderstand, and others. Regularly turning the body upside down defies gravity and brings blood to areas of the body that are starved for oxygen and nourishment.

Yoga, postures stretch and relax muscles and properly align the body, thus giving overworked muscles a chance to rest. Through proper alignment, problems can be avoided before they start, and present imbalances caused by poor posture can be addressed.

Besides its ability to strengthen the body, hatha yoga also has a relaxation component, an aspect that many people find attractive. Muscles that are chronically tense and cause pain have the chance to loosen and lengthen, thus engendering relaxation. Yoga, while it doesn't work as quickly or conveniently as popping an aspirin or prescription anti-inflammatory, will uncover the underlying causes of chronic muscle tension and pain and lead to a more permanent and ultimately healthy resolution.

Yoga and the ancient Indian healing tradition of *ayurveda* are closely connected. *Ayurveda*, which means science of life, is based on wholeness—the idea that the body, mind, and spirit are one, each affecting the other. Both yoga and *ayurveda* support the mind-body connection to health and well-being.

Since it has profound physiological and psychological affects on the body, yoga is increasingly prescribed to counteract a variety of physical problems, addictions, and postural abnormalities.

Physical Benefits

Yoga has been shown to offer the following physical benefits to the body:

Continued →

- promotes suppleness of spine and joints
- strengthens, tones, and builds muscles
- stimulates the glands of the endocrine system
- improves digestion and elimination
- increases circulation
- relaxes the nervous system
- boosts immune response
- refreshes the body by relieving muscle strain
- increases stamina
- decreases cholesterol and blood sugar levels
- invites balance and grace
- increases body awareness
- encourages weight loss

MENTAL BENEFITS

Because of its meditative aspects, both in practice of the postures and in single-pointed concentration in meditation, yoga functions as a mental discipline as well.

Yoga's ability to calm and quiet the mind has a physiological basis. Anxiety leads to a fight-or-flight response in the body, which leads to specific physiological responses, such as, the release of hormones, adrenaline in particular, that trigger shallow breathing, muscle tension, and rapid heartbeat. Yoga interrupts this mechanism by calming a busy or agitated mind, providing a stabilizing influence. Specific benefits include:

- quiets the mind
- centers attention
- sharpens concentration
- frees the spirit

History of Yoga

The Essence of Yoga

As both science and art, yoga offers the necessary tools to live fully and consciously. The ancient yogic scriptures assert that no effort is lost on the yogic path, which truly is a lifelong endeavor. Dedicated practice of yoga goes beyond the boundaries of religion and surpasses the notion that to practice yoga means legs up, head down, and a few vegetables a day. Like anything of value, practicing hatha yoga is a process; it is about wholeness, integration, stillness, and interconnectedness.

In this hurried and often troubled world, yoga serves as a tremendous resource. While yoga is most often identified today as a stress reduction method, it does far more than lessen the tension and stiffness in our bodies. When practiced regularly, yoga can be a potent tool for healing and personal transformation, opening our hearts and minds to new ways of caring for others and empowering ourselves.

The Language of Yoga

Sanskrit, the ancient Indian language, is the language of yoga. Literally translated, *Sanskrit* means mathematically and scientifically exact language. In it's written form, Sanskrit is perfectly phonetic. The Sanskrit alphabet consists of a logical array of vocal sounds, and each letter represents a basic root word. Since all Sanskrit words are built upon this guiding principle, it can be applied like a formula, making Sanskrit a relatively easy language to learn.

Historians have theorized that most Indo-Aryan languages, including English, have their origins in a language similar to Vedic Sanskrit. The first serious translations of yogic texts from Sanskrit to English in the West took place during the Victorian era.

The word *yoga* has its roots in the Sanskrit word *yuj*, meaning to merge, join, or unite. Classical yoga uses Sanskrit for the names of the *asanas* (poses or postures) and *pranayama* (breathing) techniques, and these names are still used throughout the world today. Becoming familiar with Sanskrit words as you practice yoga has some distinct advantages. Many styles of yoga, especially the Iyengar system of hatha yoga, refer to the *asanas* by their Sanskrit names, which inscribe the shape or function of the postures or reflect the names of ancient Indian gods and sages or animals and birds. Using the Sanskrit names provides a foundation for further exploration of yogic texts and philosophy and establishes a connection between the ancient art and modern practice of yoga.

THE DEVELOPMENT OF YOGA THROUGH THE AGES

Indian culture has always absorbed ideas and beliefs from many diverse sources. The history of yoga is intrinsically connected with the development of Hinduism and Buddhism. The exact origins of modern yoga are unknown, but it is thought to be about five thousand years old.

The earliest evidence of yoga practice can be traced to the highly developed civilization that flourished in the Indus Valley thousands of years before Christ's birth. In the ancient cities of Mojendro-Daro in Northern India and Harappa (in what is now known as Pakistan), stone sculptures depict seated figures in yoga positions and in meditation. The first written reference to yoga came between 3000 B.C. and 1200 B.C., with the appearance of the *Vedas*, the central texts of Indian religion and mysticism and the culture's earliest known literature. The *Vedas* later became known as the *Upanishads*, which means "to sit next to" in Sanskrit. The *Upanishads* contain the first written reference to yoga and meditation in this passage: "When the five senses and the mind are still, and reason itself rests in silence, then begins the path supreme. This calm steadiness of the senses is called yoga."

Yoga Sutras

The most widely acknowledged test on the system of yoga is the *Yoga Sytras* (sutras means "threads" in Sanskrit). Basically, the *Yoga Sutras* consist of aphorisms to guide yoga practice. While ancient they remain widely read and followed today. The work is attributed to the physician, sage, and scholar Patanjali. Patanjali, who was the first person to put the verbal teachings of yoga into writings, is often referred to as the "father of yoga." He defines yoga as the "stilling of the restless mind."

The four volumes of proverbs that comprise the *Yoga Sutras* serve as a distillation of the essence of yoga teaching as it has been passed down orally from ancient times. They offer succinct, practical statements on how to concentrate the mind through correct practice. They also discuss the ethical precepts, or yamas, that govern social responsibilities and relationships with others, including nonviolence, and niyamas, which represent the fundamentals of all yoga practice. At the core of these systematic teachings is what is known as the Eightfold Path.

THE EIGHTFOLD PATH

In second chapter of the *Yoga Sutras*, Patanjali described the eight steps of classical yoga, often referred to as the Eightfold Path. These steps offer seekers the means and methods to still the mind.

Meant to complement each other, they are fundamental to practicing meditation, correct posture, and stable breathing.

The components of the Eightfold Path include:
- yama—moral restraint
- niyama—personal discipline
- asana—posture
- pranayama—breath control
- pratyahara—control of the senses
- dharana—concentration
- dhyana—meditation
- Samadhi—contemplation

Another classic Indian text, the epic poem *Bhagavad Gita*, written several hundred years later, describes yoga as the "path of the Eternal and freedom from bondage." The Bhagavad Gita remains in wide use in India as well as other parts of the world. It details the various meanings of yoga, some of which include:

- equilibrium in success and failure
- skill in action
- supreme secret of life
- producer of the greatest felicity, serenity, nonattachment
- destroyer of pain

In his search for enlightenment, Buddha practiced yoga, and the great Indian leader Ghandi was said to have gleaned solace and resolution from yoga.

Descriptions of the postures and breathing exercises that form the core of hatha yoga were written down beginning around A.D. 1000. These writings emphasized not only the health and longevity the postures would bring to devoted practitioners, but also the significance of meditation and moral discipline.

Traditionally, disciples were men who turned to yoga in their later years, when their children were grown and their responsibilities as householders had been fulfilled. They studied under the direct supervision of a guru, or teacher, who was viewed as the embodiment of the Divine. Surrender to the guru was absolute, and his authority was not questioned. The guru-disciple relationship assumed that the aspirant was ready for the renunciation and devotion that total commitment to the spiritual life required, and the guru rejected students deemed not ready for rigors of study.

The British colonization of India introduced yoga to the West, as the British governor-general encouraged the study of Sanskrit. Subsequently, translatios of the Bhagavad Gita and the Sacred Books of the East from Sanskrit into English did much to spread Indian philosophy.

How Yoga Came to America

Hatha yoga made its debut in the United States in the mid-1800s among groups of intellectual writers interested in the esoteric philosophies of the East. These literary lions included the likes of Ralph Waldo Emerson, Henry David Thoreau, and Bronson Alcott. Later, a slim volume entitled *Light in Asia*, a Victorian-era biography of Gautama Buddha, sold half a million copies, and as a result, societies promoting Eastern thought emerged.

One of the featured attractions of the 1893 Chicago World's Fair was the appearance of Swami Vivekananda (1863–1902), one of India's most celebrated sages. While in America, he taught raja yoga; he also spent two years teaching in Detroit, Chicago, Boston, New York, and Europe. His presence was credited with further stimulating the West's interest in yoga, which opened the door for other teachers to come to this country.

Hollywood was introduced to the health benefits of hatha yoga in the 1940s, when the Russian-born yoga teacher Indra Devi migrated there.

Continued ➡

Twenty years later, the combination of the cultural changes initiated in the 1960s, including the growing interest in Eastern religions and the publication of Jess Stearn's best-seller *Yoga, Youth & Reincarnation* (Bantam Books) in 1965 caused yoga to permeate more and more of American culture. . . .

How Hatha Yoga Is Practiced in the West

Yoga Today

The more common stereotypical images of yoga—from turban-wearing swamis to snake charmers to people turning themselves into human pretzels or levitating—have gone the way of love beads and bell bottom pants. Hatha yoga, which emphasizes *asana* (practice of postures), *pranayama* (breathing techniques), and *dhyana* (meditation), is the most commonly practiced form of yoga in the West. Hatha yoga attracts people from all walks of life—children, senior citizens, women as well as men—and is readily accessible to people who aren't interested in advancing or developing a personal spiritual practice.

Different styles or forms of hatha yoga can be found in nearly every part of the United States. Many consider it as normal a form of exercise as walking or biking. It is taught everywhere, from TV to local YMCAs and YWCAs as well as at spas, gyms, community and senior centers, and private studios dedicated solely to teaching and practicing yoga.

Yoga also is increasingly embraced by the medical community. Popular health practitioners who possess mainstream medical credentials and are open to alternative practices include Andrew Weil, M.D., Dean Ornish, M.D., Joan Borysenko, M.D., and Jon Kabat-Zinn, Ph.D. Such practitioners have long encouraged patients and clients to take up yoga. Yoga is also an integral part of many stress management programs endorsed and paid for by HMOs and insurance companies. In fact, Cedars-Sinai Medical Center's Preventive and Rehabilitative Cardiac Center includes gentle yoga postures and breathing techniques to aid the recovery of patients with heart disease.

The most often cited reasons Westerners begin a yoga practice are to:
- increase flexibility
- promote relaxation
- manage stress
- complement a fitness program
- heal an injury or strengthen a weak back

Health Benefits of Hatha Yoga

Like other Eastern forms regarded as "movement arts," hatha yoga, particularly from a physical standpoint, offers both preventive and therapeutic aspects. A complete fitness program, hatha yoga will release endorphins in the brain as well as any regular exercise program. Yoga postures stretch, extend, and flex the spine, while exercising muscles and joints, keeping the body strong and supple. And when done in conjunction with breathing techniques, hatha yoga postures stimulate circulation, digestion, and the nervous and endocrine systems.

As a workout, yoga can be intense, easy, or somewhere in between. It can be practiced by anyone, regardless of age, to achieve a more limber body, increased physical coordination, better posture, and improved flexibility without incurring the potentially negative effects associated with high-impact forms of exercise.

Hatha yoga remains different from newer or more modern types of exercise. It does not aim to raise the heart rate (although variations such as Ashtanga, Power Yoga, or the flow series taught by Bikram Choudhury may) or work on specific muscle groups. Overall, the postures release stiffness and tension, help to reestablish the inner balance of the spine, renew energy, and restore health. Some postures provide the added benefit of being weight-bearing, which helps sustain bone mass (very important for women). Relaxation and breathing exercises produce stability and reduce stress and put you in touch with your inner strength. In addition, regular practice of hatha yoga can promote graceful aging. Famous yoga teachers Vanda Scavelli and Indra Devi, along with many not-so-famous people, maintain a daily yoga practice well into their eighties and nineties.

According to Mary Schatz, M.D., author of *Back Care Basics* (Rodmell Press, 1992), the psychological and physiological determinants of good health are indeed integral components of the ancient science of yoga. She writes: "Yoga provides the means to become physically fit in the context of a philosophy that encourages positive health practices and personality characteristics. The body is no longer divorced from the mind and the spirit. There is a clear correlation between yoga and the positive health practices documented in medical literature."

Some of the documented health benefits attributed to yoga include:

- relieves chronic stress patterns in the body
- lengthens, strengthens, and tones muscles
- corrects posture
- improves muscular-skeletal conditions such as bad knees, tight shoulders and neck, bunions, swayback, and scoliosis
- boosts immune function
- increases fitness levels and refines balance
- fosters healthy body awareness
- manages stress and hypertension
- improves concentration

One of the hidden benefits of studying and practicing hatha yoga is the ability to take care of yourself. If your back goes out or leg cramps keep you awake at night, a yoga posture or series of postures will help relieve the discomfort.

Hatha Yoga Systems

Because of hatha yoga's ever increasing popularity in the West, a wide variety of yoga styles have grown up around particular teachers from India or as variations on a theme developed by a Western teacher. Like individuals, styles or schools of hatha yoga have their own personalities and approaches to practicing asanas. What distinguishes the different styles is what's emphasized, be it posture, breath, aerobics, dance, slow and rhythmic movements, philosophy, or a combination of many factors.

Although the basic asanas and breathing exercises remain the same, how they are done, in what order, and where attention is focused while doing them constitute the main differences among the many schools. However, no matter which style you opt for, special clothing isn't required. All that's needed are comfortable, loose or stretchy clothes, bare feet, an empty stomach, open mind, and a few basic props.

Hatha Yoga Traditions Practiced and Taught in the West

Ananada Yoga

This method combines the physical and spiritual. Each pose is integrated with a specific affirmation to develop or heighten self-awareness. Ananada yoga also teaches a series of poses called "energenization exercises." These exercises involve tensing and relaxing different parts of the body, coupled with breathing exercises to send energy to them. Deep relaxation in the poses as a preparation for meditation is also stressed. Classes and a one-month teacher training program are offered at the Expanding Light facility in Nevada City, California, as well as other cities in the western United States and in Assisi, Italy.

Ashtanga Yoga

Consisting of 240 postures done in six successive series (*vinyasa*) linked by the breath, Ashtanga yoga represents the most intensive form of hatha yoga, requiring great stamina and flexibility.

The concentrated sequencing of postures is designed to create *tapas*, or heat, inside the body for the purpose of cleansing and detoxifying the body to bring forth *prana*, or to breathe, so it can be channeled up through the spine. Ashtanga also emphasizes strength and flexibility.

Very few teachers are certified to teach Ashtanga yoga in the West. Contact the Ashtanga Yoga Center for more information.

Iyengar Yoga

Probably the most widely known style of hatha yoga in the West, this style of hatha yoga is based on the teachings of B. K. S. Iyengar. It is regarded mostly for its rigorous scientific and therapeutic approach, concentrating on correcting structural imbalances in the physical body.

The distinguishing characteristics of the Iyengar style include the extensive use of props—blankets, sticky mats, folding chairs, wood blocks and benches, bolsters, and straps—and attention to detail, from correct posture to the placement of hands, pelvis, and feet.

Classes typically focus in great detail on only a few *asanas* so as to refine movements. Beginning students are drilled in standing poses so as to learn proper alignment and balance, which is necessary in other poses. After a foundation has been established, students are then taught *pranayama*.

Teachers undergo a rigorous certification program and are taught anatomy, physiology and kinesiology as well as yoga philosophy. There are Iyengar institutes, centers, and independent teachers throughout the world, particularly in the United States and Europe.

Integral Yoga

Based on the teachings of Swami Satchindananda, Integral Yoga emphasizes a more meditative rather than anatomical approach. It combines all the paths of yoga—*asana*, *pranayama*, selfless service, prayer, chanting, meditation, and self-inquiry—into one approach.

Kripalu Yoga

Less concerned with the structural detail of the postures, Kripalu yoga has been described as "meditation in motion." It emphasizes the student's mental and emotional states as the poses are held, while encouraging a gentle, compassionate, and introspective approach. Postures are held for a long time so as to explore and release emotional and spiritual blocks.

This inner-directed form of hatha yoga consists of three stages: willful practice, will and surrender, and finally, surrendering to the body's wisdom. Within each of the three stages, poses are offered in different intensities: gentle, moderate, and vigorous. In addition, spontaneous postures and sequences of postures are encouraged, guided by the body's internal awareness.

The Kripalu Center for Yoga and Health, located in Lenox, Massachusetts, offers certificate

Continued ➡

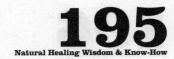

programs in teacher training, workshops, retreats, and conferences.

Kundalini Yoga

Designed to bring forth the reservoir of energy (*kundalini*) stored at the base of the spine, this style of hatha yoga focuses on arousing the *kundalini* energy, using a combination of breath, posture, chanting, and meditation to direct this energy through the energy centers (*chakras*) located along the spine.

Several breathing techniques are highlighted including alternate nostril breathing, slow diaphragmatic breathing, and the "breath of fire."

Founder Yogi Bhajan's Healthy, Happy, Holy Organization (3 HO) focuses on all aspects of the yogic lifestyle, as well as community service. There are approximately 1,500 Kundalini teachers, located primarily in the United States, Canada, Europe, Mexico, and South America.

Sivananda Yoga

Originated by Swami Vishnu-devananda, Sivananda Yoga is similar to Integral Yoga, with the same dietary restrictions and scriptural study.

Viniyoga

Originated by T. K. V. Desikachar, the style of hatha yoga called viniyoga is said to represent a middle path between the exactness of Iyengar yoga and physically demanding Ashtanga yoga. It is based on the principle of vinyasa karma, which means "an organized course of Yoga study," and combines asana, pranayama, meditation, text study, counseling, imagery, prayer, chanting, and ritual.

Yoga postures are tailored to the physical needs and limitations of each student, taking into account body type, emotional needs, cultural heritage, and interest. Emphasis is on the spine, and breath is considered more important than how the posture is done. Typically, classes are private one-on-one sessions.

Yoga College of India

Classes consist of a two-part series of twenty-six repeating postures with two *pranayatna* exercises that are designed to stretch and tone the whole body. Most poses are done twice and held for a minimum of ten seconds in a room with temperatures of eighty degrees or higher, often supplemented by moist air from a humidifier. Class concludes with a brief period of relaxation.

Founded by Bikram Choudhury, the Yoga College of India has locations in Beverly Hills (classes and teacher training), San Francisco, Honolulu, and Tokyo. Classes are also taught at private studios throughout the United States.

Hatha Yoga Traditions Based on Eastern Philosophy and Developed by Westerners

Hidden Language Yoga

Developed by Swami Sivananda Radha, who was born Sylvia Hellman in 1911, this method of hatha yoga blends postures with journal writing and group discussion to investigate the symbolic meaning of each *asana* and the posture's effect on the student's mind and body.

Hidden Language Yoga borrows from Ananda yoga and Jungian theory while using symbol and metaphor to aid students in developing deeper awareness of the psychological and mystical messages of the poses. Swami Radha established the Yasodhara Ashram, an eighty-three-acre retreat at Kootenay Bay in British Columbia, Canada, and also is the founder of the Association for the Potential for Human Development in the United States.

Ishta Yoga

Originated by South African Mani Finger, Ishta yoga (Integral Sciences of Hatha and Tantric Arts) combines *asana* with *pranayama*, visualization, and guided meditation to open the body's subtle energy channels. Individual practice consists of a mantra with a set of postures tailored to the specific needs of the student. Finger's son Alan has been largely responsible for bringing Ishta yoga to the United States.

Jivamukti

Created in the early 1990s by New Yorkers Sharon Gannon and David Life, *Jivamukti* is a Sanskrit word that means "liberation while alive in the body." This system borrows from several styles of yoga, including Ashtanga, Iyengar, and Sivananda. Spiritual teachings are taught in tandem with postures. During class teachers chant in Sanskrit and read and interpret the philosophical teachings of yoga.

Phoenix Rising

Developed by Michael Lee in 1984, Phoenix Rising yoga therapy is based on Kripalu yoga. Lee intended it as a way for people to use yoga as a tool for living. It incorporates poses to support inner awareness, mental clarity, emotional stability, spiritual attunement, and physical well-being. It features sixteen basic poses, including forward bends and backbends, inversions, and twisting poses. Phoenix Rising is done with a therapist, who gently holds the student until emotional tensions begin to surface and release, followed by a one-to-one discussion and concluded with a guided meditation.

Tri Yoga

Tri Yoga refers to the union of *asana*, *mudra* (practices similar to *asanas*), and *pranayama*. Kali Ray of Aptos, California, founded Tri Yoga, which employs three designated practices that range from basic to advanced levels with other sequences tailored to a student's individual needs. Ray is also the creator of the Devi Dance, a performance that delivers yoga, *pranayama*, and meditation accompanied by music and done in flowing sequence.

Classics consist of a spontaneous, dance-like series of poses taught at a varied pace and accompanied by background music. Sessions are completed with seated *pranayama* and meditation.

White Lotus Yoga

Developed by Ganga White and Tracey Rich, this style represents a modified version of the Ashtanga style of hatha yoga. Characterized by a flowing style of practice, postures are done in flowing sequences that are characterized as lengthy and even aerobic. Classes are taught in Los Angeles at the Center for Yoga and at White Lotus Foundation's retreat center in Santa Barbara, California, where White has been director since 1973.

Starting a Hatha Yoga Practice

Anybody who wants to can practice yoga. Anybody who can breathe; therefore anybody can practice yoga.

—T. K. V. Desikachar

How to Make Yoga Work For You

Hatha yoga has stood the test of time. It is the oldest physical discipline in existence, having been practiced for thousands of years. The original purpose of the postures and breathing exercises was to bring stability and relaxation so practitioners could prepare for the rigors of meditation, sitting still and alert for long periods of time.

Whether or not there is a clear goal in mind at the start (losing weight, relieving stress, practicing relaxation, gaining flexibility, strengthening the lower back, gaining peace of mind, enhancing overall physical well-being) dedicated, observant practice will help develop the capacity to set and achieve your goals. By its very nature, hatha yoga brings into balance the dissimilar aspects of the mind, body, and personality.

When planning to start a hatha yoga practice, you need to consider current abilities and physical limitations, as well as what you want to accomplish. Before beginning, the *Yoga Sutras* advise *vinyasa karma* (to place in a special way). One of the foremost teachers of hatha yoga, T. K. V. Desikachar explains the concept this way: "It is not enough to simply take a step as that step needs to take us in the right direction and be made in the right way . . . thus *vinyasa karma* describes a correctly organized course of yoga practice."

Ideally, your yoga practice should initially be focused on learning and becoming grounded in the basics of hatha yoga and its *asanas*. With this background, you can then center your yoga sessions around the demands of your lifestyle. If your work keeps you in front of a computer, or if you are on your feet a lot, the poses you will want to concentrate on will be different from those for someone who is preparing to run marathons or someone who has a chronic heart condition. Different people require different styles and different practices.

Finding the Style That's Right For You

Each of us comes to yoga in our own time and in our own way, much as the old proverb describes it: When the student is ready, the teacher appears. To decide on which kind of hatha yoga is right for you, you need to take into account your own personality and goals. The therapeutic aspect of yoga may be important if you are recovering from a sports injury or if chronic back pain plagues you, or the more cerebral or meditative aspects of yoga may be more appealing. If you aren't sure what you want to obtain from practicing yoga, sample classes of different styles of hatha yoga from different teachers. If a variety of styles or teachers isn't available, check your local library for videotapes to preview at your own pace and at little cost.

As there are widely differing techniques and styles of practice and sometimes confusing points of view, you will want to take the time to find the methods and teacher that are right for you and to assess intelligently and critically what is taught and how it is being taught.

In evaluating different styles, it is helpful to learn about the origins, philosophy, and founder of the particular hatha yoga tradition you are interested in. There are fewer lineages than there are teachers, and by researching the master's approach (many of whom have written books on their teachings), you can obtain vital information about the aims and philosophies of different styles of hatha yoga. By examining the cultural roots of traditional yogic teachings, you can assess them in the light of your own values, needs, priorities, and experiences.

While all styles of hatha yoga are beneficial, some have specific physical requirements. To know which style is right for you, pay careful attention to how your body responds to the postures. If you haven't exercised in a while or have tight muscles (particularly hamstring and back muscles), relying on props to gain correct alignment may be necessary. This doesn't mean that you and this type of yoga are incompatible. Give yourself time to understand the poses and your body time to get acquainted with becoming flexible in unfamiliar areas. If you aren't sure if one style is better for you

Continued ➡

than another, give it a trial run of at least three weeks before deciding. To make a fair evaluation, take careful note of how you feel after a class. You should feel centered and calm, stretched but pushed beyond your limits. Over the long haul, yoga classes should have a positive effect on your well-being.

If you have any health concerns about your health or fitness, consult your physician, qualified health practitioner, or yoga teacher before undertaking a yoga practice, especially with these specific health problems: high blood pressure, heart disease, arthritis, back or neck injury, or recent surgery.

How to Find the Right Teacher

Yoga classes and teachers vary tremendously. Each teacher instructs from his or her own experiences, thus furthering the tradition of direct transmission from teacher to student and the on-going evolution of yoga.

The American Yoga Association defines a good yoga teacher as one who:

- has spent time studying the various effects of yoga exercises, breathing, and meditation
- has a working knowledge of major muscle groups and body systems
- is able to vary techniques according to each person's individual capability
- will not confuse the yoga techniques by allowing his or her own religious beliefs to affect the class

TIPS FOR LOCATING A QUALIFIED YOGA INSTRUCTOR

- Decide what you want to learn and at what pace.
- Ask a friend for a recommendation.
- Check the local Yellow Pages, YMCAs, local newspapers, health food store and church bulletin boards, and metaphysical bookstores for information about local instruction.

If there are no instructors in your area, contact teachers in nearby areas for recommendations. Also, the yoga associations listed in the Resources section of this book can refer you to instructors in your area.

Both *Yoga Journal* and *Yoga International* magazines produce annual directories of yoga teachers and studios located in the United States, Canada, and abroad. The *Yoga Journal* list is featured in the magazine's July/August issue and is also available by mail. The *Yoga International*, published in the January issue, list is available through its regular subscription service or by special order.

Before taking a class, call the teacher to discuss her or his style and emphasize and your needs or expectations. Ask about teaching experience and qualifications.

Determine if the class size is right and if classes are conducted in an organized fashion. Are the instructions clear? Is there individual attention and gentle direction, both verbal and hands-on?

After attending a class, ask yourself whether you find the style of teaching compatible.

Various yoga institutes, centers, ashrams, studios, and independent senior teachers offer training programs. Many of them also offer certification for aspiring yoga teachers who complete a specific course of study that stresses yogic philosophy, anatomy, postures, breathing techniques, meditation, and diet. However, programs vary in content and length of study and testing. Currently, yoga teachers are not licensed or certified by any national program and are exempt from regulation by individual states. However, this may change.

The *Yoga Sutras* suggest maintaining a relationship with one teacher. This relationship will help you reach a deeper understanding and greater degree of trust in him or her. In an atmosphere of trust, the teacher will be better able to discover what it is you need to learn. Following one teacher and one direction helps you discover ways and means to avoid and overcome the various obstacles that come up in practicing yoga.

How to Be a Good Yoga Student

Like everything else in life, yoga takes time to learn and understand. It also has its share of ups and downs. One day it may seem effortless, and the next it's a struggle to bend over and reach your toes. Like any exercise program, your yoga practice should consist of warm-up poses, work toward more challenging poses, and end with a cool-down and relaxation period.

Yoga can help us stay centered when times are good, bad, and in between. Even when we think practicing is a waste of time and energy, it is not. When thoughts such as this arise, remember that the act of practice itself, sticking to our commitment, is valuable. Esther Myers, a longtime Canadian yoga teacher, explains that "yoga trains us to center and release . . . consistent practice takes commitment and discipline, tempered by compassion and self acceptance and finding the way that is right for you."

While yoga is calming and centering, it is also a vehicle for expressing and clearing strong energy and emotions, with specific poses to deal with the turmoil. While doing poses you like is important to sustaining and enjoying a solo practice, your routine should be well-rounded and should include some poses from all the major groupings of poses: standing, inversions, twists, forward bends, backbends. When beginning a yoga practice, emphasize standing postures, as they will strengthen major muscles quickly, thus providing a solid base for other postures.

Be enthusiastic. Initially, your eagerness for learning yoga may be high but may waver over time. A commitment to learning anything worthwhile requires patience and dedication, as well as renewing or reconnecting with the energy or reason for pursuing the study in the first place. Don't rely on your teachers to always pump up your enthusiasm to learn and practice.

Be open to learning from different teachers, but be careful not to take classes from too many different teachers at the same time. This also applies to attending workshops. Attending classes regularly or taking the occasional workshop is fine, but not at the expense of not developing or ignoring your own private practice. Take the time to integrate what you've learned from your teachers into your own practice before attempting more.

Be curious. Iyengar yoga expert Donna Farhi suggests one way to develop curiosity is to cultivate "disbelief" for the purpose of exploring and investigating on your own. Farhi encourages students to observe themselves carefully while in a posture. She suggests asking these questions: How does this movement affect my body? What happens if I do it another way? How am I reacting to this posture?

Without these elements, according to Farhi, there is no real learning. She urges students, regardless of where they are in their yoga practice, to regard yoga as an ongoing process rather than a single accomplishment.

Yoga can be a lifelong pursuit, but persistency, consistency, and discipline are required to gain the many lasting benefits yoga offers. This news should encourage your effort and strengthen your resolve.

There is no hurry, and the fear of loss should not concern you. The yogic scriptures state that no effort is lost or wasted on the path of knowledge.

TIPS FOR SERIOUS YOGA STUDENTS

- Be on time. This is important if you take yoga instruction seriously. Arriving ten to fifteen minutes early is advised so you can get into the proper frame of mind and warm up. Important instructions often are given at the beginning of class. Chronic lateness is a sign of disrespect to both the teacher and fellow students.
- If just starting or getting reacquainted with yoga, sign up for a beginner's class or practice only the basic postures and routines.
- Be attentive. "You're apt to learn more and grasp complex ideas more readily. Put the events of the day aside while in class. Students who are motivated and interested inspire teachers to go out of their way to help them progress.
- Be seen. Introduce yourself to the teacher, preferably before the start of class. Don't hide in the back; position yourself near the front.
- Be consistent. Your progress and the quality of class are enhanced by regular attendance. Hatha yoga, like any skill, is gained through steady, mindful accumulation of knowledge and practice. This means going to class when you don't feel like it.
- Don't compare yourself with anyone else. Individuality extends to levels of flexibility as well as body types. While it is human nature to compare, remember, yoga is noncompetitive and we all learn at different rates.
- Go at your own pace, moving gradually into each pose.
- Listen to your body. Stretching is good, pain is not. Yoga does not "go for the burn."
- Set reasonable goals, taking into account your current physical condition, degree of flexibility, and age.
- Proceed slowly when trying new poses. The mind needs time to absorb the new movements and the body to get used to them.
- Keep mind and body relaxed. When your attention wanders, bring it back gently to the yoga.
- Be appreciative of constructive criticism. Verbal and hands-on correction are typical in many of the styles of hatha yoga. Take it in the manner it was intended—to help you along the path.
- Be appropriate when asking questions. Most teachers welcome students' questions during class, as both the class and teacher can learn from them. Questions should be brief and pertain to the matter at hand. Questions not pertaining to the current subject or those of a personal nature should be asked after class.
- Be appreciative of your teacher. Offering encouragement or feedback when something a teacher does is helpful (or potentially harmful) can be a morale booster, as well as bettering the quality of his or her teaching.
- Don't give up. The initial discomfort or struggle with adapting your body to the postures eventually disappears and gives way to more positive feelings.
- The more you practice the more benefits you derive. You don't have to be an expert or master to feel and look better in a relatively short period of time.

The Importance of a Personal Practice

If you are attending regular classes, you might ask yourself why it is important to develop your own

Continued ➡

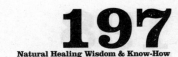

personal practice—an excellent question. Developing a personal practice goes beyond the notion of taking time or caring for yourself.

Working alone and at your own pace leads to discoveries that may not come to light during class, when you are mainly following instructions. When practicing on your own, you can spend time working on problem areas, such as lower back, shoulders, and hamstrings, or becoming more familiar with basic postures before moving on to more challenging ones.

In addition, yoga masters have determined that two years of diligent practice is required before the student fully understands the nature of the poses and begins to appreciate how they are interconnected. Patanjali wrote that the mastery of *asanas* occurs only when practice becomes effortless.

How to Establish a Personal Practice

Set a goal—whether it is stress reduction, weight loss, increased flexibility, enhanced immunity, or heightened spiritual awareness—your motivation should be personal. Remember that it takes time to perfect the posture.

Set aside a regular time to practice, as yoga frees and relaxes the body to do other things. Practice regularly, even if it's only a few minutes every day. More time, however, will deepen your practice as well as your satisfaction with it. With regular practice, tight muscles will release, and as they do, poses will become easier to do. The amount of time and effort given to practice brings equivalent results.

It may take some experimenting to determine your optimal time of day and length of practice. Steady, regular practice will help you stick to your routine on days when you don't feel like it or don't see the progress you had hoped for. As your practice develops over time, the positive effects of yoga will appear more subtle and perhaps less noticeable.

If possible, establish a regular time of day to set aside for practice. Morning or evening practice is advised. Practice when your body is most limber. Some people find their bodies are stiff in the morning, making practice more difficult. Night practice, however, may limit the kinds of postures you do as some are too stimulating and affect sleep. Whatever schedule you devise, do it long enough to see how it works, including on weekends.

Practice at the same time each day for fifteen to twenty minutes. Add another five to ten minutes to your practice every three to four weeks. The key is regularity.

Start with your favorite poses. Repeat them two or three times before moving on to the next *asana*. While in the pose, do not hold the breath. Between postures, take one or two breaths to quiet the mind.

Be patient. Some people are genetically less flexible or have tighter muscle groups than others. But this doesn't mean real progress can't be made. Stretching overly tight hamstring and neck and shoulder muscles takes some getting used to. Conversely, overflexibility presents problems as well.

When beginning, practice every other day, up to four days a week. Gradually work up to six days of practice, and rest on the seventh. Enjoy whatever time you have set aside for practice. One experienced teacher put it quite well: "It's better to practice just a little and enjoy it than to not practice at all."

How to Prepare for Practice

Have an empty or near-empty stomach. Wait a minimum of ninety minutes after eating before practicing postures and four hours after a large meal. If very hungry before class, eat some yogurt or fruit.

Wear comfortable clothing that keeps you warm, but not too warm—leotards, unitards, cotton tights, bike shorts, loose T-shirts or tank tops. Bulky or overly loose clothing will only get in the way. Practice barefoot to avoid slipping.

Set aside a special place to practice. If you use props (wooden blocks, belts, folding chair, etc.), store them together and set aside or bring to the practice area before beginning.

When indoors, set the thermostat to sixty-five to seventy-five degrees. Keep a blanket or sweatpants handy for Corpse or other complete relaxation poses and meditation. If practicing outdoors, select a shady spot with plenty of room to move. Dress accordingly.

For seated meditation, use firm blankets folded three or four times lengthwise or a firm pillow or cushion specifically made for meditation.

Minimize distractions. Turn off the radio, TV, and telephone, and set the answering machine volume to the low setting. Clear the room of pets and kids, if possible.

Locate a level surface. A bare hardwood floor is ideal, but if your feet slip, use a sticky mat. If practicing on carpet, choose an area with a tight weave, such as Berber.

How to Get the Most from Your Practice

The effects of practicing yoga are cumulative. If done every day or nearly every day, even ten to fifteen minutes will help build concentration, increase flexibility, and strengthen willpower, making it easier to practice the next day. Consistency is key. Most yoga instructors believe that there is more benefit to doing a brief practice regularly than hit-or-miss home practice sessions, sporadic class attendance, or the occasional workshop. Veteran Canadian yoga teacher Esther Myers says the value of an ongoing practice cannot be overestimated. As yoga germinates and takes root in your life, you will find the rhythm and level of practice that is right for you. The greatest and longest-lasting benefits are achieved when at least three or four yoga *asanas* are done every day.

When starting, realistically assess how much time you can devote to yoga practice. Then start with poses you find you can master easily and work toward more challenging ones.

Adjust your practice to your schedule and biorhythms. Some days will find you not feeling as energetic or flexible, even weak or tired. On those days, try doing restorative poses, such as supine poses and forward bends.

Don't practice when you have a fever. If you have a cold or other minor illness, use your judgment and restrict your practice to restorative ones.

Be aware that some poses affect mood and energy differently. Poses that are more stimulating include Sun Salutation, backbends, and standing poses. These poses are best done early in the day. More appropriate for the evening are forward bends, inversions, and restorative poses. Hero's Pose, Reclining Hero's Pose, Bound Angle Pose, and Basic Sitting Forward Bend are ideal for relaxing and recharging. Reclining Hero Pose is especially beneficial after consuming a heavy meal, as it aids digestion. (See the following section for directions for specific poses.)

One way to extend your yoga practice is to incorporate yoga throughout the day. In your daily routine, there are many ways you can practice yoga without actually doing a formal posture such as:

- Relax by exhaling and dropping your shoulders when standing or sitting. Repeat several times throughout the day.
- Straighten your spine when sitting, standing, and walking.
- Lift your chest while driving.
- Take several deep breaths that expand the diaphragm.
- When standing in line, spread your feet, straighten ankles; when walking, be conscious of touching the ground with entire surface of the foot.

How Long Should You Practice?

Most experts recommend a minimum of ten minutes of practice every day. However, to practice a range of postures and incorporate breathing or meditation, fifteen to twenty-five minutes is necessary. These brief practice sessions should also be interspersed with longer sessions of thirty to ninety minutes three or four times weekly.

To move forward in your practice, longer practice sessions of at least forty-five minutes to an hour are required. Extended practice sessions should include a specific breathing practice with a long relaxation period. However, you should never practice to the point of exhaustion. If you are overly tired or sore after a regular practice session, you may be practicing too long or attempting postures that are too advanced or strenuous.

If you're new to yoga or if you've been sedentary or you spend long hours sitting in front of a computer screen, the muscles in your legs—hamstring and calves specifically—hips, shoulders, and lower back may be sore. After practice and before retiring, take a long hot bath spiked with a couple of cups of Epsom salt to reduce the stiffness you might experience the next day. Severe muscle or joint stiffness means you've overdone it and gone past your maximum. Give your body a charge to recover by resting and, if your body permits, very light stretching. However, if you have severe pain that doesn't lessen in twenty-four hours, muscle cramps, headaches, or dizziness or any other unusual symptoms, see your doctor.

Practicing During Menstruation and Pregnancy

Inverted postures, which turn the body upside-down, should be avoided while menstruating. Some methods suggest refraining from practicing yoga postures during the first forty-eight to seventy-two hours. However, when you feel discomfort, forward bends may be done in moderation.

During the early stages of pregnancy, inversions can be continued if you have practiced them before. If pressure or breathing problems occur at any time, come out of the pose immediately. Practice of *pranayama*, without holding the breath, is encouraged as a preparation for labor.

How to Practice

Pay attention to your body. Check your alignment from head to toe for balance and stability before beginning any posture. Feet should make firm contact with the ground with toes spread. Weight is evenly distributed. Ankles are firm and straight, not rolling in. Kneecaps are lifted. Hips and shoulders are level. Chest and stomach are lifted. Shoulders roll back and down. Collarbone spreads. Chin is level. Neck balances comfortably between the shoulders. Mouth and throat are relaxed.

Pay attention to the instructions, particularly the directions for placement, as they form the foundation of the pose. Strive for correct body alignment.

- For most postures, socks should be removed before beginning. Keep the eyes open in the postures except for Corpse Pose. Relax the facial muscles and keep the eyes soft.
- Move slowly into the pose to avoid injury and

Continued ➡

to more easily feel which muscles are actively working.

- Go as far into the pose as comfortable, to a point where you can maintain the pose in correct alignment, not necessarily to its maximum. Work on the edge of the stretch, but back off if there is any pain. Listen to how your body responds.

- Don't bounce, as this shortens rather than lengthens the muscle. Bouncing creates an automatic resistance and risks injury.

- Breathe. Slow down and take the time to focus your attention on your breathing. Breath should always be taken in through the nostrils and out through the mouth.

- Hold the pose as long as even breathing is maintained. Time will increase as the body becomes more familiar with the poses and strength and flexibility increase.

- Don't hold the breath while in a pose, as it tightens the body. Use the breath, particularly exhalation, to facilitate the stretch.

- Smile when you do a posture; it helps you relax and enjoy what you're doing.

- Turn attention inward. Pay attention to how your body feels—where it's tight, strong, or tired. Practicing asanas provides valuable feedback.

- Avoid tensing muscles around the eyes, jaws, neck, throat, shoulders, and stomach. Keep your eyes open in the poses, except in Corpse Pose.

- If a pose hurts, stop and rest. There is nothing in yoga that says no pain, no gain.

- Don't tense when encountering discomfort, as this further tenses the muscles. Be calm and gentle and remain open to releasing the blocked area. If in pain, come out of the pose, and adjust the pose or add a prop to reduce the amount of stretch.

- Pay attention to your body. Trust your body's response to being in a pose. It is ego that pushes the body past the point of endurance often causing harm. Never force or push yourself into a pose or hold a pose past the point of real endurance.

Learn to distinguish between discomfort and pain. Joint pain in the neck, knees, lower back, or hips should mean to release the posture and rest. Muscles that are tight, particularly the hamstrings and the ones surrounding the hips and shoulders, will take time to lengthen and relax. As you work these muscles, begin slowly, increasing their capacity to stretch over time.

When adjusting a pose, start from the ground up. In standing poses, begin with the feet; for inversions, start with the head, shoulders, and elbows; and in seated poses, begin with the sit bones and position of the pelvis.

Don't "muscle" your way into poses through strength alone. Instead, smile, breathe, and relax and lengthen the muscles you're working.

To end the pose, come out the same way as going into it. Focus on alignment, keeping the breath steady.

Rest for a minute after three or four consecutive poses, especially when practicing standing poses. Recommended "resting" asanas are Standing Forward Bend and Child's Pose.

During menstruation, do not practice Headstand, Shoulderstand, the intense standing poses (Side Angle Pose, Intense Side Stretch and Warrior I & II), or backbends, as they reverse the flow of blood.

If you are nursing an injury or have high blood pressure, are pregnant, recently injured, or have chronic back pain, consult with your doctor and a qualified yoga instructor before beginning a yoga practice.

How to Stay Motivated

In his wisdom, Patanjali identified eleven obstacles to yoga practice:

- lack of interest
- self-doubt
- laziness
- sensuality
- false knowledge
- failure to concentrate
- pain
- despair
- sickness
- unsteadiness of body
- unsteadiness of respiration

Interestingly, only four of these obstacles have to do with physical limitations; the rest are concerned with the mind, reflecting the connection between body, mind, and spirit.

Even the most advanced yoga students have had to overcome some limitations imposed by their bodies. Beginning students, especially, must keep their expectations realistic. Achieving lasting flexibility comes in small increments over long periods of time. Conversely, don't use unrealistic expectations as a reason not to practice or to quit altogether. Every posture has a beginning, middle, and advanced stage. Props will help you to accommodate physical limitation. Holding poses for only brief periods can offer as much benefit as holding them for longer periods.

Staying Motivated

Vary your sequence or add new postures. Continue to spend time in the more familiar poses even as you add new ones.

Create space in your home for yoga, even if it's only a corner of a room. It will reinforce your commitment to a regular practice. Besides props, you might include a small bookcase to store reference books and videotapes. Add photos, candles, or incense or put up a yoga calendar for atmosphere and inspiration.

- Wear a special outfit. It offers the psychological advantage of separating yourself from the other parts of your day.

- Experiment with interesting and unusual props. Props help achieve proper alignment in postures. Try sofas, doorways, or stairs, in addition to the regular yoga props (blankets, bolsters, wood blocks, belts, etc.) Always use caution when trying a pose with a new prop.

- Find a friend to practice with and set a date and time for practice. Even if your buddy fails to show, practice anyway.

- Remind yourself why you do yoga. Don't you look and feel better—calmer, stronger, more flexible, balanced, poised—since you started practicing yoga?

- Study yoga; it's inspiring. Your local library probably has a wealth of books and videos on the subject.

- Make yoga a priority. Assigning a high priority to yoga will strengthen your commitment to regular practice. Commitment helps push through habitual procrastination and avoidance behavior. If you're a chronic procrastinator or have an extra-busy schedule, schedule time in your calendar for yoga practice. Making a date takes the hassle out of finding the time; with time scheduled in, there's no debate.

Basic Postures for Health and Relaxation

Overview

Yoga postures, or *asanas*, are the physical positions that coordinate breath with movement and with holding the position to stretch and strengthen different parts of the body. *Asana* practice is the ideal complement to other forms of exercise, especially running, cycling, and strength filling, as the postures systematically work all the major muscle groups, including the back, neck, and shoulders; deep abdominal, hip, and buttocks muscles; and even ankles, feet, wrists, and hands.

By their very nature, *asanas* affect major and minor muscle groups and organs as they simultaneously impart strength, increase flexibility, and bring nourishment to internal organs. Although most poses are not aerobic in nature, they do in fact send oxygen to the cells in the body by way of conscious deep breathing and sustained stretching and contraction of different muscle groups.

Categories of Asanas

There are a wide variety of asanas (up to 200), each one with its own distinct shape and form dictated by stretches, counterstretches, and resistance. The result is an alignment of the skin, flesh, and muscular structure of the body with the skeleton. When done with conscious breathing, the postures balance the sympathetic and parasympathetic nervous systems. These two major parts of the nervous system govern the automatic functioning of the internal organs, heart rate, blood pressure, automatic breathing, and digestion.

Yoga postures and sequences offer many benefits. For instance, forward bends, twists and inversions stimulate the entire internal system, including the lymphatic system, and boost the immune system. Other poses stimulate, calm, and energize, while others build stamina or concentration, promote sleep, alleviate PMS, or soothe digestion.

Asanas are grouped by their main physical characteristic, and each group of postures develops the body in a different yet reciprocal way. *Asanas* also are characterized by the three basic movements, including backbends, forward bends, and twisting movements.

What the Poses Represent

Through practice of the *asanas*, you learn how to sit or stand erect, stable, and relaxed without being tense and rigid or collapsing and falling asleep. One great master of therapeutic yoga declares: You should do all *asanas* with vigor and at the same time be relaxed and composed.

- standing poses = vitality
- sitting poses = calmness
- supine poses = restful
- prone poses = energizing
- backbends = liveliness
- inversions = mental strength
- twisting poses = cleansing
- balancee poses = lightness
- jumpings = agility

See Appendix, page 205, for illustrations of poses described in this section.

Continued ➡

STANDING POSES

These poses invigorate the mind and body by eliminating tension, aches, and pains. Internally, these postures stimulate digestion, regulate the kidneys, and alleviate constipation, as well as improve circulation and breathing, by developing the strength of the legs and the flexibility of the pelvis and lower back. Through regular practice, standing poses lend strength and mobility to the hips, knees, necks, and shoulders.

Standing poses are important for beginning students, as they teach the basic principles of alignment and movement in sitting, standing, and walking. In addition, they establish a firm foundation for learning other postures. Standing poses are recommended for daily practice for students of all levels because they exert a tremendous effect on the neck, shoulders, legs, and back.

Standing postures include:

- Mountain Pose (*Tadasana*)
- Tree Pose (*Vrksasana*)
- Triangle Pose (*Trikonasana*)
- Standing Forward Bend Pose (*Uttanasana*)
- Wide-spread Standing Pose (*Prasarita Padottanasana*)
- Side Angle Pose (*Parsvakonasana*)
- Warrior I & II (*Virabhadrasana I & II*)
- Intense Side Stretch Pose (*Parsvottanasana*)
- Half Moon Pose (*Ardha Chandrasana*)
- Revolved Triangle Pose (*Parivrtta Trikonasana*)

Standing poses are typically begun by jumping into them, which makes the body and mind alert and develops coordination. In jumping, the feet should land equidistant from the center and in line, and the arms should move out to the sides at the same time with the legs. People who have back or knee injuries and pregnant women should not jump into standing poses, but walk the feet outward to the sides to begin the pose. For support and to better gauge alignment, these poses can be practiced against the wall. **Caution**: Standing poses should not be practiced during the first few days of menstruation, the first three months of pregnancy, or by anyone with a problem pregnancy or high blood pressure or heart problems.

SITTING POSES

Generally, these poses are considered calming, as they soothe the nerves, eliminate fatigue, and refresh the brain. They also help regulate blood pressure and assist in recuperation from illness, as well as promote restful sleep. Sitting poses are divided into two categories: upright seated postures, which involve bending the legs into different positions, and forward bends, where the trunk bends over the legs. The primary sitting postures include:

- Staff Pose (*Dandasana*)
- Hero Pose (*Virasana*)
- Lotus Pose (*Padmasana*)
- Cow's Head Pose (*Gomukhasana*)
- Bound Angle Pose (*Baddha Konasana*)

FORWARD BENDS

Also known as seated postures, these poses stretch the lower back and lengthen the hamstrings. They are considered passive poses that encourage introspection and cool the internal body. Specifically, sitting forward bend postures soothe the nervous system and quiet the mind. They can be approached two ways—either energetically, with a vigorous breath, or calmly, with a quiet breath. When practiced with the forehead resting on a bolster or stack of folded blankets and held for several minutes,

these poses are restorative, and they are especially recommended during menstruation. They are useful after a series of backbends as they serve as a counterbalance to the body.

Forward bends postures include:

- Open Angle Pose (*Upavista Konasana*)
- Head-to-knee Pose (*Janu Sirsasana*)
- Revolving Head-to-knee Pose (*Parivrtta Janu Sirsasana*)
- Seated Forward Bend Pose (*Pascimottanasana*)
- Seated Forward Bend (with one leg in Hero Poe) Pose (*Triang Mukhaikapada Pascimottanasana*)
- Tortoise Pose (*Kurmasana*)
- Heron Pose (*Krauncasana*)

RECLINING POSTURES

These poses fall into two categories—supine and prone poses. The prone poses rejuvenate the body. Reclining poses serve mainly to stretch the abdomen and increase the mobility of the spine and hips, thus opening the groin and strengthening the back, arms, and legs.

The less strenuous of these poses traditionally are done at the end of a practice session to cool down the body and restore energy. The postures also are helpful for relieving fatigue, recovering from illness, or during menstruation. When used as a restorative series, the eyes frequently are covered and props such as folded blankets, bolsters, and belts are used to facilitate their remedial effects. When supported with props such as folded blankets or bolsters, these poses can be held for five to ten minutes each.

Reclining postures include:

- Legs Up the Wall Pose (*Viparita Karani*)
- Reclining Head-to-foot Pose (*Supta Padangusthasana*)
- Reclining Hero Pose (*Supta Virasana*)
- Reclining Bound Angle Pose (*Supta Baddha Konasana*)
- Corpse Pose (*Savasana*)

BACKBENDS

Backbends open and energize the body and mind; they develop courage, energize, and lift depression. They open the chest, stimulate the nervous system, strengthen the arms and shoulders, and increase flexibility of the spine. Since these poses are strenuous, they should be introduced gradually to a steady yoga practice. To avoid risking injury to the lower back, the legs first must be strong, and the shoulders and upper back must exhibit genuine flexibility. Backbends should not be done by those who have high blood pressure, heart disease, or other serious illness, or during menstruation and pregnancy. Those with bad backs or knee injuries should only do backbends under the supervision of a qualified yoga instructor.

Backbend postures include:

- Bridge Pose (*Setu Bandha*)
- Bow Pose (*Dhanurasana*)
- Camel Pose (*Ustrasana*)
- Upward Facing Dog (*Urdhva Mukha Svanasana*)
- Upward Bow Pose (*Urdhva Dhanurasana*)

INVERTED POSES

Along with arm balances, inverted poses reverse gravity, bringing fresh blood to the head and heart, thus revitalizing the whole body. These poses tone the internal organs and glandular system, stimulate brain function, improve circulation, and refresh tired legs.

In particular, Shoulderstand invigorates the nervous system and regulates the emotions while

activating the thyroid. To avoid straining the neck, this pose should be done with the shoulders and elbows supported by two or three firm, folded blankets, which can be staggered slightly for neck comfort. Headstand is considered the "king" of yoga postures, as it fosters poise and stimulates the brain. New students should practice Downward Facing Dog as a preparation before attempting Headstand.

Inverted postures include:

- Downward Facing Dog Pose (*Adho Mukha Svanasana*)
- Handstand (*Adho Mukha Vriksasana*)
- Headstand (*Salamba Sirsasana*)
- Shoulderstand (*Sarvangasana*)
- Elbow Balance (*Pinca Mayurasana*)
- Plow Pose (*Halasana*)
- Supported Bridge Pose (*Setu Bandha Savangasana*)

Caution: These postures should not be done during menstruation or pregnancy, or by anyone who has high blood pressure, migraine headaches, heart problems, detached retina, glaucoma, neck problems, ear problems, or hiatal hernia. Those with neck injuries should do these poses only under the direction of a qualified instructor.

TWISTS

These postures free, energize, and balance the body. Sitting twists are the most intensive, as they increase the range of motion of the spine. They promote flexibility in the spine, hips, and upper back, thus relieving backaches, headaches, and stiffness in the neck and shoulders. This group of postures also tones and stimulates the abdominal organs, thus aiding digestion and relieving constipation.

Ideally, twisting postures are done after a series of sitting poses or forward bends, which gives the hips and spine a proper warm-up. When done after backbends, they tend to relieve any lower back discomfort. They should not be done during pregnancy, with the exception of the Chair Twist (*Bharadvajasana*).

Twisting postures include:

- Seated Twist Pose (*Maricyasana*)
- Simple Chair Twist Pose (*Bharadvajasana*)
- Severe Twist Pose (*Ardha Matsyendrasana*)

BALANCE POSES

Balance poses develop lightness, strength, and agility. They also help develop body control, muscle tone, coordination, and concentration. These poses are not recommended during menstruation or pregnancy or after recent (twelve to eighteen months) abdominal surgery. Balance poses include:

- Plank Pose (*Chaturanga Dandasana*)
- Sidways Plank Pose (*Vasisthana*)
- Crane Pose (*Bakasana*)

PRACTICE SUGGESTION

Remove contact lenses when practicing reclining poses (when eyes are covered) or doing inversions.

Basic Classic Yoga Postures

After Headstand, the Lotus Pose is most familiar to Westerners. *Padmasana*, as it's known in Sanskrit, requires long and limber muscles in and around the deep ball-and-socket that make up the hip joint. Initially, this pose may be nearly impossible to accomplish, due mostly to sitting in chairs for long periods of time, which leads to the muscles and ligaments around the hip joints becoming short and tight.

Attempting this pose in its complete form without proper preparation and warm-up can result in injury, especially to the knees, because when the hips

Continued ➡

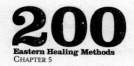

are tight there is a tendency to overstretch the knees. Lotus Pose should never be forced under any circumstances. It takes patience and practice to master. All the standing poses are excellent preparation, as are Easy Pose and Tailor's Stretch, described below.

EASY POSE (Sukhasana)

Sit on the front edge of a firm, folded blanket with legs crossed. Knees should be parallel to the floor with your weight balanced evenly on the sit bones. Move shoulders down, lift crown of head until chin is level. Hands should rest comfortably on knees. Breathe in and out slowly and deliberately. (If knees are four to six inches off the ground, support with pillows or wooden blocks.)

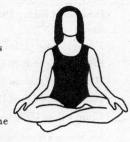

TAILOR'S STRETCH

Start in a relaxed cross-legged position. Begin moving the feet away from the groun until legs form right angles. Now hold this position and move the spine forward until an intense stretch is felt in the outside of the hip. Change the crossing of the legs and repeat.

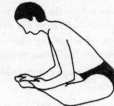

LOTUS POSE (Padmasana)

Sit in Easy Pose. Then take the right foot with the heel and bottom of foot pointing toward groin and place on the left thigh. Right hip should roll in with knee facing almost forward. Then raise left foot forward and upward and place on right thigh. Feet should move closer toward groin; move knees closer together. Straighten back, lift chest. Rest hands with palms facing up on the top side of knees. Be careful not to strain knees. Hold for ten to thirty seconds, breathing evenly.

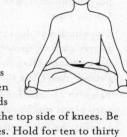

MOUNTAIN POSE (Tadasana)

The foundation for all hatha yoga postures, this pose centers and calms the mind and teaches balance. Stand straight with head centered over the legs. Bring feet together with big toes and ankles touching. Weight should be balanced evenly on both feet and toes should be elongated and not gripping. Lift the arches. Legs should extend fully, lifting the kneecaps and pulling the thigh muscles up and inward toward the bones. Then lift the hips, while moving the lower back down, tucking the pelvis under. Without tensing the stomach muscles, move them up and back. Arms should hang loosely at your sides. Raise the breastbone and relax the shoulders and flatten the shoulder blades. Stretch the neck upward and keep the head straight and chin level. Relax facial muscles, especially the muscles around the eyes. Look straight ahead. Hold for thirty to sixty seconds.

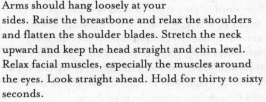

DOWNWARD FACING DOG (Ahdo Mukha Svanasana)

This pose, like many others, has a few variations. It provides an excellent method for stretching the shoulders and hamstrings and helps relieve depression, insomnia, and stress. This variation is for beginners.

With back to wall, kneel on all fours. Then place hands shoulder-width apart and six inches ahead of shoulder level. Position knees directly under the hips with heels on the wall and ball of foot on the wall. Spread toes fully. Then exhale and raise trunk, straighten knees, and move buttocks upward toward ceiling. Hold position with toes and balls of the feet spread fully. Keep head lowered. Slowly bring heels down wall and continue to spread the toes and balls of feet. To come out of the pose, return to kneeling position. Hold for thirty to ninety seconds.

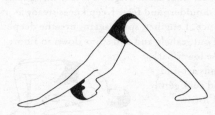

LEGS UP THE WALL POSE (Viparita Karani)

An excellent posture for relieving stress and refreshing the body, this pose also invigorates the legs and feet.

Place the long side of two double-folded blankets or a bolster parallel and about six to ten inches from the wall. Then sit at one end of the prop, facing away from it, with one shoulder near the wall and hips close to the wall. Roll toward the center of your prop, bring your legs up and parallel to the wall. The ribs closest to your waist should be supported by the bolster. Your abdominal area now should fit between the end of the bolster and the wall. Remember to maintain a curve in your neck, supporting your neck with a thin blanket or towel if necessary. Rest your arms either beside you on the floor or over your head with elbows bent. To come out, bend your knees and place your feet on the wall. Lift your pelvis slightly away from the prop. Push the prop toward the wall with your hands and press your feet against the wall to bring your body away from the wall. Then rest the lower part of your legs on the bolster and lie there for a few moments. Then roll to your right side and get up slowly.

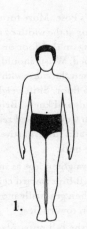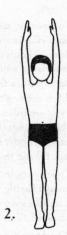

CHILD'S POSE (Pranatasana)

This relaxation is often done between asanas or asana sequences.

Start with knees on the floor. Place hands on the floor in front of knees. Then sit back, resting on the back of the calves. Hands now rest lightly on knees. Then extend hips and hands forward. Let palms rest on floor. Relax shoulders. Head can be turned so either the left or right cheek rests on the floor. Forehead can also rest on the floor. Relax in the position, inhaling and exhaling several times before coming out.

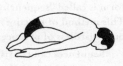

SUN SALUTATION (Surya Namaskar)

This pose invigorates the entire body with stretches and counter-stretches.

The classic sequence yoga posture, Salute to the Sun features several hatha yoga poses done in a continuous fashion. Depending on how it is performed, the posture can be mildly to very aerobic. Ideally, the pose is done in the morning. Movement should be synchronized with breathing and should be done twice in each set, alternating between leading with the left and right foot. This variation is for beginners.

First, stand in Mountain Pose and stretch the arms overhead, palms together, bending slightly backwards. Then bend forward from the hips, resting your hands on your shins, ankles, or toes, wherever your flexibility permits. If necessary, bend your knees slightly to eventually bring palms flat on the floor beside your feet. Extend the left leg back, with the knee resting on the floor. Right knee should remain at a ninety-degree angle before bringing the right foot back to join the left foot. Then lift the hips toward the ceiling to form Downward Facing Dog, with arms straight, back long and head facing downward. If necessary, move hands back a bit to lift hips. Or move hands and feet to a wider stance. Bend the arms at the elbow, then lower hips and place knees on the floor, followed by the trunk. With arms bent, extend the body in a straight line behind you. Stretch should be in lower back. Use arms to bring chest area forward; relax shoulders. Eyes look forward. Navel should be off the floor.

Now lift hips again and reposition hands until you are in Downward Facing Dog. Then bring the left foot forward between the hands. If necessary, drop the right knee and lift the foot with the opposite hand to bring it forward. Then bring the right foot forward. Both legs should be straight. If this strains your lower back, bend knees slightly. Hands should rest on shins, ankles, or toes, head moving toward the legs. With arms at your side, roll trunk up slowly. Once upright, bring arms over head with palms together and bend slightly backwards. Release and bring hands to a prayer position at the breastbone.

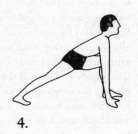

1.   2.

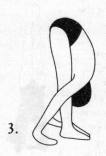

3.   4.

Continued ➡

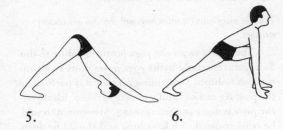

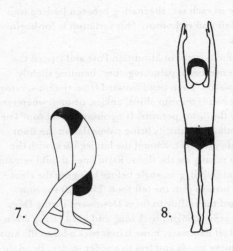

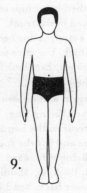

Sun Salutation

HEADSTAND (Salamba Sirsasana)

This classic posture activates the brain and develops equilibrium and inner strength.

To practice, start in Child's Pose. Move forearms out until elbows are on the floor at the width of the shoulders. Hands can be resting on the floor or fingers interlaced and hands clasped. Wrists should be resting firmly on floor. Lengthen the spine with shoulders moving downward to floor. Shift weight until you are balancing on hands and knees. Bring head between hands with crown (top) of head resting squarely on floor. Keep hands and fingers active yet relaxed. Extend the back of the neck.

To advance in the pose, straighten legs as in Downward Facing Dog Pose, lift hips toward ceiling while standing on your toes, then gradually move heels toward floor. Walk feet in toward head.

When you are ready to do the full pose, place a firm, folded blanket against a plain wall. Kneel in front of the blanket; knees and feet should line up. Interlock the fingers and move them to the edge of the blanket, facing the wall. Forearms and outer elbows should also be on the wall, with elbows under the shoulders. Forearms, wrists, and hands are parallel. Cup hands and extend the neck, placing the very top, or crown, of the head between hands. Lift upper arms and shoulders. Lift and straighten legs and elevate the hips. Walk legs toward wall until nearly perpendicu-

lar. Then swing either the left or right leg upward so it is parallel to the wall. Lift shoulders and stretch the back of neck. Stretch legs and trunk; tuck lower back inward. Feet, heels, and toes extend upward. Face and eyes should be relaxed with a soft focus. To release, extend one leg toward the floor, then bring down other leg. Rest in Child's Pose.

BRIDGE POSE (Setu Bandha)

A simple backbend, this pose opens the chest, helps to deepen breathing, and strengthens the lower back.

Lie on your back on the floor with knees bent and feet hip-distance apart. Feet should be close to the buttocks. Extend arms toward heels with palms down. Waist rests lightly on floor with feet pressing down firmly. Tuck chin slightly. Lengthen spine and lift pelvis off floor until weight is evenly distributed between shoulders and feet. Keep knees steady at hip distance. Lengthen spine again, breathe deeply. To come out, exhale and roll spine down to floor. To release lower back, clasp hands around knees and rock gently back and forth.

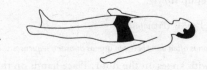

CORPSE POSE (Savasana)

This posture which represents stillness and quietness, balances the nervous system. It typically is done at the end of a practice session.

Keep two blankets handy—one to support the neck and the other to cover the front of the body should you become chilly.

Sit on the floor with the trunk upright. Lean back on the elbows with the head moving downward, trunk and legs in a straight line. Rest on the center of the back of the skull. Stretch neck and throat. Relax the eyes. Chin should be level. If it is higher than the forehead, place a blanket folded to a one-to two-inch height under the head until it touches the top of the shoulders. Shoulders move down with shoulder blades moving in. Then bend knees, lift up hips, and stretch lower back toward floor. Straighten legs and let them roll comfortably outward. Relax and extend arms about six inches from the trunk. Wrist and hands also rest on floor. Relax the abdomen. Close eyes and focus attention on the in and out breath. Let body sink into floor. Remain in pose for five to ten minutes.

To come out, open eyes slowly, bend the left leg and roll to your right side, remaining there for a few breaths. Use left hand to slowly bring you to an upright position.

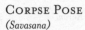

Sequencing

Moving from one pose to another without breaking form is called "sequencing," or *vinyasa* in Sanskrit. This method of practice allows for a balanced workout regardless of practice length.

Sequences can consist of related poses for the purpose of energizing (as with standing poses or backbends) or relaxing (with forward bends or restorative poses) the body or working on specific areas such as the hips, shoulders, or feet.

Whatever the purpose of a particular practice session, it should begin with two or three warm-up postures, such as Mountain Pose, Downward Facing Dog Pose, or Sun Salutation, as they stretch the spine, arms, and legs. Then you can move on to more strenuous poses that strengthen the body and increase endurance. Standing, inverted, and back-

bend poses would apply here. To wind down and settle the nerves, practice seated forward bends or supine poses. Always end with several minutes in Corpse Pose to renew both mind and body.

Minimum Practice Guidelines

According to Iyengar yoga teacher, Esther Myers, the ideal minimum practice should consist of:

- Supported Inverted Pose (*Viparita Karani*)
- Downward Facing Dog Pose (*Adho Mukha Vrksasana*)
- Triangle Pose (*Trikonasana*)
- Bridge Pose (*Setu Bandha*)
- Headstand (*Salamba Sirsasana*)
- another Downward Facing Dog
- Child's Pose (*Pranatasana*)

(See *Starting a Hatha Yoga Practice* for important information and tips about performing yoga poses.)

Props

Some schools of hatha yoga rely heavily on props, while others do not. If you are new to yoga, have limited flexibility, are practicing mainly on your own, or are taking a therapeutic approach to yoga practice, including props is quite appropriate.

The most commonly used hatha yoga props include:

- Yoga ("sticky") mat: offers a nonslippery surface for standing postures
- Two or three tightly woven or firm blankets: Woolen army-type or Mexican blankets are ideal. Used in sitting poses when there is tightness in the hips or hamstrings, for support in Shoulderstand, Headstand, and Corpse Pose.
- Two wooden or dense foam blocks (approximately 4 x 6 x 9 inches) for support in standing poses and Hero Pose (*Virasana*) and Elbow Balance Pose (*Pinca Mayurasana*).
- Belt with a buckle for Bound Angle Pose, forward bends and Shoulderstand.
- Folding chair with a flat seat for supported backbends and standing and twisting poses.

Pranayama: Working with the Breath

Prana is the breath of life of all beings of the universe.

—B. K. S. Iyengar

Yogic Breathing

As a yogic practice, *pranayama* concerns itself with various methods of conscious breathing. *Prana*, or vital force, is at the core of all life. All living beings are infused with it; without this form of energy, life could not exist. Eastern religions have long recognized that training the breath is important to mental, physical, and spiritual growth. However, many people are shallow chest-breathers, taking in only about one-third of the oxygen needed by the lungs. Chest breathing is closely linked to the workings of the nervous system. By gaining control over diaphragmatic breathing, you greatly enhance your ability to cope with stress and lessen its damaging effects. Yogic breathing emphasizes breathing through the nose and the exhalation over the inhalation.

The classic text on yogic breathing, *Light on Pranayama* (Crossroad Publishing, 1987) by B. K. S. Iyengar, instructs that the conscious breathing system of *pranayama* provides a direct avenue of communication to the self. Iyengar says that the practice of *pranayama* quickly induces the relaxation response

Continued ➡

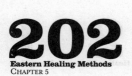

and accompanying enhancement of the immune system.

The *Yoga Sutras* declare that the more balanced and calm we are, the less prana is lost to us. When we are restless, upset, or befuddled, more *prana* exists outside the body than within, potentially leading to physical illness. When there is too little *prana* for the body to draw upon, we can feel stuck or less motivated to do what needs doing. Distinguished teacher Desikachar states: "If *prana* does not find sufficient room in the body there can only be one reason: It is being forced out by something that really does not belong there. When we practice *pranayama*, it is nothing more than reducing the 'rubbish' and so concentrate more and more *prana* within the body . . . the quality of our breath influences our state of mind and vice versa because we can influence the flow of *prana* through our breath. In yoga we are trying to make use of these connections so that *prana* concentrates and can freely flow within us."

Connection to Hatha Yoga

Hatha yoga strives to bring the body into balance, and *pranayama* lends stability to the body's energies. Yoga postures involve the most basic *pranayama* practice: paying attention to the breath. By practicing yoga *asanas*, we have the opportunity to become aware of our breathing and to affect it in some way. Yoga tests, or challenges, the way we breathe. The postures give us a new perspective on the muscles used in breathing, as they require you to twist, bend, and invert our bodies. Paying attention to the breath becomes important because for the pose to be done correctly both breath and movement must be coordinated. As a result, the connection between mind and breath is strengthened. Yoga poses automatically increase lung capacity and invigorate the muscles most directly involved in the breathing process—specifically the ribs, diaphragm, and back.

As yoga postures strengthen the body for meditation, *pranayama*, while much more subtle a practice, prepares the mind for the silence and single-pointed concentration required of meditation. A steady and correct hatha yoga practice naturally encourages the practice of *pranayama*.

Resting poses offer the most opportunity to become more aware of the muscles involved in the breathing process. They include:

- Corpse Pose (*Savasana*)
- Easy Pose (*Sukhasana*)
- Lotus Pose (*Padmasana*)

Understanding Inhalation and Exhalation

Both an involuntary and voluntary action, breathing is the act of moving air in and out of the lungs. Inhalation brings oxygen, and, therefore, energy into the body. Exhalation removes impurities from the body and creates the space for *prana* to enter the body. The out-breath is considered key because it removes any obstacles to the free flow of *prana*.

However, bringing *prana*, which is not simply air or breath, into the body involves something more. Yogic scholars believe *prana* enters the body when a positive change in the mind occurs over an extended length of time. Desikachar noted that "changes of mind can be observed primarily in our relationships with other people." He further reminds that relationships are the real test of whether we actually understand ourselves better.

Forms of Pranayama

There are five forms of *prana*, all of which have different names according to the body functions with which they correspond. The forms most Westerners practice are *prana-vayu* and *apana-vayu*. *Vaya* means "air" or "breath" in Sanskrit.

- *udana-vayu*—corresponds to the throat region and the function of speech
- *prana-vayu*—corresponds to the chest region
- *samana-vayu*—corresponds to the central region of the body and the function of digestion
- *apana-vayu*—corresponds to the region of the lower abdomen and the function of elimination
- *vyana-vayu*—corresponds to the distribution of energy into all areas of the body

Benefits

Like *asana* practice, *pranayama* practice has far-reaching, positive effects on physical, emotional, and mental well-being. It also encourages spiritual development. More specifically, mindful breathing practice:

- clears and calms the mind
- focuses attention
- develops concentration
- refreshes and renews the body
- improves metabolic function
- assists in cardiovascular function

Basic Method

Working with the breath takes time, patience, and concentration. Initial attempts at *pranayama* may be frustrating. You may find the process absorbing yet distracting at the same time. Before attempting any particular technique, breathe normally, without trying to control or change your breathing in any way. Practice this way until you are comfortable in letting your breath-flow freely. Lying down (as in the Corpse Pose or with the knees bent, feet flat on the floor) on a firm surface instead of sitting upright in a classic meditation pose may be helpful as you experiment in becoming familiar with your breathing pattern.

As you become quieter, your breath will find its own rhythm and will naturally become steadier and slower. Inhalation and exhalation will become fuller and deeper on their own. As your flexibility grows through asana practice, so will your capacity to deepen the fullness of your breath. Practicing pranayama may require a leap of faith, but through practice and patience you can master it.

Ideally, *pranayama* should follow *asana* practice, and not the other way around. At least ten to twenty minutes of rest should occur between the end of *asana* and the start of *pranayama*. Finding the ideal sitting position for *pranayama* practice also is important. Comfort is essential, so you can remain in a seated position for an extended period of time while keeping the spine straight. Most practitioners opt for Easy Pose or a variation of the Lotus Pose, either with or without back support from a wall. If your hips are tight, elevate them by sitting on a folded, firm blanket. Hands can rest in your lap or rest lightly on the knees.

In the *Yoga Sutras*, Patanjali offers these suggestions for keeping your attention on or conscious of the breath:

- Focus on a place in the body where you can feel or hear the breath; this is most easily achieved by gently contracting the vocal cords, a technique known as ujjayi.
- Follow the movement in the breath, feeling the inhalation from the center of the collarbone, down through the rib cage to the diaphragm, and following the exhale upward from the abdomen.
- Pay attention to the breath where it enters and leaves the body at the nostrils.

- Also helpful is softening the eyebrows, broadening the forehead, relaxing the eyes so that they recede, resting back in their sockets.

Should you experience any of the following signs of stress or tension as you practice *pranayama*, stop the technique immediately and resume regular, passive breathing:

- tension in the chest, neck, or shoulders
- strain in the foreheads, eyes, or throat
- a forced sound in the throat when breathing
- gasping for the inhalation
- lightheadedness or hyperventilation
- feeling tense, overstimulated, or lightheaded afterward
- more emotional release than feels comfortable

HOW TO BREATHE

- Keep mouth closed and take in breath only through the nose.
- Keep your breath slow and smooth and focus your attention inward. Pay attention to the sound of your breath. It should be steady and even.
- To even out the flow of the breath, try making a very slight, quiet sound at the back of your throat.
- Inhale and exhale should flow consistently. Avoid bringing in or expelling breath loudly or forcefully.
- Pause slightly between inhalations and exhalations.
- Do not strain or force any part of this process. Give yourself the chance to find a rhythm that is comfortable for you. Remember that the breath is connected directly to your nervous system and regulating the breath manipulates both gross and subtle energies. Shallow or agitated breathing signals a stress response.

BREATH RETENTION

The breath should be held or retained when breathing in and out fully can be accomplished with ease. The purpose of retaining the breath during *pranayama* is to quiet the mind. Retaining the breath should not interfere or disturb the inhalation-exhalation pattern. If the exhalation becomes rough or uneven, resume regular breathing.

BREATHING TECHNIQUES

Pranayama includes many techniques that are based on the Complete Yoga Breath, which includes the chest, diaphragm, and belly moved by the breath. Techniques such as *Ujjayi*, *Viloma*, and Alternate Nostril Breathing should be practiced only when the breath can be regulated with ease—ideally, when an *asana* practice has been established. Those with breathing problems such as asthma or chronic shortness of breath should practice under the supervision of a trained teacher. When practicing any form of pranayama, you must remain mindful of how the body reacts during the process.

BASIC TECHNIQUES

Reclining

Lying down is an ideal way to practice when beginning or if you are tired or ill. The spine is automatically supported; by resting in a prone position, you can relax more readily.

1. Begin in Corpse Pose. Support the head with a firmly folded blanket if there is strain in the neck or the chin is higher than the forehead.
2. Pay attention to the flow of your breath. Make no attempt to adjust or control your breathing. Inhale and exhale passively. Inhaling slowly, place one hand lightly on the abdomen. As you

Continued →

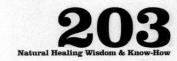

inhale, feel the abdomen expand and contract when you exhale.

3. After several cycles of inhalation and exhalation, allow the entire body to sink closer to the floor and deepen the exhalation.

Sitting

Sitting upright and comfortable is the ideal posture for *pranayama*, as it frees the upper body and aids in concentration.

1. Sit in a cross-legged position. Back and hips may be supported; if knees are higher than the hips, sit on a firmly folded blanket high enough that spine is straight and knees are lower than the hips. Spine may be supported by sitting against the wall.

2. Lengthen spine and soften the abdomen. Lift breastbone and relax the arms and shoulders. Lower back is neutral. Head rests comfortably on the base of the spine and chin points downward. Soften eyes, eyebrows, and forehead.

3. Facial muscles, eyes, and gaze remain passive. Jaw is relaxed.

4. Inhale and exhale normally, observing the breath's natural rhythm.

Extended Exhalation

This technique helps take breathing to the next level by deepening exhalation and increasing the volume of inhalation.

1. Breathe normally while paying attention to the movement of the abdomen.

2. When breath becomes rhythmic, slowly bring the muscles of the abdomen toward the spine as you exhale.

3. Let the knees and pelvis move downward as the spine and upper body move upward.

4. Keep inhalation passive as you continue the cycle.

Square Breath

This technique is very effective for steadying the breath and subsequently calming the mind. It calls for pausing briefly at the end of each inhalation and each exhalation.

1. Breathe normally until breath is steady and rhythmic.

2. Pause after the in-breath and again after the out-breath.

3. Slowly increase the length of the pauses until the inhalation, the exhalation, and the two pauses that are part of the cycle are the same length.

Meditation

Overview

The subtlest parts of yoga's Eight-fold Path are:
- *pratyahara*—withdrawal of the senses from the physical world
- *dharama*—concentration
- *dhyana*—meditation
- *Samadhi*—union with the Higher Self

Taken together, these elements represent what Westerners commonly call meditation, a natural progression from the more physical aspects of yoga practice. At its most basic, meditation is considered an effective, albeit low-tech, antidote to stress and an unfettered path to mindfulness. In the broadest sense, however, meditation can be characterized as a focusing of attention. It is very much part of the Eastern tradition, as Indian philosophy and medicine made its way to Tibet, China, Japan, and

Southeast Asia. How it was taught and practiced was altered by the cultures that absorbed it.

While the object of attention may vary, all forms of meditation have as their goal the centering of one's attention, or mental energies, for the purpose of stilling the mind. A very reliable wm to calm an overactive mind, meditation also increases physical stamina, mental concentration, and spiritual resolve. Regular meditation practice instills a sense of living in the present moment—facing pleasant and unpleasant emotions, thought patterns, fears, and cravings without distraction.

Benefits

Like the other yogic paths, meditation is nondenominational and offers many potential benefits to both mind and body including:
- stress relief
- peace of mind
- relaxation
- increased energy
- release of tension
- lower blood pressure
- mindfulness
- access to higher mindstates

Methods

There are many ways to practice meditation. The most basic and easiest mediation style to learn is to simply sit straight and quiet with eyes closed and concentrate on the breath—inhalation, then exhalation, then inhalation again, and exhalation—while not engaging the thoughts that pass through the mind. Some practices extend the observation of the breath to observing the sensations, thoughts, and emotions of the mind and body. When attention wanders, as it invariably will, meditators are instructed to gently bring their attention back to their breathing. Forcing the mind to be still only results in frustration.

Choosing a meditation method is much like adopting a form of hatha yoga or selecting a teacher. It depends greatly on what strikes a chord within and how compatible it is with your lifestyle. It is an important decision and should be made with care and consideration. Instead of accumulating techniques, stick with one style until you've mastered it.

Regardless of the method chosen, meditation requires patience, understanding, and practice. As with learning and perfecting yoga postures, meditation is a lifelong quest.

CORPSE POSE (*Savasana*)

Hatha yoga students are most often introduced to meditation through Corpse Pose, which is done at the conclusion of each practice session. This pose brings about deep relaxation, as the body is still, yet passively alert and fully supported by the floor. In the pose, muscles relax and lengthen, passive breathing—necessary in all postures—takes over, and quiet concentration builds.

POSTURES

The traditional postures for sitting meditation include:
- Thunderbolt Pose (*Vajrasana*) for Buddhist and Zen meditators
- Sitting upright in a straight chair, if you are unable to sit in a crossed-leg posture.

Whichever pose you choose, you should be able to sit comfortably with the spine and head erect, allowing for the free flow of energy throughout the body. The body should remain still and relaxed, with the mind aware yet internally focused. Sitting

on a firm cushion or folded blankets supports the hips and relieves lower-back strain.

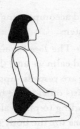

The hand position can be either resting loosely clasped in the lap; hands cupped but open, with the right hand on top of the left, resting lightly on the lap; or the thumb and forefinger touching and the hands placed on the knees.

Thunderbolt Pose
(*Vajrasana*)

While not encouraged, beginning meditators may find it easier to quiet the mind and follow the breath when lying on the floor in Corpse Pose. If you find yourself becoming drowsy or falling asleep, try meditating this way at a different time of the day.

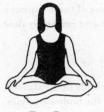 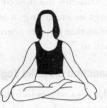

Easy Pose
(*Sukhasana*)

Accomplished Pose
(*Siddhasana*)

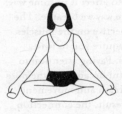 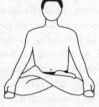

Auspicious Pose
(*Swastikasana*)

Lotus Pose
(*Padmasana*)

Establishing a Practice

Deciding when, where, and how long to practice comes first. A regular time and place, while ideal, is not mandatory.

According to Indian gurus, the best time to meditate is between 4 A.M. and 6 A.M. This time of morning is known as *brahamuhurta*, the time when the mind is infused with peacefulness and goodness and stillness exists in the outside world, as many people are still asleep. Other recommended times are 6 A.M., noon, 6 P.M., and midnight.

A quiet place free of clutter, distractions, and interruptions is essential for meditation. If this place can be set aside only for meditation, all the better. In fostering a spiritual atmosphere, you may want to set up a small shrine that holds candles, fresh flowers, sacred objects, photos of inspirational spiritual masters, and other objects of personal importance. The room should be neither too cold nor too warm; fresh air should circulate to help keep you alert while meditating.

The best way to start a meditation practice is to sit daily for five or ten minutes. After the habit has been established, gradually lengthen the amount of meditation time in five-minute increments. If you become tense or very restless, reduce the time by five minutes. You may find after a few weeks that as you meditate more, you look forward to the time you've set aside. However, should you want to expand meditation to more than an hour each day, it is best to do this in a group setting or under the supervision of a qualified teacher.

To free the body from tension, repeat the ancient mantra *Om* several times; as it is believed to represent the fundamental sound of the cosmos, the vibrations will dispel areas of tension.

—From *Pocket Guide to Hatha Yoga*

Continued ➡

Appendix of Poses

Sitting Poses

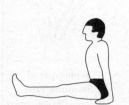
Staff Pose (*Dandasana*)

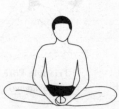
Bound Angle Pose (*Baddha Konasana*)

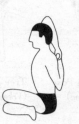
Lotus Pose (*Padmasana*)

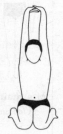
Cow's Head Pose (*Gomukhasana*)

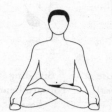
Hero Pose (*Virasana*)

Reclining Postures

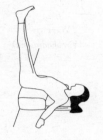
Legs Up the Wall Pose (*Viparita Karani*)

Reclining Head-to-foot Pose (*Supta Padangusthasana*)

Corpse Pose (*Savasana*)

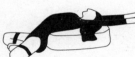
Reclining Bound Angle Pose (*Supta Baddha Konasana*)

Reclining Hero Pose (*Supta Virasana*)

Forward Bends

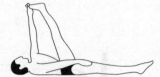
Open Angle Pose (*Upavista Konasana*)

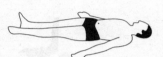
Heron Pose (*Krauncasana*)

Revolving Head-to-knee Pose (*Partivrtta Janu Sirsasana*)

Seated Forward Bend Pose (*Pascimottanasana*)

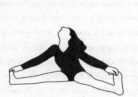
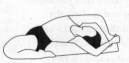
Seated Forward Bend (with one leg in Hero Pose) Pose (*Triang Mukhaikapada Pascimottanasana*)

Tortoise Pose (*Kurmasana*)

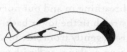
Head-to-knee Pose (*Janu Sirsasana*)

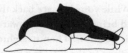
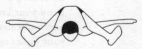
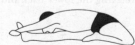

Twists

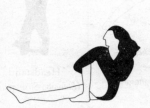
Seated Twist Pose (*Maricyasana*)

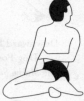
Simple Chair Twist Pose (*Bharadvajasana*)

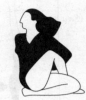
Severe Twist Pose (*Ardha Matsyendrasana*)

Balance Poses

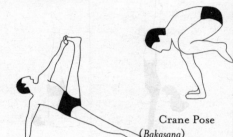
Crane Pose (*Bakasana*)

Sideways Plank Rose (*Vasisthana*)

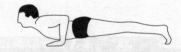
Plank Pose (*Chaturanga Dandasana*)

Backbends

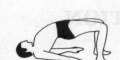
Bridge Pose (*Setu Bandha*)

Bow Pose (*Dhanurasana*)

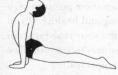
Upward Facing Dog (*Urdhva Mukha Svanasana*)

Upward Bow Pose (*Urdhva Dhanurasana*)

Continued →

Inverted Poses

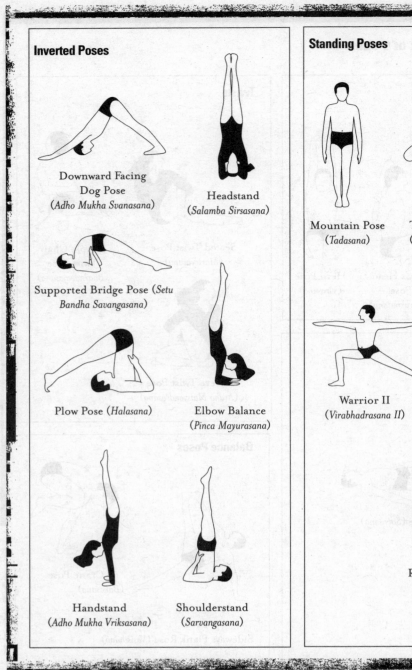

Downward Facing Dog Pose
(*Adho Mukha Svanasana*)

Headstand
(*Salamba Sirsasana*)

Supported Bridge Pose (*Setu Bandha Savangasana*)

Plow Pose (*Halasana*)

Elbow Balance
(*Pinca Mayurasana*)

Handstand
(*Adho Mukha Vriksasana*)

Shoulderstand
(*Sarvangasana*)

Standing Poses

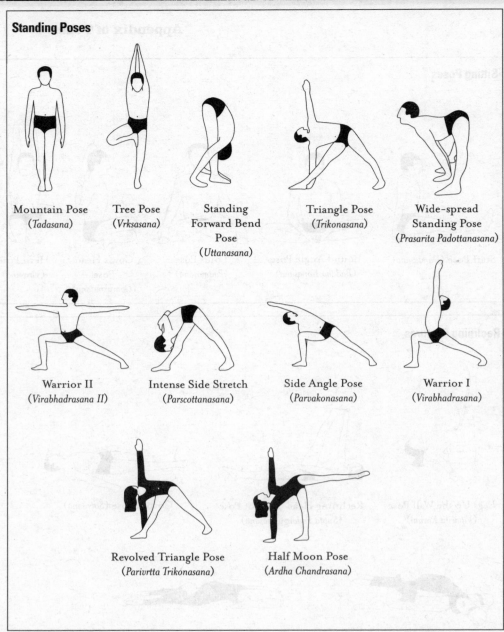

Mountain Pose
(*Tadasana*)

Tree Pose
(*Vrksasana*)

Standing Forward Bend Pose
(*Uttanasana*)

Triangle Pose
(*Trikonasana*)

Wide-spread Standing Pose
(*Prasarita Padottanasana*)

Warrior II
(*Virabhadrasana II*)

Intense Side Stretch
(*Parscottanasana*)

Side Angle Pose
(*Parvakonasana*)

Warrior I
(*Virabhadrasana*)

Revolved Triangle Pose
(*Parivrtta Trikonasana*)

Half Moon Pose
(*Ardha Chandrasana*)

YOGA FOR REJUVENATION

Helene Silver

Illustrations by Kathleen Savage

The ancient system of hatha yoga had a profound understanding of the importance of glandular health, and many yoga postures are designed to stimulate and balance the function of the various endocrine glands. . . . Practice these postures regularly to keep your glands young and healthy. If you wish, read the instructions into your tape recorder, so you can perform these postures in smooth, flowing movements without interruptions.

Knees to Chest

Lie on the floor in the resting pose, with your arms at your sides. Relax and breathe for a few minutes. Now bring both knees to the chest with your arms clasped around your knees. Relax in this position, breathing in and out normally and feeling the stretch in the lower back. Hold this position and rock gently from side to side for a minute or so. Stop rocking, and with your knees still to your chest, relax again for another minute or two, then release and straighten your knees, lower your legs slowly to the floor, and rest for a few minutes in the resting pose. This knee-to-chest posture is excellent for relaxing the lower back and easing back strain.

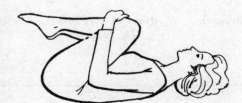

Rocking Plough

Raise your legs with the knees straight and grab your ankles, or as far down your legs as you can comfortably reach. Now, slowly pull your legs down toward your trunk, tuck your head forward, and gently rock forward and back on your spine. Rock as far back as you can comfortably go; if you are very flexible, you may be able to touch the floor behind your head with your toes. Now let go of your ankles, and if you can, bring your legs all the way back behind your head with the knees straight, supporting your lower back with your hands resting on your elbows, and relax in this inverted position. While your legs are back there, bend your knees and bring them down toward the ears and relax in this position. Then straighten your knees again, return to the Rocking Plough position, begin to rock gently, and rock forward and sit up.

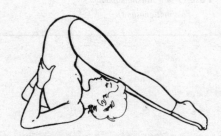

Seated Toe Pull

Sit quietly for a moment, then as you breathe out, bend forward and grab your big toes and pull on them. According to many yoga teachers, this toe-pull stimulates the pituitary gland. Release your toes and sit up. Now, as you inhale, raise your arms above your head. As you breathe out, bend forward, with your arms reaching as far down your leg as they will go and your head as close to your knees as possible. Keep your knees straight and breathe normally. Relax in this position for as long as you can, then breathe in and sit up. Breathe out and bend forward with your head toward your knees again, and relax as long as you can in the down position, breathing normally.

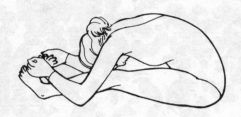

High Shoulder Stand

Lie down again and relax in the resting pose. Now bring your legs up with your knees straight and push off with your arms, supporting your lower back with your hands resting on bent elbows. Push your body up until you are in a completely vertical inverted position, with your weight on the top of the spine and the back of the neck. This is one of the most invigorating and rejuvenating yoga postures, because it reverses the effects of gravity. Support your lower back with your hands and breathe normally into your abdomen. Bend your chin into your neck to stimulate the thyroid gland. With your legs straight up in the air, rotate your ankles, first in one direction, then the other. If you are still comfortable in this position, spread your legs far out to the sides and rotate your ankles. Bring your legs back together, still breathing normally, and do a forward and back split with your legs, with first one leg forward, then the other. Come out of this inverted posture the same way you got into it, letting your legs drop back behind your head, bracing your hands on the floor, and gradually rolling back down on the spine. Pay close attention as you roll back, trying to release one vertebra at a time. Relax in the resting pose, feeling the effects of the posture.

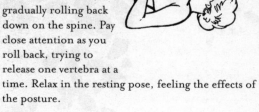

Fish Pose

The Fish Pose is a perfect complement to the shoulder stand. Lie on your back and breathe normally. Begin by doing the "easy fish." Put your weight on your elbows and arch your back, letting your head drop back so that your weight is resting partially on your elbows and partially on the very top of your head. Your back should form an arch from the buttocks to the top of your head. Let your hands rest

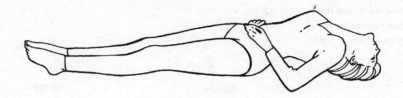

on your hip joints. This is a wonderful position for stimulating the thyroid, the thymus, and the glands in the head. This is also a wonderful opportunity to stretch the muscles in your face. No one is watching you! Repeatedly jut out your chin, open your mouth as wide as you can, blink your eyes, and stick out your tongue. Now slide back down into the resting position and relax, enjoying the benefits.

Full Fish Pose

Cross your legs at the ankles with the knees bent and pull on both big toes. Pull your toes down behind the opposite knees. Now, keeping your hands on your toes, try to drop your knees down to the floor. Feel the stretch and pull on the hip joints and thigh muscles. In this position, go into the Fish Pose once more. Push up with your weight on your elbows and the top of your head. Do your facial exercises again, breathing all the way down into the abdomen. Stretch your neck out; stick out your tongue! This is a great chance to exercise all your facial muscles again. Then slide your head and arms back down, slide your legs forward and relax, feeling the invigorating effects of this posture.

—From *Rejuvenate*

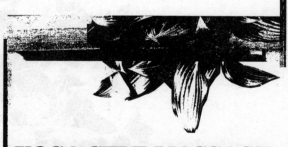

YOGA SELF-MASSAGE

Helene Silver

Illustrations by Kathleen Savage

Yoga and massage are similar in many ways. Both activate areas along the spine, directing nourishing blood and nerve impulses to the body's organs. Both help to "wake up" the joints and connective tissue and improve the circulation of blood and lymph. While massage does this through direct manipulation, yoga postures achieve the same results by targeting specific organs, joints, and areas of the body with specific postures. The gentle stretching movements of yoga help to stimulate areas that are difficult to reach and energize through walking or other forms of exercise. The following series of yoga postures provides an "internal massage" for the spine, joints, and internal organs. Use it as a warm-up before your exercise today. You may want to read the following instructions into your tape recorder and play it back while you perform the movements.

Knees to Chest

Lying on your back, bring both knees to the chest, with the arms clasped around your knees, holding one wrist with the other hand. Relax in this folded-up position, breathing in and out normally. Feel the invigorating stretch in your lower back. Now, still holding this position, rock gently from side to side to wake up the spine. Release your knees and straighten the legs, lowering them slowly to the floor, returning to the Resting Pose. Rest for a while and enjoy the feeling of relaxation. Repeat three times.

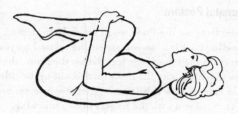

Canine Stretch

Still lying on your tummy on the floor, place your palms next to your armpits and push yourself up, with your weight on your hands and the balls of your feet. Straighten your legs and raise your buttocks in the air, as if a rope were lifting your lower spine toward the ceiling. Hold this position for a few moments. Really push up your lower back area, feeling the spinal stretch. Then bend your knees, lower your body to the floor position, and relax. Breathe in and out normally throughout this exercise; do not hold your breath. For a different stretch and a different sensation, try drawing your heels down to the floor in the raised position, rather than keeping your weight on your toes. Repeat the Canine Stretch three times, ending in the floor position.

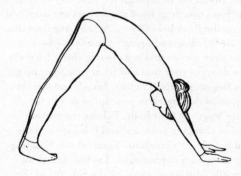

Cobra

Roll over onto your tummy. Lie flat with your toes together, your forehead on the floor, and your palms flat on the floor next to the armpits. Breathe in, slowly raising the head and neck. Open your eyes and look up through the eyebrows. Continuing to breathe in, rise farther, lifting the chest off the floor and curling the spine back as far as possible without lifting the hips or pelvis off the floor. Hold your breath in this reverse stretch, looking up through the eyebrows and jutting the shin out with the teeth together to tense the throat and neck. Hold this position for several seconds, then begin to exhale. Lower the stomach to the floor, then the chest, and

Continued ➡

finally allow the head to roll forward to the floor. Relax in a lying position on your tummy with your head to one side. Repeat this posture three times.

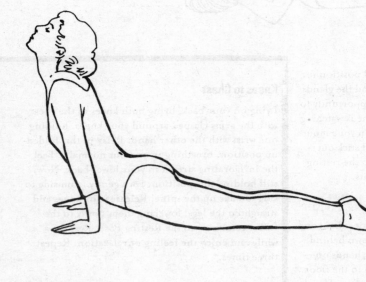

Prenatal Posture

From lying on the floor, push yourself up into a kneeling position, so you are sitting relaxed on your feet, with the tops of the feet flat on the floor, the toes touching, and the heels turned out to the sides. Take a deep, slow inhalation. Extend your arms out in front of you with the fingers lightly touching, exhale slowly, and as you exhale, bend forward until your forehead is resting on the floor with your arms extended. Relax in this position, breathing normally, for at least one minute. Repeat three times. This position, known as the Prenatal Posture, stimulates the circulation of blood to the head, making your mind alert and your eyes rested and bright.

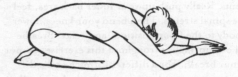

Spinal Stretch

Lie on the floor with your arms relaxed at your sides. Breathing in through the nose, slowly raise your arms over your head so that they are stretched out on the floor behind you. At the same time that you are inhaling and bringing your arms back, point your toes so that you are stretching from the waist down to your toes and from your waist up to your fingertips. Hold in your breath and feel the tension of the stretch in your spine and in the entire length of your body. Release the tension without changing position, and relax around the held breath for a moment. Then exhale, bringing your arms back to your sides. Lie flat, breathing normally, and relax, enjoying the benefits of the stretch. This lying position, known as the Resting Pose, is one of the most important postures in yoga. Take the time to experience the total relaxation that the name implies. Repeat the spinal stretch three times.

—From *Rejuvenate*

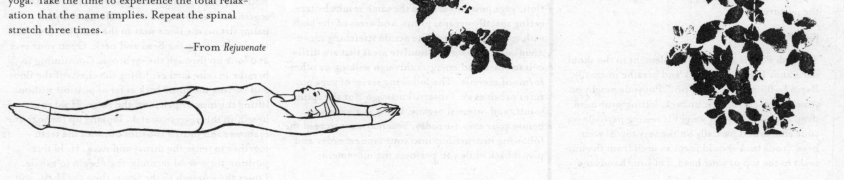

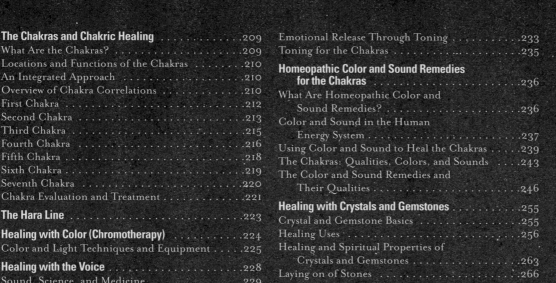

Energy Healing

THE CHAKRAS AND CHAKRIC HEALING

Joy Gardener

What Are the Chakras?

If you go to a New Age Expo or Psychic Fair or look at the classified ads in one of the Personal Transformation newspapers, you are likely to find a wide array of healing modalities including chakra cleansing, chakra balancing, and vibrational healing.

You may well wonder, *What are they talking about?* Since there is no American or International Association of Chakra Healers, there is no standardization of these terms, and those who use them may just be following their own whims. But after you have read this book, you will at least be in a better position to speculate about what they might mean. The best policy is to ask practitioners to describe their work to you.

There is a remarkable correlation among those who see and/or feel the chakras. Throughout various cultures, there is an agreement about the nature and function of the chakras, but there is variation in their precise number, color, and other details.

The word *chakra* (pronounced *shock-ra* or *chock-ra*) means "wheel" or "disk" in Sanskrit. A chakra is an invisible (to the normal human eye) center of spinning energy. Through the chakras, we are able to

receive and transmit social, sexual, and spiritual energy. The chakras have been described as spinning vortexes, or as the multipetaled lotus flower. These flowers, which are considered sacred in India, symbolize the path of development from a primitive being to the full evolution of unfolded awareness. They float upon the water, yet they have their roots in the mud, just as the flower of your crown chakra connects to the heavens and your base chakra has its roots in the earth.

Some psychics describe the chakras from the tailbone to the crown of the head as having progressively more and more segments or petals. However, the sixth chakra at the center of the brow is depicted as having only two petals, which may have something to do with your ability to understand the dual nature of the Universe. When you recognize both the male and female within yourself, you become whole. Out of this knowledge comes the merging with All That Is, symbolized so appropriately by the "Thousand-Petalled Lotus" of the crown chakra.

Some systems describe five, others six, some seven, twelve, or even thirty chakras. Some see them only along the spine, and others find them at the joints, at the hands and feet, and beyond the physical body at progressively higher points above the head. Some people experience the energy of the chakras at the front of the spine and others at the rear and some at both front and rear.

Some old pictures depict the chakras as wheels of

light located on or close to the spine. In some pictures, each chakra is shown extending out a few inches from the front or the back of the body on a stem that opens into a round flower.

Whether you think of the chakras as wheels, spirals, or flowers, it is important to remember that they are energy systems which do not have physical form. Attempting to describe such a system is like trying to describe a sound; each person who hears it will explain it in different terms and use different analogies. There may be a variety of opinions about where the sound comes from, and disagreement about whether it is pleasant or unpleasant. Yet everyone is in agreement that it does exist, energetically.

Any illustration of the chakras is merely a visual aid to the imagination, not a literal physical reality. Yet some individuals are so wedded to their particular perceptions that they will insist that their perception—and theirs alone—is the true reality. Then, of course, there are still many individuals who will categorically deny the existence of anything that they cannot see with their own eyes and hear with their own ears. Back in 1927, C. W. Leadbeater wrote in his classic book, *The Chakras*, "I know that there are still men in the world who are so far behind the times as to deny the existence of such powers, just as there are still villagers who have never seen a railway train."

For the sake of simplicity, I will limit my discussion to the seven master chakras along the spine. It is

Continued ➡

easy to see how one might reduce the number of chakras from seven to six or to five, since the functions of the first and second as well as the sixth and seventh are similar.

There are differing theories about which colors (or sounds or crystals) should be used at which chakras. Since we are dealing with energy, there is an inevitable degree of subjectivity. If three people watch the same sunset, one may describe it as salmon-colored, another as pink, and yet another as red. A fourth, whom we label color-blind, may have an entirely different perspective.

In this book, I will focus primarily on the rainbow system, with seven chakras from red to violet. I will list specific colors, sounds, crystals, aromas, color-charged waters and other colored liquids that can be used to stimulate or sedate the energy at each chakra.

Locations and Functions of the Chakras

Here are the locations of the seven chakras, and the primary characteristics of each one:

First chakra (base chakra) at the tailbone— The energy at this center is governed by whether you received unconditional love and affection as a child. When your first chakra is strong, you will be grounded and comfortable in your body, the world will feel like your home, and you will be competent at handling practical affairs.

Second chakra, below the navel—This relates to sexuality, sociability, friendliness, and desire, not just sexual desire, but the desire for anything—friends, love, material possessions, power, God. The energy at this chakra fires up those desires and gives you the enthusiasm to reach out to achieve your goals. It is also the center of physical strength.

Third chakra at the solar plexus, above the navel—This is the center of your special gift, your inner sun, and how it shines out in the world. All the digestive organs (except the large intestine) are located here, so it governs the digestion. It also relates to self-esteem and self-worth. This is the center of gut-level intuition.

Fourth chakra (heart) at the center of the chest—This chakra governs your ability to give and receive unconditional love and affection. When you experience loss, your heart will remain open if you allow yourself to feel all your emotions, including both sorrow and anger. But if you try to protect yourself from pain by putting up walls, your heart energy will close down.

Fifth chakra (throat) at the base of the neck— This is your center of communication, creativity, and opening to spirituality. Speech and singing originate from here. Writing and teaching are also associated with this chakra.

Sixth chakra (third eye) at the center of the forehead—This is about your openness to metaphysical knowledge. It relates to your higher intuition, from which all things are known.

Seventh chakra (crown) at the top of the head—From here you feel your openness to Spirit. When it is open you will experience a fullness in your meditations.

The chakras are non-physical energy centers which are located in the etheric body that surrounds the physical body. They work as energy transforming stations, enabling us to absorb energy from the environment and from other people, and transmute it into a form of nourishment for our

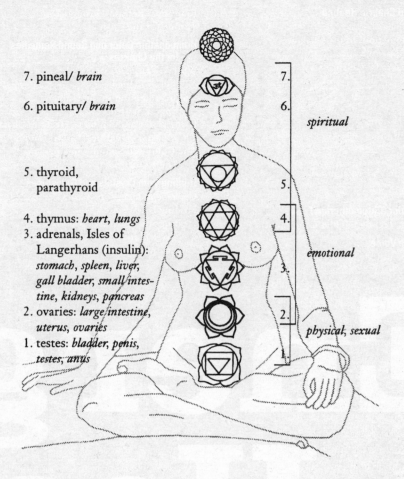

Endocrine Glands: *Internal Organs*   Energy

7. pineal/ *brain*

6. pituitary/ *brain*

7.

6.

spiritual

5.

5. thyroid, parathyroid

4. thymus: *heart, lungs*

4.

3. adrenals, Isles of Langerhans (insulin): *stomach, spleen, liver, gall bladder, small intestine, kidneys, pancreas*

3.

emotional

2. ovaries: *large intestine, uterus, ovaries*

2.

1. testes: *bladder, penis, testes, anus*

physical, sexual

own body/ emotions/mind/spirit. When we are out of balance due to fear, stress, guilt, or confusion, our ability to draw upon these energy centers diminishes. As we clear away the blocks and become balanced and clear, we become direct conduits for ongoing streams of energies from various sources which can give us phenomenal powers. The primary work of the energy healer is to help clients to clear away obstructions so that they can have easy access to these powerful transforming stations.

An Integrated Approach

Chakra Evaluation, as described in the last section of this book, provides a broad picture of the health and balance of each of the chakras. Your reactions to life challenges cause your chakras to open up or close down at the physical, emotional, intellectual, and spiritual levels. Two or three chakras relate to each of these areas, so this method of evaluating an individual's health reaches far beyond a simple physical diagnosis. Once we obtain this information, we have an excellent tool for analyzing the total human being. Various methods can be used to bring the whole person into balance and health when we understand the following interrelationships:

· **Body—**The energies of the first and second chakras are associated with sexuality and with a sense of grounding, physical connections, and the desire for and ability to attract material goods.

· **Emotions—**The energies of the second, third, and fourth chakras are associated with the emotions.

· **Mind, Intuition—**The energies of the third and sixth chakras are associated with intelligence and intuition. Women's intuition or hunches come from the third chakra. The third also relates to one's intellect and ability

to retain factual information. Scientists and mathematicians have highly developed third chakras. The sixth chakra relates to higher intelligence, which is a link to higher intuition. Someone with a highly developed sixth chakra has the ability to access the Akashic Records, the cosmic library where all things are known. In ancient cultures, a man like Pythagoras might be a brilliant architect, mathematician, and also an accomplished musician, poet, and philosopher.

· **Spirit—**The energies of the fourth, fifth, sixth, and seventh chakras are associated with spirituality. At the fourth, a person may have an experience of Cosmic Consciousness, a sense of being at one with all and everything. This is a heart-opening experience that triggers deep compassion. At the fifth chakra, a person goes through the bottleneck into a new world, embracing the things of spirit, leaving behind old, narrow ways of thinking. At the sixth chakra, a person opens to a higher level of intuition and inner guidance. At the seventh, the person feels a sense of merging with Spirit. . . .

Overview of Chakra Correlations

The following seven chapters describe each chakra in terms of its ancient names and symbol, location on the body, and the various healing modalities that can be used to influence it. This section gives descriptions of the categories that will be used to discuss each of the seven chakras.

People who have inner vision can actually see or feel the chakras. You may be able to do this yourself: lie on your back and hold your hand a few inches above your body, moving from the pubic area to the top of your head. You may feel the chakras as intense concentrations of energy, and

Continued ➡

you may see the colors of the chakras with your third eye, even if you aren't looking directly at them (it may be easier to do this with your eyes closed). You can also try to see the colors of a friend's chakras.

The first three centers are below the chest: these are called the lower chakras. The heart chakra at the chest and the top three centers are called the higher chakras (though sometimes this term is reserved just for the top two or three chakras).

The assignment of different illnesses, ailments, and emotions to particular chakras is also somewhat artificial. In fact, there is (and should be) a great deal of flow between the chakras; it's only our minds that need to put things into categories.

Some authorities believe that as people raise their consciousness, the higher chakras open and the lower chakras close. I envision higher consciousness as an opening of all the chakras.

My Spirit Guide, Dr. Laing, says, "In a highly evolved person, the chakras are like progressively larger fountains, with the yellow of personal power tumbling over the orange of sexuality, which is brimming over the small but brilliant red of a firm foundation."

Names

These are the most common names for the chakras, beginning with the ancient Sanskrit names (and their translations).

Symbol

According to Hindu tradition, each chakra has a symbol. I've given simple versions of these symbols. Each chakra is shown within a circle surrounded by lotus petals. The circle represents the spinning vortex of energy, and the lotus petals represent the segments like those of an orange, that some psychics describe at the chakras, and also the gradual awakening of the whole self, finally culminating in the fully opened lotus at the seventh chakra.

My interpretations are a combination of my research and my own intuition.

Location

There are differences of opinion about the location of the chakras, but when you consider how ancient this knowledge is and how many cultures it spans, there's a remarkable degree of agreement. The chakras are simply spinning whorls of energy which interpenetrate the body. The epicenter can be felt or seen two to three inches beyond the body, in both the back and the front. I've given the locations where I feel the greatest spin of energy, and this corresponds to the areas where most people currently describe feeling the energies.

Area of the Face

The face is a microcosm of the body. The same colors, aromas, and crystals that are used to treat the seven chakras can be used to treat the seven areas of the face.

Sense

Each chakra corresponds to a different sense such as smell, taste, and touch.

Color and Antidote

Each chakra has a particular color. Various systems assign different colors to the chakras. I've used the rainbow system beginning with red at the first chakra and ending with violet at the seventh.

An antidote counteracts the effect of a substance, as hot antidotes cold and cold antidotes hot. The colors and characteristics of the three lower

chakras can be antidoted by those of the three upper chakras, and vice versa. The center (heart) chakra is balanced and needs no antidote. These are the antidotes for the colors of the chakras:

Red antidotes blue and blue antidotes red. (Red is the color of the first chakra and blue is the first above the heart.)

Orange antidotes indigo and indigo antidotes orange. (Orange is the color of the second chakra and indigo is the second above the heart.)

Yellow antidotes violet and violet antidotes yellow. (Yellow is the color of the third chakra and violet is the third above the heart.)

This concept is essential in color healing, as can be seen in this statement from Dr. Laing: "If a baby's skin is too red, then it is overly excited. This condition should be watched closely, because it can become habitual and lead to red conditions such as heart troubles and high blood pressure in later life. If the baby's mother learns to handle it in early life, these patterns can be changed."

Dr. Laing advises, "Help the baby to relax. To do this, help the mother to relax. Impress upon her that her relaxation is good for the baby. Give her plenty of blue light. Put her under a blue lamp. Have her wear blue clothes. Listen to soothing music. Bring in blue flowers. Create a soothing environment."

When a person has characteristics of excess at a particular chakra, this may be treated by the antidote and the vibratory tools associated with the chakra that corresponds to that color. In the above example, the baby's skin is too red and he is highly excitable. These are characteristics of excess at the first chakra, which calls for the antidote, which is the color blue and all of the vibratory tools associated with the fifth chakra. He could be held under a blue light, or dressed in blue clothes. He could be massaged with oil to which a little blue chamomile oil was added for calming, or a few drops of blue chamomile oil could be added to his bath to relieve tension and anxiety. While she bathed him, his mother could tone to him, using the u as in blue) sound.

Tone and Note

Each chakra vibrates at a different frequency or vibration and on a different note. When you chant the tone on the given note, this may vibrate the chakra, awakening and opening it. If you find that you can achieve the same effect by using a different tone and note, feel free to use it.

Element

Each chakra corresponds with one of the elements such as earth, air, fire, and water.

Crystals

When used for healing, crystals are placed on the body, in the general vicinity of the chakras, though any crystal may be used at any part of the body. Healing stones can also be placed around the body, to create an electromagnetic grid. They are also used as jewelry, though most people are unaware of the vibrational influence of the stones they wear. When you understand the healing power of stones, you can deliberately wear them in the vicinity of the chakra which will most benefit, and you can avoid wearing jewelry that would be counterproductive.

I have categorized the crystals according to the chakras where they are most commonly used. The color of the crystal often corresponds to the color of the chakra, as red stones are used at the first chakra. However, black and brown stones are also

associated with the first chakra because it relates to the earth, and these are earth colors. As a general guideline, the rough stones help bring up buried, rough emotions, while the smooth stones are used to calm and soothe the nerves.

Here are some definitions that may be helpful. Technically the word crystal is defined as a solidified substance which has a regularly repeating arrangement of atoms resulting in natural external plane facets. By contrast, a rock refers to a large piece of stony material, and a stone refers to any earthy or mineral matter. Quartz is a term for minerals composed of silicon dioxide, which have six external plane facets leading to a single point (a point is a termination). The quartz family includes clear quartz (also referred to as crystals), milky quartz, amethyst, rose quartz, smoky quartz, and citrine. Gems are cut and polished stones, and jewels are valuable gems that have been prepared to be used in jewelry. Jewels and gems are usually translucent, which means that you can see light through them.

Organizing the crystals according to the chakras is the perfect way to get an overview of crystal healing. By going from the macrocosm of the rainbow to the microcosm of colored crystals, we have a perfect model for understanding color and crystal healing. Red and orange are earth colors. Thus the red and orange stones are good for connecting with earth energies. We think of the sun as yellow, and we call the nerve plexus which is located at the area of the third chakra the "solar plexus." When we lie in the sun we relax and expand and tend to feel good about life and about ourselves. The third chakra relates to your personal power; your inner sun and how it shines out in the world. Yellow stones are good for radiant relaxation, happiness, and strengthening the will power. Turquoise is a third chakra stone because it is intermixed with copper, which is yellow.

The fourth chakra relates to the color green in the rainbow, and also to pink. Green is nature's way of loving us. We breathe better in the presence of trees, and the chest is at the fourth chakra. Pink and green stones are most popular for healing the heart and lungs. Pink flowers have always been associated with love. Pink stones relate to unconditional love and the feminine mother energy. Green stones relate to protective love and the masculine father energy.

The fifth color of the rainbow is blue, which is the color of the sky. We think of going up into the heavens when we open to our spirituality. Blue stones help you to relax and to go into that meditative alpha state. They are used at the throat chakra to help remove anxiety so you can communicate more effectively. They help you to get in touch with the muse of creativity, which is like a special kind of spirit guide.

The sixth color is indigo, a purplish blue color, like sunset in the mountains. The purple stones like sugilite help to strengthen your spiritual energies. The seventh color is violet, like amethyst, which helps to transmute energies, like day turning to night. I also think of diamonds and clear quartz in relation to the crown chakra, like the stars and the snowflakes, each one totally unique, helping you to transcend or to gain insight in a variety of ways.

After using the crystals for healing, it is beneficial to cleanse them in some way. The clear quartz crystals particularly absorb energies. There are many methods for cleansing and renewing the energies of the stones. I like to hold them under cold running water for 10 to 30 seconds. Energy follows water, and this enables any negative energy that may have gotten attached to the stones to go down the drain, where they can be absorbed by the earth.

Continued →

Aromas

The most common way to use aromas in healing is through the application of essential oils, which are subtle, volatile liquids distilled from plants. These oils can be added to massage oil, or to your bath, or they can also be diffused into the room in a diffuser or various other devices that can be plugged into an electrical socket or even the cigarette lighter in your car. The aromas that arise from these oils can also be released by simply crushing a plant between your fingers, tossing a dried plant on a fire, smoking it like a cigarette, cigar, or moxa (used in Chinese medicine), or burning it as incense. Or you may just want to sit next to a flowering plant which exudes your favorite aroma.

The aromas may be categorized according to the chakras. One method is to observe the color of the flowers that the aromatic oils are taken from; another method is to take note of which parts of the body are most strongly influenced by the aroma of the plant. Please consult an aromatherapist or a good book on aromatherapy for more information on how to use aromatic oils.

Statement

The succinct phrases in this category were received during meditation when I asked my own chakras to speak and describe themselves to me. I've found that on different days (and for different people) they respond differently. These "statements" can be used as loose (and sometimes amusing) guidelines. Try it yourself.

Explanation

In this category I describe the essential energy of the chakra, often quoting from my Spirit Guide, Dr. Laing, and *The Book of Guidance*, which I chan-neled.

Balanced, Excessive, and Deficient Energy

If a child is confronted with aggressive behavior, he or she may respond by becoming aggressive or by assuming a superior attitude. These are expressions of excessive energy. On the other hand, if a child encounters indifference, she or he may respond by becoming depressed or lethargic. These are expressions of deficient energy. People with either deficient or excessive energy are imbalanced in their chakras. This is not unusual. Rather, the balanced individual is unusual in our society.

When your childhood and adolescence have been healthy and you feel well-nurtured, you may be balanced and open in every chakra. But when there is unreleased emotion such as fear or anger accumulated from years of past experience, and when there has been a lack of love and encourage-ment during the developmental period, the energy flows less freely to these centers. This may result in either excessive or deficient energy at the chakras, depending upon the personality and the kind of rejection or negative experiences that person has had. This is best explained in the section on the Development of the Chakras.

In each chakra section I have given the main characteristics of that chakra and examples of three types of individuals who have dominant personality traits in each of these chakras. These individuals represent the balanced, excessive, and deficient personality types.

Many of the examples of personality types may sound like stereotypes, but they are all descriptions of actual people. The sexes and the professions can be reversed. Not all of the characteristics need apply.

You may get a mixture of excessive and deficient characteristics in one person, or an individual may swing back and forth between excessive and defi-cient, sometimes passing through a temporary bal-ance. When the energy of a chakra is clearly defi-cient, it should be treated with the corresponding color or other vibratory tools (sound, aromas, food, etc.) of that chakra. However, if the energy is excessive, it can be treated with the antidote for that chakra (the antidotes are given on page 211).

For example, sexual energy comes mostly from the second chakra which is orange, so someone with excessive sexual energy may benefit from the anti-dote, which is indigo. This color and the vibratory tools associated with the sixth chakra will calm the sexual energy, making the person feel less compul-sive. An alternate treatment is to use yellow, which strengthens the third chakra, putting the person more in touch with his or her personal gift, which in turn enhances feelings of self-worth, making this person less desperate for sexual satisfaction.

The personality will usually reflect either the energy of the highest open chakra or the chakra with the most energy and focus. For example, I imagine that Mozart may have been a balanced second chakra personality, because while his third, fourth, and fifth chakras were certainly open, he seems to have enjoyed focusing much of his energy through his second chakra. As Laing says, "When an evolved and balanced person focuses energies through a lower chakra, the color of that chakra will glimmer in their aura, in a particularly crystalline hue."

Under the balanced personalities of each chakra, I've mentioned various religions. I have not tried to designate religions for those who are out of balance, nor have I attempted to mention every religion.

These categories are to be taken very loosely. The same religion may be practiced by people who are focused at different chakras. For example, I placed Judaism at the third chakra, because of the Jewish devotion to The Law and The Word and because of the great love that Jews have for good food. However, there is a high form of Hasidic Judaism that is full of ecstatic song and dance, which is a fourth or seventh chakra experience, depending on who practices it or how intense the ecstasy becomes.

Similarly, I put American Indian religions at the first chakra, because of their deep connection with the earth, but there are Shamans (medicine people) who express their spirituality through the sixth or seventh chakras.

When sexuality is described for a person who is balanced, this is the expression of someone who may also be open at higher chakras but their main focus is through that chakra. When I describe the sexuality of a person who is out of balance, I am referring to the person who is open at that chakra but not necessarily at the higher chakras.

Contraindications

People who have the listed symptoms should not use the color of that chakra.

Glands and Organs Influenced by the Chakra

Each chakra will have an influence over the endocrine glands and internal organs that are located in the area of that chakra. Sometimes the influence will cover a broader sphere, as happens with the first chakra, which is located at the tailbone and which rules not only the bladder, vagina, and male reproductive organs but also the blood and spine.

Illnesses and Ailments

The illnesses and ailments that are given will tend to respond well to treatment with the color and other vibratory tools that correspond to that chakra. Methods for healing the chakras will be explained briefly in the final chapter.

First Chakra

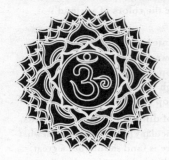

Names

Muladhara (Support)
Kundalini Center
Root Chakra
Base Chakra

Symbol

The symbol for the first chakra is a square (yantra), symbolizing the earth, the foundation. Within the square is a downward-pointing triangle, the symbol for female sexuality. Within the triangle is a linga, the symbol for male sexuality. A snake, the symbol for the kundalini, coils three and a half times around the linga. On the outside are four lotus petals.

Location

at the tailbone

Area of the Face

chin, jaw, lips

Sense

touch—as experienced by the multitude of nerve endings on the lips

Color and Antidote

red
Antidote, blue

Tone and Note

Tone, e (as in red)
Note, c

Element

Earth

Crystals

The first two chakras relate to the earth. In some creation myths, the Creator forms the four races of human beings from the four colors of the earth. Red, orange, brown, and black are considered earth colors. The orange stones are reserved for the sec-ond chakra, but the red, brown, and black stones are all used at the first chakra. Red stones are used for energy and blood circulation. Brown and black stones are used for grounding (connecting with the earth, with your body, and with physical reality). When using crystals at the first chakra, two stones are used; one at each groin point, where the thigh joins the torso. When worn on the body, first chakra stones may be placed in hip pockets.

Red Garnet. Has an arousing, invigorating energy. Good for enthusiasm and self-confidence. Place on lower back for menstrual cramps or low back pains. Red ruby can be used instead. (**Caution**: many people become overstimulated by red stones, especially when worn above the waist.)

Black Obsidian. Excellent for grounding, for people who are too spacey. If you've been running

Continued ➡

around all day and you need to get centered, or if you've been doing intensive inner healing and you don't feel stable enough to drive your car, hold a large piece of obsidian in your lap for a few minutes. Black onyx has similar properties. (**Caution**: do not use black or brown stones at your heart chakra unless you want to close down your emotions.)

Aromas

Aromas which have aphrodisiac properties are associated with the first and second chakras. For the first chakra I list the musky animalistic odors (which are not enjoyed by all) and for the second, the more subtle ones. Also for the first chakra are the aromas which promote a sense of grounding.

Patchouli. A thick dark yellowish-brown oil with a greenish tinge, patchouli is musty and pungent and—for those who like its distinctive odor—it has an aphrodisiac appeal. Can be used as a perfume. It is a stimulant and antidepressant that is commonly used in China, Japan, and Malaysia. It is useful for cracked skin and athlete's foot (the feet are also associated with the first chakra).

Geranium and particularly Rose Geranium is light green and vaguely resembles the odor of rose oil. You can use it as a perfume, placing a few drops behind your ears. It stimulates the adrenal cortex, which governs the balance of hormones, including male and female sex hormones. It is helpful for premenstrual tension and for menopause. It is also used for fluid retention, which often occurs premenstrually.

Statement

"I want stuff."

Explanation

The first chakra concerns your connection with the earth, your birthplace, your culture, your foundations. The first chakra is influenced by your earliest relationships. If there was one person (or even a dog or fairy godmother) who gave you unconditional love, you're likely to have a strong first chakra, and your survival mechanism will be good. If you didn't receive unconditional love, your first chakra may be weak, unless you have done considerable healing of your inner child.

This is the center of physical energy and vitality. It's grounded in material reality, so it is the center of manifestation. When you're trying to make things happen in the material world, in relation to business or material possessions, the energy to succeed will come from the first chakra.

Red, the color of passion, is used to arouse attention and interest. A woman who wants to be noticed should have a pair of red high heels. Passion is a source of power and self-confidence. It is an intensity of energy and even anger. It is the source of great strength, which will help you to move through challenging situations.

Sometimes anger which is repressed erupts as fever or inflammation, all of which are excessive red conditions.

Balanced Energy at First Chakra

CHARACTERISTICS

centered
grounded
self-mastery
healthy
fully alive
unlimited physical energy
can manifest abundance
able to express anger without doing harm
spiritual expression could be

Celtic
Shamanism
Hatha Yoga
Hawaiian Kahuna
sexual energy:
affectionate
able to trust and be vulnerable
sensuality is felt throughout the body

EXAMPLE

This Native American Indian medicine woman and midwife expresses her spirituality through seasonal rituals which involve specific places in nature, use of herbs, dancing, and chanting. Her eyes sparkle and though she is in her seventies she walks and laughs like a young woman. She has plenty of energy and always knows what to do.

Excessive Chakra Energy

CHARACTERISTICS

egotistic
domineering
greedy
addicted to wealth
sexual energy:
indiscriminate
focus is entirely genital
nervous sexual energy
may be sadistic

EXAMPLE

This wealthy perfectionist is the owner of a California restaurant chain. He rules his employees like a demanding general. He is nervous and chronically constipated. He owns three cars. He sleeps with many women, but he "can't get no satisfaction."

Deficient Chakra Energy

CHARACTERISTICS

lacks confidence
feels spacey and unfocused
weak
can't achieve goals
self-destructive, suicidal
sexual energy:

feels unlovable
fears being abandoned
little interest in sex
masochistic

EXAMPLE

This unskilled, insecure woman lives in a chaotic house and spends most of her time watching television. Her parents were alcoholic. She's underweight and often forgets to eat. She's chronically depressed, has no energy, and little interest in men. Life holds no pleasure for her.

Contraindications

Avoid red for all nervous and red conditions including

agitation
hyperactivity
fever
ulcers
high blood pressure
red face
swellings
inflammation
epilepsy

Caution: If you use red light on the head, limit the treatment to three minutes and apply a cool wet cloth or a blue cloth to the head during the treatment or for at least two minutes afterward. Red is

the most potent color, and the easiest to overdose with. If you feel nervous, angry, hot, or uneasy while sitting under this light, discontinue it. Sit under the blue light for a few minutes as an antidote.

Glands and Organs Influenced by the First Chakra

blood
spine
nervous system
bladder
male reproductive organs
testes
vagina

Illnesses and Ailments to Be Treated with Red

Since red is the antidote for blue, it will be used to treat blue conditions. Since it's stimulating, it will be used to treat slow and weak conditions. Since it's in the first chakra area, it will be used to treat organs which are located in the lower region of the body. Since it is red, it can be used to cleanse and build up the blood. Red is used for the following conditions:

depressed, fearful
debilitated, lack of energy
spaced out, ungrounded
low blood pressure
bladder infections
sluggish digestion
inactive, flaky skin
shock
anemia
poor circulation
impotence, frigidity
infertility
no menstrual period
after childbirth, if weak (or if there's been much blood loss)
menopause, if weak (alternate with longer doses of blue if there are hot flashes or a feeling of agitation)

Second Chakra

Names

Svadisthana (Abode of the Vital Force)
Sacral Center
Splenic Chakra

Symbol

The crescent moon symbolizes receptivity and the womb. It is the symbol of femininity. On the outside are six lotus petals.

Location

1–2 inches below navel or branching to left side of spleen

Most people have a concentration of orange energy an inch or two below the navel. But for some people (particularly those who have chosen to be celibate) this chakra will branch off to the left side of the body and settle under the left rib cage at the spleen, which is why this is sometimes called the splenic chakra. Then it will have a blue-green color.

Continued ➤

Area of Face

mouth, gums, tongue, cheeks

Sense

taste (both the second and third chakras relate to the sense of taste)

Color and Antidote

orange (below navel)
blue-green (at spleen)
(See notes under Location, above)
Antidote, indigo

Tone and Note

Tone, o (as in home)
Note, d

Element

Water

Crystals

Orange stones are used for the second chakra. The tiger's eye has a soft feminine energy and the carnelian has a strong masculine energy.

Tiger's Eye. Soothes away worries and apprehensions, especially anxieties about love and sex. If you are feeling the pains of love, this stone will remind you that you can change your energy and make it smooth. Tiger's eye makes a good gift between lovers; enhances telepathic communication.

Carnelian. This is the stone of worldly success. It will give you the courage to project yourself with warm self-confidence. Carnelian promotes self-esteem and enhances sexual energy.

Aromas

The aromatic oils that are used for the first and second chakras are fairly interchangeable. If you're looking for an oil to use as an aphrodisiac, be sure that the aroma is pleasing to both parties.

Jasmine. This is a dark, viscous oil which has a heavy, almost animal quality. The white flowers must be gathered at night, since that is when the aroma is strongest. High-quality oil is very expensive, but only a tiny amount is needed. Massage on the abdomen and lower back during childbirth to relieve pain and strengthen contractions. It is also used for postnatal depression. Jasmine strengthens the male sex organs and will reduce an enlarged prostate. Its aphrodisiac properties are helpful with both impotence and frigidity.

Sandalwood. The sandalwood is a small evergreen parasitic tree that grows in India and Australia. The oil is yellowish to deep brown and is extremely thick and viscous. It is a powerful urinary antiseptic, used to treat various infections of the urinary tract, and was formerly used for gonorrhea. Used for oily skin and acne as well as dry skin, it is excellent in aftershave lotions for barber's itch (the cheeks correspond to the second chakra). It is also an effective aphrodisiac.

Statement

"I desire" (This could relate to money, sex, God, or anything else.)

Explanation

The second chakra is about friendliness, creativity, sexuality, emotions, and intuition. It governs people's sense of self-worth, their confidence in their own creativity, and their ability to relate to others in an open and friendly way. It is influenced by how emotions were expressed or repressed in your family during your childhood.

Orange is a sociable color since it combines the physical red with the intellectual yellow, so it's good to use in living rooms and family rooms, classrooms, and social areas in hospitals. I prefer a light orange because reddish orange can be overstimulating, which can lead to nervousness. Red-orange is a great color for parties.

It's rumored that the reason why one popular fast-food chain has bright orange and pink seats is because the pink attracts customers, and the orange is friendly but keeps the customers energized so they don't want to relax and stay too long.

The second chakra is one of the centers of the emotions and it is in the area of the large intestines. Consequently, when you feel emotionally imbalanced, you're likely to experience diarrhea or constipation.

The second chakra is the center of physical prowess. In Chinese martial arts, it is called the *tan t'ien* and in Japan it is the *hara*. Students are taught to run their energy through this area, which is located 2 to 3 inches below the navel.

The second chakra is the sexual center particularly for women, because the uterus, fallopian tubes, and ovaries are located here. This may be one reason why women tend to be more emotional about sexual relations. When the second chakra has a healthy spin, it indicates that this person has a healthy sex life or at least a healthy attitude toward sex. *The Book of Guidance* says, "Fill your sexual organs with radiant acceptance. Feel your sexual desires finding union with your spiritual desires.

"Herein lies the Mystery of Mysteries, Desire itself is the Divine Motivator. Sexual energy is required to fire all other energy…

"The orange energy gives you the ability to reach out, to radiate, to extend yourself. It gives you the forcefulness to reach *up*—to your heart, and to your soul.

"Regard your sexual center as a precious fountainhead of vital energy. Explore that energy, learn to channel it, and eventually you will learn to use it as a part of your Total Self, to achieve whatever goal you seek…"

The second and fifth chakras are both related to creativity. The womb is at the second chakra, so it is a cradle of creativity, the center of gestation. Creative energy requires freedom and resists constraints, so this can lead to rebelliousness or an unwillingness to be controlled and an intolerance for authoritarianism.

Balanced Chakra Energy

CHARACTERISTICS

friendly, optimistic
concerned for others
has a sense of belonging
creative, imaginative
intuitive
attuned to one's feelings
gutsy sense of humor

clairsentient: can merge with the body and
    mind of another person and psyche them out
    in order to better understand them
may have vague memories of out-of-body
    experiences such as flying
spiritual expression could be
    Pentecostal
    Osho style yoga
sexual energy:
    extremely sensual
    highest goal is to have a wonderful orgasm
    may desire children

EXAMPLE

Mozart (as portrayed in the movie *Amadeus*) is a delightful example of a man who has a well-developed second chakra. He is friendly, jovial, self-confident, courageous, and outrageous. He actively pursues his own creativity. He writes raucous, unconventional, "immoral" operas and falls in love with a beautiful, sexy young woman whom he marries despite the fact that she is beneath his class.

Excessive Chakra Energy

CHARACTERISTICS

emotionally explosive
aggressive
overly ambitious
manipulative
caught up in delusion
overindulgent
self-serving
clairsentient (see above), but can't distinguish
    between one's own feelings and the feelings
    of other people
Sexual energy:
    obsessed with thoughts of sex
    sees people of the opposite sex exclusively as
      sex objects
    requires frequent sexual gratification

EXAMPLE

This woman works as a fashion model and sells cosmetics on the side. She is obsessed with her appearance and spends most of her money on clothes, jewelry, and perfumes. She values herself according to how much attention she receives from men. She is constantly looking at men's bodies and comparing them to her ideal of the perfect male. She uses men to get what she wants and when she feels rejected, she blows up.

Deficient Chakra Energy

CHARACTERISTICS

extremely shy, timid
immobilized by fear
overly sensitive
self-negating
resentful
buries emotions
burdened by guilt
distrustful
sexual energy:
    clinging
    feels guilty about sex
    has difficulty conceiving
    feels abused
    frigid or impotent

EXAMPLE

This fellow is shy and retiring, gentle and thoughtful. Secretly he thinks that sex is crude and often suffers from impotence.

Contraindications

excessive energy
excessive sexual energy

Glands and Organs Influenced by the Second Chakra

skin
mammary glands (milk produced through
    ovarian hormones)
female reproductive organs
kidneys

Continued ➡

Illnesses and Ailments to Be Treated with Orange

kidney weakness
constipation
muscle cramps and spasms
insufficient lactation
lack of energy
allergies (hypersensitive to environment)
repression and inhibition

Third Chakra

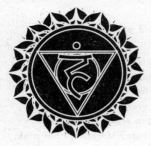

Names

Manipuraka (Jewel of the Navel)
Lumbar Center
Solar Plexus Center

Symbol

The triangle is pointing down, with swastika marks on the three sides. This is the fire wheel. This chakra is associated with the sun and the ego. It is also the center of digestion, which the Chinese call the triple warmer because heat is generated in the process of digestion. On the outside are ten lotus petals.

Location

at the solar plexus (below the breastbone, behind the stomach) or at the navel

Area of the Face

throat (which leads to the stomach and small intestines)

Sense

taste (in common with the second chakra)

Color and Antidote

yellow
Antidote, violet

Tone and Note

a-o-m (ahh-oo-mmm)
Note, e

Element

fire

Crystals

Third chakra healing stones are usually yellow. Turquoise is included here, because it contains copper which has a yellowish color, and because it is beneficial for the digestive organs, which are located in the area of the third chakra.

Citrine. Helps you to relax and feel good about yourself. Allows you to get in touch with your personal power and to express your unique gift. Strengthens the will power and improves self-esteem. Useful for those who want to break a drug habit. Aids digestion and frees up your breathing. Yellow topaz has similar properties.

Turquoise. This is a stone of peace, harmony, and beauty, in perfect attunement with Spirit. It is good for those who are afraid of power, or who

need to use power in a balanced way. Beneficial for digestive problems when worn near the third chakra. Increases your vibratory and healing powers, and enhances inner wisdom.

Aromas

In addition to the digestive organs, the nerves and the mind are also associated with the third chakra. These aromatic oils and teas are excellent for calming the nerves, soothing the digestion and stimulating the mind.

Peppermint. Used as an aromatic oil in candy and various medications, this herb is famous for settling the stomach and (as a byproduct) freshening the breath. Remember that the throat corresponds to the third chakra. Has a beneficial effect on the stomach, liver, and intestines. Massage the stomach with oil to which a few drops of peppermint has been added as an antispasmodic for colic, indigestion, vomiting, and stomach flu.

Lemon. Lemon oil relieves anxiety and depression and combats fatigue and lack of energy. Add a few drops to warm massage oil and apply to the back in light, gentle strokes. Use in a diffuser for stimulating the memory and for mental alertness. To relieve vomiting, put a couple drops on a tissue and inhale. For diarrhea, put a few drops in massage oil and gently massage the lower abdomen and lower back, then inhale from the hands with several slow deep breaths.

Statement

"I want happiness."

Explanation

The third chakra is the center of personal power. When the third chakra is open, you have found your own unique gift, the work that gives you pleasure and makes you feel fulfilled. When you're at the third chakra level of development, it's appropriate to build a positive self-image (ego). At the sixth chakra level you'll need to let go of your attachment to that image.

One way to find your gift is to consider what you most enjoyed doing when you were a child. This will give you clues about your natural inclinations. It's quite a joy to discover that what you're supposed to do is what you most deeply desire to do.

Your gift will reflect your natural skills and aptitudes, but it will also respond to training and schooling. For example, an opera singer is born with a beautiful voice but requires training to develop that skill. Dr. Laing says of people who are balanced at their third chakra, "Their personal will aligns with the Cosmic Will. These people are on their own path developing their intelligence and personal power, making unique contributions in the world."

According to Paramahansa Yogananda this chakra is ruled by the conscious mind. It is active only while awake. However, it can be trained in introspective, creative thinking which will then provide access to and influence on the subconscious mind. This helps to explain the power of negative or positive thinking.

In the martial arts the third chakra is considered the center of chi, the life force energy. So this chakra relates to physical abilities and athletic prowess.

This is the center of gut-level intuition. "I just knew it was going to rain," and "I had a feeling you were going to call," are statements that typify the third chakra intuition. (There's another kind of intuition that's found at the sixth chakra.

Yellow is the color of happiness. As an example of how this works, when I was living in Seattle I was

involved in an unhappy relationship when a psychic woman told me that I needed more yellow. One gloomy day, I had a terrible argument with this man, and I stomped out of the house and walked up the street.

As I was walking, I saw a whole rock face covered with beautiful yellow and orange flowers and I said to myself, "She said I need more yellow," so I proceeded to inhale the rich colors of the flowers. Within minutes I was filled with joy.

After that I painted my desk yellow. I liked it so well that I painted my bookcase yellow. That was so pleasing that I painted my whole room yellow.

The Book of Guidance says, "You see my sun as yellow. Through the color yellow I give you warmth and an inner glow. I radiate. This is the source of relaxation. Deep relaxation. Because you relax when you feel accepted. Then you can stop trying so hard. When you come out to the beach and lie in the sun, you relax completely because you know that nothing is expected of you. When you know that nothing is expected of you, you can just relax and be yourself. Now there is a place at the center of your body called the solar plexus. Just as my sun radiates acceptance, warmth, and relaxation from the center of your universe, you can also radiate acceptance, warmth, and relaxation from the center of your being."

Dr. Laing says, "Yellow goes straight to the soul. It is the common man. Common as the daisy and the dandelion. This soul is accessible to everyone. It is not esoteric or occult; it is ordinary.

"It [yellow] is the Middle Way. The Controller and Regulator. The Center of Strength. It is our link with the great Central Sun. It receives the radiations of the heavens and sends tentacles down to earth. It is a source of heat and energy without overstimulation. Nourishing like sunlight."

When parents have specific goals for their children, this sets up a conflict in the child's will. The child will be torn between love for the parents, and the need to develop his or her own power. If the child is loyal to the parents' expectations, he or she will probably not find his or her own unique form of creative expression. This is how people develop what appears to be a superiority complex. The superior attitude comes as a reflection of parental pride in this person's achievements. But secretly, this person feels inferior because he or she never had an opportunity to develop a true sense of self-worth.

Dr. Laing explains that in a less developed person, yellow will be mixed with red, indicating an obsession with accumulating things for one's self. Personal power will be directed in a self-serving direction and will not bring with it a sense of fulfillment.

"The third chakra relates to digestion," explains Laing. "A balance of energy here causes good digestion. A lack of energy here leads to poor digestion. Yellow relates to relaxation at meals and the flow of juices; digestive juices and bile, as well as adrenal and sexual hormones, all things that flow and radiate. Not blood because that is red and of the first chakra. But it does control dilation and constriction of the blood vessels.

"Since the third chakra rules both the digestion and the mind, it is difficult to think when too full or too hungry. But fasting will calm the mind unless there's a disorder here. Radiant relaxation comes from here. The solar plexus is the Center of Breath."

The diaphragm is located at the third chakra, so the color yellow at the third chakra is helpful for someone who is not breathing deeply because of tension or fear.

Continued ➡

Balanced Chakra Energy

CHARACTERISTICS

    outgoing
    cheerful
    has respect for self and others
    has a strong sense of personal power
    in touch with one's gift
    skillful
    intelligent
    relaxed
    spontaneous
    expressive
    takes on new challenges
    enjoys physical activity
    enjoys good food
    may have vague feelings of astral influences,
        both friendly and hostile
    spiritual expression could be
        Jewish
        Karma Yoga
        Tharavada Buddhism
    sexual energy:
        cares about one's partner
        highest goal may be to have a simultaneous
            orgasm
        sense of responsibility toward mate and
            children
        uninhibited
        relaxed
        can show emotional warmth

EXAMPLE

This man owns a large health food store and restaurant. He loves to cook and rarely uses a recipe, preferring to cook spontaneously. He derives great satisfaction from his work, and he creates a pleasant environment since he is friendly to both his employees and his customers. He's self-disciplined, reliable, and flexible.

Excessive Chakra Energy

CHARACTERISTICS

    judgmental
    workaholic
    perfectionistic
    overly intellectual
    as employer: very demanding
    as employee: resents authority
    may need drugs to relax
    superiority complex fluctuates with hidden
        inferiority complex
    Sexual energy:
        demanding
        constantly testing one's partner
        complains a lot about the relationship
        can be very affectionate
        may desire a lot of sexual activity, but rarely
            feels fulfilled

EXAMPLE

This fellow is very talented, but cannot decide how to channel his energy. He's a science teacher, carpenter, and musician. His father was a physicist and encouraged him to choose a career in science. He's a good science teacher. He drives himself very hard, but he doesn't enjoy his work. He complains frequently about his life, his job, and his co-workers. He worries about money constantly, and makes long lists of how he'll spend it when he gets it. He has many fantasies about women, but when he's in a relationship he's critical and argumentative. He has a potbelly and indigestion.

Deficient Chakra Energy

CHARACTERISTICS

    depressed
    lacks confidence
    worries about what others will think
    confused
    feels controlled by others
    poor digestion
    afraid of being alone
    sexual energy:
        insecure
        needs constant reassurance
        jealous, distrustful

EXAMPLE

This man is usually unemployed, though he's a skillful welder. He feels overwhelmed by life and can't seem to accomplish anything. He spends a lot of time smoking marijuana and hangs out at the local bar with his friends, most of whom also have deficient third chakras. His wife is a competent woman who supports him and tries to boost his ego. He's possessive of her and may become violent if he thinks she's interested in someone else. Yet he has affairs whenever he pleases.

Contraindications

People with nervous conditions and hot, red conditions should limit their use of yellow light to about ten minutes.

Glands and Organs Influenced by the Third Chakra

    the diaphragm (and the breath)
    adrenals
    skin
    digestive organs: stomach, duodenum,
        pancreas, gallbladder, liver

Illnesses and Ailments to Be Treated with Yellow

    digestive difficulties
    gas
    food allergies
    liver problems
    diabetes
    hypoglycemia
    over-sexed
    hypothyroid
    gallstones
    muscle cramps, spasms
    mental and nervous exhaustion
    depression
    difficulty breathing

Fourth Chakra

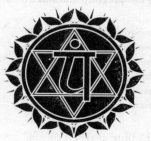

Names

    Anahatha (Unbeaten)
    Heart Center
    Dorsal Center

Symbol

Two triangles, one pointing up and the other down, representing balance. The heart is the center, with three chakras above and three below. The six-pointed star, also known as the Star of David, symbolizes the awakening of spirituality while being firmly planted on the ground.

Location

    center of chest

Area of the Face

    nose (leading to the lungs)

Sense

    smell

Color and Antidote

    green or pink
    Antidote, none needed, since it's central and
        balanced

There are two aspects of the love energy at the heart; the feminine/mother energy which we associate with pink and the masculine/father energy which we associate with green. On the rainbow, green is the color between yellow and blue. So where does pink come from? Magenta, a hot pink, is produced by combining violet (the spiritual energy of the crown chakra) with red (the grounded energy of the first chakra). A person who is balanced at their heart chakra tends to have this combination of qualities.

Tone and Note

    Tone, a (as in ah)
    Note, f#

The combined sounds of everything on earth compose a harmonic chord which is the keynote of our planet. It's the key of f (or f#), whose note becomes visible as green. This sound is good for quieting the mind.

Element

    air

Crystals

Pink and green stones and combinations thereof are associated with the heart chakra. Pink stones hold nurturing mother-love energy and green stones are associated with protective, fatherly love.

BC Jade. When your heart feels threatened or frightened, this dark green jade from British Columbia is like a loving father, reaching out to give comfort and reassurance. It is grounding, stabilizing, and protective. The Chinese say that jade (Chinese or BC) gives wisdom, clarity, justice, courage, and modesty. It will give you the wisdom to make clear judgments, the courage to follow through on them, and it will prevent you from getting big-headed about the good results.

Rose Quartz. The gentlest of stones, this pink quartz penetrates to the heart and the brain, soothing away worries. It carries the energy of unconditional love. It is comforting for those who have been hurt in love. Rose quartz helps to heal the wounded inner child. For those who wish to stop drinking alcohol, carrying a piece about the size of a quarter can help alleviate the need for alcohol.

Watermelon Tourmaline. This beautiful pink and green stone makes you feel as if you're being held in loving arms which make you feel safe enough to let yourself be vulnerable. Watermelon tourmaline helps to open dark places that have been shut down within your heart.

Aromas

Ylang Ylang. Sometimes the flowers of this small tropical tree are pink, and sometimes mauve or yellow. The oil varies from almost colorless to a pale yellow and the aroma is extremely heavy and sweet. It is used to slow down over-rapid breathing

Continued ➡

(hyperpnea) and overrapid heartbeat (tachycardia), and is useful in conditions of shock and anger. It is used to reduce high blood pressure. It is antidepressant, aphrodisiac, and sedative, helping to reduce the anxiety often associated with sexual performance. It helps to balance the male and female energies. Too much can cause nausea and/or headache.

Rose. This deep reddish-brown or greenish-orange essential oil is not distilled, but is produced by enfleurage, which requires a huge quantity of rose petals, so the cost is very high, but only a tiny amount is required. It is a gentle but potent antidepressant and is especially comforting for those who are grieving. It is an aphrodisiac and the Romans used to scatter rose petals on the bridal bed. Rosewater has similar properties and, since it is produced by distillation, it is far less expensive.

Statement

"I want to give and receive love."

Explanation

The heart chakra is the center of compassion. When this chakra opens, you transcend the limits of your ego and identify with other people, plants, animals, and all of life. This is the humanitarian center. When your heart chakra is open, you're likely to become involved with social causes. You'll care about things like ecology and saving the whales. You may find yourself working in one of the helping professions and participating in meditations for peace.

The heart chakra is your most vulnerable place. When you're hurt in life and love, the first impulse is to close your heart and say, "I'll never let anyone do that to me again." Of course, when you build a wall around your heart, you're keeping yourself locked in. Every time you experience a loss, you'll either go through a process of grieving, feeling all your feelings (especially anger and sadness), or you'll close off your heart and remain in a state of denial, becoming numb to pain as well as pleasure.

In fact, the majority of people have closed off their hearts—often at a very young age—which accounts for the alarming amount of apathy that exists in the world today. A major part of healing is to mend your heart. Your heart is at the center of your body and when your heart energy flows, your whole being is full. Then you radiate love energy to everyone around you.

Green is the color of healing. Almost all the healing herbs are green. Since it's at the center of the spectrum, green is the most balanced color. When you feel tense, it's wonderfully relaxing to go for a drive in the country or sit in a meadow of green grass. Green is nature's way of loving you.

Pink is the most powerful color for sending love to another person. When a person feels needy, you can mentally direct a ray of pink light toward them and you'll notice an immediate change, even if they are on the other side of the world. One of my clients lived with a man who constantly fought with her. I advised her to send him pink light when he was irritable. The next time he harassed her, she sent him pink light and, to her amazement, he immediately stopped arguing.

There's a common affliction of fourth chakra people. Since most of them used to be third chakra people, they're often married to third chakra people. As their fourth chakra opens and they evolve spiritually, they no longer share the same values with their mates.

Since the male sexual organs are in the first chakra, the center of physical reality, men tend to be more physically active. This energy is readily transferred to the third chakra, which is the power center. Men adapt well to becoming third chakra achievers, though this is more difficult for women, who frequently suffer from a fear of their own power.

The female sexual organs are primarily in the second chakra, which is at the seat of the emotions. This energy is readily transferred to the fourth chakra, the center of unconditional love.

The Personal Transformation Movement is basically a heart chakra phenomenon. This helps to explain why there are more than twice as many women involved in this movement. Many (third chakra) men feel threatened when their (fourth chakra) wives become involved in such activities. However, there can be compatibility between a person focused in their fourth chakra and a person who is focused in their third chakra, provided that both personalities are well balanced.

Balanced Chakra Energy

CHARACTERISTICS

compassionate
humanitarian
balanced
sees the good in everyone
desires to nurture others
friendly, outgoing
active in the community
discriminating
in touch with feelings
empathetic—instinctively aware of the joys and
    sorrows of others. May feel their aches and
    pains
spiritual expression could be
    Sufi
    Unity
    Bhakti Yoga
    Mahayana Buddhism
sexual energy:
    has the ability to surrender and merge in a
        love relationship
    desires a oneness of body, mind, and soul—
        and will feel lonely in a relationship that
        gives less than that
    strong will power, which makes it easier to
        wait for the right partner
    highest goal is to experience Divine Bliss—a
        spiritual, emotional, physical sensation—
        while in the embrace of one's beloved

EXAMPLE

This Sufi teacher lives in a huge house, surrounded by luxurious, profuse flowers. She is perpetually housing, feeding, and comforting everyone from beggars to saints. Children are drawn to her. She has endless friends and overflows with energy and love. Her lover is both affectionate and spiritual.

Excessive Chakra Energy

CHARACTERISTICS

demanding
overly critical
tense between the shoulder blades
possessive
moody
melodramatic
manic-depressive
uses money to control people
has the attitude of a martyr: "I've made so
    many sacrifices for you..."

Sexual energy:
    a master of conditional love: "I'll love
        you if…"
withholds love to get the desired behavior:
    "You wouldn't do that if you loved me."

EXAMPLE

This man is a poet and actor. He's a passionate lover, full of emotions rarely expressed except through his art. Outwardly he seems sincere and devoted, but inwardly a fire rages and he can't control his moodiness, his depressions, his grief, his fatigue. When he's alone he's miserable, and when he's newly in love, he's ecstatic. But after awhile he becomes demanding and controlling and he drives away the ones he loves.

Deficient Chakra Energy

CHARACTERISTICS

feels sorry for oneself
paranoid
indecisive
afraid of
letting go
being free
getting hurt
family members getting hurt
being abandoned
sexual energy:
feels unworthy of love
can't reach out
terrified of rejection
needs constant reassurance

EXAMPLE

This is the woman who loves too much. Because she wasn't well loved as a child, she doesn't believe she's worthy of love. She may be attractive and competent, but she chooses a mate who resembles the father or mother who was unable to give her the love she craved. Her greatest desire is to change her mate into a loving person through the power of her love. She does everything for him, but she ends up trying to control him and he often resists by pushing her away.

Contraindications

Glands and Organs Influenced by the Fourth Chakra

heart
lungs
immune system
thymus gland
lymph glands

Illnesses and Ailments to Be Treated with Green or Pink

heart pain
heart attack
high blood pressure
negativity
fatigue
difficulty breathing
tension
insomnia
anger
paranoia
cancer

Note: The best color for treating cancer is green. Ordinarily white light can be used for any ailment, because it contains all the colors. However, white light is nourishing and should not be used for cancer, because it feeds the cancer. Green is nourishing only to the healthy cells.

Continued ➡

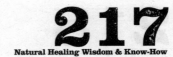

Fifth Chakra

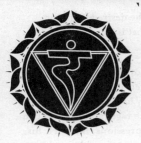

Names
> Visshudha (Pure)
> Cervical Center
> Throat Center

Symbol
The circle of unity with All That Is comes within the triangle, indicating an increasing openness to Spirit.

Location
> bottom of neck

Area of the Face
> ears
> Sense [B]
> sound

Color and Antidote
> blue
> *Antidote*, red

Tone and Note
> *Tone*, u (as in blue)
> *Note*, g#

Crystals
Fifth chakra stones are blue. They influence the throat and voice box. Since they are blue, they may be used as an antidote wherever there are red conditions such as inflammation, irritation, agitation, or fever. When used as an antidote, it is best if the stone is of at least equal size to the area being treated.

Sodalite. This blue stone with streaks of white calcite soothes all ailments of the throat and eases communication. It will help you to put your thoughts and feelings into words. It is a balancer that will enable you to keep your head in the clouds and your feet on the ground. Sodalite is invaluable for travel sickness, depression, feeling too "spaced out," and bad drug experiences. It is soothing to the third eye when doing psychic work. This stone will deepen your concentration.

Azurite. This blue stone is often found in geometric clumps, or in combination with malachite, when it is called azurite-malachite. Azurite stirs up the throat chakra and penetrates the voice box so that you're filled with the desire and ability to speak. Azurite keeps you centered and articulate. Azurite-malachite is good for bringing up the emotions (malachite) and then making you want to talk about them (azurite). Use two small smooth stones of azurite or azurite-malachite over the ovaries for menstrual cramps or ovarian discomfort, or place them over strained eyes (for example, when you've been using a computer for too long).

Aromas
These oils either have blue flowers or relate to the ears.

Blue (German) Chamomile. A fine oil is produced from this daisy-like yellow and white flower (which is also good for the third chakra). Its soothing, calming, and anti-inflammatory properties are due to azulene, the active principle which appears blue in highly distilled oil. It is beneficial for reddened skin conditions. Add a few drops to a warm bath to alleviate stress or tension. It is soothing, calming, and antidepressant. For calming babies, add a few drops to massage oil or use drops diluted in oil for the bath. For earache, rub around the ear, or apply hot compresses of chamomile. There are several different types of chamomile, but they all have similar properties.

Eucalyptus. During hot days, eucalyptus trees seem to give off a blue haze. This oil is used for cooling the body. It helps reduce fevers. Eucalyptus oil may be used in a hot or cold vaporizer to ease a tight, dry cough. It is used in gargles. It is anti-inflammatory. Add a few drops of this oil to massage oil to relieve muscular aches and pains. It can be found in most drugstores.

Statement
"I want to speak freely and openly."

Explanation
When you reach this level of spiritual development, you have to squeeze through a bottleneck. It's a struggle. Society doesn't require it of you—in fact, many people frown upon it. Most people function from their lower chakras and they can't understand the person who opens to spirituality. It makes them uncomfortable. If you open your fourth, that's extraordinary. But to open your fifth is like walking on thin ice.

The fifth chakra is the center of communication, so as you open this center, there is a desire to talk about your extraordinary experiences. When you do this, some of your old friends will fall away. But your true friends will always be there, so try to let go of the ones who are uncomfortable with you. New and wonderful friends will be magnetically drawn to your new persona. Fortunately, there is a growing community of people who have opened their fifth chakra.

Spiritual children are those who have not closed down their fifth chakra. Their parents allow them to speak freely, to sing, and when necessary, to cry and scream. They've been encouraged to trust their own perceptions and to follow their instincts.

These children may experience conflict when they enter school and encounter a new set of values. This often results in chronic sore throats or ear infections (which indicate an inability to speak freely or an unwillingness to hear what is being said to you). The blue light will comfort these children. They need to talk about the conflict they're feeling and be reassured that their reality—though it's different from the norm—is valid.

One of my students is a kindergarten teacher. After learning about the calming effect of blue, she instituted a new program. On days when all the kids are climbing the walls, yelling and screaming and acting out, she'll say, "Today's a blue day!" Then she'll bring out blue poster paint and blue play dough and blue construction paper and blue magic markers and she'll tell each child to do a project in blue. She says the effect is remarkably calming. In fact, blue classrooms are used for hyperactive children and blue holding rooms are used in prisons.

Blue can also be used effectively for the dying. Blue pictures, blue blankets, and blue flowers are calming and soothing to one who is letting go of life. If you're sitting by the bedside of a person who is dying, the tone u (as in blue) can help to calm his or her nerves and accompany that person into a different reality. Try it, and see if the effect seems beneficial. Perhaps this person will want to join you.

Balanced Chakra Energy
CHARACTERISTICS
> contented
> centered
> can live in the present
> perfect sense of timing
> good speaker
> musically or artistically inspired
> can meditate and experience Divine Energy
> easy grasp of spiritual teachings
> may be overwhelmingly prolific
> clairaudient: may hear voices or celestial music
>> from the other
> planes
> spiritual expression could be
>> Quaker
>> Spiritualist Church
>> Agni Yoga
>> Private worship
> sexual energy:
>> when all five chakras are open, can manifest incredible sexual or sensual energy, or can abstain without great effort
>> may choose to rechannel sexual energy into music, art, or meditation
>> may vacillate between seeking bliss through sexual embrace and seeking bliss through celibacy and meditation

EXAMPLE
This man is a popular writer, choosing unusual topics of a metaphysical nature just as the public becomes ready to read such material. He plays the violin for pleasure. He's highly intuitive, living fully in the present, waiting until everything feels right before making any moves. He is always at the right place at the right time. He practices T'ai Chi and meditation daily. He's devoted to friends and family, though he sometimes goes off into the mountains for weeks at a time. His wife shares his interest in combining spiritual and sexual energies, and they're both sensual and uninhibited.

Excessive Chakra Energy
CHARACTERISTICS
> arrogant
> self-righteous
> talks too much
> dogmatic
> addictive
> Sexual energy:
>> preoccupied with sexual thoughts
>> may be unconsciously macho
>> prefers partners who can be dominated

EXAMPLE
This therapist is a large, overbearing, bitter woman who has a lot of anger toward men. She's an articulate champion of women's rights, and has deep insights which make her a good therapist and writer. When she likes someone, she's a good friend, but when she turns against a person, she can be rude and abusive. She attracts sexual partners who are submissive and meek.

Deficient Chakra Energy
CHARACTERISTICS
> scared, timid
> holds back
> confused
> quiet
> inconsistent
> unreliable
> weak

Continued ➡

devious, manipulative
can't express one's thoughts
sexual energy:
can't relax
feels conflict with religious upbringing
afraid of sex

Example

This fifty-five-year-old woman was once a lawyer, but she dropped out in order to follow her spiritual master. Sometimes she has deep insights, feelings of ecstasy, and experiences a profound love of Spirit. At other times she feels like a failure and a misfit. She's in conflict about her sexuality. She's nervous and worries a great deal. She lives in a communal house and doesn't fit in. She's afraid to express her needs openly so others consider her devious and manipulative.

Contraindications

Do not use blue light for more than thirty minutes, or it may cause you to feel withdrawn and sleepy. If this occurs, follow the treatment with a few minutes of yellow or orange.

Do not use blue for the following ailments:
colds
muscle contractions
paralysis
poor circulation

Glands and Organs Influenced by the Fifth Chakra

throat
thyroid
nerves
eyes
muscles

Illnesses and Ailments to Be Treated with Blue

Since virtually every illness is characterized by inflammation, which is a red condition, blue is the most frequently used color for healing. Use it to heal all hot, red, and nervous conditions. Use it as an antidote for irritations in the first chakra area.

hyperthyroid
sore throat
inflammations
burns
skin irritations, rashes
fever
ear infections
overtired
mentally exhausted
gum inflammation, teething
ulcers, digestive irritation
nervousness
colic
back pain
hemorrhoids
high blood pressure
toxemia of pregnancy
vaginal infections
hyperactive
excitable and violent
terminal illness

Sixth Chakra

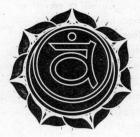

Names

Ajna Chakra (Command)
Third Eye Center
Christ Consciousness Center

Symbol

Suddenly the multiplicity of petals falls away and you are left with two huge petals. Through letting go of your attachment to the multiple distractions of the world you enter into a Divine relationship with Spirit. This is the ego self and the spirit self, the reasoning and the intuitive minds, the pineal and the pituitary, the masculine and the feminine. All dualities converge at this point. The triangle is the yoni or female energy and within it is the linga or male energy. The linga of the first chakra was black, whereas this linga is white. The linga of the first chakra was surrounded by a snake, coiled three and a half times around it, symbolizing the sleeping kundalini energy at the base of the spine. Now the kundalini energy rises to the sixth chakra; the snake uncoils and the sexual energy rises upward. The crescent moon of feminine receptivity embraces the circle above it. This circle is a golden dot which is the essence of spiritual energy. It represents being in your center. The quarter moon is an energy vortex symbolizing infinite potential.

Location

Each of the chakras can be located at the back or the front of the body, along the spine. The sixth chakra is found at the base of the skull, at the medulla oblongata. Its location at the front of the head is between the eyebrows at the third eye.

Area of the Face

eyes (the windows of the soul)

Sense

sight

Color and Antidote

Indigo (a purplish hue)
Indigo is a combination of blue and red. Red is warm, so indigo is a way of calming without cooling or slowing.

Antidote, orange

Tone and Note

mm or OM (as in home)
The sound "o" represents the sun or third eye, and "m" represents the moon or medulla. OM unifies both sides. It also combines the "o" of the second chakra with the "m" of the sixth chakra. This tone dissolves dualities and creates unity. It brings the ego self into union with the Spirit self.

Note, high a

Element

electrical or telepathic energy

Crystals

The crystals of the third eye are mystical stones which have powerful transformative properties.

Lapis Lazuli. This rich royal blue stone is usually streaked with iron pyrite. Use it at the third eye to take you deep within the vaults of your mind. Lapis facilitates hypnosis, visualization, astral travel, and understanding of metaphysical teachings. It brings your energies to a higher level during meditation when placed on the crown chakra. Polished lapis helps you to shed your ego and put your spiritual life first.

Sugilite (Luvulite). This rare stone has just been discovered in the last two decades. It combines the purple of the sixth chakra with the black of the first, bringing spirituality into every cell, integrating body and soul. Sugilite is ideal for highly sensitive, idealistic children, or adults who find it difficult to function in a less-than-ideal world. It reminds you that you are special and your gift is rare and valuable. It helps you to visualize how to bring your gift to the world.

Aromas

Juniper berries. Made from the ripe purple berries of the juniper bush, juniper oil helps overcome anxiety, insomnia, and mental fatigue. It is good for greasy hair and dandruff. It strengthens the kidneys and relieves fluid retention.

Rosemary. This pine-like evergreen helps to balance body and mind. It was used by the ancient Egyptians, Greeks, and Romans as a symbol of love and friendship because it clears the mind, stimulates the memory, and is good for the heart. Rosemary oil is used to relieve headaches, migraines, and fatigue. It was used in funeral wakes and at burial grounds because it purifies the air and prevents infections. It makes the hair shiny and eliminates dandruff when used in a rinse.

Statement

"I want to see clearly."

Explanation

The third eye is the center of psychic power and higher intuition. Through the sixth chakra, you can receive Guidance, channel, and tune into your Higher Self. This is the center that enables you to experience telepathy, astral travel, and past lives.

When this center is agitated, it often indicates that a person had early religious training that taught him or her to be afraid of the occult. Many cultures and religions have taboos against anything vaguely metaphysical. While it's true that so-called magical powers have been severely misused throughout history, the same can be said for any kind of power, particularly political power. And it is political power, including the political power of the established churches, that has outlawed or defamed practitioners of the occult, usually for the simple reason that these people were attracting too many of the churches' clientele.

The irrational guilt and fear created by these taboos make it difficult for most people to get a clear perspective so they can judge for themselves whether a teaching is beneficial or not. First it's useful to make a distinction between black magic and white magic. White magic harnesses natural energy for positive purposes. If you're in the presence of someone who practices white magic, you'll feel normal, or perhaps your energy will be enhanced. Black magic manipulates energy for selfish purposes. When you're in the presence of someone who uses black magic, your energy may be temporarily boosted, but within a short time you'll feel drained.

The energy of the third eye is, unfortunately, accessible to all people regardless of their moral and ethical values. The ability to manipulate reality is an

Continued ➡

appealing skill for those who are power-hungry, and this includes many New Age gurus. So be discerning about who you accept as a spiritual teacher. If you feel at all distrustful about such a person, pay careful attention to your perceptions.

For many people the word guru has disturbing implications of blind obedience and hero worship, and this has been a damaging pattern that many followers of gurus have fallen into. But guru is just another word for spiritual teacher. If you're fortunate enough to find a spiritual teacher you can trust, who feels like an innately ethical person, and if it feels like this person has the desire to help you to experience the fullness of your being, this can be a great blessing. A true spiritual teacher should be simply a person who has progressed further in their spiritual development than you have. Ideally it will be someone who has opened their higher chakras and achieved self-realization (balanced sixth chakra). If this is your goal, then such a person can be a great help. In every field where we seek to gain knowledge, we look for a teacher who is more experienced and more knowledgeable than we are. The same should apply to the field of spiritual development

Unfortunately, most gurus demand absolute and blind obedience. While this can be useful for a short time—to overcome attachments of the ego—when it is prolonged, it robs the devotee of his or her ability to function effectively from their own center of power (third and sixth chakras) and to be discriminating. Also it places the guru in the light of the seventh chakra, even while the guru is professing to lead the student into a deeper relationship with the Self and the Divine One.

Before the third eye opens, you see through two eyes: you experience a duality between your normal self (your conscious mind, intellect, ego) and your higher Self (your intuitive mind, or Spirit). When the third eye opens, these two images merge—like when you see a double image through the lens of a camera and then bring it into focus as a single unified image.

I don't believe in forcing yourself to shed your ego through self-denial. I believe in working with the ego until it recognizes that the fulfillment of its highest dreams is to be found through merging with the High Self and becoming One with the Divine. Then all the masks fall away: who you thought you were, who you thought you ought to be, who your parents wanted you to be. Suddenly you let go and your True Self shines forth. "I am what I am." There is no guilt, no need for illusion or pretense. You are totally in the present and you realize that you were there all along.

The pineal gland is an endocrine organ that has the essential structure of an eye. It's located in the central part of the brain, so it relates to both the sixth and the seventh chakras. It functions as a light receptor, and is believed to be responsible for ovulation occurring in response to the phases of the moon.

When the kundalini rises up the spine, it stimulates the pineal gland, which may explain the experience of seeing the Pure White Light. The third eye is the Christ consciousness center. Everyone can have Christ consciousness. Jesus said, "The light of the body is the eye: therefore when thine eye is single, thy whole body also is full of light; but when thine eye is evil, thy body also is full of darkness." Luke 11:34.

The yogis say that the pineal is the seat of memory, so when the kundalini rises this storehouse opens up and you become a witness to all your past lives, and you see into your future. You no longer require the veil of forgetfulness because you're no longer afraid of who you are—you have nothing to hide. You're flooded with compassion and forgiveness and unconditional love toward all of your selves in all of your lives and you see yourself in everyone and everything. You no longer have any karmic debts. You stand released from fear and guilt and when this occurs, you transcend the wheel of karma: you realize that it was only a reflection of your ego.

Thus you become a fully realized being. This is the meaning of self-realization. You merge with Spirit and you become the Spirit within yourself: you realize your full potential.

Balanced Chakra Energy

CHARACTERISTICS

charismatic
access to the Source of All Knowledge
receives Guidance
experiences Cosmic Consciousness
not attached to material things
no fear of death
can show the way to liberation, through example
clairvoyant: may begin with waking visions of vague colors and landscapes
experiences telepathy, astral travel, past lives
not preoccupied with fame or fortune or worldly things
master of oneself
spiritual energy could be
Essene Christian
Taoist
Vajrayana Buddhist
Raja Yoga
sexual energy:
At this level of development, one perceives oneself as essentially androgynous, and no longer requires another person for completion. A needy partner distracts one's inner bliss. Thus celibacy is a natural choice, but not a necessary one.

EXAMPLE

The Dalai Lama has conscious memory of his previous incarnations and he carries the knowledge of that lineage from birth. He is considered the incarnation of Avaloketeshvara, and it is his mission to return in human form in order to show people the way to liberation. He is kind and compassionate, a master of himself. From the time he was a young boy he demonstrated deep wisdom and remarkable abilities.

Excessive Chakra Energy

CHARACTERISTICS

egomaniac
proud
manipulative
religiously dogmatic
authoritarian

EXAMPLE

Ayatollah Khomeini is a dogmatic religious leader of Iran who persecuted anyone who did not agree with him. He was a fierce authoritarian and women were kept submissive and oppressed in his country.

Deficient Chakra Energy

CHARACTERISTICS

nonassertive
undisciplined
oversensitive to the feelings of others
afraid of success
may be schizophrenic (unable to distinguish between ego self and Higher Self)

EXAMPLE

Sometimes this schizophrenic woman believes she is Joan of Arc, and will display dynamic strength and the ability to heal by touch and to foresee future events. Then she'll sink back into a self-effacing personality, barely able to feed herself, afraid of everyone, distrustful, unable to find any direction in life.

Contraindications

schizophrenic
withdrawn

Glands and Organs Influenced by the Sixth Chakra

pineal
pituitary
brain
ears

Illnesses and Ailments to Be Treated with Indigo

pain (anesthetic effects)
diarrhea
agitation and tightness in intestines
psychic exhaustion

Seventh Chakra

Names

Sahasrara
Thousand-Petaled Lotus
Crown Chakra
Wisdom Chakra

Symbol

The fully open lotus, the flower in fullest bloom, symbolizes being totally open to the Light. You've lost all individual identity and now you merge with All That Is. You become a fully realized being. This is self-realization, the peak experience of which is called samadhi.

Location

crown of head

Area of the Face

the crown of the head, including the scalp and hair

Sense

extrasensory perception (ESP), the "seventh sense"

Color and Antidote

violet
Note: gold is also associated with the crown chakra
Antidote, yellow

Tone and Note

Tone, e (as in bee)
Note, high b

Crystals

The violet-colored stones and the clear crystals which are like the stars in the sky are favored at the crown chakra.

Continued ➡

Amethyst. This lovely violet-colored translucent quartz gives protection by allowing in only those energies that are harmonious to you and deflecting and transmuting all other energies. Use over your third eye to facilitate visualization and past life recall. Keep a cluster in your room or on your altar to calm and center your energies. Place in rooms where disharmony is felt or anticipated. If you have difficulty sleeping, hold it while you meditate before going to bed. Place a piece in wine or beer to detoxify the alcohol. Amethyst is beneficial to wear as jewelry, but not if you are nervous or hyperactive.

Clear Quartz Crystals. These hold the vibration of White Light. They absorb, transmit, resonate, and amplify energy. Crystals are good to hold while you meditate. They enhance the energy of group meditations. Placed around the home, they give off negative ions that create a sense of well-being. Be cautious about wearing clear quartz as jewelry if you aren't feeling clear, or if you're around negative people, because they can absorb negative energy and reflect it back to you. If they are kept clean, they have the ability to bring more color and light into your aura.

Aromas

Lavender. This oil is specially recommended for all ailments of the head, brain, and nerves. Several drops may be added safely to the bath water or to massage oil or used directly on the skin as perfume. Small quantities of lavender oil have been shown to calm spasms of the solar plexus. It is also excellent for insomnia, infections, allergies, fainting, headaches, migraines, influenza, insomnia, hysteria, and tension.

Frankincense. The name derives from Medieval French, meaning "Real Incense." It was the first kind of incense to be used. The essential oil comes from a resin with a somewhat camphorous penetrating aroma, familiar to Catholics, where it is used in the incense burners. This practice dates back to ancient times when it was called Holy Oil and was used by the Hebrews and Egyptians to drive out evil spirits. It has the ability to slow down and to deepen the breath, which contributes to feelings of calmness, which in turn is conducive to meditation. It is used in inhalations, massage, and bath oils for respiratory infections, chronic bronchitis, asthma, and for people who have had strokes. Steam inhalation is not recommended for asthmatics. It is believed to help those who tend to dwell too much upon their past.

Statement

"I want to be lazy." (The seventh day is the day of rest.)

Explanation

When a person enters the seventh chakra, the person you were dies. Every layer of ego attachment falls away. You die to your old self. At the fifth chakra, you may long to leave your mark for posterity. At the sixth chakra, there is no more longing; it is enough to simply be a living example.

At the seventh chakra even the desire to help falls away, though it may emerge again unpredictably. Now you become the divine madman or madwoman, utterly beyond laws and norms, totally unpredictable and unaccountable. Your behavior may be considered antisocial, amoral, and incomprehensible. But you are totally moral according to your own ethics.

You have the power to transmute matter into energy and energy into matter, which enables you to perform remarkable feats such as walking on water or appearing at several places at the same time. Food can be produced out of thin air. But

then, you're not likely to want to attract much attention, being neither a martyr, a saint, nor an egotist. So you're more likely to wander around in the Himalayas if you want to be left alone, or to wander from village to village, communicating in parables.

Your spirituality is omnipresent, and since you live constantly in The Light, there's no need for a path by which to get there, so there's no need for any organized religion.

Sexuality isn't likely to be desirable to you, though you may have evolved a form of energy exchange that's quite ecstatic though it is not focused at any particular part of the body.

The seventh chakra is the point where the silver cord detaches from the body at the time of death. The silver cord is the fine line that allows us to astral travel and then return to the body. When this cord is severed, death sets in.

Death is no stranger to the seventh chakra person.

Since there is no separation between self and spirit-self, the body is a joke; a trick of the mind. Bodies come and go, but life is eternal. Since all the bodily cells can be transmuted and renewed, you're capable of immortality and you can perform miraculous healings and raise the dead.

Balanced Chakra Energy

CHARACTERISTICS

open to the Divine
miracle worker
can transcend the laws of nature
total access to the unconscious and the subconscious
ability to leave and return to the body at will in full consciousness
ability to remain alert during and after death
almost immortal—or possibly immortal

EXAMPLE

Babaji appeared to Yogananda and to Yogananda's teacher, Sri Yukteswar, and to his teacher, Lahiri Mahasaya. He is always described as the eternally youthful saint, who appears and disappears at will. Yogananda believed that he was one of the teachers of Jesus.

Excessive Chakra Energy

CHARACTERISTICS

constant sense of frustration
unrealized power
psychotic, depressed, or manic-depressive
frequent migraine headaches
destructive
sexual expression
sometimes passionate, sometimes distant

EXAMPLE

This psychotic man imagines that he is Jesus Christ. He has delusions of grandeur as he attempts to enlist his twelve disciples. He actually does have the ability to see into the future and to read minds, but his skills are sporadic and undisciplined, and he cannot distinguish between his fantasies, or his paranoias, and reality.

Deficient Chakra Energy

CHARACTERISTICS

no spark of joy
catatonic
can't make decisions

EXAMPLE

This young boy never seemed quite normal, even as a baby. He was withdrawn, uncommunicative, and rarely smiled. When he was four years old, the doc-

tors said he was catatonic. He was quite intelligent, but unable to relate to other people. He was pale and thin. Though his parents tried to love him, he was unable to respond. He was lost in a world of his own.

Glands and Organs Influenced by the Seventh Chakra

pituitary
pineal
nervous system
brain

Illnesses and Ailments to be Treated with Violet

depression
migraine headaches
parasites
black eyes
baldness, dandruff
Note: Violet is excellent for artists and high-strung, nervous people who need grounding but find red too harsh.

Chakra Evaluation and Treatment

In some sense, everything you do (or don't do) influences your energy and your chakras. In this chapter, I will focus upon methods of healing that are specifically intended to balance the flow of energy at the chakras.

Chakra Evaluation

Before you can treat the chakras, you must determine which ones are deficient or excessive. The depth of information that can be derived will be, to some degree, dependent upon the sensitivity and experience of the practitioner. I've outlined some of the methods for evaluating the chakras.

INTELLECTUAL/INTUITIVE

This is the method which you employed when you read the previous section. It is similar to the evaluation that the practitioner comes to from simply talking with the client and considering how their symptoms fall into the categories of the chakras.

VISUAL

Those who have the gift of clairvoyance can simply look at you and see which of the mini-suns that make up your chakras shine brightly, and which are dull, cloudy or muddy. There are other visual methods:

A **colored lamp** may be used to direct colored light to different chakras. For the purpose of chakra evaluation, only the corresponding colors should be used for each chakra (red for the first, orange for the second, etc.). If you feel comfortable sitting under a particular light, as though you could sit there for a long time without any problem (but not as if there was a craving to do so), this indicates that the chakra is balanced. On the other hand, if there is discomfort, ranging from tightness or pain in the head to a simple feeling of irritability, this indicates that the chakra is out of balance. The same applies if there is a sense of craving more of that color.

The **Color Receptivity Trainer** consists of a small box mounted on a tripod, which is positioned directly in front of the eyes, at arm's length from the client. This method was devised by Jacob Liberman, author of *Light, Medicine of the Future*. Light is projected through different-colored gels. You look at a circle of colored light about 4 inches in diameter. The CRT is engineered with a timer and flashing lights. The number of flashes per minute are gradually increased. Once again, the colors that cause you discomfort provide clues about which chakras might be out of balance.

Continued ➡

Tactile/Energetic

You may **use the hands to feel the energy** a few inches above each chakra, while being sensitive to variations of temperature, vibration, and other subtle differences. Dorothy Krieger's Therapeutic Touch (described on page 223) and Pranic Healing (described on page 223) both use this method. Many body workers find that they become sensitive in this way. The tactile method may be enhanced by other tools.

A **pendulum** may be used a few inches above each chakra, to feel the relative size and shape of the electromagnetic spin of energy. Pendulums are usually made of a light, symmetrical object which dangles from a string or chain. A simple clear quartz crystal pendant works well. One method is to allow the object to swing freely, wrapping the chain around the fingers until just a few inches of chain remain. Ask the pendulum to give you its signal for a normal balanced chakra. It is liable to spin clockwise in a circular motion about the size of your open hand. Any variation on this might indicate that something is out of balance.

A **crystal** may be used to augment the vibratory energy, enabling the practitioner to feel the spin of energy a few inches above each of the chakras. My technique of Vibrational Alignment™ (described on page 223) uses this method.

Biofeedback can provide an additional source of information. For example, a simple device which senses the temperature of the fingers can be attached to two of the fingers. When a person feels agitated or fearful, the blood circulation withdraws from the extremities, and this sensor picks up the change of temperature and registers a high-pitched sound which alerts you that some kind of discomfort is being registered. This device can be coupled with the use of the CRT or colored lamp.

Measuring Chakra Openness

The size of a healthy, open chakra is approximately the size of your open hand, with the diameter stretching from the tip of your thumb to the tip of your little finger. A large person with large hands has proportionately larger chakras, but the energy emanating from and received by a smaller person is not necessarily weaker, just as a small diamond is not diminished in radiance just because it is diminutive next to a large clear quartz crystal.

The radiance emanating from an open chakra can travel a great distance. In fact, a person can consciously choose to reach out with that radiance, to affect healing for a person who is far away. Physicists are now speculating that there is a form of energy that travels faster than the speed of light, which might help to explain the apparently miraculous effects of distant healing.

In 1927, C.W. Leadbeater wrote in his classic book, *The Chakras*, "When quite undeveloped they appear as small circles about two inches in diameter, glowing dully in the ordinary man, but when awakened and vivified they are seen as blazing, coruscating whirlpools, much increased in size, and resembling miniature suns."

One theory suggests that there are seven stages of openness at each chakra. I rarely have the gift of seeing the chakras, yet I can easily feel the spin of energy. I will describe what I feel at each of these seven stages, and how I interpret what I feel. Remember that this is a highly subjective experience and three different people who have the ability to feel the energy may describe these seven stages in three entirely different ways.

First stage—My arm feels fatigued as I attempt to feel the energy at this chakra because it is lifeless, weak, and only slightly open. The chakra has barely enough energy to keep the internal organs and endocrine glands functioning. With even just one chakra this deficient, if this condition persists, the person will be highly susceptible to disease and even death.

Second stage—The energy here is slow and lethargic. The diameter of the circle is no larger than the first joint of the person's thumb. This chakra is functioning just above minimal level. This person has a low resistance to infection. Their will to live is not strong.

Third stage—The spin of energy lacks enthusiasm. The size of the spin is no greater than a silver dollar. This chakra is functional. The energy is adequate but weak.

Fourth stage—The energy spins at about the pace of the heart. The size of the spin is about the size of the palm of the person's hand. This is normal and within the range of healthy.

Fifth stage—The energy spins at about the pace of the heart. The size of the spin is about the size of the palm, plus the first digit of the fingers. This chakra feels energetic and in excellent health.

Sixth stage—The energy spins at about the pace of the heart. The size of the spin is about the size of the palm, plus the first two digits of the fingers. This chakra exudes radiance, dynamism, and enthusiastic energy.

Seventh stage—The energy spins at about the pace of the heart. The size of the spin is that of the open hand. The energy is off the scales. This person is obviously exultant and basking in the light.

Methods of Treating the Chakras

There are a wide variety of methods that help bring the chakras into balance and alignment. Once you have determined which chakras need work, any of the following modalities may be used. This list is not intended to be exhaustive, and new methods are constantly emerging.

Intellectual/Intuitive

Because the chakras are about energy, the intellect is not particularly effective for altering that energy. However, the intuition can be valuable for determining which chakras to treat, which methods to use, and for how long.

Visual/Color

When you have mastered the language of color, you will find yourself automatically applying this knowledge in your choice of clothing, jewelry, flowers, wall decorations, and every aspect of your life. Other methods of visual treatment include:

Color Breathing. You can look at a particular color or visualize it as you inhale, and imagine bringing that color into one of your chakras or internal organs. Colors may also be sent to others via the breath.

Color-Charged Water. Water may be charged by putting it in a colored glass container, or by putting a plate of colored glass against the window and setting the water in a clear glass jar in front of the color source. A few sips of this water may be taken several times a day, or it can be used externally, as a wash. The French word for water is *eau*, pronounced "o," so the names for the color-charged waters are rubio for red-charged water, ambero for orange and yellow, verdio for green, ceruleo for blue, and purpura for indigo and violet.

Juices and Other Liquids. Any colored juice can be used to enhance the energy of the corresponding chakra. Colored wines, liqueurs, and beer may also be used.

Colored Lamp. This is a lamp that shines a strong light source through colored gels or sheets of colored glass to a specific area of the body.

Phototherapy. When the client becomes comfortable with a given color by way of the CRT (described on page 221), then flashes are added, and the flash rate is gradually increased. Each eye contains 137 million photoreceptors that transform light into electrical impulses which travel to various parts of the brain which are stimulated by these impulses. Phototherapy begins by treating visual problems and then expands into the treatment of many other ailments.

Laserpuncture. This method was developed by the Russians as another method of using color for healing. Through the use of laser light, specific colored tubes are used to stimulate acupuncture points by low-energy laser beams. Some of the same principles that are used to correlate different colors for specific internal organs, for example, are used in laserpuncture.

Audio/Sound

Toning and Sounding. Toning is the sustained, vibratory vocal sounding of single tones—usually vowels—without melody, rhythm, or words. Sounding is the free-form use of sounds without any particular structure. By making vibratory sounds with your voice, you can tune up your chakras. The sounds which correlate with the chakras are given on my cassette tape, *The Healing Voice*.

Tuning Forks. Each fork is U-shaped, with a stem at the bottom of the curve of the U. A person can hold a fork by the stem and then strike the fork against something like the bone of the knee, and this will set off a vibratory frequency. A set of seven tuning forks is used, and each fork is tuned to one of the seven notes of the scale. A simple chakra tune-up consists of striking each of the seven forks, beginning with C and holding the fork to the corresponding chakra, beginning with the first chakra.

Musical Instruments. Various instruments may be held or suspended directly above the chakras that need work. Crystal Bowls and Tibetan Bowls of varying sizes can be used to tune up the chakras, much as the tuning forks described above. Other instruments that have a profound effect upon the chakras are gongs, Tibetan bells, and the didjeridu, a long hornlike instrument originated by the Australian Aborigines.

Sound Tables. There are various massage-type tables with speakers installed, for example, at each of the seven chakra areas. Appropriate music for awakening, stimulating, or calming the chakras is piped in through each chakra section.

Aromas

Aromatherapy. Many of the volatile oils have a tendency to favor a particular internal organ or endocrine gland, and this—together with the color of the flower or the oil itself— gives us clues about which chakra will be most influenced, though all of the oils may be used at various parts of the body. See each chakra chapter for aromas that may be used in conjunction with each of the chakras. There are many ways to receive the benefits of aromatherapy, including using a dif-fuser, bath oil, massage oil, or incense.

Movement

There are specific exercises—both ancient and modern—which are designed to influence the health of the chakras. One of the oldest is called the Tibetan Rites and it is described in *Ancient Secrets*

Continued ➧

of the Fountain of Youth. An excellent modern book which gives movements and a vast array of other information about working with the chakras is *The Sevenfold Journey*. Once again, any movement, particularly yoga and various forms of martial arts, will have an influence upon the chakras. Martial arts are particularly useful for developing the second chakra.

Energy Healing

Pranic Healing. *Prana* means "to breathe forth" which refers to the life force that vitalizes the etheric body and nervous system. Prana is a Sanskrit term for vitality and magnetism. An important function of the chakras is to vitalize the dense physical body, including the endocrine glands. Pranic healing attempts to heal the physical body by directing prana to one or more of the etheric chakras, which is then believed to vitalize the corresponding organs and endocrine glands. The healer uses her/his breath to draw extra prana into their own body, and then sends that prana through their own chakras to the corresponding chakras of the client.

Therapeutic Touch. This method, developed by Dorothy Krieger, RN, uses the secondary chakras at the palms of the hands to feel the energy emanating from the body, particularly at the chakras, a couple of inches away from the physical body. Then the practitioner directs energy through their own hands, working entirely in the energy field without actually touching the physical body, to increase or decrease energy to bring it into balance.

Healing Touch and Reiki. Healing Touch, developed by Janet Mentgen, RN, is similar to Therapeutic Touch, also using hand-scanning to feel the energies, but it involves actually placing the hands on the chakras. Reiki, developed by Dr. Usui in Japan, involves placing the hands directly on the chakras and other parts of the body.

Combined Methods

Vibrational Healing. The Vibrational Healer balances the body's electromagnetic energy using vibratory tools such as color, light, sound (toning), gemstones, and aromatic oils.

Vibrational Alignment™. In this form of Vibrational Healing that I have developed, the practitioner uses their hand or a long clear quartz crystal to feel the spin of subtle energies at each of the chakras to determine: where the client is holding unfinished business (first and second chakras); issues of self-worth and fear of power (third chakra); unresolved traumas from the past (fourth chakra); and sources of mental and spiritual confusion (higher chakras). Once the reason for the illness is understood, the practitioner uses the vibratory tools to help the body find its own healthy harmonic resonance.

—From *Pocket Guide to Chakras*

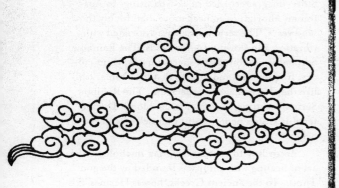

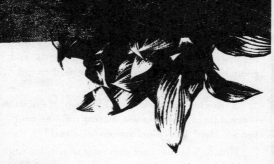

THE HARA LINE
Diane Stein

The hara line holds and maintains our life purpose, why we have incarnated for this lifetime. Clear understanding of this purpose leads to productivity, fulfillment, and peace of mind in one's life. Energy blockage on this emotional body hara level obstructs our intentions and accomplishments and our awareness of this purpose. More and more, the emotional body comes to the forefront as central to any level of healing, from the physical body to the core soul. The hara level is vitally important for today's healers and healing.

The first hara chakra is a clear-colored (all colors, no color) center above the head, which I call the transpersonal point. It is a chakra familiar to many women who have placed it on the kundalini channel. This is the soul's first manifestation into matter, the first opening of energy from the Goddess/Void. It carries the individual's reason to incarnate into her body, mind, emotions, and spirit. The transpersonal point separates the soul from its Goddess source, giving it a personal reality and a life on Earth. Other names for this center include the Soul Star. Ch'i Kung calls it the source of Heavenly Ch'i. Some clear gemstones activate this center.

Next is a pair of silver chakra centers located behind the eyes. I call these vision chakras. The eyes can be used as lasers in healing, as well as for visualization and for manifesting our needs through visualization. They are considered minor centers but are important for psychic healers. Some of the gray, iridescent, and silvery gemstones open and develop these chakras.

The causal body chakra follows, located in the base of the skull at the back where the neck meets the head. Some healers see this very major center as a light silvery blue, while others perceive it as resembling crimson yarn wrapped around a golden skein. Gemstones for this center include both crimson and silver-blue. The causal body is described as all-potential (the Nonvoid or Goddess within) and the transformer of nonphysical information/light into consciousness, as in channeling, automatic writing, and working with spirit guides. The chakra must be activated and balanced to bring mental commitment to one's life purpose, but this should be done only with all the hara line chakras together. Causal body activation manifests one's spiritual life purpose, as embodied in the entire hara line, into earthplane, physical reality.

The next hara line chakra, also a major one, is the thymus chakra. I perceive this center's color as aqua or aquamarine, and I see it as connecting the hara line and emotional body to the kundalini line and etheric double. The center connects our emotions to our physical body. On the physical level, this chakra protects the immune system, which is clearly effected by the emotions, and on an emotional level is our wish to live and maintain this incarnation. The center holds our drive and passion to fulfill the task we incarnated to accomplish in this lifetime. It is obviously a vital center, central to most of today's healing issues and dis-ease sources.

You can find the thymus chakra. It is located on the chest, between and about three inches above the nipples on the breastbone. When you find it, you will know immediately; it is painful and sensitive to pressure. Gently pressing this point "brings oneself wholeheartedly awake to the grief we have carried for so long and the vastness which awaits a merciful awareness." Meditating on the sensations that come while touching this point opens and releases grief (which may include anger, resentment, fear, or other feelings). Aqua gemstones also activate this center, and much healing happens along the way.

Next, below the thymus is the diaphragm chakra, at the level of the physical diaphragm muscle, just above the solar plexus. Its color is lime green, and it is activated by some of the green or yellow green gemstones. I perceive this center as providing a clearing and detoxification of any obstructions to the fulfillment of one's life purpose. This is a cleansing of the entire hara line and can be a quite intense, deep emotional purging. Healers who have experienced this chakra have called it the "garbage chakra" or the "vomit chakra." The process is ultimately positive but may not seem so at the time. Go through it by simply allowing it to happen. Watch the sensations and let them go, not fighting, resisting, or trying to change them. Welcome the clearing and send love.

The next primary center on the hara line is the hara chakra, or the hara itself. Known in Asia from ancient times, it is located about two and a half inches below the navel, above the kundalini belly chakra. Its color is golden to orange brown but may deepen in healing, even turning hot and red. In Asia, all energy work starts and ends at this center, which is the source of incarnation and the place that the life force emanates from. The hara chakra connects one's will to live with the life-sustaining energy of the Earth at the Earth chakra (see below). Strength, power, life force, and regenerative ability also originate from this center when the chakra is fully grounded to the Earth.

The deep ruby or maroon perineum chakra is next. This energy point is located (on the emotional body) between the openings of the vagina and the anus, where episiotomies are performed in childbirth. This is the energy gate through which the Earth Ch'i life force is brought into the body and held for distribution at the hara center. In Ch'i Kung it is called "the gateway of life and death." The perineum is the place of activating and anchoring one's life intention and purpose into physical plane reality. Only a few gemstones activate this chakra.

A pair of small chakras is located behind the knees. Called movement chakras, they direct one's movement forward on one's life path. People who have resistance or difficulty in fulfilling their life purpose may have pain in their knees, and the color-matching gemstones are usually tan or forest green. Below the knee chakras, on the soles of the feet, is another chakra pair. These are called grounding chakras, and their color is brown. These chakras center one's life purpose into physical direction and manifestation.

The energy line begun at the transpersonal point moves vertically through the body and enters deep into the Earth, as deep as the person can ground herself into the planet and root her intention for being here. The chakra that roots the hara line into Goddess Earth is called the Earth chakra, or Earth Star. I see its color as shiny black, and some black gemstones help to activate it. The chakra anchors the incarnation/lifetime into earthplane reality, makes this planet one's home, and places one's life purpose into an Earthly context. This

Continued ➡

ending of the hara line is the grounding and ballast for one's lifetime and life purpose.

Besides the chakras, the hara line itself is comprised of a double flow of energy. One channel moves from the perineum chakra up the back, over the top of the head, down the face to the upper lip. In acupuncture and Ch'i Kung this channel is called the Governor Channel. The second energy flow starts at the lower lip and descends down the front of the body to end at the perineum. This is called the Conception Vessel. Auxiliary flows move energy through the legs and arms into these channels. Ch'i Kung is the ancient energy discipline that develops the hara channels and chakras, similar to the way that yoga works with the kundalini line.

The emotions are central to today's healing issues and needs, and the hara line chakras offer access to achieving profound emotional healing. Gemstones that match the hara line chakras provide direct entry into the emotional body and through it to the outer aura bodies for core soul healing. The ability to have that access is a major healing breakthrough.

—From *Healing with Gemstones and Crystals*

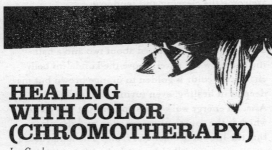

HEALING WITH COLOR (CHROMOTHERAPY)

Joy Gardner

Color is where the mind and the universe meet
—Cezanne

Color is such a source of joy and delight! Now we are beginning to appreciate how powerful colored light can be. John Ott's experiments have shown that the color of light affects something as basic and vital as the sex of your babies, and the size of their genitals—to say nothing of the health of their teeth, and their ability to be agreeable rather than hostile.

Your energy field or aura precedes you wherever you go, and all your perceptions are colored by that aura. Your ability to deeply appreciate color is an indication of how open your channels are. You may be like the person who sees life through rose-colored glasses, or the one for whom all perceptions must pass through a gray fog.

There are abundant examples of people who have reached a state of ecstasy or enlightenment, who describe their experience in terms of color.

A woman who has been told that she has just three months to live attends a workshop on death and dying, finishes all her unfinished business, and begins to live her life fully. Living one day at a time, puttering in her garden, she exclaims, "Each morning I awake with such gratitude! I sleep with the curtains open so that when I open my eyes I can see the bright-colored flowers in my window box, winking at me in the sunlight!"

A man has been fasting in the desert for seven days, with nothing to eat or drink but water. He returns home sunburned, dirty, and radiant. "The colors!" he raves. "The colors are so bee-uu-ti-ful!"

A woman gives birth at home after fourteen hours of labor. She holds up her newborn daughter, looking up with gratitude at the faces of her two midwives and her husband. "You are all so beautiful! There are bright colors all around you!"

"And around you and your baby!" smiles one of the midwives, marveling at the pink, magenta, and green lights dancing around the new mother and child.

A man has a transcendent LSD trip. He stops in the middle of a city at night, staring into the neon lights. "Man! The colors are out-of-sight!"

Now let's look at how your aura can "color your world." A man—we'll call him Bill—has most of his savings invested in stocks, and the market takes a huge plunge. The same day his dog gets run over by a truck and his girlfriend breaks up with him. "It's been a gray day," Bill says morosely to a friend. He has no outlet for his emotions, and he seriously contemplates suicide.

Another man, Ralph, has major investments in stock, and the market takes a huge plunge. He doesn't worry too much about it; what goes down must come up. The same day his dog gets run over by a truck. He finds the dog and lovingly buries him and cries over the grave. Later that day his girlfriend breaks up with him. In his heart, he forgives her. But when he meets his close friend that night, he suggests a game of racket ball. He allows himself to take out his anger on the ball and wins the game. At sunset he takes a walk alone. The colors of the sunset are incredibly bright, and he finds himself saying aloud, "I'm so glad to be alive!"

Life is not measured by what happens to you, but how you react to those events. When the chakras are clear and open, you are like a master of martial arts, standing totally relaxed, able to respond instantly and appropriately to whatever comes your way. You are in a state of ready alertness, totally alive and in the moment.

Contrast this with the state of fear (gray), which constricts every muscle and blood vessel, leading to a deficiency of chi (energy), so the flesh loses its healthy hue and elasticity and becomes sluggish, unable to respond.

Red is the basic color of illness. It is the color of infection, repressed anger, fever, and overexertion. Blue is the antidote to red, and it is the primary healing color. Blue is calming, soothing, cooling. Sitting under blue light will help you overcome (or prevent) anxiety and ulcers. It will take away a fever. But don't stay under blue light for more than 30 minutes or you may feel withdrawn and depressed.

If you are "feeling blue," if your energy is depressed, lacking in vitality, if you have a deficiency of passion (red) and need some energy to cheer you up, you might enjoy some red light. You might even drink some red wine and go to the red-light district! If you are a lady and you want some action, get out those red high heels and strut your stuff.

But don't get too carried away, and don't let anger build up inside you for too long, or you are likely to see red, and then there will be no stopping you.

There are many ways to bring color into your life. You can absorb it as colored light; you can apply it to injured bone or tissues in the form of a handheld laser; you can wear it as colored clothing or jewelry; you can ingest it as food, juice, or colored water; you can take it in through your eyes; or you can visualize it through inner vision.

Antidotes

An antidote counteracts the effect of a substance, as hot antidotes cold and cold antidotes hot. The colors and characteristics of the three lower chakras can be antidoted by those of the three upper chakras, and vice versa. The center (heart) chakra needs no antidote because it has both green and pink. Green is for protection and pink is for vulnerability. So if the heart is overprotected, pink is useful. If the heart feels too vulnerable, green can be comforting.

The concept of antidotes is most useful in dealing with red and blue conditions. When the first chakra has excessive energy, it manifests in conditions that we associate (literally or figuratively) with red, such as inflammation, irritation, body heat, anger, jealousy, and rage. Blue (the color associated with the throat chakra, the first of the three chakras above the heart) can be used to calm and cool the energy of the first chakra or any excessive red condition such as a burn or inflammation.

On the other hand, when the fifth chakra (the throat chakra of communication) has excessive energy, it manifests in blue conditions such as withdrawal, chills, numbness, extreme shyness, and lack of communication. Red can be used to stimulate and warm the energy of the fifth chakra or any excessive blue condition such as the sensation of extreme cold.

The concept of antidotes blurs with the orange and yellow rays, as it does with the indigo and violet rays. Indigo and violet are both purple colors that contain elements of red and blue. Indigo has a greater predominance of blue, and violet has a stronger proportion of red. When orange (the color of the second chakra) is excessive, it becomes red-orange. Then indigo or violet (the colors associated with the sixth and seventh chakras) can be used as antidotes. When yellow (the color of the third chakra) is excessive, it can also become red-orange, and it can be calmed with indigo or violet. Indigo is calming (since it is more blue than red), and violet is more stimulating (since it has more red than blue).

When the sixth chakra is overstimulated, orange is a good antidote. In truth, I have never experienced a problem with excessive crown chakra energy, but if it was a problem, yellow would be the antidote.

This concept of antidotes is essential in color healing, as can be seen in this statement from Dr. Laing:

If a baby's skin is too red, then the baby is overly excited. This condition should be watched closely, because it can become habitual and lead to red conditions such as heart trouble and high blood pressure in later life. If the baby's mother learns to handle it in early life, these patterns can be changed.

Help the baby to relax. To do this, help the mother to relax. Impress upon her that her relaxation is good for the baby. Give her plenty of blue light. Put her under a blue lamp. Have her wear blue clothes. Listen to soothing music. Bring in blue flowers. Create a soothing environment.[2]

History of Color Healing

Story-images recorded in cave paintings by Australian Aborigines go back more than twenty thousand years. The serpent is always associated with vibration and flowing energy fields. The Rainbow Serpent is portrayed as a spectrum of various colors, frequencies, and powers that look remarkably like the electromagnetic spectrum. The Rainbow Serpent is attracted to menstrual blood. During fertility rituals people paint themselves with red ocher.[3]

According to ancient Egyptian mythology, the art of healing with color was founded by the god Thoth. To the ancient Greeks, he was Hermes Trismegistus, literally "Hermes thrice-greatest," because of his various works on mysticism and

Continued →

magic. In the Hermetic tradition, the ancient Egyptians and Greeks healed with colored minerals, stones, crystals, salves, and dyes and painted their sanctuaries with healing colors. The ancient Greeks used color to restore balance. Colored garments, oils, plasters, ointments, and salves were employed to treat disease.

In Rome of the first century C.E., Aurelius Cornelius Celsus followed the doctrines established by Pythagoras and Hippocrates, and included the use of colored ointments, plasters, and flowers in several treatises on medicine.

Avicenna (980–ca. 1037) was an Arab physician and disciple of Aristotle. In his *Canon of Medicine* he spoke about the vital importance of color in both diagnosis and treatment. He developed a chart relating color to temperament and the physical body. He taught that red moved the blood, blue or white cooled it, and yellow reduced pain and inflammation. He prescribed potions of red flowers to cure blood disorders, and yellow flowers and morning sunlight to cure disorders of the biliary system.

Avicenna wrote also of the possible dangers of color in treatment, observing that a person with a nosebleed, for example, should not gaze at objects of a brilliant red color or be exposed to red light, whereas blue would soothe the condition and reduce blood flow.

Theophrastus Bombastus von Hohenheim (1493–1541) was a Swiss doctor known as Paracelsus. He was familiar with the secret teachings of the Rosicrucians though he was not believed to be a member of that society. Paracelsus is credited with transforming western medicine by improving pharmacy and encouraging scientific experiments, which earned him the title of the Father of Modern Medicine. He considered light and color essential for good health and used them extensively along with elixirs, charms, talismans, herbs, and minerals.[4]

Augustus Pleasanton studied the effects of color in plants and animals and in 1876 he published *Blue and Sun-lights*, stating that the quality, yield, and size of grapes could be significantly increased if they were grown in greenhouses made with alternating blue and transparent panes of glass. He also claimed to cure certain diseases and to increase fertility and the rate of physical maturation in animals. He used color to alleviate human disease and pain.

In *The Principles of Light and Color*, published in New York in 1878, Edwin Babbit used red as a stimulant for the blood, and yellow and orange as nerve stimulants. He claimed that blue and violet were soothing to all systems and had anti-inflammatory properties. Babbit prescribed red for paralysis, consumption, physical exhaustion, and chronic rheumatism; yellow as a laxative, as an emetic and purgative, and for bronchial difficulties; and blue for inflammatory conditions, sciatica, meningitis, nervous headache, irritability, and sunstroke.[5]

Investigations into the therapeutic use of color were carried out in Europe during the early twentieth century. In Austria, Rudolph Steiner (1861–1925) related color to form, shape, and sound, suggesting that the vibrational quality of colors is amplified by certain forms, and that combinations of colors and shapes have either destructive or regenerative effects on living organisms. In the Waldorf Schools inspired by Steiner's work, classrooms are painted and textured to correspond to the moods of children at various stages of their development.[6]

Color and Light Techniques and Equipment

Dinshah P. Ghadiali (1873–1966) was born in India, and in 1917 he became a United States citizen. He studied chemistry, physics, and electricity in addition to his spiritual practices. In 1891 he was initiated as a fellow in the Theosophical Society.

He developed a method called the Spectro-Chrome System that uses "tonation," treatments with just one color on a given area (or areas), directly on the flesh, for one hour. He used five color filters of red, yellow, green, blue, and violet, and then combined them to obtain the following colors:

Red and yellow = orange
Yellow and green = lemon
Green and blue = turquoise
Blue and violet = indigo
Violet and yellow = purple
Red and violet = magenta
Red and blue = scarlet[7]

Initially he used five glass slides, screening them carefully because each filter had to be a polychrome of suitable proportions to generate appropriate colors when they were mixed. They had to be broad spectrum filters with a preponderance of the primary color. They are called filters because their purpose is to remove (filter out) specific parts from the complete spectrum of white light.

After Ghadiali's death, his son, Darius Dinshah, changed his name to reflect his father's more famous first name, and carried on his father's work by writing *Let There Be Light*. In his book he explains that the intensity of the light source does not make a difference in results. Sunlight may be used by placing large filters over a window, but this can be done only when the sun is shining at a particular angle. A skylight is not acceptable. A treatment can be done outdoors, just by exposing the area, and covering it with the appropriate filters. He recommends closing the eyes during a treatment unless the treatment is intended for the eyes. (This is in direct contradiction to the Syntonics method. Personally, I like to look into the colored light for brief periods.)

Another primitive method is to work indoors, place the filter over the desired area, and shine a flashlight on the area, or tape filters over the head of a flashlight. He emphasizes that anything can be used, and gives many examples in his book.

If you want to pursue the therapeutic usage of color healing, Dinshash's *Let There Be Light* is an invaluable resource. It catalogues 331 color schedules with specific tonations for more than four hundred health conditions.

This was the method used by Dr. Kate W. Baldwin (1855–1935), senior surgeon at Philadelphia Woman's Hospital, during the last three of her twenty-three years at the hospital. The following is taken from an abstract of a paper she presented at a clinical meeting of the section on eye, ear, nose, and throat diseases of the Medical Society of the State of Pennsylvania, and published in the *Atlantic Medical Journal* of April 1927.

Each element gives off a characteristic color wave. The prevailing color wave of hydrogen is red, and that of oxygen is blue, and each element in turn gives off its own special color waves.

If one requires a dose of castor oil, he does not go to a drugstore and request a little portion from each bottle on the shelves. I see no virtue, then, in the use of the whole white light as a therapeutic measure when the different colors can give what is required without taxing the body to rid itself of that for which it has no use, and which may do more or less harm. If the body is sick, it should be restored with the least possible effort. There is no more accurate or easier way than by giving the color representing the lacking elements, and the body will… appropriate them and so restore the normal balance. Color is the simplest and most accurate therapeutic measure yet developed.

For about six years I have given close attention to the action of colors in restoring the body functions, and I am perfectly honest in saying that, after nearly thirty-seven years of active hospital and private practice in medicine and surgery, I can produce quicker and more accurate results with colors than with any or all other methods combined—and with less strain on the patient.[8]

A contemporary physician in Ohio, Teresa E. Quinlin, reports similar results and is equally enthused about the Spectro-Chrome method. "My experience with the lamp is nothing short of stupendous. Burns, infections, pain, and cancer have all had remarkable improvements and successes. A case of the West Nile virus turned around in 72 hours using the color lamp, acupuncture, essential oils, reflexology and the blood type diet. Migraines and fibromyalgia, if not cured, are lessened dramatically. Three cases of ulcerative colitis and/or Crohn's disease are in remission (biopsy proven in two cases). The list goes on."[9]

Light Box. A light box should be large enough to accommodate a floodlight or lightbulb. The bottom is constructed so that different colored plates of glass can be inserted and removed.

The box that is shown has three side boards, each eight by eleven inches. The fourth side, where the glass or plastic filters slide in and out at the bottom, is eight by nine inches. There is no board at the top; this is where the flood lamp is inserted and clamps in. The bottom board is six by eight inches with a five-inch-diameter round hole that supports the glass and allows the light to shine through. The box is made of hardwood so it is less susceptible to heat and does not become a potential fire hazard if the light is left on and the floodlight is too close to the side. The wood is three-fourths inch thick; this is not necessary, though it gives a firm surface for clamping the light and hanging the chain. The box hangs from a chain, which allows the height to be adjusted, and the chain is fireproof. I'm sure this model can be improved upon.

The goal of color healing is to strengthen and purify each color in your aura. I believe that high-quality German glass gives the purest color and the

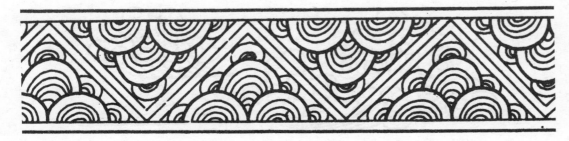

Continued ➡

highest vibratory intensity. In my experience, other kinds of glass are less monochromatic and less effective. Glass or strong plastic is needed if you want to put crystals inside your lamp. Glass can be obtained at stores that sell stained glass.

The lamp may be hung from the ceiling so the light will shine through the glass onto the person seated or lying below. Hang the box so the bottom is six to twelve inches above the part of the body that you are treating.

Colored Lamp. A wire frame may be constructed around a lightbulb or floodlight, along with a clamp that holds a plastic gel, so the light shines through the plastic. The whole fixture can be clamped in a suitable place that allows light to shine on the appropriate part of the body.

Colored Lightbulb. Ordinary incandescent lightbulbs are available in red, yellow, pink, green, and blue. They can be inserted into a regular lamp or light fixture. At night or in a darkened room, they will give off a good dose of colored light. Even Christmas lights may be used.

Stained Glass. Leonardo da Vinci wrote, "The power of meditation can be ten times greater under violet light falling through the stained-glass window of a quiet church." The power of colored light was understood long ago, and may account for the popularity of stained-glass windows in churches.

Colorpuncture. This technique is described in Peter Mandel's book *Practical Compendium of Colorpuncture*. Mandel employs three sets of opposite colors, comparable to the Chinese yin-yang opposites, to determine the nature of an illness and its treatment. He uses the meridian system and many acupuncture points, but instead of needles, he uses the gentle impulses resulting from light in concentrated form in a kind of flashlight with a pyramid focus tip. He claims that this light spreads out in a fanlike form from the body surface to the tissue below. If a patient experiences discomfort with a particular color, he replaces it with its complementary one. Discomfort indicates an excess of the color and its corresponding vibration in the body.

Syntonics. This form of light therapy is used by Dr. Jacob Liberman, based on the work of Dr. Harry Riley Spitler. It works on the concept that most dysfunction is caused by an imbalance between the sympathetic and parasympathetic portions of the nervous system. Filters are divided into three categories: one kind stimulates the sympathetic nervous system, another stimulates the parasympathetic nervous system, a third acts as a physiological or emotional equilibrator.

The practitioner chooses the appropriate color and sets the color dial. The client looks into the box. The color can be arranged to either glow steadily or flash at a designated tempo. As an optometrist, Liberman used Syntonics to treat a vast array of vision problems and vision-related learning problems.

Then he devised his own technique for treating addictions and emotional problems. He would call out pairs of colors (red and blue, yellow and violet, lime and turquoise) and ask the patient to select the set she felt most comfortable with. If she chose red and blue, but preferred blue to red, then red was probably the color she needed for deep healing. The colors that were most disturbing to the patient seemed to represent painful experiences in her life.

At this point I noticed that the behavior of patients with addictive personalities becomes more addictive or less addictive depending on the colors at which they looked. For example, an alcoholic would look at one of the colors to

which he was receptive (comfortable with) and be fine; a color to which he was slightly unreceptive might elicit an urge for him to drink juice or soda; a color with which he was most uncomfortable would cause him to want to drink alcohol. It was now becoming clear to me that when situations in life trigger fear or discomfort, our inability to be present with these feelings as well as to deal with them forces us to protect ourselves by avoiding, or numbing out, the situations and going into an addictive behavior pattern....

Since the degree of receptivity varied from color to color for each patient, I eventually decided to arrange the colors for treatment from least unreceptive (least uncomfortable) to most unreceptive (most uncomfortable). Starting the treatment with a color that was only mildly uncomfortable allowed patients to gradually develop an authentic security in their ability to go through this process. This would then transfer to their ability to handle stressful situations in their lives....

Although the technology of phototherapy is, in itself, very powerful, its true power blossoms only when the awarenesses that it stimulates can be expressed in the presence of a loving, compassionate human being. In other words, the interaction between the patient and the facilitator is primary....

One of my most important clinical discoveries was that the colors to which people were unreceptive correlated almost 100% of the time with the portions of their bodies [according to the rainbow system of the chakras] where they housed stress, developed disease, or had injured themselves. For example, a person might be uncomfortable looking at the color blue, and during the case history I would discover that this person had chronic sore throats, significant dental problems, [and] difficulty with verbal expression....

Additionally, I noticed that once patients had resolved the emotionally painful issues triggered by the colors, then looking at these colors, which were originally uncomfortable, actually stimulated feelings of joy and euphoria.10

Low-Level Laser Therapy. This therapy is now being used for healing by doctors, dentists, veterinarians, acupuncturists, and laypeople. In Europe it is used for treatment of traumatic, inflammatory, and overuse injuries, pain and healing of arthritic lesions, reduction of abscesses, and treatment of persistent nonhealing wounds such as cold-sores and ulcers. Healing with light and use of low level laser therapy can encourage the formation of collagen and cartilage in damaged joints and the repair of tendons and ligaments.

Infrared light is emitted through some handheld portable low level lasers and other instruments. It has been shown to speed up bone repair by stimulating fibroblastic and osteoblastic proliferation.11 Cell membranes become more permeable, ATP levels increase, DNA production goes up,

and overall cell metabolism becomes more efficient. This seems to be highly stimulating to the cells because they respond rapidly with an increase in density of the capillary bed, reduction of pain and inflammation, stimulation of nerve regeneration, muscle relaxation, and increased muscle tone. There is also an indication that laser light therapy helps increase immune system response.12

In addition, low level laser therapy can be used to reduce inflammation and pain by stimulating the release of anti-inflammatory enzymes and endorphins that are natural pain-killing chemicals. It enhances lymphatic draining and releases tight muscles that create chronic pain, joint problems, and decreased mobility. When applied in the correct frequency, low level laser therapy appears to be antiviral, antifungal, and antiherpetic.13

Lasers that were once so cost prohibitive that only hospitals could afford them are now in the range of a midpriced computer. Soon I expect that no health professional will be without one, and they will be as common as computers in our homes.

Visualization and Color Breathing

For this visualization, close your eyes and picture a color. If it is difficult for you to see yellow, imagine a lemon. Color visualization is most effective when combined with color breathing, as described below.

The colors of the first three chakras, going from bottom to top, are red, orange, and yellow. These are associated with the earth. Visualize these colors arcing up from the earth like half rainbows and entering each of the corresponding chakras. The heart chakra at your chest has two colors: pink and green. Think of one or both of these colors coming directly across the horizon, toward your heart. The top three colors (blue, indigo, and violet) are associated with the heavens. Visualize each of these colors arcing down from the heavens like inverted half rainbows, entering each corresponding chakra.

Imagine you want to bring yellow to your third chakra. Begin by getting a clear mental picture of something yellow. Perhaps you can imagine a lemon. Inhale through your nose and visualize a band of this color arcing up from the earth and flowing into your solar plexus (below your breastbone). As you exhale through your mouth, fix it there.

If you want to send that color to someone else, begin by breathing in the color a few times and fixing it at your own chakra. When you feel that you have enough for yourself, you can send it. The third and sixth chakras are power centers, so they are good transmitting stations. The lower three colors may be sent through the third chakra at the solar plexus, pink and green are sent directly from the heart, and the top three colors may be sent through the third eye.

For example, if you are sending orange, inhale and bring the color to your second chakra (which is orange). Exhale and fix it there. Repeat this several times until you feel you have enough orange. When you are ready to send the color, inhale and bring the orange to the surface of your second chakra,

Continued ➡

and then bring it up to your solar plexus (without trying to absorb it), and then as you exhale, direct it like a beam of orange light to the person who needs the color. Send it from your solar plexus to the appropriate part of the person's body.

As you exhale, you can also tone, which gives additional vibratory energy. (See Healing with the Voice, page 228.) Repeat this process three times, then ask the person how it feels. If the results are good, continue until she feels she has had enough (usually six to twelve times). If there is no significant response after six times, it probably is not the color she needs. If she actually feels worse, send the antidote, which, for the second chakra, would be indigo or violet.

Color visualization can be done in the presence of the person you are sending it to or at a distance. The same technique can be used, but instead of directing the color to a person who is directly in front of you, visualize him in your mind and direct the color to that visual image or to a photograph or drawing of him. You may want to focus the color at a particular area of his body. This is remarkably effective, because color healing is energy healing, and energy does not require a person's physical presence. You would not be able to receive verbal feedback about the treatment, so just trust your intuition.

When you send color healing (or any form of energy) to another person, it is best to get his permission first. Not everyone wants to be healed, or even to feel good. However, if a person is unconscious, or unable to speak, or too young to communicate, you can begin by mentally asking permission. Then, unless you feel a definite resistance, you can send healing energy.

One exception pertains to using pink light for self-defense. Pink light is extremely potent. Pink is the energy of love, and when you send pink light in earnest, you must be able to forgive the person you are sending it to. If a person is belligerent, irrational, or irritable, sending pink light is a powerful form of self-defense. It is literally disarming. As soon as she feels the ray of love and forgiveness, she is likely to change her behavior. This may be an invasion of her privacy, but other forms of self-defense would be far more invasive. Here is one example.

One of my students was working at a health food store, and a fellow came in who had had too much to drink. He was being generally obnoxious, insulting the customers and knocking boxes off the shelves. When she asked the man to leave, he ignored her. She was about to call the police when she remembered the pink light. Despite his behavior, she was able to feel compassion as she sent him a strong wave of pink light directly from her heart to his. Within a minute, the man picked up the boxes, apologized for his behavior, and walked out of the store.

Color-Charged Water

Water can be charged with a particular color and then taken internally or externally. For example, the color of the second chakra is orange, and this chakra is in the area of the large intestines. If there is constipation, it is beneficial to take a few sips of orange-colored water (ambero) before each meal.

When I first heard about color-charged water, I found it hard to believe. The water doesn't look any different after it has been charged. But I am open-minded, and when I got constipated, I decided to give it a try. I could not believe that a few sips would make any difference, so I drank about half a glass before each meal. By evening, I had diarrhea! Since then, I have taken color-charged water more seri-

ously, and it has proven effective for many ailments.

To charge the water, pour into a colored bottle or jar (for example, a green wine bottle or a blue water bottle) and set it on a windowsill so that the light will shine through the glass and into the water. (I would advise against charging all of your drinking water in a blue bottle unless you want to slow down your digestion or unless you have ulcers.) Alternatively, you can put a plate of colored glass or a plastic filter against the window and set the water in a clear glass jar or bottle in front of the color source. Or cover the jar with a thin piece of colored cloth. Allow it to stand for one to four hours (four hours may be stronger), and then refrigerate. Take a few sips two or three times a day, as needed.

In cool weather or when refrigerated, red-, orange-, and yellow-charged water will last two to three weeks. In warm weather without refrigeration, it will lose its charge after three or four days. The other colors will last indefinitely. In fact, green, blue, or purple jars will help preserve oils, herbs, and so on.

The French word for water is eau, pronounced "o." The following French names are used for colored waters.

Red—rubio
Orange and yellow—ambero
Green—verdio
Blue—ceruleo
Indigo and violet—purpuro

Color Healing for the Face

The face is a microcosm of the body, and Dr. Laing explains that the same colors used to treat the chakras can be used to treat the seven areas of the face that correspond to the seven chakras.

1. Red—chin, jaw, lips
2. Orange—inside of mouth, gums, tongue
3. Yellow—throat, leading into intestinal tract
4. Green—nose, leading into respiratory tract
5. Blue—eyes, which are windows to the soul
6. Indigo—ears and third eye
7. Violet—crown chakra

Here are some examples of how to apply this information: During their forties most people experience a waning of sexual energy (second chakra). At this time there is often a deterioration of the gums. This can be treated with a tincture made from calendula (also known as pot marigold, an orange flower) or by rinsing the mouth with ambero (orange-charged water).

When the eyes are overstrained, which may occur when you work too hard and don't take enough time for sleep and meditation, the fifth chakra suffers. This condition responds well to placing a smooth blue stone over each eye or by allowing blue light to shine upon your closed eyelids for ten minutes.

How to Use Color in Your Daily Life

Given the opportunity, your mood will affect your choice of clothes. When you understand the power of color, you can consciously alter your mood. For example, you may be feeling somber and withdrawn and attracted to gray or black. But if you want to cheer up, you would be wise to wear orange, yellow, or pink.

Black, however, is the color of mystery, so if you are in a pleasantly mysterious mood, don't hesitate to wear it. Gray is a neutral color; it doesn't commit you to any particular feeling, so if you are feeling withdrawn, it will leave you that way. But if you are feeling good, gray gives you the flexibility to move through different moods and associate with various kinds of people. You can accessorize neutral colors with colorful scarves, belts, and jewelry.

The color of your underwear can have a strong effect. Red or orange underpants can stir up sexual feelings. Light blue underpants can calm sexual feelings and counteract nervous itching. Red or orange undershirts can cause tension in the back and should not be worn when you have back pain.

The color of clothing can also be used to create a particular impression on those who behold it. Deep purple robes are worn by royalty and religious figures to create an impression of power and devotion. By contrast, bright red is often worn to convey the message of sexual availability.

A masseuse can use pink, green, or yellow sheets on the massage table to encourage clients to breathe deeply (all of these colors strengthen the lungs and diaphragm). In bed, an erotic atmosphere can be created with orange or red sheets and blankets. A cheerful atmosphere can be enhanced with yellow. But a nervous or hyperactive child should never sleep with red, orange, or yellow. A calming green or blue is most desirable.

An argumentative family changed wall-to-wall carpeting from orange to blue, and members got along better afterward. Operatic composer Richard Wagner composed uplifting spiritual music in a room with violet curtains. The color of a room or of furniture influences your mood and health. Yellow cupboards in a kitchen create a cheery atmosphere that is also good for digestion.

Colorful decorations and paintings on the walls will raise the spirits. You can change them when your mood changes.

Color in Nature. Nature is full of color, and you can take advantage of her beauty. The way you landscape your home and whether you live near trees, parks, or water can have a profound effect on your well-being. Nature gives a perfect balance of colors, allowing you to choose your favorite colors from her vast array. Be sure to bring in some of your less favorite colors as well, because those are the ones you probably need most. If bright red is distasteful to you, begin with a shade that is less disturbing to you.

I have chosen to live in Hawaii. Seeing large, brilliantly colored flowers all year long—rich reds, outrageous oranges and radiant yellows—feels like a continuous blessing. On clear days, when the sun is bright, the ocean is a brilliant blue. Some days, it is a deep royal blue. Other days it turns emerald green. Sometimes the water close to the coral turns turquoise, while the water farther from shore becomes a rich blue. I inhale those colors and feel as if I am being fed by them.

You may experience being fed by nature if you have been in the city for too long, and you go for a drive in the country and stop to gaze at a meadow of green grass. Breathe in that green and exhale all the dirt and pollution of the city from your lungs. Within a short time, you will feel charged and refreshed. Green feeds the heart chakra, including the lungs. The green of the trees and plants fills the air with oxygen, and those same trees and plants absorb the carbon dioxide that you exhale.

If you are feeling tense after a hard day's work, sit in a comfortable chair outdoors, put up your feet, look at the sky, and soak up that expanse of blue. It is truly remarkable that wherever you live on this planet—even in the depths of big cities—the blue of the sky is usually available to you. You can go for a drive and look at the blue expanse of a lake or ocean. Blue is calming and feeds the higher chakras.

When you feel exhausted, you can lie out in the sun and soak up the yellow rays, which feed the third chakra. When the season is right, a bouquet of

Continued ➡

bright yellow daffodils will cheer up any room, because yellow is the color of happiness.

People who call themselves Breatharians claim not to need food of any kind. I believe that in ancient times there were Beings of Light who simply fed on the colors of nature. I have experienced this on several occasions with rainbows. The first time occurred when I was on a long trip and I was exhausted after driving all day.

I saw a bright and perfect rainbow and pulled off on the shoulder to admire it. I thought how marvelous it would be if I could just gaze at the yellow in the rainbow and inhale its energy. On an impulse, I tried it. Then I watched with amazement as the yellow—and only the yellow—of the rainbow turned exceedingly pale. Feeling recharged, rather mind-boggled, and a bit guilty for possibly diminishing someone else's pretty rainbow, I got back in my car and drove away, fairly convinced that it had been an odd coincidence.

Since then I have had this same experience on several occasions. Sometimes just the color I concentrate on will fade, and sometimes the entire rainbow or section of the rainbow that I'm looking at will fade. It seems that the greater my need, the quicker the colors fade. I don't do this for entertainment, because it is sad to see a rainbow fade, and I don't like to deprive myself or others of the opportunity to witness such a blessed sight. I have done this with one or more people, and others have found that they, too, can derive nourishment from the colors of the rainbow.

The Book of Guidance says, "Think of a rich green meadow, and as you draw in your breath, inhale the green of the grasses directly into your heart. In ancient times, people did this constantly and automatically. They looked into the expanse of blue sky, and they drew this color into their spirits. They looked at the yellow of the sun, and they drew this warmth into their place of happiness."[14]

Color in Food and Drink. In Asian cuisine, the cook often strives to include the four basic colors. When a meal looks appetizing, it is pleasant to eat and easier to digest. A meal that contains the colors of the first four chakras will usually be nutritionally balanced. For example, a meal with tomatoes, carrots, corn, and steamed greens would be pleasant and nutritious. It is good practice to steam the greens until the color is at its brightest; when the greens darken, flavor and nutrition diminish.

The color of food often indicates which parts of the body it will heal. For example, the first chakra is red and relates to the blood. Most of the blood-cleansing foods that tone the liver and lymph glands, eliminating toxins from the blood, are in the red family: red cabbage, cherries, cranberries, blackberries, and red clover tea.

Yellow foods are good for the liver and gall bladder. A flush made from olive oil and lemon juice is excellent for cleansing these organs. Dandelion root tea strengthens the liver and gall bladder.

Endnotes

1. *Paul Cezanne: The Man and the Mountain*, video, a Glashaus Film Production in association with RM Arts, 1985.

2. Dr. Laing, author's Spirit Guide, received 1976, Eugene, Oregon.

3. Robert Lawlor, *Voices of the First Day-Awakening in the Aboriginal Dreamtime* (Rochester, VT: Inner Traditions, 1991), 114–116.

4. Manly P. Hall, *The secret Teachings of All Ages* (Los Angeles: Philosophical Research Society, 1988), CXXXIX.

5. Health Research, *Color Healing, An Exhaustive Survey Compiled from 21 Works of Leading Practitioners of Chromotherapy* (Mokelumne Hills, CA: Health Research, 1956), 1–34.

6. Helen Graham, *Discover Color Therapy* (Berkeley: Ulysses Press, 1998).

7. Darius Dinshaw, *Let There Be Light* (Malaga, NJ: Dinshaw Health Society, 2003), 14.

8. Ibid., 7–8.

9. Teresa E. Quinlan, M.D., personal communication with the author, Columbus, Ohio, May 2003.

10. Liberman, 1991,188–189.

11. Jan Turner and Lars Hode, *Low Level Laser Therapy* (Grangesberg, Sweden: Prima Books, 1999), 21.

12. Melyni Worth, Ph.D., "Low Level Laser Therapy Provides New Treatment Possibilities," *World Equine Veterinary Review*, 3, no. 3 (1998).

13. Turner and Hode, 1999.

14. Joy Gardner, *The Book of Guidance* (Winlaw, B.C.: Healing Yourself Press, 1985), 18–19.

—From *Vibrational Healing Through the Chakras*

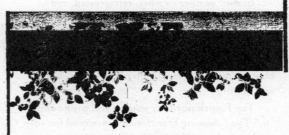

HEALING WITH THE VOICE

Joy Gardner

The mystics of numerous cultures agree upon the absolute power of sound. We begin with sound, we are held together by sound, and someday we will return to the cosmic Music of the Spheres.

Sound is the original mystical experience of creation. The Sufi master Hazrat Inayat Khan, a musician of great renown, comments on the Bible and other great works:

We find in the Bible the words, "In the beginning was the Word, and the Word was God"; and we also find that the Word is Light, and that when that light dawned the whole creation manifested. These are not only religious verses; to the mystic or seer the deepest revelation is contained in them....

It teaches that the first sign of life that manifested was the audible expression, or sound; that is the Word. When we compare this interpretation with the Vedanta philosophy, we find that the two are identical. All down the ages the Yogis and seers of India have worshipped the Word-God, or Sound-God; and around that idea is centered all the mysticism of sound or of utterance. Not alone among Hindus, but among the seers of the Semitic races too, the great importance of the word was recognized.... Sanskrit is now a language long dead, but in the meditations of the Indian Yogis, Sanskrit words are still used because of the power of sound and vibration they contain. . . . .[1]

In 1986, I was privileged to attend a social dance of Coast Salish Indians. It was delightful to be among young and old, with men and women, gathered in a circle around a big drum, each person keeping a constant rhythm with one stick, chanting familiar songs while everyone, including children and old people, danced the simple and graceful steps passed on for generations.

Knowing the power of unifying the communal heartbeat, and the way song and dance give expression to the emotions and the soul, virtually every culture has made use of song and dance, chant and procession, to carry their voices and spirits to the deity of their choice.

The Shoshone, the Coast Salish Indians, and the Huichol Indians of Mexico believe (or used to believe) that the chokecherries won't come back, the salmon won't run, and the sun won't rise unless they chant their prayers of thanks and perform their seasonal rituals. Modern thinkers tend to look upon such ideas as being superstitious or cut off from reality.

Yet when the last traditional Shoshone, the last Coast Salish Indian, the last Huichol Indian, the last of the great trees, and the last of the ancient oil reserves are wiped from the face of the earth, will it surprise us if the salmon do not return (as has happened already in many places), if the chokecherries do not bloom, if the earth shifts on her axis and (as the Hopi predict) if the moon turns the color of blood?

How shall we prevent—or survive—these catastrophes?

Through song. Through finding the voice within. Because if the ancients of every culture can be trusted, life begins with the Word. Through the breath and the Word, we breathe our thoughts into Life. Through the vibratory power of Word and Song, we enter the matrix of vibration from which all of life emerges.

My indigenous friend Craig Carpenter says, "When we sing, we give thanks. And when we give thanks, then miracles begin to happen."

I know this to be true. My life has become a perpetual giving of thanks, and I am constantly amazed by the coincidences, the synchronicity, and the miracles that constantly unfold upon my path. I hear the same testimony from friends and students who take time to meditate, and to give thanks for the blessings of their lives—with words, song, prayer, and silence.

When we believe that we have no one to thank for our good fortune except ourselves, when we neglect to sing and give thanks for what we have; when we believe we are totally separate individuals living in a meaningless universe that has no connection with the Great Mystery or the cosmos, when we believe our songs have no impact upon the universe, then our lives feel empty, and we forget about miracles.

By changing our thinking, remembering to be grateful for all we have, and giving voice to our inner songs, we have the ability to increase our own magnetism, to influence the earth's magnetism, and to create—to give rise to—miracles. I know it. I have seen it.

The way the Australian Aborigines understand (or understood) reality is that energy ordinarily moves very fast. But when it gets an idea, it slows down. When it slows down considerably, it comes into physical manifestation.

The Word is the bridge between energy and material manifestation. Energy becomes sound, and sound transports us into material reality. The spoken or sung word is the most vibratorily powerful manifestor, which is one reason why radio and television are more powerful than newspapers. Native people understand (or understood) the power of using the voice, especially in song, to create and perpetuate the reality they desire.

I believe that when we continually praise life—give thanks for what we have—the energy around us is enlivened, and we become more potent manifestors.

For most North American Caucasians, song and dance are gone from our lives. Too often life is about money: dead paper scalped off proud trees, and precious metals gutted out of sacred places.

Living on this planet today, we are at a painful and thrilling turning point. We can either turn toward a caring, soulful way of life, discovering our

Continued ➡

inner personal and communal songs, crying out for guidance and miracles, or we can become apathetic and indifferent.

Sound Healing is the therapeutic application of sound frequencies to the body/mind of a person with the intention of creating a state of harmony and health. **Toning** is the use of sustained vocal tones, on the out-breath, without the use of melody, rhythm, or words (toning OM, for example). **Sounding** is making improvised sounds without specific melody, rhythm, or words (though melody, rhythm, and words may emerge spontaneously).

Sound, Science, and Medicine

We do not live in a void. The seemingly empty space around us is full of invisible sound and light waves. We influence that space and are influenced by it. Most of us are unaware of our effect upon it and its effect upon us. Yet we can become intelligent and active participants in this cosmic drama. We can learn to work the miracles that were once reserved for Shamans and esoteric schools of healing.

Sound is the key.

Let us begin in the womb. For eighteen weeks your cells have been growing and multiplying. You can feel, move, and even respond to stimuli.

Then something dramatic happens that changes you forever. Suddenly *you can hear!* The ear is the first organ to develop in embryo.[19]

Here is quote from my own book (currently out of print), *Healing Yourself During Pregnancy.*

One of my clients told me that there were certain passages from the Bible that he early loved and easily learned by heart. Later his mother told him that those were the passages that she had read aloud, over and over, during her pregnancy with him

With my first child, I was in labor for thirty-six hours. The last several hours were filled with painful contractions. I had been trained in the Lamaze method, and I made good use of the pant-and-blow technique consisting of three short pants followed by a long blow. For several days after my son was born, he had a peculiar habit of taking three short pants followed by a long blow![2]

John Ortiz, Ph.D., director of the Institute of Applied Psychomusicology, a licensed psychologist in central Pennsylvania, and author of *The Tao of Music*, cites many sources for current research in the effects of music on healing.[3] Music is now making its way into the hospital wards of premature infants. Researchers found that lullabies rapidly cause an increase in oxygen saturation levels as well as heart and respiration rates.[4]

Autistic and developmentally disabled children benefit significantly from the use of music, displaying better pragmatic skills[5] and increased positive participation in social activities with less disruption.[6] They are better able to focus, they show fewer symptoms of boredom,[7] and they have better recall.[8]

While adults tend to have a negative reaction to the driving beat of heavy metal music, it seems to be beneficial for adolescents who are overcome by anger, fear, and feelings of hopelessness.[27]

Adults also benefit from the effects of music. Several studies show an increased ability to tolerate pain.[10] As mentioned elsewhere, Dr. Mitch Gaynor, oncologist, had the same experience with many patients with cancer, and with a woman who had fibromyalgia.[11] Many of my clients have thrown away their pain medications. Here is the story of one of my students, Karen McDaniel:

In late 1998 a recurring foot infection took me back to the large university medical center where I had previously received a pancreas/kidney transplant (having had Type I diabetes for 35 years). The third day, an intern announced that the toe next to the big toe on my right foot was completely dead and needed to be amputated immediately.

The surgery went smoothly, and with the prayer support of caring friends I was able to send healing energies to my right foot. The only problem was that the throbbing pain proved unbearable, in both the amputation site and in the "phantom toe." High-powered pain relievers with codeine couldn't touch this pain that kept me edgy and unable to sleep.

I had attended Joy Gardner's Vibrational Healing Intensive a few months previously, and I thought she might be able to help. So I called and she offered to spend five minutes each day for the next couple weeks, toning directly into the toe, over the phone. (She was in Hawaii, and I was in Ohio.)

On our first call, I held the receiver down to my foot and I could feel her tones reaching out to make contact with my toe. Then they changed and the sounds seemed to become the voice of the toe, expressing outrage and distress. This went on for some time. She finished by sending peaceful, healing tones, which soothed and quieted the throbbing pain.

After that session, the pain was less sharp and less insistent. On the following days, she repeated similar toning, and by the third day, the pain was gone by the end of the session. It did return after a few hours, but with less intensity. Each day, the alleviation of pain improved, and the pain-free time increased.

A comical incident occurred one day when Joy was in the midst of a toning session. I was diligently holding the telephone receiver at my foot when along comes the Chief Surgeon making his rounds, followed by his flock of white-coated minions. I insisted on completing my sound treatment and they all stopped in total amazement to hear the sounds pouring out of the phone toward my foot!

After a few days I had enough strength to try some light toning for myself in between Joy's treatments. Luckily I was in a private room.

By the second week, I stopped asking for other pain relievers. When I was back at home, I toned for myself during the rare times when the pain recurred. My body seemed to instruct me when the toning needed to change, and I began doing

what felt like a knitting-together tone, going in and out, like a needle and thread. In the end, my skin—which was not expected to heal well, due to diabetes and immune-suppressant drugs—healed beautifully.

Musician Jim Oliver concurs that the body is capable of responding to sounds that the ears do not necessarily hear. He put specific sounds into a pair of headphones and set them on a client's ankles with positive results. He believes that the blood cells quickly carry the resonance throughout the whole body.[12]

During the 1990s researchers produced many reports about the tranquilizing effects of music on physical and mental health. But few studies used rigorous methodologies or adequate sample sizes, and results were inconsistent. Also there was disagreement concerning the type of music that should be offered to patients. In 1994 an abstract by Karen Allen and J. Blascovich was reported in the *Journal of the American Medical Association* titled "Effects of Music on Cardiovascular Reactivity Among Surgeons." In this study the surgeons' cardiovascular responses to music were calmed as they performed stressful tasks while listening to self-selected music as well as experimenter-selected music. The study concluded that familiarity with and control over selection of music produced positive physiological response, whereas the music that was presumed to be sedative did not produce consistent results.

In a second study from the State University of New York at Buffalo, Karen Allen, a psychologist, and Lawrence Golden, a cardiologist, followed elderly patients undergoing eye surgery at an ambulatory clinic where they would go home on the same day as the surgery. This process was known to be stressful, especially for older patients who were not accustomed to such procedures. Forty patients were selected. Twenty-one had drug-controlled high blood pressure, ten in the experimental group and eleven in the control group. They did not stop using their medications.

One week before surgery, their blood pressure and heart rate were taken as a baseline. At that point there was no significant difference between the two groups. On the day of the procedure, the same vital signs were taken before, during, and after the surgery. Participants in the experimental group were given stereo headphones, a cassette player, and a choice of twenty-two types of music including soft hits, classical guitar, chamber music, folk music, and popular singers from the 1940s and 1950s. No more than three individuals selected the same type of music. Control group participants were left to rest quietly without headphones or music.

Both groups showed significantly higher heart rates and blood pressure at the clinic than the baseline measurements when they arrive. The experimental group was provided with music, and diminished physiological effects occurred within five minutes. During surgery, the patients provided with music had heart rate and blood pressure values similar to the baseline rates taken one week previously. The control group had persistent elevations in blood pressure similar to preoperative levels. Patients with music reported a dramatic reduction of stress and increased coping abilities, whereas those without music did not.

When participants using music were interviewed, they repeatedly mentioned the word *control* noting that when they entered the facility they immediately felt as if they were relinquishing all personal control. Given a choice of music helped restore a small amount of personal control. It also blocked out "the chatter of the doctors and nurses." In the previous study reported in the *JAMA*, sur-

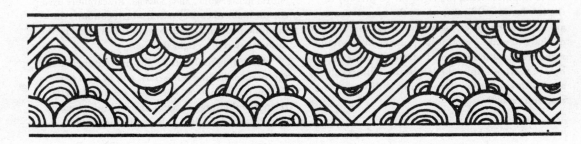

Continued ➤

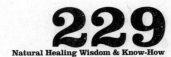

geons also felt strongly that the ability to control the type of music enhanced their abilities to perform cognitive tasks and influenced reactivity.[13]

A study at Michigan State University in 1993 allowed experimental subjects to select music from one of four categories: New Age, mild jazz, classical, and impressionist. Control subjects were given only magazines. After just fifteen minutes, the experimental group showed an increase in blood levels of interleukin-1 from 12.5 to 14 percent. Interleukins are a family of proteins associated with blood and platelet production and lymphocyte stimulation. They help protect cells against invasion by AIDS, cancer, and other diseases. In this study, participants showed decreased levels of cortisol by as much as 25 percent. Cortisol, a steroid hormone associated with the adrenal complex, is related to stress and susceptibility to inflammatory diseases. The scientists concluded that preferred music "may elicit a profound positive emotional experience that can trigger the release of hormones which can contribute to a lessening of those factors which enhance the disease process."[14]

In 2004 researchers at Ohio State University took thirty-three heart patients who had undergone bypass surgery or angioplasty. These procedures carry a risk of cognitive impairment. The patients were given fluency tests before and after two separate sessions of exercising on a treadmill. During one session they heard Vivaldi's *Four Seasons*. While all the participants felt better after working out on the treadmill, the verbal fluency after listening to the music increased by more than double.[15]

Other studies show that music can be used to alleviate depression, anger, and loneliness, and improve awareness and insight.[16] It can increase motivation, endurance, and psychological well-being and physical comfort, as well as alleviate anxiety and enhance relaxation.[17]

One of my graduate students, Cynthia Mitchell, a former theater teacher at Duke University in North Carolina, was hired by the Health Arts Network at Duke Hospital to sing for the patients. She would go into a room, chat with the patients (and their families, if present), and inquire if they had any special song requests. After singing a familiar song or two, she would tune in on the energies of the patient and ask permission to improvise a special song. Using her intuition to sense the sounds needed, Cynthia would watch as the patient's breathing slowed and deepened, her face relaxed, and tension left her body.

One evening, as she was passing an intensive care room, the nurse on duty asked Cynthia if she would come in and sing for her patient. The woman's heart rate had been dangerously high (between 120 and 94) all night. Cynthia came into the room, tuned in on the woman, and knew exactly what sounds to make. When she finished singing, as she turned to leave, the nurse put her hand on Cynthia's shoulder. There was a look of amazement on her face as she whispered, "While you were singing, her heart rate dropped by twenty points!" A few hours later, before leaving for the night, Cynthia stopped by to check on the woman and the nurse told her gratefully that the woman's heart rate had stabilized at 74.

How does sound affect the emotions? One explanation is that when it passes through the ear, it activates the vagus nerve that extends from the ear down into the larynx and through the entire intestinal tract, where its fibers control gastric and pancreatic secretions. This is in the area of the third chakra, which is an emotional center. The vagus nerve also has inhibitory fibers that pass through the heart,[18] which is in the area of the fourth chakra, another emotional center.

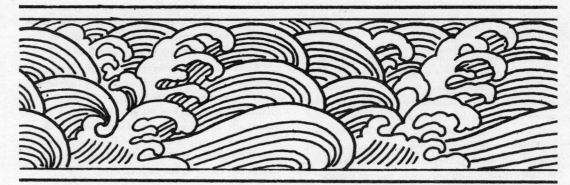

In fact, sound is a kind of food for the brain and the body (to say nothing of the soul). Dr. Tomatis, a French physician, psychologist, and auditory neurophysiologist, found that the brain requires three billion stimuli per second for at least four and a half hours per day *just to stay awake!* He claims that the ear produces over 90 percent of the body's total charge.[19]

Surely this explains why so many young people seem to be addicted to music with a driving beat. It literally acts as a stimulant. When you need a shot of energy, music can give it to you. During the 2003 invasion of Iraq, the soldiers in the United States army listened to CDs inside their tanks as they attacked. One popular song selected for the occasion was "*The Roof is on Fire*," by the Bloodhound Gang, which includes the following verse:

The roof the roof the roof is on fire
The roof the roof the roof is on fire
The roof the roof the roof is on fire
We don't need no water let the motherf——r burn
Burn motherf——r burn.[20]

What better way for young men to overcome their dread of taking human lives than to listen to loud, incessant, aggressive music in an isolated cage that resembles a booth at a video parlor?

Dr. Tomatis claims that the ear is the conductor of the entire nervous system. Through the medulla (the brain stem), the auditory nerve connects with all the muscles of the body. Thus muscle tone, equilibrium, flexibility, and vision are all influenced by sound.[21] This helps explain why, when yoga is accompanied by toning, it becomes possible to stretch longer and deeper. It also explains why most people like to hear music while they exercise.

According to Dr. Tomatis, high frequency sounds (3,000 Hz and above) increase the electrical potential of the brain.[22] The music of Mozart has also been credited with increasing mental powers, as made popular by Don Campbell in his book, *The Mozart Effect*. He cites a study by Frances H. Rauscher, Ph.D., and her colleagues in which thirty-six undergraduates from the psychology department scored eight to nine points higher on a spatial IQ test after listening to ten minutes of Mozart's Sonata for Two Pianos in D Major. The effect only lasted for ten to fifteen minutes, but the team concluded that there was a strong relationship between listening to this music and spatial reasoning.[23]

Don Campbell points out that the right ear relays auditory impulses more quickly to the speech centers in the brain than does the left ear. Nerve impulses from the right ear go directly to the left (rational) brain, where the speech centers are located. However, nerve impulses from the left ear have to make a circuitous journey through the right brain, which is devoid of speech centers, before they end up at the left brain. This results in a subtle loss of atten-tiveness and ability to respond verbally.

Consequently Campbell advises situating yourself so that a person is slightly to your right while conversing, and holding the telephone to your right ear to improve listening, focus, and retention of information.[24]

Dr. Tomatis became acutely aware of how important the voice is in charging the body when he was called to a Benedictine monastery in France where the monks were well known for sleeping little, eating a simple vegetarian diet, observing silence, and chanting six to eight hours a day. This monastery had just been taken over by a young abbot who was convinced that chant served no useful purpose and had eliminated it. Within a short time, seventy of the ninety monks complained of feeling inexplicably fatigued.

The doctors who were brought in tried prescribing more sleep and adding meat to the diet, but this only made things worse. When Dr. Tomatis arrived, he promptly prescribed a return to their usual schedule of chanting. Within five months, most of the monks returned to their normal health and vigor.[25]

Gregorian chants are a collection of chants taken from various cultures and standardized into the Catholic Mass by St. Gregory (pope from 590 to 604 C.E.). They differ from ordinary music because the timing is not according to meter, but depends upon the ability of the singers to chant on a prolonged exhalation. The training takes four years before a novice is brought into the choir.[26]

Because the chants are based on the breath, they have a powerful effect on the listeners, who soon find themselves taking deep breaths, which in turn slows down their hearts and reduces their blood pressure. Tomatis explains, "If you put an oscilloscope on the sounds of Gregorian chant, you see that they all come within the bandwidth for charging the ear. There is not a single sound which falls outside of this."[27]

Listening to Gregorian chants helps create a state of calm and an increase in energy, memory, and concentration. I often listen when I am writing because it keeps my mind calm and prevents my body from holding tension. Tomatis explains that music in relatively low frequencies (such as shamanic drumming) affects the more primitive areas of the brain, creating a hypnotic state, whereas the Gregorian chants stimulate the cortex, making you feel alert.[28]

A study of thirty-two choir members in Irving, California, in 2001 confirmed the benefits of singing in a choir. They performed Beethoven's choral masterwork, *Missa Solemnis*. Researchers used cotton swabs to collect saliva, which contains the immune protein Immuno-globulin A, used by the immune system to fight disease.

According to the study, the protein increased 150 percent during rehearsals, and by 240 percent during performance. The boost seemed directly related to the singers' states of mind, which many participants described as happy or euphoric.

Continued ➡

"Afterward, I'm floating," said Morris, age sixty-one, a member of the choir. "I feel terrific. There have been many times going into a concert when I'm fighting a cold or have a sore throat, but I managed to show up and do the performance, and I'm higher than a kite when it's over."

Education professor Robert Beck, who coauthored the study with Thomas Cesario, concluded that, "The more passionate you feel while singing, the greater the effect."[29]

Resonance and Entrainment. The principles of resonance and entrainment are basic to understanding how Vibrational Healing works. In 1665 Dutch mathematician Christian Huygens (1629 to 1695) was working on the design of pendulum clocks. He found that when two clocks were mounted on a wall near each other, even though the pendulums were swinging at different rates, they would eventually end up swinging in sync with each other. He discovered that the powerful rhythmic vibrations of one object will cause a less powerful object to lock into the vibration of the dominant source.

Similarly, when individual pulsing heart muscle cells are brought close together, they begin pulsing in sync with each other.[30] In sound healing, the practitioner may begin by expressing sounds that feel similar to the client's depressed or angry energy. Once the client feels a sympathetic vibration, he is more likely to resonate with the sound healer and to fall into alignment when she makes soothing and relaxing sounds.

The vibratory tools of sound, crystals, and essential oils are so powerful and so coherent that they can entrain the vibrations of depressed organs or tissues in the body. When just the right sound, crystal, or oil is chosen, it can remind the body of its own healthy harmonic resonance.

The same effect can be achieved when you strike a tuning fork that vibrates at 100 cps and bring it near another tuning fork of the same frequency, the second instrument will start vibrating without being struck. Then the two objects are in resonance with each other. External rhythms can also be used to affect the rate of the heart, respiration, and brain wave activity.

Every organ, bone, and cell has its own healthy resonant frequency. Sound healer Shari Edwards has the remarkable ability to hear these frequencies, and she has assigned a hertz frequency to each of the muscles, organs, and tissues of the body. Shari can also produce these sounds with her voice and has devised a machine that reproduces these sounds.

She and I were both teaching at a healing convention many years ago. When we met again, I had sustained an injury in which a boulder fell on my left thigh. It never fully healed, and my thigh had a large depression. I had the feeling that Shari could help me so I explained my situation to her, and we went to her room to give it a try.

When I showed her my thigh, she reached out and placed her fingertips on the depression. Then she opened her mouth and a distinct sound came out. She used her machine to measure the frequency of the sound and it calibrated at a particular hertz. Then she looked it up in her booklet and sure enough, the sound she made was the exact frequencey for the thigh muscle.

Shari set me up with a pair of headphones and dialed in the sound I needed, and I sat there listening to the repetitions of this one sound. Half an hour later, she asked me to take off the headphones and stand up. We looked at my thigh, and we were both amazed and delighted to see that the depression was 80 percent gone.

Shari was applying the principle of *resonance* by invoking the sound of a healthy thigh muscle. When the less healthy muscle heard that sound, it presumably was stimulated to emulate its own healthy manifestation. When we hear a statement and respond by saying, "That resonates for me," we mean that it rings true, and it has a healthy harmonious vibration.

Shari was also using the principle of *entrainment* by encouraging my weak thigh muscle to lock in to the stronger healthy vibration of her machine. If you have a relatively weak voice, you have probably experienced entrainment while singing with stronger vocalists. It takes too much energy to sustain a tune at a weaker vibration, so your voice just naturally wants to lock in and sing along with the stronger voices.

Bodily Harmony. Dr. Peter Guy Manners works with sound in his medical practice in Worcester, England. He writes, "Experimentation indicates that human beings, as all objects, are radiating sound waves; therefore their fields are sonic fields."[31]

We are inclined to believe that reality is limited by what we experience with our five senses. It is difficult to believe that there are sounds we cannot hear and vibrations we cannot feel. Yet we know that infrared and ultraviolet light rays are invisible to our eyes, and there are subsonic and supersonic sounds that we cannot hear, and ultra high frequency (UHF) and extremely low frequency (ELF) vibrations we cannot feel.

The seawater crocodile senses electrical vibrations more than one hundred yards away. The shark has electrosensors covering its snout that sense the vibrations of creatures hiding under the sand. Sharks have a hearing-feeling sense (scientists call it a lateral line) through which they can sense the vibrations of moving prey.[32]

We are all vibrations, and every part of the body has a frequency. Dr. Manners defines harmony within the body and describes how to use sound to detect the source of bodily disharmony. He explains that just as each of us has our own unique shape and size, we each have our own distinct pattern, or collection of tones. "Within the human body any deviation from this harmony would result in ill health. . . . We can easily see that each organ will have its own sonic (or sound) field. If properly detected this should provide information on processes going on in a particular organ."[33]

Discoveries by Dr. Raymond Royal Rife in the 1930s show how potent the right tones can be for eliminating disease. He found that every cell has its own vibratory frequency, and every cell within a specific organ system has a common vibratory resonance. Rife is best known for his amazing microscope that magnifies living cells at hundred thousand magnifications. While observing the internal workings of a living human cell, he took a Ray-O-Vac tube and a frequency generator, and charged the cells with different frequencies. Eventually he found a resonance that exploded the cells.

Armed with this knowledge, Rife started curing cancer. For cancer of the breast, for example, he could take a biopsy of cancerous tissue and put it under the microscope and then observe the cells while he adjusted his frequency generator until the cells exploded. Once he knew the frequency that would obliterate the malignant cells, he put his patient next to the tube and directed it to her breast, and when the treatment was complete the cancer cells would be gone without affecting the rest of the breast or body.[34]

Perhaps Rife's work inspired the development of the German lithotripter, which translates as

"stone crusher." This remarkable medical machine destroys kidney stones and gallstones by selectively attacking them with the appropriate sound resonance that mimics the sound frequency of the stones, causing them to break up. The machine passes high voltage electrical shock waves through a spark gap under water. The shock waves produce a compressive force, and the brittle stones start to crumble into small sand like particles that are passed out in the urine. Kidney, ureter, or bladder stones can all be treated in this painless procedure that takes two to three hours.[35]

Dr. William Tiller, a Guggenheim Fellowship recipient from Stanford University, writes in *Radionics, Radiesthesia and Physics*, that each gland of the body has its own healthy waveform, so one can scan the waveform of a gland to detect abnormalities. Then "if energy having the normal or healthy waveform of the gland is pumped into...the gland [it] will be driven in the normal or healthy mode."[36]

This helps explain why exercises in this section such as Toning for the Pain in Your Body and Toning with Bodywork are effective. Toning brings healthy waveforms into imbalanced or diseased tissues and organs, reawakening healthy vibrations within the body.

A physically sensitive healer can send out sounds, as a bat uses radar, to scan the wave field of each gland, checking for imbalances. Intuitively, he can find sounds to charge the glands with healthy energy, thereby restoring their healthy harmonic frequency.

Dolphins use sound for echolocation, and presumably this same skill enables them to detect abnormal areas of the body and to direct sound to those areas. This probably accounts for the seemingly miraculous healings that some people experience after swimming with dolphins. During my workshops on the Big Island of Hawaii, we swim and kayak with wild dolphins. No experience can compare with having these huge mammals voluntarily swim next to you in the ocean and look you in the eyes. The depth of their consciousness and compassion is undeniable.

Once I swam with a student who was pregnant though her belly was not noticeably enlarged. We were approached by nearly a dozen dolphins including two baby dolphins, swimming alongside their mothers. I was amazed to see a baby dolphin break away from its mother and swim in circles directly under this pregnant woman for at least five minutes. How did the baby dolphin—and its mother, who allowed it to swim alone—know that this woman was pregnant? Probably by sound, just as doctors use ultrasound to examine the fetuses of pregnant women....

Toning

A tone is a distinct sound that maintains a constant pitch and is identifiable by its regularity of vibration. Toning is the sustained, vibratory sounding of single tones, often vowel sounds, without the use of melody, rhythm, or words. These sounds may cause vibrations that create overtones that reverberate in a way that can be highly penetrating.

Overtones are sounds that emanate from a single musical note and have a high frequency. Many overtones are higher than your ears' ability to hear, so these are called subliminal sounds and may explain why toning has the mysterious ability to put people into a trancelike state or to invoke profound emotions. This book will not teach you how to make overtones deliberately, but overtones tend to occur when you tone, especially in a group.

Continued ➤

A tone may be high-pitched (having many vibrations per unit of time) and piercing or it may be low-pitched (having fewer vibrations) and soothing—or anything in between. A specific tone will have a fairly predictable effect on the person listening (and the person making the tone). High, piercing tones tend to speed up the heart, and low, soothing tones tend to slow it down. Harsh tones tend to create feelings of anxiety, while rich, mellow tones tend to elicit a sense of deep inner peace. Some tones stir up strong feelings, and others pull you out of your emotions, into a meditative state.

Pleasant low-pitched tones tend to produce a grounded, earthy sense of well-being. Low tones can help you get into your body and accomplish things. Pleasing, high-pitched tones can help release stress and day-to-day worries, producing a euphoric, deeply relaxed feeling.

Most people have heard the toning of the syllable OM, which is believed to create an energy of harmony and unity. Regardless of their religion, people tend to experience a quiet centeredness when OM is toned repeatedly, especially when it is done in a rich and sonorous voice.

During true spiritual expression, whether in a church or a synagogue, under a tree or on a mountain, people experience direct communion with their God or Creator. Toning, chanting, and droning are practices that virtually all cultures have used, particularly in their religious services. Whether you grew up chanting AMEN, OM, or AMEIN in your church, mosque, or synagogue, or whether your army, tribe, or football team made hollers or whoops, you have in all these ways experienced some form of toning.

We are seeing a spontaneous emergence of the intuitive use of sound. People are using toning for spiritual expression, enhancement of community feeling, and physical and emotional healing. People are listening to and expressing their inner voice in new and exciting ways: toning with tai chi, yoga, spontaneous dancing, lovemaking, toning at men's groups, and wailing at women's groups.

Even the cry of an infant can be a form of toning. Although infants are nonverbal, they can fully express distress, happiness, love, and anger. Simply through the use of vibratory sound, they persuade us to pick them up, feed them, comfort them, or change their diapers. If you have ever been an infant then you already know how to tone.

But most children in our culture learn how to censor their emotions, words, and every sound that comes out of their mouths. They learn to make only sounds that are socially acceptable. As a child, I was taught not to make loud noises of any kind: boisterous laughter, painful crying, and screaming with pleasure.

I grew up feeling secretive and shy about using my voice in a forceful and passionate way. I harbored a desire to sing, yet singing was only for people who had great voices. When I auditioned for the school chorus, I barely got in. I took two or three singing lessons, but my teacher was not terribly impressed. My main vocal achievements for the next twenty years consisted of improvised lullabies to my babies and then singing songs like "I've Been Working on the Railroad" during long trips in the car with my boys.

I didn't get over my fear of singing until I started toning. It's not necessary to have a beautiful or powerful voice to tone, and it's not possible to make mistakes!

The first person I heard tone was my friend Laeh Maggie Garfield, who wrote *Sound Medicine*. It was a loud, intense sound that shocked me. But it also vibrated deeply within me. I never imagined that I would be able to make such sounds or that I would want to!

The next time I heard toning was when I taught at a women's retreat in California, where I attended a workshop with Dhyani Ywahoo, author of *Voices of Ancestors*. She held a huge crystal in each hand and made powerful unearthly sounds that awakened something within me. It would be years before I could give myself permission to make such sounds.

But eventually I did. Then I helped others do the same. I find that it is easier for people who are not trained as singers to let themselves make uninhibited sounds than for singers who are trained to believe there is a right and a wrong way to make sounds.

I still felt shy about *sounding* (another word for *toning* or making improvised sounds) in public, but I would tone with my students as we made sounds for the chakras. Sometimes the whole room would reverberate with overtones bouncing off the walls and ceiling—as if there were a chorus of angels on the rooftop.

Gradually I overcame my shyness. The feedback I received about my toning was so positive that it gave me confidence. The sounding took on a life of its own. It seemed to have its own intelligence, and I learned to trust it. During meditations or talks or healings I would be overwhelmed by the desire to make sounds. I just had to open my mouth and the sounds would come pouring out of me. Eventually I produced a CD called *Altered States of Planet Earth*. It combines my spontaneous sounds that I call Shamanic Sounding with Alejo's didjeridoo, a long instrument made originally by the Australian Aborigines by hollowing out a small tree.

Toning with Laughter. Laughter is a form of toning. One Zen master told his students that if they would say "HO! HO!" vigorously for five minutes each day, they would never die. According to Laurel Elizabeth Keyes, author of *Toning, The Creative Power of the Voice*, the *H* and *K* sounds such as *HI, HAH, HOH, HU, KAH* and *KOO*. stimulate the glandular system. They are produced by tightening the abdominal muscles and forcing the breath against the roof of the mouth, thereby creating strong vibrations in the adrenal, thymus, pituitary, and pineal glands. We conceptualize laughter as a repetition of *h* sounds such as *ha-ha-ha* or *he-he-he*.[37]

Norman Cousins provides yet another way of using laughter for healing in *Anatomy of an Illness*. He had a rare life-threatening disease, ankylosing spondylitis, characterized by a gradual deterioration of collagen, the fibrous substance that holds the body together through the connective tissue in every part of the body and particularly the spine.

Cousins was familiar with research showing that repeated stress leads to illness and disease. He reasoned that if distress causes disease, joy and laughter should cause healing, so he arranged to have funny movies and hilarious old TV programs shown throughout the day in his hospital room. He discovered that ten minutes of good belly-laughing provided a full two hours of pain relief. Eventually Cousins cured his disease with a combination of laughter and massive doses of vitamin C.[38]

Abdominal Breathing. Toning expands the abdomen and lower lungs, pushing stale air out of the lungs, enabling you to absorb more fresh oxygenated air. You don't need to have strong breath control, but since toning requires deep breathing, it contributes to health and a sense of peacefulness, helps eliminate the effects of stress, and can help prevent (and sometimes heal) heart disease, asthma, bronchitis, and senility.

Shallow breathing contributes to a lack of oxygen. The habit of shallow breathing begins in early childhood, when children are forced to be quiet, to be still, to hold back their feelings. When you're scared, you literally hold your breath. You don't let a single sound escape, not even a sigh. When you're afraid, angry, excited, or sad, you tend to take very shallow breaths, because taking a deep breath would expand your heart or abdomen, and that's where you hide those intense emotions. That's why children so often complain of tummy aches when they're emotionally upset, and why adults consume so many little tablets for indigestion.

American women rarely breathe from their abdomens, because they believe they look better with flat, rigid stomachs instead of relaxed, rounded ones. Women (and men) with rigid stomachs often have trouble with indigestion and may have trouble getting in touch with their feelings.

If you feel inhibited about making sounds, you're not alone. One way to overcome this resistance is to start humming. Follow the exercises and hum instead of toning. When you get comfortable with humming, make a louder hum. As you notice that nothing terrible happens, you'll be able to make increasingly louder sounds.

Here's an exercise to strengthen your diaphragm and give you better control of your breathing. Stand up, with your feet shoulder length apart. As you take a deep breath, feel your lower abdomen (below your navel) and then your upper abdomen (above your navel) expand, like a balloon. Your shoulders will rise slightly. Hold your breath to the count of five and then—without exhaling—contract your entire abdomen. Push it out again. Then exhale and relax your entire abdomen. Practice until you can do this easily Next, inhale as before and hold your breath. Contract your abdomen and push it out as before, then repeat. Exhale and relax your stomach. Continue practicing until you can contract and push out your abdomen ten times while holding your breath.

How to Tone. The human voice is one of our finest tools for healing the body and spirit. Yet it weighs nothing, costs nothing, and you don't even have to carry it in your pocket.

When you're ready to tone, you can stand, or sit upright in a firm chair with your feet on the ground, or sit on a cushion on the floor in the tailor or cross-legged position. Be sure your spine is straight. Relax your jaw (you might open and close your mouth a couple times, as if you were yawning). Inhale through your nose. Feel your lower and then upper abdomen expanding. Before they are fully expanded, feel your breath continue up into your lower and then upper lungs as they, too, expand. Your shoulders will rise slightly. Feel your shoulders relaxing.

Relax your jaw; just let it hang open. Release your breath through your mouth while making a long sustained sound, preferably a vowel sound. This is the tone. Allow the sound to continue as long as you exhale. When you run out of breath the sound will stop. Inhale deeply through your nose as you bring your breath all the way down to your lower abdomen. Continue this process for as long as you like.

It is not necessary to concentrate too much on taking complete breaths. After the first few breaths, just relax and enjoy the process. Here are some exercises you can experiment with:

· Tone a long vowel (A, E, I, O, or U) at a comfortably low pitch for as long as your breath allows. Repeat several times. Tone the same vowel at a medium pitch. Repeat several times.

Continued ➡

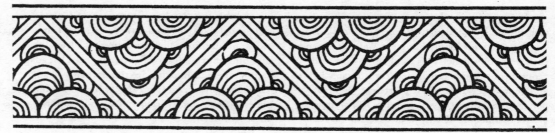

Tone the same vowel at a comfortably high pitch. Repeat several times. Do the same with a different vowel.

· Tone a syllable (a single uninterrupted sound formed by a vowel and one or more consonants such as "OM") at a comfortably low pitch for as long as your breath allows. Repeat several times. Tone the same syllable at a medium pitch. Repeat several times. Tone the same vowel at a comfortably high pitch. Repeat several times. Do the same with another syllable, such as "RA."

· Let go entirely and play like a kid. Beat on a tabletop, hit a cup with a spoon, or bang pots and pans together. Get silly. Loosen up.

· Make up a song in a pretend language that sounds Indian, Chinese, or Greek.

· Get a drum that gives off lots of reverberations. Hit the drum repeatedly and try to imitate or blend your tones with the sounds.

· Get a Tibetan bowl or a quartz crystal bowl or a tuning fork, and make spontaneous sounds or chant the following Tibetan or Egyptian sounds.

The Tibetans have a sound for each chakra that can be chanted individually, or you can chant all of them on one breath: *LAM* (first chakra), *VAM* (second), *RAM* (third), *YAM* (fourth), *HAM* (fifth), *OM* (sixth and seventh).

Dr. Mitch Gaynor, oncologist, has had excellent results reducing stress and pain for his patients by having them play a Tibetan or crystal bowl while chanting the Tibetan seed sounds.[39]

The ancient Egyptians had sounds that were later adopted by the Rosicrucians. In one exercise, *AUM* is repeated twice at a low pitch. Then *RAH* and *MA* are sounded at a high pitch. Then *AUM* is repeated twice at the same low pitch.[40]

When using toning during a healing session, your client will probably be lying down. If she wishes to participate in the toning, it's perfectly all right to tone while lying down, but she may prefer to stand or sit while toning, and then lie down again.

Most of this book is directed toward self-healing, but all the exercises can be used in a client-practitioner or friend-friend context. In this section I address the Sound Healer. With some of the exercises, such as Toning for the Pain in Your Body, your client may feel too inhibited to make his own sounds. Once you become proficient at making sounds for yourself, you may be able to tune in on your client's emotions and give voice to his feelings—which may inspire him to begin making sounds for himself. Most people feel less self-conscious after hearing someone else make outrageous sounds, because there is less fear of being judged.

If you sense that a client is holding onto an emotional sound that she cannot get in touch with, you might say, "I feel the impulse to make a sound, and it may not be very pleasant. Is that all right?" If she says "yes," then you can add, "Feel free to join me."

When sounds are released, memories often come flooding up into awareness, so be prepared to do counseling in conjunction with this work.

There are three basic sounds:

1. **Cleansing and Releasing**. These sounds express emotions and help release stress and tension. Moaning and groaning are cleansing sounds that come naturally when aches and pains and strong emotions are being released.

    High-pitched, penetrating sounds or even fierce screaming can help break up energy blockages that may have led to emotional and physical armoring. Sharp, intense sounds combined with sweeping gestures can purge negative energy. If you feel the impulse to make sounds for your client, go ahead and release those sounds. You may feel a blood-curdling, terrifying scream, and your client may be amazed to find herself joining you. This could go on for several minutes and might actually end in laughter! Releasing a scream that has been held in for decades can be a joyous, liberating experience.

    Sounds can also be used to cleanse the energy in a room. When people are angry, brooding, and unable to release heavy emotions, they tend to leave negative energy behind. A dark cloud seems to hover in the energy field of the room, even after they are gone. The same technique can be used to clean the energy in a room.

    Many people are reluctant to make "negative" sounds in a room, partly because they are afraid of leaving their "bad energy" behind. I have found that the opposite is true. Unexpressed emotions linger in the energy field of a person or a room, whereas even the "worst" emotions, when fully expressed (without causing harm to others), leave the energy revitalized.

    While you are making releasing sounds for your client, you may see him twitch, jerk, or tremble briefly as negative thought patterns and holding patterns are released. Don't be alarmed; this is perfectly natural.

2. **Soothing and Relaxing**. These sounds bring body and spirit back into their natural harmony and alignment. Through toning, you can provide a soothing environment for the release of tension. Humming can be calming to the nervous system and may help your client take deeper breaths.

    You may feel inspired to sing words of support and encouragement, or even to break into familiar bars of music or pop tunes. Trust the impulse; it often turns out to be surprisingly appropriate.

3. **Regenerative**. Sit in silence with your client and allow your energy to align with his, so that you can feel the resonance that he is lacking. This may happen spontaneously while you are talking or while he is toning. Once you feel the needed resonance, allow your voice to provide that sound. When regenerative sounds are for survival or for resolving sexual issues, they tend to be low and full-bodied (corresponding to sounds for the lower chakras). When they are for healing the emotional body, they usually fall in the mid-range (corresponding to the middle emotional chakras). When they are for opening to spirituality, they tend to be high and ethereal (corresponding to the higher chakras).

    You may notice tears rolling down your client's face. He may experience a wave of heat rushing over him, or a cool breeze. He may feel goose bumps on his skin. His heartbeat may slow down or increase. He may have a sensation of a great weight being lifted from his shoulders.

    Sometimes—particularly toward the end of a session—you may have an impulse to sing silly songs: popular songs, hillbilly songs, rock and roll, sentimental songs. These often turn out to be just the right thing, and the laughter that follows may be just the right ending for your session.

Emotional Release Through Toning

The following exercises are specially designed to help you get in touch with your emotions. Toning is one of the most powerful tools for releasing pent-up, repressed emotions. Sound bypasses the intellect and has the inherent ability to trigger physical or emotional reactions: Your eyes and nose may water, phlegm may come up from your chest, you may cough, your sinuses may feel aggravated, you may feel tightness in your neck, shoulders, and chest, your heart may beat rapidly or feel painful, your body may twitch, you may feel dizzy or nauseous. Buried memories may come flooding into your consciousness.

These symptoms are signs that the toning is working for you, stirring up emotional and physical blockages that have been preventing you from breathing and living freely. If you are accustomed to holding in your feelings, you may be afraid that something terrible is going to happen if you lose control. Releasing control for a while can lead to becoming relaxed and healthy. Having too much control leads to illness, including heart attacks, high blood pressure, and arthritis.

Some people are afraid that once they open up, they'll become violent or crazy. I can assure you that I have never met anyone who became mentally or physically ill as a result of expressing their emotions. However, I have met innumerable people who became both mentally and physically ill as a result of suppressing their emotions.

Still, there is a fear—no matter how irrational—that once you open the box of repressed emotions and let them out, you will never get it closed again. After over thirty years of helping people with emotional release, the only problem I've seen occurs when people get scared and try to close the box.

If you are unaccustomed to releasing emotions, and if it is intensely disturbing to you, you may want to have someone present that you feel comfortable with, who can hold and comfort you if the need arises. *If you know that you have a lot of pain to release, and you're not sure that you can handle it—alone or with a friend— seek the help of a trained counselor or therapist, and ask this person to work with you as you do these exercises.*

There are other precautions you can take. Before you begin working, sit quietly and take ten deep breaths. Tell yourself, "I give myself permission to temporarily lose control. I will not do harm to myself or to anyone or anything else." Repeat this three times. It is like making a pact with your subconscious. I have never seen anyone violate such an agreement.

Continued →

If you feel upset during or after these exercises, just sit quietly and bring ten deep breaths all the way down to your lower abdomen. Watch it expand each time you inhale. This will help to calm and ground you. People usually feel considerably lighter and better after doing these exercises. They breathe better, their sinuses open, and they feel empowered. Most people delight in discovering that they enjoy making sounds as their voices become stronger, fuller, and more vibrant.

If you would like to do these exercises but find that you just can't do them—if you can't even begin to open your mouth and make loud sounds—you may have been punished for being noisy when you were a child. Punishment can take the form of a harsh look or a strap. Very sensitive children respond to a sharp glance as if they'd been hit.

Even if you weren't punished, you may have internalized the idea that it is bad, naughty, inconsiderate, or obnoxious to make loud noises. For a child, it is a matter of survival to be accepted by her caregivers, so most children learn to behave in a way that is acceptable to adults. Even after we are grown, when we behave in ways that our caregivers did not approve of, it triggers that old fear of abandonment. So when someone asks you to make loud noises, even if you think it's a good idea, you may find that you simply can't do it.

One way to overcome this resistance is to start humming. Follow the exercises and hum instead of toning or groaning or making loud noises. When you get comfortable with humming, make a louder hum. As you notice that nothing terrible happens, you will be able to let yourself make louder noises.

The important thing is to *release* any pent-up feelings that you may have, and to *express* your emotions. As you're doing this, you may find yourself yawning, screaming, crying. Your body may jerk, shiver, or tremble. You may want to pound on the bed with your fists or stomp your feet. If you are standing, you may want to fall down on the mat. Just make sure you have plenty of padding under you.

Just let it happen. If your body is twitching and jerking, this is good. It means that your body is finally breaking free of its armoring, and you will probably feel much better afterward. Give yourself as much acceptance as you possibly can, and let yourself release whatever needs releasing. Exaggerate your sounds. If you notice that your voice is beginning to sound like a siren, make a loud siren noise. If you're starting to sound like a howling dog, then *become* a howling dog. If you sound like a baby crying, then become a baby calling out desperately for its mama. Don't worry about sounding silly. Try not to judge yourself.

Welcome the emotions, no matter how painful or how wonderful. Emotions that are pent-up are limiting or poisoning you. Instead of shying away from the exercise because it seems to be making things worse, try going more deeply into it; instead of doing it for five minutes, try it for ten. You may get worse before you get better, but this is almost certainly going to help. By the end of the session, you are likely to notice a distinct change for the better.

Dr. Elisabeth Kübler-Ross did groundbreaking work with teenagers in high schools where there were serious problems with violence. She persuaded certain school boards to put in soundproof screaming rooms with mattresses on the floors and walls, so kids could go in and beat the mats and scream their heads off. When students had a physical outlet for their emotional pain, they no longer needed to numb themselves with drugs and alcohol, and they had less need to be aggressive with other students. Screaming is a form of *sounding*—making uninhibited sounds without specific words. . . .

Adults, too, can benefit from some form of emotional release. When we are in stressful situations, we automatically start pumping adrenaline and other hormones for fight or flight. That adaptation served us in primitive times when we had to kill an enemy or run from attack. But in modern times, we become civilized and learn to suppress these instincts.

When you stifle your natural impulses, these hormones turn into toxins that get stored in your body and gradually build up to create chronic physical problems. I have no medical evidence of this, but I have helped innumerable people to relive traumatic incidents from childhood. When they can scream and curse and hit the mat, the incidents come back with perfect clarity, as if they happened yesterday.

The release of old repressed emotions enables clients to experience a sense of anticipation and joy in life they hadn't felt since they were infants. When they express and then let go of emotional pain that plagued them for years, their physical pain falls away. They stop drinking alcohol and using harmful medications, whether they are street drugs or pharmaceuticals.

Toning is a remarkable way of letting go of emotions that have become trapped in specific parts of the body. It is also a way of restoring harmony so that the ailing part can find its natural interrelationship with the whole body, allowing the energy to flow freely….

Toning Exercises

Groaning and Moaning. This is a short emotional release exercise that you can do while you're in the shower or driving on a back-country road. A shower is ideal, because the water (preferably cool or cold water) is continuously bathing your electromagnetic aura and literally showering you with healthy negative ions. This is an excellent way to start the day or to wind down after work or after an argument or any stressful encounter. It gives you an opportunity to express your feelings without doing harm to anyone.

Start out by thinking about all the nasty things that have happened to you in the last week or month. Really get into it. Scrunch up your mouth and eyes and make ugly, disgusting faces like a six-year-old. Give yourself permission to be gross. Begin making low, groaning, moaning sounds. Feel sorry for yourself. Exaggerate it. Dramatize your feelings. Make loud, complaining, disgusting noises. Let your voice dredge up all the frustration, annoyance, and grief that you feel about anyone or anything.

After doing this for a while, your voice will go into a higher register. It may go up and down. As you release tension and begin to feel better, your voice will tend to go higher for longer. At some point, you will feel a definite release and a leveling off. You may sigh or tone a long note. You will know when you are finished. This typically takes five to ten minutes, but varies from person to person (the first or second time may take much longer). Just continue until you feel complete.

Toning for the Pain in Your Body. Focus on a painful part of your body and think of three words

that describe the pain. Write them down. Think of a metaphor for the pain such as, "My hip feels like a rusty machine with the gears locked." Write that down.

Now give a sound to the first feeling. If the sound doesn't come spontaneously, begin by toning on a low note and slowly raise the pitch until you find a tone that resonates with the pain. Continue making sounds until you feel a release, as if you've given yourself an inner massage. This may take five to ten minutes or more with each feeling.

Here is how the exercise worked with one of my clients. John had a pain in his shoulders. His three words were: "Tight . . . scrunched . . . heavy." I wrote these down and then I asked him for a metaphor by saying, "It feels like. . . ?" He responded, "It feels like I'm carrying the whole world on my shoulders." I wrote this down. Then I read the first word aloud. I asked him to move around and make sounds to express feeling tight. He had a little trouble doing that, so I told him to, "Begin by making low sounds and slowly raise the pitch until you find a sound that feels tight. It might be a weird sound." Then I realized that he might feel self-conscious making such a sound, so I offered to demonstrate. I went into my own body, and it wasn't too hard to remember having a tightness in my own shoulders. I scrunched up my shoulders and made a strange gutteral sound that seemed to express the tightness. We both laughed and then it was easier for him. He rolled his head around on his neck and opened his mouth and made a powerful OOOO sound, which he continued to make until he felt a release.

He did a similar process with the word "scrunched," this time making little barking sounds. With the word "heavy" he leaned over in a stooped position like an old man and made deep gutteral groans of pain. When this was complete, he stood up much straighter than before.

I asked him to make sounds for "I'm carrying the whole world on my shoulders." Suddenly his chin jutted forward and his shoulders came up again as he made short, fast panting sounds. He did this for several minutes, then shook himself off like a dog coming out of the water. "My God!" he exclaimed. "I feel totally different! The pain is gone. I never get that much relief from a massage."

This exercise works so effectively because it gives our bodies and voices an opportunity to express the pain, resentment, and frustration that we normally suppress. It's a great relief to be absolutely authentic. It takes a load off your shoulders.

Toning with Bodywork. It is rewarding to give yourself permission to make sounds while you are giving or receiving a massage, or any kind of bodywork. This section is directed to the masseuse, but the person receiving the work will also benefit from making sounds.

As I said earlier, there are three basic sounds: (1) cleansing and releasing, (2) soothing and relaxing, and (3) regenerative. Sounds may be released through the mouth into the air while you are massaging your client, or—if you want to direct the sound to a particular part of the body—you can cup your hands to create a kind of megaphone, with the mouthpiece at the circle formed by your thumbs

Continued ➡

and index fingers. Place your clasped hands directly on the painful part of your client's body and put your mouth to the mouthpiece, toning directly into the body. Some practitioners prefer to tone with their lips about a half inch from the body or to tone through the clothing or through a piece of cloth placed on the body.

Ted came to me because he had a serious case of lethargy and depression. Ordinarily I would begin by encouraging him to talk about what had been happening in his life, particularly the events preceding the feelings of depression. On this occasion, he had barely started talking when I had an impulse to press on his stomach. Asking for and receiving his permission, I started kneading the area around his solar plexus. Following my intuition, I found myself making gagging sounds, pushing firmly on his abdomen and gagging repeatedly (cleansing and releasing).

Ted broke into intense heaving sighs and released a well of tears (his own cleansing and releasing). "I've been feeling nauseous lately," he explained. "I'm feeling sick to my stomach about my family situation." He explained that his grown son wanted to come and live with him.

Though there was plenty of room in his house, it felt like an invasion of his privacy. Once he got in touch with his gut feelings, he realized that he wanted his son to make other arrangements.

I asked Ted to lie down, and I placed my hand gently on his solar plexus, mentally directing blue light to the area as I toned UU several times (soothing and relaxing). Then I directed yellow light to the same area as I toned AOM (regenerative). (See Visualization and Color Breathing.)

When I saw Ted two weeks later, he said that his depression "evaporated" after our session. "I had a great talk with my son, and it felt good to acknowledge my own needs, and my son seemed to respect me for that. It seems to be changing the whole dynamic of our relationship."

Another example involves a sixty-five-year-old man who got a new weed-trimmer and spent all afternoon enthusiastically whacking weeds. By evening, the muscles in his right forearm were so traumatized that he could barely make a fist, and his energy was completely depleted. The next morning he didn't feel any better, so he came to see me.

I asked if I could massage his forearm. He agreed, and as I worked on loosening up the muscles I seemed to be mentally reaching into that part of his arm. Feeling a strong impulse to make a high-pitched sound, after receiving his permission, I gave voice to the sound that seemed to be stuck in there. Suddenly I realized that the sound I was making was probably on the same pitch as the weed trimmer (which he confirmed).

By giving voice to that sound, I was initiating a process of cleansing and releasing. Then I made a low, deep tone as a kind of antidote, to calm his energy (soothing and relaxing). Within a few minutes, the pain was gone and much of his strength restored. The next day he called to say that his arm was fine and he was feeling energetic again.

Sounding can be combined with bodywork in a variety of ways. Find a friend who is open-minded. Offer to give her a massage in exchange for being able to experiment with sound. Before the massage, ask permission to make absolutely any sounds you feel like making. Encourage your friend to do the same. When you finish the session, sit down and give each other feedback about how it felt to work together.

Most people enjoy this kind of massage, but if your friend does not respond favorably, don't be discouraged. It's a matter of personal preference. Just find another friend and try again....

Toning for the Chakras

You can derive great benefit from using your voice to vibrate and strengthen your own chakras. You can also tone for others, to energize their chakras. According to Dr. Alfred A. Tomatis, we charge the brain when we speak or sing, and the greatest charge comes from the higher frequencies. So the most effective way to charge the brain, which in turn charges the whole body, is by using a rising curve in your sound.[41] The exercise below follows that pattern.

When toning for a given chakra, place your fingertips lightly over that area. Begin by trying the tones that I give in the chart, then experiment with different notes and tones until you find a sound that causes a vibration beneath your fingertips.

There are many systems of toning. For the sake of musicians, I have given the C major scale as a guideline for moving through the chakras, beginning with middle C at the tailbone, and ending with B at the crown. If you are not a musician, don't be intimidated by this. The main guideline is that—as you go up through the chakras—each tone should be higher than the previous one (and not necessarily by just one note). In my practice, I do not necessarily use the scale of C major, and I use different notes at different times. But I always use low notes for the low chakras, and progressively higher notes for the higher chakras.

The most important factor in toning for the chakras is to make a tone (the combination of a sound and note) that—for you—vibrates the chakras. There are no right or wrong tones, and you do not have to be musically inclined to be good at toning. People who have no ear for music have wonderful results.

The following chart gives the color, note and tone for each chakra, and an "as in" word to clarify how the tone should sound (example: E as in red).

Chakra	Color	Note	Tone	As In
First	red	C	E	red
Second	orange	D	OO	home
Third	yellow	E	AOM	amen/home/mom
Fourth	green/pink	F	AH	amen
Fifth	blue	G	UU	blue
Sixth	indigo	A	MM	mom
Seventh	violet	B	EE	glee

Endnotes

1. Hazrat Inayat Khan, *The Mysticism of Music, Sound and Word, The Sufi Message, Volume II* (Delhi: Motilal Banarsidass, 1988), 157–158.

2. Joy Gardner, *Healing Yourself During Pregnancy* (Berkeley, CA: Crossing Press, 1987), 22–23.

3. John Ortiz, PhD, "Sound Psychology: the Tao of Music," *Positive Health Magazine*, .

4. J. W. and J. M. Standley, "The Effects of Music Listening on Physiological Responses of Premature Infants in the NICU," *Journal of Music Therapy*, 32 (1995): 208–27.

5. E. M. Buday, "The Effects of Signed and Spoken Words Taught with Music on Sign and Speech Imitation by Children with Autism, *Journal of Music Therapy*, 32 (1994): 189.

6. D. L. Nelson, V. G. Anderson, and A.D. Gonzales, "Music Activities As Therapy for Children with Autism and Other Pervasive Developmental Disorders," *Journal of Music Therapy*, 21 (1984): 100–116.

7. L. L. Morton, J. R. Kershner, and L. S. Siegel, "The Potential for Therapeutic Applications of Music On Problems Related To Memory and Attention," *Journal of Music Therapy*, 27 (1990): 195–208.

8. D. M. Ricks and L. Wing, "Language, Communication, and the Use of Symbols In Normal and Autistic Children," *Journal of Autism and Childhood Schizophrenia*, 5 (1975): 119–221.

9. M. A. Wooten, "The Effects of Heavy Metal Music on Affect Shifts of Adolescents in an Inpatient Psychiatric Setting," *Music Therapy Perspectives* 10, 1992, 93–98.

10. L. M. Bailey, "Music Therapy In Pain Management," *Journal of Pain and Symptom Management* 1 (1986): 25–28. See also S.L. Beck, "The Therapeutic Use of Music for Cancer-Related Pain," *Oncology Nursing Forum*, 18 (1991): 1327–1337. See also H. M. Heckman and J. B. Hertel, "Pain Attenuating Effects of Preferred Versus Non-Preferred Music Interventions," *Psychology of Music* 21 (1993): 163–73.

11. Mitchell L. Gaynor, MD, *Sounds of Healing—A Physician Reveals the Therapeutic Power of Sound, Voice, and Music* (New York: Broadway Books, 1999), 14–16.

12. Jim Oliver, notes from CD: Harmonic Resonance (New York: The Relaxation Company, 1995).

13. Karen Allen, PhD et al, "Normalization of Hypertensive Responses During Ambulatory Surgical Stress by Preoperative Music," *Psychosomatic Medicine*, 63 (2001): 487–92, www.psychosomaticmedicine.org/egilcontent/full/63/3/487.

14. Dale Bartlett, Donald Kaufman, and Roger Smeltekop, "The Effects of Music Listening and Perceived Sensory Experiences on the Immune System as Measured by Interleukin-1 and Cortisol," *Journal of Music Therapy* 30 (1993): 194–209.

15. Susan Aldridge, PhD, "Music with Exercise Boosts the Brain," Heart and Circulation Center, .

16. T. K. Cordobes, "Group Songwriting as a Method for Developing Group Cohesion for HIV-Seropositive Adult Patients with Depression," *Journal of Music Therapy* 34 (1997): 46–67. See also G. Wijzenbeek, and N. van Nieuwenhuijzen, "Receptive Music Therapy with Depressive and Neurotic Patients," Music Therapy and Music Education for the Handicapped (St. Louis: MMB Music, Inc., 1993), 175.

17. S. Boldt, "The Effects of Music Therapy on Motivation, Psychological Well-Being, Physical Comfort, and Exercise Endurance of Bone Marrow Transplant Patients," *Journal of Music Therapy* 33 (1996): 164–88. See also J.M. Standley, "Music Research in Medical Treatment: Metaanalysis and Clinical Applications," *Journal of Music Therapy* 23 (1986): 56–122.

18. Bradford S. Weeks, MD, "The Physician, The Ear and Sacred Music," *Music Physician for Times to Come, An Anthology* compiled by Don Campbell (Wheaton, IL: Quest Books, 1991), 41.

19. Tim Wilson, "Chant: The Healing Power of Voice and Ear; an interview with Alfred Tomatis, MD," in *Music Physician for Times to Come*, 13, 17.

20. Michael Moore, *Fahrenheit 9/11* (video documentary), Dog Eat Dog Films, June 25, 2004. See also Bloodhound-Gang, "The Roof is on Fire Lyrics," Bloodhound-Gang/ 4B8AFCFD3214FA7548256D250006E497, January, 2005.

21. Don Campbell, *The Mozart Effect* (New York: Avon Books, 1997), 53.

22. Alfred Tomatis, *The Conscious Ear* (New York: Station Hill Press, 1991), 125.

23. Don Campbell, 1997,15.

24. Ibid., 50.

25. Weeks, 1991,19,13–14.

26. Ibid., 47

27. Wilson, 1991,13,17.

28. Ibid., 18–21, 23.

29. Maria Jo Fisher, "Joy of singing in a choir could be preventive medicine, researchers say," *Knight Ridder/Boston Globe*, March 31, 2001, 5.

30. Howard Richman, "The Entrainment Transformation Principle," www.soundfeelings.com/products/alternative_medicine/music_therapy/entrainment.htm, October 16, 2004.

31. Laurel Elisabeth Keyes, *Toning, The Creative Power of the Voice* (Marina del Rey, CA: DeVorss & Co., 1973), 99.

32. Shark exhibit at Monterrey Bay Aquarium in Monterrey, CA, November 1991.

33. Keyes, 1973, 99–100.

34. Barry Lynes, Dr. Royal Rife, *Tie Cancer Cure that Worked—50 Years of Suppression*, (Qyeensville, Ont: Marcus Books, 1987).

35. Kay Gardner, *Sounding the Inner Landscape: Music as Medicine* (Stonington, ME: Caduceus Publications, 1990), 29. See also B.M. Stone Clinic, "What Is Lithotripsy," www.geocities.com/hotsprings/villa/5556/litho.htm., January 9, 2005.

36. *The Varieties of Healing Experience: Exploring Psychic Phenomena in Healing*. Transcript of Interdisciplinary Symposium of October 30, 1971. Academy of Parapsychology and Medicine, Los Altos, CA: 1973.

37. Keyes, 1973,108.

38. Norman Cousins, *Anatomy of an Illness* (New York: Bantam Books, 1991), 30–43.

39. Gaynor, 1999, 46–50.

40. Dr. H. Spencer Lewis, *Sanctum Invocation and Vowel Intonations*, a cassette tape from record S-33, Rosicrucian Supply Bureau.

41. Wilson, 1991, 19, 25.

—From *Vibrational Healing Through the Chakras*.

Continued ➡

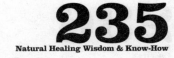

HOMEOPATHIC COLOR AND SOUND REMEDIES FOR THE CHAKRAS

Ambika Wauters

What Are Homeopathic Color And Sound Remedies?

Color and sound affect the core of our being, and we touch soul forces with these remedies. People have responded to them with improved levels of health and well-being, greater happiness and joy, and more resolve to deal with their underlying problems. Such remedies open channels for our own sweet natures to reveal themselves to us.

There are ten homeopathic color remedies, which are made by exposing colored theatrical gels and Indian silks to sunlight and water. The colors are red, orange, yellow, green, turquoise, indigo, violet, magenta, pink, and spectrum, which is made from all the colors.

Homeopathic sound remedies are made by placing tuning forks of specific musical notes over pure water in a crystal bowl and then potentizing the water. This potentization process is the same as the process described above for using coffee as a remedy. The dilutions for color remedies are 6X (six dilutions in ten drops of alcohol and water), 12C (twelve dilutions in one hundred drops of alcohol and water), and 30C (thirty dilutions in one hundred drops of alcohol and water). The sounds remedies are potentized to 6X.

Color remedies have been available to the general public since 1998, when the book *Homeopathic Color Remedies* was published. Responses from all over the world brought unusual demands for these remedies to be used in different environments and conditions. They have been used in substance abuse treatment, in veterinary practices, with austistic children, and for relief from many physical and emotional problems never foreseen when they were originally made.

Sound remedies were first created in 2004 at the School of Spiritual Homeopathy in Chicago. The students and teacher proved their effectiveness over a period of several months. They are now in clinical use.

The History and Early Provings of Color and Sound Remedies

I made the original color remedies during the winter solstice of 1989 in the Lake District of northern England. They were the result of an offhand inquiry made during a tutorial with homeopath Ian Watson. I asked how homeopathic remedies were made, and he replied that remedies could be made

out of any substance on our planet. When asked if they could be made out of color, he said theoretically that was possible. Then he suggested that I try making some and see if they worked.

After Ian Watson provided the original impetus to make the first batch of color remedies, I was left wondering how to do so. Shortly after this tutorial, I had a dream in which I was shown how to make the remedies. So I gathered all the equipment I needed: distilled water, theatrical lighting gels in full-spectrum colors, beakers, and small cosmetic mirrors that could be tied around the containers. Since I couldn't find any pink filters, I used a pair of pink silk tights to wrap around the containers as a source of that color.

So it was that I made the first batch of color remedies on the winter solstice—the day with the least amount of light in the northern hemisphere—December 21,1989. Where I lived, in the north of England, there are only five hours of available light at that time of year. That day, the sky was overcast and the weather so dreary that I had no idea whether the color would be absorbed into the water, nor did I know whether the remedies would have any healing effect. I preserved the first remedies in vodka, which was the most appropriate fixative, as pure alcohol was impossible to obtain.

As I wondered how I was going to find anyone to "prove" them (validate their effectiveness), two friends from homeopathic college, Dave Evans and Greg Conform, came to visit and asked if they could have a drop of color to test. I gave them each a drop of pink and sent them home after tea and a chat. The next day, Dave called to tell me he thought I should continue to look into these remedies. He reported that two patches of eczema in the creases of his elbows, which had persisted for a long time, suddenly disappeared overnight and, coincidentally, he had a fight with his partner, which was unusual as they shared a normally tranquil relationship.

Hahnemann said, in his treatise on homeopathic provings, that the best people for proving a remedy were those who lived together and shared the same conditions, having followed the same daily routines, eaten the same food, and drunk the same water for long periods of time. I was fortunate to have two communities near me that were willing to support the proving process. They were full of self-aware, open people who helped me discover how homeopathic color remedies worked. One was a large Buddhist community in Ulverston, in the Lake District, and the other was an Alexander Technique school in Kendall, also in the Lake District. Both produced ample volunteers for my project.

The original provings were amazing but confusing. All provers were given a single dose of a color remedy using a 30C potency. They were not told either the substance or the color. A volunteer from the Buddhist center, who had suffered from rheumatoid arthritis for forty years, was relieved from pain as a result of taking one dose of Indigo 30C. However, she immediately developed boils

along the liver meridian of both legs. I realize now this resulted from detoxification of her liver, but at the time was mystified by what happened. Her detoxification followed the homeopathic rule of "healing from the top down and the inside out."

When I asked another prover, who took a dose of the same color, if anything unusual had happened to him, he told me that six women had fallen in love with him that week. I asked him whether this was part of his normal experience, and to what he attributed this experience—both good homeopathic questions. He said that he felt his confidence was extremely high while on the remedy. This same prover also dared to dive off nearby cliffs into the sea, which was something he had feared more than anything. He felt, while on the remedy, that he could do anything he wanted.

This original proving of indigo 30C led me to conclude that this remedy affected the pituitary gland. It gave people some control over their minds that could affect healing. One prover, who was a sedentary, cold woman in her fifties, suffered great emotional distress while on the remedy. She felt acutely detached and disconnected before taking the remedy, and the remedy exacerbated her symptoms. She went to her general practitioner and asked to be given drugs to alleviate her misery after taking the homeopathic remedy. These did not work because her suffering was psychological, not physical. What finally gave her relief was being massaged and touched by other people. So the solution to her suffering came from the proving.

After this I began a period of differentiating the remedies, determining how they worked and what their symptom pictures were. I investigated which colors helped certain symptoms and exacerbated others. My colleagues and I were looking to establish perceivable pictures of each remedy and each level of potency. It became clear that the 6X (six dilutions in ten drops of water) potency worked well on physical levels, 12C (twelve dilutions in one hundred drops of water) was a portal into the emotional sphere, and 30C (thirty dilutions in 100 drops of water) was a one-time remedy for many physical conditions as well as for the higher mental and emotional symptom pictures.

The provings revealed that indigo (blue) increased suffering for depressive people. The expression to "have the blues" seems to come from a deep unconscious knowledge about this color. Indigo leads to clarity of mind and detachment, improving thinking, but it also cools passions and provides mental focus. It proved to be healing for the unhappy woman mentioned earlier because it forced her to ground her energies and listen to her needs for personal contact, leading her to start having regular massages. It forced her to reach out and ask for help, something she had never done before.

After this experience, however, it was decided that the best way to test these imponderable remedies was in clinical provings. This testing period lasted for nearly eight years and helped us more fully understand color remedies. The sound remedies, which were made in 2004, were eventually proved in clinical situations also.

Students at the School of Spiritual Homeopathy initially proved the sound remedies. A group of twelve people participated in making these remedies. Sandra Applequist, a sound and vibrational healer and a student at the school, shared her tuning forks of the entire musical scale and acted as proving mistress. She muscle tested each fork to determine how many times it should be placed over the pure water when a remedy was being made.

After taking a sound remedy, each prover shared his or her experience. We were able to col-

Continued ➡

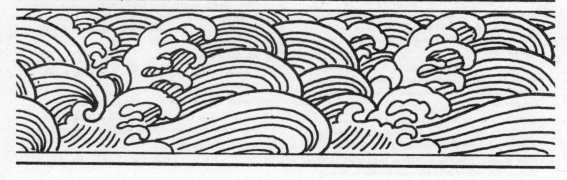

late the information quickly to find each note's theme and to understand the healing nature it provided.

The provers shared many collective experiences as a group. The first sound remedy proved was the note D, which is affiliated with the sacral chakra. After everyone in the group took the remedy, which was administered in drop form, they all began to giggle, then laugh with more and more gusto; we all sat at our desks, laughing for a long while. The note D remedy had triggered the sense of joy and happiness associated with this energy center that is resonant with joy. The group bonded with one another during this first shared experience, and from that point they continued to enjoy doing the provings.

The sound remedies are distinct from the color remedies, which work on the etheric, or energy, field; rather, their affinity is to the astral body. (See page 241 for more information on the etheric and astral bodies.) They focus their action on longings and desires, mentality, and focus. The color remedies are more about our energy itself, whether there is enough, how it is balanced, and how to soothe, tonify, and stimulate it.

There were instant and immediate reactions to the sound remedies. They did not need time to be absorbed or to work their way into the system. As a consequence, they have never been potentized past their original potencies of 5–7X. Anyone who takes them has an immediate response, even though it may be subtle. Sound remedies do not last for very long, but they work deeply and turn around our thinking and perception quickly. We have found them to be far more potent than the color remedies and their use is distinct as well.

Differences between Color and Sound Remedy Provings

After taking the color remedies, the provers experienced a variety of symptoms. With the sound remedies, nearly everyone had the same response. They worked more collectively and less individually than the people taking color remedies. Some of the color remedies produced very clear physical characteristics, while others seemed to work more subtly on emotional and mental levels.

For instance, a very interesting thing happened to all the provers who took homeopathic color remedy pink. They all dreamed of being with their mother, or of motherhood. These dreams were always soothing and comforting. One woman, who was pregnant and contemplating a termination, decided to go ahead with the pregnancy after taking the color. Pink was obviously about mother love, and it triggered this response in her.

The group taking sound remedies experienced collective laughter and hunger, and felt unified throughout the proving. They would stay together as a group, unable to leave one another, even if they had to go to the toilet or wanted to eat. They would walk like ducks in a row down the street, happy to be together. They were inseparable. When difficult experiences emerged in the provings, it happened to the whole group, not just to one person. It was as though the color individualized people and the sound communalized people.

The homeopathic color remedies differ from conventional color healing, which uses light and pigment applied to the skin or through the eyes, because they go deeper into a patient's energetic economy (mind, body, and spirit) and have a specific affinity with the etheric field of energy. The most obvious information learned about the colors was that they work in relation to the chakras, or energy centers of the body. These are nonanatomical energy points located in the subtle energy sheath we call the aura. The chakras channel vital energy into the physical body and act as conductors, or filters, from the etheric body.

The sound remedies act on the astral field, which lies next to the etheric field. It is the interface between the energy body and the higher mind of the Ego, or "I am" principle, that defines our individuality. The astral body is the repository of our longings, desires, thoughts, and attitudes. If these are positive, more energy flows into the etheric field and our energy is vibrant. The more negative or fear-based these are, less energy filters through into the etheric, creating depletion and lack and often leading to illness and weakness.

Advice on Using Homeopathic Color and Sound Remedies

The color remedies are now seventeen years old and are ready to be used by both homeopaths and the lay public. The sound remedies are three years old and just finding their way into clinical use. They are gentle, safe, and effective in treating physical, mental, and emotional symptoms. Many of the original problems encountered at the beginning have been eased with time and experience. In the beginning, I was a student, unsure of myself and not aware what I was facing. Now, I am a fully qualified homeopath with years of clinical experience behind me. As I developed my skills, working with the sound remedies has been easier and more efficient.

In the field of vibrational medicine, homeopathic color and sound remedies fit somewhere between flower essences and homeopathic plant remedies. They are similar to the flower essences, as they work to rebalance disharmonious energy states. They work best when used in conjunction with deep-acting homeopathic mineral, plant, or hormonal remedies. Color and sound remedies support the action of constitutional treatment. These remedies also work well on their own, particularly for spiritual insight and emotional harmony. There are many practitioners around the world who have had outstanding results working with the color and sound remedies by themselves, in spite of the fact that they know very little about homeopathy.

One colleague in Ireland, Monica O'Malley, has had outstanding results working with addiction, and severely handicapped children. She is a healer who works with Syntonic light therapy in addition to using the homeopathic color remedies. There are other practitioners who use just these remedies and see results.

These remedies are not meant to replace deep-acting homeopathic care or medical treatment. Many people inquire whether these remedies can cure long-standing chronic disease. They cannot do that. Please be advised that it is best to consult a homeopath or doctor regarding deep-acting and long-standing chronic diseases. Color and sound remedies work by opening an energy field so healing can happen and, in this respect, make good support remedies for other forms of deep-acting treatment. On their own, however, they are not strong enough to treat serious conditions and should never be used in this way.

Color and sound remedies easily transform energy states, such as moodiness, fatigue, exhaustion, confusion, or anger. They can be used to increase energy and to provide tonification and soothing, but cannot reverse pathology on their own. They offer support and gentle healing, and can create a positive response. Ascribing more to these remedies than they can actually do would not serve healing. We recognize that sometimes people need stronger treatment for their conditions. These remedies also support other modalities....

Color and Sound in the Human Energy System

Color captured the imagination of Sir Isaac Newton, one of the greatest scientific minds in history. He explored color, endeavoring to learn what it is, and his conclusions about the nature of light and its components, which we call the visible spectrum, are still honored by the scientific community today.

We owe our understanding of the fundamental properties of light to Newton, but color was understood and used in healing for thousands of years before his discoveries. We know the early Egyptians used crystals to focus color onto parts of the body for healing purposes, balancing mind, body, and spirit. They also loved sunlight and knew of its healing properties. They worshipped the sun and created healing chambers where light was directed, like today's lasers, onto the body. They understood color's physical and emotional properties, even developing some color pigments that we can no longer replicate; they also respected its esoteric aspects. Color had symbolic meaning for them, as is seen in their ancient tomb drawings.

Many peoples have also used sound as a healing agent. Tibetans have used singing bowls to heal the chakras for unknown numbers of generations. Metal alloys were blended and forged to create singing bowls (bowls that produce a warm tone when struck or stroked with a soft mallet) with perfect pitch. They knew that the proper mixture of certain metals would directly affect the chakras and open the field for healing.

Today, we are again using color and sound to reawaken our deepest potential for healing, as well as for personal growth and self-development. Color and sound can expand our consciousness, heal our wounds, and help us develop new ways of looking for solutions. They are gentle, effective, and provide us with a wonderful tool for balancing our systems.

We now have an advanced technology that allows us to break down color into energy; lasers and crystal spectography are techniques that enable us to use color more directly. We are developing the wisdom to know how to use light and sound as medicine in both allopathic and homeopathic forms that are kind to the body and loving and supportive to our being. New advances in the use of light and sound go directly into our energetic field. This book is dedicated to explaining the power of homeopathic color and sound and how they can be used for healing the human energy system.

Color, Life, and the Electromagnetic Scale

Color is fundamental to life. Its vibrations are necessary for physical growth and healthy development. When people are deprived of light and color, they do not grow, either mentally or physically.

Color exists in the form of oscillating light waves, which, when viewed through the light spectrum, are broken down into components of white light. When we look at the energy emanations that come from cosmic rays as they enter the earth's atmosphere, we see that white light is only a small portion of a greater energy.

Modern scientists use the electromagnetic scale to measure the cosmic forces as they penetrate our earth's atmosphere. At one end of the electromagnetic scale, there are gamma rays, which may be found in the nether regions of the cosmos. These rays oscillate at a particular speed and vibrate at a fixed rate. The vibrations slow down as the rays enter the earth's atmosphere, and the gamma rays are transformed into X-rays, with their own fixed patterns of movement and vibration. As this energy

Continued ➡

slows down even more, it is transformed into ultra-violet light. In the next step of deceleration, the energy becomes white light, which further breaks down into the colors of the spectrum. As these waves of energy slow down even more, they turn into infrared waves, then microwave, radar, FM radio, television, short wave, and finally AM radio waves. The electromagnetic spectrum consists of wavelengths ranging from light to radio (sound) waves.

Sound also exists in waves and is measured by its rate of frequency and its level of vibration. We know there are sounds so low- or high-pitched that the human ear cannot register them. However, animals can register many of these sounds. When people are exposed to these extreme sounds, they can suffer from serious conditions. We want to eliminate overstimulation from both high or low sound and light frequencies.

Measuring Energy Waves with the Electromagnetic Scale

The electromagnetic scale is measured in meters. Some electromagnetic waves, such as radio waves, are hundreds of meters long. Others, such as visible light rays, are much shorter, about 0.0000005 meter in length. An energy wave is like a rope that is continually oscillating up and down, creating peaks and troughs, and the energy vibrations are perpendicular to the direction of their propagation. Energy wavelengths reflect the distance a wave travels in one cycle of vibration, between two crests of a trough. A vibration's frequency is the number of waves that pass a point in one second. The energy, or brightness, of a wave of light is proportional to the amplitude from the crest of one trough to a zero, or center, line. White light is a mixture of many wavelengths.

As we work with the vibratory frequency and oscillation of energy waves, it is apparent that various remedial substances fall within the same vibrations as specific colors and sounds. For instance, antimonium crude and Berberis vulgaris are a mineral and a plant remedy, but both substances fall into the field of yellow vibrations and both resonate with the musical note E. The symptoms these plant and mineral remedies address share a psychological and physiological pattern, both with the color remedy of yellow and the musical note E. Every substance we have on earth falls into a ray of the spectrum. We can identify its ray by seeing what color the plant or mineral is, but also by what symptoms the substance addresses. For example, a remedy that works on the adrenal cortex of the kidneys will be in the orange or orange-yellow ray of light.

A mineral remedy will have a deeper and longer-lasting effect than a plant remedy, which will, in turn, last longer than a color or musical sound remedy. However, color and sound remedies help bring harmony to the mind, body, and spirit—a person's energetic economy—by virtue of their similar vibratory frequencies. How colors and sounds resonate in our body at specific frequencies is discussed in the section on chakras

All medicines fit into the light-emitting energy range of the electromagnetic scale. Homeopathic color remedies, which are made from natural substances, reflect one or another color of the visible light spectrum. They also resonate with the sound remedies. All substances, or remedies, are part of the continuum of light, sound, energy, and vibration. Knowledge about this scale helps us understand the healing properties of our medicines.

Cases of Using Color and Sound to Heal Energy

As you study the qualities that relate to each color and sound, you will begin to understand which remedies each patient needs for their healing. For example, you may see a person who appears "out of it." They hover in the realms of the cosmic forces and are not fully incarnate. This person lives in the color violet and the note of high C. They lack the red of life energy and the vibration of middle C, which is grounded. They can show pale shades of blue or violet when you look into their energy fields. There is not enough physical energy in their field. Their lower chakras are weak because they live in another realm of existence. They would do well to have the lower sound remedies and the hotter colors, which would ground their spirit and help them connect with the world around them.

Colors and sounds can be quick and effective in treating this person's energy, bringing back their natural vitality and returning them to the flow of life. These patients do well when treated with such homeopathic remedies as camphor or coca, which fit into the violet ray or high C. Using these color and sound remedies strengthens their earth forces and brings them into a space where they can relate to life more easily, as opposed to staying separate and isolated.

Giving this person the energy of violet or high C, which will exacerbate their disconnection, follows the principle of like curing like. An alternative treatment method, the traditional color healing choice, is to give them the color red or middle C, which will bring their vibration down to earth quickly. Both sets of remedies will serve their healing process, releasing tension from their upper centers and allowing their spirit to come into their body.

At other times, we see people who are too earthbound, too fired by the passions of life. They lack refinement, and their bodies are plagued with the diseases of the lower vibrations, which fall into the red or orange part of the spectrum. Their pathologies tend toward inflammatory processes, as well as poor distribution of their vital energy. When we give them hot colors, their energy is freed, allowing their higher centers of spirituality to thrive. Again, you can give them either red and/or middle C, following the homeopathic approach, which will inflame them and burn off some of their lower vibration energy, or you can follow traditional color healing methods and give them blue or violet and/or high C, to raise their energy to a higher chakra.

All homeopathic remedies have their place on the electromagnetic scale of color and sound. We look at energy in relation to our patients' needs, to help facilitate their healing and balance. As we explore the nature of their symptoms, we can see whether their etheric forces, or chakras, need to be addressed with color or sound remedies.

Symptoms can be addressed with constitutional homeopathic remedies, herbal tinctures, or even vitamins. Constitutional remedies are specific to a person's totality of symptoms, whereas a color or sound remedy addresses the field that is out of balance and helps to create flow and vitality again where it has been arrested. Homeopathic sound and color vibrational remedies, used with other remedies or alone, help people do more than heal a symptom; they help people move forward in their life. They open the chakras so healing can happen. They are like an energetic vitamin pill for whichever chakra or subtle body needs addressing.

Balancing Energy Universally

The electromagnetic scale contains the energy we need to balance not only ourselves, but all life forms on our planet. Where a person's energy fits on this scale can give us information about what needs healing and how we can best provide that. This is where vibrational medicine becomes part of the universal energy forces. It can also be applied to animals, plants, and the environment.

As we look at what needs healing, we determine where the source of imbalance lies. If it is in a person's etheric body, we need to examine which chakra is in need of balance. If energy needs to be rejuvenated through stimulation, either a color or sound remedy is an excellent way to begin the healing process, as it opens the space for healing to happen. These remedies are so gentle they can do the job of bringing balance to the system and can also support other forms of healing.

If a person needs more cerebral energy or more spiritual insight to think about the situations in their life, then treatment should begin with a sound remedy, which encourages healing in the mental realm. In the past few years, it has been shown that the power of the mind truly plays a considerable part in whether people will heal or not.

Sound remedies clear mental stagnation, reflected in negative thought forms, which may appear as self-hatred, self-loathing, or obsessional fears that are self-limiting beliefs. A sound remedy can shift congested thought forms, help release unhealthy desires, and eliminate phobic aversions, thus allowing energy to flow into the etheric and physical bodies with more ease and clarity. As energy moves down into the etheric and physical bodies, assist it with color remedies.

As we use these energetic forces for healing, our planet's vibrational field also will move to a higher vibration. These truly are remedies for the future. However, it takes time and understanding to accept that something as ethereal as light and as simple as a musical note can affect the human energy system and our world with such a profound impact.

It is interesting that most of the remedies we use in homeopathy fall into the color range of yellow to lime green, or the musical note E. We do not need to use the lower vibrations of red and orange as often. It is also interesting to note that in healing the chakras, the energy center that needs healing the most often is the solar plexus, which resonates with the color yellow and the note E. This means many people are working on old childhood issues of loss and abandonment, seeking their center, owning their power, and trying to move into the heart chakra, where love, peace, and joy reign. This is the transition the whole planet is undergoing at this time. It is part of our collective evolution.

The solar plexus chakra deals with issues of personal power, self-worth, and confidence. Its primary focus is on knowing our worth, finding our freedom, and the right use of power. In acupuncture the solar plexus represents the fire element and relates, at a psychological level, to healing the wounds of an unloved childhood and cultivating a strong sense of Self. When we work to strengthen this chakra, we know who we are and who and what is for our highest good. As we grow in spiritual consciousness, we lay the past to rest and move forward in life with clarity about our purpose. We come to know that we are worthy of the love we say we want. We know what our value is.

On a universal level, working with this chakra is about transforming ideas of power into the reality of love. This comes when we kindle the flame of love within ourselves through healing, reflection,

Continued →

and meditation. In terms of vibrational medicine, this means we are moving from the brilliance of the yellow light and the note E to the neutral and soothing color of green, a color associated with the heart chakra and the musical note G. We are all dealing with this level of inner development.

Using Color and Sound to Heal the Chakras

Chakra means "wheel of light." It is a Sanskrit word describing the vortices of energy that filter the life force through the different layers of subtle bodies. They are cone-shaped in appearance, with the apex of the cone pointing in toward the body and the funnel out toward the environment. The chakras act as conductors for the electromagnetic field. This field, when fully functioning in each chakra, gives us a sense of well-being and balance. We feel in the flow of our lives as well as open and receptive. We are mentally alert, emotionally in touch, and physically resilient, with the vitality we need to meet our challenges.

At this stage in our evolution, the human energy system possesses eight major chakras and twenty-one minor chakras. (All the acupuncture points are minor chakras.) These chakras, or energy centers, filter energy into the physical body from the etheric field surrounding the physical body. This energy stimulates the endocrine system, which, in turn, release hormones into the bloodstream. These affect our growth, development, and balance, and have a profound effect on our mental and emotional well-being.

The Subtle Bodies of the Human Energy System

All living things are comprised of an energy system; in humans it is called the human energy system. It is made up of several subtle bodies, or sheaths of highly refined energy. Each surrounds the body and fits into the aura, or greater outer sheath, which protects us from environmental and psychic attack. Our aura keeps our spirit intact and helps us maintain our energy field by allowing energy to flow through our system.

The aura is divided into four subtle bodies: the physical body; the etheric, or energy, body; the astral, or mental, body; and the egoic body, which is the Higher Self, or godlike aspect of our being. The subtle bodies correspond to organs of our physical body as well as to specific emotional and spiritual aspects of our personality, and they resonate with different life challenges. We study these bodies because they help us develop a clear and

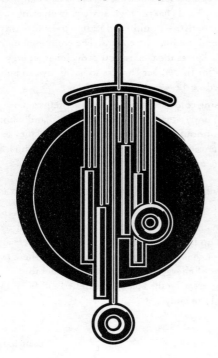

conscious image of how energy works, how the body and spirit function together, and how we can fulfill our destiny through coming to know ourselves in our totality. Health is a function of balance in all the subtle bodies.

The study of sound remedies has opened up a new vista in learning how the etheric, astral, and egoic bodies influence our health. This information has come from a study of anthroposophy (the study of man) and the work of Dr. Rudolf Steiner. He was a pioneer in the field of Spiritual Science, teaching how these bodies affect our nature and how to bring healing to their imbalance.

THE PHYSICAL BODY

The physical body deals with a person's cellular, metabolic, and systemic activities. It is our flesh and blood, bones and ligaments; in other words, it is the mineral matter of our being. It is also the vessel that holds our spirit. It is not, however, who we are or what we think and feel, no matter how much science tries to reduce our habits and behavior to biochemical reactions.

The physical body is especially influenced by (1) genetic predisposition (what we inherit from our parents and ancestors); (2) miasms (root causes of chronic diseases); and (3) our mobility and expressive patterns, which reflect our attitudes about ourselves, others, and life. These attitudes actually reflect our soul nature and resonate through all the subtle bodies.

When we address genetic predisposition in homeopathy, we look at the chronic diseases that run through a patient's life as well as in their family history. This information suggests appropriate remedies to help cleanse cellular stagnation and chronic dysfunction in the physical body. With these remedies, we can also prevent the taint of chronic diseases from being passed down to the next generation by treating people before they have children. It is one of the most profound aspects of homeopathy.

The chakras and color remedies are associated with five specific miasms: the root chakra and color red correspond to the psoric miasm, the sacral chakra and orange are related to the sycotic miasm, the solar plexus chakra and color yellow relate to the syphilitic miasm, the heart chakra and green relate to the tubercular miasm, and the throat chakra and turquoise correspond to the cancer miasm. These taints, which affect the nature of miasmic dysfunction or genetic predisposition, are found only at a cellular level, and are entrenched in a person's physical body. They are shifted only by deep-acting homeopathic remedies called nosodes, which are able to clear the miasm from the cells. These are powerful tools for healing but should be administered only by a professional homeopath.

The emotional, mental, and spiritual components to our being are connected with color and sound through the etheric, astral, and egoic sheaths. In this regard, the body has no mind of its own, but is a reflection of the higher bodies, which act as conductors for energy. The more we come to the core of our being, where we are color and sound, the more we resonate with these remedies and the more they impact our being.

Physical health allows a person to use their body to assimilate everything that is external to it, such as their physical surroundings—geology and climate—and nutrition. The body requires self-discipline and activity. It functions well when the senses are open and there is an alertness and ability to respond, with free play of the limbs and with extensive possibility of movement. Our body is the tool we use to perceive the world around us. It is also the

instrument we need to fulfill our tasks on this earth plane.

Illness, according to Dr. Rudolf Steiner, educator and philosopher, can be the consequence of disinterest in the world or an inability to assimilate experiences. Illness is a form of inner disassociation, a lack of interest or desire to learn. The lesson from illness is that it teaches us about ourselves and what we need to do. The way to health becomes a function of participating in the things that give us joy and make us happy.

The physical body corresponds to the mineral kingdom and is deeply connected to the earth. Too much earth energy in a person can lead to obsession, melancholia, delirium, and inflammatory processes. Too little can lead to anxiety or excessive head activity, which can produce exhaustion, coldness, and degeneration. Keeping the body in harmony with the elements and the world around it leads to a healthy life.

Color and sound remedies can assist the body in staying strong, resilient, and flexible by adding a vibrational dimension that nourishes the energetic field, allowing more energy to flow into the physical sheath. They can also cool and soothe the body when it is overly stimulated or when there is too much energy passing through it. Health is a function of balance, which requires tonification, stimulation, and soothing in proper proportions.

THE ETHERIC (ENERGY) BODY

The etheric, or energy, body corresponds to the layer of vital life force energy that surrounds the physical body. It acts as a conduit for energy to work its way into the physical body, where it can be utilized for metabolism and a well-functioning body. In homeopathy this is called the vital force. The etheric body provides the fuel that drives the physical body. This life energy is channeled through the chakras, or energy centers, of the etheric sheath, or layer. These centers affect the body's organs and glands and stimulate them to release hormones into the blood.

The chakras, which correspond to physical systems, inner emotional qualities, and life issues, exist in the etheric body. They develop and become functional in seven-year periods, starting at conception and continuing through the years until they are open and fully expansive in our late forties.

The physical and etheric bodies are strongly linked. They work as a unit, with the etheric forces moving and propelling the body toward physical growth, mental development, and spiritual realization. In the etheric realm, color remedies dominate, while the sound remedies help to filter energy from the astral body (the next layer of subtle energy) to the etheric and physical bodies. Whereas work on the astral field helps us establish positive and clear thinking, work on the etheric body gives us abundant energy for our physical needs. Just attending to the needs of the physical body does not cultivate the higher centers.

THE ASTRAL (MENTAL) BODY

The astral body is more refined and subtle than the etheric body. It works mainly with our mental processes, corresponding with sound, music, and ideas. It is directly related to our thinking, especially to our desires and aversions. Our astral body will expand or contract depending on how we think, what we like, and what we dislike. The channel for developing our thinking, it also works on our spirit.

If our thinking is strictly material, without any spiritual affinity, then our astral forces will be coarse and underdeveloped. When we begin to consider the realm of spirit and the enormous influ-

Continued ➜

ence the spiritual hierarchies have in our lives, we start the process of cultivating our astral body. It grows as we develop. Developing clear and focused thinking expands our capacity to connect with the spiritual forces that guide our lives as well as the energy that sustains us. When our astral body is not aligned with our etheric or physical bodies, we experience a form of anxiety separation. We feel we are not connected or centered in our own being.

Sound remedies work closely with the astral body. When it is balanced, it expands and fills the etheric and physical bodies. The power of the subtle bodies is that they work together to propel us forward in life. The strength of the astral body is that when we think positive thoughts and self-affirmations, there is an abundance of energy available to us. When we think negative thoughts and lack a sense of our worth, we have little energy to work with.

The Egoic (Higher Self) Body

The egoic body is the highest part of our consciousness and defines who we are. It forms as we mature. It is that part of us that recognizes our own uniqueness, goodness, and sense of worth. When we know who we are and that we are worthy of love, kindness, and respect, we begin to develop and cultivate our egoic body. This is known in metaphysics as the "I am that I am" principle. It takes us beyond the time-space continuum into the realm of the eternal, where every positive thought and generous act becomes etched into the cosmic forces working for the good.

When we connect with this aspect of Selfhood, we experience what the Buddhists call our own true goodness. We become intimate with ourselves and retract our projections onto the world. We become responsible and self-aware and make an effort to work for the good of the world. We are no longer victims of circumstance when we know our true selves. As this subtle body develops, we learn to accept our karma and thus become empowered. The consequence of this is that the very presence of our being helps to make the world a better place. Work on the egoic forces is facilitated through meditation, reflection, and solitude.

Color and sound remedies work quickly and efficiently on people whose egoic sheath is developed. These remedies also help those in the process of developing their egoic body.

What Do Chakras Do?

The chakras are nonanatomical in character and exist in the etheric body. They penetrate all the other subtle bodies but work primarily in the physical body through their corresponding hormonal gland. For instance, the brow chakra is located in the area of the pituitary gland, and the throat chakra is located near the thyroid gland.

In this book the chakras are called by their English names, which correspond to their location in the physical body. Their traditional names are in Sanskrit, which may be difficult to remember, though the translation of their meaning and purpose is beautiful. For instance, in Sanskrit the sacral chakra (located in the pelvic region) is called Svadistana, which means "my own sweet abode."

The chakras relate to traditional Hindi gods and goddesses of folklore. Chinese, Indian, and Tibetan medicine provide a wealth of information about the different functions ancient people ascribed to the chakras. Yoga practices also refer to the chakras, and there are now many books written about them. What makes chakras interesting to us in the West is that they are the repositories of our biography; they carry our attitudes and beliefs about ourselves that define our energy field. If we believe we are worthy, our energy field will show an

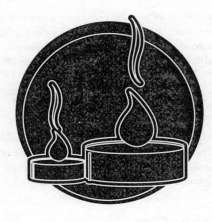

expanded field that is open to receiving the goodness around us. If we do not believe we are worthy, we will struggle against all odds to prove otherwise.

The archetypal qualities of each chakra are described in an upcoming section, "The Chakras: Qualities, Colors, and Sounds" and then related to corresponding physical problems and mental and emotional issues that affect each chakra. A person's chakras can be treated with constitutional homeopathic remedies, homeopathic color remedies, and flower essences to redress imbalance.

The chakras correspond to specific colors and sounds that resonate at the same energetic frequencies as they do. The sounds and colors stimulate them, which encourages healing in the psychological archetypes, emotional issues, and life challenges that correspond to each chakra. By working to heal the physical characteristics and the emotional issues surrounding an illness, we can rebalance the chakra system, dissipate congested energy, and create vitality and resiliency. Healing our minds helps the chakras; healing the chakras helps our bodies. The action of healing is from the inside out and from the top down. This is known as the Law of Cure and is universal in all forms of traditional healing.

Color and sound healing balance whichever energetic bodies are out of synch or in distress. For example, if a person suffers from a lack of confidence, which is a solar plexus issue, we use homeopathic yellow or the note E to stimulate that chakra. In doing so we encourage the chakra to expand, and with this expansion a person's sense of worth grows. This helps people feel better about themselves and go forward in life doing positive things for themselves and others.

This is similar to acupuncture, which stimulates the points on a particular meridian in the body to increase the charge to the area deficient in energy. When the physical area is stimulated, psychological and emotional areas are also charged.

As opposed to the previous example, when people are too deeply steeped in issues of personal power, also a function of the solar plexus, they may surround themselves with too much yellow. You may notice they wear it, paint their favorite rooms that color, and even drive a car that color. Too much yellow means the egoic forces are too strong, and they need a complementary color to bring balance into their lives. The complement of yellow is violet, the color of spirituality. Giving violet to a person with an inflated ego, to wear or to take as a remedy, helps reduce their inflated ego forces and releases rigid energy, which can become fixated in the energy system. In nature, yellow blossoms are offset with violet and purple. The colors support one another, as they do in the field of the human energy system.

Blocked energy can be shifted by chakra massage (refer to my book *Healing with the Energy of the Chakras*, Crossing Press, 1993), reflective meditation, and appropriate affirmations. Cultivating a positive

sense of one's worth is essential. Knowing that you are worthy of the love you seek and the things you want in life strengthens the chakras and creates a resonant field, so that what you long for materializes in your life. Chakras are attuned to positive thought forms.

It is always best to seek ways of healing that offer deep-acting transformation without being either invasive or aggressive. Homeopathic sound and color remedies provide a gentle, safe, and effective way of transforming life energy when it is stagnant or blocked. They work to address the centers and do not have either aggravation or strong detoxification effects.

The chakras are made of subtle etheric energy, and their function is to filter life energy in and out of the body, from the most substantial form of energy needed for our everyday survival to more refined levels of mental and spiritual energy.

Chakras are formed, healed, or destroyed as the life force melds itself into forms that resonate with our belief system. If we are contracted, closed, and intense, our chakras will display the same qualities and be unable to perform their function. If we are open, expansive, and loving, our chakra system will be the same and energy will be abundant and flowing.

If they are out of balance, chakras can be healed through positive thought, conscious and alert movement, and touch. However, sustaining the high vibration necessary to change old existing attitudes or patterns may require persistent efforts on our part for many years. It may require therapy, healing, and homeopathy to transform old patterns that limit our belief in ourselves. Sound and color remedies, along with flower essences, are good tools for transforming old problems that linger in our energy centers.

Color and sound remedies can increase a chakra's power and energy and help it regain cohesion and function if there is congestion or weakness. These remedies work well after trauma, injury, or separation, as they help create a unified field. When color or sound is homeopathically potentized, it acts as an energetic stimulant to the chakra and helps it regain balance and harmony to continue its job of filtering energy into the physical body.

Since a homeopathic color or sound remedy is pure energy, it is also easily assimilated into the chakra itself. When we can assimilate energy easily, we can find our balance easily. When a chakra is overcharged and drains energy from other centers, then the complementary color is best indicated. For instance, a person exhibiting symptoms of an overcharged sacral chakra—high anxiety, overeating, and frenetic activity—would need indigo to reduce this drain and stabilize the chakra. The complementary color balances the chakra and provides an energy source for the weaker chakras so harmony can be restored in the system.

Using color and sound remedies helps a person resolve physical problems and emotional and mental issues without great struggle or despair. Balance is experienced as well-being, inner harmony, and what in homeopathy is called "being well in oneself."

Following the Flow of Energy Through the Chakras

Energy flows freely from the cosmos and enters the human energy system at the crown chakra. It also comes up from the core of the earth and enters at the root chakra. A vortex is formed where these two streams of energy meet. It acts as a funnel for energy, creating the electromagnetic field in and around the body.

Continued ➡

This energy flows throughout our subtle bodies while we are alive. It has a dynamic movement and is constantly circulating through us. When a person dies, this energy flow ceases. The chakra itself is the conduit of the life force; it filters energy into and out of the physical body. After death it fades away until the subtle bodies have completely dissolved.

The chakras constantly filter the energy flowing through our bodies. When energy becomes stagnant, such as when a person's spiritual forces are not developed or the person has no sense of who they are or their own innate worth, then chronic illness can occur. Stagnation can trigger miasms, which is our genetic predisposition and the root of chronic disease. Homeopathy helps to clear our miasms, and it furthers our self-development and self-actualization; it helps enhance our self-love, and cultivates compassion for our suffering. It helps heal our chakras, which continue to grow and expand as we grow internally.

A block in one chakra, which may result from a limited belief or a pattern of arrested development, limits the flow of energy moving in and out of the other chakras. This will affect the entire energy body. Such limitations are experienced as weakness, malaise, low energy, self-doubt, fear, and anxiety. These limitations, along with long-term dysfunction, allow disease to take over.

If, for instance, an excessive amount of energy is flowing in and around the solar plexus, the higher and lower chakras will be weakened, which can result in massive egotism and an ungrounded sense of reality. The ego will become strong based on an inflated sense of itself. The chakra above, which is the heart chakra (or love center), will be underdeveloped because relationships would not be considered as important as self-aggrandizement. This person would place money or power before love and intimacy.

In this scenario, it is likely that the root chakra would be weak, with a limited sense of reality, and the sacral chakra would be overly expanded, with a sense of greed or gluttony.

When a relationship is based solely on a desire for self-aggrandizement rather than deep, intimate connection, the heart chakra shrinks and the solar plexus expands. This reflects a person who tries to be more than they actually are, focusing on issues of personal power and manipulation, often at the expense of others. The etiology of this in early childhood is not feeling loved and having to create a false sense of one's self to survive.

In another example, someone blocked at the throat chakra would have an overly full heart chakra and a weak brow chakra. This person would be very sensitive to emotional pain. This could manifest as having an inability to express their personal feelings, having limited ideas about themselves, and being unable to think wisely about who they are and what they are doing in life. This energetic pattern is often found in creative people and in many healers. Energy is blocked in the heart and those deep feelings cannot reach the throat to find expression. The flow of energy to the brow chakra is weak, and, as a result, clear and effective thinking and self-reflection is limited.

The flow of energy to the physical body becomes limited when either the sacral or root chakra is blocked. If issues of belonging, connection, pleasure, and well-being are not reconciled in a wholesome way, then energy becomes stagnant in these lower centers. As a result, the physical body can become weak or age prematurely.

Each chakra is supplied energy for its own particular function. The energy varies in terms of quality and quantity. However, it is the same flow of energy that comes from the heavenly and earthly forces. Each chakra needs to perform its own function, and it is dysfunctional for one energy center to do the work of another. Systemic problems arise when one center is robbed of the energy it needs in order to support an adjacent blocked chakra. It is not appropriate, for instance, for personal power to replace our need for well-being and pleasure.

Just as certain boundaries in life serve to enhance social organization and protect our individual sense of Self, so boundaries in the human energy system serve to allow each chakra to do its job in a well-defined way. Each boundary helps differentiate one energy center from another. Emergency compensation can help a center repair itself, but the long-term effects of this will weaken the totality of the system.

For example, when a person uses their sexuality (a sacral chakra function) to enhance personal power (a solar plexus function), it reflects a deep dysfunction, and eventually physical pathology of some sort will materialize in this lower center, such as in the reproductive system. Homeopathic color and sound remedies, such as orange or the note D, can strengthen the sense of ease and enjoyment and take pressure off the reproductive organs, and yellow or E can strengthen the solar plexus and develop a healthy, functioning sense of selfhood.

People who are unable to express themselves appropriately (a throat chakra issue) may have a very strong or overcharged heart chakra. They use their heart center to contain the love they find difficult to express to others. They may tire easily and suffer from weak hearts in later years. They can use turquoise or the homeopathic sound remedy G to strengthen their throat chakra and green and pink or F to strengthen their heart chakra when they feel drained. Psychologically, these people need to create relationships where they can express their love fully.

We are always working with the totality of our being, which helps us to realize we are capable of more than our limited ways of coping and managing in our daily lives. People who are confined to only one way of coping or operating in the world may need to examine what is blocked in their lives that creates an inflexible and rigid energy field. If identifying with a particular way of being, such as being a healer or homeopath, a businessperson, a teacher, or a priest, is our only way of expressing ourselves in the world, we need to see what other function is weakened and put some light (that is, color or sound) into that area of our lives.

These vibrations can help us expand our sense of life and enjoyment. Being too strongly identified with a particular way of being limits us and dampens our energy field. It creates a rigidity in our energy centers. Being more flexible in our thinking, less critical, and slower to judge others may create a more flexible and viable energy system as well.

A thought form or attitude about joy, ease, pleasure, or creative expression may need to be transformed for healing to happen in our chakras.

Using color and sound remedies can open a channel for personal transformation. Color helps replenish a low energy supply so that the work of reevaluating our lives is easier and more joyful. Sound helps us make clearer choices as we think about what and who is best for us.

As energy flows into the chakras, it stimulates the ductless glands associated with them. The stimulation of the gland releases hormones into the bloodstream and affects our health and well-being. It also opens blockages. This, in turn, feeds the body's organs and tissues, stabilizes the emotions, and helps, ultimately, to fulfill each individual's divine potential. Chakras, like homeopathic remedies, function in a broad spectrum, spanning the breadth of physical and emotional development on to the reaches of karmic destiny and spiritual growth. When we add color or sound to a chakra, we increase the intensity of vibration in that center, which stimulates the energy moving in and through the entire energy body. This has a powerful effect on a chakra's functioning. Potentized remedies have the advantage of lasting longer than direct applications, and they are easier to repeat.

For instance, when a person is in the midst of emotional separation from their partner, the heart chakra becomes weakened. We may call this grief a form of energetic starvation. The heart chakra loses its tonicity as external input of energy (from the relationship) ceases to be a sustaining element in this person's life. When this happens, the solar plexus chakra takes over temporarily to help this person rebuild their confidence and regain a stronger sense of their personal power and self-worth.

Through self-actualization, the internal mechanism of loving one's self creates energy that nourishes the heart. Eventually the heart center, which has had time to heal, becomes capable of functioning again, and love flows in and out of this chakra, becoming its sustaining force again. The locus of power here has shifted from external sustainability to internal sustainability, which not only brings healing but intensifies the quality of their energetic field.

Traditional Color Healing and Homeopathic Color Remedies

Color can be applied to the human energy system through the use of colored lights or colored clothing, eating certain foods, direct application of color to the eye, or inner visualization techniques. Homeopathic color and sound remedies are given in pill form, and are taken orally.

In addition to general color light healing, homeopathic color remedies directly influence the chakras for a substantial length of time, both stimulating and balancing the whole energetic system. Depending upon a color's potency, the length of time required for healing will vary. Low potencies will need to be repeated more often than higher ones. They can be repeated three to five times a day. Higher potencies will stay in the system longer than low ones. A 30C potency can last for weeks before needing to be repeated. It depends entirely on how depleted the chakra is of energy. If it is greatly depleted, the remedy will need to be repeated twice daily or every day. If the chakra can hold color on its own, it may not be repeated more than once.

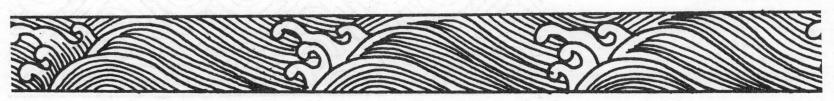

Continued ➜

Dosages are at the discretion of the practitioner. Color remedies increase the flow of energy in a chakra, and work physically, emotionally, and mentally during the time they are active. When the old symptoms return—although to a lesser degree than their original strength—it's best to repeat the remedy.

We know from provings that color and sound remedies have a direct effect on body temperature and fluid retention; they can increase or release irritability and promote tranquility or create irritability. They assist with expressing emotions and enhancing levels of confidence and self-worth, and they influence feelings of love and hate. Depending on the potency and color, remedies can restore vitality and joy. They directly affect energy levels in people who were completely exhausted and shut down from chronic and even terminal disease. When given the color remedies, these patients made a remarkable shift on all levels of their being.

Orange 6X and Saccharine officianalis 30X have been used for deep depression in suicidal patients. These remedies revived the patients' energy and spirit almost immediately. This has become a prescriptive formula for deeply depressed patients who are unable to make healthy decisions or positive moves in their lives, and whose energetic systems is almost completely shut down.

Traditional Sound Healing and Homeopathic Sound Remedies

We have known from ancient times that sound—be it the use of bells, singing bowls, chanting, or toning—has a profound healing effect on our energy. Music is one of the most evocative and powerful forms of stimulation, relaxation, and rejuvenation that we have. Specific types of music, such as Indian ragas and Native American chanting, can alter our consciousness.

Homeopathic sound remedies consist of potentized notes of the musical scale that resonate with their specific chakra and directly influence the energy field related to it. The notes clarify the mind and transform our attitudes about ourselves. The sound remedies heal at a profound level by clarifying our perceptions of the world within and around us. Strengthening the astral body, which influences our emotions, and working on our aversions and desires helps clarify our sense of our right to happiness, well-being, and joy.

Sound remedies can stimulate deep levels of joy and laughter, release anxiety and a sense of separation, and help us form clear speech and profound thought. They tone the mind, helping us find ease and pleasure, and deepen our inner knowing and receptivity to spiritual guidance and protection.

Sound remedies can be used in conjunction with homeopathic color remedies or as individual remedies on their own. They are kept purposefully at a low potency because they are very strong and powerful. At this point in their evolution, they do not need further potentization.

Symptoms and the Subtle Energy System

It is vital for a practitioner to understand that when a patient complains about certain emotional or physical problems, the person is alluding to an imbalance in their subtle energy system. For example, we know that pain refers to an imbalance in the astral forces, and low energy or vitality refers to an imbalance in the etheric forces.

As we look for the basis of a person's health problems, it is essential to find out what they are experiencing on the emotional level. The Energy Assessment in this book reviews each chakra to help determine where a patient is functional or dysfunctional. If we look at personal problems as a

causative factor in a patient's life, without recognizing that each person creates their reality by virtue of their attitudes or thoughts, we are doing our patients (and ourselves) a serious injustice. By not helping them take responsibility for their destiny, we are limiting their ability to expand their inner development and spiritual growth. Encouraging a person to come out of the victim archetype and learn to unconditionally love themselves, for example, is what homeopathic healing can offer.

When we address a person's problems and overcompensatory tendencies, we help them value their own truth in honesty and integrity. This can assist them in making healthy decisions for themselves, such as where they want to go and what they hope to do to fulfill their highest potential. We are, in effect, serving their higher consciousness (the egoic body). External circumstances can seldom be changed, but attitudes about experiences can. By changing the way we think about a situation, we release ourselves from its ties and get closer to living in freedom and love.

It lightens the burden on practitioner and client alike to come to this level of truth. This way, we literally shine light on dark areas of our unconscious and bring insight and healing into our lives. We act as facilitators when we show our patients where we see blocks and support them with the appropriate remedy to shift the balance in them from suffering to health.

Unearthing Emotional Issues Related to the Chakras

Each chakra in the etheric body focuses on a different level of emotional expression when facing different life issues and challenges at the various stages of development. This provides us with a hierarchy of awareness that helps us see individuality and personal empowerment emerge in terms of sustained physical vitality, deepening emotional truth, and the capacity to meet challenges in a mature and consistent manner.

Chakras develop throughout our lives. As we grow internally, so do they; as we become more physically present, our chakras become more resilient. The first three chakras (root, sacral, and solar plexus) are formed during the first twenty-one years of life. If they remain underdeveloped, certain healing work will need to be done to expand them to increase that person's physical vitality, enhance their personal empowerment, and strengthen their emotional well-being.

For instance, an arrested development of personal power and a failure to experience who a person truly is suggests a weakness in the solar plexus chakra. We will likely see a lack of confidence or self-esteem; ideally, this would have formed in youth, but unfortunately, the individual lacked unconditional love or a proper education to nurture a sense of well-being and self-identity. This person does not know their heart's true desire, nor do they know who they are at a core level.

Such a person often turns out to be the victim of power plays or manipulation or sometimes they may become very manipulative themselves to compensate. This may be overtly evident in a weak or impaired personality with an inability to stand up

for themselves. They may look like children well into their adulthood. From their stories, we can discern the damage to the first three chakras. They may be plagued with irrational fears, be afraid to express themselves, or have phobias or obsessions that mask their fundamental weakness and lack of strength.

People with damage to their first three chakras may also be hateful or resentful, and intense negative emotions may block their personal power. If this remains a chronic state and the person cannot break free of their limitations, they will fail to grow and thrive. We will eventually see pathology express itself in an under-functioning digestive system, such as poor assimilation, liver problems, and gallstones. We could see diseases in the liver, the seat of anger, or in the gallbladder, where timidity about love is reflected and where frustrations can fester and solidify into stones.

If such problems are treated allopathically and steroids are administered, then a slow and steady deterioration is predicted, as a person became less and less capable of harnessing their inner resources to deal with the world, both physically and mentally. They would not find the energy to face their emotional challenges and might turn to antidepressants or recreational drugs. Allopathic drugs create so much weakness that people are left bereft, weakened, and incapable of harnessing their strength. This is a problem that healers and doctors see every day.

Instead, there are homeopathic remedies that address these problems and their pathology. There is a direct correlation between the colors and sounds and the homeopathic remedies used. These can be found at the back of the book. Reliance on allopathic medication is a diminishing return in terms of vitality, insight, and holistic treatment.

It is important to look at the energetic and emotional causative factors in any case where there is imbalance. If we treat only a patient's pathology without looking at the deeper underlying issues, we are not helping them in the long run; we are merely providing a quick fix for their problems. We may even be suppressing their physical symptoms with a treatment that does not consider the more serious underlying emotional and mental issues.

In our example of a solar plexus chakra imbalance, homeopathic healing can strengthen the patient's inner psychological state, as well as the chakra, by reinforcing egoic strength. Color or sound remedies can do this energetically, directly stimulating the solar plexus and thus increasing the flow of energy through the chakra into the ductless gland, in this case, the pancreas, which in metaphysics is known as the seat of joy.

Other homeopathic remedies address the underlying weakness as well. Sound, color, and deeper-acting homeopathic remedies stimulate digestion at both the physical and emotional levels. Homeopathy offers the choice of working at many levels to help the patient through their difficulties. However, the remedies must have a parallel resonance with the patient's body, mind, and spirit.

Following the Law of Cure, balance first reappears at the mental and emotional levels, as people

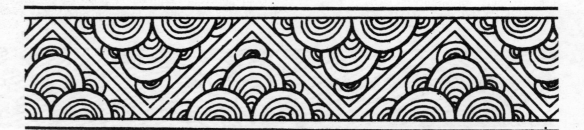

Continued ➡

gain greater self-confidence and faith in their ability to get on with their life. They begin to live the kind of life they wish for and become stronger in creating healthy boundaries, standing up for themselves, and saying no to what does not work for them.

Healing then moves into the physical arena, and the pathology begins to disappear. Physical pathology begins to clear when the egoic and astral forces are reconciled and can channel sufficient energy through the etheric body to heal the physical body.

We have seen in the provings that color and sound remedies transform the energy of under-functioning chakras and help heal emotional as well as physical dysfunction. Throughout all the provings, patients repeatedly made statements that they were "better able to cope" and "stronger in myself." This signifies that their chakras and their subtle bodies were more functional, and the patients had more control over how they used their energy.

Emotions are not the only cause of physical distress, but they do play a very large part in the healing process. There are often hidden issues in a person's life that are deeply rooted in their energetic and subtle bodies. These become triggered by stress and then appear on the surface as symptoms.

Emotional issues come up to be healed, and it is a great sign of healing when emotions that have been deeply suppressed begin to surface. It is a sign that the vital force is reanimated. In homeopathy, our philosophy is "better out than in." We want physical and psychical toxins released from the field. That gives tranquility to the physical and subtle bodies; then healing can happen.

Healing Ungroundedness in the Root Chakra with Color and Sound

If people are ungrounded and disconnected from the realities of their physical life, this is reflected in their energy system. This ungroundedness will show up as a lack of vital heat in their metabolism, which we would see as red and orange light. They will lack strong, vital energy in their lower chakras, and their other centers will appear weak and depleted.

They may either shun the colors and sounds that are associated with these chakras or they will have a strong desire for them. Their desire for these colors is how they compensate for their energetic depletion.

Often by asking people which colors they like and dislike we can determine which chakras are in need of treatment. Asking about the emotional issues that correspond to these chakras can confirm a diagnosis; in most cases, the colors and related qualities are identical.

Healing can be administered in the form of a homeopathic color or sound remedy. The potencies range from 6X to 30C. Depending upon the patient's degree of disconnection and separation, the remedy they will need can be repeated over a period of time. As the color or sound remedy is ingested into the system, it stimulates the chakras that correspond to the color and musical note remedy, and it creates a resonant field where healing takes place.

As the person's energy becomes more balanced, they will need less stimulation and fewer doses of the color or sound remedy. This is an indication that the remedy is working and healing is under way.

The patient's emotional behavior will indicate when their chakra has been stimulated. This is true with both color and sound remedies. The patient may show signs of irritation, anger, or frustration,

or may suddenly appear more relaxed, at ease, or empathic and understanding. They may develop a stronger appetite for more earthy things, such as food, exercise, sex, or material items. Irritability is a life sign and one of the signs that the system is awakening or coming out of its anesthetic state of passivity. This should not be suppressed.

If an ungrounded person, who had little interest in food, suddenly develops a strong appetite, it indicates the remedy is working. Patience, order, stability, a concern for physical security, and a desire to make their dreams come true are also signs of grounding. These are aspects of the root chakra and are associated with a strong vital force. Anger could also be a symptom that indicates they are becoming grounded.

The issues related to each chakra and the color and sound that correspond with them are given in the charts at the end of this book. Grounding and survival, as well as family or tribal issues, are related to the root chakra, whose color remedy is red and sound remedy is the note C. When a person is tired and worn out, orange or D are the remedies to consider. These work on the sacral chakra and help with rejuvenating physical energy.

These therapeutics are guided by emotional issues, and the color or sound remedy is administered accordingly. It is a simple and easy system to follow, neither complicated nor complex. It moves beyond the general physical symptoms and becomes anchored in life issues and developmental stages in an individual's life. However, it does require that the practitioner be attuned to the emotional reality of their patient.

Since we are constantly evolving and growing, we may need different sound and color remedies at different stages of our life. Classical homeopathy prescribes a constitutional remedy, which is an individual's signature remedy. With color and sound remedies, we can use the entire color spectrum or musical scale, depending on what needs to be addressed in a person's energy system. There is no one remedy as in classical homeopathy; there are many, which can be used at different times, to deal with different challenges.

We can facilitate the process of change and transformation when we acknowledge our emotional truths and take responsibility for ourselves. If we suppress and deny our issues, then we will become susceptible to physical pathology. Suppression ages us and makes our energy stagnant. When we become physically ill, it is difficult to sort out our emotions, which, by the time we are facing physical crisis, may be confused and entangled. Staying in touch with our feelings is important. This connection is a barometer for our responses to life around us.

Transforming Limited Beliefs and Attitudes

Every day in private homeopathic practices, people seek help for deteriorated health. They are often very unhappy about some aspect of their lives. And they often subscribe to the victim archetype by not doing what they want with their lives, afraid to explore the realm of possibilities that can give them happiness and satisfaction. They are stuck, fixed in a pattern of limited self-belief. They are also fixed in an archetypal response to situations they feel they cannot or will not change.

Their energy levels may be as low as their spirits. They are out of balance and out of alignment with their destiny. And their personal colors may be dark, dull, and generally unhealthy.

When you hear people say that they will wear only a certain color and would never consider

another, you know they are limited in their beliefs. What is it that they get from this one color? When they say a certain color makes them feel anxious or fearful, you know that they are unwilling to make a life change. This is an indication of blocked energy. The same is true about choices in music. What is it that we seek in sad music? In any music that we listen to repeatedly? Are we soothed or satiated by these sounds? There are so many responses to music—it is important to be aware how it affects us.

Exploring the attitudes and archetypes affiliated with the chakras helps people open up to the realm of possibilities for how they can transform their lives. Using color and sound remedies changes both a person's inner and outer vibrations, bringing healing to negative and fixed attitudes and beliefs. One of the things we witness when people begin to heal is a shift in the way they look at color and sound. Their choices for both expand and become more balanced.…

The Chakras: Qualities, Colors, and Sounds

This section discusses the chakras, their individual qualities, and the colors and sound remedies that work with them.

The Root Chakra — Red and Middle C

The root chakra's primary quality is a sense of grounding, defined as a realistic way of engaging and connecting with the world around us. It means we are present in ourselves, aware, alert, and resonant with our surroundings. When we are grounded, we lie in our bodies, not hovering over them, which we do when our spirit is disincarnate. We also tackle life's challenges in a positive, wholesome way that allows us to validate ourselves no matter what happens. Health in this chakra assures our ability to manage life's essentials by securing what we need to sustain life, such as food and shelter, for ourselves and our family. Survival is the main issue of this chakra. It relates to how we connect to our family, community, tribe, and nation. It also relates to organizational and administrative skills. This is the chakra where we distill order out of chaos. Via this chakra, we build, we connect, we develop, and we participate in life as fully as we can.

Patience, the ability to see projects and relationships through to their natural conclusion, is also an aspect of this chakra. We persevere and do not give up. A strong sense of grounding and determination is required to stay on track and develop our patience. People who are not grounded lack patience. They are easily victimized and frustrated and give up too soon.

Another quality the root chakra provides is the ability to create a wholesome structure for our life that is both meaningful and fulfilling. This means we allow life to unfold in healthy and creative ways that we can pursue. Structuring our time and energy so that we can make the best use of our gifts and skills helps us fulfill our destiny.

Stability is an essential quality of a healthy root chakra. Constant dramas or crises only deplete and drain our vital energy. Stability and consistency help us hold the fort when everything and everyone around us is in despair or panic. Leading a stable life, which is both rhythmic and routine, keeps us stable and on course during change.

The root chakra also offers a sense of security, which is vital. If we don't feel safe, we will never settle in, settle down, or settle into ourselves. Many people have no deep sense of inner or outer security in their lives. They live with constant threat or

Continued ➔

peril, which drains away precious life energy, creating a weakened immunity system and opening the door for illness to take hold. It is essential to feel safe in one's self and in the world in general. No one should feel threatened in their own private haven, even if it's just a small room where you can be yourself and rest. A person with little or no inner security cannot thrive.

In order to ground our creativity, we need to believe that we can manifest our dreams into reality. We must learn to trust life and believe that we are here on earth to fulfill a higher purpose. The ability to manifest our dreams into reality is a very important aspect of the root chakra.

The root chakra's functionality can become impaired whenever there is uprooting or drastic change in one's life. Dysfunction can be the result of war, poverty, divorce, separation, abuse, or disease. Cultivating trust, hope, and the belief that we are meant for joy, happiness, and goodness keep the root chakra open and expanding.

The Roots of Desease

When homeopaths describe the roots of disease, they refer to miasms, or genetic predisposition for disease, which are reflected in the root chakra. In homeopathy, five miasms are considered to be the root causes of disease: psoric, sycotic, syphilitic, cancerous, and tubercular. A person with a psoric predisposition will be overwhelmed by struggle and conflict and want to give up. Someone with a sycotic predisposition will want to conquer their environment and will run the risk of becoming ill from excess work. Those with a syphilitic predisposition will be unusually creative and then begin to destroy themselves in their attempts at success. Those with a cancerous predisposition will design their lives so that they remain unfulfilled or unexpressed. A tubercular miasm reflects itself in restlessness and longing. (Refer to a classical homeopathy guide for a discussion on the miasms. They are too complex to discuss in this book.) Our predispositions also mean that certain types of situations will make us susceptible to particular imbalances. How we respond is governed by our miasmatic, genetic inheritance and whether these tendencies have been treated homeopathically.

The root chakra, which stores our genetic inheritance, governs the adrenal cortex and the medulla of the kidneys. When we need to draw upon our reserves of energy, we call up what the Chinese call ancestral chi, or energy, which is stored in the adrenal cortex of the kidneys.

Whenever we fall into our chronic patterns of response, which have accumulated over generations, we are activating our "roots." This can be either positive or negative. If, for instance, people find themselves victims of life, they may need to harness their strength and reserves to create a new and better life. We have the ability to transform the victim archetype to one of mother, nurturer, healer, and giver. The choice to change is always ours.

This core vitality and strength goes beneath our primary responses and gives us the ability to rebuild a structure, create better security and more stability, and patiently reestablish order in our lives. It allows us to refashion our dreams so we are able to manifest what we need and see what we desire.

The root chakra is also related to issues of family and tribe, and the attitudes that maintain their continuity. The issues of this chakra are not related to higher consciousness as much as to survival patterns that kept the family alive. We need to ask ourselves whether we still need to be in survivor mode, or whether we can ease down into life, enjoy ourselves, create a stable and centered existence, and live creatively and productively.

Determining Color and Sound Remedies for the Root Chakra

The color red and the musical note middle C are remedies we would use to treat any dysfunction of this chakra. They can be given in low potency, repeated twice a day; when stability becomes apparent, then one 30C remedy can be administered. If there is real fear about survival, then use both the color and the note at the same time.

To determine whether a person needs the note or the color, ask whether this person needs the energy of grounding or needs to reflect on survival. If it is both, then give both. If they need more energy, then the color remedy would precede the sound remedy. Give the remedy that offers the primary solution, and when they stabilize, use the other remedy.

THE SACRAL CHAKRA—ORANGE AND THE NOTE D

The qualities of the sacral chakra, which is located two inches below the navel and two inches into the pelvis, revolve around ease, pleasure, sexuality, creativity, and abundance. They relate to the manner in which we choose to live on the physical plane, and, ultimately, how deeply and lovingly we value ourselves. These life issues reflect how we feel about ourselves, including our bodies, our pleasures, and the things we cherish. These attitudes create vitality, good health, and physical well-being, and give us a sense that we are entitled to pleasure, wealth, beauty, and abundance.

Another aspect of this chakra is focused on how we look after our physical body in terms of cleanliness, beauty, care, exercise, proper eating, rest, and time for relaxation. Physical vitality and the ability to move freely and joyfully are also governed by this center. Pleasure is an issue for most people, and it is reflected in the ways that we open ourselves to seeking joy, happiness, and creating a standard of physical well-being.

If we are plagued by guilt and feel we must suffer, and feel burned out often, then we do not have a healthy second chakra. We wind up giving away what we want or going without pleasure because we feel our duty lies in sacrifice. We then live out a martyr's archetype.

The good we are able to enjoy strengthens and fortifies this chakra. Pleasure supports life and gives us the will and the energy to do the tasks we have set for ourselves. We choose the things we want, as well as the jobs we do.

Pleasure sustains us when life is challenging, and it recharges us for our work. It stimulates expansion at every level. How we view our right to pleasure is what defines this chakra's function.

Sexuality is part of this chakra's strength and vitality. Dysfunctional or disconnected sexuality is an indication that this center is not balanced. Problems with fertility, menstruation, or reproduction, including difficult births, suggest a person has unhealthy ideas and attitudes about sexuality. Other problems, such as premature ejaculation, impotence, and low libido, also reflect an imbalanced sacral chakra.

In general, this center is universally dysfunctional, because of the way the world generally views sexuality. Sexuality is cut off from the heart and is used as a commodity throughout the world. When people's worth is measured by their material wealth and what they have, not who they are, their sexuality will be dysfunctional.

At an energetic level, people who are dependent on constantly recharging their sacral chakra energy will repeatedly grasp the external validations of sex and money as a way of reaffirming themselves. This suggests weakness and fear at their core, as well as a lack of personal identity.

This chakra becomes strong through a rhythmic, intentional life that honors a person's body, mind, and spirit. It implies balance in all things, from what we eat to the levels of physical engagement we partake in. Learning to enjoy ourselves and finding down time from demands and stress soothes our nervous system and replenishes this chakra.

This chakra controls the sense of appetite, so eating disorders and greed are reflected here. Interestingly, this chakra also controls the body's fluid balance. In homeopathy, we look at retentive emotions as a causative factor in fluid retention. This center also governs emotions. When people swell up, it is often suppressed emotions that they are unwilling to experience that are creating the condition.

The sacral chakra also controls our sense of abundance. A person may overemphasize or underemphasize wealth and material possessions, which raises the question of how someone feels about experiencing life's goodness. One must deeply honor one's self to value one's self above any material possessions and enjoy the beauty and power of the physical world.

Determining Color and Sound Remedies for the Sacral Chakra

Many physical illnesses that revolve around fatigue and exhaustion respond well to homeopathic orange and the note D. These are the resonant color and sound for the sacral chakra. They regulate and stabilize the energy flowing into the physical body through this chakra, helping people regain their health and vitality.

Orange can be used whenever there is a need for more physical vitality. It energizes this chakra and is good for people who are depleted and low of energy. When orange is combined with pink, a sense of well-being is created. Pink is associated with mother love and brings order to this center. The note D stimulates vitality and joy; it can be used by itself or together with orange where there is serious dysfunction.

THE SOLAR PLEXUS CHAKRA—YELLOW AND THE NOTE E

The solar plexus chakra relates to our sense of personal worth: knowing who we are without any veils to disguise our true nature.

Self-worth, self-esteem, confidence, and personal power are all qualities that are associated with this chakra. They reflect a deep sense of personal

Continued ➤

identity. The stronger their sense of self, the more a person takes command of their life and makes healthy choices. People who make unhealthy choices in their lives and get caught in compromising situations where they become manipulated, treated badly, or abused may have issues with personal identity. When patients speak of situations in which they cannot stand up for themselves or fight for their rights, we know they need to fortify the solar plexus chakra.

An unhealthy solar plexus chakra is reflected on a physical level by problems with the gallbladder, liver, stomach, small intestine, and pancreas. Hyperacidity, ulcers, and digestive disorders all indicate that a person is blocking feelings of aggression, fear, or anxiety. They are literally swallowing their feelings and not putting a stop to abuse in their lives.

Another aspect of the solar plexus chakra is freedom of choice. This means having the awareness to know that we can choose what we want and how we want to do things. People who have given over their power to choose and allow others to make their choices have given away their power. Calling our power back from all the projections we have created is a way in which we strengthen our solar plexus chakra and ourselves. Calling our power back empowers us and makes us whole.

Cultivating the power to live out our destiny requires a sense of purpose and worth. When we buy into any form of invalidation because of our age, sex, race, or sexual preference, we are diminished. When we collude with a negative image of ourselves we give away our power.

When we forget who we are, such as in a difficult job or a challenging relationship, and we fail to speak our truth, we weaken this center. We must believe in our worth and know that we are good and loveable and that we deserve to be treated in a loving way.

Determining Color and Sound Remedies for the Solar Plexus Chakra

Yellow and the note E can help transform the energy of the solar plexus chakra. It focuses on issues of self-worth, confidence, personal power, and freedom of choice. Yellow can energize this chakra and provide a deeper sense of power, authority, and mastery in dealing with situations. It can provide energy to the digestive system and help tonify the liver, gallbladder, stomach, and pancreas. The musical note E can be used to reflect on issues of Selfhood and ideas about power and worth. The note helps the mind form clear ideas about who we are and what we feel we are worthy of having in this life.

THE HEART CHAKRA—GREEN AND PINK AND THE NOTE F

The heart chakra is concerned with all aspects of love, peace, and joy. It works on two levels. One level is the heart itself and the other is the heart protector, which acts as a shield against whatever is negative and hurtful. The heart protector corresponds to the pericardium in the physical body. This shield also acts to protect the purity and innocence of the human heart from exposure to harsh or unloving experiences. The heart protector provides a safe refuge and sanctuary for the heart to reside; it sustains the core of our being from pain and abuse.

The heart protector's core energy is made from the fabric of our experiences of love, whether that is family love, personal friendship, partnerships, love of nature, love of animals, or spiritual love. For those who have experienced deep abandonment and unloved lives, energy channeled from the spirit realm often acts to shield the heart from breaking.

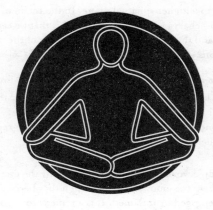

Love doesn't always have to be personal to sustain us. Love from many sources can keep us going forward in life. What we do need to acknowledge is that this love is all from the one Source.

All experiences that contribute to love, be they personal or impersonal, strengthen the heart protector. When we experience things as heartfelt, the inner chambers of our heart, the Holy of Holies, resound in joy.

Our heart's innocence and purity make us vulnerable. It takes love to strengthen us, sustain us, and protect us in the world. But love can send us soaring to the heights or bring us down so low we ache with pain. And when the heart has been too open or too closed, emotional pathology may result.

After a heart operation, people heal quickly when they are able to cry and release blocked emotions. The tears act to release pent-up energy that has been locked in the heart for a long while. Love keeps the two-way valve of the heart open and flowing.

The heart chakra is in the center of our energy system, just as the heart is the center of the body, and love is the center of our lives, providing the core strength that keeps us moving forward in life. Love asks us to forgive those who hurt us, move forward in our own way, and discover our own path. If love is what drives us forward, it will surely come to us in return. When we allow love to be that guiding star in our life, we draw to us those experiences and people who fulfill our yearning for love.

As we mature, we find higher levels and more refined ways of expressing and experiencing love. The expression of love may acquire a very different appearance than the one to which we were accustomed in our youth. Love of the heart transcends all barriers, all situations, great distances, and even death. Love endures in the soul and leaves an indelible mark that builds up the spirit and nourishes us. The ultimate truth is that love heals.

Determining Color and Sound Remedies for the Heart Chakra

The colors of the heart chakra are green, for peace and balance, and pink, for universal mother love. The musical note F is the sound for this center. Both these remedies can help heal a broken heart and fortify the heart center when it is challenged.

When used to soften the heart center, green and pink create calmness and tranquility and ease tension in the heart. Green has been used for cardiac edema and angina. Pink keeps the emotions around the heart soft, gentle, and loving. The musical note F allows us to think about love, how we can open the channel for love to reach us and transform our life.

THE THROAT CHAKRA—TURQUOISE AND THE NOTE G

The throat chakra focuses on communication and our need to be expressive and creative. It rules our ability to share our feelings and find the right words to convey our heartfelt emotions, as well as our ideas and thoughts. Our relationship to truth—both our personal truth and the higher truth of God—affects this chakra's tonicity and functionality.

This chakra governs our integrity and willpower and affects how we cultivate our personal forces of strength, flexibility, and resiliency. At a physical level, this applies to what we eat, drink, and smoke, and whether we choose to say no to what is harmful and bad for us. All substance-abuse issues pass through the narrow opening of the throat and destroy the will. The use of bad language, cursing, and gossip also weaken this center. We need to use our will to meet the difficult challenges we face in our development.

The throat is a center for truth in all regards. That applies not only to how we communicate with others, but our ability to find what is moral, right, and truthful in ourselves. In metaphysics, this center is called "the mouth of God," because it is from here that we channel our highest good. It is said that angels whisper in our ears and bring us healing and guidance. The sense of hearing is a throat chakra function.

If we cannot cultivate a strong will or we are too busy with external affairs and fail to hear our inner guidance, this chakra becomes congested and blocked. If we allow slander, negativity, or invalidation to corrode our sense of Self, we are not valuing the precious life energy we have been given or our true nature.

Right use of will is a very important aspect of the throat chakra. When we abuse alcohol or tobacco, or when we use drugs, either recreational or allopathic medicine, we weaken our will and diminish our ability to protect ourselves against what is harmful and damaging to our core. If we persist in abusing our systems, we will find it increasingly difficult to harness our will for purposeful tasks. We will give up on ourselves and the things that really mean something to us. When this chakra is balanced, there is space for feelings to be expressed and for thoughts to arise freely.

It is through the throat chakra that we are linked to a higher source of light and truth. This is the point where we channel our Higher Self. Energy enters the back of the throat center and projects onto the front of the throat. This is where communication is expressed to the world. When we commit to being truth tellers, our integrity levels soar and our throat becomes a channel for truth, clarity, and vision.

Integrity is our ability to "walk our talk." This means that we do what we say we are going to do, to the best of our ability. Vital moral impulses work through us and find direct expression in our lives—in our relationship with others, in our work, and in the things that anchor us on this earth plane. Having integrity refers to our ability to relate to the world from the place where we are whole and complete. This is reflected in the timbre of our voice, as well as in the words we speak.

Children who have been abused, people who have been taught not to speak their truth, or those who have taken many drugs over a prolonged period of time have a very weak throat chakra. It takes a strong act of will to control our negativity, express our thoughts and feelings from a place of personal power and responsibility, and ask for what we want and what we believe is ours. Proper communication skills, which allow us to say what is in our heart in an appropriate manner, help to strengthen this chakra.

Determining Color and Sound Remedies for the Throat Chakra

The color associated with the throat chakra is turquoise. It helps strengthen this center and seal

Continued ➡

off energy, which tends to dissipate as a result of blocked emotions. Turquoise can be used for physical problems with the jaw, mouth, and throat. It is also excellent for people who cannot express their emotions. The musical note G opens the ears and throat and allows for clear, resonant thinking. It can help us clear the patterns of fear associated with speaking our truth. This note can expand our hearing so that we are tuned to our higher truth.

THE BROW CHAKRA—INDIGO BLUE AND THE NOTE A

The brow chakra is located between the eyebrows, and in yoga it is known as the control center. It functions as an antenna, allowing us to perceive such things as safety and danger. In a normally developed brow chakra, which begins to bud in early adolescence and becomes fully functional by the time of our Saturn return at age twenty-eight, you will find such qualities as discernment, wisdom, knowledge, intuition, and imagination taking hold. When a person is endangered, especially if they had angry or volatile parents or unsupportive siblings in childhood, this chakra will develop very quickly, even prematurely, to help them see their way through crises and adapt to change. Some of the strongest clairvoyants are those who grew up in unsafe homes or countries.

The brow chakra controls many vital functions and is our conscious link to our life choices and how we function in the world. Our imagination, an aspect of the brow chakra, is used to visualize what we want in our future. It helps us see what action we need to take and how we want events to unfold. It helps us make our dreams become reality. This is the realm of imagination.

The intuitive function of the right brain allows us to know the truth about people and situations. It helps us develop wisdom from our life experiences. Wisdom is this center's chief goal. It reflects our capacity to acquire wisdom from negative experiences in our lives and distill it into a moral impulse that can be a guiding light. We can cultivate wisdom by looking at the difficult and challenging times in our lives and asking ourselves what we learned. This way, we build a treasury of wisdom out of our hardships. It is said in the Bible that wisdom is more valuable than gold.

Knowledge about how to live a happy and useful life also contributes to a well-functioning brow chakra. Knowledge helps us upgrade our lives and move to the next level of creative expression and fulfillment. Discernment is another function of this chakra. It helps us to pick and choose who and what is best for our highest good. Like wisdom, discernment comes with time and experience. It is ultimately the way we can find our truth and stay on track with our lives. Saying no to what is painful and hurtful gives us a stronger sense of self and more energy to do what we know is right for us.

The brow chakra's five qualities—imagination, intuition, discernment, knowledge, and wisdom— make it the center of control for 90 percent of our vital functions. Those who have a highly developed brow chakra are able to master their lives. A weakened solar plexus, for example, will drain energy from the brow chakra, so energy spent proving our worth stops us from using our higher creative powers in a positive way. However, by placing positive thoughts and affirming our worth in this chakra, we not only strengthen the brow chakra but all the other chakras as well.

The brow chakra is important for developing our spiritual path. By living fully in this chakra, we learn the universal truths that govern human interaction. From here, we are better able to direct our

energy to a higher spiritual plane. In the realm of the brow chakra we form clear thoughts that we can act on and that will lead us to good results in the situations we face in life.

Determining Color and Sound Remedies for the Brow Chakra
Indigo blue is the color of the brow chakra, and the musical note A is the sound remedy. This is the color and sound of universal healing; they also represent detachment and are both cooling and remote.

Indigo works on the senses, especially the eyes. It can help the emotions detach when they become overly engaged or inflamed. It is a remedy for cooling what is heated, including a fever. The note A is for developing wise and grounded thinking about one's self, or about situations that require clear and focused thought.

THE CROWN CHAKRA—VIOLET AND THE NOTE B

The crown chakra sits at the top of the head. It influences pituitary and pineal functioning and governs our communion with the spirit realm, which is the highest Source of consciousness. Its function is to help us live in bliss, peace, and beauty. It strongly influences our aesthetics and helps us create harmony. It also connects us to that place within ourselves where tranquility and serenity live.

When the crown chakra is impaired, we see such health problems as epilepsy, brain tumors, strokes, and disjointed mental patterns develop. Whenever there are physical problems in this area, there will be problems facing emotional issues about growth, maturity, and natural development. People with these problems often may wish to remain in an undifferentiated, amorphic state, not wanting to grow up or mature or have to take personal responsibility for themselves. They wish to remain childish, tied to their parents, particularly their mother, and not face the responsibilities of an adult life.

Meditation helps to stabilize this area and can show a frightened mind the truth of what is real. This chakra is known as the "thousand-petaled lotus," and it governs illumination and enlightenment, the goal of all spiritual practice. The crown chakra controls spiritual truths and higher consciousness.

Issues of spiritual growth that surface are often resolved in this chakra. The more we attempt to live our own lives and fulfill what we feel to be our higher purpose, the more we may experience difficulties, invalidation, and hardship. Each test is there to affirm our strength, clarify our resolve, and create trust in a Higher Power. The road to individuation is fraught with peril, yet something within us drives us to grow, tell our truth to those who can listen, and define ourselves in this world and with the spirit realm. That is what energy in this chakra can do to support our growth and healing.

Stabilizing the crown chakra takes time; it must move slowly. Invasive therapies or harsh medication can shock and overwhelm the nervous system, which is profoundly affected by the crown chakra.

Determining Color and Sound Remedies for the Crown Chakra
Violet is the color of the crown chakra; it provides stability to this center. The musical note B also can be used to stabilize crown chakra energy. They both provide peace, act as an anesthetic, and help to control pain. Violet can also promote sleep and restful awareness. The note B helps us to think about our spiritual connections and reflect on spirit working in our life.

THE ALTA MAJOR CHAKRA—MAGENTA AND THE NOTE C

The alta major chakra sits a foot above the head and relates to our link with the collective unconscious. This chakra holds information about our past and present incarnations and the contractual agreements we made with our Higher Self before this incarnation. This center is undeveloped in most people and will open up in the new age as we all become more aligned with healing and protecting this planet.

This chakra is our telepathic link to the akashic records, which are the repository of all knowledge and activity from all time. The alta major chakra acts as a communication link with the spirit realm, and when it is in balance we know and love ourselves, and the world around us, at a deep and profound level. The more we love who we are, the more we accept our oneness with the Creator and the more we have clear intentionality about our role in making our world whole, beautiful, and complete.

Determining Color and Sound Remedies for the Alta Major Chakra
The color of the alta major chakra is magenta, which incorporates the properties of red, green, and violet. The musical note is high C. This color and sound give us spiritual understanding and a sense of creative purpose in our lives. They allow us to be repositories of the collective unconscious and to find guidance from higher spiritual realms.

Magenta provides wisdom and insight into a situation and helps us look at the bigger picture. High C helps us to think universally, focusing our awareness on a larger horizon than we have normally been used to.

The Color and Sound Remedies and Their Qualities

The qualities of the color and sound remedies can lead you to discover which remedy would work best for you or your client. We use the qualities to understand the deeper nature of our problems, and if we are lacking in one particular quality we have the opportunity to cultivate that in our life. We can use these qualities as benchmarks for our development and growth.

RED AND THE NOTE MIDDLE C

Red and the note middle C are the sound and color of the root chakra, which deals with survival, administration, organization, structure, and security. This center focuses on the emotional qualities of patience, stability, structure, security, and the ability to make our dreams come true. If a person is able to live sufficiently from this center, they are ready to create the next level of their life, a level that relates to pleasure, sexuality, financial abundance, and well-being.

RED

Red is the color of life. It flows through our bodies. It is found in all forms of nature, from the red clay of the earth to the garish feathers of a desert cardinal flying from cactus to cactus. We value red for its vibrancy; we love it as a metaphor for courage, vitality, and even danger.

Red has the slowest vibration and most dense energy field of any color. It also has the longest wavelength and the lowest energy level of all colors. It is a heavy color with no respite from engagement. Red forces us to notice it, whatever its form may take. When we see red, we are pulled into it and connected with it, whether we want to be or not.

Continued ➔

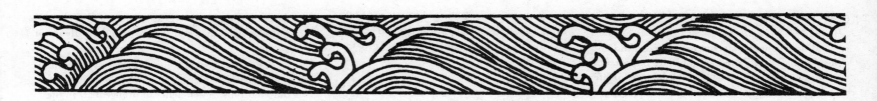

We notice red; it is the first color the human eye will see in a series of colors. It is used to alert the senses and to convey messages of caution. It is believed that very early man could see only red, yellow, and black—the colors of warning. As we have evolved, our ability to identify color has developed, but red remains the primary color that the eye distinguishes from all others.

Red relates to the planet Saturn and governs our physical and material existence. It is the first color to intrude on the senses when one has been in a darkened space. It is believed that, of all colors, babies see red first because it is the color that has surrounded them for many months.

Red carries the greatest emotional impact of any color. It is the color of passion, lust, and violence. It pulls us in and heats us up. It warms our feelings. It is impossible to be impassive and remote in its field. Long exposure to red is said to quicken the heart rate, cause adrenaline to be released into the bloodstream, and give a sense of warmth. Red stimulates our senses, and people sitting under red light for more than a few minutes report a heavy, leaden feeling, irritation and anger, and a quickening of the pulse.

When things are painted red, they appear nearer than they truly are. Red has the effect of making spaces appear small and congested. It is a color that demands attention and says, "Here I am. Look at me; see me." Its conspicuous power makes it the obvious color to wear when giving commands. It is used in military uniforms because it is believed to charge the blood and lend courage. This color is linked to combat, aggression, and a martial spirit.

Color has long been used in medical diagnoses, and red suggests inflammation and a quality of disorganized blood, seen especially on people's faces when they are excited or frightened. Red is also associated with body heat. In China the word for blood translates as "blood red." The first association with this color is that of our own blood.

Red feeds and nourishes the blood. It is associated with the heart and is used in healing to enhance circulation. It is also associated with the physical, carnal aspects of life. Too much red has been known to raise blood pressure and create irritability and anger. We have an expression in English that when we are angry "we see red." This could be the result of elevated blood pressure, which inflames the blood vessels in the eye and actually creates an optical vision of red.

The bond between earth, life, and red is found in every culture on our planet. Rituals involving blood, for both men and women, are found in all tribal societies. Tribesmen in Kenya drink the blood of their cattle for nourishment and strength. They honor red as the essence of life. They also wear red-dyed robes to honor life. Graves found in prehistoric sites in East Africa were painted with red ochre. The poet William Butler Yeats said that red was the color of magic in every country and has been so since the very earliest times. Red is synonymous with life.

Esoterically, red represents the final stage in alchemy before turning base lead into gold. It had great import for the old alchemists, who were the precursors to homeopaths. Anger is often thought to be the final step before enlightenment, with alchemy corresponding to the inner stages of awareness.

Red is associated with iron and can be given whenever the blood is lacking that mineral. It is indicated for anemia or any immunodeficiency disease, whether it is given with colored lights or in homeopathic potency. Red works well when people need to be earthed, or grounded, to bring them out of their mind and into their body and feelings.

When people are recovering from illness or when they have been uprooted from their ordinary life through loss, shock, or trauma, this color helps them regain their footing, becoming grounded. Red stimulates a person's sense of their right to existence. It is also indicated whenever healthy boundaries have been violated. It enhances our sense of place and promotes passions that we need in order to choose a meaningful and fulfilled life. Red suggests independence and freedom.

People who need red are infirm and weak, low in their life force, or too involved with the spirit realm and not "on the ground." It is a color with great vital energy. It can be used homeopathically for people who have inflammations on the phyical level or deep emotional suppression that keeps them disconnected from their reality.

Too much red can create hemorrhage and an overflow of feeling, and it is to be used cautiously. It is suggested that a medium potency be given and the patient be observed over a period of three to four days before repeating the remedy.

When we use homeopathic remedies such as ferrum, or cinnabaris, which is mercurius sulphate, we would not use red as a support remedy, as these remedies contain large quantities of this color. Mercurius sulphate is a red mineral that has all the characteristics of a person with an abundance of red in their energy field. Its picture contains violence and manipulation and reflects an emotional person who is suspicious and seeks to hold onto power, in other words, a person who is very red by nature.

Mercurius sulphate creates inflammation of the bones, burning pains, and swollen glands, which can inflame and indurate. Mercurius sulphate patients fear murder and being murdered, poverty, dirt, and ugliness. This reflects a deeply dysfunctional root chakra, having an excess of red energy congested and blocked in this chakra.

It would be best to use one of the higher colors to help decongest the red energy in this patient's chakra. It is evident with mercurius sulphate that, at a certain level, there is also an impaired crown chakra where spirituality is not being nurtured and the moral impulses are not connected with a higher spiritual consciousness.

Red can also be combined with plant remedies, especially those that survive in winter and have a healing effect on the vital force, such as Helleborus, Bryonia, and Arnica. These remedies possess a high vital force that is capable of restoring vitality in those who are weak or prostrated. Carbo vegetalis and Carbo animalis also possess red energy and can be used in conjunction with red to awaken, enliven, and restore low vitality.

Red should not be given to someone who is unable to express their rage or anger. It will stimulate these emotional forces they have blocked or deeply suppressed and may create an explosive reaction. For example, in the original provings, red 30C stimulated one woman's emotions right before her menstrual period to the point that she tried to stab her husband with a fork. Her emotions ran high and she had no filter to control herself. Red needs to be given with caution to someone with emotional issues, certainly not above a 12C potency and not repeated frequently. The patient should be warned that they could become very irritable.

Homeopathic red can be used very successfully to stimulate the birthing process and gently help bring new life into the world. It stimulates the cervix to dilation. Conversely, it should not be given to anyone who is terminally ill and ready to pass over. They would need green for peace or violet for spirituality.

Wherever people are slow to react to life, need grounding, or lack strength, red is the color to consider. It can be given to sick people in very low potency to help their vitality if they are infirm and their vital forces are slow to reactivate. However, in treating the elderly, do consider using magenta, as it is a more appropriate remedy.

THE NOTE MIDDLE C

When the note middle C was being proved as a remedy by four women at the same time in the same room, they all experienced a feeling of stony heaviness, solidity, and a lack of mentality. These were intelligent and active women who, after taking the remedy, became slow and lethargic and felt like they had "turned to stone." They had trouble thinking and sat very still for long periods of time without speaking or connecting with one another. The women reported feeling strong, present, and unyielding. One woman said she felt she had lost her "mind" because she had no thoughts.

This is the homeopathic signature of the middle C sound remedy, and it suggests widespread use for people who are slow to move, slow to think, and slow to react. It would be an excellent remedy for those who have problems recovering from chronic illness or who have suffered a head injury and are slow to regain their clarity and get "up to speed" in their life. This may prove to be an excellent remedy for head injuries.

Middle C is also useful for treating Alzheimer's disease, where the mental functions deteriorate quickly and the ability to think clearly slows down. It can be used when memory is impaired, mental energy is low or lacking, or when people need to ground their mental processes, because it relates to rhythm, organization, rules, and regulations.

This remedy, as with all sound remedies, works on the astral forces, which control thinking, aversions, and desires. It can be used to help people who fail to think about their lives and need more mental stimulation. Middle C helps to focus thinking on survival issues since it corresponds to the root chakra.

This musical note has helped people who felt disconnected from their homes and families. It works to reestablish the links between Self and home, Self and community, Self and country, Self and the earth. Whenever there has been an interruption in the cycles and rhythms of one's life, this remedy helps to reestablish those basic rhythmic patterns of existence within ordinary life. This sound remedy can be used after a divorce, separa-

Continued ➡

tion, house move, or any other fundamental change in one's life.

Middle C helps a person focus their mind on the essentials of life, who and what are important to their well-being, and how grateful they are for life. This sound remedy is made in only one potency, 5X, and can be given two or three times daily for a few days. It supports mental healing, gratitude, and self-acceptance.

RED AND MIDDLE C USES

Red and middle C can be used together or separately for the following conditions.

Physical Problems

Red and middle C can help people with poor circulation; constipation; piles, rectal and urinary troubles; problems with the feet, knees, or legs; childbirth; slow onset of labor; anemia; weakness; slow recuperative ability; immunodeficiency diseases, HIV, and AIDS; or dementia.

Contraindications: Red and middle C should not be given to people with high blood pressure or who are violent and aggressive by nature. Keep the potency of red under 12C initially to see how people respond. When you feel that their vital force is able to handle 30C, move to the next potency. Watch for changes before repeating and do not repeat this color too often. Move to middle C if there is irritation with red. Do not give these remedies at night. You can use red and middle C together when someone is really deeply traumatized and disconnected. Red and middle C would have the effect of bringing their consciousness back into their body and making them very present.

Emotional Issues

Red and middle C address issues of lack of grounding and feelings of disconnection, not belonging to home, family, community, or the planet. These remedies work for people who are spaced out. It is suited when there are feelings of detachment with little or no affect or emotional expression, or a lack of emotional awareness.

These remedies can be used for unstable people who have no structure to their life, who are unable to patiently await their goodness to unfold, who have trouble settling in a place, or who are unable to see a horizon in their life. Red and middle C can be used for deep depression and anxiety about survival. It is good for suicidal tendencies and long-term unhappiness.

Contraindications: Do not give red or middle C to people with a history of violence. Do not give these remedies at night.

Mental Issues

Red and middle C are good for people who are absorbed in spiritual practices and do not think about the practical realities of life, people who are very detached and live in another sphere of reality, dreamers, and indolent people who are unable to work or support themselves.

Contraindications: Do not give red or middle C often to people who suppress rage and channel their feelings into rationality. Do not give these remedies at night.

Spiritual Issues

Red and middle C can be used for people who are locked into giving their spiritual energy to others, who do not feel they have a right to their own life, who are enslaved and unable to freely live their lives, and who need spiritual courage to make the next move in their life. At this level, red and middle C give courage and help people find the inner resources to break destructive and unwholesome patterns.

These remedies also can be used for abandoned babies, those put up for adoption, and adults who were orphaned at a young age. These remedies help all those who were abused and lost their connection to their right to their own life.

RED AND MIDDLE C ESSENCE

The quintessential quality of red and middle C is imploded, congested, or compacted energy—energy turned in on itself, not connected with an external presence or reality. Red is hot. Middle C is the base note. These remedies provide energy that is contracted and full of vitality, but potentially explosive. The energy is intense, dense, and slow moving.

Red provides heat, shelter, strength, and nourishment. Middle C gives stability and steadiness in the face of change. It forces people to think about themselves and their situation. These remedies relate to the mother archetype and the life force found in our blood. People who comprise this archetype ask to be contained, held in, or held back. For example, someone with the victim archetype has little or no stability, and red and middle C can act as stabilizers. They help ground, anchor, and connect....

Orange and the Note D

The second chakra, known as the sacral chakra, is the center of joy, creativity, and pleasure. It governs ease, movement, pleasure, sensuality and sexuality, well-being, and abundance. It is ruled by the archetype of the empress/emperor, who lives abundantly in the material world and enjoys the good things of life. This archetype is a metaphor for pleasure, as are orange and the note D.

The sacral chakra and its corresponding archetypes are associated with people who have a healthy appetite for life. Orange and the note D both govern a person's appetite, as the advertising industry so clearly knows. Observe the way cheap junk food advertisements are printed in orange. They appeal to the appetite on a subliminal level. Conversely, too much orange or vibration of the note D in a person's system reveals a sign of greed, an indication that the person feels they are not enough and need to compensate for those feelings. This manifests at a psychological level as wanting or needing more. This may manifest as desiring more food,

more experience, more sex, or more money, but all reflect a belief that what they have in their life is not enough.

The sacral chakra controls the water element of the body and is essential in regulating the flow of our emotions. A deficiency of orange or D in the human energy system is also linked with allergies; this means that the energetic sheaths that protect us from invasive assault are weak and need fortifying. We have also found in the provings that the craving for chocolate relates to emotional suppression and a deep longing for love. This has been transformed when the homeopathic orange or note D remedy has been given.

Patients get a tremendous sense of joy and well-being from these color and sound remedies. One prover said she laughed all day and found herself giggling for no apparent reason. This is why it has been used so successfully for depressed and suicidal patients. The two remedies have been used to treat low spirits and have been successful in lifting the energy of chronically depressed patients.

Orange and the note D provide us with a vibration that stimulates our sense of joy and enlivens our physical vitality. They restore a sense of humor. These remedies also help people who are deficient in sexual energy to regain a sense of pleasure, nourishing and stimulating the sexual organs and getting the hormones flowing again. This serves both people who have depleted their sexual center from overuse or who have not had any sexual contact for a long period of time. It is also useful when people have negative attitudes that inhibit their sexual function, or lack a sense of ease and joy in relation to their bodies. These remedies relate directly to a sense of pleasure. They can be given as a tonic when vitality is low, especially after an illness. They should never be given at night because the energy of the remedies will keep people from relaxing into sleep.

These two remedies can be used to stimulate lazy bowels and to help relieve slow onset of the menses. They can be recommended for girls with irregular periods, such as homeopathic pulsatilla types or calcium carbonicum constitutionals. However, they are not suggested for women who have a tendency to flood during menstruation.

Since orange and D both govern the water element in the body, they can be used as active diuretics to stimulate urination and ease PMS. Provers repeatedly mentioned frequent urination and a need to cry over things that disturbed them when taking the remedy. Water imbalance is directly related to suppressed emotions, and orange and D seem to activate the body's ability to release fluid and reanimate feelings. It is much gentler than the violent emotions released from using red.

Orange and D stimulate physical energy. They can also be considered for infertility if a couple is having trouble conceiving. These remedies, along with good constitutional treatment, can stimulate fertility and help bring on pregnancy. They are life-enhancing and life-promoting. It is suggested that they be used around the time of ovulation and given approximately five times daily for five days.

These remedies can cause emotional upsets and displays of anger if used too frequently, especially by people whose tempers run high and who anger quickly. In the provings, people enjoyed being social more than usual and liked to be close to one another. In the proving of D, the people taking the remedy all wanted to stay together and eat together, and they actually all ordered orange food in a restaurant. They were more friendly than usual while taking the remedy. A high sociability factor

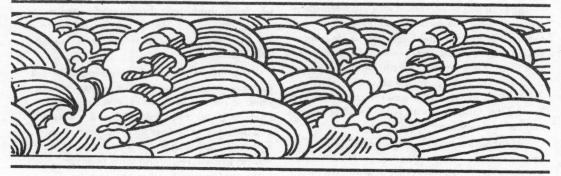

Continued ➡

fits closely with this chakra and orange and D can help shy people overcome their timidity.

ORANGE

Orange, in its various shades of coral, apricot, sienna, and umber, is the color for people who are enthusiastic about life and are eager to participate and engage with others. It is the color of vitality, and, in shades of pale orange and apricot, it represents the sensual side of our nature and addresses our love of pleasure. On the whole, it is a warm, positive, and vibrant color that lifts flagging energy and gives a bright, affirmative quality to those who wear it or decorate with it.

Orange has only one negative association; it can represent excess or indulgence, and people sometimes need the higher colors to balance lusty appetites. Orange combined with turquoise or pale blue can create a spiritual balance. Many churches throughout the world combine orange, or terracotta, and blue in their buildings. This signifies heaven and earth. It is a mixture of the physical and the spiritual. This is also seen in jewelry from the Native Americans and Tibetans, who often mix turquoise and carnelian or coral.

Psychologically, orange behaves like yellow, sharing depth, intensity, and brightness as an aspect of its nature. Orange is cheerful, expansive, rich in energy and vibrancy, and extroverted. This suggests that a person who has the heat and warmth of orange about them would also be confident, be powerful, and have an abundant sense of self-worth and self-esteem.

In Europe, there were no words for orange until the Middle Ages, when the fruit of the same name arrived from Arabia. Previously, things that were orange were perceived as an aspect of red. For instance, red hair, red clay, and even fire, which is distinctly orange, were called red. The color is also associated with the metals of copper, brass, and bronze. They all have an orange tint to them. In ancient alchemy, tin was the metal that corresponded with the sacral chakra. It is the metal linked with orange.

Orange energy is found in amber, citrine, quartz, and topaz, which is a Sanskrit word for fire. Many birds and mammals have orange coloring. It is also a color that is suggestive of food, and many highly nutritious foods are orange. One of the provers felt like redecorating her kitchen while taking the orange color remedy. She wanted to paint her walls orange. Color analysts know that decorators who use orange have a high success rate, mostly because it makes a space feel warm and inviting.

The color stands for fecundity and, in the Middle Ages, it had a sexual connotation. In an earlier bridal custom, brides were adorned with orange blossoms, which symbolized fertility. In fashion, orange is in constant demand and found in different shades and hues all year long because it addresses our sensuality.

When orange is mixed with pink in the homeopathic color remedies, it opens people up to a sense of fun and enjoyment. Some homeopathic nitric acid or nitrogen patients, who had difficulty allowing themselves to feel joy, benefited from using orange and pink in combination. When faced with a long and boring task, pink 3X and orange 12C in combination help to bring a sense of pleasure back into a person's life. Again, do not give these remedies at night, as they cause sleep disturbances.

THE NOTE D

The musical note D brings joy and laughter as a tonic for overly serious people. In the provings, an entire group of near strangers started laughing out loud and enjoyed one another in a moment of ease

and delight immediately upon taking the remedy. This remedy is used to stimulate sweetness and joy in a person bereft of these qualities who may have suffered too long.

The note D engenders laughter and happiness and can be used for people who are joyless, uncomfortable in social situations, or are too strict in allowing themselves pleasure. It can be used to help people reflect on the nature of pleasure in their lives and how they want that to manifest. It can aid people who have experienced loss or separation. It supports people when times are challenging and their energy is low. It can be used as a tonic for the astral forces when illness has required prolonged rest and recuperation.

ORANGE AND D USES

Here are ways orange and D can be use therapeutically for healing.

PHYSICAL PROBLEMS

Consider orange and/or D for bowel problems, infertility, menstrual period irregularity, slow onset of menstruation, anorexia, or appetite disorders, including people who have little or no appetite or have food cravings for chocolate and sweets. These remedies are good for people who have postviral conditions, including difficulty recovering their natural vitality after their illness. They are good for postoperative recovery and after dentistry, emotional shock, or trauma. Orange and D are excellent for menopause, myalgic encephalomyelitis (ME, also known as chronic fatigue syndrome), multiple sclerosis (MS), and other autoimmune diseases, such as HIV and AIDS.

Contraindications: Orange and D should not be given to people who have excessive anger or rage. Nor do they suit someone with an abundance of energy, as the person may become overstimulated and restless. These remedies should not be given at night.

Emotional Issues

Orange and D suit people who are depressive or feeling low emotionally. They have been used successfully along with Saccharine officianalis in 30C potency to help people who feel suicidal. They have been used on their own for depression and emotional "funk" for people whose feelings were blocked at a subconscious level and needed releasing. Both remedies also bring people into the present if they tend to feel spacey, allowing them to refocus their awareness into their physical body.

The note D, because it works on the astral, or mental, plane, helps people think positively about the things they enjoy and like doing. It helps people connect with their sexuality and desire for pleasure and their right to abundance. Orange is known as the "laughing color," as the provers found themselves happy and laughing much more than usual. Interestingly enough, everyone wanted "more." Therefore, it could be considered a remedy for overindulgence, binge eating, and excess.

During the provings, people cried more while on these remedies, releasing pent-up feelings that had been dormant. All the provers said that their sense of well-being was increased while on orange and the note D.

Contraindications: Neither orange nor D should be used with hyperactive people, nor should they be used at night.

Mental and Spiritual Issues

Orange and D are suited for anyone lacking a sense of their own well-being. These two remedies offer people who have a negative attitude about their bodies and sexuality an opportunity to open up and develop a healthy degree of self-acceptance. They bring an

awareness of the nature of pleasure and stimulate an appetite for the good things in life. They increase interest in sexuality and abundance. D can nourish creativity, playfulness, and fun, and it helps people find what is simple and delightful in life.

Contraindications: Orange should not be given to people who are persistently restless or anxious, nor should it be used at night. D should be used only during daytime.

ORANGE AND D ESSENCE

The essence of both orange and D as homeopathic color and sound remedies is a joyful, very physical state of being that nurtures life and its more pleasurable aspects. This essence resonates with joy, health, and vitality, and it can bring people who are locked up with excessive overintellectualization into the present. These remedies help people to feel their emotions if they are cut off from their feelings. They can also help release negativity and feelings of despair....

Yellow and the Note E

Yellow is the brightest of all colors in the visible spectrum, and it contains more light than any other color. The musical note E and yellow relate to the solar plexus chakra. They both convey power and presence, a sense of worth, and healthy self-esteem. Both are associated with the sun and with the metal gold.

Yellow is a warm color that gives off heat, though it is less intense than orange or red. Yellow and E can lift the spirits and give people a sense of ease and lightness; they can also help people connect to their power, deepen their sense of freedom, and acknowledge their self-worth. Most people respond to the color and the note, which represent hope and faith in the future, in a positive manner.

At a deep level, yellow and the note E affect our sense of self-worth. This is reflected in our confidence levels and the ways in which we value ourselves in relation with others. Our self-esteem and personal power show that we know who we are and what we want from life. These qualities are best represented in the warrior archetype. The dysfunctional archetype represented here is the servant, who has a diminished sense of self and weakened levels of personal power.

The association of yellow and E with the solar plexus chakra implies that a person has a healthy ego. However, too much of either the note or the color leads to an overly developed ego, and too little suggests taking a cowardly approach to challenges, or, as the slang implies, this person is a "yellow belly." From time to time, a person may need a hero's dose of courage. Yellow and E can stimulate the energy in this chakra for that. They also help balance the chakra if someone is overly inflated. Yellow given with its complement color violet works well for high levels of inflation.

Yellow lights up a drab and dull environment. It can bring a sense of radiance to clothing or a dull wardrobe. Too much yellow or too much emphasis on the note E suggests that a person is overly concerned with power and self-aggrandizement. New shades of yellow, recently developed by the automobile manufacturer BMW, suggest power and prowess on the road. They have names like Dakar Yellow (named for a challenging car race) and are reminiscent of endurance rallies.

Yellow symbolizes enlightenment because it is the color that contains the most light. The note E represents the intellect, the brighter part of the mind. Yellow has the highest reflectivity of all colors and appears to radiate outward, or to advance. The note E exemplifies the faith and hope of warmth and love, which is emotional light.

Continued ➡

In the provings, people with fears and anxieties had an affinity for yellow and E, which helped them get over periods of doubt and worry. These remedies helped end a bout of gallbladder colic in one prover who had suffered for several days with distressing symptoms before taking the remedy. Yellow generally strengthens people who have low self-esteem and helps others make clear and intelligent choices. All provers said this remedy made them feel better about themselves and boosted their confidence. One prover became pregnant while on yellow.

YELLOW

Yellow is a primary color and cannot be made by mixing other colors. For instance, orange is a combination of yellow and red; green is a combination of yellow and blue. Yellow is more closely associated with light and bright spirits than any other color.

Yellow is a diffuse and radiant energy, and if a person is not well centered, it can create an aura of confusion and make it hard to locate boundaries. Because there is so much light within this color, it can cause people to become disoriented and "spaced out," not knowing where their center is. In terms of personal development, yellow is associated with a lack of personal identity.

This color is also connected with our personal power and prowess. Through its association with gold, it relates to qualities of worth and value. It is the color of the solar plexus chakra, which represents our sense of self-worth, self-esteem, confidence, personal power, and freedom of choice.

Many body secretions are yellow and so are many foods and vitamins that we ingest. This suggests the presence of sulphur, which is a homeopathic remedy that works on the egoic forces in our personality. Sulphur is bright yellow in color.

Yellow directly affects our digestion and stimulates the stomach, pancreas, liver, and gallbladder. Too much yellow in a person's system produces jaundice or an oversecretion of bilirubin, which signifies a weakened gallbladder and liver. Too little yellow in a person's system suggests that they are not assimilating nutrients properly, and they may have problems with absorption.

Yellow is associated with the fire element required for proper absorption of nutrients. Like the sun, the color yellow implies that, when we are well in ourselves, we too shine and our systems function well. Physically and psychologically, the ability to digest our nutrients and our life experiences defines our state of health.

In food, this energy level signals the presence of vitamin A and C. Different shades of yellow evoke either the astringency of lemons and citrus or the richness of butter and cheese. In nature, yellow is caused by carotenoids and sometimes by the presence of melanin.

In the animal world, yellow is a color of warning. It is seen in tropical fish, insects, and exotic poisonous frogs. The subdued yellow of the big cats acts as a perfect camouflage for hiding in the tall, parched grasses of the bush. Such animals, like the lion and tiger, who display yellow coats, often have great presence and power.

In the early Sung dynasty in China, yellow was adapted as the imperial color, to be worn only by the emperor, his retinue, or someone wearing imperial regalia. Buddhist monks wear yellow as a sign of humility and renunciation. It is a color seen more in the Orient than in the West. In the West, yellow has been used to describe cowardice among soldiers.

THE NOTE E

The note E has been used to support clear and intentional thinking when people need to make wholesome choices for their lives. It fosters a sense of Selfhood, which may have been arrested or never developed. If a sense of Self is weak, then the organs of digestion will also be weak. The note E stimulates both the digestive process and the mental process of claiming one's power, and strengthening a sense of personal identity. The musical note E helped a woman who lacked confidence speak out about the things she had held bottled inside her for a long while. It gave her clarity of mind, focus, and ease in expressing her intellectual ideas.

YELLOW AND E USES

Here are some cases that describe the use of yellow and E.

Physical Problems

Yellow and E relate to the digestive organs and are most suited for treating stomach, liver, gallbladder, and pancreas symptoms. These remedies help to decongest blocked energy in the abdomen and are considered for any type of gastric colic. They can be helpful with diabetes, stomach disease, hepatitis A and B, and cancer of the liver or other digestive organs. They have been known to work on gallbladder colic, eliminating pain and congestion. They can be excellent remedies for assimilation problems, such as celiac disease, and can be used concurrently with other remedies that further enhance assimilation.

Both yellow and the note E stimulate the right eye and improve eyesight. According to Chinese theory, the eyes are controlled by the liver. Provers noted improved vision and were able to read without glasses when on these remedies.

When the vital force is low, yellow and E help unblock congestion and shift energy. They are extremely useful for colds and weakened lungs because they act as an astringent and work to unblock and decongest the bowels.

When there is an excess of yellow in the system, it is wise to use the complementary colors of purple and violet, or the note high C. When new babies are born with weakened livers and an excess of bilirubin in the blood, they are jaundiced. The standard treatment in hospitals is to place these babies under ultraviolet light for a few hours every day to break up the congestion in the blood. Homeopathic violet and high C can also help with this.

Contraindications: Yellow and the note E should be used as an astringent or a decongestant. They should be used in daytime only, as they can cause sleep disturbances.

Emotional Issues

Yellow and the note E can be used for issues of confidence, lack of a sense of worth, low self-esteem, or a shaky sense of personal identity. It is particularly well suited to people who give their energy and life force over to others too easily and are too open in their solar plexus chakra. These remedies strengthen the ego and help people develop their individuality. Where there is emotional weakness or vulnerability, they stimulate confidence and encourage personal empowerment.

Contraindications: People with an excessively developed ego should not use yellow and E, unless they balance it with homeopathic violet or high C, as they can increase their sense of self-importance. They should not be used at night.

Mental and Spiritual Issues

Yellow and E represent gut level intellect. These remedies stimulate the mind to help it become clear and focused. They help to transfer "gut knowing," which comes from the solar plexus chakra, to a higher mental level. They can be used to help increase memory and thinking ability, and they provide a rich potential for clarity and effectiveness. These two remedies help a person identify where they are weak and how they can grow in wisdom and maturity. They support empowerment, responsibility, and accountability, and in that way, promote moral impulses.

Contraindications: Too much yellow or E can cause a dissociated feeling from an overexpansion of the mind. Use during the daylight hours.

YELLOW AND E ESSENCE

The essence of yellow and the note E is their remarkable brightness and diffusion of energy. The color is radiant and the sound clear. They help people shine on an inner plane and claim their power and worth. The energy resembles gold on the material plane and, therefore, relates to earthly power and worth. On the spiritual plane, the energy represents lightness of mind, a willingness to transcend the limited ego, and an opening to the power of a higher plane. Yellow and E help people feel good about themselves and let their inner light shine....

Green and the Note F

Green is the most neutral of all colors, being neither hot nor cold. It sits in the middle of the spectrum and offers respite from the heat of red, orange, and yellow and the chill of blue, purple, and violet. It is the most prevalent color in nature, and it relates to nature's healing power, bringing ease and rest to frayed nerves. Green and the note F correspond to the heart chakra, and they are associated with the transpersonal issues of love, joy, peace, and unity.

People who do well with these two remedies, together or separately, are those who are undergoing volatile change and need emotional balance in their lives. These are the most balanced and neutral of all remedies. These remedies are also good for people who are resistant to change and seek or need stability.

In the provings, both the color and the note bestowed a deep sense of peace on people who were restless and out of sorts. They soothed fractious nerves when people felt agitated, providing both relaxation and tranquility. Some provers reported restorative sleep as well. When taking the remedies, people felt at ease in tense situations, with no need to hurry. The remedies also helped to relieve pain in the lumbar region of the back and behind the heart.

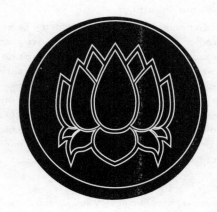

Continued ➔

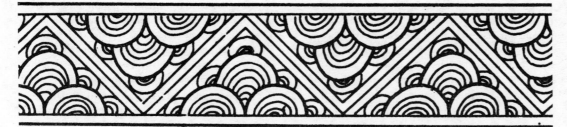

Green and the note F correspond to the emotions of love and are linked with the planet Venus, which is associated with love and beauty. Green was worn at medieval weddings to signify love, fidelity, and peace. This color gives peace of mind and helps restore balance to ailing hearts.

Green and F are both natural detoxifying agents that release fluids from the body and help drain edematous tissue. They act as diuretics for congestive heart problems and have been used successfully for cardiac edema when given as homeopathic remedies.

Associated with the heart chakra, these remedies work together with homeopathic pink, combining natural tranquility and motherly love. The note and the color can be given together with homeopathic pink. These forces represent the totality of love, care, and unity in our lives. Pink represents the universal quality of love that transcends the baser emotions of the three lower chakras.

Green and the note F are essential energies in supporting life and can sustain our efforts toward inner growth and greater harmony. That is why they are recommended for those in need of balance and tranquility.

GREEN

Green is the easiest color for the eye to see. The lens of the eye focuses green light almost exactly onto the retina. It is a tonic for the eye, which explains why eye shades and sunglasses are often tinted green to ease harsh glare. Green has been used since ancient times as a respite for sore eyes. Medieval engravers kept a piece of green beryl to contemplate and relax their eyes after long hours at work, and in ancient Egypt, the green stone malachite was crushed and made into an unguent to protect the eyes.

There are many shades of green, each suggestive of one of the color's different aspects. Most common are lime green, which contains the fire of yellow, and blue-green, which carries the creative energy of indigo and the stillness and detachment of turquoise.

Green has a duplicity at both the physical and emotional levels. It is both the color of life and the color of decay. It is associated with nausea, poison, envy, and jealousy. It is also the color of rebirth in spring and eternal peace. Its dual nature is linked with its ability to fit at both the top part of the visible spectrum and at the bottom part. It is made from a mixture of yellow and blue and is known as a secondary color because it is made of two primary colors.

As the energy of decay, plants do not grow well under green light. Fluids drain out of them, they become lifeless, and they begin to rot and decay. Green is also associated with infection in the body, and when this color is administered in homeopathic potency, it helps drain the body of pus and poisons. When given during one woman's menstruation, she reported passing large clots along with copious urination. In the provings, green was noted for symptom of frequent urination, which several provers experienced. Green is an excellent diuretic, eliminating toxins from the body. It is used for cardiac and cellular edema.

THE NOTE F

The note F represents the qualities of love and peace at the higher level of the astral plane, where desires can be quelled and aversions soothed. It helps bring balance to the emotions, which, if not disciplined, create damage and drama. F works on the heart chakra by helping us value what and whom we love. It helps us reflect on the nature of love in our life and gives us the ability to hold love as the central theme of our life. It stimulates the intelligence of the heart to be thoughtful and introspective. It serves higher consciousness by creating the platform for us to affirm our worth and honor our choices for love.

GREEN AND F USES

Here are ways to use green for physical, emotional, and mental issues.

Physical Problems

Green and F have been used successfully to drain excess fluid from the body. They act as a diuretic and help with edema, inflammation, and congestion. These remedies have been used to soothe PMS symptoms, such as when women develop engorged breasts, retain fluid in the ankles and belly, or feel highly emotional. They can be used for inflammation of the testicles or breasts and for soft tissue swelling. Both remedies can be used for both tired eyes and for headaches where there is a feeling of congestion.

Green can help women who have cystic breasts. It helps ease pain in the left breast. It has also been used, along with other heart remedies, for congestive heart failure to tonify the heart and stop fluid retention. The relief is quick, but not long-lasting.

F has been used to ease stressed nerves and provide a sense of deep tranquility after an emotional upset. It helps a person relax and calm down.

Contraindications: If there has been a serious loss of fluid from diarrhea, vomiting, or kidney failure, Green or F would not be indicated. These remedies should not be given at night since patients may need to urinate frequently.

Emotional Issues

Green and F have been used successfully on patients who have a serious lack of equilibrium in their emotional lives, who barely manage to cope with problematic situations, whose inner resources are drained, and who are tired and exhausted. It is especially good for people undergoing major life changes. Green and F help restore emotional balance and provide an opportunity to detach.

These remedies are good for fatigue and can be used whenever people are overly tired, overworked, and have trouble attaining a restful state. They help to restore peace and harmony to a stressed economy.

Contraindications: Green and F should not be given to people who need stimulation, as they are more of a tranquilizer and sedative than a stimulator. They are not to be given late at night because they may encourage urination.

Mental Issues

Green and F are excellent for people who suffer from nervous tension. They are good for those who are high strung and hysterical. Since they can soothe shattered nerves, these remedies help create a more balanced nervous system so that a person can think clearly and develop positive impulses. They make a person feel happier.

Contraindications: Green and F should not be given to indolent people who need energy. Again, they are not indicated for night use because of their diuretic effect.

GREEN AND F ESSENCE

Green and F essentially provide balance and harmony. They help restore energy to people who are exhausted and worn down without overstimulating their body. These remedies help a body release fluid, which is another form of retained energy. They give the heart stability and ease distress throughout the mind, body, and spirit. Since they relate so closely to the heart chakra, they are associated with the qualities of love, friendship, family, unity, and joy, and can help when life becomes stressful…

Turquoise and the Note G

Turquoise is a name the French used to describe the beautiful sea around the Turkish coast. Turquoise and the note G represent creativity and self-expression. They correspond to the throat chakra and represent our innate ability to express ourselves, communicate our truth, and tap into our willpower.

This color and note are associated with spiritual values and healing. Many churches are painted terra-cotta and turquoise, and much heartfelt music is written in the note of G. Santa Sophia, the great mosque in Istanbul, is made of thousands of tiny turquoise mosaics. Often the muezzin, who calls the faithful to prayer in Islam, chants in G. Turquoise and G are linked with the vast expanse of sea and sky, which engender feelings of beauty, depth, and freedom. These are the color and sound used most often in spiritual healing to connect people with their souls.

Turquoise and the note G have a calming effect on the body and are said to be able to bring down high blood pressure. These remedies are best used when people are able to relax and have time to express themselves creatively.

This color and sound nourish the soul forces working in the throat chakra. When worn as an ornament, a turquoise stone is thought to enhance creativity and promote healing. The note G opens the channel to hearing your inner voice. Turquoise and G both show a strong connection with the mouth and throat also. One prover developed a tooth abscess while proving this color remedy, which, in homeopathic terms, suggests that it could heal this condition. Turquoise has been used for this as well as for mouth ulcers, problems with the tongue and teeth, and an ulcerated throat.

TURQUOISE

Turquoise and pale blue are the colors most often chosen to express beauty in clothing and decoration. The Virgin Mary's cloak was reputed to have been pale blue, and she is often depicted as the Queen of Heaven wearing her blue cloak. Turqoise and pale blue are considered the same vibration in terms of the chakras.

The supreme Greek and Roman gods, Zeus and Jupiter, are represented by turquoise. It is associated with spirituality in the Native American and Tibetan traditions. Both cultures highly prize the stone, which they frequently use in rituals. They say it represents heaven and earth in one substance. The color has been linked with royalty and led to the term "blue bloods."

Continued ➡

In the provings, turquoise appeared to have a definite link with excess catarrh, which diminished when turquoise was taken. For example, a large, overweight woman began to lose weight while on the remedy. It is possible this color remedy stimulated her sluggish thyroid gland.

THE NOTE G

Affiliated with the throat chakra, G helps people speak up for themselves and express their truth. Wherever they have felt unwilling or unable to speak up and ask or demand what they felt they needed, this remedy supported their inner process. G allows the energy of self-expression to be communicated in a thoughtful and mindful way. It helps people think about what they want to say. It helps people gather the will necessary to move forward in life. Musicians who have used homeopathic G have reported that their music became more attuned and creative, their voice clearer, and their expression more open and vivid.

TURQUOISE AND G USES

Here are ways to use turquoise and G in healing.

Physical Problems

Turquoise and G can be used to heal inflammation, particularly around the throat and mouth area. These remedies can help clear up a cold or sore throat quickly. They help balance the thyroid and parathyroid, whether underactive or overactive, and can be given along with other deep-acting homeopathic remedies, including Thyroidinium. Turquoise and G are good for obesity when the thyroid is underactive and the patient has low energy, tires easily, and is apathetic.

These remedies also can be used for teeth and gum problems, and they work successfully in alleviating toothache. They can be considered for mouth ulcers, ear infections, sore throat, and bronchial inflammations.

Contraindications: Turquoise and G are not recommended for a person currently taking drugs or antibiotics. It would be best to wait for a few weeks until these drugs have left the system. They can be given both at night and during the day.

Emotional Issues

Turquoise and G can be given to people who have problems with self-expression. They open the throat chakra so that a person feels comfortable expressing their truth, their feelings, and their intentions. These remedies create healing on the emotional level by releasing pent-up emotional tension, and allowing it to flow freely into words or creative outlets. They stimulate communication skills and strengthen people's ability to speak up for themselves. Musicians, artists, and people who are sensitive to the inner meaning of life have benefited from taking turquoise and G, both separately and together. Turquoise has been helpful for singers and people who speak publicly.

Drugs, overeating, smoking, and drink weaken the throat, and this, in turn, weakens the will. Any time the will needs to be engaged to achieve some task and is weak or shows decreased function, these remedies are indicated. For instance, if someone wants to quit smoking, begin a diet, or reject any other personal addiction, turquoise or G would strengthen their resolve.

Contraindications: These remedies are not a substitute for communication, but they do help resolve tension where it is blocked.

Mental and Spiritual Issues

Turquoise and G relate to a person's ability to hear and express their truth. These remedies can help

people who resist speaking up for themselves, or those who fear repercussions. They may also aid people who have very fixed ideas and have trouble hearing the opinions or feelings of others. They open our channel for hearing as well as expressing our truth. These remedies work to strengthen the will so a person can clearly express their intentions.

People who are very critical of others, who gossip and speak maliciously, can benefit from this color and note. Since so much negative energy is channeled through the throat, this color and note strengthen it and make it less likely that energy will drain away and dissipate into negativity. These remedies are good for anyone who has problems differentiating the truth.

Contraindications: None.

TURQUOISE AND G ESSENCE

The essence of turquoise and the note G is their ability to stimulate the expression of truth, both the higher truth of God and our personal expression of it. They stimulate our creativity and clear a path for us to express ourselves in the highest and most joyful ways. They help define a person's individuality by strengthening their will. They work on the throat chakra and are associated with all the organs of speech, hearing, and ingestion. . . .

Indigo and the Note A

Indigo is a color of beauty and grace. It carries the energy of the cosmos in it and is reminiscent of an evening sky on a winter day. This energy is both cool and detached. It symbolizes the intellect of the mind and detachment from the emotions. Indigo and the note A are used for healing the mind and the senses, relieving what is inflamed and impassioned. Indigo and the note A relate to the brow chakra, or, as it is known in yoga, the control center. The brow chakra is the seat of the pituitary gland, which stimulates growth and controls reproductive cycles.

This color and note have the ability to lower blood pressure, cool a fever, and enhance clarity and lucidity. The color and note both work to promote detachment from overheated emotions. Indigo and the note A are closely associated with the qualities of wisdom, discernment, knowledge, imagination, and intuition. These are the qualities of the brow chakra.

Indigo and the note A represent the energy of universal truth. This energy may be slightly cold and a little merciless, but it is able to cleanse and calm the spirit by cooling the passions that inflame the mind. If these remedies are used too much, they may destabilize people by detaching their spirits from their bodies. This energy can keep people fixed in the realm of the mind, where they remain in their intellect and forget the world around them.

Indigo and A both calm frayed nerves and anxious states. When people are too strongly engrossed or engaged in their problems, these remedies promote cool, unemotional mental clarity and control. This can help people step back from a menacing situation and reevaluate their possibilities, better able to see what is wholesome and good. This discernment is particularly strong with homeopathic A.

These remedies are not suited to anyone suffering from depression because they are too cool and detached. These people need hotter colors and lower notes, which will reanimate their ability to feel, not remedies that detach them from their feelings. The coolness of indigo and the note A help when a person wants to think clearly and express their ideas fluently.

Indigo is used to tonify the lymph, and it works well on mucous surfaces to remove inflammation. The note A soothes and helps regenerate life energy. Both remedies give a feeling of exhilaration and courage, which can increase physical strength. They act as a tonic for general health.

At a psychological level, Indigo and A can be used to cleanse and clear the body's psychic currents. They can purify and stabilize fear and repressed feelings. Indigo and A are useful for people who need to create healthy boundaries to protect them from intrusive people and experiences. These remedies give a clear mental framework and help people resolve emotional difficulties by thinking with greater clarity and in a more expanded way.

Both the color and the note stimulate the senses and can be used with eye, ear, and nose problems. They help clear headaches and soothe itchy scalps. They are both best given at night or early in the morning when the light is still a deep blue. They have a strong relationship with dawn and dusk, when the sky is a beautiful shade of indigo.

INDIGO

Indigo is an anesthetic, providing soothing and cooling relief from the pain and irritation of inflammation. It is known as the universal healing color. It is ethereal, more a color of the intellect than the passions.

While on indigo, one of the provers had a sense of things being very chaotic, and she couldn't find obvious things she had left in front of her. She made writing mistakes and felt very disoriented for the first hour after taking the remedy. This suggests, in the homeopathic fashion of like curing like, that indigo could be useful for people with dyslexia and confused states of mind. The remedy also seemed to produce a clear picture of mental control, and those who took it in the provings felt they could control their lives with a greater degree of conscious mastery.

THE NOTE A

The note A has been used for helping with long periods of concentration, when the mind can become weary and tired. It stimulates thinking and promotes focus. This remedy is excellent before taking an exam or writing a report. The note A helps us reflect on our problems so that we can find wholesome solutions to them. It helps us think in a positive and holistic way about who we are and what we are doing. If there is some issue that needs resolution, this remedy helps a person look at the bigger picture without getting emotionally tied up or becoming afraid of looking at the realm of possibilities.

INDIGO AND A USES

Here are ways these remedies can be used for healing.

Physical Problems

Indigo and A act as an anesthetic and help relieve pain. They are natural blood purifiers and help alleviate lymphatic congestion that causes inflammation. Both can be used effectively for swollen joints, boils or carbuncles, or skin irritation, or to soothe the internal organs. Indigo is useful for congestive problems in the pelvis, and is even considered for sterility problems in both men and women. It is used for mental instability, fever, and tuberculosis, and it has been useful in treating asthma, epilepsy, and chronic diseases with degeneration.

Contraindications: None. Remember, these remedies cool and soothe; they do not stimulate or energize.

Continued ➡

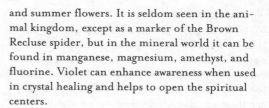

Emotional Issues

Indigo and A have a profound influence on calming the emotions. They are good for anxiety and fearful states or when the emotions run high. They cool, clarify, focus the mind, and relax emotional states where people become hysterical or overly involved in other people's problems. These remedies support detachment and ground a person in realistic thinking. People find they are more analytical as well as more observant on these remedies. They are also good for insane and agitated states, when people are unable to take conscious control of their actions and speech.

The note A is more mentally oriented than indigo, and it supports people in sorting through their emotional baggage. It helps people think about their lives and seek out what is important to them and what they wish to accomplish.

Contraindications: Neither of these remedies is good for depressed states and can make a person more depressed and dissociated from their feelings and body. Be aware of this before prescribing to people on antidepressants.

Mental and Spiritual Issues

Indigo and A are very good at helping a person organize their thoughts. They represent mentality and help the mind elucidate matters that weigh heavily. They are good tonics for tired and weary minds, and they help restore balance where clarity has been lost.

Contraindications: These remedies are not suggested for people who analyze constantly and who are always in their heads. It would only accentuate that tendency.

Indigo and A Essence

Indigo and A are essentially coolants, and they bring order to strongly heated and chaotic states, whether physical, emotional, or mental. They assist the mind in maintaining control. Their clear, soothing energy nurtures consciousness, wisdom, truth, and integrity….

Violet and the Note B

Violet is a mystical color that represents spirituality and beauty. It is soft, inviting, and very gentle. This color and the musical note B are associated with serenity, beauty, and the realm of spirit. They work on the crown chakra, located at the top of the head. They link the personality, or smaller self, with the Source, also known as the Higher Self. They both enhance our intimate relationship with our higher nature, where that place of "peace beyond all peace" can be experienced. This is the place of inner stillness and quiet where the Self abides, deep within our being.

Violet and B soothe and bring comfort to the soul forces, and they also act as an anesthetic and purifier on the physical level. However, violet can create confusion and dissonance for the ego, and it requires a well-grounded person to stay anchored in himself or herself when taking this remedy.

Violet and B are associated with the pineal gland, located in the top of the skull. Scientists are still baffled by its function. Esoteric healers and Asian teachers share the belief that this gland's function is to open the spiritual center, known as the crown chakra. The pineal gland responds to light similar to the way an eye does. It is made of tiny light-sensitive rods and cones. This light sensitivity is thought to control many physical functions, such as women's menstruation and reproductive cycles. Other pineal functions include the feeling of jet lag, fatigue associated with our intake of light, and the production of melatonin.

Tibetan lamas practice specific yoga postures and say mudras and prayers that stimulate the pineal gland to secrete an essence they call nectar, a substance reputed to enhance feelings of ecstasy and bliss. This takes many years of devotion and practice.

Violet and B created an "otherworldly feeling" for many of the provers. Violet created nausea, disorientation, and headache in some provers, which means it would be useful in treating those conditions in people who suffered from these symptoms. It has been used to palliate pain in cancer care, giving relief and peace.

Violet and B can be used by the elderly, as it is a vibration to which they are more closely attuned. They are also good for people who have difficulty finding a spiritual path in life. These remedies help them attune to a greater understanding of their purpose in life, as well as develop a more refined sense of beauty and serenity.

Both remedies can be used to treat epileptic seizures and alcoholism, along with deeper-acting homeopathic remedies. Violet was given to an artist who was unable to see or paint violet or purple until he took the remedy. He suffered from seizures and was a recovering alcoholic. Whenever he attempted to paint these colors, they appeared as a muddy brown. After taking homeopathic violet, he was able to paint a natural violet color.

It has been found that people may lose their sense of ego identity when exposed to too much violet or B. If people are not grounded in their personal identity, they easily become susceptible to the influence of others. They find it difficult to make decisions and be affirmative, and they can become touchy and irritable. They can become ungrounded in their spirituality and afraid of moving forward. However, violet is a gentle color and can give great comfort to those who are overly sensitive.

Violet

It is traditionally felt that violet represents the spiritual aspect and purple stands for the temporal element of power represented by the Catholic Church. Purple was a color reserved only for nobility, both in ancient Rome and Byzantium. It was very expensive to make and required the use of thousands of tiny mollusks to obtain the color. The expression "to the purple born" comes from Byzantium, where all queens were required to give birth to future emperors in a room completely swathed in purple silk. This may have actually been quite hygienic, as purple and violet are both anesthetics. Purple is now worn by high-ranking officials in the Catholic Church at specific times during the liturgical year.

Violet is found in nature in beautiful spring and summer flowers. It is seldom seen in the animal kingdom, except as a marker of the Brown Recluse spider, but in the mineral world it can be found in manganese, magnesium, amethyst, and fluorine. Violet can enhance awareness when used in crystal healing and helps to open the spiritual centers.

A highly evolved spiritual teacher in India who complained of chronic pain in his feet and legs was treated with homeopathic violet. He was given violet 6X in a split dose, and all of his pain disappeared. He resonated with the violet ray so strongly it seemed to be the best medicine to give him.

Violet has also been used by headache sufferers who were troubled by spiritual and ethical problems. These sufferers had conflicts between higher spiritual ideals and their emotions. Violet relieved the pain, and the headaches never reoccurred.

The Note B

The note B is very gentle and tender. The people who proved the note B came away with a very gentle, loving feeling. They were not very determined or aggressive and acted quiet, ungrounded, and submissive in their approach to situations and other people. They were easily irritated when they could not make up their minds. This indicates that B could aid people who dither and are passive in their approach to life.

The provers of violet did not want to connect with their problems, understand difficult challenges, or get involved. They wanted to be left alone to watch fantasy videos and stay secluded. Conversely, this remedy can assist with shyness and timidity and when people are frightened of exposing themselves to strangers and act introverted. It helps people feel spiritually connected and part of a greater whole and supports people on their spiritual path.

Violet and B Uses

Here is how violet and B can be used for healing.

Physical Problems

Violet and B, because of their connection with the crown chakra, can be used to help brain disorders, such as alcoholism, epilepsy, and neurosis. They are particularly good for stopping pain and can be used for menstrual cramps, headaches, and any pain around the head and shoulder area.

Contraindications: Violet could make people who are too sensitive feel uneasy and irritable. Magenta may have better results, as it carries the red and green rays. It is suggested that if there is mental or emotional instability, a small amount of violet can be used, but once the patient becomes restless or uneasy, it is best to stop the treatment. Violet and B are best given at night.

Emotional Issues

Violet can be used to open realms of spiritual understanding, ease impacted emotions, and bring the gift of inner peace. It soothes nervous conditions in which a person feels fractious and out of sorts. Violet and B can bring emotional stability to violent minds and relief to neurotic states of anxiety and chronic worry.

Contraindications: These remedies should be used in limited dosage. The remedies can be used alone or together, with time for observing the patient's response before giving a second dose. Caution should be used with hypersensitive people or people who are taking prescription medication.

Continued →

Mental and Spiritual Issues

Violet and B give a person a spiritual outlook on life. They can both ease egotistical streaks and narcissistic tendencies. These remedies can be useful for anyone trying to grow emotionally. However, too strong an identification with the spiritual plane can limit a person's individuation, or healthy ego development. Violet and B can cause a person to surrender their ego too readily. Finding a balance and staying grounded with this color is important.

Contraindications: Use judiciously with people who have a weak ego or who are taking prescription medication. They can become very sensitized, even temporarily insane, from too much violet light.

VIOLET AND B ESSENCE

Violet and B are energy fields that connect us to our higher spiritual nature. They both reflect the divine light within us and help us connect to the beauty around us and our innate serenity. They are gentle and healing, cleansing a person's aura and attuning them to the spiritual aspects of life. . . .

Pink (No Musical Note Applies)

Pink is the color of joy and universal mother love. It is a favorite color with young children and is associated with the heart chakra. Pink is closely associated with gentleness, sweetness, and naivete. It represents the purity and innocence of the human heart and helps open our capacity to give and receive love. Pink is found in the aura of babies, visible through Kirlian photography. It is the color that reflects the joy of life.

Pink is about inner and outer rosiness, and it indicates that there is vitality and life within us. Pink has been associated with little girls, but is now a color that is finding its place in men's fashions. When it is worn or used in decoration, it is linked with the softer, sweeter side of life. This color is positive, loving, and a sign of the purity and innocence of the human heart. It represents joy and tenderness.

In the provings of pink, all the provers had a dream associated with motherhood. They dreamed that either they were physically close to their mothers or were pregnant, giving birth, or holding a baby. This was not specific to women; men also had dreams of being held by their mothers or loved and cherished by their mothers. These dreams about mother love suggest that pink be used when we feel disconnected from love.

In the provings, pink also made everyone feel well. People found their problems were less acute, and they could manage them better. They all reported feeling well in themselves. Even provers who had serious family, financial, or health problems responded well while on the remedy. It also had a specific physical action on skin problems, relieving dry eczema, acne, and skin rash. These conditions, at an esoteric level, are thought to be reflections of feeling unloved.

PINK USES

This is how pink can be used in healing.

Physical Problems

Pink can be used for heart problems and is excellent for reviving vitality without the aggressive energy of red or orange. It can help people overcome shock, such as the trauma of childbirth, injury, or grief. It is a general toner and helps people through difficult times of change when they feel tired, fed up, or exhausted. Pink can be used for any skin condition, which suggests a person may be somatizing feelings of rejection and being unloved into physical pathology.

Contraindications: None.

Emotional Issues

Pink is associated with love. Whenever there is a hardening or an emotional closing down, this color remedy can be used to add a soft and gentle quality to a person's life. It is good for heartache, loss, and emotional suffering, especially in association with the loss of feminine love. Pink is not just a woman's remedy. It can be given to either sex at any age, wherever there is grief or loss of love. When combined with orange, it adds vitality and a sense of joy to any situation.

Contraindications: None.

Mental Issues

Pink can add a soft emotional element to the harsh light of the mind. It offers a sweetness and a refreshing quality to mental activity.

Contraindications: None.

PINK ESSENCE

Pink is the color of love. It offers us the bloom of roses, the sweetness of youth, and the joy of the heart. It suggests something childlike in us that relates to eternal youth, innocence, and motherhood. It fills us with a sweet, gentle, and humorous light. . . .

Magenta and the Note High C

Magenta is a regal color. Dr. Rudolf Steiner calls it the color of ultimate creativity. The color is a mixture of green, red, and violet, and it encompasses the energy of red's life force; green's peace, harmony, and neutrality; and violet's serenity and beauty.

Magenta and high C correspond to the alta major chakra, which sits about a foot above the crown chakra. This energy center is concerned with our higher purpose in life. This chakra represents the collective unconscious and the bonds of humanity that make us all one.

MAGENTA

Magenta is reserved for special occasions and creative ventures. Whenever we want a depth of understanding that supports our deepest spiritual nature, homeopathic magenta is the color of choice.

The esoteric issues of the alta major chakra correspond to the contracts made with our guardian spirits before incarnation. This color links us to the distant memory of past lives and also to the spiritual realm, where guidance, protection, and love are given to us.

In the provings, homeopathic magenta helped people gain insight into their problems. It added a spiritual dimension to the way they perceived situations. It seemed to elevate those who were too grounded in their thinking, and ground those who were too "airy" in their approach to life.

Magenta has been given to victims of abuse and to children who had neglectful parents. In all cases, it helped the person reestablish links with their Higher Self and gain wisdom and insight.

Magenta is used in color healing to stimulate a person's adrenals, heart, and sexuality because it is made in part with red. Magenta is said to strengthen the heart muscles and stabilize the heart rhythm. This color should be considered whenever there is fluid retention and also when the patient may need the extra vitality that they would receive from red. It can be considered a tonic for elderly people. Also, it is felt that many female disorders are helped by magenta. It has a diuretic effect as well, because of the green component, and helps release excess fluid from the system.

This color remedy was given to a woman who had developed weeping sores on both her legs at a crisis point in her thirty-year marriage. She had not responded to any other remedies. She could not see a future for herself if she stayed in her marriage, and she did not know what to do. This color helped her focus and helped her find a horizon. When she took the remedy, her wounds began to heal and she found the sense of freedom she needed to think about what she wanted from life.

THE NOTE HIGH C

The note high C corresponds to the alta major chakra. It is the end of one scale and the beginning of another. It provides a way of thinking about spiritual realities, and it encompasses past, present, and future in its totality. It offers a visionary way of thinking, with both sides of the brain involved, and helps a person maintain a clear horizon with hope, trust, and faith in the future. High C is more than just the energy of this center: it is the logos for it. With this note, the realms of spirit and humanity blend together. This note opens up new ways of looking at ourselves in relation to all of life, both visible and invisible.

MAGENTA AND HIGH C USES

Here are ways magenta and high C are used in healing.

Physical Problems

Magenta and high C can be used as good heart tonics. They can also be used for impotency, frigidity, and low libido. These remedies help stabilize the nerves when they are stretched from too much tension. Magenta stimulates sexuality by increasing circulation and the rate at which the heart pumps blood. It can also be used as a remedy for slow or late onset of the menses, infertility, or endometriosis.

Contraindications: Magenta should not be used on hysterical patients.

Emotional Issues

Magenta and high C are given when a person lacks insight, or when their emotions are too strongly engaged and they need an overview of the presenting problem. These remedies suit people who have trouble envisioning a clear horizon.

Contraindications: None.

Mental and Spiritual Issues

Great thinkers gravitate to magenta and high C. These remedies awaken latent creativity and also stimulate the vital physical and sexual realms. This energy can be transmuted into creative expression. These remedies elevate thinking toward higher realms of awareness while maintaining a grounded and realistic approach to life.

Contraindications: None.

MAGENTA AND HIGH C ESSENCE

The essence of magenta and high C is creativity and insight. These remedies combine the best of the vital force contained in red, the peace and tranquility of green, and the beauty and bliss of violet. They enhance our acceptance of what is universal in mankind and stimulate our creative powers.

Spectrum and the Chord

Spectrum and the chord are compiled by using all the color remedies to create a rainbow, or spectrum, and all the musical notes to create the chord. They have a very strong affinity with immunosuppressive diseases or diseases that weaken a person's entire energetic system.

If a person's immune system is affected, these remedies can boost energy. Spectrum was first used with a fifty-six-year-old woman who suffered from full-blown AIDS. She had previously had cancer

Continued →

and was so depleted that she could do nothing herself. She took spectrum I2C five times daily for several weeks. After the first week, she reported that she was able to do her housework, wash her hair, and dress herself for the first time in nearly a year. She had the energy to resolve many of the issues in her life that she had ignored. She said goodbye to those she loved and had the energy, right up to the last days, to take care of herself. She lived an extra six months and had a peaceful passing. Since then, the remedy has been given to anyone with serious energy depletion problems, HIV, AIDS, or other immunosuppressive diseases, with successful results.

SPECTRUM

Spectrum can be given over a long period of time without aggravation, and it seems to have a restorative effect when used for times of stress and exhaustion. It can be used as a travel remedy as well and gives energy whenever it is used.

Spectrum also helps eliminate the effects of drugs (such as repeated doses of allopathic medicine) from a person's aura, and, after taking it, people have had increased levels of vitality and awareness. Any substance abuse case, where the body is weakened or depleted of vitality, will reveal an auric field that is ash or gray. Spectrum revitalizes the entire energetic system and brings color back into a person's aura. It is useful for drug rehabilitation or alcohol recovery.

THE CHORD

The chord inspires holistic thinking and clarity in all endeavors. Like spectrum, it is a broadly used remedy, focusing intelligence on resolution and refinement. It is given in a low potency and needs to be repeated as needed. This sound remedy can open the realms of creative thinking and help expand the way a person looks at any situation.

SPECTRUM AND THE CHORD USES

Here are ways spectrum and the chord can be used for healing.

Physical Problems

Spectrum and the chord boost energy. They work in autoimmune deficiency and immunosuppressive conditions and have been used successfully with AIDS, HIV, chronic fatigue syndrome, postviral syndrome, glandular fever, alcoholism, and drug abuse. They also help with pregnancy, labor, and postpartum care. Any degenerative disease responds to these remedies because they give people energy to heal. People who have been ill a long time have more vitality with their use. This healing energy also benefits anyone with a long-term chronic disease, where severe pathology exists.

Contraindications: Spectrum should not be given at night, so as not to disturb sleep.

Emotional Issues

Spectrum and the chord provide relief to people with nervous exhaustion and emotional upset. They help people handle change and trauma in their lives.

Contraindications: None.

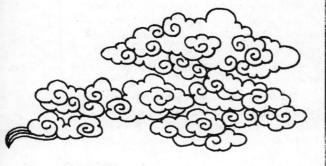

Mental and Spiritual Issues

Spectrum and the chord revive tired minds and are excellent to take after working with large groups of people or in other situations where energy can be drained. They establish peace and balance after long hours of engagement in a project.

Contraindications: None.

SPECTRUM AND THE CHORD ESSENCE

The essence of spectrum and the chord is the energy of all the colors and all the notes, which revitalizes a worn-out, fatigued system. These remedies contain all the vibrations within the visible spectrum and musical scale, to provide energy for a person's spirit as well as their body.

—From *Homeopathic Color & Sound Remedier*

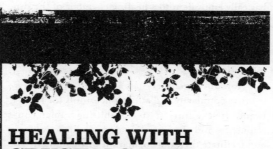

HEALING WITH CRYSTALS AND GEMSTONES
Sirona Knight
Additional illustrations by Eddie Clough

Crystal and Gemstone Basics

Grown during the cooling, formative stages of Earth's development, crystals and gemstones are gifts from nature. According to modern physics, they consist of naturally balanced, solid-state energy fields. Because of their energetic properties, crystals and gemstones have a wide range of technological, scientific, and metaphysical uses.

Many cultures around the world, including Chinese, Native American, and Celtic, have traditionally revered and used crystals and gemstones as tools for healing and spiritual purposes. Mythology and history abound with accounts of stones being used in myriad ways, from healing common ailments to protecting the wearer. For example, the purple gem amethyst has been purported to protect against intoxication, to have a sobering effect on passions, and to quicken the intellect. Mentioned in Exodus as one of the stones in the twelve-jeweled breastplate worn by the High Priest Aaron, brother of Moses, amethyst is still worn today by bishops in the Catholic church.

Because of their extremely high and exact rates of vibration, crystals and gemstones play important roles in modern technology, ranging from the liquid crystal diodes on our calculators and clocks to the use of diamonds for precision cutting of optical lenses. The technological uses of crystals and gemstones impact almost every facet of our daily lives, with new uses being discovered all the time. Computers, credit cards, fiber-optic phone lines, and laser technology—which enable everything from new surgical techniques to the playing of compact discs—are just a few of the examples.

Crystals and gemstones are both minerals. Minerals are defined as homogeneous, naturally occurring, inorganic solids. As a result of the orderly arrangement of its atoms, each mineral has a composition that can be expressed in a chemical formula, and a characteristic crystalline structure. The atoms which make up minerals and all matter in the universe are in constant motion. This

motion affects the physical structure and energetic field of each stone.

A mineral can be a single element, such as gold, or a complex compound of several elements, such as quartz crystal. The distinctive qualities and properties of each mineral are due to its chemical composition and the patterned arrangement of its atoms. A particularly interesting example of this patterning and its effect is the element carbon, which occurs in nature as several minerals, two of which are graphite and diamond. Identical in chemical composition but with different atomic patterns, they are at opposite ends of the hardness scale, with diamonds being the hardest of minerals and graphite being the softest.

Mineral deposits form in three ways: by precipitating out of a low-temperature solution; forming at depth under great heat and pressure; or crystallizing from hot liquids or gases of magmatic origin. How a mineral originates greatly impacts the patterning of its atoms. For example, it takes a tremendous amount of heat and pressure to create a diamond from carbon, whereas the formation of graphite requires very little heat and pressure.

A rock is an aggregate of minerals. Like minerals, rocks form under a variety of conditions. Mineralogists know where and in what types of rock a particular mineral is likely to be found, and what other minerals are likely to occur nearby. An example of this is tourmaline, which is largely found in deposits of the coarse-grained granitic rock, pegmatite.

What Is a Gemstone?

The main difference between crystals and gemstones is that gemstones have ornamental value. To mineral collectors, the term *gemstone* has become the commonly accepted name for all ornamental stones of value, eliminating the previous distinction between so-called precious and semi-precious stones.

Three qualities set gemstones apart from other minerals: rarity, durability, and beauty. Many mineral species qualify as gemstones, which are graded by gemologists according to the following characteristics: vividness of color, "fire," transparency, luster, and hardness. Gemstones are generally free from flaws and therefore prized for their beauty.

A gemstone becomes a gem when it is cut, shaped, and polished for use as an object of adornment. The final form becomes a faceted stone, a cabochon, or a carving. To create a faceted stone, a gemologist cuts the stone with the intention of bringing out its brilliance and sparkle. The cabochon cut emphasizes a stone's color and pattern by polishing it highly until it's rounded or flattened, rather than faceted. This method is often used on star and cat's eye–type gemstones. Carving is a way of working with larger gemstones such as quartz, turquoise, and jade. In this process, carvers sculpt the stones into a variety of shapes, for example, animals, Goddess figures, and cameos.

What Is a Crystal?

The Earth is composed of 85 percent crystal. The word crystal originates from the Greek word *krystallos*, meaning ice. This stems from the early belief that crystals were pieces of ice, frozen so hard they never melted. Indeed, crystals, in particular clear quartz, do look like ice, as one of their primary characteristics is transparency.

Another defining quality of a crystal is geometric regularity and a repeating internal pattern of its atomic structure. This repeating characteristic is referred to as crystal symmetry. If you rotate a crystal on one of its axes in such a way that the same configuration of faces appears more than

Continued ➡

once during the course of rotation, this is an axis of symmetry. A plane of symmetry is a place on a crystal where, if it were cut in half, each half would be a mirror image of the other. Crystals also have a center of symmetry meaning that every face of the crystal has a similar face lying parallel to it on the other side. This concept is akin to the human body, which also shows symmetry in that all the elements making up the left side are repeated on the right side, i.e., eyes, hands, ears, legs, and so forth.

The structure of a stone and the shape of its external faces and how they relate to one another also define it as a crystal.

Formed from a gaseous, liquid, or molten state in a process called crystallization, crystals are a large classification of stones including topaz, citrine, and fluorite. Some stones, such as diamonds, rubies, and sapphires, are both crystals and gemstones. For a more complete list of crystals and gemstones, refer to the section Healing and Spiritual Properties of Crystals and Gemstones. Lead, glass, and synthetic crystal are not included in this chapter because they do not contain the same healing and/or spiritual properties possessed by natural crystals.

Quartz is the most common crystal—it can be found in all classes of rock, under all sorts of conditions, and in all parts of the world. The most notable quartz specimens come from Arkansas in the United States and Brazil in South America.

The occurrence of single crystals is rare; crystals generally occur in groups which have developed together in rock fissures, on flat surfaces known as druses, or in cavities called geodes. Sometimes crystals develop together in clusters, either in contact or actually interpenetrating one another. Additionally, different types of crystals can grow together— for example, white quartz is sometimes the host stone for emerald. A host stone is a mineral or rock that is older than the stones in it.

In the study of crystals and other minerals, certain characteristics determine classification. These include:

- Texture—The surface appearance of a homogeneous rock or mineral aggregate. The degree of crystallization, the size of the crystals, and the shapes made by the interrelationships of the crystals or other components all contribute to the texture of a mineral.
- Hardness—The resistance of a mineral to abrasion or scratching.
- Luster—The surface appearance or the manner in which it reflects light.

Crystals always grow according to simple mathematical laws and fall within six basic systems, or lattices. These are as follows:

- Isometric—Also referred to as the cubic crystal system; these crystals are blocky or ball-like in appearance, with similar, symmetrical faces. Characteristic forms are cubes, octahedrons, and dodecahedrons.
- Tetragonal—Often long and slender, even needle-like, these forms include four-sided prisms, pyramids, and dipyramids.
- Hexagonal—These crystals are prismatic or columnar in the forms of three- or six-sided prisms, pyramids, and rhombohedrons.
- Orthorhombic—These are short, stubby crystals with a diamond-shaped or rectangular cross section.
- Monoclinic—Mostly stubby, these crystals have tilted matching faces at opposite ends, suggesting a distorted rectangle.

- Triclinic—Usually flat, these crystals have sharp edges and contain no right angles on the faces or edges.

Energy Fields of Crystals and Gemstones

Throughout the history of humankind crystals, especially quartz, and gemstones have been highly valued by spiritual leaders, healers, and scientists. Plato's writings referred to extensive use of crystals in Atlantis, and Edgar Cayce, famous seer and healer, often used quartz crystals in his work.

Irish mythology tells the tale of Art, son of King Conn, who was placed by the goddess Creide in a chamber of crystal, a place where all the rays of the sun converged. The hero remained in the crystal chamber for a month, after which he had acquired a new strength and energy, enabling him to face the worst of perils. The crystal chamber was basically equivalent to a healing chamber of the sun.

According to legend, Merlin the Magician resided in a crystal cave with the goddess Viviane, where he stayed protected until awakening from his magic sleep.

Now once again, crystals and gemstones are gaining popularity and attention as tools for the twenty-first century, a time of shifting human consciousness and change. Crystals can help activate and facilitate this transformation through their ability to amplify and balance energy fields such as the ones surrounding your body.

We are more than our physical bodies. We also have an energy body that stores information and roams at will each time we release a thought. Physical form in essence is comprised not of matter, but of energy. Everything that exists is an external manifestation of an energy form, a rate of vibration.

Crystals and gemstones have extremely high and exact rates of vibration which can be precisely manipulated to augment, transform, transduce, store, and focus other rates of vibration. Crystals are used for these purposes in communications, computers, optics, laser technology, audio-visual equipment, microcircuits, and in the equipment used for broadcasting radio and television signals. These same vibrational qualities of crystals can be used to modify thoughts, emotions, and the energy fields of human bodies and other physical forms by first effecting change on the subtle energetic level—just as shamans, healers, and mystics have been doing for ages.

Crystals restore balance in your body, allowing your body to breathe again in a meaningful and harmonious way. All life, in order to exist and be meaningful, must be in a state of balance. When life becomes polarized in one direction or the other, there is an imbalance and interference with the natural pattern of living. Quartz crystals, blood, and water all have an affinity for each other because they all share common elemental properties.

Crystals store energy, a certain rate of vibration, a specific matrix structure, color, memories, as well as sound, fragrance, light, emotions, dreams, and specific experiences. The form and development of quartz crystals is governed by morphogenetic fields. Crystals consist of atoms arranged in a patterned and orderly fashion, and are living entities in their own right. They exhibit a naturally balanced, solid state energy field, which makes them invaluable in electronic equipment. Crystal energy affects our totality like each breath of fresh air.

Quartz crystals have piezoelectric properties, meaning they emit an electrical charge when pressure is applied to them. Piezoelectronics use crystals in radio transmission, sonar equipment, and aircraft frequency control. Crystals also have pyroelectric qualities, meaning they produce an electric charge when heated.

The piezoelectric and pyroelectric properties of crystals are used in: oscillators, which control radio frequencies in electronic equipment; capacitors, which modify energy capacity and block excessive flow; transducers, which transmit energy from one system to another; condensers, which store a continual charge from an energy force field in solid form; energy force fields, used as sonic protection against static, and around an area or individual; and body balancers, which alter the body's vibration or frequency by passing ions through the crystal's molecular structure.

These are the same qualities that allow quartz crystals to modify thought and emotions and to heal our bodies and other physical forms by first effecting changes on a subtle, energetic plane. For example, the basis of crystal healing relies on the principle that disharmonious energy can be harmonized. Crystals and gemstones can amplify and transform thoughts, and increase powers of meditation, intention, visualization, and affirmation.

One early conception of crystals was that they were the living brain cells of the Earth Mother Gaia. If this is true, we are destroying countless cells for use in stereos and computers, as well as objects of adornment and metaphysical tools. As mentioned earlier, crystals and gemstones represent gifts from the Earth, and should be treated as such. When harvesting crystals and stones, please be aware of the finite nature of these gifts. Often a one-time harvest, they are being dug up at an ever-increasing rate. Crystals and gemstones, as with anything in nature, represent the eternal connection between human beings and the Earth. As with all relationships, this connection works best when it's in harmony and balance.

Healing Uses

Crystal Healing

As the growing field of psychoneuroimmunology indicates, our state of mind has a great influence on our state of health. The physical, mental, spiritual, and energetic go hand in hand. Energetic disturbances or blockages occur whenever there is injury, illness, or trauma in your life. During the healing process, you remove these blockages, restoring a healthy energy pattern to that part of your body. Every injury and emotional hurt takes a little bit of light out of your energy field. Crystal healing restores that light, renews the energy, and gives you an opportunity to be healthy again.

Through pain, your body receives the signal to pay attention. Dis-ease or illness begins on an energetic level before being transferred into the mental and physical levels. Pain is a by-product of energy blockages. One extremely effective method of removing these blockages is by using crystals.

Crystal healing, based on the transfer of energy from the crystal into the body, and vice versa, is an extremely effective method of removing these blockages. Crystals are silicates, which constitute the largest and most common class of minerals found throughout the world. Quartz crystals contain silicon and oxygen, a combination found in most minerals on our planet. Our bodies also contain silicon dioxide, suggesting a genuine physical connection with crystals. In addition to silicon and oxygen, water is often present in many type of quartz crystals. The human body is made up mostly of water.

The atomic similarities between crystals and the human body allow for the communication and transfer of energy, often benefiting our well-being. For example, carrying a crystal in your pocket or

Continued →

wearing one in a pendant that is cleared and programmed on a regular basis increases the strength of your energy field. This in turn shields you from negative thoughts and emotions emanating from other people. Your intention directs the energetic activity of the crystal. Crystal healing is effective on its own, or you can combine it with other healing methods, such as nutrition therapy, therapeutic massage, visualization, and hypnosis.

Utilizing color and light enhances crystal healing. Begin practicing with colors by gathering colored objects like small panes of glass, pieces of fabric, or paper. Focus on the color and practice pulsing the hue into the stone to charge it with a specific color essence. The following is a list of colors with their corresponding healing properties:

Blue: Used when you begin a healing work, blue cleans out any negativity. Imagine a brilliant electric blue or cobalt blue light or wave of energy washing out your stone and your energy field.

Green: After flushing the energy out with blue, green sets up new healthy patterns in the energetic field. See or sense forest green or bright kelly green, the color of health, abundance, and nature, and pulse this color into your stone and into your entire being.

Gold: Gold fuels the new healthy pattern. Visualize and/or sense the gold of the sun warming and energizing the new healthy pattern. Pulse this hue into the stone and your energy field.

White: This color is used for awareness of your higher self and spiritual path.

Rose: For a sense of love, use rose, especially when dealing with emotional issues in the healing.

Remember, you are a catalyst or channel for energy in the healing process. When doing healing work, the more you can step aside and move out of your ego the better the results.

Gemstone Essences

As an alternative vibratory aid, gemstone essences help balance your body and energy. You can purchase them or make them yourself at home. Sometimes the stone is ground into a powder and then mixed into a tincture, but this is not necessary in order to access the healing qualities within the stone.

Make crystal and gemstone essences or tinctures by placing a crystal or gemstone in a glass of water for several hours. After you remove the stone the liquid will be imbued with its essential properties. The elixir can be drunk or applied topically. You can place a few drops of the essence on a piece of personal jewelry, or on a crystal for healing or enhancing meditation. When you wear the jewelry or use the crystal, the gemstone essence is transferred into your body, and will remain until the essence is washed off or cleared from the stone.

Marcel Vogel used quartz crystals to charge or "structure" water and other liquids such as wine and fruit juice. You can try this yourself by first clearing and programming a quartz crystal. An appropriate program would be to fill the crystal with energy, light, and love. After programming, place the crystal in the liquid for at least two hours. Drink the beverage and notice the difference in taste. The liquid generally tastes smoother and has a noticeable sweetness.

GEMSTONE ESSENCE RECIPES:

Aquamarine Essence: For a gently cleansing gemstone essence, place a cleared and programmed aquamarine stone in a glass of spring water. Let the glass sit outside in the moonlight for at least three hours. Remove the stone from 1 the liquid and drink it.

Amethyst Essence: Use a stone that has not been set, placing it in a small, clear glass bottle. Mix two parts spring or distilled water to one part grain alcohol. Cover and set in direct sunlight for at least six hours. Use a few drops at a time to deepen meditation, enhance your receptivity to spirit, and as a remedy for internal parasites.

Emerald Essence: Use two parts distilled or spring water with one part 180-proof grain alcohol, and add a well-colored, uncut emerald crystal that has not been placed in a setting. For four ounces of liquid, use at least one carat of rough stone, to a maximum of four carats. Bring the mixture to a gentle boil in a Pyrex pan or glass coffee pot, then cover and simmer for thirty minutes. When the mixture cools, put it in a clear glass bottle with a stopper and place it in direct sunlight for at least six hours. Store the tincture in a green glass bottle. Use two to nine drops of tincture in a glass of water or wine. Used for balancing body, mind, and spirit, emerald essence is especially healing for heart, spleen, and sacral centers, and acts as an internal stabilizer and tranquilizer.

Self-Healing Techniques

You can use crystal healing techniques on yourself as well as other people. Following are four techniques for self-healing:

Technique #1: Hold your crystal in your left (receiving) hand and close your eyes. Visualize a brilliant white light emanating from the crystal into your hand, up your arm, and into your entire body. See the light fill and surround your body, until it seems as though you are wrapped in a cocoon of white light. Breathe in the light. Small, clear, and rutilated quartz balls are excellent for this technique. Be sure to clear your crystal when finished.

Technique #2: Hold your crystal over your solar plexus, pointing up. Visualize or sense a ball of golden energy coming from the crystal into your solar plexus area. Feel the golden light warm the area, and then with your breath, expand the light outward into your head and limbs. Expand the light outward about an arm's length distance from your body, surrounding yourself with warm, golden light. Bathe in the light for about ten minutes. Clear your stone when you are finished.

Technique #3: Breathe while asking yourself about any sensations and impressions in the problem area. Try to sense the color and texture of the area, and if there are any feelings, sounds, or images contained there. Place the crystal on your body, and fill it with your awareness of the illness or pain. Do this as many times as it takes to remove all of the pain or illness. Clear the stone when you are done.

Technique #4 (Seven-Step Vogel Self-Healing Technique): Hold your healing crystal with both hands in front of you. In your mind's eye, go to the problem area.

Make an effort to find the root cause of the problem. Breathe deeply and rhythmically, and focus on as many details of the problem as you can.

Release the problem and cause, using the pulsed breath technique. With your mind, transfer the problem or blockage into the crystal.

Visualize the healed area alive, flowing with energy, and whole.

Fill the area with white light and thoughts of love, harmony, and well-being.

Clear and clean the crystal.

Repeat the procedure three times.

Treating Common Ailments

The solar plexus and the heart region are the two major energy centers in the body. The solar plexus acts as a window to the past, and the heart region is a window to the present and future. Use any of the following techniques to move the energy up through the solar plexus and through the heart area, continuing upward through the chakras (see chart, page 63). You can also work along meridian lines and acupressure points with the crystal. The most effective healing distance is 1 to 1 ½ inches above the skin.

Headaches: For headaches, place a pain reliever, such as white willow, on your healing crystal. Place the crystal on your forehead and draw your breath in and pulse your breath out. The essence of the pain reliever will be absorbed by your etheric body, and you will feel relief.

Another method is to place the healing crystal (citrine is the best for headaches) directly on your forehead, back of the neck, temples, or wherever the pain is located. Breathe the pain into the crystal, and then clear the crystal using the pulsed breath technique, salt, or smudging. Repeat three times or until the pain subsides.

Muscular Pain (Including Lower Back Pain): Many of us experience lower back pain because of the frustration of not being supported or the inability to achieve what we desire. Because most people spend several hours a day sitting down, this frustration locks in and becomes focused in the solar plexus. Stress and anger fuel the problem by causing blockage in the solar plexus which prevents emotions from flowing.

Working with another person, use the seven-step Vogel Healing Technique, focusing on the area between the base of the spine and the skull. Rotating the crystal clockwise, draw in your breath, and release the locked energy along the spine. Repeat this procedure three times. When working locally, place your hand directly behind the problem area.

Injuries and Wounds: If you have just suffered an injur, position your healing crystal, with its tip pointing toward your head, on the area of injury. Leaving the crystal in place for a few minutes will generally reduce pain and swelling of the tissues. As it absorbs the pain and imbalance of the injury, clear it with the pulsed breath technique and reprogram it repeatedly, until the pain, bleeding, swelling, and redness subside.

Chakra Balancing and Layouts

To balance your chakras using a clear quartz crystal, first clear and clean your crystal. Then program it for balance. Hold the crystal over each of your seven chakras (at the crown, third eye, throat, heart, solar plexus, just above your navel, and sacral areas) checking for blockages of energy. The chakra area should vibrate and feel warm when working with crystals and stones. If it feels lifeless, pulse your breath through the crystal with the intention of opening the chakra area. Use the mental command "Open." Do this process slowly, and remember you are dealing with very real energies, even if they are subtle. Balancing your chakras helps restore health and clear the mind.

CHAKRA LAYOUTS

The following layouts provide a framework; feel free to adapt them according to your own intuition. Clear and program each of the stones before using it, and clean and clear the stones after you are finished. To determine which stones work best on specific areas, my suggestion is to try at least two different types of stone on each chakra. Stone types and placements will vary, depending on the person.

Continued ➡

Stone Color, Chakra, and Sound Relationships

Stone Color	Chakra	Sound (Note)
Red	First	C
Red-Orange, Orange	Second	D
Yellow-Orange, Yellow/Gold	Third	E
Yellow-Green, Green	Fourth	F
Blue-Green, Sky Blue	Fifth	G
Dark Blue, Indigo/Violet	Sixth	A
White/Clear	Seventh	B

Healing Layout

The purpose of this layout is to facilitate healing, first on an energetic level, which then carries over to the physical. Two stones for each chakra position are suggested. Try one stone, and then the other, testing which one works best for you. Place your cleared and programmed stones in a basket or on a cloth next to you. Lying comfortably on your back, begin placing the stones on your body, from the lower chakras up to the crown. Breathe deeply and visualize or sense a bright golden or white, warm and healing light radiating from the stones and filling your body. Allow the stones to remain in position for at least fifteen minutes, and then remove them, one by one, in the reverse order you placed them on your body, from the crown down to the base.

Crown (Top of head)—Clear Quartz or Rutilated Quartz

Third Eye (Between and above eyebrows)—Amethyst or Moonstone

Throat (Center of base of neck)—Sodalite or Lapis Lazuli

Heart (Center of chest)—Rose Quartz or Jade

Solar Plexus (Below breastbone)—Gold Calcite or Carnelian

Navel Chakra (Just below navel)—Red Jasper or Bloodstone

Root or Base Chakra (Between genitals and anus)—Onyx or Hematite

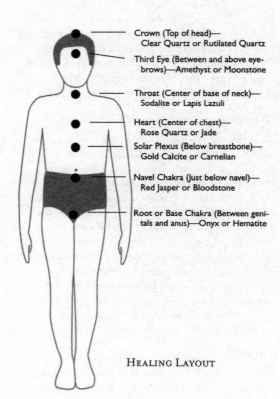

Crown (Top of head)—Clear Quartz or Rutilated Quartz

Third Eye (Between and above eyebrows)—Amethyst or Moonstone

Throat (Center of base of neck)—Sodalite or Lapis Lazuli

Heart (Center of chest)—Rose Quartz or Jade

Solar Plexus (Below breastbone)—Gold Calcite or Carnelian

Navel Chakra (Just below navel)—Red Jasper or Bloodstone

Root or Base Chakra (Between genitals and anus)—Onyx or Hematite

Healing Layout

Meditation Layout

The purpose of this layout is to enhance personal meditation and communication with the divine. Again, there are two suggested stones for each chakra. Lay the stones out beginning with the root

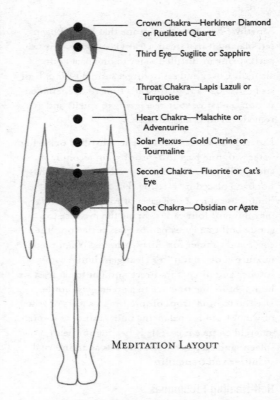

Crown Chakra—Herkimer Diamond or Rutilated Quartz

Third Eye—Sugilite or Sapphire

Throat Chakra—Lapis Lazuli or Turquoise

Heart Chakra—Malachite or Adventurine

Solar Plexus—Gold Citrine or Tourmaline

Second Chakra—Fluorite or Cat's Eye

Root Chakra—Obsidian or Agate

Meditation Layout

or base chakra, and finishing at the crown. Breathe deeply and meditate as usual. Allow the stones to remain in position for at least half an hour, up to eight hours, leaving the stones on your body while you sleep if you desire. Remove the stones in reverse order.

Crown Chakra (Top of head)—Herkimer Diamond

Third Eye (Between and above eyebrows)—Sugilite or Sapphire

Throat (Center of base of neck)—Lapis Lazuli or Turquoise

Heart (Center of chest)—Malachite or Aventurine

Solar Plexus (Below breastbone)—Gold Citrine or Tourmaline

Sacral Areas (Below navel)—Fluorite or Cat's Eye

Root or Base Chakra (Between genitals and anus)—Obsidian or Agate.

Marcel Vogel Healing Technique

Originated by Dr. Marcel Vogel, my friend and teacher, this remains the most effective healing technique I have seen demonstrated or personally experienced. When working with another person the primary intention is to help your partner bring her body into balance, so her energy field flows in a healthy, natural pattern. Your role is to act as a conduit for healing energy.

The Eight Healing Motions

The healing crystal is always held with the operating tip pointing out and up. In this position the crystal generates a field of energy that oscillates with the energy field surrounding the body.

Most people prefer to hold the healing crystal in the right (sending) hand, but this is not an absolute rule. Try both hands and see which one works best.

Finger positions and hand motions influence and enhance the effectiveness of your crystals. Generally, position either your index or middle finger on one of the crystal tip faces. This regulates the intensity of the energy field emanating from the tip of the crystal. As you move your finger closer to the tip, the field becomes narrower, and as you slide your finger down toward the base of the crystal, the

field becomes broader.

Your thumb acts as a sensor, and with it, you can vary the vibrational rate of the crystal and the frequency of oscillation released through the crystal, by moving your thumb up and down the surface of the crystal.

Four basic hand motions are used with crystals: a clockwise, circular motion that moves energy into the treatment area; a counterclockwise, circular motion that pulls energy out of the treatment area or withdraws the charge; a steady motion, with slight movements, while finding the optimum position for greatest field strength; and an up and down motion, and back and forth (stitching) motion which creates an oscillating field vibration.

When you are working in a circular motion, you are visualizing light, and when working with the crystal in an up and down motion, the focus is on vibration and sound.

The energy emanating from a charged crystal forms a spiral. When you rotate the crystal, the spiral flows outward and becomes stronger with each spin, building up a greater linkage between you and the focus of your crystal.

Healing Dialogue

Establishing rapport and trust by communicating with your partner plays an integral part in any healing. Start by asking the key question, "Do you want to be healed?" Although this may seem obvious, sometimes a person doesn't really want to resolve a problem, be it spiritual, emotional, or physical. Everyone deals with personal issues at their own pace, so be sure you receive an affirmative response. If you receive a negative or fearful response in any form, whether verbal, physical, or psychic, it is not wise to continue the healing.

Preparing for a Healing

After receiving the affirmation from your partner, the next step involves merging with divine energy. Whatever your preference—the Spirit, Divine Mind, Oneness, or Cosmic Consciousness—link yourself with this energy to facilitate the highest possible benefit from the healing. Now is the time for prayer and asking for divine guidance and help in the healing.

Ask your partner to remove all jewelry, belts, and coins from her pockets, and any metal objects from her body. Your partner should avoid wearing clothes with metal buttons, zippers, or hooks during the healing, as the metal creates a "false" energetic field in those areas. Be sure to clear all jewelry before putting it back on at the conclusion of the healing session.

Provide a stool or chair for your partner to sit on, one which gives you access to both the front and back of her body. Because this healing method is very powerful, she may go limp during the process, making it essential that she be supported in some way.

Build a state of equilibrium by creating an envelope of energy around yourself, which looks like a cocoon of white light, edged in cobalt blue. This serves as a form of protection, especially important when working in stressful situations. While you are building this field of energy around you, send thoughts of harmony, love, balance, and inner strength to your partner. This will increase your partner's energy field prior to the healing work, and prevent you from being drained during the procedure.

Crystal Healing Process

Begin by handing your partner the healing crystal. Ask her to breathe her energy into it. This creates a union between you and your partner, within the crystal. Also, the more actively your partner partici-

Continued ➡

pates in the healing, the better the results will be. While your partner merges with the healing crystal, continue gently questioning her regarding the problem, and how long it has lasted. Next ask whether she is ready to release the problem and let go of the root cause of the imbalance. Give praise and encouragement if you receive a positive reply.

Now take your healing crystal back and slowly scan your partner's etheric field by holding the crystal in your right hand, tip pointed toward her and slightly upward. Place your left hand on her back, opposite the crystal. Your left hand serves as an anchor. If you prefer, you can work with your hand and the crystal about an inch away from the surface of the body. Scan the body with your crystal, using small circular motions, combined with slow, up and down motions, to gather energetic information. Notice any sensations you experience or sudden energetic messages.

Breathing with your partner, use your breath to obtain a clearer indication of the energetic flows and streams of her body by breathing deeply and rhythmically. Continue to move your left hand in unison with your right hand, like a shadow. Move the crystal along the chakra line, and notice any areas that seem hot or cold, dark or gray. These are generally places of energetic imbalance. Be sure to ask your partner what, if any, trauma occurred in these areas, or if she is having discomfort or pain in these particular places.

After scanning the body, move your healing crystal over the thymus, or witness, area, 3 to 5 inches below the throat chakra. Take a deep breath and hold it, and at the same time use a counterclockwise twist of the crystal, and then rotate it slightly, to enter your partner's subtle energy body. Resume breathing, remembering to synchronize your breathing with your partner. You and your partner may feel a tugging sensation when you connect with the etheric body. This is completely normal. Use diagonal and horizontal stitching motions with the crystal, and then move on to small clockwise circular motions over the body's surface. The stitching motions tie the energy field together and can be used all over the energy body.

Next, hold the crystal on the problem area and have your partner see and sense the problem as clearly as possible. Increase in speed the small circular motions with the crystal. Ask her to draw in a deep breath with you and hold it; give the voice command to release the problem. Release your breath together with force by pulsing it through your nose. Your healing crystal is at its optimum effectiveness when you draw your breath in and hold it. By holding your breath, you build and strengthen the charge to its maximum potential.

Shake off the buildup of unwanted energy from your healing crystal using a snap of your wrist while pulsing your breath. While doing this, visualize a clear, cobalt blue light washing through your crystal. Go back to the same area and repeat the "release" process two times.

Next, use clockwise circular motions to fill the area with energy and light, moving through the colors blue, green, and gold in succession. Finish by using large, circular and up and down sweeping motions with both of your hands holding the crystal, 4 to 6 inches from the surface of the skin. Visualize her body being filled with bright, white light, and direct your positive and loving thoughts her way. This builds a new, healthy pattern of energy in your partner's etheric body.

Exit the etheric body at the same place you entered (the witness area) with a small, clockwise twist of your wrist. Stand your partner up slowly and give her a big hug. Marcel Vogel always emphasized ending each crystal healing with a warm, compassionate hug. Have your partner drink six to eight glasses of water each day for the next two days as a way to flush out the toxins released during the healing session. Be sure to clear your crystal after the healing, and before putting it away.

Crystal Grids

Crystals and gemstones, positioned in specific geometric patterns, produce unified energy fields called grid systems. Grid systems manifest a certain energy vortex that results in higher octaves of energy and light becoming more pronounced within them. In this way, a grid acts as the meeting ground between this planet and other energetic dimensions, opening a communication link for accessing healing energies, information, and knowledge from the many realms of existence.

Every time you form a grid, you create an energy mandala or light pattern that facilitates a healing and spiritual experience. Placing the grid stones in harmonious positions is imperative. When you point two or more of the grid stones at a specific area, this focuses healing energy on that area. Pointing stones inward adds healing energy to the grid, while pointing stones outward disperses the negative energy from inside the grid. Rely on your common sense, intuition, spiritual guidance, and experience when deciding how to position and use stones.

Each kind of crystal and gemstone has its own healing and spiritual uses as listed in the following chapter. When you begin placing stones together in grids, the energies of the stones blend, producing a synergistic effect. When creating a crystal grid, clear quartz is often preferable because it is easier to program than other crystals, but using different kinds of stones produces an unlimited number of patterns and healing effects. The choice depends on your intentions and needs.

Clear and program each crystal or gemstone. Having a specific intention when you program a grid serves to strengthen the energy mandala and vortex. You can also use breath, music, drumming, chanting, color, scent, and textures to amplify the grid energy and effect. Another way to enhance the energy is by holding crystals or stones of similar types and sizes in your hands while laying or sitting in a grid.

Often a grid contains a focal crystal, which is usually the crystal placed at your head or feet. Using your breath, begin at this focal point, and visualize or sense an energetic silver or gold thread connecting the grid stones in a clockwise circle. Do this three times to strengthen the grid field. When you are finished with the grid, pull up the grid stones in the reverse order in which you laid them down, and be sure to clean and clear your stones before putting them away.

When you use clusters in grids, the energy mandala will take on a more complex pattern. Be aware of this when positioning and connecting your clusters. You can use pyramids, obelisks, and other cut shapes in grids, but remember, like clusters, they add more dimensions to the field or energy mandala.

Multipurpose Healing Grid: Eight clear quartz crystals placed around you in an oval; two each at your shoulders, hips, knees (psychic entry points), one positioned at your head and one at your feet, as shown in the layout. Infuse the crystals with healing color, visualizing and/or sensing blue, green, gold, and then white light radiating from the stones. Mentally connect the crystals with a gold or silver thread of light in a clockwise pattern, starting at the focal crystal, which is the crystal placed at your head. Use your breath to move the energy and light through the crystals.

Grid for Body, Mind, and Spirit Balance: Three crystals. Connect the stones with a silver or gold energetic thread in a pyramid shape, starting with the focal crystal, which is the crystal in front of you.

Meditation Grid: Twelve crystals, plus focal crystal (thirteen total), placed in a circle as shown. Hold your focal crystal in your hands, and connect the stones in a clockwise pattern, starting at the focal crystal.

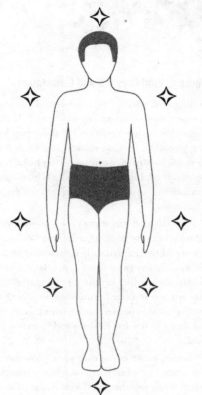

Multipurpose Layout

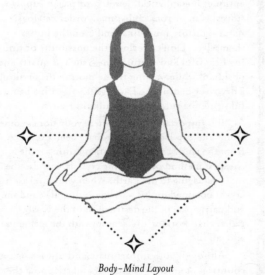

Body-Mind Layout

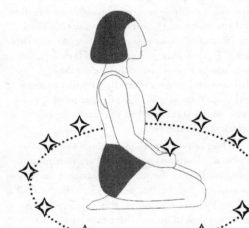

Meditation Layout

Continued →

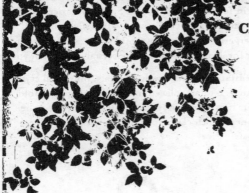

Choosing and Caring for Crystals and Gemstones

Siroma Knight

Where to Find Crystals and Gemstones

Finding and purchasing crystals and gemstones is an adventure, often an enjoyable one. Many inexpensive stones are available for those just beginning to collect and use stones, and of course, there are more expensive stones, costing hundreds of thousands of dollars, such as the famed "pad-paradschah," an extremely rare orange variety of corundum.

Crystals and gemstones are a good investment, not only because of their enduring beauty, but also because of their spiritually nourishing and healing qualities. Many gemstones appreciate in value quickly, depending on the type of stone, the setting, cut, carat weight, and so forth. Keep in mind that the most expensive stone is not necessarily the best stone to use for healing and spiritual purposes.

Stones often come into your possession at a time when you need them—as gifts, through bartering, or by purchasing them. Some of the sources for stones are rock shops; gemstone and mineral shows; New Age stores, fairs, and events; antique, metaphysical, jewelry, or pagan supply stores; gem or rock clubs; mail-order catalogs; natural history museums; and even the mines themselves. Don't overlook the possibility of finding beautiful and useful stones, such as quartz and obsidian, while walking in the mountains or along a dry river bed. If the Earth gifts you with a beautiful stone, be sure to give thanks in return.

It is important to know where your stones come from, and by what means they have been excavated from the land. For example, strip mining is the cheapest method of extracting crystals, but also the most damaging to the Earth. When you purchase a crystal obtained in this way, you indirectly condone and participate in the destruction of the Earth, rather than working in harmony with the elements and land.

Although both unfortunate and unwise, many countries are pitting the Earth and stripping the land away for gemstones and crystals in order to meet the incredible market demand. Because most of the stones near the surface have already been mined, mines are now being dug deeper into the Earth. For instance, ten years ago Herkimer diamonds were found just inches below the soil, whereas today miners must dig fifty feet or more to find these same stones. This deeper mining costs more, which is reflected in the escalating prices of crystals and gemstones.

When selecting personal stones, ask the salesperson all the questions you feel are pertinent to buying and using the stone. If you don't like any of the answers you receive, perhaps you should find a different source for stones. Buying a crystal or gemstone should be a positive experience, and never rushed or forced.

The following list provides tips on what to look for when purchasing crystals and gemstones:

- Damage—the less damage (imperfections, cracks, chips) the better. Chipped tips on quartz crystals are the worst sort of damage.
- Clarity—Depending on the type of stone, clarity is usually a desired characteristic, especially in clear quartz. Clear points, which are very clear quartz, crystal points, make excellent pendants, healing tools, and wands.
- Shape and configuration—Odd and unusual shapes cost more, for example, tabbies, which are flat healing crystals.
- Rarity—When particular mines close or the mineral becomes scarce, the cost escalates. Rare stones are the most costly.
- Inclusions—The rainbows, patterns, or landscapes inside the stone that are desirable for various ritual and ceremonial uses.
- Spiritual Qualities—Generators, healing crystals, record keepers, meditation, and channeling stones used for esoteric, meditation, and energy applications. See "Types of Quartz Crystals" and "Healing and Spiritual Properties of Crystals and Gemstones."

How to Select Personal Stones

All crystals and stones are naturally tuned to particular frequencies, vibrations, and harmonics of energy. When you are in attunement with a stone, you will experience sensations of balance, harmony, clarity, and wholeness.

Choosing stones is an intuitive act. Take a deep breath and notice which stones feel good to you. If a stone feels right, it's probably the right one for you. If it doesn't feel right, try another one.

To increase your sensitivity to the energies of crystals and gemstones, first wash your hands, dry them completely, and rub them together vigorously and rapidly several times to build up a surface charge. Pick up the crystal or gemstone and feel the energy. Your hand may actually stick to the stone. This indicates that you and the stone are in harmony.

One effective means for selecting personal stones is simplified kinesiology. Working with another person, extend your right arm at shoulder height. With your left hand, hold the crystal or stone on your witness area at the thymus, where your physical and subtle energy bodies meet, and ask the question, "Is this a good stone for me to use, wear, or carry?" Continue by asking for more specific information, such as, "Is this a good stone for me to use for healing? For meditation? For channeling?" After each question, have the other person press down firmly on your extended arm, while you resist. If your arm remains strong, you have made a wise selection. If your arm becomes weak, choose another stone.

Another way to test how in sync you are with a particular crystal is by holding the crystal in your right hand and drawing in a deep breath. Hold your breath until you feel your body vibrate or oscillate. As you exhale and relax, point the tip of the crystal (the dominant tip, if it is double terminated toward the palm of your left hand, and at a distance of five to nine inches, begin to move the crystal slowly up and down. You should feel a tingling sensation in your left hand, reflecting the

movements of the crystal. The feeling you experience may be akin to a slight breeze flowing across the surface of your skin. First, move your hands closer together, and then about an arm's length apart, all the while noticing the difference in the sensations from the crystal. The stronger the tingling sensation or breeze, the stronger your connection with that particular crystal.

As you work with crystals and gemstones, you may experience or intuit a variety of sensations. Following is a list of examples:

- Tingling or energetic charge in your hands or across your skin
- Electric charge or humming sensation
- Sweating or dampness, a slickness when rubbing the stone
- Heat
- Cold
- Vibration or pulsing
- Flow of energy or heat from the crystal tip
- Twitching in your fingers and thumbs
- Breeze or cool wind across your skin
- Sound or audible humming in your ears
- Glowing light or a visible or sensed field of energy
- Scent or odor
- Immediate sense of balance and being centered

Types of Quartz Crystals

Attunement Crystals—These serve as "tuning forks'" in meditation, influence and increase the vibration of energy within a certain sphere or area, and key to specific harmonics of energy. They are usually very clear and simple.

Cluster—A group of connected crystals usually joined at the base. One or more crystals growing from the same host stone.

Crystal Pairs—Twinned crystals, used for uniting energies and communicating with the divine.

Dead Crystals—Irradiated stones that are vibrationally dead and therefore useless. Most smoky quartz sold in the U.S. is white or clear quartz from Arkansas that has been irradiated. When purchasing stones, don't hesitate to ask the salesperson where the stones come from, and if they've been treated in any way. Look for genuine smokies from Nevada, California, Washington, and Montana.

Devic Crystals—Elemental devas use crystals as dwelling places. These crystals are usually formed in such a way as to allow entrance into the stone. Best kept in a special, secluded spot, and used primarily for multidimensional communication and travel.

Double-terminated—A crystal with two points, one on each end. Energy moves in both directions in these stones, but usually one of the points is dominant, meaning it projects more energy than the opposite end.

Fire Crystals—Intense energy crystals that seem to radiate a fire from within, and act as a long-lasting source of energy.

Generator—A large quartz, hand-sized or larger, used to generate energy. Often used in crystal

Continued ➜

grids or to create ley lines, which are energetic lines that crisscross the Earth's surface.

Generator Cluster—A very large group of connected crystals, used to generate great amounts of energy. Excellent for manifesting goals and ideas.

Geode—A hollow stone, lined on the inside with crystals. Also crystals layered on the top and bottom of a stone.

Goddess Crystal—Quartz crystals with a five-sided C-face (located on the tip, this is the largest of the crystal's six faces). Two sides are longer and form an arrow point.

Healing Crystals—Usually palm-size crystals that exhibit a balanced field of energy, and elicit a like response of harmony when employed for treating imbalances in the body.

Hydro Crystals—Quartz with one or more water bubbles. The trapped water is hundreds of thousands to millions of years old. Adding the elemental quality of water is extremely useful in healing, due to the fact that the human body is mostly made up of water.

Penetrator—A crystal that grows through and extends out of a larger crystal. These are ritual and ceremonial stones of initiation and rebirth.

Library Crystals—Stones with the capacity to receive and store large amounts of information. Very useful when learning, studying, or doing research work. Often these crystals already have a great deal of knowledge embedded in them. These crystals feel very dense or heavy and often have multiple pyramids and windows in them.

Phantom—An image within the quartz, created by inclusions, that echoes the shape of the outer crystal. Excellent stones for healing.

Rainbows—Inclusions within a quartz crystal that resemble a rainbow when the crystal is placed in the sun or under a bright light. Used for meditation, crystal gazing, and ritual. Double rainbows are very rare and particularly useful for out-of-body, shapeshifting, and channeling work.

Record Keepers—Crystals with three-sided pyramids which are within the stone, etched into it, or raised above its surface. Considered to carry the wisdom of the ancients.

Power Rods—Long, thin crystals that respond quickly and powerfully to thought-forms and project them in a laser-like beam of energy. Used to motivate change.

Reverse-sceptered—A crystal with a small, fine, and delicate tip, and a larger stone at its base.

Ritual Crystals and Gemstones—Consecrated stones such as initiation pendants and talismans, used primarily for ritual.

Sceptered Crystal—Quartz with a primary crystal and another crystal growing on the tip.

Scrying Crystals—Usually large quartz crystals with very clear centers. Often spheres, pyramids, obelisks, and similarly shaped quartz crystals are used for scrying or crystal gazing Singing Crystals—Stones that seem to sound when they are used in certain applications, such as meditation, healing, or ritual.

Skeletal Quartz—Stones with small openings and channels into the layered interior. These crystals work especially well for communicating with angels, ancestors, and otherworldly beings.

Transmitting Crystals—Quartz that transmit a wide spectrum of spiritual light, which serve as tools to amplify and project thought-forms or light from place to place.

Watchtower Crystals—Very clear, single-terminated and fine-pointed quartz crystals that are tuned in a specific manner and used exclusively for guarding the Four Corners: North, East, South, and West.

Natural, Polished, Cut, and Synthetic Stones

The energetic and healing effects of a stone differ depending on whether it is polished and cut or in its natural state. Certain stones need cutting and polishing to bring out their properties, while others work better in their raw, uncut state. Some healers work primarily with polished stones, while others feel natural stones, or a combination of polished and natural stones, work best. Use your own intuition and judgment when choosing a polished, cut, or natural stone. The stones you are drawn to are probably the most appropriate ones. Cut and polished stones are usually more expensive than natural stones.

In general, gemstones transmit their energies more intensely when polished, while clear quartz remains very powerful both in its natural and cut state. Cutting and polishing an amethyst crystal often increases its energy and effects. Also, garnet and ruby are highly effective when cut and set properly in jewelry.

Unlike natural stones, synthetic crystals are not beneficial for healing or energy balancing. Simulated gemstones do not contain all of the elements found in natural stones. Because they are grown in the laboratory they do not interact with your body's energy in the same way as natural stones, and are solely attuned to the person(s) who manufactured them. Worthless for purposes of therapy and healing, I do not recommend using simulated gemstones or crystals for anything but occasional adornment—but be sure not to allow synthetic stones to touch your skin. Also avoid using all irradiated and heat-treated stones, as they can be harmful and are definitely useless for healing or spiritual applications.

Care and Programming of Crystals and Gemstones

Cleaning and Clearing

Crystals and gemstones constantly collect energy from their surrounding environment. This buildup is a record of the energy of each person who has come in contact with the stone.

Whenever you obtain a new crystal or gemstone, clean and clear the stone before using it. Cleaning the stone is crucial when you use it for healing and spiritual work. This is particularly important if you use someone else's crystal: if you do not clear it first, instead of getting a clear channel you will pick up the other person's vibration. By using the cleaning and clearing methods outlined in this chapter, you will be assured of starting with a clear energetic channel, using your crystals and gemstones to their fullest spiritual and healing potential.

Following are some tips for physically cleaning your stones:

- A soft toothbrush or vegetable brush is good for loosening dirt particles, particularly when cleaning clusters.
- Avoid soaking stone clusters, geodes, and soft stones, as they can break apart and crumble.
- Keep crystals and stones in a container or a natural cloth bag between cleanings.
- Do not click the stones together as you clean them because they will chip and crack.
- Avoid extreme temperatures and sudden changes of temperature when cleaning stones. This can crack them, particularly if a weak point exists in the stone.
- Use soap only as a last resort, and use only natural soaps and detergents, nothing synthetic.
- Be aware of magnetic fields, EMF fields, and polarities within your house as these will change the resonance in the stones.

Salt and Water

One simple method for purifying the energy in a crystal or gemstone is to use salt. Traditionally, metaphysicians used salt to break up energetic patterns, because the crystals of salt absorb and clear the energy of everything that comes into contact with them. When using salt for clearing your crystals, use natural sea salt rather than salt processed with chemicals. Follow these steps for using dry salt to clear the energy in your crystals and gemstones:

1. Fill a container large enough to hold your crystal with dry salt.

2. Put the crystal into the container, submerging it completely in the salt.

3. After a few minutes, remove the crystal from the salt, and hold it in your hand. Use your intuition to check into the crystal. The energy field should feel cleaner.

4. Dispose of the used salt—do not use it, either in your salt shaker or bath.

In the case of stones which have had major energy patterns imprinted in them, you may need to use this technique in conjunction with other clearing methods to ensure that the crystal is indeed free of unwanted energy. Some experts suggest that the crystal be packed in salt for twenty-four to forty-eight hours. This isn't necessary, because as soon as the crystal makes contact with the salt, the energy is transferred.

Another method is to place the stone in salt water for a few minutes to twenty-four hours. I have found that a few minutes is sufficient, and that leaving stones in longer pits them or breaks them apart. Another quick way to clear your stone is by holding it under cold running water for a minute, tip downward, and visualizing white light washing through it.

Smudging

Smudging is a traditional cleansing technique used primarily by Native American shamans. They use the smoke of certain herbs, including sage, cedar, and sweet grass, to purify their bodies and lodges. The purpose of smudging crystals is essentially the same. The smoke of the herbs cleanses the energy of the stone.

Smudge sticks made of these herbs can be found in metaphysical or New Age stores, and are reasonably priced; or you can collect and dry your own sage, cedar, and sweet grass. You can also smudge your stones with sandalwood incense, or

Continued →

copal, a resin, which have a purifying effect on energy. Following is a basic method for smudging your crystals and gemstones:

1. Light the smudge stick or incense, and blow on it softly until it starts to smoke. Hold a fire-proof dish or container under the burning smudge, as pieces of the burning herbs may drop off.

2. Take the crystal in your hand and pass it through the smoke, making sure the smoke completely surrounds it.

3. Continue moving the crystal through the smoke until it feels clean to you. The number of times you need to pass the crystal through the smoke depends on the strength of the energetic charge in the crystal. As always, trust your intuition when smudging your stones.

Pulsing Technique

The pulsing method uses breath and intention to clear the stone. Breath is the staff of life, while intention forms the foundation of all spiritual and healing work. Cradle the crystal or stone between the thumb and middle or index finger of your left hand; place the thumb and index or middle finger of your right hand on either end of the crystal or stone. By using both hands, you create a flow of energy, or natural circuit. When working with spheres, clusters, or similarly shaped stones, simply cup the stone between the palms of your hands, with your right hand on top.

Your intention is one of clearing; hence in your mind's eye visualize an image, or sense a feeling of clearing or clarity filling the crystal or stone. As you breathe in deeply, visualize whatever symbolizes clarity to you, and then pulse your breath out, sharply through your nostrils only, not your mouth. Your pulsed breath becomes a carrier wave for the image or sensation of clearing that occupies your awareness as you breathe out.

Dr. Marcel Vogel taught me several ways to clear crystals. Dr. Vogel was one of IBM's most prolific Senior Scientists, with over 100 patents in his name. He was a man of unlimited creativity and faith, who was recognized as an authority on the therapeutic use of crystals. One helpful method for clearing crystals is to breathe in and visualize or sense a laser beam of white light moving from your forehead or third eye to the stone. As you pulse your breath out, fill the stone with cleansing light. Another useful method is to breathe in and visualize or sense a black void with a single point of white light in the center. Place this image into the crystal or stone with your pulsed breath.

Rotate the crystal or stone in your hands as many times as you feel necessary for thorough clearing, repeating the pulsing technique each time. In this manner, you clear the major axes and faces of the crystal or stone.

The pulsing technique effectively clears crystals, stones, and metals, which makes this technique particularly useful for jewelry, healing crystals, and pendulums, as well as crystal and stone tools. Personal jewelry that is worn regularly should be cleared at least once a day, and any stones used for healing, meditation, or divination need to be cleared immediately after the work is finished. By pulsing, you can return jewelry, crystals, and gemstones to their normal vibrational state, ridding them of any residual energy or undesired charge.

Demagnetizing Devices

Another method for clearing crystals and gemstones is by using a demagnetizer or bulk eraser. These devices are available at most electronic supply and stereo stores. In much the same way that you would use it to demagnetize tape heads, draw the demagnetizer along the outer edges and faces of the stone to erase any unwanted energy or residual charge. Cover each face.

There is a great deal of speculation about the desirability of using electronic devices to clear crystals and stones. This method of clearing is my least favorite, but it is effective and practical for clearing a large number of stones in a short period of time. Used in tandem with salt water, demagnetizing devices are very effective.

Amplifying

Holding the crystal in your right hand, with the tip pointed outward, snap your wrist in a whipping motion, directing the energy of the crystal into the ground. This motion stimulates the crystal into full activity. If you visualize cobalt blue light flowing through the crystal while doing this, it also has the effect of clearing the stone. Because the motion is easy and quick, this method is especially effective during healing procedures, when the stone builds up negative energy. Be sure to point your crystal toward the ground. In this way, any unwanted energy is absorbed and transformed by the earth.

Charging and Programming Crystals

Crystals act as simple computers and can be tuned and programmed to your vibration. Through this vibration, you communicate—receive and send—a charge from another person or object. Just by holding a stone, you charge or imprint it with your energy. You can store any pattern of thought that you choose in your crystal. For example, if you want to expand your awareness, place that thought-form into the stone, and carry it on your person. This process is a simple way to access and develop your personal abilities, such as concentration, healing, meditation, relaxation, and goal achievement.

Intention and breath are the key components in charging and programming crystals. Your indwelling breath diminishes the charge, while your outgoing breath amplifies it. The ideal intention when working with crystals and stones is one of love and well-being. By directing your intention and breath in specific ways, you set up a vibrational field or charge within the crystal. This transfer charge is stored within the crystalline lattice, and carries a magnetic quality that can be erased, just as it can be programmed.

The programming procedure is simple. While holding your cleared crystal in your right hand, point it toward the palm of your left hand, at a distance of eight to twelve inches. Close your eyes, take a deep breath and hold it a few moments. At the same time, focus your attention and awareness on the tip of the crystal. Visualize and verbalize what program you wish to put into the crystal. As you exhale, sharply pulse your breath through your nostrils, not your mouth. This transfers your feelings and visual messages to the crystal. Repeat this procedure three times for a six-sided crystal, cluster, or sphere, four times for an eight-sided crystal.

This charging or programming process links the crystal to the vibration of your body. Every living form has its personal vibration, like a signature. The rhythmic vibration of the crystal, which resonates with the vibration of your etheric body (your subtle energy body that surrounds you), is similar to your heartbeat, but much faster and more delicate.

The strength of the crystal charge or program depends on your level of concentration and clarity of intent. Staying focused on the task at hand is the key to crystal programming. If you find your mind wandering, stop what you are doing and regain your center and focus. Take a deep breath and turn your mind to oneness, which will help you to regain your focus.

Your breathing acts as a carrier wave. You program the crystal by imprinting a thought-form onto this carrier wave, which is absorbed by the stone. Thought is rhythmic energy, and displays distinct repeating patterns. When you program a crystal with specific thought patterns, the stone reflects this pattern when you use it in any application, be it healing, meditation, prophecy, protection, or astral projection.

To check if your crystal is charged and programmed, rub one of the faces with your index or middle finger. You should feel it stick slightly to the crystal. It may feel as if the crystal is sweating or vibrating.

The crystal will hold the charge or program until you clear it or reprogram it. For this reason, clearing and cleaning your crystals after you use them is standard procedure. Otherwise you remain connected to the crystal and any energies that permeate or influence it.

You can charge crystals with a permanent program. For instance, the crystal you wear can be programmed with a non-erasable program of love, well-being, and protection. To do this, simply clear the crystal and then charge it with that program, first along one axis, then along a second axis at right angles, and finally along the third axis, creating a three-dimensional program. To check whether the program is indeed permanent, try clearing the crystal in the usual ways, and see if the program remains. If it does, go ahead and repeat the procedure to reinforce the original program.

Once you have set the primary program in place, you can then imprint the crystal with secondary programs, depending on its use and your intention. Remember, your intention is what is most important. Don't be overly concerned with whether your crystal is perfectly charged and programmed. The depth of your connection with the crystal determines its effectiveness.

Elemental and Sensory Charging Techniques

You can charge crystals and gemstones with the natural energy of the four elements—earth, air, fire, and water, as well as with sound and light. The following are ways of charging your stones with the energies of nature.

Sunlight: Place the crystal outside in the sun, on a fireproof surface. Avoid setting clear stones on the window sill, as they magnify the sun's rays and can actually burn a hole in the sill, and possibly start a fire. Depending on the charge you want to put in the crystal, you may want to set it out several days in a row until the sun's energy is firmly lodged within it. If you want only the sun's energy in the crystal, remember to bring it in each day before the sun goes down, otherwise moon and star energy will also be imparted to the stone.

Continued ➡

Never place your crystals or stones in fire, as this will damage them, both physically and energetically.

Moonlight: One method for charging your crystal with moonlight involves placing the crystal out at night for an entire cycle of the moon (twenty-eight days). Another method is to leave the crystal out only during the full moon, new moon, crescent moon, and so forth, depending on the kind of energy you want it to absorb.

Starlight: I suggest you try this technique on a New Moon because the stars are much more visible. Also if possible, select a spot on the beach, the mountains, or in the desert where there are no extraneous lights. Begin with a cleared stone. Select a favorite star in the night sky, for example Sirius. Stare or gaze at the star while holding your crystal or gemstone cradled in both hands. Slowly lift the stone in front of you with your left hand until the light from Sirius shines through it. Gaze at the crystal absorbing the star energy for about five minutes, and then switch the crystal to your right hand. Allow the starlight to shine through it for five more minutes. Use your breath to pulse the light and qualities of the star into your stone. This charging technique works best with clear quartz crystals because of their clarity and ability to absorb light.

Earth, sand, soil: Bury the crystal or gemstone in the earth, sand, or soil. The longer you leave it buried, the stronger the charge. Leaving the stone in the earth for a full year is particularly effective, as the natural seasonal cycle becomes embedded in it. If you have a favorite spot out in nature, bury the stone there. It will collect the energy from the site, and you can tap into this energy when using or carrying the stone.

Air, incense, oils: Place your stones outside during a strong wind to charge them with the element of air. Burn incense and pass your stones through the smoke. Sandalwood, copal resin, sweet grass, and pine smoke are particularly useful, and can also clean any negative energy from stones. To charge your stones with oil essences, place one drop on the tip of the crystal. Stones may become gummed up with oil, so be sure to clean them with a sea salt solution after use.

Water, ocean, lakes, rivers: Submerge the crystal in the water of the ocean, lake, or river having the energy you want to impart to the crystal. The longer you leave the crystal in the water, the longer the charge will last.

Sound charging: Use music, chanting, singing, drumming, and other sounds to enhance the healing or spiritual properties of your crystals and gemstones. One way of doing this is to place your stones next to your stereo speakers.

—From *Pocket Guide to Crystals & Gemstones*

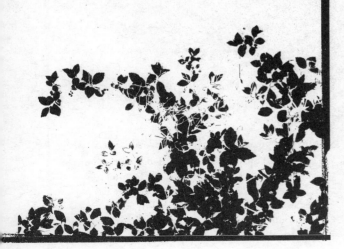

Healing and Spiritual Properties of Crystals and Gemstones

Agate, Blood Agate, Red Agate, Banded Agate, Moss Agate, Blue Lace Agate, Brown Agate, White Agate, Black Agate, Green Agate

Color: Variegated and banded, translucent and sometimes transparent, white to gray, brown, blue, black.

Healing and Spiritual Uses: A kind of chalcedony comprised of microscopic quartz crystals, agate is excellent for emotional and physical balancing, digestion, grounding, building healthy energy patterns and self-confidence, longevity, protection, self-honesty, scrying, reducing stress, and blood circulation.

Amazonite, Amazonstone (Feldspar)

Color: Blue-green, green.

Healing and Spiritual Uses: Finding personal truth, luck, prosperity, successful completion, growth, soothing energy, creativity, psychic ability, and receiving energy.

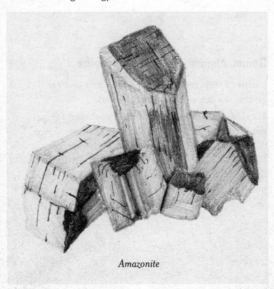

Amazonite

Amethyst

Color: Light to dark purple, dark purple-red, deep violet to pale lavender to almost clear.

Healing and Spiritual Uses: Spiritual development, divine connection, mental clarity, healing, balancing and controlling temperament, love, divination, wisdom, courage, psychic growth, dreaming, protection, and invulnerability. Curbs the urge to drink alcohol, helps to overcome addiction, and increases hormone production. Beneficial for the circulatory and nervous system, relaxation, astral travel, doubling out, which is being in the physical world and in an "other" world at the same time; seeing beyond illusions, and banishing nightmares.

Aquamarine

Color: Green, pale blue-green, aqua.

Healing and Spiritual Uses: Form of beryl utilized for clarity of perception and eyesight, releasing old patterns and conditioning, flow of creativity, inspiration, peace of mind, multidimensional experience, protection, courage, centering, purification and cleansing, calming and soothing energy, reducing fears, and sharpening intuition.

Aventurine

Color: Green, red, blue, brown.

Healing and Spiritual Uses: Positive participation, growth, healing, general well-being, activating the imagination, creativity, prosperity, good luck charm, and travel amulet. Strengthens eyesight, increases perception, and calms emotions.

Azurite

Color: Blue, blue-green (with malachite), copper flecks.

Healing and Spiritual Uses: Copper-based, called the "jewel of wisdom," azurite is beneficial for amplifying healing ability and energy, gaining insight, mental clarity and control, enhancing meditation, and prenatal strength.

Benitoite

Color: Pink, white, purple, blue, or translucent.

Healing and Spiritual Uses: Benefits the pituitary gland, improves intuition, communication with the Earth, growing patterns, and gardening.

Beryl, Heliodor

Color: Yellow, white, blue, gold, green, blue-green.

Healing and Spiritual Uses: Relieves stress and provides clarity. Helpful for discarding unwanted memories and habits. Strengthens circulation, boosts the immune system, clears eyesight. Enhances verbal communication and expression, reawakens love, romance, and self-responsibility.

Black Tourmaline

Color: Black.

Healing and Spiritual Uses: For ancestral communication, working with the shadow self, purification, protection. Repels negative energy, diffuses stress and tension, and boosts the immune system.

Bloodstone

Color: Deep or dark green with red inclusions in the form of flecks, or spots.

Healing and Spiritual Uses: Type of quartz beneficial for creativity, strength, vitality, circulation, building energy, higher knowledge, courage, purification, detoxification, divination, weather prediction, shrinking tumors, and strengthening the heart.

Calcite

Color: Shades of gold, white, black, green, gray, yellow, blue, brown, and red.

Healing and Spiritual Uses: All-around healing stone, place in bath water as a healing and calming essence. Use for mental clarity, boosting memory, adjusting to transition, transforming negativity, learning, meditation, concentration, and astral projection.

Carnelian

Color: Translucent or clear, dark red or orange-red to reddish brown, gold-red, and brown.

Healing and Spiritual Uses: A kind of chalcedony excellent for enhancing sexuality, accessing fire energy, building power, motivation, activating energy and creativity. Helpful for past life awareness, fertility, purification, lower back problems, prosperity, protection against injury or falling, courage, mental focus, and strength.

Chrysocolla

Color: Blue and green, resembles turquoise.

Healing and Spiritual Uses: For tapping into your inner voice, sacred communication, digestion, ulcers, arthritis, hypertension, stress. Beneficial for self-confidence and musical ability.

Continued ➡

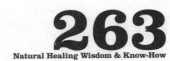

Chrysoprase

Color: Apple green, bright green.

Healing and Spiritual Uses: Quartz excellent for humility, personal insight, adapting to new environments or situations, creativity, fertility, and mental wellness. Relieves gout, strengthens eyesight, aids in cultivating the art of invisibility, out-of-body experience, psychonavigation, and shapeshifting.

Citrine

Color: Gold, brown-gold, pale to dark golden-yellow.

Healing and Spiritual Uses: Enhances mindfulness, intellectual reasoning, mental quickness, clarity. Relieves headaches, increases motivation, dispels negativity. Beneficial for manifesting goals and ideas, insight, personal empowerment.

Clear Quartz, Rock Quartz

Color: Clear, with or without inclusions.

Healing and Spiritual Uses: Called "the stars within the earth"; excellent for healing, doubling out (see "Amethyst"), balancing energy, sight, clarity, higher consciousness, spiritual enlightenment, meditation, divine guidance, perseverance, scientific applications, storing, releasing and regulating energy, purifying, unblocking energy in the body, mind, and spirit.

Diamond

Color: Clear, refracting all of the colors of the rainbow.

Healing and Spiritual Uses: Associated with lightning; the hardest substance of nature; used for healing, strength, power, good fortune, sexuality, love, insight, inspiration, protection, personal development, catalyzing and amplifying energy, multidimensional awareness, clarity, endurance, memory, and prosperity. Amplifies the energy of the wearer, be it positive or negative.

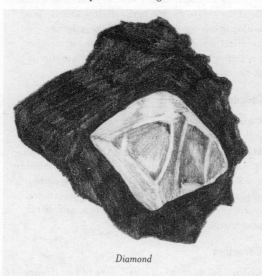

Diamond

Emerald

Color: Light to deep green, and all shades in between.

Healing and Spiritual Uses: A kind of beryl excellent for psychic clarity, divination, growth, enhancing sexuality, healing, inspiration, cleansing, gastric problems, cultivating patience, equilibrium of body, mind, and spirit, meditation, wisdom, managing diabetes, back problems, and neutralizing radioactivity. Boosts the immune system and raises consciousness.

Fluorite

Color: Translucent in shades of blue, purple, pink, red, white, brown, yellow, gold, or colorless.

Healing and Spiritual Uses: For self-discipline, harmony, balance, empowering female energy, other world experience, cancer remission, arthritis, enhancing sexuality, spiritual awakening, out-of-body experience, projecting a sense of peace and tranquillity. Benefits teeth and bones.

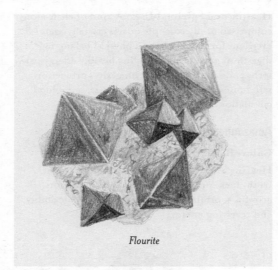

Flourite

Garnet, Almandine, Pyrope, Rhodolite

Color: Deep red translucent to deep emerald green, shades of yellow and brown.

Healing and Spiritual Uses: Employed for prosperity, physical strength, love, passion, imagination, flow of ideas, friendship, and creativity. Benefits the circulatory system. Helpful for accessing past life and future life experience, good luck in business, cultivating compassion, calming anger, and sharpening perceptions.

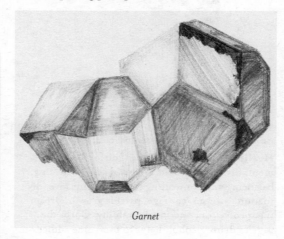

Garnet

Hematite (Iron Oxide)

Color: Steel gray to iron black, sometimes with red spots.

Healing and Spiritual Uses: Excellent for grounding, enhancing the circulation of bodily fluids, manifesting light and energy, protection, astral projection, strength, and working with the shadow self. Boosts low self-esteem. Helpful for kidney problems, tissue regeneration, headaches, hysteria, and feelings of vulnerability.

Herkimer Diamond

Color: Clear, sometimes with tiny black specks on surface.

Healing and Spiritual Uses: Propitious for dreaming, higher love, stimulating psychic centers, and empowerment. Reduces stress, provides a natural filter for negativity, and assists in recalling past-life experience.

Jade, Jadeite, Nephrite, Serpentine

Color: Green, yellow, orange, blue, pink, red, lavender, white, brown.

Healing and Spiritual Uses: Considered the concentrated essence of love, beneficial for protection, divine love, connection with Earth, removal of toxins, purity, calming nerves, ridding yourself of negativity, developing the capacity for receiving and giving love, meditation, and spiritual awareness. Helpful for kidney and bladder disorders, and assists in childbirth.

Jasper

Color: Red, yellow, gold, brown, green, variegated and mottled.

Healing and Spiritual Uses: Member of Chalcedony family excellent for gem essences, endurance, cleansing, fortitude, prayer, protection, quick thinking, and neutralizing stress.

Kunzite

Color: Pink and pink-white.

Healing and Spiritual Uses: Stone with high lithium content beneficial for mental disorders, circulatory system, receiving love, joy, building tolerance and gratitude, releasing old hurts and unwanted memories, and balancing mental and emotional bodies.

Labradorite, Spectrolite

Color: Blue.

Healing and Spiritual Uses: A kind of feldspar employed in magic, ritual, and ceremony. Elevates consciousness, enhances psychic ability, and assists in regeneration, sexuality, and protection. Helpful in psychonavigation and shapeshifting, and divine communication.

Lapis Lazuli

Color: Deep blue, often with flecks of pyrite or mottled with white calcite.

Healing and Spiritual Uses: For psychic development, divination, protection, self-knowledge, wisdom, creativity, magical power, prosperity, doubling out (see "Amethyst"), shielding, and shapeshifting. A thought amplifier, helpful for respiratory or nervous disorders. Boosts energy and the immune system, expands awareness, and is propitious for personal empowerment.

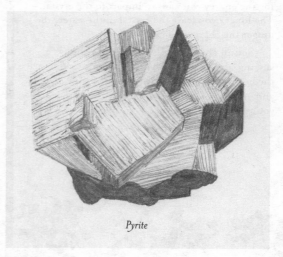

Pyrite

Lepidolite

Color: purple, some with pink tourmaline crystals.

Healing and Spiritual Uses: Called the "stone of peace" and rich in lithium, excellent for out-of-body experience, increasing psychic ability, acceptance, awareness, peace and tranquillity, relieving stress, soothing anger and diffusing negativity, good luck, restful sleep, and pleasant dreams.

Continued ➡

Malachite

Color: Bright green to light green, variegated.

Healing and Spiritual Uses: For magic, will-power, communication with nature, visions, rapport with animal kingdom, shapeshifting, moving energy, sound sleep, divine communication, and balance. Used for tissue regeneration and healing. Stimulates the optic nerve, balances dyslexia, and neutralizes radioactivity.

Moldavite

Color: Deep green.

Healing and Spiritual Uses: For transformation, shapeshifting, personal metamorphosis, cleansing, and personal attunement. Stimulates psychic senses, accelerates spiritual growth and development, and encourages motivation and change.

Moonstone

Color: Milky and translucent, pale blue, green, and gray.

Healing and Spiritual Uses: Connection to female energy, receptivity, tidal flow, cycles, multi-dimensional awareness. Beneficial for balancing emotions, the reproductive organs, and healing. Enhances sensitivity, intuition, clairvoyance, open-mindedness. Employed in farming, divination, artistic pursuits, and dancing. Brings good fortune, fruitfulness, and true love.

Obsidian, Apache Tear

Color: Black transparent or semitransparent, flecked with white or striped.

Healing and Spiritual Uses: Volcanic stone for protection and working with the shadow self. Sharpens inner and outer vision. Used for divination (obsidian mirrors), ritual tools, past life regression, good luck, letting go of old patterns and memories, and in ceremony and ritual.

Onyx

Color: Black, white, or translucent, with layers of red, yellow, brown, or pink.

Healing and Spiritual Uses: Story-telling stone, beneficial for building life patterns, creating structure in your life, accessing physical memories, and alleviating mental and emotional stress. Strengthens energy, lessens fear and worry, and allows for communication with underworld energies.

Opal, Fire Opal, Star Opal

Color: Milky or white with multicolored patterns inside, opaque, clear, transparent, yellow-brown.

Healing and Spiritual Uses: Containing up to 30 percent water and called the "eye stone," excellent for harmonizing energy, eye disorders, accessing cosmic energy, activating creativity and wisdom, gaining balance and inspiration, doubling out (see "Amethyst"), intensifying emotional states, business, protection, and lucid dreaming.

Peridot

Color: Clear, pale green.

Healing and Spiritual Uses: For balancing energy, emotional tranquillity, healing, insight, clairvoyance, personal empowerment, vision, clarity of purpose, and enlightenment. Enhances digestion, stimulates tissue regeneration, and boosts confidence.

Rhodochrosite

Color: Orange and pink with white veins or stripes.

Healing and Spiritual Uses: Employed in matters of the heart, and accessing your inner child. Helpful for asthma, respiratory illness, kidney disorders, and alleviating irrational fears and worries. Enhances dreaming and promotes restful sleep.

Rose Quartz

Color: Light to medium pink mottled with white.

Healing and Spiritual Uses: Excellent for emotional balancing in relationships, friendships, and higher love. Helpful for spiritual awakening, compassion, personal attunement, forgiveness, self-acceptance, adapting to changes, tapping into the inner voice, restoring faith, and fertility. Raises low self-esteem, assists in healing, and enhances creativity.

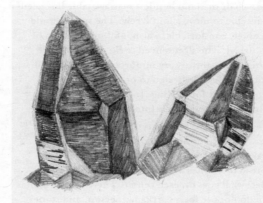
Quartz

Ruby

Color: Deep red to bright purple-red, shades of pink and lavender.

Healing and Spiritual Uses: Builds inner strength, amplifies inner energy, enhances personal empowerment, insight, creativity, physical and mental strength, and activates the life force. Beneficial for building energy and drive. Aids the heart and circulatory system, and is excellent for doubling out (see "Amethyst"), clarity, friendship, passion, and protection.

Rutilated Quartz, Venus Hair, Fleches d'Amour

Color: Clear to pale yellow with needlelike rutile inclusions.

Healing and Spiritual uses: For healing, directing energy, balance, insight, sustaining good health, and creating positive life patterns. Boosts the immune system, elevates energy, enhances sexuality and self-esteem.

Sapphire, Star Sapphire

Color: Deep blue, shades of black, gray, green, and yellow, star sapphire with aqueous inclusions, which create a five-pointed star on the stone's surface.

Healing and Spiritual Uses: For psychic development, enhancing focus, creativity, providing serenity, calming emotions, diffusing negativity, healing, especially eyesight, easing stress and tension, and dispelling fear. Excellent for concentration, meditation, divine communication, divination, doubling out (see "Amethyst"), astral projection, aligning body, mind, and spirit, and good fortune.

Smithsonite

Color: Shades of pink, purple, blue, yellow, and green.

Healing and Spiritual Uses: Named for James Smithson, founder of the Smithsonian Institute, beneficial for healing, enhancing relationships, sexuality, unity, evoking emotion, and sparking romance. Strengthens feelings of security and clarity. Accesses innovative thoughts, ideas, and multi-dimensional awareness.

Smoky Quartz

Color: Medium to dark brown and chocolate brown-black.

Healing and Spiritual Uses: For grounding, centering, connecting to the Earth, healing, and building prosperity. Neutralizes negative influences and balances the nervous system. Helpful for radiation-related illnesses. Used for crystal scrying.

Sodalite

Color: Blue, sometimes with gray or white veins.

Healing and Spiritual Uses: Helpful for lymph circulation, mental clarity, and boosting the immune system. Enhances objectivity, vision, clairvoyance, balances the metabolism, and neutralizes radiation.

Sugilite

Color: Purple, sometimes with darker veins.

Healing and Spiritual Uses: Employed in dreaming, divine communication, channeling, out-of-body experience, multidimensional awareness and travel. Enhances psychic abilities and helps to charge the energy body.

Tanzanite

Color: Clear, shades of blue and purple-blue.

Healing and Spiritual Uses: Excellent for insight and helpful for discerning the truth. Used in divination, channeling, divine communication, astral projection, and psychonavigation. Enhances psychic abilities and expands perception.

Tiger's Eye, Cat's Eye

Color: Light to dark brown with fibrous inclusions.

Healing and Spiritual Uses: Quartz stone used for balance, invisibility, strength, insight, and inner knowledge. Instills the confidence to accomplish your goals and recognize inner resources. Helpful for protection, mental focus, concentration, and shape-shifting.

Topaz

Color: Bright yellow, brown-yellow, shades of green, blue, and brown.

Healing and Spiritual Uses: Enhances insight, knowledge, intention, loyalty, higher love, and creativity. Helpful in unmasking deception in others, recharging energy, balancing and warming, healing, problem solving, and scientific discovery. Assists in artistic pursuits, calms the nerves, eases tension, and is excellent in gem essences, or for treating eyesight problems.

Tourmaline

Color: Green, pink to salmon (rubelite), blue, opalized.

Healing and Spiritual Uses: Strengthens energy body and boosts the immune system. Used for regeneration, creativity, and growth. Beneficial cleansing and purifying properties for the body that are helpful in polarity work and healing. Employed for divine communication and spiritual awakening.

Turquoise

Color: Sky blue to soft and deep green or green-blue.

Healing and Spiritual Uses: Excellent for ritual and ceremony, for gaining wholeness, knowledge, elemental wisdom, communicating with devas and ancestors, and promoting personal attunement. Stimulates motivation and healing. Beneficial for respiratory problems, greater self-realization, and endurance.

Continued →

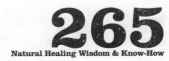

Watermelon Tourmaline, Rainbow Tourmaline

Color: Multicolored bands of pink, green, and purple.

Healing and Spiritual Uses: For inner peace, harmony, balancing and energizing body, mind, and spirit, polarity work, and problem-solving.

Zircon

Color: Clear in shades of blue, green, yellow, red, and brown.

Healing and Spiritual Uses: A look-alike for diamond, excellent for personal reflection, calming nerves, teaching patience and reserve, and improving tolerance.

—From *Pocket Guide to Crystals & Gemstones*

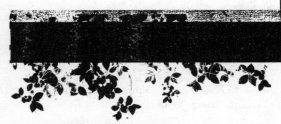

LAYING ON OF STONES

Diane Stein

The technique of using crystals and gemstones on the receiver's body for healing is called laying on of stones. It is a powerful method of cleansing negative energy, clearing and balancing the chakras, effecting emotional release, and bringing light and healing into all the aura bodies. Cleared, programmed, and dedicated stones move the receiver's vibration into alignment with the planet and the universal grid. This results in a freeing of life force energy in the chakras and aura, a healing of the Body of Light, and a transformation of negative or dis-ease energy into health. Laying on of stones also affects the chakras on both kundalini and hara line levels.

The process may be done with clear quartz crystals only, colored gemstones only, or a combination of both. I prefer a combination. The stones may be used alone or with a hands-on healing, and again I prefer both. The stones are placed upon the receiver's body from feet to head. The healer then begins using her hands as usual, starting at the head and moving toward the feet. Use gemstones with colors matching each chakra's color, the hara chakra stones appearing between the kundalini centers. The stones can be any combination of forms—faceted, raw, tumbled, eggs, strings of beads, etc. Clear crystals can be used at any chakra, with or without colored gemstones.

Energy in this type of healing needs to move in one direction through the body, either Earth to sky or sky to Earth. If the energy is Earth to sky, all of the crystals or gemstones that have points are placed with the points turned toward the receiver's crown. The effect of this direction is to move the receiver's energy to a higher vibration or more spiritual level. If the direction is from sky to Earth, it is the opposite, with the crystals pointing toward her feet. This direction moves life force energy from crown to feet, for grounding and rooting into Earth. A number of patterns can be used for placing crystals and gemstones on the body, but following the line of the central channels is basic, all that is actually required.

To place the stones, put colored gemstones on the chakras, matching their colors to the chakra colors. Put clear crystals in the receiver's hands, above her crown, below her feet, and in a circle around her body a few inches away. The crystals around the body should point toward the receiver. Clear crystals can also be used at each chakra, surrounded by the colored gemstones. They can be placed between the kundalini chakras so that they are over the hara chakras to activate the hara line, or colored stones can be placed over the hara chakras, as well.

To begin, the receiver lies on her back on a padded floor or massage table, with pillows under her head and knees for comfort. The healer may use a chair or stand beside a massage table but needs to be able to move about freely. The space should be quiet, comfortable, warm, and not likely to be disturbed. The stones need to be cleared before using them—this is very important. Use only stones that have been dedicated to positive energy and programmed for healing. Invite the participant's spirit guides and angels into the session.

Start by placing the crystals below the receiver's feet, in her hands, and above her head. Then go chakra by chakra, moving from feet to crown. Spread the stones where you can reach them and select what goes on each center. There may be stones you do not use for a particular person, and stones that are drawn to a chakra where their colors don't logically match. Let yourself be guided; there are no real rules. A stone whose energy is not needed for the session or is inappropriate for the receiver's energy will roll right off or roll to another place where it is better utilized. Allow this to occur. If you "forget" to place a stone, it is because its energy is not useful for that person or healing. If the receiver says a stone feels uncomfortable take it off; the energy isn't right for her needs.

When the stones are all in place, the healer has two options. She can next go to the receiver's head and begin a hands-on healing. She must place her hands carefully so that she does not scatter the stones. Her other choice is to sit beside the receiver quietly and simply wait, allowing the stones and spirit guides to do the healing. As the receiver's chakras and aura absorb and are balanced by the crystal and gem energies, the stones begin to roll off one by one. The receiver may say that something now feels uncomfortable or feels finished; move that stone from her body. Sometimes all the stones seem to jump off at once, though the receiver is lying perfectly still. It can startle and is often funny when this happens. Do not replace them.

When all the stones are off, or you or the receiver feel finished with those that remain, the healing is over. Allow the receiver to lie quietly for a while without the stones. While she is doing this, the healer can gather up the stones from the table and floor and clear them again before putting them away. Clearing the stones before and after each healing is necessary. After clearing, I keep mine in a protective pouch.

A laying-on-of-stones healing can be quite intense. There is often a major energy shift during this type of healing. More frequent emotional releases, past-life and this-life trauma openings, and other transformative events happen when gemstones and crystals are used than would occur without them. The healer's role in this is to wait for the release to end and to be entirely nonjudgmental. After a session, there may also be a physical and emotional detoxification process that can continue for up to a week. Be aware of what is happening and, again, allow it. The changes are always positive and are usually gentle.

—From *Healing with Gemstones and Crystals*

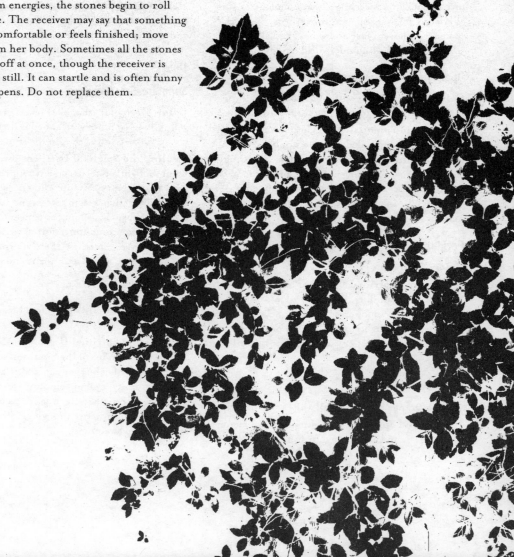

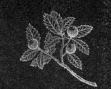

Flower Essences

BACH FLOWER ESSENCES

Rachel Hasnas

Dr. Edward Bach and His Philosophy of Healing

We each have a Divine mission in this world, and our souls use our minds and bodies as instruments to do this work, so that when all three are working in unison the result is perfect health and perfect happiness.

—Dr. Edward Bach

The Bach Flower Essences were developed in England in the late 1920s and early 1930s, by renowned British researcher and physician, Dr. Edward Bach. They are considered the first in what is now considered vibrational medicine. Bach, a brilliant physician, bacteriologist, immunologist, and pathologist, eventually turned from the orthodox medicine of his day to that of homeopathy. It was his understanding that to truly cure disease, the treatment of symptoms was not adequate. One needed to get to the root cause of disease for any cure to be lasting.

It was Dr. Bach's belief that a negative state of mind was at the core of any illness. It was not enough for him to treat the body alone. Body, mind, and spirit all needed to be considered in regard to healing. He was concerned about the treatment of the whole person. It became his dream to develop an entirely new system of medicine based upon his insight. He soon gave up his lucrative medical practice and began his search which took him back to the English countryside. He intuitively knew that there, among the flowers and trees of the field, he would find the healing properties that he was seeking.

One morning, while walking through a meadow, his highly developed sense of intuition made him realize that the dew on the plants, heated by the sun, now held the healing properties of the flowers it laid upon. As he continued his work, his intuition became so sensitive that, by holding a flower or tasting a petal, he could immediately sense what its healing effects were. In this way, one by one, he found and developed the 38 different flower essences that have come to be known today as the Bach Flower Essences.

Dr. Bach was a deeply spiritual man. His philosophy about disease was tied into his philosophy about life. He wrote in *Ye Suffer From Yourselves*, "Disease of the body, as we know it, is a result, an end product of something much deeper. Disease originates above the physical plane, nearer to the mental. It is entirely a result of a conflict between our spiritual and mortal selves. So long as these two are in harmony, we are in perfect health: but when there is discord there follows what we know as disease."

It was Dr. Bach's belief that we are more than physical beings—we are spiritual beings in truth, each coming into this world with a certain purpose or mission to fulfill. When we become out of sync with our spiritual purpose, disharmony arises. This can come about by interference of other people—allowing them to push us off our course—or by our own moods, fears, or hesitations. Dr. Bach further wrote in *Ye Suffer From Yourselves*, "Whatever errors we make, it reacts upon ourselves, causing us unhappiness, discomfort, or suffering. . . The object being to teach us the harmful effect of wrong action or thought: and by its producing similar results upon ourselves, shows us how it causes distress to others, and is contrary to the Great and Divine Law of Love and Unity."

As we can see from his writings, he considered disease beneficent and purely corrective—a message from our soul that changes need to occur in our lives if we are to find and maintain our health and happiness. He goes on to write that disease "is the means adopted by our own Souls to point out to us our faults: to prevent our making greater errors: to hinder us from doing more harm: and to bring us back to the path of Truth and Light from which we should never have strayed."

It was his contention that in order for health to exist, there must be perfect harmony between body, mind, and spirit. And it was this harmony alone that needed to be reestablished for any lasting cure to be effected. To this end he developed the flower essences—to release the emotional and mental

Continued ➔

disharmony within us, to facilitate being true to our soul's purpose once again, thereby restoring our system's equilibrium. As he wrote in *The Twelve Healers and Four Helpers*, "It is not possible for us to be ill unless we are not in harmony with our true nature. But whatever condition is behind our trouble, whatever fault there is in our nature it matters not, because these remedies will help us to correct that fault and thus curing the root-cause of our illness and give back to us bodily and mental health."

Thus it would seem from Dr. Bach's writings that the presence of germs, or even our genetic make-up, although they may play some part in the development of illness, are not the true cause of lack of health. This is a profound insight and one that brings to us a whole new way of looking at health and healing.

Dr. Bach wrote, "These [negative states of mind], if we allow them, will reflect themselves in the body causing what we call disease. Not understanding the real causes we have attributed disharmony to external influences, germs, cold, heat, and have given names to the results, arthritis, cancer, asthma, etc.: thinking that disease begins in the physical body."

The old model of looking at the human body as merely a machine may be on the verge of extinction—and long overdue. Our materialistic view of life is being challenged with the recognition of a spiritual component that has, for too long, been overlooked. We are living in exciting times!

Bach Flower Essences Defined

You are about to begin a sacred journey, a journey of self-discovery. . . one that opens you to personal growth and emotional healing. I'll be sharing with you concise information on Dr. Bach's flower essences—their use and effect—gleaned from my personal and professional experience, to give you a deeper and richer understanding of the energy in each and to facilitate your selection of the appropriate flower essences with confidence.

You'll soon learn how the flower essences can assist you in just about any area of your life where you find yourself emotionally out-of-balance. When you're having difficulty in coping with the situations you face in these stress-producing times—whether it's worries and fears, lack of self-esteem, or even depression, the flower essences can help. And as we are now beginning to recognize, these negative emotional states may be the catalysts to the eventual development of disease.

It is interesting and exciting to note that traditional Western medicine is now taking notice of the mind-body connection, and beginning to recognize that emotions play a much greater role in the body's health than was believed or understood before. For several years now, studies by psychoneuroimmunologists are being conducted in leading universities and research centers countrywide, establishing a firm link between the mind, emotions, and the body. It has now been proven that negative emotions do have an ill effect on our well-being. Psychoneuroimmunology is a relatively new branch of medicine which has been studying brain chemistry in relation to stress. It appears from these studies that adverse neurotransmitters are produced by the brain when we are under stress, deleteriously affecting the immune system, our body's first defense against disease. The longer this biological process continues unchecked, the more vulnerable we become to the onset of any number of disorders.

We know that high blood pressure, ulcers, migraine headaches, heart disease, allergies, and asthma have all been linked to stress. As far back as May 24, 1983, this link was reported in an article in the *New York Times* entitled "Emotions Bound to Influence Nearly Every Human Ailment." It stated, "Virtually every ill that can befall the human body—from the common cold to cancer and heart disease—can be influenced, positively or negatively, by a person's mental state." It appears that Dr. Bach was well ahead of his time, with modern medicine only now catching up!

Before we explore the 38 Bach Flower Essences in depth, a short introduction to what they are and how they work is needed for those not familiar with them.

Please remember, the flower essences are an adjunct modality to be used along with traditional medical treatment. They work as catalysts in restoring and balancing your body's own healing system.

Simplicity, Humility, Compassion

These three words are inscribed on the plaque which hangs over the door of the Bach Center in England. They are more than just words acknowledging Dr. Bach's contributions to humankind. They also have a powerful message for all who are open to hear. The flower essences can teach you the true meaning of these words, as they assist in bringing inner peace and a sense of well-being into your life.

Simplicity—The flower essences teach us that things don't have to be complicated. These natural preparations, carefully made from the essences of flowering plants, offer a complete, effective, safe, yet simple system of gentle stress relief—a system that allows you to be involved in your own healing process. It was Dr. Bach's intention that his system be so safe and simple that anyone could use it at any time, even during pregnancy. To paraphrase his words, he wanted it to be so simple that when an individual was hungry they would go to the garden and pick some lettuce, and when they were afraid they'd take a dose of Mimulus (one of the 38 flower essences he developed to counteract known fears).

Humility—As you begin selecting your flower essences, you'll find as I have, that this is a journey of self-discovery, for you are learning about the personal issues and conflicts inside yourself that are the cause of disharmony within you. Humility becomes crucial, for it allows you to be open to self-reflection which ultimately can lead to personal growth. To be honest with yourself and admit that change may be needed takes great courage and strength. Yet this is a necessary step on your journey to wholeness. By looking within and being in touch with your feelings, recognizing your negative states of mind, you'll be better able to select the essences that relate to you. You will understand the issues that have been holding you back from living life in a richer, more meaningful way.

Compassion—Dr. Bach's flower essences were developed out of his love and compassion for humanity. He felt a calling, even as a young boy, to be able to help people heal. As you work with the flower essences personally, you'll find yourself recognizing certain flower essences that could be helpful to others you know. You will begin to see the flower essences, not only as facilitators of change in your own life, but as special gifts to be shared from your deepening sense of love and compassion, as did Dr. Bach.

The Bach Flower Essences contain certain properties taken from 38 specific flowering plants and trees that Dr. Bach determined to have special healing attributes, with the addition of pure spring water and brandy, added as a preservative. Like other natural medicine, they take effect through treating the whole individual, not the disease or symptoms of disease. Therefore, they are never selected for any specific symptom or condition. The negative emotional state determines the selection.

As an example, two people, each with the same disease—perhaps high blood pressure—would more than likely each benefit from a different flower essence. One may have developed the condition because of an impatient nature, the other from an overly critical one. Hence, a different flower essence, with its unique vibration, would be appropriate for each individual. The person who is overly critical, and takes the Beech flower essence for this state of mind, would experience increased tolerance. The individual who is impatient, and takes the Impatiens flower essence for this state of mind, would experience more patience. Their own potential for self-healing will be reinstated, freeing the physical system of the stress that was originally creating these conditions.

In the cases of these two individuals the flower essences were selected for their particular negative emotional states. They were not chosen for their symptoms or conditions. The Bach Flower Essences work by transforming (rather than suppressing) negative attitudes or emotions into positive ones.

The Bach Flower Essences are a form of energetic or vibrational medicine, as it is now termed. The energy or vibration taken from the flowers gently affects and enhances our system on subtle levels. In *Vibrational Medicine*, Dr. Richard Gerber defines this energy medicine as, "That healing philosophy which aims to treat the whole person—the mind/body/spirit complex—by delivering measured quanta of frequency-specific energy to the human multi-dimensional system. Vibrational medicine seeks to heal the physical body by integrating and balancing the higher energetic systems which create the physical/cellular patterns of manifestation… Vibrational medicine is a healing approach which is based upon the Einsteinian concept of matter as energy, and of human beings as a series of complex energy fields in dynamic equilibrium."

With his great sensitivity, Dr. Bach was also aware that we have a series of energy bodies within our physical body. He wrote in *Heal Thyself* that, "Materialism forgets that there is a factor above the physical plane which in the ordinary course of life protects or renders susceptible any particular individual with regard to disease, of whatever nature it may be. Fear, by its depressing effect on our mentality, thus causes disharmony in our physical and magnetic bodies and paves the way for (bacterial) invasion. The real cause of disease lies in our own personality. . . ."

The flower essences were created to work on these subtle bodies, for it is here where our system's equilibrium has been disturbed by our negative attitudes and emotions, with the mind-body connection coming into play. And it is here where the flower essences can balance and restore our system's homeostasis once again.

As you go through your selection process, remember to choose your flower essences solely with regard to the out-of-balance emotional or mental states you may be suffering from—such as impatience and being overcritical. There are many other stress-producing emotions that the Bach Flower Essences bring balance to, such as fear, bitterness, lack of self-esteem, denial or repression, resentment, apathy, guilt, to highlight several more. Dr. Bach felt that all known negative emotional states are addressed by them and considered his flower essences a complete system.

It cannot be emphasized too strongly that Dr. Bach believed that it was our negative states of mind that were the root cause—the very breeding ground of disease—and, if left unchecked, the catalyst for

Continued ➡

eventual illness and symptom manifestation. Dr. Bach wrote, in *Free Thyself*, "This disharmony, disease, makes itself manifest in the body for the body merely serves to reflect the workings of the soul; just as the face reflects happiness by smiles, or temper by frowns. And so in bigger things; the body will reflect the true causes of disease (which are such as fear, indecision, doubts, etc.) in the disarrangement of its systems and tissues."

By selecting the appropriate flower essence that remedies the particular negative emotion, the healing properties contained in the essence act like an antidote. A flower essence has the ability to gently and safely release negative emotional states by flooding the body's system with the positive vibration it carries. Over time, emotional balance is again restored. It is important to state again that the flower essences never repress emotional imbalances. Rather, they are catalysts for their release.

The flower essences don't have the effect of tranquilizers or antidepressants, aren't considered herbs or vitamins, and won't interfere with the effects of other medication being used. Because the flower essences are so safe and gentle, you cannot overdose in their use. Dr. Bach's self-help system is totally safe, natural, and harmless, without need for any concern over the possibility of side effects. And when kept in a cool, dark place, the flower essences have an indefinite shelf life. As this system of healing is a very individualized modality; there is no specific length of time as to how long you need to take them. Many flower essence users report that they feel the effects within two to six weeks. Individual sensitivity is a factor here; thus, the reaction time is different for each individual.

Know that a commitment to the flowers essences is important for them to be effective. If you are not committed to using them consistently, you'll think they don't work. Most flower essences need to be taken from one to two months. Only you can determine when your issues have been released. If you stop too soon, and your issues reappear, just continue to take them for a while longer. Another factor in your reaction time to flower essence use is how long you have been dealing with a particular emotion or issue, and how deeply ingrained into the personality it has become. The more deeply ingrained, the longer will be the reaction time.

The question of the Bach Flower Essences being a placebo comes up many times. This placebo effect has long been an accepted phenomenon in medical practice, although little understood. The answer to this question is a definite no. It is not just mind over matter that produces the flower essences' positive effects. A placebo study was done by Michael Weisglass, Ph.D. at the California Institute of Asian Studies in 1979. His study showed the flower essences to have a much greater effect on those who actually took them, in comparison to the control group—those who were not given the flower essences, but only thought they were taking them. In his research he found that the flower essences operated independently of the belief system of the user.

Young children and animals have no awareness that they are being given any special medicine to bring about any emotionally related changes. In my work with them I have found the flower essences to indeed have a marked effect in bringing about relief. This will be further illustrated with case studies in later sections on the use of the flower essences with children and animals.

The next section will assist you in identifying the flower essences you may need. The indications which describe the out-of-balance emotional state(s) and/or personality trait(s) that each flower essence addresses are clearly and simply presented. As you read through this information, it is sug-

gested to keep paper and pen handy to make note of which flower essences speak to you. Choose the ones that relate to your specific emotional issues and character traits that cause you problems.

It is recommended that no more than seven flower essences be used at any one time. It is not unusual at first to find yourself feeling you could use almost all of them. The key to limiting your selection to only seven is to focus on the issues that are the most intense for you right now—the ones that cause you stress on a daily basis. Of course, it's important to choose the appropriate flower essences to benefit from their effects. However, it is also reassuring to know that no harm can be done if you make a wrong selection. In this case, nothing happens. You will only respond to those that you need.

Indications for the 38 Bach Flowers

1—Agrimony

Botanical Name—*Agrimonia Eupatoria*
Vibration—*joyfulness*

Indications: Agrimony is indicated for those who do not acknowledge their feelings of pain and torment, but repress and deny their feelings, putting on a brave front, a cheerful facade. "Everything's fine," they say. Many times these individuals turn to alcohol or drugs to help mask feelings that are too difficult to face. Be aware, however, that substance abuse does not always have to be a part of the Agrimony personality to indicate the need for this flower essence. Other avoidance techniques can come into play: an addiction to TV as in the couch potato syndrome, overeating to numb emotional pain, as well as any other activity to ensure the repression of feelings. The Agrimony Type is driven to avoid torments at all costs. They shy away from confrontations and arguments, needing to keep the peace at any price.

Agrimony is suggested for use when in counseling, as it facilitates openness in getting in touch with what has been repressed or denied and releases buried issues, allowing emotional healing to take place.

Examples: This flower essence profile relates very much to the personality of Marilyn Monroe. Some other well known personalities that reflect the Agrimony profile are the TV character from *All in the Family*, Edith Bunker, who always seemed to be in denial regarding her feelings, and TV news anchorwoman Jessica Savitch, who died in an automobile accident. Since her death it has been revealed that her personal life was filled with deep emotional torment. She turned to drugs and alcohol to ease her pain.

2—Aspen

Botanical Name—*Populus Tremula*
Vibration—*fearlessness*

Indications: This flower essence, one of several available for treating states of fear, is indicated when the source of fear is *unknown*, such as with feelings of foreboding, uneasiness, apprehension. Use it when you don't really know what it is you're afraid of, yet you are experiencing feelings of fear. Nightmares, fear of the dark, and sometimes even a fear of God or the supernatural can bring on the Aspen state. Anxiety and panic attacks are also states that are relieved by this flower essence. The mark of the Aspen profile is the inability to put your finger on exactly what it is that is causing your fear, anxiety, or apprehension—the source being very vague and unclear.

Examples: The form of fear that Ebenezer Scrooge experienced with the appearance of the ghosts of Christmas past, present, and future in Dickens's *A Christmas Carol*, describes a facet of the Aspen state perfectly.

3—Beech

Botanical Name—*Fagus Sylvatica*
Vibration—*tolerance*

Indications: The indications for this flower essence are extreme criticism and intolerance of others—constant fault finding and judging. In most instances, feelings of intolerance are verbalized, but this doesn't have to be the case. The Beech Type may just observe and ruminate at how annoying others seem to be. There's a constant condemnation concerning others when in the negative Beech state. One is unable to accept others as they are. This flower essence is indicated for those with intolerance, as well as feelings of prejudice towards others—being judgmental to the extreme.

Examples: Jesus exemplified for us the most positive aspect of the Beech state, when he uttered, "Father forgive them, for they know not what they do." Felix Unger, the movie and TV character from *The Odd Couple*, is a perfect example of the out of balance state that Beech addresses, with his constant criticism of roommate Oscar. The comedians Don Rickles and Joan Rivers, and not to forget Carroll O'Connor in his role as Archie Bunker from TV's *All in the Family*, all beautifully portray the negative Beech state in their performances. By the way, Beech is the perfect flower essence to take before going to a family reunion—both for dealing with the possible intolerance of your relatives, and their possible intolerance of you!

4—Centaury

Botanical Name—*Centaurium Umbellatum*
Vibration—*self-determination*

Indications: In the negative Centaury state, the ability to refuse others' requests is difficult, if not impossible. These people are easily taken advantage of. The desire to serve others is really an admirable attribute although not when it is constantly at one's own expense. Being a doormat is not healthy. In fact, resentment develops when personal needs are always put aside. Centaury Types find it hard to let others know they are feeling resentful, and continue to allow others to use them. This cycle will persist, creating even greater resentment. They will hurt themselves in the process with the underlying negative emotions that result. Centaury Types don't like to make waves, to displease others, to be disliked; they find it extremely difficult to stand up for themselves. This behavior is classic co-dependency, and many have found Centaury helpful in releasing their victim issues.

It is as important that each of us is able to take care of ourselves, as it is to serve and help others. This is the lesson of the Centaury state. When giving to others is detrimental to their own welfare, this flower essence enables individuals to be able to say, "No—I'm really sorry, I'd love to help you out, but it's not possible now—maybe another time." Centaury allows us to do this gently and feel okay with it and know, "I can do what I need for myself. I don't always have to sacrifice my needs for others." We each need to learn to honor the spirit in us, as well as in others. It is our right and duty, actually, to consider and take care of ourselves. If we cannot love and nurture ourselves, how can we honestly love and nurture anyone else truly from our hearts? Dr. Bach indicated that Centaury Types are on the

Continued ➡

road to being of great service—although their motives are good, they are being passively used instead of actively choosing their own work.

Examples: When I think of the indications for Centaury, Cinderella always comes to mind. This fairy tale character is really the perfect example of the Centaury profile— always willing to please others at her own expense—always willing to serve and never say no. Again, we turn to Edith Bunker, portrayed by Jean Stapleton, as an excellent illustration for the Centaury profile, always putting her own needs last, if considering them at all.

5—Cerato

Botanical Name—*Ceratostigma Willmottiana*
Vibration—*inner certainty*

Indications: The indication for this flower essence is an extreme lack of self-confidence in decision making, which leads to constant dependency on others' advice. "I need to make a decision, but I don't have enough confidence in myself. I'd better check with Mary and John, also Sally and Jim, and find out what they think I should do." Cerato people check it out, they are told what to do and then maybe a day or two later, realize that the advice was wrong and they should have gone with their own feelings, after all. Cerato is indicated for those who lack confidence in their own judgment—always seeking advice and reassurance from others before they can act. Cerato releases this deep-seated reliance on others, bringing an inner confidence and ability to rely on one's own discernment. This Type is exemplified by the psychic junkie—always going from one consultation to the next, looking for answers that really lie within.

Examples: Kirstie Alley's portrayal of Rebecca in the TV show *Cheers*, illustrates the Cerato profile, with Rebecca always going to the rest of the characters for advice.

6—Cherry Plum

Botanical Name—*Prunus Cerasifera*
Vibration—*composure*

Indications: This flower essence addresses the fear of losing control in some way. These Types wish to harm themselves or others by taking unneeded risks or acting rashly. Cherry Plum aids in restoring self-control and helps bring an awareness of what's really in one's best interest. It is highly recommended in times of extreme emotional crisis, when there is danger or threat of suicide. There are many other situations—or Cherry Plum states—where there is a tendency to lose control, such as in temper outbursts, abusive behavior towards others, out-of-control gambling, and credit card use, as well as substance abuse. In fact, Cherry Plum is helpful for risk taking of all sorts. It has also been extremely successful in treating obsessive-compulsive behavior.

Examples: Kurt Cobain of the rock band Nirvana was in an extreme Cherry Plum state when he committed suicide. Musicians Janis Joplin and Jimi Hendrix, with their history of substance abuse and loss of control, are other examples of Cherry Plum Types who are out of balance.

7—Chestnut Bud

Botanical Name—*Aesculus Hippocastanum*
Vibration—*capacity for learning*

Indications: Chestnut Bud would be indicated for those who do not seem to learn from past mistakes, and continue to repeat the same old habit patterns that cause difficulty for them. In this state there seems to be a lack of observation. As an example, let's take a situation in which Chestnut Bud would be indicated. In this case scenario, an individual is constantly attracting unhealthy partners many times over—perhaps an alcoholic, or abuser. Each time the dysfunctional relationship is ended, like magic, the identical personality type, with a different name of course, appears at the doorstep, and once again, is invited in! Old patterns are hard to break. However, when you are ready to face the destruction they cause you, Chestnut Bud is waiting to help you learn from the past and act with more wisdom in the present. This flower essence is also highly recommended in releasing addictive behaviors.

Examples: Jerry Garcia, from the Grateful Dead Rock Band, would exemplify the out of balance state with his on-again, off-again use of drugs which eventually destroyed his health and led to his death. Nicole Simpson is another illustration of the Chestnut Bud profile, returning several times to an abusive relationship.

8—Chicory

Botanical Name—*Cichorium Intybus*
Vibration—*selfless love*

Indications: The indications for this flower essence are represented perfectly by those who exhibit the Mother Hen syndrome—the over-possessive, over-nurturing types—female or male—who tend to smother those they love, as well as want absolute control over their lives. They can also be martyrs but expect to be rewarded for any perceived sacrifice, and will be filled with self-pity if none comes. They are often heard to say, "And after all I've done for you, this is how you treat me!" The love they so generously give has invisible strings. They are possessive, self-centered, and demanding in their strong need for attention and appreciation, and are not above manipulation to get what they want. The Chicory Type, once in balance, gives love freely, no longer requiring anything in return.

Examples: The character Cliff (the mailman), from the *Cheers* TV show, had a mother who portrayed the Chicory profile to a T, with her constant need for attention and manipulation of her son.

9—Clematis

Botanical Name—*Clematis Vitalba*
Vibration—*creative idealism*

Indications: The profile for the out of balance state this flower essence treats is that of excessive daydreaming and lack of concentration. The Clematis Type appears to be lost in another world, and finds it hard to be in the here and now.

Dr. Bach called Clematis the flower essence for "polite suicide," as he felt these individuals had lost interest in daily living, letting life simply slip by. In the Clematis state, there is a strong need to escape from life on some level. Preoccupied with their fantasy worlds, these individuals are not really happy with their lives. Yet, they take no action to create change for themselves. These people are often highly artistic, but lack the ability to express their gifts in practical and material ways. They tend to lack energy and appear listless, and are often drowsy during the day. They would rather be alone, do not like confrontation, and avoid this by withdrawing. Clematis is highly recommended for grounding—to bring focus to the present and to encourage taking an active role in life. For many children with learning disabilities, Clematis is frequently used with great success.

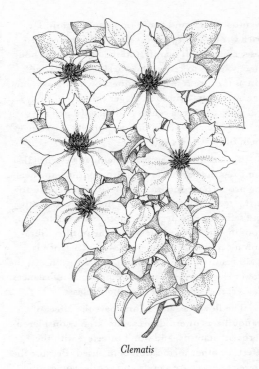

Clematis

Examples: For those familiar with the fictional character Don Quixote, it is easy to recognize the out-of-balance Clematis state he personified. Rip Van Winkle is another character who was, without doubt, in the Clematis state!

10—Crab Apple

Botanical Name—*Malus Sylvestris*
Vibration—*purity*

Indications: Crab Apple is the flower essence for cleansing. It is also indicated for those who feel unclean, or dissatisfied with their body image. There may even be feelings of self-disgust regarding the body. Crab Apple Types don't accept themselves as they are, many times blowing out of proportion a particular physical flaw they perceive they have—"My nose is too long, I'm too fat, my hair is too thin," and the list goes on.

Crab Apple can be extremely helpful in treating anorexia and bulimia, as those who suffer from these conditions have an obsession with their weight. This flower essence is also a great help for women during the end stages of pregnancy, when they look in the mirror thinking, "My God, I look like a beached whale. Where did that waistline go?" As Crab Apple is a cleanser, it is also recommended for pregnancy in general, as the body is now cleansing two life systems.

In cases of rape and incest, Crab Apple is indicated, as these victims experience feelings of being soiled and unclean. Crab Apple assists in releasing the toxic emotions of shame, guilt, self-loathing and disgust, so as to pave the way for the process of emotional healing to begin.

Examples: Again, we look to Felix Unger, the character from the movie and TV show, *The Odd Couple*, who is also an excellent example of the out-of-balance Crab Apple state. His name should be Mr. Meticulous! It would also seem he was a bit obsessive about his health with the nose spray, and his extreme concern for dirt and germs.

Michael Jackson is an extreme example of the Crab Apple Type, with his obsessive concern for his appearance.

Millionaire Howard Hughes also exemplified the Crab Apple profile to the nth degree. Toward the end of his life he became obsessive-compulsive over germs to such an extent that anyone or anything entering his home had to be sterilized!

Continued ➡

Princess Diana was another illustration of the Crab Apple state, with her reported past struggle with anorexia.

11–Elm

Botanical Name—*Ulmus Procera*
Vibration—*right responsibility*

Indications: The negative Elm state is usually temporary. It comes about when there is too much to do and not enough time or energy available to do it, and the feeling of being overwhelmed is experienced. This state usually affects responsible people who normally are able to handle their affairs. When our plate becomes too full, quite suddenly we may experience exhaustion, and feel overwhelmed and inadequate to handle everything. The flower essence Elm brings a confidence that you can accomplish all you need to, in the right time and place.

Examples: The nursery rhyme character, The Old Woman Who Lived in a Shoe (and had so many children she didn't know what to do!) is a prime example of the Elm state!

12–Gentian

Botanical Name—*Gentiana Amarella*
Vibration—*faith*

Indications: The indications for this flower essence are feelings of despondency that come with setbacks and delays—with situations not going as planned. "Why can't things ever go right?" you wonder. The out of balance Gentian state is a "what's the use, anyway" kind of feeling. When this occurs often enough, one begins to feel tired and depressed, with a loss of faith. For these feelings of discouragement due to life's inevitable setbacks and delays, Gentian seems to melt away those negative feelings. It brings a knowing that it will eventually work out. In most instances in life, we have very little control over the progress of a situation. Once we've done our part, we need to let it run its course as it will, and not allow ourselves to be unduly discouraged. We need to keep the faith that all is indeed working in divine order! This flower essence also aids children with learning disabilities, as their progress in school, many times, is a struggle, often producing feelings of discouragement and failure.

Examples: The Hunchback of Notre Dame portrays this state so poignantly; the constant setbacks in his life created discouragement and frustration for this poor soul.

13–Gorse

Botanical Name—*Ulex Europaeus*
Vibration—*hope*

Indications: Dr. Bach noted that Gorse individuals looked as if they needed sunshine in their lives. The indications for the Gorse state are feelings of hopelessness and extreme despair. One feels as though nothing more can be done. The feelings experienced here are deeper and more pervasive than in the Gentian state.

Examples: We can look to Shakespeare's *Romeo and Juliet* for the most definitive portrayal of this state. Both these lovers went into such a state of hopelessness, they chose to end their very lives.

14–Heather

Botanical Name—*Calluna Vulgaris*
Vibration—*empathy*

Indications: The key indication for this flower essence is a total preoccupation with self. These individuals are caught up with their own troubles, and are often hypochondriacs. They find it difficult to be alone, with an uncontrollable need to talk about themselves, and they are usually poor listeners. Unfortunately, they tend to alienate others, as friends and family often feel drained by the negative Heather's self-involvement. Most of us want relationships of mutual sharing—a two-way street, so to speak. Yet, Heather's sense of loneliness and great need for attention makes it hard to be able to give as well as receive. They're much too needy to consider others most of the time. This flower essence releases the extreme self-involvement of this state and brings awareness of being supportive to others—caring about others' needs and not just their own.

Examples: We can again look to the *Cheers* character, Cliff—himself this time—for an example of the Heather Type, in his constant self-absorption.

15–Holly

Botanical Name—*Ilex Aquifolium*
Vibration—*divine love*

Indications: The negative Holly state is portrayed by extreme feelings of hatred, suspicion, envy, jealously, and revenge. Holly assists us to open to a deep inner love that all possess within, as it releases these negative states of mind. This flower essence aids in releasing very negative and poisonous emotions, as it frees our true loving nature, making forgiveness possible. In many instances of divorce, which can bring up deep feelings of rage and hatred, Holly can assist in release and eventual forgiveness. Feelings of paranoia can also be treated with this flower essence.

There is an important point that needs to be addressed here, before continuing with the remaining flower essences. You do not choose Holly if you feel you want to be more loving—unless you are dealing with the aforementioned negative emotional states of the Holly profile. You do not take any flower essence to receive the positive quality it holds. You choose a particular flower essence only if you are experiencing the negative state that the flower essence addresses. Holly can open your natural loving nature, but only if you relate to the indications of the negative Holly state. This is true for all the flower essences, and important to remember in your selection process.

Examples: Again we turn to Ebenezer Scrooge, the main character portrayed in Charles Dickens's *A Christmas Carol*. This time it is Holly's profile that is revealed so well in the Scrooge we first meet as the story unfolds. He's depicted as cold-hearted, suspicious, and unable to care for anyone but himself. Another illustration is that of the character, J. R. Ewing, from the TV series *Dallas*. He was also unloving, suspicious, envious, jealous, vengeful.

Terrorists, assassins, and recently, the unabomber, are other examples of the out of balance Holly state—to the extreme, as was the biblical character, Cain, the brother of Abel—all committing deplorable acts of cruelty and violence.

16–Honeysuckle

Botanical Name—*Lonicera Caprifolium*
Vibration—*capacity for change*

Indications: This is the flower essence for those who seem lost in the past, longing for the good old days. The sense of nostalgia experienced prevents these individuals from living in the present in a productive and meaningful way. Many older people find themselves in this state, especially as partners and friends pass away. There doesn't seem to be much to live for anymore. Honeysuckle releases dwelling on past memories, and brings a new lease on life. It enables one to go out and meet new friends and develop new interests. Life becomes meaningful and vital again.

Holding onto the past is not just an issue with the elderly. It can arise at any age, depending on life circumstances. Many times, with divorce, it may be difficult not to think of the past and what was, preventing one from moving on in life. This flower essence is also excellent for young children who experience separation anxiety, as well as homesickness, making it difficult in going off to school, sleeping at a friend's, going away to camp, and other related situations of separation.

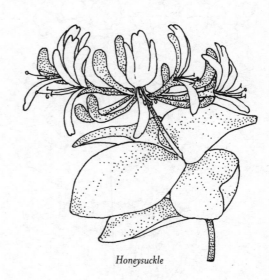
Honeysuckle

Examples: Dorothy, from *The Wizard of Oz*, is a wonderful illustration of this state. I can still see her clicking her little red shoes together and repeating, "There's no place like home, there's no place like home!" The character, Blanche DuBois, from Tennessee Williams's *A Streetcar Named Desire*, is another outstanding illustration of the Honeysuckle Type—lost in nostalgia for her lost youth and barely able to function in the present. Charles Dickens's book *Great Expectations* provides another superb example of this state. In this story, a character by the name of Miss Haversham, who was jilted just before her wedding many years ago, continues to wear her wedding gown, which is now in tatters, seemingly living in her memories of what was to be. It would appear she certainly has refused to get on with her life!

17–Hornbeam

Botanical Name—*Carpinus Betula*
Vibration—*inner vitality*

Indications: This is the flower essence for that Monday morning feeling—where you feel that your get-up-and-go has gotten up and gone. In this state you find that once you get started, you're fine. It's just that initial effort that seems so hard. There seems to be a weariness on some level. Your energy is a bit sapped. Many times, it is more on a mental level than physical one, and boredom may be at the root. Hornbeam assists those who feel a need for revitalization, and also helps with procrastination. This flower essence is also recommended for those who feel they may not be strong enough physically, with the need to strengthen the body, to build up their muscles.

Examples: The body builder types, such as Arnold Schwarzenegger, would exemplify this state, as does the Biblical character Samson, who experienced a loss of vitality after having his hair cut off by Delilah!

Continued ➡

18–Impatiens

Botanical Name—*Impatiens Gladulifera*
Vibration—*patience*

Indications: To get right at the heart of the matter quickly— Impatiens is for impatience! This personality type is a very independent, assertive, action-oriented individual who finds it difficult to work with others who are slower, and is intolerable of others who don't have the same energy drive, speed, and quickness of movement and perception. For this Type, "I want it done yesterday" isn't even soon enough! These individuals are easily irritated and restless, and don't take time to smell the flowers, coffee, or pizza!

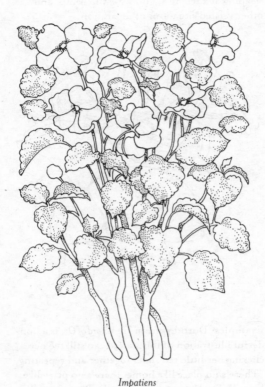

Impatiens

Examples: New York City taxi drivers exemplify this negative state, par excellence. The White Rabbit, from Lewis Carroll's *Alice in Wonderland*, really gives you the sense of the impatient nature that this flower essence addresses!

19–Larch

Botanical Name—*Larix Decidua*
Vibration—*self-confidence*

Indications: The indications for this flower essence are low self-esteem and lack of self-confidence. Feelings of inferiority run deep in this Type. These individuals feel that success can never be theirs, and many times, don't even make the effort. As they anticipate failure in the end, theirs is an attitude of "why even bother." Larch puts us in touch with our own specialness. It brings awareness that we each have our own gift to share. This is another excellent flower essence for children with learning disabilities, as many have very little self-worth.

Examples: The roles played by Woody Allen in many of his movies illustrate this profile—all are characters who exhibit very little self-esteem and suffer from inferiority complexes.

20–Mimulus

Botanical Name—*Mimulus Guttatus*
Vibration—*courage*

Indications: The indications for this flower essence are fears of known things—those you can name and put your finger on—such as fear of illness, fear of death, fear of not being financially secure, fear of loneliness, fear of intimacy, fear of public speaking, fear of animals, to mention a few of many possible fears. Phobias have also been successfully treated with Mimulus. This is the flower essence chosen for those who are extremely shy and timid individuals—characteristics which in most cases stem from a fear of being judged and rejected by others.

Examples: Little Miss Muffet, the nursery rhyme character who was frightened away by the spider who sat down beside her, is an example of the Mimulus state. Clark Kent, the alter-ego of Superman, portrays perfectly the profile of the Mimulus state. His persona is one of a timid and fearful man, seemingly lacking any courage. The Cowardly Lion from *The Wizard of Oz* is another illustration of the Mimulus state.

21–Mustard

Botanical Name—*Sinapis Arvensis*
Vibration—*cheerfulness*

Indications: This flower essence addresses another form of depression—one that comes upon us unexpectedly, and for no apparent reason, and then just as suddenly disappears. Mustard is for depression from an unknown, unconscious source, bringing feelings of doom and gloom. For those individuals who experience this state, Mustard eventually will bring to consciousness what it is that is causing the depression. This flower essence is excellent in cases of the "Postpartum Blues" which affects many new mothers.

Examples: The writings of Edgar Allan Poe, with gloom and doom soaking the pages, exemplify the negative Mustard state without peer!

22–Oak

Botanical Name—*Quercus Robur*
Vibration—*endurance*

Indications: This profile reflects very strong, capable, and self-reliant individuals who rarely seek help from others, possessing enormous endurance. However, sometimes they are too strong for their own good. They find it difficult to let go, ask for support, or take a break. Many of these individuals fall under the heading of workaholic—refusing to take time to rest, or heaven forbid, to play once in awhile! In the extreme, even when ill, the Oak goes to work, ignoring the body's need for rest. The out of balance Oaks are very hard on themselves—with nose to the grindstone at all times. Being so dedicated and determined are admirable traits. Yet, if abusing the body and not considering its needs are continued, there eventually will be a price to pay.

There is another important point to mention before going further. The flower essences do not change the basic personality type. Their effect is to bring balance to the negative state. An Oak will always be an Oak, but now in equilibrium—no longer pushing beyond endurance, as before. This holds true for all the flower essences.

Examples: Abraham Lincoln was a genuine Oak. Reading about the hardships he encountered on the road to the presidency, one is amazed at this man's strength and endurance in the face of all the obstacles he surmounted. *Star Trek's* Captain Kirk is another depiction of the Oak Type—married to his ship the Enterprise, nothing could stand in the way of his dedication to her and his crew. He was responsible and hardworking to a fault in his role as captain and willing and able to withstand whatever challenges came his way. Mel Gibson's portrayal in the movie *Braveheart* is another quite profound example of this flower essence Type, as is Gloria Estefan, the pop singer whose back was broken and against all odds, has made a comeback. The biblical character Job, as well, is another illustration of the Oak Type, as he persevered in the face of all obstacles.

23–Olive

Botanical Name—*Olea Europaea*
Vibration—*regeneration*

Indications: The indication for this flower essence is that of extreme exhaustion going far beyond the Hornbeam state. Here we have a situation where the physical system is totally depleted of energy, as during any major life-threatening illness, such as with cancer and AIDS, or after an operation, or even after childbirth. Olive is also of great help during emotional traumas, where the sense of loss is so extensive, one's physical energy has been depleted. It is suggested for any situation where major recovery and recuperation is indicated either emotionally or physically.

Examples: Greta Garbo's portrayal of *Camille*, in the movie of the same name, illustrates the Olive state, as she languishes from a terminal illness, her vitality all but depleted.

24–Pine

Botanical Name—*Pinus Sylvestris*
Vibration—*forgiveness*

Indications: The profile for this flower essence is that of the perfectionist. Nothing is ever good enough for the Pine, who feels there's always room for improvement. This perfectionism is only directed at themselves, however, and not expected of others. Self-criticism is the issue here. While beginning my studies of the Bach Flowers, my teacher remarked that Pine Types probably grew up with Beech parents who were intolerant of anything less than perfection. If their child brought home a 99 on a test, why wasn't it a 100? We can see, from this scenario, the potential for psychological damage. If children are constantly criticized in the formative years, they will most likely develop the feeling that nothing they do is really approved of.

Personal satisfaction is something hard for the Pine to relate to. Coupled often with this striving for perfection are feelings of guilt for not doing better. Many times, with the Pine profile, these individuals may blame themselves for others' mistakes. They are extremely apologetic. Out of balance Pines put much pressure on themselves with their demand for perfection at all times, setting high standards, yet feeling they can never attain them. By taking Pine, things are put into perspective. The Pine Types begin to realize they have done their best, and the pressure of feeling their efforts have not been good enough is released. Remember, the flower essences do not change the personality—selecting Pine doesn't change the desire for perfection, an intrinsic part of the Pine individual's personality, but brings balance to the pressure of the negative state.

Examples: The character Diane, portrayed by Shelley Long in the TV show *Cheers*, is the perfect example of the Pine Type. This character is unremittingly hard on herself, never feeling satisfied with her accomplishments—the perfectionist.

Continued ➡

25—Red Chestnut

Botanical Name—*Aesculus Carnea*
Vibration—*solicitude*

Indications: The indications for this flower essence are major anxiety and overconcern for loved ones. Fears for the welfare of others are haunting and pervasive, bringing much stress in dealing with these constant worries. And constant is key here, as many of us worry from time to time about those we care for. But the Red Chestnut state is one of extreme fear—being overwrought and wrapped up in these stressful feelings continually—such as the mother, fearing for her child's safety constantly, or a wife, waiting for her husband to return from work. He's a half hour late. She finds herself imagining the worst. He must have had a car accident, and is now lying on the road critically wounded!

Examples: TV sitcom *All in the Family's* Edith Bunker again is used as a wonderful illustration, this time for the Red Chestnut state, as Edith is portrayed as constantly overwrought with concern for her family.

26—Rock Rose

Botanical Name—*Helianthemum Nummularium*
Vibration—*steadfastness*

Indications: Dr. Bach saw Rock Rose as the flower essence for emergency situations. It assists in releasing absolute terror and panic that usually emerges in any crisis. This flower essence is also excellent in calming the aftershocks of nightmares. The Rock Rose state is usually brief, and often related to a particular situation of extremity.

Examples: The character Ichabod Crane, from Washington Irving's *The Legend of Sleepy Hollow*, experienced and exemplified the Rock Rose state to the extreme while attempting to escape from the terrorizing specter of the headless horseman!

27—Rockwater

Vibration—*adaptability*

(There is no botanical name for 27 since it is the only remedy that is not a plant.)

Indications: This is the only Bach Essence not made from a plant or tree. It comes from healing waters where Dr. Bach worked and lived which he found to have special healing properties. Rock Water Types are those individuals who are self-denying, sometimes to the point of martyrdom. They have high ideals, and tend to be rigid in their disciplines. When out of balance, Rock Water Types can be too rigid and hard on themselves, slowly but surely squeezing the joy from their lives. The Rock Water sets an example for others, not by proselytizing, but by living and being the example. There is a strict adherence to a living style, or a personal, religious, or social discipline. The positive Rock Water deserves admiration. However, when out of balance, their personality traits can be potentially harmful to them. This flower essence brings balance to the overly rigid ideals of the Rock Water, instilling a sense of gentleness towards themselves.

Examples: Mahatma Gandhi personifies the Rock Water state in balance so perfectly. He had high ideals and followed a particular path in life, holding strongly to his convictions and beliefs. Several other examples of the Rock Water state are: Joan of Arc, Saint Francis, and Mother Teresa.

28—Scleranthus

Botanical Name—*Scleranthus Annuus*
Vibration—*balance*

Indications: "Do I buy a Chevy or a Toyota? Do I choose teal or silver? Do I want a 2-door or 4-door?" Decisions, decisions, decisions! When faced with choosing between two things, and we find we cannot make up our minds, then it's time to turn to Scleranthus. People of this Type are very indecisive in their lives—vacillating back and forth in making their choices—they waffle. This flower essence is also helpful for those who have a tendency towards mood swings, experiencing extremes of joy/sadness, optimism/pessimism, etc. Scleranthus is the flower essence for balance on many levels, and also extremely helpful for motion sickness.

Examples: Shakespeare's *Hamlet* exhibited the Scleranthus state in his "To Be or Not To Be" soliloquy.

29—Star of Bethlehem

Botanical Name—*Ornithologum Umbellatum*
Vibration—*restoration*

Indications: The indications for this very special flower essence are deep feelings of grief due to the loss of a loved one, either through death or separation of any kind, as well as any physical or emotional trauma we've experienced. The trauma may have occurred many years ago, or yesterday—any trauma, including physical or emotional abuse, an accident, or trauma from an operation. It seems that the body holds on to shock and trauma long after the fact. Many times, even years later, delayed effects may manifest as physical symptoms, nervous breakdowns, anxiety attacks, depression, etc. For many, true healing can only begin after the release of any trauma. The vibration of this flower essence works at the cellular level and releases any traumatic experience from the cellular memory itself. Star of Bethlehem is highly recommended for survivors of incest, physical/sexual abuse, rape, and those suffering from post traumatic stress disorder. Both mothers and infants can also be helped in releasing the trauma of the birth process.

Examples: *Gone With the Wind's* Scarlett O'Hara was in a Star of Bethlehem state after losing her beloved home Tara, as was Olympic figure skater Nancy Kerrigan after her physical assault.

30—Sweet Chestnut

Botanical Name—*Castanea Sativa*
Vibration—*release*

Indications: This is another flower essence that treats depression—a depression that is more profound than that of the Gentian or Gorse states. In the Sweet Chestnut state, one feels as though plunged into a black hole filled with darkness and despair, unable to go on. Yet, so weakened by despondency, there is no energy left to end it all. This state is probably the most severe depression that can be experienced. It leaves a sense of isolation so great that even God seems out of reach. Sweet Chestnut brings solace when the limits of our endurance have been tapped.

Examples: Shakespeare's *Hamlet* is again used to now illustrate the profile of Sweet Chestnut. The angst that Hamlet experienced in his soul-searching soliloquy, "To Be or Not To Be," gives us a sense of the depths of his emotional pain.

31—Vervain

Botanical Name—*Verbena Officinalis*
Vibration—*restraint*

Indications: Those people who are strong-willed individuals, always having to be right, and also needing to convince others of their stand fit this profile. They will argue to the death defending their beliefs and opinions! This is the personality Type of the teacher, the prophet, or the proselytizer. There is high personal energy in Vervain individuals, and a tendency to be a bit on the hyper side at times, making them predisposed to burnout. When out of balance, the need to sell their opinions to others becomes a problem. They force their beliefs on all those they encounter, thus alienating themselves. Vervain Types in balance are special teachers who stimulate and inspire those whose lives they touch—without using that 2 by 4! They live their truths and are a model for others.

Examples: Dr. Martin Luther King beautifully exemplifies the balanced Vervain Type in his "I have a dream" speech. President John F. Kennedy also typifies the positive Vervain Type in his moving address to the country, as he admonished us to "ask not what your country can do for you, but what you can do for your country." We can also recognize the Vervain profile in former First Lady Eleanor Roosevelt, a great humanitarian; actress Jane Fonda, with her stand on the Vietnam War some years ago; evangelist Billy Graham, and lawyer Johnnie Cochran, in his defense of O. J. Simpson. Talk show hostess Oprah Winfrey is another inspiring example of Vervain, as well as the fictitious character Robin Hood, who robbed from the rich to give to the poor as he lived by his beliefs.

32—Vine

Botanical Name—*Vitis Vinifera*
Vibration—*right use of authority*

Indications: "I am in the position of authority and control here. We do it my way and there is no room for discussion." This dictatorial statement could have easily been made by a Vine out of balance. This personality Type is domineering, controlling, and inflexible. They believe their way is the only way, and brook no interference. On the positive side, when in balance, Vines are born leaders, organized, in control of themselves, and very together. They are capable individuals who take charge and get things done. Many look to the Vine for leadership and direction. Rigidity is not healthy, nor is shouldering the entire responsibility, as Vines tend to do. This flower essence brings flexibility and the willingness to listen to others, and creates a beneficent leader who is appreciated, respected, and looked up to, rather than avoided, feared, and disliked.

Examples: When the Vine is out of balance, we have the dictator—a Napoleon, a Hitler, a Saddam Hussein, who all exemplify the negative Vine profile. Called Chairman of the Board by his friends, Frank Sinatra appears to have the qualities of a Vine. The popular ballad "My Way," which was written especially for him by Paul Anka, captures the very essence of Mr. Sinatra and his life, and is an amazing portrayal of the Vine Type. My sense is that Elvis Presley, forever immortalized as the King by his adoring fans, was a Vine personality, as well as having exhibited traits of the Agrimony, Crab Apple, and Pine Types. Many biographies have been written, portraying Elvis as a man who held a tight rein over his entourage, was addicted to drugs and alcohol, was overly concerned about his appearance

Continued ➡

and subsequent weight gain, and was a perfectionist in his work.

33—Walnut

Botanical Name—*Fuglans Regia*
Vibration—*unaffectedness*

Indications: There are many uses for this remarkable flower essence. It is one of the most often selected of all 38, and for good reason. Walnut's indications are for all transitional periods in life—teething, puberty, beginning a career, marriage, becoming a parent, the empty nest syndrome, divorce, retirement, and menopause, to give several illustrations of major life changes. Walnut is for any time or period in life that requires adjustment to new situations. It brings to us an ease and more confidence to move through these transitions smoothly and with less stress. It assists us to more easily break the links or ties with the past that may bind us to the old ways—as in a relationship that isn't working out, yet we fear making the break and going it alone.

Walnut is known as the "Link Breaker," and is another flower essence that assists in releasing drug dependency. It also enables individuals to steer their own ships, and not be influenced by others who disagree with a course they have chosen (as with the dominating Vine Type father, or possessive Chicory Type mother who may do their best to control or manipulate their adult children's path in life according to their personal agenda). Walnut assists in remaining true to convictions and in being master of one's own life. It helps individuals to not be swayed by what others think is best for them. Perhaps the course of history would have been changed if Walnut had been available to Adam and Eve!

This flower essence is a protection against all outside influences, and has been used successfully in treating allergies for this reason. It is also a wonderful support for all those who work in the healing field—counselors, body workers, nurses, etc., as it also protects against any client's potentially draining energy.

Examples: Dr. Bach was a strong Walnut Type. He cared so little for what the medical establishment thought of him that he jeopardized his medical career to remain true to his calling. The singer and actress Madonna is another marvelous illustration of the Walnut Type. She certainly appears to be unaffected by the influence of others, and has been charting her own unique, if sometimes outrageous, course in life.

34—Water Violet

Botanical Name—*Hottonia Palustris*
Vibration—*humility*

Indications: Water Violet individuals are proud, aloof, independent people who go through life doing their work quietly, preferring to be left alone. They are gentle souls who do their own thing—not easily influenced by others, nor do they have the need to influence others. The problem with the out of balance Water Violet is their tendency towards isolation. No person is an island. We are all connected on some level, and need human contact for our growth. Those who relate to the Water Violet profile, as well as to Oak and Rock Water, may feel there is no need for change. These three personality Types have many worthy qualities. This is true so long as balance is maintained. Stress to the system begins once balance is lost. Water Violet finds it uncomfortable relating with others. There is a tendency to become loners and shun

contact which prevents them from truly knowing themselves. In addition to this pervading quality of detachment, the Water Violet profile may have feelings of superiority involved—which is actually well-founded. Water Violet is a special teacher and leader. Others look to them for their sense of calmness and self-assurance. They have gifts to share with humanity.

Examples: The TV and movie character Mr. Spock, of *Star Trek* fame, shows many of the Water Violet tendencies especially with his detached demeanor. Jackie Kennedy with her strong sense of pride, represents another Water Violet profile, as does actor James Dean, known by his peers as a loner. The actress Greta Garbo is remembered by many not only for her great dramatic talent, but for her extreme sense of privacy. In her inimitable accent, she reportedly spoke the following words, "I vant to be alawn," words that will always be a testament to her personality. And these are the very words that are at the heart of the Water Violet profile.

35—White Chestnut

Botanical Name—*Aesculus Hippocastanum*
Vibration—*tranquility*

Indications: The White Chestnut state is expressed during those times when the mind seems to race on and on, or it feels like a record has gotten stuck in the groove—repeating the same obsessive thought many times over. Peace of mind is nowhere to be found in this state. We find ourselves plagued by unwanted thoughts, and can't seem to focus or concentrate on anything else.

In this state as well, sleeping patterns may be disrupted. We are unable to shut off the mind when going to sleep, or may wake up in the middle of the night as the mind continues to work overtime. Sometimes we wake well before it's time to start the day and are unable to go back to sleep. White Chestnut assists in releasing these persistent, unwanted, and sometimes obsessive thought patterns, as it brings a stillness and peace to the mind. This flower essence is another often used for children with learning disabilities, as an aid in concentration.

Examples: Shakespeare's *Lady MacBeth* was suffering from the White Chestnut state, in her obsession with washing her hands to remove imagined blood stains, as she continually repeated, "Out, out, damned spot!"

36—Wild Oat

Botanical Name—*Bromus Ramosus*
Vibration—*purposefulness*

Indications: "What is the meaning and purpose of my life? What direction am I to go in?" For those with these questions, Wild Oat, known as the "Pathfinder," may be the catalyst in discovering the answers. Wild Oat's profile includes dissatisfaction, boredom, and feeling unfulfilled in our present work. There's a futile kind of feeling that doesn't go away as we continue on the same road. It's true that we all need to support ourselves, yet, hopefully, we can also find what it is we love to do. Wild Oat assists us in handling and dealing with present circumstances by releasing the attached stress and restlessness. It helps us find contentment in what we're doing or, if necessary, opens us to the courage needed to leave so we may go out and find what our calling is.

Examples: The character Walter Mitty exemplifies the Wild Oat state, with his constant changing of occupations and search for his path.

37—Wild Rose

Botanical Name—*Rosa Canina*
Vibration—*inner motivation*

Indications: The profile of this flower essence is that of apathy and resignation. These Types feel that their lot in life can never change, and have totally accepted their circumstances as irreversible. The Wild Rose individual feels as though there is no hope left to live a richer life. There isn't even depression anymore—just a pervasive numbness, as though the spark of life has just about gone out. Many who suffer from life-threatening disease are prone to this state, as well as invalids and the handicapped, and those who see themselves as victims of abuse. This flower essence brings the realization that there are choices, and it's not too late to have a more meaningful life.

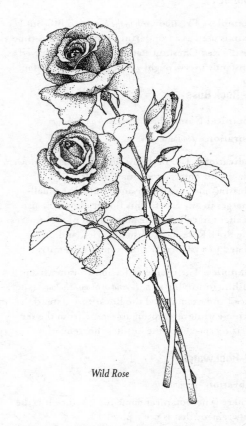

Wild Rose

Examples: Willy Loman, in Arthur Miller's *Death of a Salesman*, exemplifies the apathy and resignation of the Wild Rose state. The baby duckling in Hans Christian Andersen's story, who faces almost insurmountable rejection, also exemplifies the Wild Rose state.

38—Willow

Botanical Name—*Salix Vitellina*
Vibration—*personal responsibility*

Indications: The last but definitely not the least of the 38 individual Bach Flower Essences is Willow. The indications for this flower essence are bitterness and resentment. Willow individuals feel that life has given them a raw deal—whether it be their mother or father they blame, or the universe itself. They see themselves as victims. Willow personalities take no responsibility for their lives, blaming others, or circumstances and events, for the causes of their misery. We all need to realize that on some level, we—not others—are responsible for the place we are in. At age thirty-five or forty, we need to stop blaming our parents for any hurts or actions that took place thirty years ago or perhaps, what they didn't do for us. It's time to grow up and get a life! At some point we need to finally release the blame we hold. We're only hurting ourselves with the toxins produced in our bodies by these negative

Continued →

emotions. We need to forgive and let go of the past. We also need to understand, although it may be difficult to see, that our parents or anyone else we may hold grievances against have been doing the best they are capable of, even if we perceive it has been hurtful. This is not to excuse wrongful behavior. Yet eventually, for our own peace of mind and state of our health itself, we need to move past what was. Willow assists in releasing bitterness and resentment. It brings awareness of our responsibility for our own life, and helps us to see that all we experience are lessons and opportunities for our personal growth—even when we may not be given any reasons as to why we need to go through these lessons.

Examples: Tonya Harding, Olympic figure skater, appears to experienced the Willow state in her resentment of her rival, Nancy Kerrigan, as well as the Holly state by her subsequent attack on Nancy.

Regrettably, a deeply poignant illustration of the Willow state, as well as Holly and Star of Bethlehem states, was televised nationally. With the tragic murders of Nicole Simpson and Ron Goldman, many of us were witness to their families' extreme emotional turmoil and loss—clearly depicting the indications for the Bach Flower Essences Willow, Holly, and Star of Bethlehem.

We have now completed the Indications for each of the 38 individual Bach Flowers. If you wish to obtain a deeper understanding of Dr. Bach's insights into healing, as well as the indications for each of the 38 flower essences in his own words, I highly recommend reading *The Bach Flower Essences*, as well as *The Original Writings of Edward Bach*.

One final Bach Flower preparation—Rescue Remedy— remains to be addressed. As there is so much to share regarding this extraordinary combination formula, the next chapter is devoted to an in depth exploration of Rescue.

Thus we see that our conquest of disease will mainly depend upon the following: the realization of the Divinity within our nature and our consequent power to overcome all that is wrong; secondly, the knowledge that the basic cause of disease is due to disharmony between the personality and the Soul; and thirdly, our willingness and ability to discover the fault which is causing such a conflict; and fourthly, the removal of any such fault by developing the opposing virtue.

—Dr. Edward Bach, *Heal Thyself*

Rescue Remedy: Dr. Bach's "Emergency" Formula

In addition to the 38 individual flower essences that Dr. Bach developed, there is also one special combination of his flower essences that was created specifically for Emergency Stress Relief, known as Rescue Remedy. This outstanding preparation is composed of five of the original 38 flower essences, and can be used with great success in any emergency situation. The five flower essences comprising Rescue Remedy are Clematis, addressing dizziness or loss of consciousness; Cherry Plum, addressing loss of mental and/or physical control; Impatiens, addressing emotional tension and/or pain; Rock Rose, addressing panic and terror; and Star of Bethlehem, addressing emotional or physical trauma and/or grief and loss.

Rescue Remedy is highly effective and always brings instant relief in cases of extreme stress when a person is close to the edge. This is the only Bach Flower Essence that has an immediate Reaction Time, with its effects felt usually within 15 to 20 minutes. It may also be taken as often as needed without fear of overdosing, as all the flower essences are totally safe and gentle, natural and non-toxic preparations.

Any crisis condition warrants its use. To illustrate, some of the many possible crisis situations that Rescue Remedy eases are: anxiety attacks, grief, shock and trauma, panic and hysteria. Even minor incidents that cause stress and anxiety, such as arguments, exams, public speaking, job interviews, visits to the doctor or dentist—all are addressed and feelings calmed with Rescue Remedy. Once you've personally experienced its amazing effectiveness, you'll want to keep Rescue Remedy available for any emergency situation that should unexpectedly arise. Rescue Remedy also comes in a cream formula, with the addition of Crab Apple, the flower essence for cleansing. It is used for burns, cuts, rashes, insect bites and stings, bruises, and even helps with blemishes. It is also wonderfully soothing for tired eyes, as well as easing nipple soreness that many mothers who breast feed sometimes experience.

Several actual experiences with Rescue Remedy taken from my client files are now presented as illustrations of its remarkable efficacy.

CASE HISTORIES:

Kim woke in the middle of the night, finding herself extremely nauseous. As she rushed to the bathroom feeling she might vomit, she also experienced dizziness. She had been using the Bach Flowers for some time, and always kept a bottle of Rescue Remedy in the medicine chest. She immediately reached for it and sank down to the floor, feeling faint. She managed to put several drops in her mouth, and within minutes, the dizziness passed. Although still nauseous, she was unable to throw up. She put four to five drops of Rescue Remedy into a half glass of water and brought it back to bed with her. She sipped every few minutes, and within fifteen to twenty minutes her nausea abated enough for her to be able to go back to sleep. When she awoke the next morning, her experience of the previous evening seemed like a bad dream. She later called me to share her delight at how helpful Rescue had been.

Sue was experiencing a major anxiety attack when she called me. She was restless and pacing, feeling overwhelmingly agitated and unable to calm herself. I suggested she put several drops of Rescue Remedy into a half glass of water and sip every five minutes. I asked her to call me back in a half hour. When she called back, she was amazed at how calm and relaxed she now was. Whatever she had been experiencing was totally gone. She told me how glad she was that she had taken my advice in our last consultation, when I recommended she have Rescue Remedy on hand for unexpected crises.

Ann recently reported this incident to me—one concerning her mother. They bowled together, and one day her mom began to feel dizzy. Ann is "hooked on Bach," and always carries Rescue Remedy in her purse just in case. Well, it really came in handy in this situation. Ann gave her mother some Rescue Remedy in half a glass of water, advising her to sip every five minutes. She did as instructed, and within about fifteen minutes or so, her mom was feeling up to resuming her bowling. Her dizziness was completely gone! Ann's mother now carries her own bottle of Rescue Remedy in her purse.

When Jim came for a recent Bach consultation, he mentioned that his dog, Hercules, was afraid of thunderstorms. He wondered if the flower essences could also help his pet. I suggested he administer some Rescue Remedy the next time it stormed. An opportunity soon arose, and Jim called to let me know that Hercules now lives up to his name!

Vicki had recently lost her father. She had been in deep emotional pain over her loss for several weeks when a friend and client of mine told her about the Bach Flowers. Vicki came to see me and soon was using Rescue Remedy, at first taking it as often as she felt the need, then eventually four times a day. Within the week, she reported that her grieving had eased up considerably and she was much more comfortable. Where she was finding it hard to cope with everyday life before, caused by her depression over her dad's death, she was now able to resume her normal routine.

Tom, my brother-in-law, had come to visit several summers ago. I couldn't help but notice his swollen hand. I had never seen anything like this before—it was three times its normal size! When I asked what had happened, he said he had been stung by a bee earlier in the day. I told him I had something I felt could help his discomfort, and asked if he'd allow me to put some Rescue Remedy cream on his hand. He agreed and within the hour, the swelling had been markedly reduced. We put on a second application and by the time he left, his hand was almost back to normal. He was amazed with the results and asked me to order some for him. I have to honestly admit that I was almost as amazed, as was Tom, by the dramatic change.

Lyn, after a recent consultation, learned to always keep Rescue liquid and cream on hand. She recently called to let me know how helpful they had been after badly burning her arm and how glad she was that she remembered to use them. She first made a compress with the liquid, and held it on her arm for about one-half hour. Initially, the throbbing pain was unbearable, but soon after applying the compress, the pain quickly subsided. She then applied some cream on the effected area and bandaged it. The next morning she discovered how beautifully it had healed. A water blister had developed, which she broke. Once again she applied the cream, and again bandaged her wound. All pain had disappeared and by the next day, it was well on its way to total healing.

Esther, a new friend with whom I had shared my work with the Bach Flowers, had recently gotten some Rescue cream not knowing how soon she'd need it. One morning, just as her eight-year-old son Adam was leaving for school, he fell against the storm door, badly banging his forehead. He sustained a large bruise which was beginning to swell. Esther immediately reached for the Rescue cream and generously applied it to Adam's wound. After waiting a bit to determine if her son was okay, and not in need of further medical attention, she sent him off to school. He agreed to take the Rescue cream with him and apply it several more times. Esther reported that she was amazed when she later saw her son. She could find no evidence of the bruise or any swelling that had earlier appeared. She remarked to me, "It seemed like a miracle!"

Mary, another Bach Practitioner, shared this experience with me. Her elderly mother had fallen and bruised her shoulder. She called Mary for advice as it was bruised. Mary told her to apply Rescue cream to the area which she did, as well as place a bandage on it. The next day, Mary came by to check on her mother. It seems her mom had only applied the Rescue cream to a portion of the bruise where she had bandaged it. When Mary removed the bandage, the skin here was completely free of discoloration. However, the surrounding area that hadn't been treated was still black and blue!

Marc, my son, had badly cut his finger late one evening. It really needed a few stitches, but as it was after 11 p.m., we decided to treat the wound with Rescue. We first made a compress with the liquid. Once the bleeding stopped, we applied the cream and bandaged it. The next morning we again applied the cream with a fresh bandage. Within

Continued →

three days the cut had completely healed with no evidence of it ever being there. The cut had been pretty deep. It was remarkable that it had healed so quickly, and without any scarring.

I could go on and on in sharing the remarkable effects of Rescue Remedy liquid and cream. The above experiences should suffice in giving you a pretty good picture of the many situations that Rescue assists with. If you try no other flower essence, I deeply urge you to at least experience Rescue Remedy. It is my opinion that no medicine chest should be without it. Carry Rescue in your purse and glove compartment of your car for any unexpected emergency situation that arises.

Bach Flower Preparation and Use

You should now have a firm handle on those essences which relate to your emotional issues and negative states of mind, and are ready to experience for yourself the remarkable efficacy of this very special self-help system.

Once you have your flower essences on hand, there are many different ways to use them. You may take your drops directly from the concentrate bottles. However, I would like to recommend an easier and more economical way of taking them, especially when taking several flower essences at once. You can combine your flower essences together in a Personal Dilution Bottle.

As the flower essences are homeopathic in nature, it is possible to dilute them one time without changing their strength. For some, this concept may be difficult to accept, and bring concern that the potency is weakened by diluting. Let me reassure you that this is not the case with the Bach Flower Essences. Know that they may be safely diluted according to directions that now follow without disturbing their original potency.

You will need a one-ounce amber dropper bottle into which you place two or three drops of each flower essence selected. The *only* exception is Rescue Remedy. Because it is a combination formula, you will need to use four to five drops of Rescue. Remember—it is suggested that no more than seven flower essences are to be used at any one time. Rescue is considered one flower essence when combining it in your dilution bottle. If you are in need of more than two or three of the flower essences in Rescue, it may be helpful to use Rescue itself, rather than the individual ones, to keep the number of flower essences from exceeding seven.

Sterilize the bottle before you prepare it with your personal formula. Boil both the glass bottle and rubber dropper top for at least fifteen minutes. It is perfectly safe to boil the rubber top, and it will not be harmed by boiling. It is not necessary to re-sterilize your bottle after the initial preparation, so long as you continue to use the same flower essences. When your bottle is empty, simply add the water, flower essences, and preservative as before. However, when you find the need to change any of the flower essences you have been using, it then becomes necessary to again sterilize your bottle to ensure the removal of the vibration of previous flower essences.

After placing your flower essences into your bottle, add a teaspoon of one of the following as a preservative: either apple cider vinegar, brandy, or vegetable glycerin may be used. As the flower essences are not to be refrigerated, but simply kept in a cool, dark place, they need a preservative to prevent spoilage. Now, fill the rest of your bottle with spring water and shake well. You are ready to begin your flower essence use.

The dosage is at least *four* drops from your dilution bottle under the tongue for a minimum of four times daily. If you choose to take the flower essences directly from the concentrate bottle, you need to take *two* to *three* drops from each bottle that you are presently using. If you are using Rescue, it's *four* to *five* drops of the concentrate. You can see how much more convenient it is to take your drops from a single bottle with all your flower essences combined than it would be to do so from several different bottles. You may also place a few drops from the concentrate into a half glass of water. Each sip is considered a single dose. Again, I remind you, in most cases you probably won't feel the effect of the flower essences immediately, with the exception of Rescue Remedy. The other 38 individual flower essences usually need to be taken for a one to two month period, with your personal commitment to use them regularly before you may begin to feel their subtle effects. And reaction time does vary with each person.

In regard to limiting the number of flower essences to the general recommendation of seven, one of the most helpful and effective ways to do this is by using an Intensity Scale. This simple technique may be done by noting on a piece of paper the flower essences you wish to take. Review each one, determining how often you are experiencing their indications. Is this once a week, every few days, or every day? You will then need to rate all tentative selections. Give each a numerical value between one and ten, depending on how intense each issue is for you. Give the highest value to the most stressful.

To illustrate this process, perhaps you've related to ten flower essences, and Mimulus is among them—for the constant fears you feel. This issue is one you face daily. You would give Mimulus a "ten." Another of the ten flower essences you are considering may be Cerato—for your inability to make your own decisions. Yet, you notice that although you have a need to go to others for advice, sometimes you are able to make your own decisions without asking others' opinions. Cerato would be a "six" perhaps. You continue this procedure with all ten flower essences. Once you've rated each one, simply select those with the highest numbers. These represent your most intense issues. Hopefully, this process will have narrowed down your selections to the recommended maximum of seven. If you are unsuccessful on the first try, simply repeat this process until only seven remain.

One of the most common occurrences with Bach Flower usage is referred to as the "Peeling Effect." When you feel you are ready to stop taking your original selections—and this is something only you can determine—you'll probably discover, as have so many others, that different issues have now surfaced and are now also ready to be released. It seems that in our healing process, as one or more surface issues are resolved, other underlying and deeper issues may begin to emerge into consciousness. A helpful analogy is that of the onion with its many layers. As the top layer is peeled, the next layer is revealed, and then another, until the core is reached. The uncovering of deeper, unresolved emotional issues is a normal and continuing process in your personal growth throughout life. As this peeling effect occurs for you, simply repeat the selection process in choosing new flower essences that relate to the issue or issues now being revealed. Simply re-read the indications for each of the flower essences previously presented, for further assistance with your new selections.

For those who are alcohol sensitive and wondering if they can safely use the flower essences which contain a significant amount of alcohol in the concentrate form, the answer is absolutely yes. There are several ways to prepare and use the flower essences, dispelling the alcohol, if this is a question or concern for you. By putting the drops directly into hot water, the alcohol is totally evaporated. Making the dilution bottle as previously instructed is another way to reduce the alcohol content. Do not select brandy as your preservative. Also, the flower essences may be directly applied to the pulse points of the skin, itself. And one last possible application suggested for alcohol sensitivity—mist the flower essences into the air from a spray bottle. Any one of these alternate ways of using the flower essences has been found to be just as effective as taking them by mouth.

Another possible circumstance to be aware of, although very infrequently experienced when using the flower essences, is something called the "Healing Crisis." In any healing process, in some cases, it appears that a situation will get worse before it gets better. This takes place in traditional medical treatment, in counseling, in all healing modalities. A common illustration of this is a simple fever. We have all experienced how this condition seems to reach a certain point before it can break. In simplest terms, this is what is known as a healing crisis.

As the flower essences bring up our emotional issues for release, sometimes an individual may feel an issue growing more intense instead of easing, at the outset. If this happens to you, know that this experience is very short-lived, usually disappearing within one to two days at the most. The Bach Flowers themselves do not cause any side-effects. This healing crisis is but a part of the healing process itself. The following suggestions will help you to move past this situation. You may use Rescue, along with the other flower essences you are using, to ease what is taking place and push through the crisis. You may also decide to stop taking whichever flower essence you sense may be causing you this emotional discomfort. And know that this is an option—you may not be ready to deal with this particular issue at this time. And this is okay, as your healing process is very personal and not to be judged, even by you! Honor your feelings, and if you are too uncomfortable, discontinue use for awhile. You may also want to continue taking Rescue for a few days until you feel all discomfort has passed. Please be gentle with yourself. Don't force any healing. Go at your own pace. Know that you are in charge of your own healing process here. And again, I repeat—this healing crisis is *rarely* experienced.

Dr. Bach developed his flower essences not only for acute emergency situations, and for the healing of deep-seated emotional issues and negative states of mind but also for one's personality make up, to prevent the manifestation of disease in the future. Therefore, it is helpful to know which of the flower essences relate to your *personality*. The flower essences that address the personality and long-standing feelings that may cause an individual to go out of balance are called "Type" flower essences. These have the ability to transform your character flaws or weaknesses into your greatest strengths.

Type flower essences are those that relate to our Basic Nature. Most of us usually have several, as we are diverse beings, and there is usually a combination of flower essences which represent our unique complexities. You probably recognized several of your own Type flower essences while going over the 38 Indications, ones that spoke to you, that you identified as parts of your personality characteristics. Our Type flower essences are ones we will never outgrow, and have the ability to open us to our most positive states of being.

By taking the flower essences that depict your personality, you are assisting your system's harmony

Continued ➡

and balance at all times. This is a key concept with Bach Flower usage. By taking your personality Type flower essences, even if the characteristics addressed by them are in balance for you, you are ensuring the continuation of this state. And this is an important concept in assisting you in your healing process. Take the time to discover your Type flower essences, and use them even when you feel balanced, as a preventative.

Dr. Bach felt that if individuals could determine their personality Type flower essences, these would then be the only ones needed, regardless of what was taking place in their lives, and the emotional responses to these situations. This is possible because the Type flower essences bring one's basic disposition into balance. Any ensuing conflict or disharmony, therefore, would also be balanced easily.

One last factor that needs to be addressed in regard to flower essence use is the question of "Integrity." Many have brought up the question of the feasibility of giving the flower essences to others without their knowledge or approval (more likely, to help themselves more than the person they'd like to give the flower essences to. Perhaps they are dealing with a Beech or Vine Type!) Although the flower essences are effective regardless of the awareness of an individual, this question is really one of ethical principles.

Without the intent to preach here, I personally do not believe we have the right to force change on another, or to take actions along these lines without another's approval, even if it may be for their own good. Just as Dr. Bach believed that no one has the right to interfere in our life, he also believed that we do not have the right to interfere in another's life. He stated in *Free Thyself*, "God gave us each our birthright, an individuality all our own...He gave us each our own particular path to follow...Let us see to it that not only do we allow no interference, but even more important, that we, in no way whatsoever, interfere with any other single human being." As we take our freedom to be ourselves, we need to give this same freedom to others. When we share the Bach Flowers with others, it must be with their awareness and approval. Although I have stated my feelings regarding this question, and also shared those of Dr. Bach, you are, of course, free to determine your own position with this issue.

However, there are several situations where receiving another's approval is not possible, as with an individual being unconscious, or mentally incompetent, as well as with young children under our care. They are all unable to help themselves. In situations such as these, with our positive intention of bringing relief to others we may be responsible for, there would be no breach of integrity in our use of the Bach Flowers. To administer the Bach Flowers to an unconscious individual, simply moisten the lips with several drops of the essence, apply to the pulse points, or mist the room with a spray bottle containing at least eight drops of each of the flower essences you wish to use.

Bach Flowers for Common Life Situations

The remaining sections are devoted to bringing to you many of the diversified uses of the Bach Flowers, from various emotionally challenging "Life Situations" we all have in common to flower essence application with animals and even plants! Cases from my own practice will be presented as illustrations for you, to assist you in your own understanding and use of the Bach Flowers.

There are many difficult and stressful life situations that we all will face at one time or another as a part of the human condition. There is no way of avoiding them. A loved one dying, facing our own mortality, a painful divorce, the loss of a career, a diagnosis of cancer or other life-threatening diseases, are just a few of the many devastating emotional traumas we may experience. Although we cannot always prevent the course that our life may run, we do have help in dealing with the repercussions of emotional stresses we may encounter—with the Bach Flowers.

Bereavement

In times of deep grief and loss experienced with the death of a loved one, the flower essences most often indicated are Walnut for the state of transition; Star of Bethlehem for grief and loss, and possibly shock and trauma, if the death was sudden; Honeysuckle for nostalgia and living in past memories; Willow for resentment towards the one who died and/or the situation itself; and Sweet Chestnut for deep depression. Agrimony may also be indicated if there is denial and repression of feelings of grief. If the loss is emotionally devastating, bringing on physical exhaustion, there may also be a need for Olive. And Rescue Remedy itself (which also contains Star of Bethlehem) is extremely helpful.

Death and Dying

In facing our own death and the issues that confront us, or in assisting another who is making this final transition, many of the same flower essences are indicated as for the loss of a loved one. It is sad that there is so much avoidance and fear surrounding the death experience. We do ourselves a terrible disservice in our culture. Many people find themselves isolated and alone in their final days, with friends and relatives tiptoeing around the truth, caught up in their own denial and fear. The following flower essences are generally suggested to bring comfort to the dying. Agrimony assists with denial and brings the ability to face our deepest feelings over death. Aspen eases the fear of the unknown. Either Gorse or Sweet Chestnut may be indicated for feelings of hopelessness or extreme anguish when confronted with death. There may be a need for Holly during the initial phase when anger and rage may surface. Mimulus brings courage and releases fear. Olive may be indicated where total exhaustion from infirmity is experienced. Red Chestnut is needed when there is overconcern for how loved ones will manage without them. Star of Bethlehem comforts feelings of grief and loss. Walnut is always indicated for this time of major transition. Wild Rose may sometimes be needed if apathy or resignation sets in. And Willow may be a consideration when feelings of bitterness or resentment develop.

Divorce

During and after a divorce the flower essences most often indicated, especially for those deeply hurt, are Star of Bethlehem for grief and loss; Mimulus for fear of being alone; Honeysuckle for living in the past; Walnut for breaking links with the past life, and the state of transition; Holly for rage and hatred towards the ex-spouse; and perhaps, Willow for bitterness and resentment; Larch for lack of self-confidence in making it alone; and, for possible depression, Sweet Chestnut or Gorse, depending on the severity of the depression. Olive may also be indicated for the total exhaustion possibly caused by this emotionally stressful situation. Pine is another consideration, when there are feelings of guilt and self-blame involved that are unwarranted.

Loss of Career

With the loss of a career, the flower essences most often indicated are Rescue Remedy for anxiety and panic; Mimulus for all known fears that may come up in this situation; Wild Oat for considering a new direction in life; Impatiens for impatience while going through this transition Walnut for the state of transition itself; Larch for lack of self-worth; either Holly or Willow for feelings of rage or bitterness; as well as Star of Bethlehem (which is also in Rescue Remedy) for grief and loss. Gorse may also be indicated for feelings of hopelessness.

Life-Threatening Illnesses (AIDS, cancer, heart desease, etc.)

The flower essences most often indicated are Rescue Remedy for the terror and panic; Mimulus for fear of death; Gorse for hopelessness, or Sweet Chestnut for extreme anguish; Wild Rose for apathy and resignation; Olive for physical exhaustion; and Crab Apple, as a cleanser. Holly or Willow may also be indicated for feelings of rage or bitterness, as well as Agrimony for denial.

The life-challenging scenarios just presented are examples of some of the many different emotional states that can come up during such experiences. Not everyone will experience them in the same way, nor need the same flower essences, nor are these states described definitive. These situations have been generalized so as to give you a deeper understanding of the various negative emotional states possible and the 38 flower essences, including Rescue Remedy that address them.

The illustrations that now follow are of clients I have counseled during similar life challenging situations. They are presented as more specific and individualized illustrations, to bring further clarity and understanding in your use and practice of the Bach Flowers.

CASE HISTORIES:

Barbara, a woman in her early sixties, had just lost her husband. His death triggered deep depression, with feelings of abandonment and fear. She withdrew into herself, unable to continue with daily life. Her daughter Joan became increasingly worried over her mother's emotional state and felt her mother needed help in overcoming her bereavement. Fortunately, Barbara agreed to seek help and an appointment was set up for a Bach Flower consultation. When I saw Barbara, her deep emotional pain was evident. Her face was pale with dark circles under her eyes. It was hard for her to talk without dissolving into tears. She expressed deep grief, as well as fear of being on her own now. Her husband had been her strength, she advised. She didn't know if she could manage on her own. She also expressed resentment at her husband dying and leaving her alone—"How could he do this to me?" she bitterly cried. (In my studies of death and dying, I have come to learn that it is not uncommon for those who experience the death of a loved one to feel deep resentment towards the one who died. It appears this is part of the grieving process itself—one of the stages that needs to be moved through).

After listening to Barbara share her feelings over her situation, I suggested the following flower essences which related to the negative emotional states I felt she was experiencing: Star of Bethlehem for her deep grief; Mimulus for her fear of being alone; Larch for her lack of self-confidence on making it on her own; Willow for her resentment towards her husband for leaving her; Walnut for the state of transition; Honeysuckle for clinging to the past and Sweet Chestnut for the deep depression she was in. I explained what each flower essence addressed, asking if she related to these states and was willing to be involved in this self-help treatment. She agreed with my recommendations. I asked her to call me in four to six weeks to follow up on her progress.

Continued →

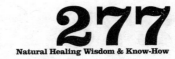

Barbara later called as requested and reported that she was doing much better since taking the flower essences. Her depression and grief had eased a great deal, she felt less fearful and more confident in her ability to manage her life, and the feelings of resentment towards her husband were not as strong. She seemed surprised at how helpful the flower essences had been. She remarked that she didn't exactly understand how they worked yet, she was experiencing great relief. I felt she should continue with these original seven for another month or two, and then we'd speak again to determine if any changes would be indicated. Barbara agreed.

When we spoke two months later, Barbara was doing even better. She had been taking the flower essences for almost four months now and some changes were indicated. She felt she was over her issue of resentment towards her husband and was no longer living in the past. Her deep depression had lifted although feelings of grief still surfaced from time to time. She decided it was time to drop Willow, Sweet Chestnut, and Honeysuckle but still felt the need for Star of Bethlehem, Larch, and Mimulus. I felt she was well on her way to recovery from the emotional devastation of her husband's death.

(Note: In cases of divorce, also experienced as a deep loss for some, many of the above flower essences would also be extremely helpful. Many of the emotional states that are felt are quite similar.)

John, a twenty-five-year old, had seen me in the past concerning his issue of breaking free from a domineering father. He was making good progress with this, having moved away from home, when a major crisis erupted in his life. The company he was working for was downsizing, and he had lost his job. He was quite depressed as well as concerned over how he would support himself. He felt going back home would negate the progress he had made with his father. His fear and anxiety were overwhelming and he felt discouraged. After going over his present issues together, the following flower essences were suggested for John's current state of emotional stress: Walnut, which was originally recommended for helping him break away from the dominance of his father. It seemed this issue wasn't completely released yet. Walnut would also assist now with this period of transition. Wild Oat would be helpful for a possible new life direction; Mimulus for his fear; Gentian for his discouragement and feelings of setbacks taking place in his life; and Rescue Remedy, for his state of general anxiety (Rock Rose, one of the flower essences in Rescue, assists in cases of terror and panic, and John was in a panic state; Impatiens assists in easing impatience, which John was certainly experiencing with finding another job as quickly as possible). John related to the indications of the suggested flower essences, and without hesitation agreed to try them. As he had already experienced success with the Bach flowers, he was more than willing to do so for his current situation.

I saw John some six weeks later and he seemed like another person. Many of the negative emotional states he had experienced after losing his job had abated. He was now attending school at night for a master's degree. He realized he needed to further his education to work in a field he really loved. Meanwhile, he found another job, although only temporary, in order to secure the funds to continue with his schooling and support himself. He felt he had a new future to look forward to. He no longer felt discouraged and saw the loss of his job in a new light. It provided him with the opportunity of making some changes he would not have had the courage to do before. We both agreed that he didn't need Wild Oat, nor Gentian or Rescue, as he had

found his direction, was no longer discouraged, nor was he dealing with constant anxiety. He wanted to continue with Walnut and Mimulus, and Larch was now added, as he felt his self-esteem needed a boost in regard to finishing his master's degree.

There are other common life situations that may be stressful at times. I refer to marriage, becoming a parent, moving to a new home, and a change in career by choice, …as several examples. As we all know from personal experience, life is filled with change—life itself being a cycle of maturation. Change may be experienced as either positive or negative. Yet, regardless of how change is seen, there is always stress involved, with fear of the unknown assailing most of us.

Marriage

The Bach Flowers can be incredibly helpful in assisting us through whatever changes we may go through, by releasing stress and emotional issues that may arise during these times. When getting married, most feel some apprehension, indicating Mimulus. Marriage is a time of transition. For this, Walnut is also indicated. And often, feelings of overconcern and worry for the new partner crop up, indicating Red Chestnut. New brides and grooms may feel overwhelmed as well, with the added responsibilities that marriage presents, and Elm may be indicated.

Birth of a Child

The birth of a first child, although usually a joyous time for most of us, may also be a time of stress emotionally. Again, Walnut is indicated, with the transition from couple to family, and the adjustment to this major change in their lives. Elm may also be indicated, as many a new mother and/or father feel overwhelmed by this added responsibility. Fear of being a good parent, as well as lacking self-confidence in raising a child may come up, indicating Mimulus and Larch. Overconcern and worry for the health and safety of the baby may also be an issue, indicating Red Chestnut. And many times, the father may feel resentment over all the love and attention his wife now gives their offspring. He may feel somewhat neglected, indicating Willow.

Moving

When a move comes up, even a planned one, this change can still bring stress. Of course, Walnut is always indicated, to help in breaking the old links to the past. Nostalgia and homesickness for the old home sweet home can be treated with Honeysuckle. With packing and unpacking and feeling overwhelmed by all the work still to do, Elm is indicated.

Changing Careers

Even by choice, a career change is always an anxious time. For fear of failure, Mimulus is indicated. Wild Oat may be indicated if there is uncertainty over career direction. Larch may be needed for lack of self-esteem and not feeling up to the challenge. Walnut is always indicated for any major change in life, to ease transitions.

Retirement

Retirement, as well as aging, can be a stressful time. This is another major time of transition, and Walnut is once again indicated. Wild Oat is another consideration when these individuals feel they no longer have any purpose in life, or possibly even Wild Rose, if apathy sets in. Star of Bethlehem may be indicated, if feelings of grief and loss arise when the person feels forced to retire, as well as the need for Willow, for resentment. Honeysuckle may also

be indicated for living too much in past memories, that prevent opening up to the opportunities life now presents. And Mimulus may also be indicated, when there is fear of no longer bringing home a salary and of loss of health.

As before, the common life scenarios just presented are illustrations of some of the many different emotional states that can come up during such experiences. Not everyone will experience them in the same way, nor have the need of the same flower essences. These situations have been generalized, to give you a deeper understanding of the various negative emotional states possible under such conditions and which of the 38 flower essences address them. Similar situations as described above now follow.

CASE HISTORIES:

Sally, a new mother, was having a problem in adjusting to the birth of her first child. She reported feelings of constant worry over the infant's well-being and was also feeling extremely overwhelmed with its continual care. She was in a state of exhaustion from lack of sleep when I saw her. She also expressed fear of not being a good enough mother, that she would hurt the child emotionally in some way. It seemed she also lacked confidence in her ability to care for her baby adequately. She was filled with anxiety and quite upset. After listening to Sally's plight, the following flower essences were suggested: Red Chestnut for overconcern; Elm for feeling overwhelmed; Olive for her extreme exhaustion; Mimulus for her fears of not being an adequate mother; Larch for lack of self-confidence in her role of mother; and Rescue Remedy for her extreme state of anxiety. Sally agreed with my evaluation of her emotional state, and was willing to try the recommended flower essences. She would call me in four weeks for a progress report. I heard from Sally within three weeks! The flower essences were already making a difference, and she couldn't wait to share her news. The extreme anxiety had totally disappeared, and her fear was lessening. She was also feeling more self-confident in her new role as a mother. Her overconcern was also easing up. Although she was still exhausted, it wasn't as extreme as before. She was still feeling overwhelmed however. Sally felt she no longer needed Rescue Remedy on a daily basis, nor Red Chestnut. She did feel the need to continue with Elm, Olive, Larch, and Mimulus for a while longer.

Tom had just retired when he came to see me. His wife Nancy was a client of mine, and when she realized Tom was in an emotional crisis, she asked if he would try the flower essences. He was experiencing a mild depression and appeared listless, withdrawing into himself. When we talked, he expressed sorrow over the loss of his youth, stating that he didn't know what he'd do with the rest of his life. There wasn't anything he felt he could do, and he seemed to long for the "good old days." After hearing his words, I suggested the following flower essences: Walnut for his state of transition; Wild Oat to bring a new path into view; Wild Rose for his sense of apathy and resignation; Star of Bethlehem for his sense of loss, and Honeysuckle, as it seemed he was stuck in the past. Tom related to the indications of these flower essences, and agreed to using them. I would speak with him in four weeks.

When we again spoke, Tom was no longer listless. He told me that he had taken up golf, something he had always wanted to learn, but never before had the time. He remarked that he was a bit surprised at his change in mood over the last few weeks. He had taken his retirement harder than he thought he would. He said it made him feel that his life was over. He now realized that although he was

Continued ➡

"getting on in years," he was still strong and healthy. And he now had the time to do many things that his work schedule had previously prevented. I noticed a complete change in Tom's energy. We went over the flower essences he had been taking, to determine if any changes were indicated. He no longer felt the need for Wild Rose. He said he was now taking his life back and was grateful for his change in attitude. He decided he'd continue with Honeysuckle, Star of Bethlehem, Walnut, and Wild Oat for a while longer however, as he was still experiencing feelings of nostalgia, loss, stress in adjusting to the life change, and he was still a bit uncertain as to what he wanted to do with the rest of his life. He also told me that although he knew the flower essences really helped his wife Nancy, he really didn't think they'd work for him.

Bach Flowers for Women's Issues

I feel it important to now focus on certain issues that pertain to women alone—issues that are not common to men. These issues can embrace not only the unique biological factors that at times put women at the mercy of their hormones, such as with PMS, pregnancy, childbirth, and menopause, but the mental challenges women also face in fully actualizing their own potential in what is still considered a "man's world." Although women have been slowly gaining ground in obtaining the same rights that men have, regretfully, true equality has not as yet been reached. While changes are indeed taking place, the effects of male chauvinism continue to be felt, with women struggling to take their rightful place beside their male cohorts. Lamentably, women are still seen by some men as inferior.

The movie *Tootsie*, starring Dustin Hoffman, attempted to bring to greater awareness the unfairness that women face in our society with the sexist attitudes of men that continue to prevail. While pretending to be a woman, Tootsie was faced with situations in which her worth as a female was disregarded, as well as being disrespected by men. For the first time in his life, he could relate to what it felt like in being a woman. He experienced this inequality firsthand. And it made him angry. Unfortunately, many women have to deal with what Tootsie did. The once familiar roles of women are expanding with issues of self-worth, respect, and a sense of personal accomplishment going beyond the roles of wife and mother.

The confusion surrounding a woman's role in today's changing world is a cause of emotional stress for many women. They often find themselves caught up in not only being wives and mothers, but taking on the added load of careers. "Supermom" has become a term applied to more and more women, and the pressure that women find themselves under is not so easily dealt with. Once considered primarily male concerns, heart disease and other stress-related illnesses are now on the rise in women.

Some of the possible challenging situations that many women may have to deal with, and the many Bach Flowers that can bring balance to the negative emotional states and stress produced by these experiences are now explored.

Abusive Relationships

Self-esteem is usually at the heart or this situation, with many women seeing themselves as helpless victims of male dominance. Often, these women were emotionally or physically abused as children, creating feelings of little self-worth. If there was no actual personal abuse, most likely they were privy to the abuse of their mothers. It then seems natural to accept abuse from male partners later on in their own relationships.

For women caught up in abusive relationships, the following flower essences are often indicated: Agrimony for denial; Centaury for being too passive and sacrificing one's own needs; Chestnut Bud for not learning from the past; Gorse for hopelessness; Larch for lack of self-worth; Mimulus for fear; Pine for guilt and feeling somehow deserving of abusive treatment; Star of Bethlehem for grief and trauma; Walnut to help break the link with the past and free oneself from an abusive partner; Wild Rose for resignation that nothing can be done to change the situation; and Holly for rage and hatred.

Incest and Rape

These reprehensible acts can totally disempower a woman. The effects can be felt for her entire life with the damage to her sense of dignity and self-worth possibly scarring her forever. In our society, in cases of rape, there is still the lingering inclination to blame the woman, creating deep feelings of guilt and shame that somehow she brought it on herself. With incest, the young female is taught to see this act as one of receiving love from the adult male, creating great sexual confusion as well as guilt and shame.

For women who have been victims of incest or rape, the following flower essences are often indicated: Star of Bethlehem for grief and trauma; Crab Apple for feelings of shame and disgust, and feeling unclean; Gorse or Sweet Chestnut for hopelessness or deep anguish; Holly for rage and hatred; Pine for self-blame; White Chestnut for constant unwanted thoughts; Mimulus or Rock Rose for fear or terror; and Olive for emotional exhaustion.

Anorexia/Bulimia

Eating disorders are much more common and prevalent in women. In our culture, there is so much emphasis placed on a woman's body, with Hollywood and Barbie dictating a quite unrealistic ideal for most women. Unfortunately, many women allow themselves to be taken in by this projection and hurt themselves in the process.

For women who suffer from eating disorders, among these anorexia and/or bulimia, the following flower essences are often indicated: Agrimony for their silent torment; Cherry Plum for loss of control expressed in their compulsive-obsessive behavior; Chestnut Bud for not learning from the past; Crab Apple for self-disgust; Gorse for hopelessness; Olive for exhaustion from gravely depleting the body; Larch for lack of self-worth; Mimulus for fear of obesity; Pine for not being "good enough"; White Chestnut for constant obsessive thoughts; and Walnut to withstand the influences of others.

Pregnancy

For most women, pregnancy is embraced as a joyful time. However, this time in a woman's life can be wrought with great emotional fluctuation created by the hormonal shifts taking place in her body, affecting sleep, energy level, and greater emotional sensitivity. During this very special time in a woman's life, the following flower essences are often indicated:

1ST TRIMESTER

Hornbeam for loss of vitality; Rescue Remedy for morning sickness; Mimulus for fear; Scleranthus for hormone imbalances; Willow for resentment, in cases where the pregnancy is unplanned; Red Chestnut for fear of the baby's welfare; White Chestnut for an inability to sleep; and Walnut for this time of transition.

2ND TRIMESTER

It is recommended to continue with Scleranthus and Walnut. Rsecue and Hornbeam may no longer be needed once into the fourth month, as nausea and fatigue usually abate. Many of the others suggested may also not be needed once into the 2nd trimester.

3RD TRIMESTER

By the seventh month, Beech may be needed for supersensitivity to others; the indications for Elm may now come up—feeling overwhelmed at the prospect of having a baby; Impatiens may be also needed, especially in the ninth month, as the due date creeps up along with feelings of impatience; Crab Apple will probably be needed now, to help deal with body image in the final stages of pregnancy; a need for Mimulus may again be evident, with fear of going through the birthing process now developing; Red Chestnut, as well, may be needed for overconcern of safety for the baby; it is suggested that Walnut be continued throughout pregnancy; and the need for Rescue Remedy may also become evident now, with feelings of general anxiety and nervousness over giving birth.

DURING THE BIRTH PROCESS

It is highly suggested to make up a dilution bottle of the following flower essences to assist with the emotional ups and downs while giving birth. And don't wait for the last minute to prepare your bottle! Add Rescue Remedy, Olive, Elm, Beech, and Walnut as previously directed. This combination will be of great help during delivery. Remember—the flower essences may be taken as often as needed, without concern of overdosing or harming mother or the baby in any way. In fact, the baby will be also greatly assisted in its birthing process.

AFTER BIRTH

The flower essences recommended after giving birth are: Olive for total exhaustion; Red Chestnut for overconcern for the infant; Elm and Larch for feeling overwhelmed, and lacking confidence in the new role of mother; Mustard for postpartum depression; Walnut to be continued in this state of transition of becoming a mother; and possibly Mimulus for fear of not adequately caring for the baby.

PMS (Premenstrual Syndrome)

Many women experience emotional ups and downs and sometimes physical symptoms such as tender breasts and bloating just prior to their monthly period, due to hormonal changes in their bodies. The flower essences suggested for most women troubled by PMS are: Rescue Remedy for general tension and feelings of anxiety; Scleranthus for mood swings; Beech for hypercriticalness; Willow for feelings of resentment; Mustard for depression from no apparent cause; Hornbeam for feeling fatigued; and possibly Crab Apple for feeling unclean as bleeding begins.

Women who experience PMS may want to take some of the above mentioned flower essences (take only those which relate to the emotional discomfort you are feeling) just during this time. If you are already using other flower essences for current emotional issues in your life, simply stop these for a few days and substitute the flower essences needed for the stress caused from PMS. Once your period is over, resume using your original combination.

Menopause

This is a time in life that can be particularly challenging for many women—and a time of possible deep fear. In our youth-oriented culture, aging is

Continued ➜

unfortunately seen as something to dread, and even more so for women. We only have to look at the movie industry where leading men continue in these roles far into their senior years (as did Cary Grant and Clark Gable, for example), while leading women are very quickly given character roles once their prime is considered over. As men age, they become "distinguished," while women become "old ladies." Women seem to lose their value more quickly than do men. And sadly, menopause is viewed as the end of the productive years for women in more than one way. This can be one of the greatest emotionally challenging times that a woman may face. Especially in our patriarchal society, where menopause is saturated with negativity—instead of seen as an initiation into the Wise Woman years.

The flower essences suggested to help a woman through this time of major transition are: of course, number one, Walnut for transitions; Star of Bethlehem for grief and lost youth, and the possible trauma that is felt by some women; Mimulus for fear of aging, fear of illness, fear of abandonment, fear of loss of sexuality, etc.; Honeysuckle for longing for the good old days, and being stuck in the past; Scleranthus for mood swings caused by hormonal changes, as well as hot flashes, and one of the most highly recommended of the flower essences for this life passage; Gorse for hopelessness; Wild Rose for apathy and resignation; Willow for bitterness and resentment; Wild Oat for new life direction; and Rescue Remedy, which is extremely helpful for hot flashes, as well.

Self-Empowerment

In the workplace, as well as in the home, women are no longer accepting unfair and unequal treatment, nor the unwarranted demands of others. Centaury enables a woman to recognize her own power, to be more assertive and not easily taken advantage of, both on the job, as well as in the home, when often exploited by family demands. Elm is wonderful for the Super Mom, relieving feelings of being overwhelmed, and helps prioritize what needs to be done. Oak is extremely helpful for the single mom who is raising a family and also working full time, and the career woman as well. Both can seem to struggle against formidable odds. Pine helps with women who are too hard on themselves, ever striving for perfection, as well as feeling guilty for the shortcomings of others. Vervain assists the overachiever, the woman who burns her candle at both ends and always feels keyed up, unable to relax. Mimulus releases fears of not succeeding or of success itself and instills courage. Gentian eases feelings of despair with setbacks and delays regarding career progress. Wild Oat assists in determining the correct path in life, and career direction if uncertain. Walnut helps with charting one's own course, and staying with it, despite what others may think. Willow assists with releasing resentment and bitterness when feelings of unfairness arise. And Larch is highly suggested for the woman who has low self-esteem, feels she won't succeed, and needs to be more confident that she can.

Please remember, these illustrations of possible women's issues and the flower essences that have been suggested for the probable emotional states that could arise are generalizations. Let us now look at some specific and individualized illustrations.

Case Histories:

Sherry had just been through an emotionally devastating divorce. She had lived with a man who had been emotionally and mentally abusive. She was in a state of severe depression when I saw her. There was deep-seated anger and rage, not only for her former husband but for herself as well for staying in an abusive relationship. She was having difficulty in

functioning, with her depression preventing her from going on with her life. A rash had begun to develop on one of her legs which had become irritated by her constant scratching. Once I had a picture of Sherry's emotional state, I suggested the following flower essences to ease her stress: Star of Bethlehem for the emotional trauma, grief and loss she was experiencing; Walnut for the state of transition she was going through; Centaury for allowing another to take advantage of her, and not standing up for herself; Sweet Chestnut for the angst she was suffering from; both Willow and Holly for the bitterness and rage she expressed; and Wild Rose, as she appeared apathetic, her spirit seemingly all but gone. As I explained why I had chosen each, she was in agreement with my assessment. She would take these and call me in four weeks.

When I next spoke to Sherry, she advised that most of her depression had lifted, and she was beginning to make plans for a new life. She was still dealing with her feelings of bitterness and resentment, and felt there was a great deal yet left to process from all the years of abuse. Her feelings of grief and loss were less intense, although still present. What amazed her the most, however, was that the rash on her leg was healing. She stated that the flower essences really seemed to have made a difference in her emotional state. She would continue to take Star of Bethlehem, for her grief and loss; Willow and Holly for lingering feelings of bitterness and rage; Centaury, as she related to the personality type this flower essence represents, and wanted to be more self-assertive in the future. She would also continue with Walnut, as the transition was not over. She no longer felt the need to continue with Wild Rose or Sweet Chestnut, as she no longer felt apathetic or deeply depressed as before. Jointly, we agreed to add Wild Oat, as she had mentioned she wasn't quite sure of her new direction regarding work. She had been a housewife and mother for almost twenty years, not needing to work outside the home. She was now faced with finding a career. And since she was a bit apprehensive with both being on her own and going out to work, we also agreed that Mimulus was in order—for her fears.

Marge was beginning her change of life. She was sure her menopause had begun, as she was beginning to experience hot flashes and her period was two months late. It had only been a month since her symptoms began that Marge came to see me. She explained that she wasn't sleeping well, waking several times each night because of the hot flashes, and becoming exhausted. She was also becoming cranky and irritable and upset over her lack of patience. For the most part, she seemed to be accepting of this natural progression of her life and only concerned by her emotional discomfort that was causing a strain in her daily life. I suggested the following flower essences to ease Marge's situation: Rescue Remedy for the general stress and anxiety she was feeling (and Rescue contains Impatiens for irritability and tension, and Cherry Plum for feeling out of control), as well as to help with the hot flashes; Walnut for her state of transition; Scleranthus for the hormonal changes taking place; Beech for her temporary state of intolerance; and Olive for her exhaustion. I asked Marge to call me in four weeks for a follow-up. When she did, she reported that she was much calmer than before, less irritable and grouchy. She was also sleeping better. When she was awakened by a hot flash, she would just take some drops from her dilution bottle, and very quickly she'd able to go back to sleep. Her emotional distress was definitely easing. We then discussed which flower essences to continue with. She felt she would stay with all five for the present, and be in touch later on.

Elizabeth is a survivor of incest and child abuse. She was working with a therapist at the time that she came for a Bach consultation. This was initiated by recently becoming aware of early childhood memories that had been repressed, memories that were now causing her great emotional pain. When she heard about the Bach Flowers, she felt they might be another healing technique to work with, along with her therapy, in moving through a very distressful time. As we spoke, I could see how her childhood abuse had gravely affected her adult life. She had been in an abusive marriage and, when that finally ended, in several other abusive relationships. She had very little self-esteem and found it extremely difficult to take care of her own needs, always sacrificing them for others. She shared how hard it was to confront others when she felt unfairly treated. She could never let on that she was unhappy. Her early-life experiences had created a woman who saw herself a victim of others, undeserving of much, if any, consideration by others— whether it be in a relationship or at work. Elizabeth, however, was now ready to face her issues and desperately wanted to finally free herself from her past conditioning—from feeling and being a victim. The following flower essences were recommended: Agrimony for hiding her torments behind a brave front, as well as her inability to confront others; Star of Bethlehem for the trauma she had experienced as child and the grief now surfacing; Chestnut Bud for not falling into the old habit pattern of victim and reprogramming her old tapes; Centaury, the flower essence for those who allow others to take advantage of them, to give her the ability to now consider her own needs just as important as others; Walnut for protection against the influence of others, and to break the links from the past; Pine for her guilt feelings of "somehow it was her fault" for being abused; and Holly for her deep-seated feelings of rage and anger at what had taken place as a child. Elizabeth expressed great hope that the flower essences would be of help to her. She was to call me four weeks later.

When Elizabeth got back to me, as scheduled, she laughingly told me that her boss was beside himself! She was no longer the meek and mild woman he knew. She has begun to speak up for herself, to his consternation. She also shared that she's been having bouts with some depression, getting in touch with her childhood trauma. She understands, however, that this is part of her healing process and it needs to be released before her healing can be completed. I questioned if her emotional discomfort was manageable. She affirmed it was, and didn't feel the need to discontinue Star of Bethlehem (which is the one bringing up her feelings of deep grief, as well as releasing the emotional and physical trauma she suffered). She also didn't feel a need, at this time, to make any changes and said she wanted to continue with all the original flower essences as she feels they have been truly facilitating her healing process.

Bach Flowers for Children

It appears that the flower essences are even more effective with children! The baggage that most carry is a great deal lighter, as well as more short-lived, than that of adults, making for a faster reaction time in children. You will find that the Bach flowers are of great assistance in so many situations that children are subjected to. Many times, the emotional distress that affects our children goes unrecognized, as in a divorce. It is common, often, for both parents to be so caught up in their own emotional turmoil that they fail to notice the devastation that their children may be experiencing.

Continued ➡

There are other times, as well, that parents may neglect to take into consideration the difficult emotional states their children may be going through. Fear of separation, even going to sleep at night, hyperactivity, the threat of a new baby, as well as learning disabilities are all very stressful and emotionally difficult situations that children may be faced with. The Bach Flowers can be of great assistance for your children's negative emotional states, as they are with your own.

Divorce

The Bach Flowers that are usually indicated to assist children with the emotional difficulties that come up during divorce are: Walnut for this difficult state of transition that children experience; Star of Bethlehem for the trauma and emotional sense of grief and loss; Scleranthus for when children are put in the position of choosing which parent they want to live with; Pine for the sense of guilt that many younger children feel that somehow they are to blame, that they were bad, and are now being punished. It's unfortunate that most young children are unable to understand the reasons for divorce, with their ability to discern or judge not yet well-developed, and magical thinking playing a large role in their world. Willow, for feelings of resentment towards one or both of their parents; Holly for anger and rage over the disruption of life and breakup of the family unit; Elm for feeling overwhelmed with the situation, and the many changes encountered; Honeysuckle for nostalgia and living in the past, and not accepting the current situation; Mimulus for feelings of fear that come up with the uncertainty of what now lies ahead; Gorse or Sweet Chestnut for depression, a feeling of hopelessness or extreme angst, and possibly Olive, if the trauma is particularly emotionally and/or physically depleting.

Separation Anxiety

The Bach Flowers that are usually indicated to assist those children who experience the emotional difficulties of separation are: Walnut to assist with the transition of separation from the parents (it is the "link breaker"); Honeysuckle to ease nostalgia and homesickness; Mimulus and Aspen for feelings of anxiety and foreboding; Rescue Remedy, the emergency combination for times of crisis and great anxiety (contains Rock Rose for terror and panic, and Star of Bethlehem for grief and loss); Chicory for overly possessive children; and Larch to boost self-confidence.

Sleeping Problems

The Bach Flowers that are usually indicated to assist children with sleeping problems, often caused by fear of being left alone or threat of nightmares are: Rock Rose, Mimulus, and Aspen for terror, fear, and apprehension; Chicory for children who tend to be manipulative, and have a great need for attention; White Chestnut to help in relaxing the mind; Vervain for hyper children who are easily wound-up and find it hard to relax; and Rescue Remedy, the all-purpose crisis formula (which also contains Rock Rose for terror and panic).

Hyperactivity

The Bach Flowers that are usually indicated to assist children who are hyperactive are: Vervain for the unusually active child who finds it hard to settle down; Impatiens for children who are keyed up and always in a rush; and Rescue Remedy itself is very helpful in bringing about a state of calm and relaxation once again.

Allergies

There are two flower essences that are especially helpful with allergies—Walnut and Crab Apple. Walnut is a protection against the effects of outside influences. Pollen is certainly an outside influence. And Crab Apple is a cleanser for the system.

Children are not alone in suffering from the effects of allergies. I recently had the most amazing experience with Walnut at one of the Bach Seminars I present countrywide. My assistant for this seminar had advised me that she didn't know if she'd be able to work with me the whole weekend. She had an extreme sensitivity towards environmental pollution, as well as being highly allergic to many substances. She hadn't been able to sleep in hotels. This would be her first attempt in several years. Although she had tried many different types of medication, nothing seemed to help. Without giving it much thought, I asked her if she'd like to try Walnut, explaining how effective it has been for allergy relief. As I always travel with the complete set of the Bach Flowers, I was able to make a dilution bottle for her on the spot. She was agreeable to giving it a try, and took Walnut throughout the day. When I saw her the next morning, she rushed over in great excitement and said to me, "It's a miracle! I was able to sleep undisturbed last night. I had no allergic reactions. Nothing has helped me before. I am amazed!" I was also amazed. I had never seen the flower essences work so quickly before (excluding Rescue Remedy, of course). We have since kept in touch, and her allergic reactions seem to be a thing of the past.

Sibling Rivalry

The Bach Flower Essences that are usually indicated to assist children who experience difficulty relating with other children in the family, whether it be the birth of a new brother or sister that threatens their position, or sibling rivalry itself, are: Walnut for the transition of no longer being the only child; Willow for feelings of resentment towards the sibling; Vine for bossy and aggressive children who always need to be in charge and have their way; Cherry Plum for the loss of temper, poor impulse control, and physical aggression; Chestnut Bud for the child who does not learn from past behavior; Holly for the child who has feelings of anger and rage, as well as envy and jealousy; and Larch for a poor self-image and lack of self-esteem. Many children with issues of sibling rivalry have feelings of inferiority, as well as jealousy, that are masked by their aggressive behavior.

Learning Disabilities

There are many issues that arise with children who have special problems. They are extremely sensitive little souls who realize they are different from other children. Many times this perceived difference brings on deep feelings of low self-esteem and possible depression. Limitations in learning can also cause frustration, guilt, and anger, as well as apathy.

The Bach Flower Essences that are usually indicated to assist children with learning disabilities are: Larch for low self-esteem, feeling inferior; Clematis and White Chestnut, as many are caught up in daydreaming and not in the present moment, seeming to be inattentive and forgetful, as well as unable to concentrate and focus. These two flower essences are excellent for grounding and concentration: Wild Rose for the child who becomes apathetic, appears listless, and seems to have given up; Chestnut Bud, which is helpful for learning from past mistakes, learning new lessons, and decreasing forgetfulness; Gentian for the despair caused by setbacks and delays that come with their progress (two steps forward, one step backward); Gorse and

Sweet Chestnut may be indicated for deeper depression (feelings of hopelessness or extreme anguish); Agrimony for denial, concealing painful feelings from themselves and others (this can create a state of restlessness); Centaury, as many of these children allow themselves to be exploited and bullied by other children; Walnut for children easily influenced by other children or affected by their cruelty; Pine for feelings of guilt and self-blame; and Impatiens for tension, frustration, and impatience with themselves for not accomplishing tasks as easily as other children. It is common that many children with learning disabilities also suffer from hyperactivity. Several of the already noted flower essences indicated for this state may be applicable as well.

Behavior Problems

There are many other situations in which the flower essences can be of great assistance in treating unwanted or troubling behaviors in children: Vine for the child who is a bully and refuses to listen to authority; Cherry Plum for the child who has poor impulse control, is aggressive, and physically acts out, including temper tantrums; Mimulus for the shy, timid, and fearful child; Chicory for the child who is demanding and in need of constant attention; Walnut for transitions and changes, which are usually uncomfortable and create issues of adjustment—as when teething, starting school, puberty, moving, etc.; Mimulus and Cherry Plum have also been effective with bedwetting, addressing the emotional issues of fear and loss of control; Larch and Centaury for low self-esteem and allowing others to victimize them; and Aspen for hypersensitivity.

As before, the above illustrations are but some of the many different situations with their corresponding negative emotional states that may come up with children. Not all will experience them in the same way, nor have need of the same flower essences, nor are these states described definitive. Here are more specific and individualized illustrations presented for your future practice and use.

CASE HISTORIES:

Tina's mom was beside herself in relieving her five-year-old daughter's constant nightmares and resultant bedtime anxiety. Tina would awaken several times a week, screaming in terror. It had escalated to the point that Tina would no longer sleep alone. Tina's terror was now also causing a strain on the whole family. Her mother finally called for help. The flower essences we selected to help Tina over her fright and terror were: Rescue Remedy for her general state of anxiety (and Rescue contains Rock Rose for panic and terror, specifically); Mimulus and Aspen for her fear and apprehension; and Chicory for her recent possessive and clinging behavior. Tina was to be given this combination at least four times daily, and especially before going to bed. We also felt it best, for the first few nights, to allow Tina to sleep with her mom. Once the nightmares began to subside, Tina would again sleep in her own bed. Within the first week, the nightmares began to ease. By the end of the second week, they had just about stopped. Tina was no longer in a state of panic at bedtime, and was now able to stay in her own bed. Whatever had produced her nightmares seemed released. It was agreed to continue with these flower essences for another month. Once discontinued, if the nightmares should begin again, both Tina and her mom knew what to do.

Timmy was a bright five-year-old who was very attached to his mom. He would become quite upset whenever she left him with anyone. The situation worsened when, for the first time, he was to start

Continued ➡

school. While waiting for the school bus, he would begin to cry, and when it was time to get on, still crying, he would cling to his mother in panic. This was not only a stressful situation for Timmy, but for his distraught mother. As she had been using the Bach Flowers herself, she felt they would also be helpful for her son. After describing the situation to me, we felt the following flower essences were indicated to help relieve Timmy's intense emotional state: Rescue Remedy for the emotional crisis precipitated by going to school; Mimulus and Aspen for his extreme fear and apprehension; Honeysuckle for the separation anxiety he was feeling; and Walnut for this stage of transition with beginning school. It was also suggested that Timmy's mom add some Red Chestnut to her dilution bottle to ease her worry and concern for Timmy's current plight, as this was a difficult time for both of them. Little by little, as each day passed, Timmy was less panic stricken. It took almost a month for Timmy to be totally adjusted to the change in his life and no longer exhibit any apprehension of fear when going off to school. After two months, the flower essences were discontinued, and as it turned out, no longer needed.

Jordan was five when he was diagnosed with minor learning disabilities. He had a very short attention span and was also somewhat hyperactive. It was recommended by the school that he be placed in a special class for a year or two to receive the extra help and attention needed for him to catch up with his peers. Although Jordan had learning disabilities, he was aware enough to realize that something was wrong with him, and that he was in a special class. This seemed to affect him greatly, and his self-esteem plummeted. I became familiar with Jordan when his mother called, deeply concerned over her son. At the age of seven, she told me, he was talking about not wanting to live anymore. She had immediately gotten him into therapy, but also felt the Bach Flowers were another avenue to try, as they had been so helpful with her emotional issues. After discussing Jordan's situation and his current emotional state, the following flower essences were selected: Larch for his low self-esteem; Gorse for his state of depression; Vervain for his hyperactivity; Clematis and White Chestnut for his inattentiveness and lack of focus; Willow for his feelings of resentment for being different, and Star of Bethlehem for the trauma he suffered (being teased by other children). As Jordan had been suffering from these emotions for almost two years, his response to the flower essences took almost two months. Although his progress was slow in the beginning, by the end of the second month his turn around had begun. His depression had disappeared, with his self-esteem rising. His schoolwork was also improving. His mother and I felt it a good idea to continue with these same flower essences for a while longer.

Lisa had been an only child for four years when her baby brother was born. This became a traumatic event for Lisa, as she had been the little princess of the family, and now there was a prince! Her mother thought she had prepared her daughter for the appearance of her new brother, and was quite shocked at Lisa's behavior. She wanted no part of her brother, and seemed very resentful, as well as in need of more attention than ever before. And she began to exhibit regressive behavior, pretending she was also a baby. Of course, Lisa's mom was well aware of what was going on. Lisa was evidently jealous of her new baby brother, and experiencing difficulty in accepting the change in her life. Despite her awareness, Lisa's mom was quite concerned over the situation, and soon called to inquire about flower essences for Lisa. The following are those

selected for Lisa's distressing feelings: Walnut for her transition from only child to sister; Willow for her feelings of resentment; Chicory for her need of attention and possessiveness of her mother; Star of Bethlehem for the trauma and grief of no longer being #1; and Larch for low self-esteem and self-confidence. Lisa began to respond almost immediately to the flower essences. Her neediness subsided, and she began to take an interest in her new baby brother. Her feelings of resentment seemed to be replaced by wanting to mother him instead. She took delight in helping to feed him and play with him. She no longer saw him as a threat to her position in the family. This was also helped by her parents' awareness, and they made a strong effort to make sure she received her share of love and attention as well. After four weeks, it was decided to discontinue all but Larch and Walnut to assist Lisa with her self-esteem, as well as moving through her transition.

The flower essences are chosen for children as they are for adults—by noting the stressful emotional states being expressed and the child's personality Type. These are your guides to the flower essence or combination of essences needed to address the current situation. The dosage is the same with children as with adults, and is administered four times daily. You may make a dilution bottle or place at least four drops of the concentrate into milk or fruit juice. A baby who is being breast-fed can also receive the effects of the flower essences when the mother is taking them herself. Also in regard to infants—it is highly recommended to give all newborns Star of Bethlehem (or Rescue Remedy, which contains Star of Bethlehem), for release of the birth trauma that all experience.

Bach Flowers for Animals and Plants

We love them dearly and we know they love us every bit as much. They're our pets, our beloved companions, and we do everything in our power to protect them and keep them safe.

In this final section we will now turn to treating animals and plants, as the Bach Flowers facilitate emotional healing for all of God's creatures. The healing vibrations contained in the flower essences are effective for restoring emotional balance and harmony in all living things—from the Human to the Animal, as well as to the Plant Kingdom. And as with children, the Bach Flowers bring relief to animals and plants in a much shorter time.

One may wonder, "How do I determine which flower essences are needed by my pet? I can't communicate with them!" This is true. However, by being empathetic to their moods and possible emotional distress—and we all have this ability—we can get a pretty good feeling as to what they may be suffering. As all of us who have animals already know and don't need to be convinced of, our pets certainly have emotions. We know when they are happy or when they are distressed.

To determine which of the flower essences may be needed for particular crisis situations that our pets may be experiencing, we need to put ourselves in their shoes, so to speak. What would you be feeling if you were in the same situation? It most likely is the same for your cat or dog, or whatever other animal is sharing your life. And many times, when you are going through a particularly difficult period emotionally, your pet will be experiencing the same stressful state(s) that you are. It's also reassuring to know that a wrong selection cannot hurt your pet, nor are there any side-effects.

The following illustrations of many of the possible stressful states that animals may face are now provided to give you an understanding in selecting the appropriate flower essences that treat these states:

Agrimony assists with the torment that many animals face when a wound or injury is slow to heal.

Aspen is a great help with very nervous and easily frightened animals.

Centaury aids the runt of the litter who always seems to be pushed around by its bigger brothers and sisters.

Cherry Plum is for the very aggressive animal who may threaten to bite and seems uncontrollable.

Chestnut Bud is excellent in training. It prevents the same mistakes being made over again.

Chicory assists with animals that demand a lot of attention, and also for those who are too possessive of their owners.

Clematis is helpful for the animal that is always sleeping.

Holly assists with animals who seem jealous, and is also good for nasty temperaments.

Larch is extremely effective for the animal who seems to lack self-esteem and is low in the pecking order.

Mimulus helps with fear, as with thunderstorms, for example, and is also for the very timid and shy animal.

Olive is extremely helpful after an illness or operation.

Rock Rose treats extreme panic and terror.

Star of Bethlehem is for any trauma, shock or grief an animal may experience. It is especially helpful with animals who have been victims of abuse.

Vervain, and also Impatiens, are very effective with high-strung, nervous animals.

Vine is used for the animal who won't accept authority, and also for the boss animal who dominates other animals it lives with.

Walnut is always indicated for any change taking place in an animal's life, such as a move, a new owner, a new pet introduced into the home, as well as a new child.

Water Violet is used with aloof animals who tend to be loners and is the personality Type for most cats.

Wild Rose is needed when an animal appears listless and apathetic.

Willow is excellent when feelings of resentment may crop up, as with a new pet or birth of a baby.

And the final selection—for all emergency crisis situations:

Rescue Remedy—When in doubt as to which flower essence may be needed, Rescue is always helpful in just about any situation that may arise for animals. I give my animals Rescue on a daily basis as a general balancer and de-stressor. And don't forget to give your pet some Rescue before a visit to the vet, which always produces great anxiety. You will be amazed at how Rescue eases your pet's panic attack.

The following illustrations are cases from my practice in which the Bach Flowers have been used with remarkable results with animals in distress. Know that the flower essences are not only a wonderful assistance in regard to maintaining general emotional well-being, but are also extremely effective in modifying behavioral problems.

CASE HISTORIES:

Rocky was adopted by the Smith family at about six weeks of age. He was a normal, healthy, friendly, and playful kitten. Several weeks later, the Smiths'

Continued →

two young sons left for camp. When they returned home at summer's end, dramatic changes in Rocky's personality abruptly took place. This once friendly, easy-going kitten had became a recluse, hiding under the bed and only coming out to eat dinner. This became his way of life. No one could go near him except Mr. or Mrs. Smith, and even with them he was extremely nervous. They had their suspicions that one of their sons had traumatized the kitten in some way, although they could never get either of them to 'fess up to any foul play. Rocky remained in his shocked and fearful state for over two years, until Mrs. Smith learned of the Bach Flowers. She was extremely encouraged and hopeful that they would help Rocky's plight. In discussing the case with them, we began the task of selecting the essences we felt were appropriate for his emotional condition—one dominated by extreme fear, suspicion, and terror. After carefully considering Rocky's emotional state, we selected the following six flower essences that addressed what we felt he was experiencing: Rock Rose, for extreme terror and panic; Mimulus, for fear; Aspen, for apprehension (as his fear was so extreme, we felt it best to touch all bases); Scleranthus, for emotional instability; Holly, for suspicion and mistrust; and Star of Bethlehem, for whatever shock and trauma that had caused the radical change in Rocky's behavior. Six weeks passed before any noticeable changes occurred, and when they did, they were dramatic. A turnabout in his behavior had begun. While Mrs. Smith's mother was visiting, Rocky actually came out from hiding, approached her, sashaying his way across the room, and let her pet him. He then went to the kitchen door, requesting to be let out. Mrs. Smith's mother commented to her, "I had forgotten you had that cat, haven't seen him in ages!" and proceeded to open the door for him. Mrs. Smith told me that she was in shock for the moment! This was the first time since Rocky's out-of-balance emotional condition had developed that he had appeared with unfamiliar people present. His new lease on life was initiated. Rocky no longer stayed in hiding under the bed, and except for one of the Smith boys (and this is a major clue as to which one may have traumatized him!), he no longer displays fear towards people. Rocky is now a happy, healthy, mostly well-adjusted cat. (Let's be honest, how many cats are totally well adjusted!) Mr. Smith, who was a skeptic at first, was quite impressed with the change in Rocky; so much so that he now takes the flower essences himself.

A woman recently called concerned about her horse Baby. He had become apathetic and listless, and she was worried about his health. I suggested she give him Wild Rose for his seeming apathy and resignation. A few weeks later, she called me back to report that Baby was up and about, and back to his normal self.

I received another call from a man, someone I had helped in the past, and had recommended the use of Rescue Remedy. He was calling to share a wonderful story in which Rescue had been extremely helpful. Recently, his colt Black Beauty had caught his hind leg in a fence and had cut some tendons. After first calling the vet, he then began to treat the colt every fifteen minutes with Rescue, as it would take a while for the vet to get to him. About an hour later the vet arrived and was amazed that he was able to stitch and dress the wound without a tranquilizer. The wound had to be treated and dressed for three months, and he continued using Rescue before each treatment to keep Beauty calm, as well as administering Rescue to the horse daily to assist his healing process.

Bobbi, a client of mine herself, called one day about her cat Angel, who wouldn't use the litter box. She certainly wasn't living up to her name! Angel would normally relieve herself outside the house. It became a problem, however, when she was unable to go out because of rain or snow. When this took place, she would use the bathroom rug instead of the litter box. Bobbi had tried numerous times to train Angel to use her box, to no avail. She felt this couldn't go on much longer. Bobbi was now turning to the flower essences before giving up her pet. Chestnut Bud was suggested, for failure to learn from past mistakes and repeating the same mistake many times over. This flower essence has been extremely effective in training many animals, as well as correcting any bad habits, like scratching on the furniture. I am happy to report that Angel is now using her litter box, and a good thing for her. She was on the verge of losing her home, and possibly her very life. Bobbi was quite amazed, as well as extremely grateful, at how helpful Chestnut Bud was and how quickly it worked. Within two days, Angel had been retrained. Bobbi was greatly relieved, as she deeply loved her cat, and had been distressed at the possibility of giving Angel up. I suggested she continue using Chestnut Bud for a while longer, and also to use Rescue Remedy everyday and always, as a general balancer.

The Bach Flowers help with all animals—even with birds and fish. I have had the personal experience of rescuing several birds that my cats, regrettably (for me!), brought home from time to time. They are lucky enough to still be alive thanks to Rescue Remedy. I have learned firsthand, many times over, why it's called the emergency first aid treatment. I place a few drops (I always make a dilution bottle because of the great amount of brandy in the concentrate, which makes it difficult for animals to accept) on their beaks and rub some on their heads. I then place them in a box I have filled with some grass and put them in a safe place. Every half hour I give another dose. As they recover, I make arrangements to bring them to a local bird sanctuary to complete their healing process. I'll never forget the time when one of my rescued baby birds, after seeming almost dead, hopped onto the edge of her box and sang her little heart out! I had put her in an upstairs bedroom safely away from her predator and had closed the door. Several hours later, I began to hear her chirping. When I went to check on her, I found her amazingly well. And Rescue Remedy even works with fish. A friend of mine has tropical fish that almost died. She was able to bring them around by placing several drops in their fish tank.

Sammy, my good friend Linda's dog and faithful companion for many years, suddenly refused to eat or drink. Linda became very concerned and called me for help with the Bach Flowers. I soon learned that Linda's cat—a playmate of Sammy—had died two days ago. These two animals had become inseparable friends. I strongly felt that Sammy was mourning the loss of his friend. With Rescue Remedy in hand, off I went to Linda's. Once there, we began treating the dog with Rescue. I had made a dilution bottle and continued giving him several drops every fifteen minutes. When I left, I told Linda to continue treating Sammy with the Rescue, and I'd call the next day to see how he was progressing. When I spoke to Linda the next morning, she said Sammy had eaten a bit, but was still languishing. I brought over Sweet Chestnut and Wild Rose to be added to Sammy's dilution bottle—for his anguish and listless state. After about two weeks on the flower essences, Sammy was his old self again. And Linda had also gotten another kitten as a new playmate for him.

Karen had two dogs, one from birth, Bo, and the other, Floyd, only recently adopted. She called

one day, hoping the flower essences would help, relating the following situation to me. Bo had always been a timid dog, and not all that affectionate. Floyd, on the other hand, was quite possessive, and very jealous. He was forever picking on Bo and gave him no peace. The flower essences that were indicated for the emotional states of Bo and Floyd were: Mimulus for Bo's timidity, and Water Violet for his aloofness; Chicory for Floyd's possessiveness, Holly for his jealousy, and Vine for his domineering behavior. After about three weeks, Linda reported that changes had begun to take place in both dogs. Bo is much more affectionate and no longer cowers in the presence of Floyd, with the help of Water Violet and Mimulus. And Floyd has become much more tolerant of Bo, his domineering behavior and possessiveness slowly diminishing with the help of Holly, Vine, and Chicory. I suggested that these flower essences be continued for

The Bach Flower Essences— Keyword Indications
Rachelle Hasnas

The Bach Flower Essences	Keyword Indication(s)
Agrimony	mental torment behind brave front
Aspen	unknown fears, anxiety
Beech	intolerance
Centaury	weak-willed, subservient
Cerato	no confidence in decision making
Cherry Plum	fear of loss of control
Chestnut Bud	failure to learn from the past
Chicory	selfish, possessive love
Clematis	disinterest in the present moment
Crab Apple	sense of uncleanliness
Elm	overwhelmed by responsibilities
Gentian	despair from setbacks, delays
Gorse	hopelessness
Heather	self-involvement
Holly	hatred, envy, suspicion
Honeysuckle	nostalgia, living in the past
Hornbeam	low vitality
Impatiens	impatience
Larch	low self-worth
Mimulus	known fears
Mustard	sudden depression
Oak	bravely endure all obstacles
Olive	extreme exhaustion
Pine	perfectionism, self-blame, guilt
Red Chestnut	overconcern, anxiety for others
Rock Rose	panic, terror
Rock Water	self-denial
Scleranthus	indecision, vacillation
Star of Bethlehem	grief, shock, trauma
Sweet Chestnut	extreme mental anguish
Vervain	overenthusiastic, opinionated
Vine	domineering, inflexible
Walnut	easily influenced by others
Water Violet	aloof, proud
White Chestnut	obsessive thoughts, restless mind
Wild Oat	uncertain of path in life
Wild Rose	apathy, resignation
Willow	bitterness, resentment

—From *Pocket Guide to Bach Flower Essences*

Continued ➜

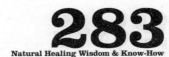

awhile longer. I also advised that it may be possible that Bo is a natural Mimulus Type, and that Floyd is a Vine Type. Both might do well to continue with these flower essences as their personality essences on a permanent basis.

Administering the flower essences to animals is as easy as placing a few drops of the concentrate in their drinking water or food—four drops of Rescue, and/or two drops of any of the other 38 flower essences that you have selected. And don't worry about your other pets who may not need the same essences and drink or eat from the same bowls. The flower essences will not affect them if they do not need them. Remember, a wrong selection does nothing. A dropper bottle dilution preparation may also be made to administer directly into the animal's mouth. The directions are the same for animals as for humans. It is suggested however, not to use alcohol as a preservative in your pet's dilution bottle. Its taste seems to be an unwelcome one for pets.

Seven flower essences is also the generally recommended limit for your pets, as with you. Larger animals (horses, etc.) can be given the flower essences with the aid of a large dosage syringe available from livestock supply companies. As with humans, the flower essences are administered four times daily. In cases of extreme stress or crisis, they may be given every fifteen minutes. And remember, there is no danger of overdosing. From my personal experience with my own pets, they seem to know that the flower essences are helping them, and easily accept taking them.

The Bach Flowers may also be used for plants, and are highly effective in many situations. Although plants may not appear to be very conscious or to have feelings, my understanding of this was radically changed by reading Peter Tompkins's book, *The Secret Life of Plants*, many years ago. According to Tompkins's information, plants actually respond to perilous circumstances, and possibly may experience feelings of fear as well as other stressful states.

This book describes an experiment that was done where electrodes were attached to a group of plants to see if it was possible to monitor electrical impulses produced by them in various situations. In one situation, one of the experimenters purposely killed one of the plants in the group. While this was taking place, unusual electrical activity was picked up. A day or so later, different individuals, including the perpetrator, would go into the room where the murder took place, while one of the researchers monitored any activity. When the experimenter who had done the deed entered the room, the needle went off the page!

This and various other experiments described in this book appear to point to the fact that plants, indeed, have consciousness—more than we would imagine. It would therefore seem beneficial, from what we know of the Bach Flowers, to make use of their efficacy with our plants as well. And from my personal experiences in doing so, as well as that of many others I know, this appears to be extremely helpful. The following are illustrations of generalized situations in which flower essences may be effectively used for plants.

Whenever transplanting, Rescue Remedy is recommended for the shock and trauma experienced from this procedure. For insect infestation, Crab Apple is highly recommended. When moving plants to another location, Walnut is suggested for this state of transition and change. For plants that have been attacked by a pet, Mimulus is the flower essence to use. When a plant appears drooping, some Hornbeam will perk it up. And for cut flowers, to assist in keeping them fresh longer, Rescue is also recommended.

I have been adding Rescue to cut flowers for years now, and they definitely keep longer. Once a month I spray some Rescue on all my houseplants. My plants are just thriving, all lush and vibrant. The following experience is presented now to give you a more specific illustration of the help available for plants with the use of the flower essences.

I recently had an occasion to see how incredible the flower essences are with plants in crisis. This past June, I had planted three azaleas in my front garden. After a few days, one of the new plants began to wilt and looked pretty pathetic. It looked like I might lose it. I quickly made up a combination in a bucket, using eight drops of each of the following flower essences: Rescue Remedy for the crisis situation (and it also contains Star of Bethlehem, for shock and trauma), Hornbeam and Olive for sapped vitality and major exhaustion, Wild Rose for its listless appearance, Walnut for just being transplanted and its state of transition, and Centaury, as it seemed quite weak. I first poured a bucketful around the base of the plant, and then every half hour I sprayed its wilted leaves. When I checked on it the next morning, it hadn't seemed to respond. I didn't give up, though, and continued to spray it throughout the day. The next morning, I could not believe my eyes. It had perked up and now was as strong and healthy looking as the other two just-planted azaleas. It was an incredible feeling to be able to bring the plant around again. At this writing, it is the end of August, and the azalea plant is absolutely thriving!

—From *Pocket Guide to Bach Flower Essences*

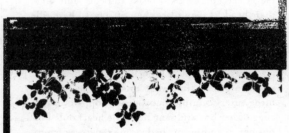

FLORAL ACUPUNCTURE

Deborah Carydon, C.F.E.P. and Warren Bellows, Lic. Ac.
Photography by Deborah Craydon

The New Topical Use of Flower Essences

Flower essences work therapeutically when taken sequentially over time. Because it is difficult to see your own darkness, it is useful to work with a trained practitioner who can listen while you describe your current conditions and match essences in a harmonic combination for you to use over the following month or so. Traditionally the remedy is taken internally, a few drops several times a day. When treatments are repeated over time, layers of chronic behaviors and patterns that could take years, or even a lifetime, to overcome transform themselves. Practitioners include those who use flower essence exclusively as well as physicians, acupuncturists, chiropractors, naturopaths, bodyworkers, and others in the health care professions. Most of these practitioners speak highly of the results these simple drops have on their clients.

The expectation for the remedy is that the person will feel better emotionally. Dr. Bach's original intention for healing all disease through his tinctures has been replaced with the idea that flower essences heal the emotional body. Part of this reasoning is for the protection of the companies that produce flower essences sold in the United States under the category of nutritional supplements. It is also partly that flower essences are affected by the life force of the person who makes the remedy. Flower essences are made by floating freshly picked flowers in a bowl of pure water in the early morning-tide hours in full sun. Pure intention on the part of the flower essence maker is essential for the resulting mother tincture to fully capture a clean imprint from the flower. The person who makes the flower essence, then, must learn to potentize the flower essences in the way that Dr. Bach intended.

In every age there have been healers whose faith transcends the physical substance they offer to those who are ill. Like the wine and wafer at a Christian communion, to those who believe, the healer's remedy makes them well. Or was it the kindly eye and gentle touch?

As flower essences have grown in reputation among healers, many have begun to incorporate them into topical applications such as creams, bottled sprays, and massage oils. What can be said of the repeated use of flower essence creams for a person with fibromyalgia who within a year is free of pain and well? Or someone who places compresses containing specific flower essences on his or her back when it is out of alignment and hears it click back into place after twenty minutes? Or a painful tooth a dentist is unable to fix, yet a flower essence compress heals without recurrence of symptoms? One has to wonder how this is occurring and why applying flower essences to the organ of the skin may be so successful.

In order to grow faith to fit into the shoes of master healers like Dr. Bach or Paracelsus, properly made flower essences, emanating the pure vibration of flowers, act as perfect training wheels. Holding a vibrational octave (meaning that the remedy holds the vibrational imprint of the flower rather than actual physical substance), the essences enable healers, including self-healers, to experience minor "miracles."

Healing with the Human Energy Field

Hanna Kroeger, a master herbalist from Boulder, Colorado, who died in 1998 in her mid-eighties, effected the same kind of cures Dr. Bach did. She said that for healing with the word, a kindly touch was also necessary. Touching a shoulder, for instance, while saying the words, "Don't worry, you'll be okay," was what was needed, she said, provided the healer's faith and life force were strong enough. Touching the physical body with the pure "word" of a flower essence is a way for healers to learn how the body responds to pristine floral messages. Placing the pure imprint of the flower on its corresponding body site using the five-thousand-year-old Chinese acupuncture system creates an exponential effect; outer nature is greeted by its inner counterpart through the sacred doorways of the physical body. . . .

The Five-Element Theory of Acupuncture

The Tao of Acupuncture

The Five-Element style of acupuncture originated some three thousand to five thousand years ago through the healing arts of the ancient Taoist tradition. The Taoists believed that the role of the individual was to become an embodiment of the marriage of heavenly and earthly forces. They saw

Continued ➡

that heavenly influences united with earthly matter created a dynamic tension through which the soul's emergence into the world takes place. Since this emergence occurred through the vehicle of time, the Taoist goal was to live a healthy long life in order to accomplish this task. Acupuncture is one of the many tools they developed toward this end.

Being an agrarian society, the Taoists were closely aligned with the forces of nature. They saw man and nature as woven together from a single fabric and believed that to touch one or the other was to affect both. They understood the building blocks of reality to be composed of varying levels of subtle energies that precipitate into substance. A descending hierarchy of Original Source Energy steps down through spiritual, mental, and emotional levels respectively, solidifying into matter as manifested through the physical body. The Taoists understood this descending movement of spirit into matter was seen as being counterbalanced by an uprising movement of information and intelligence from the various levels into the soul. The revolution of this twofold circuit defines the soul's emergence into the world along a "middle path" of health and balance. The Taoists envisioned the purpose of evolution as the perfection of this circular relationship of the spirit's descent with the soul's ascent.

The Taoists mapped all the major energy lines or meridians on the body. While the meridians can be likened to electrical circuits in a house, they provide electricity not only to your physical body but also to your emotional, mental, and spiritual bodies. The meridians are punctuated at intervals by vortices, called acupuncture points. The mode of stimulating the vortex is by lightly puncturing it with a very thin needle; this creates an energetic resonance that affects the health of the physical, emotional, mental, and spiritual functioning of the particular meridian that has been activated through stimulation of one of its points.

For instance, to use the Liver Meridian as an example to describe these varying levels, there is a vibration from the Original Source that downloads into the spiritual energy known as hope. This vibration is housed within the Liver Meridian. When the Liver Meridian is stimulated, it accesses hope and helps you mentally to plan and see the future. On the emotional level, Liver energy expresses itself as assertiveness, the energy required to implement your plans. On the physical level, this vibration from the Source manifests as the organ of the liver and affects the health of the eyes. According to Chinese medicine, the Liver Meridian vibrates to the megahertz of the color green in the visible spectrum—the hue that reveals itself in springtime through trees and plants. (Wood is the element and spring is the season associated with the Liver Meridian.)

Man being Nature, the Taoists knew that the way to live a long, healthy life was to live according to Nature's laws. The most basic law is that life constantly moves and transmutes in phases. One of the ways to stay healthy is to recognize these energetic phases inside yourself and to know when it is time to move from one phase to the next. The role of an acupuncturist is to help you facilitate this movement when you find you are stuck in one phase by stimulating the acupuncture point or points that mirror your condition.

There are more than three hundred acupuncture points on the body. The Taoists gave each of them a name, identifying them as portals into the body at the various energy levels to which they access. Some of these names are *Soul Door, Heavenly Palace* (soul-spirit level doorways), *Not at Ease, Thought Dwelling* (mental-level doorways), *Wail of Grief, Abdomen Sorrow* (emotional-level doorways), and *Root of the Breasts, Sea of Blood*, or *Knee Yang Border* (physical-level doorways). However, the Taoists named most of the points in reference to landscapes in nature, such as *Greater Mountain Stream, Outside Marsh*, and *Penetrating Valley*.

Acupuncture utilizes a stainless-steel needle or the burning of moxa (dried mugwort) to stimulate the acupuncture points on a specific site. This book shows you how to apply outer floral nature in the form of flower essences to the energy portals of the acu-points that connect to your inner nature. Each flower essence is an energetic key that unlocks a specific acu-point to communicate between the worlds. This communication creates the possibility of knitting together the fabric between man and Nature, a fabric which has been rent apart in modern times. Through these kinds of treatments, we envision the possibility of a new marriage between man, cosmos and the natural world.

The Five Phases and Their Corresponding Elements

The Five-Element theory of acupuncture is also called the Five-Phase theory, as it identifies five phases of evolution in the material world that are circular beginning to end. The Five-Element theory helps you to identify what phase of your journey you are currently in and helps you to move appropriately from that phase to the next by stimulating a specific acupuncture point. When you are healthy, you move through each of these five phases in a graceful, timely manner, and your body, as a result, receives the gift of long life.

The following are the five phases and their corresponding Element.

Winter the Element of Water, which holds the potential for all life

Spring the Element of Wood, which creates identifiable forms and boundaries for this life

Summer the Element of Fire, which warms what is formed, creating joy through relationship

Late Summer the Element of Earth, which supports and nurtures this vitalized life

Fall the Element of Metal, which brings value and meaning to this process

WINTER PHASE (A SEED IN THE GROUND)

Element Of Water

In the Winter phase, your energy is hidden deep within your body. Like night, it is cool, dark, and condensed. A contracted yin stage, it is static and receptive in the way that plants and animals remain dormant or sleep for long periods during the cold months. Contained in this stage, however, are the regenerative forces that are gathering potential through this long rest.

Water holds the potential for all life; it is mercurial in nature in that it imprints information. In its larger aspect it contains the entire recipe of the cosmic "soup" that births life itself. In relation to you as individual, water carries your potential in seed form as well the entire book of your encoded hereditary information. By allowing the Water Element to flow through you, you naturally follow the course of your destiny.

SPRING PHASE (A SPROUT EMERGING)

Element Of Wood

Spring is a yang or active rising phase that gives your seed potential a protective form for action in the world. Through the formative forces of the sun, which sends new information via light, your body is given definition as it grows and becomes individualized.

In the spring, snow melts: the liquid sap in trees and plants utilizes the renewed sun forces to shoot quickly upward. What was hidden in seed form awakens, sprouting up toward the light. Plants and burgeoning new tree branches become visible. Wood is imprinted with identifiable bark patterns that delineate to the world its particular species. It also creates boundaries for the protection of the rising interior tree sap. Ring patterns on the core of a fallen tree record the evolution of the life of that individual tree. Through experiencing the Element of Wood, you enter into the outer world as a defined individual.

SUMMER PHASE (A BLOSSOMING FLOWER)

Element Of Fire

In the Summer phase, your energy is radiant, forming a relationship through warmth with all aspects of life, including your environment, other people, and the various parts of your own system. This high-noon stage represents the zenith of your yang, or active, outward-emerging forces. Your substance, fully formed, now radiates rarefied fire that awakens your conscious awareness in the way that your heart rules as the sun of your body.

Summer accumulates fire forces that precipitate the blossoming of trees, shrubs, and flowers. Warmth and joy spread from these blossoms as Nature expresses herself in her fullest array. When a forest accumulates old wood, lightning is Nature's way of creating fires to clear the brush below.

Fire's enthusiasm for relationships merges, jumps boundaries, and burns carefully made wooden structures of creatures and men. Communal warmth is formed as humans bond together to build new structures and new plant species emerge from the cleared forest floor. Allowing fire in your life assures that you find joy in appropriate and mature relationships.

LATE SUMMER PHASE (FRUIT)

Element Of Earth

In the Late Summer phase, your energy begins to coalesce out of brilliance. Spiraling downward in a descending yin cycle, you begin to gather the fruits of your outward journey. At this stage, these fruits are picked as tangible nourishment from the ground that supports you. Your thoughts gain substance and your spirit becomes enveloped in a concrete form that reflects your achievements. At harvesttime, your energy is filled with flavor, density, and fullness.

What burned so brightly at midday as radiant ephemeral flowers, now gives way to actual substance in the rounded forms of fruits. The earth's atmosphere in late summer usually produces the hottest months, having collected warmth from the sun's zenith. Fruits swell at this time, ripening into palpable physical forms that provide nourishment and sustaining food for your system. By allowing yourself to experience the Element of Earth, your goals achieve substance.

FALL PHASE (FALLING LEAVES)

Element Of Metal

The Fall phase provides evolutionary thrust through an ongoing interactive process of creating new inspiration, inherent within its rising quality, as well as releasing substance that is no longer needed, inherent in its aspect of falling. Autumn is a stage of gathering or receiving yin—a quiet period of reflection in which your energy both rises into the clarity of cosmic possibilities and falls into matter carrying this higher imprint. Like the evening-tide, when you go through a transmutation of extracting

Continued ➔

nutrition from your activities of the day, this stage of letting go of what no longer serves you prepares you for rising into the deeper dreaming mode of sleep.

Metal is the fifth or quintessential Element. Falling leaves and the clarity of the sky in autumn are images of its synthesizing aspects. Each leaf pattern is a formative code from the universal tree of life. As a leaf falls to the ground, it alchemizes earth by disintegrating into ash, cosmic intelligence. Metal ores are precious for their ability to refine and transform substance. Phone wires, jewelry, and the gold standard are symbols of the value and meaning metals create through their presence on earth. By allowing yourself to experience the Element of Metal, you extract the finer meaning of your life.

PHASE CIRCUIT

Winter snows melt as warm weather approaches. Quickly rising sap forms new plant matter into hardened, identifiable species in the spring. The sun brings ethereal blossoms into flower in the summer. Flower petals waft away, revealing slowly ripening fruits that are harvested in late summer. Fruits and leaves fall to the ground, alchemizing earth with cosmic substance refined by earth in autumn. Seeds of fruits and flowers, covered by leaf humus, sleep through the cold winter until spring comes again.

The Twelve Meridians and Their Corresponding Elements: Connecting the Circuitry

There are twelve main meridian circuits that serve as transmitters of *chi*, or life force, which animate the physical as well as the emotional, mental, and spiritual substance of your system. They are meandering lines that run in left-right pairs vertically up and down the body. Their pathways and directional flows vary. All together, they map the organ of your skin, including the limbs. The name of a meridian is derived from the body organ that it oversees. Each of the twelve meridians is paired, and each pair works in alignment with one of the Elements and phases. The twelve meridians, like fixed stars of the twelve zodiacal houses, carry archetypal forces. The Taoists called the organizing energy of the meridians Officials (for instance, they called the Heart Meridian the Monarch).

There are twelve basic roles the body needs to participate in for optimal functioning in life's play. Each of the twelve meridians is characterized by one of these roles and transmits the archetypal light of each through the meridian circuits. In order for the Elements-phases to be in dynamic movement, they receive formative forces via light-encoded information from the twelve meridians. The twelve, according to their phase activation sequence, are as follows.

KIDNEY-BLADDER: ELEMENTS OF WATER (WINTER PHASES)

Kidney Meridian

The Kidney Meridian is like a deep well or underground spring that is the keeper of your spiritual, hereditary, and constitutional "seeds." It generates, motivates, and regulates your destiny, providing you with purpose and direction when you follow its flow.

Without the sun to warm it (Element of Fire), water is frozen and cold, qualities associated with the emotion fear. Following your destiny requires courage to flow in deep places where you are unable to see the direction your path is leading. Activating the Kidney Meridian recalibrates your body's ability to access faith that allows you to follow this flow.

Bladder Meridian

The Bladder Meridian acts as a fluid container for the wellspring of the Kidney Meridian. It controls the floodgates and time-releases properly distributed amounts of Kidney's raw energy to your system. It sends fluid essences to your organ system, lubricating and nourishing all functions.

Budgeting your reserves, the Bladder Meridian creates boundaries that help you to manage your physical, emotional, and spiritual resources. When fear takes over, the ordered release of the Water Element can malfunction, flooding your system and causing overwhelming emotions and a scattering of your consciousness. Activating the Bladder Meridian closes the floodgates and reestablishes faith that following the deep flow of your destiny will take you where you need to go.

GALL BLADDER–LIVER: ELEMENTS OF WOOD (SPRING PHASES)

Gall Bladder Meridian

The Gall Bladder Meridian translates your seed potential provided by the Kidney Meridian into visible manifestation of an integrated personal identity. The Gall Bladder rules your eyes, ligaments, tendons, and sense of time, all of which enable you to stand up and see what is happening in the present moment. Like the Element of Wood, the Gall Bladder Meridian is a quickly moving energy; it makes immediate clear decisions that define how your seed potential is to be specifically structured into an identifiable form.

Structure needs flexible material to withstand strong winds. Irritation and anger can be the result of impatience for action. This impatience may cause you to make inappropriate snap judgments. In these situations, the Gall Bladder can reconnect you to the virtue of hope and its embedded understanding of how the larger picture emerges over time.

LIVER MERIDIAN

The Liver Meridian creates a protective environment that supports the unfolding of your integrated personality into the world. It helps you envision the future and set goals, and it smoothes the pathway of chi into this future. Like an immune system, the Liver Meridian foresees potential problems, wards off attacks, and acts as a blueprint for a rhythmic rising of your soul's strategic plan.

The Element of Wood can sometimes be thorny and hard. Impediments to your quickly growing forces can result in passionate anger or sharp self-righteousness. If the Liver Meridian becomes stagnant, depression may arise through the experience of feeling stuck and being unable to reach your goals. At these places, activating the Liver Meridian stimulates the quality of forgiveness for your own blindness as well the virtue of hope, reestablishing a smooth path to your future goals.

HEART–SMALL INTESTINE–PERICARDIUM TRIPLE WARMER: ELEMENTS OF FIRE–SUMMER PHASES

Heart Meridian

The Heart Meridian is the switchboard that directs the harmonious working of all your meridians to function in a unified manner. It contains insight and understanding through its sunlike nature, controlling chaos, maintaining oversight, and encouraging cooperation with radiating compassionate love. Like the physical organ of your heart, which sends blood throughout your body, this meridian maintains mastery over your whole system of meridians by sending source light and warmth that enlivens your seed potential and physical form with spirit essence. When you lose connection to this sun, you dim your ability to see the whole picture. Without warmth, your energy may become either dictatorial, controlling others, or soft, allowing others to control you. Activating the Heart Meridian reconnects you to the loving fire of your spirit.

Small Intestine Meridian

The Small Intestine Meridian acts as a transformer, raising the energy of your sun or heart-fire forces into usable form. Like a caterpillar becoming a butterfly, the Small Intestine stores the rarified jewels of your fire forces into icons or information packets for alchemical transformative action. Sorting pure from impure, the organ of the small intestine uses enzymatic action to transform matter into refined substances that can easily enter and nourish your body. On the mental level, this meridian helps you sort and discriminate among different levels of reality. This discrimination helps you set priorities as well as embrace appropriate levels of relationship with various people in your life.

Compression of your alchemical fire forces may create mental confusion, making relationships difficult to sort through. An inability to learn or change in reaction to life's experiences may also occur through lack of warmth in your operating system. Activating the Small Intestine Meridian reboots your ability to achieve transformation through fire, allowing magic to result from the qualities of love and joy.

Pericardium Meridian

The Pericardium Meridian radiates warmth to the cool waters of the Kidney Meridian, circulating and activating deep inner fire within all the meridians. Joy and pleasure result from the penetration of your heavenly fire forces into the interior organs of your physical body via the meridian circuits. Also called the Heart Protector, the Pericardium is like a hinged door that opens to receive love and closes when your heart needs to be protected. On the emotional level, the Pericardium is a guardian that allows access to the inner voice in your heart. This inner voice can counsel you on what is or is not appropriate intimacy and vulnerability.

Damage to this fine warmth network can cause the Pericardium door to shut, creating a state of shock throughout your whole system, or to remain open, blurring your discernment of appropriate boundaries. Activating the Pericardium Meridian heals the polarization of these two states and naturally opens your heart again to experience loving joy.

Triple Warmer Meridian

The Triple Warmer Meridian keeps all the fire forces transmitted by the Pericardium moving. When the Kidney forces send water through the circuits warmed by the Pericardium, the Triple Warmer Meridian radiates heat in the form of light and moisture. It transfers this Fire-Water energy to the "three burning spaces," alchemical transmitters of chi located over the heart, solar plexus, and lower abdomen. Resembling a network of Fire and light, the Triple Warmer acts as thermostat and temperature regulator of these three burning spaces, creating an overall environment of warmth for the "house" that is your body. This warmth radiates as perspiration on the physical level; on the emotional level, it creates joy and connection in your outer relationships with others.

If any floor of your house loses its heat source, your ability to function outwardly is made much more difficult. Symptoms such as spaciness, disconnected thought patterns, and inept social inter-

Continued ➡

actions may result. Reactivating the Triple Warmer Meridian reconnects your "wiring" so you can again smoothly negotiate with harmony and joy in the outer world.

STOMACH–SPLEEN: ELEMENTS OF EARTH (LATE SUMMER PHASES)

Stomach Meridian

When your chi is infused with the Water Element, brought to visible form through the Element of Wood, and warmed with higher forces through Fire, it needs nourishment from Earth to sustain its evolution. The Stomach and Spleen Meridians are pathways that ground spirit in your body.

When you ingest physical nourishment through the mouth, the Stomach Meridian helps you to assimilate and digest the combination of Earth and cosmic sustenance. The Stomach Meridian is the circuit that locates where this nutrition is needed and brings in the necessary substances from outside to nurture life forces. The organ of the stomach receives food and begins the process of breaking it down for assimilation. The Stomach Meridian receives, holds, and ripens the fruits of your infused substance, enabling you to feel satiated and nourished. Its mental aspect facilitates an ability to access your needs, manage tasks, and provide service to yourself and others.

Lack of feeling nourished can cause anxiety. Food may be used as a substitute for not feeling supported. Mentally you may find yourself ruminating excessively. Activating the Stomach Meridian restores the ability to nourish yourself, transforming anxiety into motherly expressions of empathy, compassion, and understanding toward the larger world as your own sense of being fed is stabilized.

Spleen Meridian

The Spleen Meridian distributes to all of your meridians the nutrition that the Stomach Meridian provides. Like birds that distribute the seeds of fruits they have digested, the Spleen transports and delivers the infused riches of your physical, emotional, and spiritual harvest in their fullest expression. Mentally, a balanced Spleen Meridian will express itself by helping you create healthy daily routines. It also helps you be dependable in your service to others.

If you feel your life is lacking satisfaction, it may be that your internal source of nourishment is being inappropriately distributed to others. Lacking a model for self-nourishment may cause starvation on an emotional level. Stimulating the Spleen Meridian restores a balance between too little and too much, into a perfect portion that sustains and satisfies.

LUNG–LARGE INTESTINE: ELEMENTS OF METAL (FALL PHASES)

Lung Meridian

The Lung Meridian brings meaning and value to all the meridian circuits. It ministers by acting as a channel for sovereign cosmic forces to inform, inspire, and integrate the body/mind. Through rhythmic breathing, the organ of the lung tunes your "radio" to receive resonance from higher frequencies. As food is important to the stomach, air is crucial for the Lung and keeps you alive (as the most refined substance, the Element of Metal correlates to air or ethers). A healthy Lung Meridian enables you to maintain balance, receive inspiration, and experience self-worth.

Impediments to your breathing may indicate grief or deep feelings of loss that create gravity, weighing you down. Guilt arises when you feel unable to live up to your own or others' high standards. At the opposite, overinflation of the Lung forces may make you feel arrogant or better than others. Stimulating the Lung Meridian brings balance between gravity and levity, enabling you to feel an inspired connection to the cosmos as well as to those around you.

LARGE INTESTINE MERIDIAN

The Large Intestine Meridian helps you operate at the highest frequency by taking in the cosmic forces that it receives from the Lung Meridian and refining them. It also eliminates what doesn't support your highest worth. The organ of the large intestine takes in trace minerals (refined substance in crystalline from) and water (the life principle) to bring about evolution into your next phase and releases all other substances that are no longer needed. Overseeing quality control, this meridian searches for what is needed to propagate right living, releases what is impure, and manages a proper accounting of your accumulated worth. On the mental level, a healthy colon enables you to live according to your own standards, complete tasks set for yourself, and experience self-value.

An inability to let go on an emotional level creates stagnation leading to feelings of grief and heaviness in the body. Activating the Large Intestine Meridian enables you to transform matter and rise phoenixlike to your next phase.

The Generative Circuits: Conception Vessel and Governing Vessel Meridians

The twelve main meridians can be thought of as rivers or streams on the body landscape. The Conception Vessel and Governing Vessel are central channels running vertically through the body's midline, front and back, and they can be visualized as great seas of energy from the Source. They are the major reservoirs that are utilized by the other meridians; together with the twelve already described, they comprise the fourteen major meridians of the body.

The Governing Vessel Meridian is the main operating system in the body that governs with masculine force. Descending spirit energy enters the Governing Vessel at the tailbone and rides up the spine, which transmits your electromagnetic energy to your body. Its path courses up over the middle of the head and face, exiting under the nose at the top of the lip. From here it descends deep within the body to the perineum on the floor of your torso, where it alchemizes into the Conception Vessel.

The Conception Vessel Meridian is the pathway for your ascending feminine soul forces to give birth within you. From its genesis at the perineum, it rises up the front of the body to the bottom of the lower lip. At this point it cascades downward inside the body to the coccyx, uniting with the entry point for the Governing Vessel.

Together, these two comprise a lemniscate (figure-eight pattern) for your energy to continually enfold, recharging your system as it cycles from yang to yin and back again, in a constant dance of receiving spirit and giving birth to your soul. Damage to this circuit compromises your ability to regenerate. It is significant that twelve of the flower essences originally made by Dr. Bach activate one or the other of these central generative vessels.

Application Methods

The twelve main meridians are paired on the left and right sides of the body. When you apply a flower essence to a point on one of the twelve main meridians, it must also be applied to a point in the same location on the other side of the body. This means that whenever the directions describe floral acupuncture method for a prone treatment, or easy-application method, the essence must always be applied to both sides of the body, despite the fact that the body map photos in chapter four often illustrate only one side of the body and its location. The Conception Vessel and Governing Vessel Meridians, located on the midlines at the front and back of the body, are an exception to this rule, as they have only single points of entry.

Applying Flower Essences to Acupuncture Points

To apply a flower essence, you will need cotton balls or cotton swabs, a small clear glass bowl, and water to dilute the essence. Follow the steps outlined here.

INFUSE WATER

Put 2 to 4 drops of the flower essence of your choice into a small, clean glass bowl filled with 4 to 6 ounces of water. (Infusing water with the flower essence dilutes it to the correct potency for most people. In general, we recommend this method for everyone using flower essences for self-healing.)

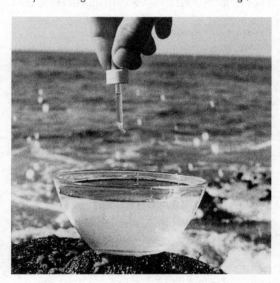

HOW TO APPLY

Dip a cotton ball or swap (the applicator) into the infused water. Rub the applicator in a large circle around the direct acupuncture site indicated on the body map (on both the left and right sides of the body, except for the Conception Vessel and Governing Vessel Meridians). Don't worry if you're not sure where the precise location of the site is. Covering a large area around the site will ensure its application: The flower essence and its direct acupoint are in vibrational resonance with each other and will lock in, or find each other.

An alternative application method is to use the stock dilution. If the treatment described above seems too weak or not effective for you, you can apply 1 drop of the flower essence directly from the stock bottle (the dilution or the bottle you buy from the store) to the acu-point. This procedure may work better for certain constitutions; it is much stronger, however, so try the infused-water technique first. Take care to keep the glass dropper from touching the skin if you choose this method. Flower essences are delicate substances, and contact

Continued →

with your skin may dilute their effects when the dropper is replaced in the bottle. (Simply dip the dropper in alcohol to clean the tip if this does occur.) When you apply it this way, rub the flower essence drops in a wide circle around the acu-point with your finger or a cotton ball to ensure that the direct site is covered,

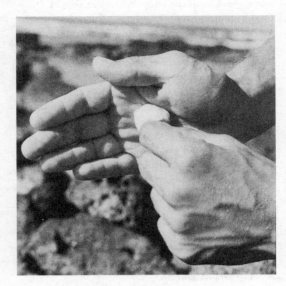

After Applying the Flower Essence

For a traditional treatment, lie down on your back after applying the flower essence to the acu-point and rest for 20 to 45 minutes. (Lying on your back rather than in the lounge position on your side tends to help you stay awake, so you will receive the treatment more consciously.) Three-quarters of an hour is the optimal time for activation of chi to the site; however 20 minutes is refreshing if you have limited time to rest.

For those who don't have the time or inclination to rest during the day, following one of the application methods described above before bedtime also works well. This can be a simple way of treating your body while also getting your rest. When you wake in the morning, it is helpful to scan your body for any changes. The more consciousness you bring to the process, the more helpful conjoining the modalities of flower essences and acupuncture becomes.

Traditional Treatment Rhythms

Your body will most likely inform you how often you need a particular floral acu-treatment. You may want to do a treatment once a day for a week, or once a week for a month. You may need to do it only once before moving on to a new treatment. (Twice a day is the recommended limit for this type of application.) Let your body inform you how often to repeat and how long to continue a particular treatment. For instance, if you think you need to do it for a week and at midweek you "forget," trust that your body is assimilating the previous treatments and resume when your body prompts you to do so.

Other Application Methods

Easy Treatment Method

Instead of lying down and receiving a formal treatment, you can also apply the infused flower essence water on the direct site with a cotton ball and simply go about your day. If you choose to do so, it may work best to repeat the application two to three times a day. This heightens the effect and assures its efficacy while enabling you to maintain your daily rhythms. You can add 2 to 4 drops of the flower essence to a small glass bottle filled with spring water to carry with you during the day for easy application away from home. Health food stores often sell one-ounce bottles with glass droppers.

These bottles are ideal, as you can use the glass dropper to apply the infused water to the site. (Be sure not to touch the end of the glass dropper to your skin when you apply it this way.)

Patch Method

Another treatment method you might find useful is to infuse water with a flower essence according to the instructions (at left). For this treatment, diluting the flower essence in water is better than using drops directly from the stock bottle. Using two standard-size adhesive bandages, dip the soft cushion of the bandages into the infused water to moisten, and affix to each acu-point on the left and right sides of the body (or to the single point if you are applying it to the Conception Vessel or Governing Vessel Meridians). You can use this method for a traditional prone treatment or for the easy treatment method. Again, let your body tell you when to remove the adhesive strips. Twenty minutes may be enough for you, while someone else may want to leave them on for a longer period of time.

Using Intention to Heal

Floral acu-treatments work, no matter what way you choose to use them. However they work best with conscious awareness. If you simply go about your day after putting them on your body, it is helpful to use conscious intent by keeping in mind the quality of the essence and description of the acu-point. The treatments may act in subtle ways, and if you choose to be mindful of the process, you will be awake to witness these shifts in your thoughts, feelings, and physical body. If you simply feel better, and this is your goal, remembering to offer gratitude to the particular flower and acupuncture point on your body for facilitating this renewal, also enhances the effect of the application.

Notes for Professional Practicioners

The treatments described above are easily adapted to fit into your healing practice.

Acupuncturists and Acupressurists

The recommended method of application is to use the flower essence infused into water and apply it directly to the site with a cotton swab. However, if you feel your client can handle the potency of the stock dilution applied straight from the bottle onto the acu-point, do so. It's very helpful to gauge the potency effects of using infused water or the stock dilution by treating yourselves. Once you experience the dilution level effects in your own body, you will be able to discern which potency is correct for the individual needs of your clients.

You can use the flower essence treatment on its own, or you can insert the acupuncture needle or massage the site subsequent to the flower essence application. For a potent treatment, insert a gold acupuncture needle just subcutaneously on the point after applying the flower essence. The vibration of gold is a particularly powerful connector of flower essence to acu-point. Giving the client a dosage bottle of the flower essence with instructions on how to apply it at home once a day for a week extends and may deepen, the effect of the treatment.

Massage Therapists and Body Workers

Infuse 2 to 4 drops of a flower essence into a small amount of massage oil. Massaging this mixture into the appropriate acu-point works well.

The Flower Essences of Dr. Bach and Their Acupuncture Points

The simplest way to release an emotion is to focus on it. Using conscious intention and deciding to be present in the moment, you touch not only the negative aspect of your discomfort but also the hidden positive aspect. A union of opposites occurs that sparks the creation of new life forces. Knowing where you are at any given moment is the secret to keeping your system operating at optimal levels. Learning to get in touch with the specific geographic location of an imbalance in your body can lead to an awakening or an ability to heal yourself.

As you read the following thirty-eight descriptions of the flower essences and their acupuncture points, some may stand out for you. Listening to your body for "sparks" when reading about certain points or flowers is a good way to gain information about where you may want to start with treatments. Applying floral liquid light in the form of essences to locations on your meridian system may also give you "keys," and help you understand that your ultimate goal is to be able to use your own conscious awareness as the light source to locate and open locked points on your body without the use of this book.

It is important to remember that while the body map photographs show only *one* acu-point, the twelve major meridians are paired on the *left and right* sides of the body. When you apply an essence to an acupuncture point, *it must also be applied to its mirrored acupuncture point, in exactly the same location on the other side of the body.* Doing so ensures that the treatment is balanced. The only exceptions are the body maps showing the Conception Vessel and the Governing Vessel Meridians. Because these meridians are located on the body midlines, the acu-point you see in the photograph is the only point of application.

Note To Practitioners Of Traditional Chinese Medicine (TCM)

The numbers next to the acupuncture points in this text follow the Five-Element system of acupuncture as described by J. R. Worsley. These numbers sometimes differ from the acupuncture point numbers used in TCM: for instance Bladder 54 in Five-Element annotation is known as Bladder 40 in the TCM system. For those of you who practice TCM, the appropriate TCM acupuncture point number will be found as a note at the end of the Aspen and Olive descriptions (the two acu-points that have different notation numbers). Also, note the slightly different location of Liver 14 (Gorse) in the two systems (explained at the end of the Gorse description).

Agrimony Flower Essence

Agrimony is the "sleeping beauty" remedy that helps you awaken to the outer world. It is used when you are cheerful outwardly and yet feel inwardly tormented. A membrane can form between your inner and outer world when you witness dysfunctional behavior that is repeatedly discounted by those around you. Eventually disbelief in your own perceptions and a wish to please others can cause the doorways to your heart to shut, concealing truth even from yourself. Using Agrimony as an essence helps you open into a world where things can be seen in their true light.

Agrimony is a rose family plant with light-filled yellow flowers on a towering stalk. Though cheerful and beautiful in outward appearance, Agrimony seeds produce burrs that cling to your clothes as you walk by— thus the dual message of this plant.

Continued ➡

AGRIMONY ACUPUNCTURE POINT

Pericardium 6, *Inner Frontier Gate*

Inner Frontier Gate connects the Heart Protector or Pericardium Meridian to the Triple Warmer Meridian. The pericardium acts as a doorway into your heart that allows you access to your most intimate feelings. The Triple Warmer Meridian is the gateway that opens you to the world at large. *Inner Frontier Gate*, therefore, unites you not only to your intimate friends but also to the world at large. This is the site to use when the gate to your heart has been shut. Bringing a feeling of protective warmth, it gives you courage to see the damage that has occurred and helps you begin speaking your truth again.

SYNTHESIS

The pericardium is like a cradle that holds the heart. When this membrane has been damaged, your childlike joy disappears. You feel tortured in the Agrimony state because your heart has become permanently shut. Applying Agrimony essence at *Inner Frontier Gate* enables light from the world to flood the inner sanctum of your heart, restoring joy.

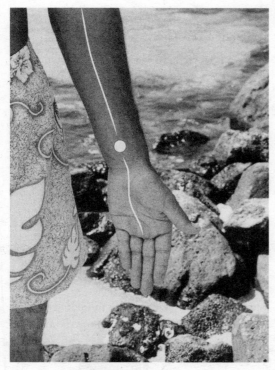

Agrimony Acupuncture Point, Pericardium 6, Inner Frontier Gate.

Aspen Flower Essence

Aspen is a remedy for unknown fears. This state can be caused by early childhood trauma seeded in your cells or can be a short-term condition that results from your life taking an uncertain turn. Often the Aspen state is precipitated in childhood by frightening episodes that happened when you least expected them. Using Aspen releases this state of inner quaking, connecting and grounding your finer energies so you experience trust and confidence in the future.

The Aspen is a small tree with silver, papery bark. Its rounded leaves grow vertically like little paddles on their branches, causing them to quiver continually at the slightest breeze. In the fall, the leaves of Aspen forests turn into a symphony of gold that imparts a tremendous sense of light and courage.

ASPEN ACUPUNCTURE POINTS

Bladder 54, *Equilibrium Middle*
The Bladder Meridian is ruled by the Element of Water, which is associated with the emotion of fear.

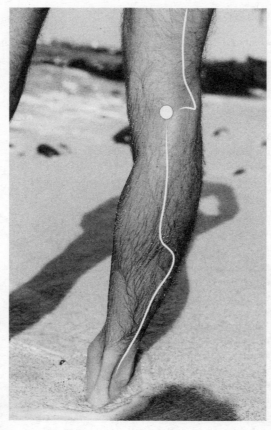

Aspen Acupuncture Points, Bladder 54, Equilibrium Middle

Equilibrium Middle is the Earth point on the Bladder Meridian. At times, when you are unable to see around a corner, fear and anxiety may take hold of you due to lack of faith in what lies ahead. Using the Earth point on the Bladder Meridian establishes "river-banks," or a container for your Water Element. This containment gives you a secure sense of being held in the present moment and helps dissolve negative pictures you may have for the future.

SYNTHESIS

In the Aspen state, your body quivers. When you apply Aspen to *Equilibrium Middle*, located behind the knees, your legs stop shaking, so to speak, and you can stand calmly upright with faith and security in the direction that your life is taking.

TCM practitioners: Bladder 54 in the Five-Element notation is Bladder 40 in TCM.

Beech Flower Essence

Beech flower essence is used when you feel critical and judgmental of others. When you find yourself using harsh words to create boundaries for yourself, the cause is often having too loose a connection to the physical body. Using Beech flower essence brings you into the body and gives you a feeling of rootedness that grounds and supports your real nature. When you feel secure again, it is natural to experience the beauty of others and the world.

The Beech tree has weak roots and is easily blown over in high winds. Beech forests tend to create pristine environments for themselves with a strong tree canopy, preventing light from entering and excluding other shrubs and trees from growing below. Known as a planetary tree of Venus, lovers often carve their initials into its soft, vulnerable bark.

BEECH ACUPUNCTURE POINT

Gall Bladder 41, *Foot above Tears*
A major self-esteem point, *Foot above Tears* connects above and below, holding a strong vertical energy so you can stand upright in your truth. The strong, rushing energy of this point, connecting your crown to your roots, helps you access your core identity. As the Wood point on the Wood Meridian,

its fast-moving energy is like the first day of spring and the quickening experienced by plants at this time, as they come into their fullness.

SYNTHESIS

The gall bladder excretes bile, an acidic substance originally manufactured in the liver that breaks down fat. In people, a bilious personality is expressed in an acerbic tone that breaks down others through sarcasm and judgments. *Foot above Tears* helps the body to experience flexibility, giving you tolerance in the present moment. Like Beech flower essence, it brings you into the body, where you can remember your true essence. Conjoining these two helps you overcome the need to create false barriers by using unkind words for protection.

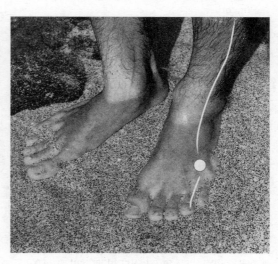

Beech Acupuncture Point, Gall Bladder 41, Foot above Tears

Centaury Flower Essence

Centaury is useful when you find yourself giving too much of your energy and service to others, leaving yourself depleted. The "put your foot down" essence, Centaury teaches you to nourish yourself. By saying no to outside requests because they are beyond your actual resources at the moment, Centaury helps you learn the value of gathering abundant reserves that can make your life forces a magnetic source of healing for others through your presence alone. By replenishing sustenance for yourself, you naturally distribute comfort that satiates and feeds others.

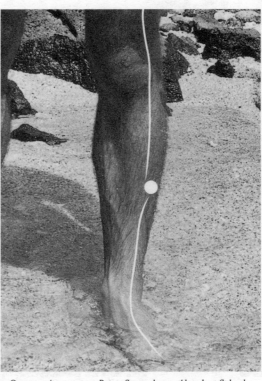

Centaury Acupuncture Point, Stomach 40, Abundant Splendor

Continued ➡

Used for healing since ancient times, Centaury is a gentian family plant. Its herbal constituents are bitter, and in the past it was widely used as a stomach tonic. Its star-shape magenta flowers are light-sensitive, opening in the morning hours when the sun is out and closing by midday.

CENTAURY ACUPUNCTURE POINT

Stomach 40, *Abundant Splendor*

Abundant Splendor connects the Spleen Meridian to the Stomach Meridian. The Spleen Meridian distributes nutrition to all of the meridians while the Stomach Meridian supplies the ingredients for this distribution. If the stomach and spleen aren't working together, you deplete your resources when serving others.

SYNTHESIS

Life can be bitter, like the Centaury plant, when you neglect to mother yourself. Uniting Centaury with *Abundant Splendor* allows your body to feel fully nourished. On the mental level, this partnership supports your ability to discern when to be in the world and when to retreat gracefully to replenish yourself.

Cerato Flower Essence

Cerato is a remedy for establishing heart-based wisdom that reflects your own truth despite what others tell you. In Dr. Bach's time, this essence was described as helpful to intuitive people who distrusted their own knowledge, following others' advice against their own better judgment. Today, learning to trust intuitive perceptions is gaining wide acceptance and expanding Cerato's influence so that it has become the most popular single flower essence made worldwide, according to Dr. Bach's indications. Cerato has the ability to establish your heart as a cognitive organ of thinking and listening.

Originating in Tibet, Cerato was found naturalized by Dr. Bach in an English garden. Its bright blue, five-petaled flowers are small and grow in clusters as an ornamental shrub. Its unusual color attracts attention as one of the few of its kind in the flower kingdom. Glimpsing Cerato in nature can cause your heart to leap with happiness, similar to the beneficent impression of a flock of bluebirds.

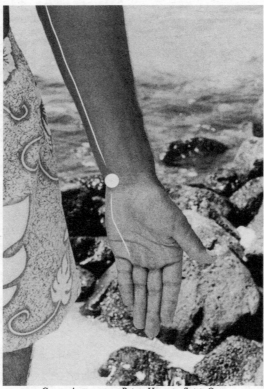

Cerato Acupuncture Point, Heart 7, Spirit Gate

CERATO ACUPUNCTURE POINT

Heart 7, *Spirit Gate*

Spirit Gate is the Earth and source point for the Heart Meridian. It is the gateway for your heart fire to access your entire system. As the Earth point on the Heart Meridian, it calms and grounds you when you need to be able to hear the voice of your heart, the voice that informs you of your truth at the moment. As the source point, this site is self-regulating—it balances either overactive or underactive heart-fire—making it an ideal "rescue" spot to apply Cerato's higher energies.

APPLYING CERATO DIRECTLY ON YOUR HEART

In general, Cerato's energy transcends the meridian system. It has the ability to access new heart forces that inform your mind of a new way of thinking that is holographic. Beyond right-brain or left-brain functioning, holographic thinking originates in the heart as a cognitive organ of listening; it functions beyond polarity and brings higher awareness. The most effective way to use Cerato for this purpose is to put 2 drops into a bowl of warm water and, using a cloth dipped in the solution, rub it in a wide circle around your heart.

For a refreshing treatment, you can also rest with the compress cloth (well wrung) over your heart for 20 to 45 minutes.

Cherry Plum Flower Essence

Cherry Plum is a remedy for fear of losing control of your temper or even losing your mind. In extreme cases, this energy can feel suicidal. In much milder forms, Cherry Plum is useful for addressing temper tantrums in children. As it releases pent-up forces, Cherry Plum's sweet, deeply calming energy facilitates an ability to surrender and trust in the ultimate goodness of life. It is also helpful in stabilizing faith in your own perceptions.

Cherry Plum is a rose family tree that can grow quite large and produces small, sweet, orange-red plums in summer. Its peeling, papery bark looks bright cherry-red when lighted by the setting sun. When it blossoms in spring, its small white blossoms completely cover the tree in a hazy cloud.

CHERRY PLUM ACUPUNCTURE POINT

Governing Meridian 14, *Great Hammer*

Great Hammer calms excessive anger or red forces when they rise up from below; it also forcefully injects your spirit back into your body. Useful for emergencies, it helps you to come immediately into yourself, sending back down excessive heat that threatens to overwhelm you.

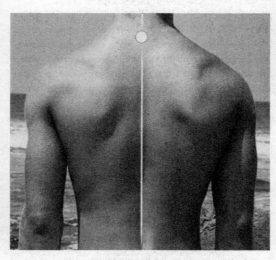

Cherry Plum Acupuncture Point, Governing Meridian 14; Great Hammer

SYNTHESIS

The Cherry Plum state comes on quickly and feels beyond your ability to control. The marriage of Cherry Plum and *Great Hammer* allows the body to experience release of this state at the moment it happens and circumvents unpleasant experiences.

Chestnut Bud Flower Essence

Chestnut Bud is indicated when you continually repeat patterns, as though your life lessons are enfolded in tight configurations that seem to enact themselves over and over. This essence has been shown to be helpful for those with learning disabilities or obsessive-compulsive disorders. At the deepest level, however, Chestnut Bud has the ability to contact your core essence and help it blossom in fullness into the world.

This essence is made from the buds of the White Chestnut, a large tree that produces branches of large, sweet-smelling white flowers. Each of Dr. Bach's chestnut tree preparations addresses a different state of anxiety. He captured the essence of the bud of the Chestnut in order to bring forth soul forces that are still enfolded and birth them into the world.

CHESTNUT BUD ACUPUNCTURE POINT

Conception Vessel 20, *Flower Covering*

Flower Covering, centered over the thymus gland, which helps to build the immune system, holds enfolded your most precious spiritual essence. The Conception Vessel can be visualized as a lotus plant growing out of mud, up through water, and becoming a bud in the sunlight. This vessel brings understanding to your soul of the trials you experience in life. *Flower Covering* can be thought of as the place on the Conception Vessel where the lotus bud opens. Activating this site brings your ultimate quintessence or flower out into the world.

SYNTHESIS

Dr. Bach's deep intuition created this essence from the large, juicy Chestnut Bud as a way to bring you into an experience of life at a higher octave. Conjoining Chestnut Bud and *Flower Covering* gives the body a visceral experience of this unfolding that creates a sense of new peace.

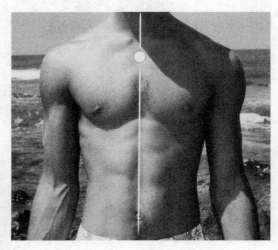

Chestnut Bud Acupuncture Point, Conception Vessel 20, Flower Covering

Chicory Flower Essence

Chicory is used when your mind is focused on thoughts of self-pity. Feeling that the world is not fulfilling your needs, you may refuse to take up your life tasks until what you perceive as your requirements are met. Usually those around you also suffer the consequences of this refusal through

Continued ➡

negative attention-getting and excessive demands. Not finding what you seek in the world, you may feel in this state of frustration as if your search will never lead to a place that is comforting and familiar. Chicory opens the doorway to your real home.

Chicory flowers are a beautiful shade of pale blue growing successively up tall stalks on plants often found by roadsides. The flowers open in the early morning and close by noon, and may remind you of heavenly eyes that close too quickly for you to see them properly. If you long for their usual pale blue color, you will also find that they close up upon picking them.

CHICORY ACUPUNCTURE POINT

Stomach 29, *The Return*

The Return is a point you can utilize when you have worked through many of your old patterns yet find that you need a final push to let go. Feeling ultimately starved for the food you've been missing along your path may be the impetus for this leap. *The Return* is the site that effects this letting-go and brings you "home" to your center. Like receiving a sumptuous banquet after you have been away for years, support and nourishment rush in.

SYNTHESIS

The Chicory state is like *The Return* in that it can be one of the last steps you must take before going to the next stage. Self-pity visits until you realize that life hasn't served your needs, not because you are a victim but because evolution requires you to create this sustenance out of your own forces. Once you have reached this stage, you go home to yourself and begin to create your own destiny. Cojoining these two gives your body the ability to make this leap.

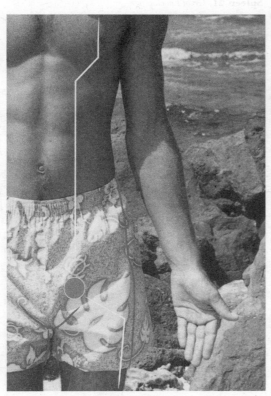

Chicory Acupuncture Point, Stomach 29, The Returdn

Clematis Flower Essence

Using Clematis as an essence brings you back into your body when you are unable to experience life in the present moment. In this state, you may experience feelings of being ungrounded, including an expanded sensation in your head, which makes it difficult to focus your thoughts. The quiet wish to leave this world for a more beautiful place in your dreams can be precipitated by your emotions as a

way of avoiding the pain of taking on challenges in life. Clematis helps you bring your head out of the clouds and grounds the gifts and talents that will lead you to your destiny.

Clematis is a vine with small, white flowers that elevate your mood into a gentle dreaming state. Unable to grow on its own, the Clematis climbs on trees and shrubs, looking down on earth from a bower of white blossoms. It is also called Traveler's Joy, indicating the uplifting sense it brings to those who pass by.

CLEMATIS ACUPUNCTURE POINT

Bladder 58, *Fly and Scatter*

Fly and Scatter connects the Kidney Meridian to the Bladder Meridian. The Kidney Meridian gives you access to your overall purpose and the willpower to accomplish it. The Bladder Meridian acts as the bank where this information is stored so you can draw from it when you need it. When the Bladder Meridian is disconnected from the Kidney Meridian, the bank where your wealth is stored is closed for the holidays, and you are unable to withdraw this valuable essence from your account.

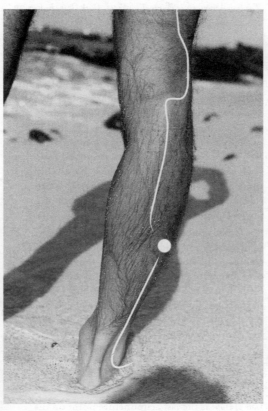

Clematis Acupuncture Point, Bladder 58, Fly and Scatter

SYNTHESIS

The gifts that you hold in the Clematis state are not grounded into your physical body, resulting in a weakening of your whole system. Uniting Clematis with *Fly and Scatter* enables the body to come out of its "away for the holidays" mood and make conscious use of all the wonderful gifts you have received.

Crab Apple Flower Essence

Crab Apple is a remedy that is used to purify feelings of being unclean. The impression that there is something impure in your life stream can grow to large proportions through your thoughts, affecting not only the way you see the world but also the way others see you. As this feeling of contamination is cleared from your system with the help of Crab Apple, physical cleansing also often follows. In using Crab Apple, there can be a sense that a state of original paradise has returned to you after having long been absent.

Crab Apple trees, charmingly gnarled and unkempt-looking, produce pink-tinged white blossoms of immaculate beauty that can take your breath away in the spring. The tree is a study in paradoxes: The fruit is as tart as the flowers are fragrant and heavenly. The trunk gives an ancient impression while the flowers retain a youthful freshness that returns spring after spring.

CRAB APPLE ACUPUNCTURE POINT

Large Intestine 18, *Support and Rush Out*

Support and Rush Out is one of the six "window to the sky" points on the body, which means its function is to instigate and support profound transformational change on all levels. This point helps you access the unconscious reason behind your inability to let go of toxic physical, mental, or emotional states. Once this reason is understood, you experience support for positive coping mechanisms and let those that are keeping you feeling unclean "rush out."

SYNTHESIS

Cojoining Crab Apple and *Support and Rush Out* enables you to accept the support offered by the wisdom of your body as well as to feel young and fresh again by letting go of what doesn't support you.

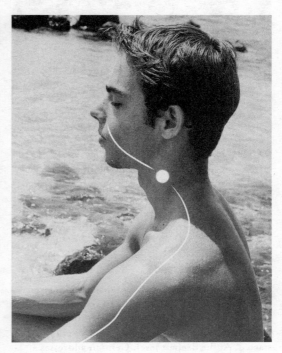

Crab Apple Acupuncture Point, Large Intestine 18, Support and Rush Out

Elm Flower Essence

Elm is the flower essence to use when you feel overwhelmed in your life, such as when you are consumed with many projects going on at once. Your energy may spread out to the periphery of your field in an attempt to encompass the myriad details. This scattering of your forces can result in a sensation of trying to keep your feet on the ground while being blown back and forth by the demands coming toward you from all directions. Elm brings your energy out of peripheral awareness into your body, where it establishes a strong central core of energy that holds you upright. Now strongly rooted to the earth, you feel secure and able to undertake all of your tasks with joy.

A tall, majestic tree, the Elm can grow to a height of one hundred feet. Its small purple flowers blossom for only a few days in the spring, and its wide overall shape makes it a good shade tree. Dutch Elm disease has decimated the Elm in many places in recent years and is a vivid example of the tree's vulnerability in environments of low vitality.

Continued ➜

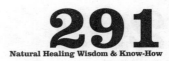

ELM ACUPUNCTURE POINT

Conception Vessel 8, *Spirit Deficiency*

Spirit Deficiency is the name of the acu-point that is located in the navel or umbilicus. Activating this point connects you to your core and, by holographic association, to the core of the earth, grounding your energies. Your spirit is "deficient," or starved, when this connection is severed. As the physical location of your original connection to your mother at birth, *Spirit Deficiency* is a major plexus for reestablishing stability between your soul/spirit energy (residing on the Conception Vessel Meridian) and your body.

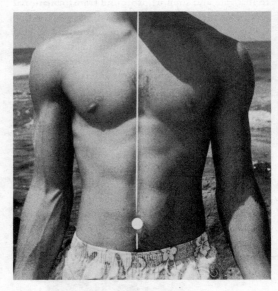

Elm Acupuncture Point, Conception Vessel 8, Spirit Deficiency

SYNTHESIS

When you go in many directions at once, you may lose a sense of your center. Applying Elm at *Spirit Deficiency* gives you an immediate compass to reorient yourself. When this fulcrum is reestablished, your body is able to welcome its various parts back home.

Gentian Flower Essence

Gentian is useful when you have been making progress on your path, yet suffer a setback. As an essence, Gentian brings into proportion the resulting disappointment that you are back where you started. At the deepest level, Gentian addresses a state of mind of ongoing disillusionment with the world. There may be a feeling that your journey through life is colored with deep disappointment at what you find on your path. Using Gentian helps open the door out of what may seem to be a long, dark hallway and lifts you into a higher, brighter reality.

The Gentian plant grows low to the ground. Its purple, cupped flowers make an ascending chord that comes directly out of the earth facing skyward, nestled in long, oval leaves. Gentian carries an impression of sounding a very low note, like an ancient sage or grandfather. It likes to grow on high hills in proximity to the sky.

GENTIAN ACUPUNCTURE POINTS

Kidney 21, *Dark Gate;* **Kidney 22,** *Walking on the Veranda;* **Kidney 23,** *Spirit Seal*

The Upper Kidney Meridian points oversee movement toward your highest aspirations to bring attainment of your destiny. *Dark Gate* opens the way to the beginning of the end of the darkness you have been walking through. *Walking on the Veranda* resurrects and refreshes you after the long journey. *Spirit Seal* puts a stamp on your achievement, sealing in the new phase you have reached.

SYNTHESIS

Disappointment sounds a very low note that can project deep into your essence. Transcending this state by combining Gentian with the three upper Kidney points for retrieval of your essence refreshes and revivifies your body/mind at a new octave.

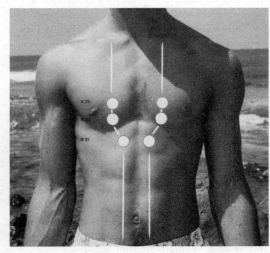

Gentian Acupuncture Points, Kidney 21, Dark Gate; Kidney 22, Walking on the Veranda; Kidney 23, Spirit Seal

Gorse Flower Essence

Gorse is used when you feel hopeless and are unable to envision a way out of a situation. Very often this feeling is caused by a lack of faith and fear that you don't have adequate resources to face the darkness you are witnessing. Gorse restores tremendous light to the system that counters this darkness. When the fiery forces you use to assert yourself and reach your goals stagnate, you may experience the sinking feelings of despair and depression. When this stagnation is released, hope returns in the form of positive pictures of the future.

Gorse is a broom-family plant that grows in sandy places and acidic soils in thicketlike, impenetrable scrub. Covered with strong thorns, its golden pea-shape flowers proliferate, giving the Gorse bush light that is almost overwhelming. The allure of its bright flowers contrasts with its fierce unapproachable thorns, which make the Gorse impossible to pass through.

GORSE ACUPUNCTURE POINT

Liver 14, *Gate of Hope*

Gate of Hope is the last acupuncture point on the Liver Meridian, and its influence goes directly to the organ of the liver. This site calms excess rage and opens suppressed liver functioning. Accessing this point mentally stimulates remembrance of the hopeful future you visualized for yourself and clears obstacles to realizing your goal. Like springtime, you rise up and start to grow again.

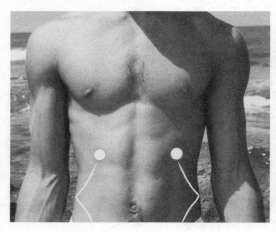

Gorse Acupuncture Point, Liver 14, Gate of Hope

SYNTHESIS

The Gorse state is very heavy. You sink down when you are unable to successfully visualize anything but darkness ahead. Using Gorse on *Gate of Hope* is like opening a cork of something bubbly and delicious that has long been stopped up. Celebrating, you can now see a bright future.

TCM practitioners: Note that the Worsley Five-Element placement of Liver 14, *Gate of Hope*, is slightly lower than the TCM location. The location is on the inferior edge of the thoracic cage on the nipple line, and lies halfway between Ren 11 and Ren 12. The point is just inferior to the middle notch found along the rib.

Heather Flower Essence

Heather is helpful when you think incessantly about yourself and your problems. A deeper aspect of this state is to be constantly speaking about your problems to others. A form of mild hysteria, this state can occur when you feel alone in witnessing what appears to you to be a dysfunctional world. If attempts to express this to others fail, you may feel desperate and exiled. Using Heather effects a release from this aloneness, helping you see and feel a part of the larger world once again.

The beautiful pink-flowered Heather grows as a spreading shrub in lonely, windswept places. Approaching it you may experience a feeling of gladness in your heart, like seeing a dear friend who has also traveled these out-of-the-way roads. By establishing itself in these remote spots, Heather sends you a message that even while you travel far from home, your beauty is remembered and unites the hearts of those who have met you along the way.

HEATHER ACUPUNCTURE POINT

Spleen 21, *Great Enveloping*

Great Enveloping is the last point on the Spleen Meridian and the "mother of all uniting points." The Spleen Meridian rules your mental processing and distributes your thoughts properly when they begin to go around and around obsessively. The "give yourself a hug" point, *Great Enveloping* knits together the tapestry of all your meridians in one great embrace.

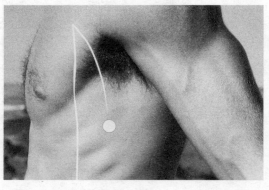

Heather Acupuncture Point, Spleen 21, Great Enveloping

SYNTHESIS

In the Heather state, you call attention to yourself, uniting others by causing them to think about you over and over. Bringing together Heather and *Great Enveloping* gives your system exponential help to feel ultimately held through the combined distribution of nourishment to the entire community of your body, mind, and spirit.

Holly Flower Essence

Holly is a remedy used to reestablish love forces in your heart when you feel jealous or angry. It may seem that others receive love that you lack. Anger is

Continued ➤

a creative stage—higher than depression, which locks you inside— its active presence means that you may be very close to breaking through into manifesting what you seek. Using Holly fires this quest for love and can burst through barriers into your inner heart chamber, where your passionate desires for igniting this flame are realized.

One of the most beautiful ornamental trees in the world, Holly produces small, white, waxy flowers that proliferate on its hardwood branches surrounded by shiny, spiked dark green leaves that make them a trial to pick. The glossy red berries are delightful to the eye in winter when they shine through its snow-capped branches, making Holly look like an incarnation of love.

Holly Acupuncture Point

Heart 5, *Penetrating Inside*

The heart is like a royal chamber that sends fire to the whole kingdom of your organs. *Penetrating Inside* is the point that allows you to return your own loving warmth to your heart when, through bitterness, you have locked it out. In this state, you witness love everywhere but inside yourself. This site allows a passageway for what belongs to you to reenter and take its rightful place.

Synthesis

When you need Holly, your state can be described as one of "divine madness," with rage and anger as unwelcome guests. Aware that you are not yourself, you may be perplexed not only by how you came to be in this situation but also about how to fix it. Using Holly on *Penetrating Inside* magnifies your ability to solve this mystery by reuniting your own loving warmth forces with your heart. In this way, you feel like yourself again and are able to experience love in your life.

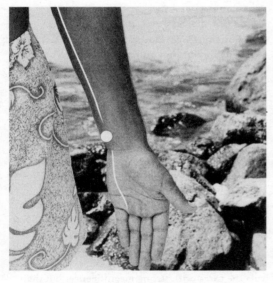

Holly Acupuncture Point, Heart 5, Penetrating Inside

Honeysuckle Flower Essence

Honeysuckle is used when you find yourself continually pulled into the past in nostalgic remembrance of better times or into regret about how things could have been. When this longing is present, you are unable to go forward into the future. Honeysuckle clears this backward pull so preparation for a new octave of experience can begin.

The Honeysuckle is a climbing vine that tumbles about, covered in bouquets of twelve or so long rose-colored buds that burst open into white flowers. Its scent and sweetness often draw children, who know to pluck the flower and suck its honey. The joy in smelling and tasting the flowers can become a heightened tactile remembrance of past summer days.

Honeysuckle Acupuncture Point

Lung 3, *Heavenly Palace*

Heavenly Palace is a "window to the sky" point that allows you to let go of past beliefs that have inhibited and constrained you from expressing yourself fully in the present moment. Activating *Heavenly Palace* downloads a whole new level of inspiration and values into your system, bringing about a major shift in perspective. Sparking vibrancy and tracing new patterns, this point enables you to experience life at a whole new level.

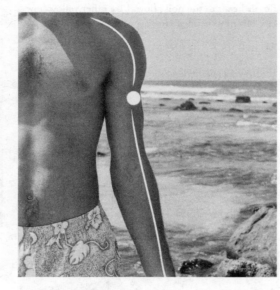

Honeysuckle Acupuncture Point, Lung 3, Heavenly Palace

Synthesis

Regret and continual thoughts of past events takes up space that could be utilized for experiencing pleasure and joy in the present. Conjoining Honeysuckle and *Heavenly Palace* allows your body to breathe out, releasing the past, and breathe in fragrance that comes through being in the moment.

Hornbeam Flower Essence

Hornbeam essence is indicated when weariness for life descends upon you as soon as you wake up in the morning. Related to tiredness connected to your destiny, this state can make your body feel dense and hard, or "wooden," as though your soul's experience of your daily tasks has transferred repetitive monotony to your physical body. Using Hornbeam refreshes your body, sparks new interest in your tasks, and revivifies inspiration to find a connection to your true destiny.

The Hornbeam is of medium height, with long, rounded leaves that make it a good shade tree. The *horn* in its name indicates its extreme strength and the toughness of its wood. The swirling pattern on its bark resembles muscles and mirrors its hard interior nature. Hornbeam wood was used in the past to make many manual work objects such as cart wheels and butchers' mallets.

Hornbeam Acupuncture Points

Bladder 1, *Eyes Bright*; Bladder 67, *Extremity of Yin*

Eyes Bright and *Extremity of Yin* are the first and last points, respectively, on the Bladder Meridian. Like a "body spritzer," the combined use of these two sites floods your Bladder Meridian with revitalizing water, thereby rejuvenating your whole system. Through activating *Extremity of Yin*, your depleted yin, or feminine, forces are charged with renewed yang or masculine energy. *Eyes Bright* helps you witness the replenishment of what has become desiccated and hard.

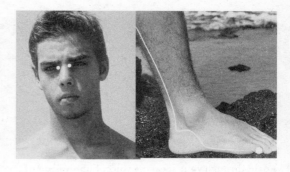

Synthesis

Used as an essence, Hornbeam helps infuse new inspiration when your life forces have reached their lowest ebb. Marrying Hornbeam with the first and last points on the Bladder Meridian makes your body suddenly flexible again, as it floods with vital water.

Impatiens Flower Essence

Impatiens is a remedy for feelings of irritation and impatience. Time, which should flow smoothly, feels out of sync instead, bumping into you, jangling your nerves, and trying your emotions. Using Impatiens soothes and softens this jarring energy, helping you bring your energy inside yourself. By moving your energy field from without to within, harmony and the natural flow of timing can reestablish themselves in your body.

Like little magenta orchids standing out from watery bright green stems and leaves, Impatiens flowers bloom and reseed themselves very quickly in moist areas, producing many flowers in rapid succession. Their seedpods broadcast as they burst open, as if they are impatient to make future plants. The plant's whole energy is one of bright clarity of purpose.

Impatiens Acupuncture Point

Gall Bladder 37, *Bright and Clear*

Bright and Clear joins together the Liver and Gall Bladder Meridians. The Liver Meridian smooths your energy when it is ragged, enabling you to visualize yourself achieving your goals in the future. The Gall Bladder Meridian reveals to you who you are in the present moment. When the gall bladder loses its sense of timing, it is because it is not connected to the liver and is unable to get to its future tasks, causing you to feel irritable and impatient.

Synthesis

The beautiful impatiens plant is in a hurried state. Desire to move quickly into future tasks can blur events in the present moment. Like a car when its

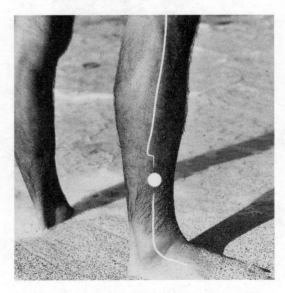

Impatiens Acupuncture Point, Gall Bladder 37, Bright and Clear

Continued ➡

timing belt is off, your internal engine no longer runs smoothly. Conjoining Impatiens with *Bright and Clear* allows you to hold simultaneous awareness of the present and the blueprint for the future. In this way, time as well as your nervous system are bright and clear again.

Larch Flower Essence

Larch is a remedy for enhancing self-confidence, particularly in relation to coming forth into the world through your speaking voice. Suppression of your authentic voice can be of long standing dating from an early age when your core essence was denied by people and influences outside yourself. When you feel energetically held down and unable to speak your truth, Larch will help you stand upright and express yourself. Larch resurrects your unique expression, banishing this stagnation, and brings your creative capacities into the world.

Larch is a deciduous pine tree that loses its needles in the winter. In spring, the female flowers are red and look like charming miniature trees. Its green needles grow out of the bark in circular sprays from a central point. The miracle of its resurrection quality is that although it belongs to the family of evergreen trees, which symbolize immortality, Larch follows the cycle of death and rebirth like other broad-leaved deciduous trees.

Larch Acupuncture Point

Triple Warmer 15, *Heavenly Bone*

Heavenly Bone is a powerful point. The energy of the Triple Warmer Meridian travels in a deep pathway from the acu-point on the shoulder into the heart before it travels back again into the throat. In addition to physically releasing shoulder tension, the function of this point is to send warm fluids to lubricate the heart, open its truth, and bring that truth to the surface through the voice box in the throat. If you have shut down your heart and voice to speak your truth, this point will instill you with the courage to shed the "hand that is holding you down" and speak authentically.

Synthesis

In the Larch state, your core essence is suppressed—like the Larch tree in winter, which holds in its seed potential, its evergreen needles that will sprout in the springtime. Larch helps you raise budding forces up and send them out, giving voice to who you are, in the same way that *Heavenly Bone* helps you stand up and deliver that which has been within you and waiting to resurface.

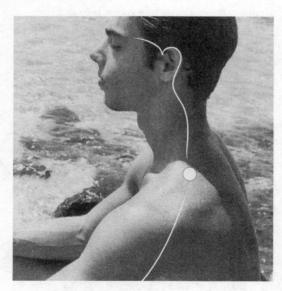

Larch Acupuncture Point, Triple Warmer 15, Heavenly Bone

Mimulus Flower Essence

Mimulus is indicated when you suffer from specific fears that may attach themselves to various physical activities or emotional themes in your life with repetitive insistence. Using Mimulus causes these fears to evaporate, vanishing what seemed darkly real and restoring a sense of calm and happiness that is the real you. Mimulus brings back the part of you that is naturally resilient and effervescent.

Mimulus establishes itself near streams or riverbanks, where it appears to gather happiness from the chatter of the bubbling water, nodding its bright flower heads to the noisy flow. Like other yellow flowers, Mimulus exudes a feeling of brightness and light.

Mimulus Acupuncture Points

Kidney 24, *Spirit Burial Ground; Kidney 25, Spirit Storehouse*

The upper Kidney Meridian points connect you to the storehouse of your essence when fear has closed down your ability to access these resources. *Spirit Burial Ground* is the energetic point for exhuming and resurrecting your spirit when fear has banished it. *Spirit Storehouse* is the site where you retrieve your gifts from spirit, realigning you to your original blueprint and the natural fearlessness that exists when these gifts are present in your life.

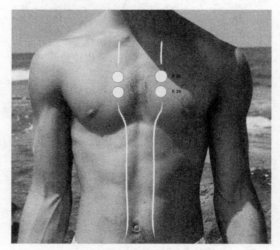

Mimulus Acupuncture Points, Kidney 24, Spirit Burial Ground; Kidney 25, Spirit Storehouse

Synthesis

The Mimulus state can feel unfamiliar, as though you are visited by emotions that have no relation to your real self. The success of uniting Mimulus to the two upper Kidney Meridian acupuncture points reveals that in this state, your immobility results from the stored quality of your spirit self. The union of Mimulus to these two points brings about a reversal of this condition and resurrects your core essence.

Mustard Flower Essence

Mustard is a remedy for the kind of depression that feels as though you are under a dark cloud with a weight on top of your head. This type of depression occurs when you witness something that feels too threatening for your conscious mind to process. Mustard's fiery forces of light burn deep down through this mantle of fear and bring to awareness what has been causing your depression. In this way, through your own conscious light, the depression is released.

Mustard is one of the first plants to herald the end of the gray snow and rains of winter. Covering entire fields and valleys with its bright yellow flowers, its presence indicates that the days of darkness will soon be gone. Its seeds are well known for their fiery spice through their use as a condiment that enlivens the palate, aiding your ability to digest what you take in.

Mustard Acupuncture Points

Kidney 20, *Through the Valley; Kidney 21, Dark Gate*

The Kidney Meridian is the storehouse of your resources, including your life's potential. *Through the Valley* gives you the faith and courage to walk through dark places when you can't see where you are going. By opening the acupuncture point Dark Gate, you pass through the last barrier or door that heralds the beginning of new light. The ability to get on with your destiny is set in motion.

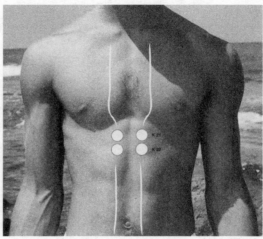

Mustard Acupuncture Points, Kidney 20, Through the Valley; Kidney 21, Dark Gate

Synthesis

Conjoining Mustard to *Through the Valley* and *Dark Gate* effects a release of the dark season your soul has been traveling through. Like the light-filled promise of mustard fields at the end of winter, combining Mustard to these two Kidney Meridian points enables you to digest the last aspects of this journey and make your way into the light of spring.

Oak Flower Essence

Oak flower essence is indicated when you feel weighed down by duty and responsibility. A typical sign of this condition is ignoring exhaustion and using your will to push the body beyond its limits. Using Oak enables your body to let go and surrender.

As you release your personal will, you activate a wellspring of energy that raises you up out of gravity. The ability to envision future possibilities is restored as you enter the river of life that is flowing unimpeded toward your destiny.

Oak trees are responsible citizens of the forest, providing food and homes to many creatures. They are hard to transplant once their acorns have sprouted on the forest floor, as too much water will damage their roots. Like mighty kings, Oak trees rule the forest with strong magnificence, but their branches are inflexible and break in high winds. Oak trees live to an advanced age, when their branches dry out and succumb to gravity.

Oak Acupuncture Point

Kidney 1, *Bubbling Spring*

Bubbling Spring is the first point of the Kidney Meridian, located on the soles of both feet. Connecting to this point, you experience a strong upward-rushing energy that floods the body with a renewed sense of joy and purpose. *Bubbling Spring*, as a major wellspring point, is the energy gateway that revitalizes the entire spectrum of your body, mind, and spirit and supports your ability to manifest this essential nature in the world.

Continued ➡

SYNTHESIS

The purpose of the Kidney Meridian is to keep you connected to your divine purpose. Oak types have materialized their existence and lost their connection to this wellspring, becoming hardened and dry as a result. Reuniting the Oak temperament with the Water Element of the Kidney Meridian releases the downward pull of the lower will, creating levity that raises feelings of duty into joy and reunites you with the flow of life.

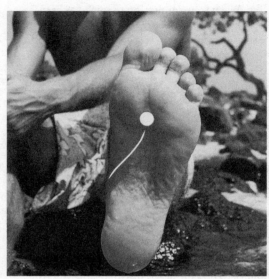

Oak Acupuncture Point, Kidney 1, Bubbling Spring

Olive Flower Essence

Olive is a remedy for long-term exhaustion. Being involved in the details of daily life can be demanding. While you may refresh yourself, residual effects can accumulate that require restoration to a higher octave. Olive helps you find this higher ground. Its use deepens your connection to your eternally peaceful self and gives you wings to fly there.

The Olive tree is small, grows in climates of intense heat, and gives its fruit into old age. The dove brought an Olive branch to Noah in his ark and foretold the end of his suffering as he found land again. The fruit and oil of the Olive have long sustained generations of people with health-giving properties.

OLIVE ACUPUNCTURE POINTS

Bladder 37, *Soul Door;* **Bladder 38,** *Rich for the Vitals;* **Bladder 39,** *Spirit Hall*

Olive's main activation sites are the three major wing points on the upper Bladder Meridian that line up along the inside of the shoulder blades on your back. *Soul Door* is one of the entryways into your body that reconnects you with the highest octave of your soul. *Rich for the Vitals* is a point that nourishes

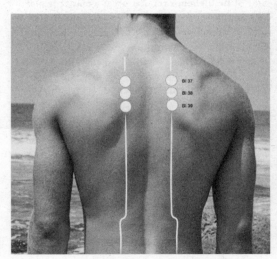

Olive Acupuncture Points, Bladder 37, Soul Door; Bladder 38, Rich for the Vitals; Bladder 39, Spirit Hall

every level of your body, mind, and spirit. *Spirit Hall* connects to the spiritual aspect of your heart, giving you an overview, like the bird's-eye view of the dove that flies high enough to see new land.

SYNTHESIS

Olive, like these three upper Bladder points, gives you wings to fly to a higher octave, so you can see your life from an elevated perspective. Olive partnered with these three Bladder Points gives your body a direct experience of the activation of these wing points and the rush of vitality connected with this opening.

TCM practitioners: The TCM notations for the Bladder points are as follows: Soul Door, Bladder 42; Rich for the Vitals, Bladder 43; and Spirit Hall, Bladder 44 (Outer Shu of Lung, Pericardium, and Heart).

Pine Flower Essence

Pine is a remedy for self-forgiveness and recovery from guilt that keeps you bound and imprisoned. There is an aspect of guilt that has to do with looking down on yourself from above in self-judgment. Using Pine helps you climb down from this height, bringing with you the gift of self-love. Pine is especially helpful in quickening the intervals between making mistakes, forgiving yourself, and inevitably making new ones to forgive—a technique that is useful for attaining success in life!

Pine trees are evergreens and symbolize the part of you that never dies. They love to grow in cool, high, mountainous regions and climb into the higher, rarefied air. Walking in a Pine forest cleanses, clears, and refreshes your spirit with its liquid green, clean scent.

PINE ACUPUNCTURE POINT

Lung 1, *Middle Palace*

Middle Palace is the first point on the Lung Meridian and connects to Gate of Hope—the last, or exit, point on the Liver Meridian. The liver has to do with forgiveness and envisioning the bigger picture that is beyond judgment, while *Middle Palace* activates an ability to witness your stellar nature and experience self-worth.

SYNTHESIS

When using Pine as an essence, you can almost hear a sigh of relief from your body, which has been wondering why your feeling life has been beating it up for so long. Joining Pine to *Middle Palace* helps your physical system experience what it's like to be in the present moment without the debilitating guilt that has kept your capacity for creative action locked away.

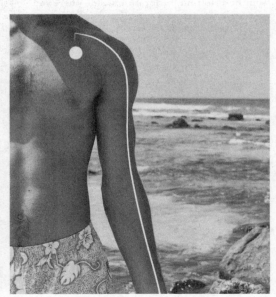

Pine Acupuncture Point, Lung 1, Middle Palace

Red Chestnut Flower Essence

Red Chestnut is a remedy that is used to overcome anxiety about someone you love. This anxiety may center on something real that you are afraid of reoccurring, or it may be based on an irrational fear that you hold for them. Red Chestnut has the ability to take the energy that you have projected onto the one you love and bring it back to you. In this way, both of you feel clear again to envision fresh positive outcomes.

Red Chestnut is a beautiful medium-size tree that blossoms with large bouquets of pink-red flowers that are attractive from a distance. Up close, they exude a scent and stickiness that feel slightly overwhelming, in the way that sympathy for a loved one can be cloying.

RED CHESTNUT ACUPUNCTURE POINT

Conception Vessel 12, *Middle Duct*

Middle Duct joins ten major meridians together and is located at the midpoint over the solar plexus, the seat of your power. This site calms down the anxiety that may come when you project your energy onto someone else. It allows you to knit back together the fabric of your various energy systems as well as to reestablish your boundaries.

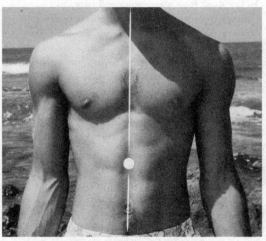

Red Chestnut Acupuncture Point, Conception Vessel 12, Middle Duct

SYNTHESIS

Living in a loved one's shoes can make you to feel powerless and out of control. When you come back into yourself, your strength returns and life events tend to straighten themselves out for all concerned. Joining Red Chestnut to *Middle Duct* aids this transition, returning to your body the governing energy that it was lacking.

Rock Rose Flower Essence

Rock Rose is a remedy for experiences of fear and panic at the threshold of an experience. This threshold can be a positive psychological one that is new to you and feels like a terrifying risk, or a real physical experience that is life-threatening. Rock Rose activates courage to flow through this threshold and instills trust that you will not only survive the experience but blossom once you are through it.

A short plant that grows on grassy meadows, the yellow flowers of Rock Rose radiate light. Its flowers are flat and papery like poppies; they bloom with unusual brightness and fade quickly.

ROCK ROSE ACUPUNCTURE SITE

Conception Vessel 4, *First Gate*

First Gate is a point that connects directly to the kidneys and activates them. The Kidney Meridian holds the imprint of your life essence and is connected to the emotion of fear because of its deep,

Continued ➡

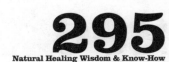

cold nature. The Conception Vessel helps you to give birth to your feminine soul forces. Stimulating this point enables you to retrieve your life forces and move with courage through this "first gate" upward into life.

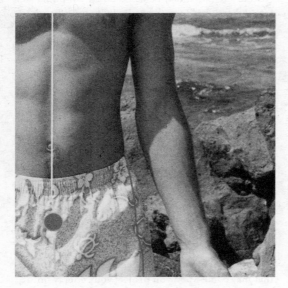

Rock Rose Acupuncture Site, Conception Vessel 4, First Gate

SYNTHESIS

In the Rock Rose state, you need tremendous courage to cross over into unfamiliar territory, trusting that all is well on the other side of the experience. Uniting Rock Rose and *First Gate* releases a reservoir of fresh patterns from your Kidneys, enabling your body to feel safe to birth itself through this place.

Rock Water Essence

Rock Water is a core remedy for releasing hardened soul forces so you can flow again with the stream of life. Growing up in a harsh environment or being overly sensitive can cause you to form a shell of protection. This hardening may numb your feelings, causing you to be harsh on yourself and others. Rock Water lifts the stone barrier that blocks your energy flow so life becomes easy again and events in your life can transform into new creative possibilities. Rock Water is also useful for breaking up specific issues that feel like a boulder in your path.

Rock Water is made from a sacred well in England that has been known for centuries for its special healing capacities. The water is collected and potentized in the same way the flower essences are made. This well is surrounded by rocks that have been broken down over the years by the action of the deep spring, making the water deeply mineralized.

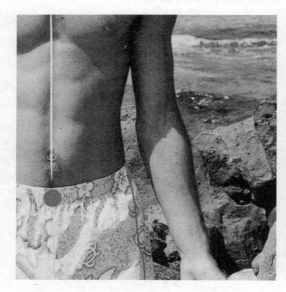

Rock Water Acupuncture Point, Conception Vessel 5, Stone Gate

ROCK WATER ACUPUNCTURE POINT

Conception Vessel 5, *Stone Gate*

Stone Gate breaks open the barriers to the expression of your life forces. These life forces, ruled by the Triple Warmer Meridian, accumulate in the lower "burning space" that is located in the core of your body behind this point. This point combines your internal fire from the heart with your internal water from the kidneys and washes away all the constrictions as it sends this enlivening Fire-Water through your whole system.

SYNTHESIS

Rock Water is a core essence for the state of denial. Conjoining Rock Water with *Stone Gate* pries the rock off the cell where your life forces have been imprisoned, bringing about a miraculous resurrection of vibrancy that has been missing from your body.

Scleranthus Flower Essence

Scleranthus is a remedy to use at times when you are unable to determine where you stand in relation to actions you should take. Indecision may cause you to consider one option, then its opposite, wavering back and forth. Acting on left brain–right brain coordination, Scleranthus helps you recognize the geographic location inside yourself that reveals where you stand. This fulcrum of knowing is then mirrored in the outer world through certainty in your actions.

Scleranthus is a low-lying plant that forms a mat close to the ground and bears tiny green flowers. Its geographic location is difficult to find—here one day, eaten by rabbits the next. The common name of this plant, knawel, means "knot of tangled threads," much like the wandering psychological state that it helps to heal.

SCLERANTHUS ACUPUNCTURE POINT

Gall Bladder 24, *Sun and Moon*

Sun and Moon unites what is inside with what is outside, creating conjunction between your active yang, or sun, forces and your receptive yin, or moon, forces. Decisiveness is dependent on inner certainty. By locating where you stand inside, your outer actions become decisive as they align with your inner knowing.

SYNTHESIS

Using Scleranthus helps you come together, creating synthesis between your feminine and masculine sides. Applying Scleranthus to *Sun and Moon* assists your body to find the location inside where you

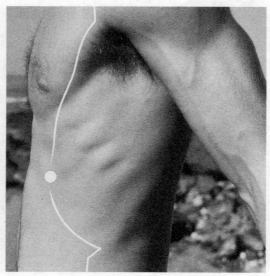

Scleranthus Acupuncture Point, Gall Bladder 24, Sun and Moon

stand, which can then be mirrored in the outer world by the action that is proper for you to take.

Star of Bethlehem Flower Essence

Star of Bethlehem is a core remedy for rebirthing out of long- or short-term shock. This state has a direct impact on your heart, keeping you from feeling fully present or properly nourished. Star of Bethlehem imparts spiritual milk to your soul, feeding it heavenly food for which it has been starving. When your connection to spirit has been reestablished, your heart is again able to open and experience new life as it is born through you.

Star of Bethlehem is a tiny white lily- or onion-family plant that pushes itself out of the ground even through ice and snow. To reach it, you must bend down, sometimes on your knees, to gaze at its exquisite beauty. Pristine, it carries the signature shared by other lily-family flowers of being heavenly in nature. Its white color indicates nourishment from spirit.

STAR OF BETHLEHEM ACUPUNCTURE POINTS

Conception Vessel 14, *Great Deficiency;* **Conception Vessel 15,** *Dove Tail*

These two Conception Vessel Meridian points link directly to the Heart and Pericardium Meridians. Shock freezes the heart, disconnecting you from your spirit and disabling it from conducting life forces to your body. *Great Deficiency* reestablishes communication with the organ of the heart and also reboots the pathway to your Pericardium or Heart Protector. *Dove Tail* goes straight to the pericardium, allowing you to experience joy and pleasure once again.

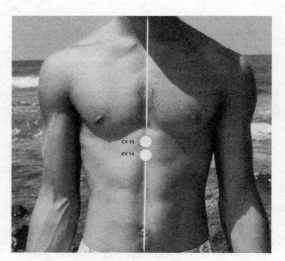

Star Of Bethlehem Acupuncture Points, Conception Vessel 14, Great Deficiency; Conception Vessel 15, Dove Tail

SYNTHESIS

Star of Bethlehem's reputation as a master healer can now be seen in its larger scope. It reactivates both Pericardium and Heart Meridians through the Conception Vessel, allowing you to rebirth soul forces that have been disabled through shock.

Sweet Chestnut Flower Essence

Sweet Chestnut is a remedy for the deepest form of anxiety, in which you feel alone in your suffering. Called the "dark night of the soul," this state is a harbinger of new light arising. When you are seemingly abandoned by the spiritual world, this state requires that you release your hold on your old reality and trust what is coming. Sweet Chestnut gives you the ability to surrender. By letting go, you allow light forces to descend and lift you into the higher reality your soul has been longing for.

The Sweet Chestnut is remarkable for its stature and resilient nature. It blooms prolifically with

Continued ➤

whorls of long-stemmed creamy flowers that, like other chestnut varieties, are sticky and smell overly sweet. Its nuts, encased in spiked green cases, open to reveal smooth brown nuts that provide delicious, nourishing food.

Sweet Chestnut Acupuncture Point

Governing Vessel 1, *Long Strength*

Long Strength is the first point on the Governing Vessel Meridian and one of the entry points used to inform the body of descending yang or masculine spirit. The Governing Vessel feeds the Conception Vessel, where the soul rises in the body and ascends as the feminine yin force. *Long Strength* is used to jump-start and revitalize your body when you have suffered far too long.

Synthesis

Dr. Bach's original description of feeling alone in the Sweet Chestnut state is illuminated by understanding the function of its acupuncture site counterpart, *Long Strength*. This site reestablishes the flow of your ascending masculine spirit energy up your spinal column, following the pathway of the Governing Meridian. Using these two together gives your body a jolt that can charge your system into a new light-filled octave of awareness.

Acupuncture Point Location

Governing Vessel 1, *Long Strength* is located at the underneath tip of the tailbone just between your buttock cheeks. To apply Sweet Chestnut to this site, apply a cotton ball dipped in the flower essence solution to the base of your tailbone.

White Chestnut Flower Essence

White Chestnut is an anxiety remedy that alleviates distress when your mind is going around and around. This mental chatter tends to make you see problems from every point of view. There may be an uncanny sense of being in the shoes of everyone around you and experiencing, one by one, their views of your problem. White Chestnut brings you back into your own shoes, releasing the sense of being imprisoned and quieting your mind so peace can be restored.

The large white flowers of the White Chestnut tree proliferate on stalks that stand out from the canopy, creating an alluring appearance. Upon your approach to the flowers, however, their overly sweet fragrance may overwhelm your senses the same way your state of anxiety overwhelms your system.

White Chestnut Acupuncture Point

Conception Vessel 1, *Meeting of Yin*

Meeting of Yin is the nodal point for the fertilization of your ascending feminine soul forces, yin, by your descending masculine spirit, yang. When this first point on the Conception Vessel Meridian is disengaged from its masculine counterpart, which resides on the Governing Vessel Meridian, your soul loses its ability to inform your head and your mind goes around in circles.

Synthesis

The experience of your mind going around and around can be puzzling. It is an unwelcome state, and yet you may be unable to stop it from happening. Applying White Chestnut to *Meeting of Yin* quiets this state and reveals its origin as the disconnection of your soul energy from your spirit essence.

Acupuncture Point Location

Conception Vessel 1, *Meeting of Yin* is located on the perineum, between the legs on the floor of the torso. To apply White Chestnut to this site, apply a cotton ball dipped in the flower essence solution to the floor of your torso, midway between the anus and genitals.

Note: We have chosen not to illustrate the acupuncture point locators for Sweet Chestnut and White Chestnut due to the sensitive nature of their locations.

Vervain Flower Essence

Vervain is a remedy for those with fiery ideals. Your ability for strong inspiration may keep you above the crowd, firing your body into idealistic actions that eventually burn your own forces with their intensity. Those around you may feel controlled by your lack of freedom to change what you see as the ultimate truth. Vervain helps you release steam, granting your body a renewed ability to flow with life as it is. Floating down to earth, you can see things from a more grounded and peaceful perspective.

Vervain plants are all stem, with few leaves and tiny pink flowers that peek quietly out at intervals up the stalk. Growing to a height of three to four feet, the thin stems give the impression of tension as they blow stiffly in the wind. Its pretty flowers are so tiny that they call you to come and appreciate them at close view.

Vervain Acupuncture Points

Gall Bladder 18, *Receive Spirit;* **Gall Bladder 34,** *Yang Mound Spring*

These two sites combined connect the crown area of your head to your roots. *Receive Spirit* is the landing pad that allows your unique individual expression to download into your body. *Yang Mound Spring* is the Earth point on the Gall Bladder Meridian; it creates grounding for your unique expression to form roots through the Element of Earth.

Synthesis

Receive Spirit and *Yang Mound Spring* illumine the Vervain dilemma of seeing everything idealistically from above or out of your body and trying to relate this point of view to others, an attempt accompanied by frustration and impatience with the disconnection between above and below. Uniting Vervain to these two points gives the body an immediate feeling of refreshment and a rush of new vitality.

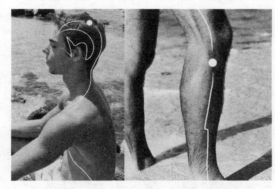

Left: Vervain Acupuncture Points, Gall Bladder 18,
Receive Spirit
Right: Vervain Acupuncture Points, Gall Bladder 34,
Yang Mound Spring

Vine Flower Essence

Vine is a remedy that helps you overcome the pattern of using your life forces to control others. This control—whether masculine and forceful in nature or the harder-to-discern feminine sort (the passive-aggressive approach)—manipulates and constrains your own life forces as well as those of others through the tension required to hold people and things in their allotted space. Vine helps you to rise to your higher life's purpose by allowing those around you their freedom. Through the sacrifice of your own will, your evolution is supported again by

the flow of greater life as it blesses all who accept this streaming goodness.

The grapevine is unlike other plants that repeat their life cycle through the four seasons in the same manner through the centuries. To produce a spectacular vintage requires a growing season that marks a particular beneficence from nature. To this end, winegrowers manipulate vines in all manner of ways, and vines manipulate growers, who worry constantly about how their grapes are faring. In the end, grace from nature and a special turning point in time create a wine that shines forth in a certain year.

Vine Acupuncture Point

Large Intestine 20, *Welcome Fragrance*

Welcome Fragrance is the last, or exit, point on the Large Intestine Meridian, and it leads to the first or entry point on the Stomach Meridian, *Receive Tears*. *Welcome Fragrance* effects a release of your false motives and welcomes in the "fragrance" of your quintessential self. Letting go of the attempt to refine others, you harvest a new season for your soul. As this released energy travels to, and connects with, the Stomach acu-point *Receive Tears*, you are able to allow the earth to support and welcome you at a new level.

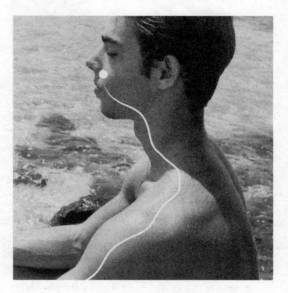

Vine Acupuncture Point, Large Intestine 20, Welcome Fragrance

Synthesis

Controlling others creates tension for your body. Applying Vine to *Welcome Fragrance* releases this tension, allowing you to experience a new communion with life. *Welcome Fragrance* (located to the left and right sides of the nostrils) is aptly named in relation to vintners, who gauge a wine's qualities by its scent.

Walnut Flower Essence

Walnut is a remedy for making a transition and freeing yourself from the influences of those around you. Working at the threshold level, you can use Walnut for physical or psychological transformations, such as giving birth or getting married. Its ability to facilitate exponential leaps in consciousness makes it an important all-purpose remedy that can help you re-create your life at a new level of experience.

Walnuts are large trees with long oval leaves; they blossom with hanging green-brown male catkin flowers (the female flowers are small, green, and pear-shape). Substances extruded from this tree create acidic soil, so it often stands alone. The nut resembles the human brain, with two clearly delineated sides and a bridge between them.

Continued ➜

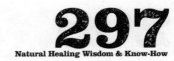

WALNUT ACUPUNCTURE POINT

Small Intestine 16, *Heavenly Window*

Heavenly Window is a "window to the sky" point that opens you up to the vision of yourself as a transformed individual. The small intestine sorts pure from impure substances for transformation into usable energy. This site flips the switch that turns on the transformer energy you have assiduously built, making you capable of moving to the next level. A "graduation" site, it gives you perfect vision of yourself as unique.

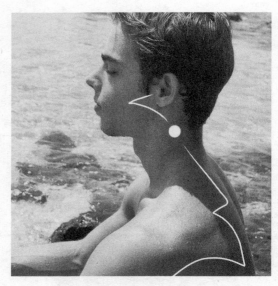

Walnut Acupuncture Point, Small Intestine 16, Heavenly Window

SYNTHESIS

Conjoining Walnut to *Heavenly Window* gives the body the experience of releasing itself from the cocoon stage of creative chaos and breaking free in the form of a butterfly.

Water Violet Flower Essence

Water Violet is a remedy for a delicate condition of soul that finds comfort in being alone. Accomplished and self-sufficient, you may draw those around you to your singular gifts. Water Violet helps you engage more fully in the world and share the fragrance you exude. Your disdain for physical existence and need to retreat are softened by new warmth for embodied fullness.

The pale violet-pink flowers of the Water Violet, an aquatic plant, hold their heads up above the water on slim, erect stems while their leaves and roots are fully submerged. Not able to accept direct sunlight, the leaves photosynthesize light through the liquid medium in which they live.

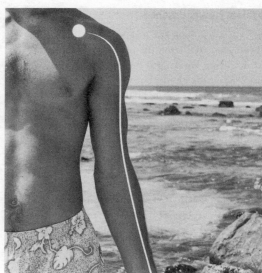

Water Violet Acupuncture Point, Lung 2, Cloud Gate

WATER VIOLET ACUPUNCTURE POINT

Lung 2, *Cloud Gate*

Cloud Gate is the turning point where the Lung Meridian brings its energy and information out of the ethers into your body. When lung energy is too inflated, you may have a tendency to be other-worldly, creating a disconnect between yourself and others. This point brings your life forces down out of the clouds and roots them into the earth, creating a unified spectrum between levity and gravity.

SYNTHESIS

Water Violet types have a disdain for Earth. Feeling too sensitive for gross matter, they have a tendency to retreat in this state. Joining Water Violet to *Cloud Gate* deflates this elevated view of life and lets the body breathe out, joining others in a grounded manner.

Wild Oat Flower Essence

Wild Oat is the remedy that addresses questions regarding your work or life's destiny. It may be that you are searching for your destiny or questioning your next move in regard to it. Or you may be fully engaged in your life task, yet it feels joyless. Using Wild Oat helps you connect the dots to arrive at the juicy juncture where you find passionate renewal through fulfilling a task you feel you were meant to do.

Wild Oats grow very tall; their drooping green panicles sway in the wind. They give an impression of freedom as they move this way and that in the breeze. Unlike many other grasses that plod along the ground, Wild Oat stands out and is easy to see from a distance.

WILD OAT ACUPUNCTURE POINT

Governing Vessel 4, *Gate of Life*

Gate of Life is where the hereditary Water forces of the kidneys unite with the spirit Fire seeded in your heart, combining into Fire-Water. This site warms the waters of your destiny like a house with plenty of hot water available. A fulcrum or nodal point where the spine holds the upper body straight, this is a common place for lower back pain, often caused by caving in to stress and tension in relation to over-work.

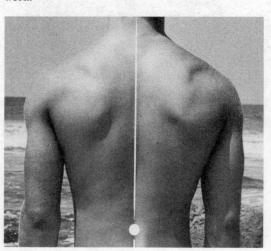

Wild Oat Acupuncture Point, Governing Vessel 4, Gate of Life

SYNTHESIS

When your life droops like Wild Oats in the wind, applying Wild Oat essence at *Gate of Life* will help your body stand tall again. There is a voltage switch that turns on at this site as your masculine spirit energy, seeded on the Governing Vessel Meridian, lights up with Fire-Water, sending vitality surging through your system.

Wild Rose Flower Essence

Wild Rose is a remedy for long-term exhaustion and resignation. Having suffered much, you may no longer expect to recover from the onslaught. Deep feelings of sadness may make your heart feel heavy. Using Wild Rose restores your spirit. Bringing solace to your heart, it uplifts you again into love for life. Enthusiasm is returned to you after a long bout in the wilderness.

The Wild Rose is a beautiful bush that produces pink or white roses with five fully open petals. All roses hold something precious that sparks the heart with love for life. The English Wild Rose holds this promise of resurrection into new life with exponential force.

WILD ROSE ACUPUNCTURE POINTS

Governing Vessel 10, *Supernatural Tower;* **Governing Vessel 11,** *Spirit Path*

The Governing Vessel Meridian oversees your entire system and directs the Heart Meridian on how to conduct your system harmonically. The combination of *Supernatural Tower* and *Spirit Path* ignites your Heart to envision a master template of your life's purpose. *Supernatural Tower* enables you to view this original purpose, while *Spirit Path* connects directly to the organ of the heart and helps you stay connected with this purpose while on your current path.

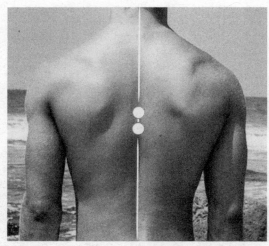

Wild Rose Acupuncture Points, Governing Vessel 10, Supernatural Tower; Governing Vessel 11, Spirit Path

SYNTHESIS

In the Wild Rose state, your head and upper body hangs down, crestfallen. Applying Wild Rose to *Supernatural Tower* and *Spirit Path*, the back heart sites, allows you to raise your head again and gaze with passionate wonder at the beauty of life in front of you.

Willow Flower Essence

Willow is a remedy for feelings of resentment. Bitterness can accumulate when you are unable to establish proper boundaries in giving to others. This may build up a dam of frozen rage that inhibits your ability to experience joy. Willow helps unleash this frozen anger so your forces can burn again with the passionate rose tones of love. When you are flowing with life, forgiveness toward others is a natural expression of this upwelling movement.

Willow grows quickly near flowing water. Its vitality and fast growth make it ideal for marking boundaries. In earlier days, people wove its flexible branches together for fencing. The Willow sprouts vigorous, beautiful branches filled with long, oval, green leaves that are remarkable for their resiliency as they flow and bounce in the wind.

Continued ➡

Willow Acupuncture Point

Liver 4, *Middle Seal*

Middle Seal is the Metal point on the Liver Meridian and a site you can use to address arthritic conditions. In ancient China, a letter bore three identification wax seals, the middle seal indicating the insignia of the emperor or empress. The *Middle Seal* acu-point accesses your interior emperor/empress and retrieves your ability to wield ultimate authority through your own internal power. By reconnecting to your authentic self, this site helps you to release the stones of indignation and to forgive the actions of others. Forgiveness is the sweet balm that releases calcified energy (the Element of Metal).

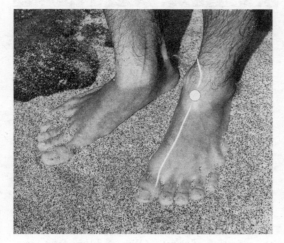

Willow Acupuncture Point, Liver 4, Middle Seal

Synthesis

The Willow state accumulates bitterness when you are unable to galvanize fire to stand up for your own best interests. By harboring what you perceive as external insults or injuries, you internalize these experiences, causing stones of locked energy to accumulate that may lead to arthritic conditions. Applying Willow to *Middle Seal* accesses your ability to release these hardened accumulations and joyfully accept your own power.

Special Treatments

As we conducted the research for this book, the following special treatments evolved naturally. They work best with the method of infusing water to dilute the flower essences and lying down to rest for 45 minutes after application, but you can also use them as overnight applications, with good results. Another option is to use these treatments two to three times a day, without resting, while you continue your activities. Do what appeals to you and trust your body's ability to guide you on which method is best for you. (For application instructions, see page 287.)

We suggest that you do these treatments once a day for seven days with rest, or two to three times a day for seven days when putting the essences on the acu-sites without taking a rest period. Certain constitutions may find that doing the treatments three times a week rather than every day works more smoothly. Observe your body to know what is best for you. If you unfailingly remember to do the treatment each day, it is an indication that your body is benefiting from this rhythm. If you find yourself forgetting to do the treatment, it may mean that your body is digesting previous treatments. If this is the case, trust that your body knows what it is doing and adjust your rhythm of applying the treatments accordingly. Consult the body site map for each essence to determine the specific acupuncture point for application.

Anxiety: Rebirth

Sweet Chestnut, White Chestnut, Red Chestnut, Chestnut Bud

The following treatment is useful for the gradual release of long-term anxiety. We recommend that you reread the four descriptions of these essences in this chapter to understand how the soul and spirit aspects of their acu-points may be helpful for anxiety. We suggest you use each Chestnut remedy once a day for seven days in the order listed below, starting with Sweet Chestnut and ending with Chestnut Bud. Using these four essences may bring a welcome release for the body, since there is suffering in these conditions. If you feel you're not done with a certain essence after a week, extend its use until you feel ready to move on to the next one. Chestnut Bud can, in certain cases, feel less relaxing because it is bringing out into the world precious aspects of yourself that have been bottled inside for a long time. Be kind to yourself, and use each treatment according to your comfort level. If strong emotions surface, you can slow down the treatments, giving yourself time to digest the changes, and resume when you're ready. If you're ready to release stored tensions despite any discomfort you may experience, keep the same rhythm and the state will pass quickly. (Each person will have unique sensations; discomfort is less common than deep relaxation and is usually short-lived, so trust in the process.)

Week 1 Sweet Chestnut—Reclaiming Spirit

Week 2 White Chestnut—Reclaiming Soul

Week 3 Red Chestnut—Reclaiming Power

Week 4 Chestnut Bud—Rebirth

Depression: Restoring Light

Mimulus, Mustard, Rock Rose

You can use this treatment when you experience depression, sadness, or a downcast state of mind. Reread these three descriptions to see how each may be helpful to restore happiness. It is simple and can be applied once with good results if the depression is mild, or it can be used long-term if needed. Using it for seven days is a good general treatment; if your depression is of long-standing, however, using it for thirty days may be what you need.

For this treatment, use all three essences at once. Put 2 to 4 drops of each essence (Mimulus, Mustard, Rock Rose) into a single bowl of warm water; dip a cloth in the solution, wring out well, and apply directly to the sites for all three essences indicated on the body site maps. (Since these sites are close together, using a clean washcloth rubbed over the whole area is an easier way to cover the sites successfully than the cotton-ball method of application.)

Fire and Water: Connecting Your Destiny With Your Passion

Holly, Wild Oat

Dr. Bach considered Wild Oat and Holly to be the two "polycrests" of his system. By this he meant that these two flower essences effect positive changes for any type of condition and can be utilized when it is not clear precisely what is needed in a particular case. Applying both of these flower essences at the same time to the Gate of Destiny acupuncture point (located on the Governing Vessel Meridian on the lower back) is a treatment for opening the way not only to your destiny but also to passion for your destiny task in life. The Gate of Destiny acupuncture point is where the Element of Water (Wild Oat) ascends and the Element of Fire (Holly) descends. When the two streams meet at this site, Fire-Water is created and provides a potent spark for your entire system, charging it with light and warmth.

For this treatment, put 2 to 4 drops each of Wild Oat and Holly into a bowl of water, dip a cotton ball into the water, and apply to Gate of Destiny. It is recommended that you lie down for 45 minutes on your back and rest after this treatment.

Rescue

Cerato, Cherry Plum

This is a treatment you can use when you need to retrieve and center yourself during or after an experience of shock. Cerato connects your heart to your head, while Cherry Plum brings you back into your body. Together they make a good emergency treatment.

To use, put 2 to 4 drops each of Cherry Plum and Cerato into a bowl of water and apply with a cotton ball in a wide circle around your heart as well as to the nape of your neck. (See the Cherry Plum body map for the exact location of Great Hammer, which is the direct acu-point for Cherry Plum.) You can apply this treatment straight from the bottle you buy from the store to get a quicker result. The stronger concentration of essences may be more effective. Take care not to touch the dropper to the skin when you apply essences to skin zones, as oils from the skin may compromise the efficacy of the remaining flower essence when you put the dropper back in the bottle.

Flower Coronation

Olive, Star of Bethlehem, Wild Rose

This is a wonderful all-purpose treatment that connects your Pericardium Meridian (Heart Protector) to your Heart Meridian and activates your back heart area and "wings" at the shoulder blades. Flower Coronation sends up renewed energy and light into your head, opening the cranial plates. There's an impression during this treatment of fragrance or grace around the crown, thus the name. It is a good treatment for long-term exhaustion, as the combination of the lily (Star of Bethlehem) and rose (Wild Rose) activate the whole heart complex, while the Olive and Wild Rose raise up and renew your life forces.

For this treatment, put 2 to 4 drops each of Wild Rose, Star of Bethlehem, and Olive into a bowl of water. Using two or three cotton balls, apply to the body following the body site maps for the specific essences. Lie down to rest for 20 to 45 minutes. (Olive and Wild Rose are difficult body sites to reach by yourself; you will most likely need someone else to rub the essences on your back at these sites). You can also infuse water and simply apply the essences to these sites before going about your daily routine, or place a compress on the sites overnight. Every day for seven days is a good rhythm for this treatment application.

Flower Essences, Acupuncture, and Self-Healing

It is important to note that flower essences are a form of self-healing. You can buy them at health food stores, where they are sold as nutritional supplements. They are completely safe and bring wonderful results. They do, however, require your mental participation, since they often bring to the surface what may be bothering you at subconscious levels. This process occasionally may include uncomfortable periods where your emotional, mental, and physical symptoms intensify and "get worse" for a short period (this is classically called a "healing crisis"). After this short period, you generally feel better than before and experience life at a higher octave. For this reason, flower essences are

Continued ➔

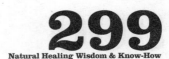

utilized mainly by those wishing to take responsibility for their own well-being. In general, they don't appeal to and are not used by those who require supervision for health-related conditions unless when they are given for use by a health care professional.

If you are someone who consults with health professionals, we recommend that you show this book to them. Using these treatments under professional guidance may provide the support you need for your healing journey. This may also be the best way for you to increase your confidence in learning how to incorporate self-help techniques in the future.

Connecting the flower essences of Dr. Bach to acupuncture sites is a new modality. As more people utilize these treatments, the larger shared body of humanity absorbs this information, which downloads into the planetary ethers as new possibilities for well-being. If initial use of these treatments causes you discomfort, you may want to discontinue their use and experience them in a professional setting.

—From *Floral Acupuncture*

HOW TO MAKE YOUR OWN FLOWER ESSENCES

James Green, Herbalist

It has been my recurrent experience and observation that floral vibrations that have been infused in water that is sitting on the Earth in a clear glass bowl, floating blossoms in the warm sunlight of a clear blue sky, can profoundly affect the subtle disposition of an ailing (or even more promising, a preailing) being. Like a music master's hand tuning the eager strings of a perfect Stradivarius, the pristine clarity of a flower's uplifting vibrations adjusts the tone of one's thoughts and respondent feelings, bringing them back in harmony with the richness of one's true nature. When our thoughts and feelings are in line with our spirit's unique path, we resume our journey as a vital creator of a prosperous, healthful, joyous life—the intrinsic dynamics of a human beings essence.

The life work of Dr. Edward Bach (1886–1936) pioneered understanding of the subtle energy and actions of flower essence medicine. Dr. Bach created a bouquet of subtle, water-infused floral essences, each of which embraced and treated a being's subtle nonphysical nature, ultimately relieving manifested physical symptoms. More importantly, the essences helped individuals establish ease in their life, thereby preventing unpleasant physical manifestations entirely. Edward Bach's vision was to develop a system of herbal medicine that anyone, when feeling out of sorts, could use to diagnose and prepare his or her own medicines, and treat himself or herself, thereby allaying illness before its physical symptoms are made manifest. In a short period of seven years, Dr. Bach succeeded brilliantly, and developed a system of herbal therapeutics the core of which is pure simplicity. I'm convinced that the principles underlying this and other forms of subtle energetic medicine will guide the practical course of mainstream medicine and the art of self-medicating in the very near future.

One can illustrate Dr. Bach's insight and technique for treating an individual whose illness has progressed to the manifestation of physical symptoms by reprinting a short quotation taken from his book, *The Twelve Healers and Other Remedies*: "Take no notice of the disease. Think only of the outlook on

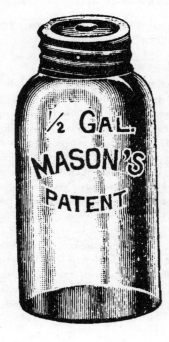 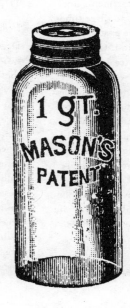 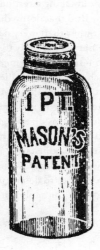

life of the one in distress. The same disease may have different effects [varying states of mind or moods) on different people; it is these effects that need treatment, because they guide to the real cause…as one becomes well by gaining increased happiness and interest in life, the disease goes, having been cast off by the increase in health. Health and disease are caused by how we think, how we feel within ourselves. Health and disease are the consolidation of mental attitude."

This section explains how to prepare a flower essence infusion for one's personal use….

Methods of Preparation

There are three stages in the preparation of flower essence infusions before a dose is administered to an individual: the first preparation is what I will refer to as the Mother Essence; the second is the Stock Water; and the third is the Medicine Water.

There are two basic methods for preparing the Mother Essence: the sun method, used for flowers that bloom during the late spring, summer, and early autumn when the sun is often overhead, full and hot, and the boiling method, used for the flowers and twigs of plants that bloom at times other than when the sun is at the most intense phases of its solar cycle.

Wildflowers growing in their natural habitat rather than cultivated flowers are preferable (with the exception of Cerato, Olive, and Vine found in Dr. Bach's materia medica).

Each individual essence should be made with blossoms gathered from as many different plants of the same kind as possible.

About the Equipment

When preparing flower essences by either the sun method or the boiling method, all equipment to be used must be first sterilized by placing it in a container of cold water, slowly heating it, and gently boiling it for 20 minutes, then carefully drying it and wrapping it in a clean cloth. Dr. Bach felt it was important to tend to these details.

Simply, one first prepares a Mother Essence from wildflowers by using either the sun method or the boiling method; from this essence one prepares the Stock Water; from this one prepares a Medicine Water; from which one takes daily doses.

Preparing the Mother Essence by the Sun Method

Equipment

· One thin-gauge, plain glass bowl, approximately 8 fl. oz. (Do not use an etched, cut glass, or otherwise ornate bowl or a Pyrex-type ovenproof glass bowl.)

Continued ➡

- A quart jar with a lid to carry water to the flower site
- A 30 ml (1 oz.) amber dropper bottle with a glass pipette

Method

1. When the dropper bottle and pipette have cooled from the sterilizing process, fill half the bottle with brandy (or half fill many bottles with brandy; you will be creating a relatively large amount of Mother Essence), cap it tightly, and label it with the name of the flower to be prepared. Note on the label that this is the Mother Essence. Dr. Bach preferred to use brandy as a preservative, considering it a purer and more natural agent than rectified spirit.

2. Decide beforehand which plant community you are going to harvest, and choose a perfectly sunny morning when there are no clouds in the sky that might obscure the sun's light, therein immersing the bowl and its contents in the most animated energy of Earth's crystal clear air element.

3. Take your bowl, jar, and dropper bottle and arrive at the site a little before 9 A.M. (Pick the flowers at about 9 A.M., so they are floating in place as the sun is gaining intensity during the hours between 9 and noon. By 9 A.M. the flowers will be freshly opened in full bloom, and most airborne, pollen-spreading creatures will have not yet arrived.)

4. Sit with the flowers for a few minutes and focus on your intent; honor and extend gratitude to the plant community. You'll probably be feeling pretty good right now; you couldn't be in a better place than you are at this moment.

5. Place the bowl on the ground near the flowering plants, thereby connecting the subtle essence to the stabilizing energy of the Earth element. Choose a location for the bowl that is well away from trees, bushes, tall grasses, fences—anything that might cast a shadow over the bowl of basking flowers as the sunlight brushes across the Earth's surface.

6. Fill the bowl to the brim with the water you transported in the jar, or water from a clear stream, if one is nearby. Empty any unused water from the jar. Do not drink from this jar; it needs to remain sterile, as it will be used again later.

7. Pick some leaves, preferably from the plant you are preparing, or from some broadleaf plant, and place them on the palm of your hand. A Mullein leaf or one of similar dimensions is ideal.

8. Select the most perfect blossoms and carefully pick the flower heads just below the calyx (the external, usually green part of the flower that attaches to the stem) from as many plants or bushes of the same kind as possible. Let the flowers fall onto the leaf in your hand.

9. Quickly, carry the flowers to the bowl and float them on the surface of the water, thereon uniting everything with the fertile, receptive energy of the water element. Continue this process until the surface of the water is thickly covered. Overlap the flowers, but make sure each flower touches the water. (Throughout this process avoid casting your shadow over the bowl and avoid touching the water with your fingers. Eliminate the human vibrations as much as possible from the flower vibrations in the subtle infusion.)

10. Leave the bowl in full sunshine for 3 to 4 hours to absorb the resplendent energy of the fire element.

11. After about 4 hours, there will be slight signs of the petals fading, giving evidence that their subtle properties (vibrations) have been transmitted to the water. With a stalk from the plant you are preparing, or with a rigid portion of grass, lift the flower heads from the water. Do not touch the water with your fingers. The water will be crystal clear and full with minute, vibrant bubbles. Many herbalists confess to feelings of elation at this point.

12. Pour this Mother Essence into the jar that has been previously emptied, and from this fill the remaining half of the labeled dropper bottle (or as many bottles as you wish to prepare with this mother load). Cap it tightly.

Preparing the Mother Essence by the Boiling Method

Equipment

- One 4-quart enameled pot and lid
- Two 1-quart jars
- A 30 ml (1 oz.) amber dropper bottle with a glass pipette
- A funnel
- 2 or 3 pieces of filter paper

Method

1. Sterilize the jars, funnel, and dropper bottle in the enamel pot. When this equipment has cooled from the sterilizing process, half fill the dropper bottle with brandy, cap it tightly, and label it with the name of the flower to be prepared. Note that this is the Mother Essence.

2. A sunny morning is chosen whenever possible. For the same reasons you chose 9 A.M. for the sun method, gather the flowers and twigs at that time.

3. Decide beforehand which plant community you are going to harvest and take the enamel pot, covered with its lid to keep out any dust and debris, to the location. Sit with the flowers and focus on your intent; communicate with the plant community.

4. Fill the pot about three-quarters full with flowering sprays, including the leaves, buds, and twigs. Also gather two extra twigs of the same species of plant. These will be used later.

5. Place the lid on the pot, grab the extra two twigs and the pot filled with flowering sprays, and quickly return home.

6. Upon returning home, cover the plant parts with approximately a quart of cold water. Use rainwater, stream water, pure well water, bottled spring water, or, if nothing else is available, tap water that has been allowed to sit in an open container overnight. (Dr. Bach didn't like the energy of distilled water; he referred to it as "dead water." If you want to use distilled water, let it first sit in a clear glass bottle in the sunlight for a day. This should resurrect it.)

7. Place the pot uncovered over heat, and bring the water to a gentle boil. If necessary, press the flowers beneath the water with one of the twigs you brought home with you to prevent touching the water with your fingers.

8. Boil the plants over low heat for ½ hour.

9. At the end of a half hour, remove the pot from the heat and set it outdoors to cool.

10. When it is cold, remove all the twigs, leaves, and flowers, using one or both of the extra twigs as tools to help you. Do not touch the water with your fingers.

11. Cover the pot with its lid and allow the water to stand long enough for any sediment to settle to the bottom of the pot.

12. Line the funnel with a filter paper and place this in one of the two empty jars.

13. Fill the other jar carefully with the flower water from the pot. Pour slowly not to disturb the sediment.

14. Pour the liquid from this jar into the filtered funnel that is sitting in the first jar. This will take a while. Often, there is much sediment and you may need to filter the liquid twice.

15. From this filtered water, fill the remaining half of the labeled dropper bottle containing the brandy.

16. Cap tightly.

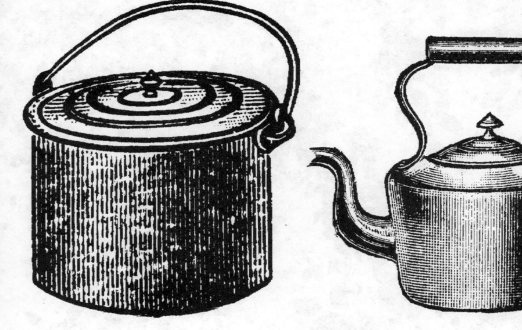

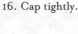

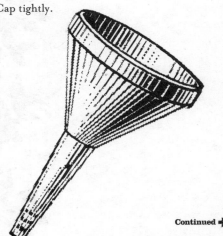

Continued ➤

Preparing the Stock Water

This is the second stage in the preparation of a flower essence infusion. Later, from this Stock Water, a person's Medicine Water is prepared.

To prepare a Stock Water from a Mother Essence which has been prepared by either the sun method or the boiling method:

1. Sterilize and dry a 1-oz. amber dropper bottle.

2. Label it with the name of the flower essence. Note that this is the Stock Water.

3. Fill the bottle with brandy.

4. Add merely 2 drops from the Mother Essence bottle.

5. Cap it tightly and succuss it (shake it vigorously) for a few moments.

Preparing the Medicine Water

This is the third stage in the preparation of the flower essence, and it is from this one the individual takes the doses suitable for a human, an animal, or a plant.

1. Determine which essence or combination of essences an individual requires. (Using 2 or 3 in combination is ideal, and from my experience, I recommend using no more than 5 at a time.)

2. Into a sterilized dropper bottle, put 2 drops from the Stock Water of a selected essence, or 2 drops from each of the essences selected for use in combination (making a compound essence).

3. Add a teaspoonful of brandy as a preservative to inhibit the water from going cloudy.

4. Fill the bottle with water.

5. Cap it tightly and succuss it.

6. Label with the flower(s) name and note it as a Medicine Water. Include the recommended dosage. . . .

Preservation and Storage

The Mother Essences and the Stock Waters, when prepared as directed above, will retain their strength indefinitely. If they are kept for several years, a slight sediment may form at the bottom of the bottle; this is not harmful. Sometimes, over a lengthy period of time, the rubber bulb on the dropper top will soften and lose its tone; it should be replaced with a new sterilized one.

When using the boiling method a large quantity of sediment may form. This should be filtered twice. Then, even though you have filtered the liquid a couple of times, after some months more sediment may form again at the bottom of the Mother Essence bottle; this should be re-filtered and rebottled.

The Medicine Water will be preserved quite adequately during the relatively short time it is used by the individual.

It is best to sterilize the bottle each time it is refilled.

—From *The Herbal Medicine-Maker's Handbook*

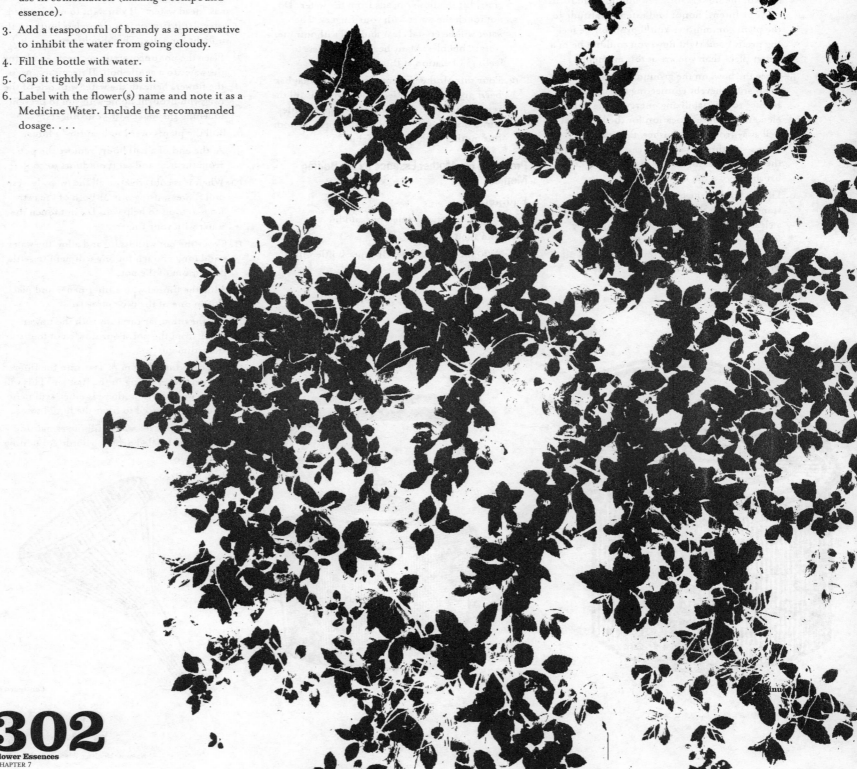

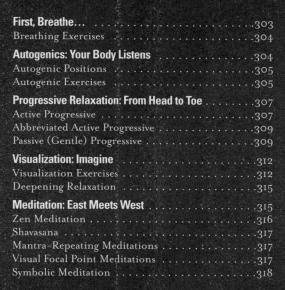

Mind-Body Healing Techniques

FIRST, BREATHE...

L. John Mason, Ph.D.

When you were born, you took a deep, full breath. Learning to breathe deeply again is the first step in learning to relax, and the deep, diaphragmatic breath is the core of the relaxation exercises discussed in this book. It is also used in the treatment of asthma, in the practice of yoga and meditation, and as a method of relaxation in childbirth.

Place one hand just below the rib cage (above the stomach). Take a deep breath, and as you inhale, notice the movement of your hand. Does it move in or out? Does it move at all? If you breathed properly, your hand moved outward. Be aware of how deeply you breathe.

We have been taught to hold our stomach in and our chest out. Unfortunately, this posture inhibits healthful breathing. In proper breathing, the diaphragm (the muscle that separates the lung cavity from the abdominal cavity) moves slightly down to create a vacuum in the lung cavity. As a result of the downward movement, the abdomen is forced forward.

Imagine that your lungs are divided into three parts. The deep, full breath begins with the diaphragm moving downward and the lowest part of the lungs filling with air; the middle part fills; then the chest expands; and finally the upper part of the lungs fills with air. The shoulders may move slightly upward. Take another deep breath and try to imagine this progression. Is this the way you usually breathe?

Take another deep breath. Do you inhale through your nose or through your mouth? How do you exhale? Do you exhale fully and completely? In breathing for relaxation, remember to breathe in through your nose and fill your lungs completely. Breathe again, inhaling through your nose. Visualize your lungs filling slowly with air; feel the movement of your abdomen. Then, exhale through your mouth and feel the warm air leave your body. You may find it uncomfortable to breathe exclusively through your nose. *Don't be confined by a rigid pattern—do what feels right.* But begin to breathe the deep, slow, healing breath instead of the rapid-shallow-shoulder-chest breath.

Inhale and hold your breath for ten seconds, feeling the tension in your throat and chest. Exhale through your mouth with a slight sigh; feel the "sigh of relief" release the tension. Sighing may not feel comfortable at first—give it a fair chance, as this may be a way for you to instantaneously release tension. The quietest or calmest time of the breath is between the exhalation and the inhalation. If you can feel the stillness at that moment directly after exhaling, at the end of the sigh, then you are learning how to relax. Inhale again; exhale with a slight sigh. As you exhale fully and completely, feel all the tension leaving your body, melting away. *Be aware of the quiet time of the breath.* Whenever you find yourself in a stressful situation, remember this feeling, and try to re-create that moment of peace and calm.

Why the deep, full breath? Breathing properly is healthful; it increases the amount of oxygen in the blood and strengthens weak abdominal and intestinal muscles. When you are tense or upset, your breathing becomes shallow and irregular, and your heart rate tends to accelerate. When you are relaxed, your breathing deepens and your heart rate decelerates. Breathing is the easiest physiological system to control. If you can breathe the deep, slow breath inherent in relaxation, then you can trigger the rest of the characteristics of the relaxation response. Once you become aware of your breathing patterns and know how to use breathing to reduce tension, you may gradually notice how you hold tension throughout your body.

The proper breath is the basis for a variety of breathing exercises. It can be learned quickly and may be easily integrated into your busy day. Don't wait for a stressful event to practice deep breathing. When people become tense, they often forget to breathe and develop a pattern of locking up the chest muscles and the diaphragm. Take a deep, slow breath and you may be surprised to discover how quickly your tension melts away.

Take at least forty deep breaths every day. (*This is a very important technique to try. Please work with this for two weeks to give it a fair chance to benefit you.*) To remind your-

Continued ➡

self to practice deep breathing, associate it with something commonly done during the day. If you are in a busy office, and the telephone seems to ring incessantly, don't grab the phone on the first ring. Let it ring an extra time and take a deep breath. Exhale fully and completely. Remember the quiet time of the breath and pick up the phone—relaxed and free of nervous tension.

All the time you spend driving from place to place can make you tense and edgy, and if you find yourself in a traffic jam, you may be grinding your teeth by the time you arrive home. If you drive a great deal, try taking a deep breath and relaxing at each stop signal, or use billboards and highway turnoff signs as reminders. Every time you inch forward in rush hour traffic, instead of frantically beeping your horn at every stop, take a deep, full breath and exhale fully and completely. As you breathe, check your shoulders and your forehead to see if they are tense. You really don't need to drive with your shoulders or your forehead.

A dramatic but not unusual story was told to me by a man who had attended one of my stress-reduction lectures. He had a very high-pressure job and was going through a difficult custody fight for his son. The added pressure of the legal battle made it almost impossible for him to function well at work. He was having difficulty meeting deadlines and relationships with his co-workers were rapidly deteriorating. After signing up for the entire five-week course, he attended the introductory lecture. I didn't see him at the second and third lectures and began to wonder what had happened to him; the course had been closed and he had been very insistent that I allow him to enroll. When he didn't show up for the fourth lecture, I decided to call him at work. He told me the following story:

I had recommended that clock-watchers put a piece of tape on the office clock; every time they turned to check the time they would be reminded to take a deep, full breath. After the first lecture he realized that he was constantly looking at his watch while working. He placed a piece of tape (in his case it was bright blue) on his watch and took a deep breath when he checked the time. Exhaling fully and completely, at first very difficult to do, became easier with each day. Even though he couldn't attend the second lecture because of work responsibilities, he continued to practice deep breathing. On the ninth day of practice he actually counted the times he took a deep breath and was amazed to discover that he had taken fifty-three deep breaths in just one workday. On the tenth day of practice he was approached by an office secretary who commented on the change in his personality; she wanted to know what drug he was taking because it had obviously helped him so much. She didn't believe that deep breathing had effected such a radical change, but when he showed her the tape on his watch she finally believed him. Breathing cues, combined with proper deep breathing, had worked for him; he apologized for not returning to class, but he felt that deep breathing exercises were enough to keep him relaxed and free from tension.

The simple deep breathing exercise may not be enough for you—but if you learn how to take a deep, full breath and exhale fully and completely, you will have mastered the first technique for relaxation. If none of the breathing cues is appropriate for your lifestyle, find a recurring event in your daily schedule to use as a trigger for deep breathing and relaxation.

Breathing Exercises

Practice these initial exercises to control tension. They may or may not be enough. Try each one three times a day for a week; you will probably find that one or two feel most comfortable for you. Pick a quiet spot for your practice session. If this is impossible and you are in a noisy place, just try to concentrate on the exercise and shut out the distractions. Always get into a comfortable position before attempting any exercise.

1-to-8 Count

Take a deep, slow breath and close your eyes. Exhale fully and completely, making sure to get the last bit of air out of your lungs. Breathe in again. As you inhale, try to see the number 1 in your mind; at the same time focus on the inhalation. Hold your breath for three seconds. Exhale, and as you breathe out the air fully and completely, mentally say "two" and visualize the number 2 in your mind. Breathe in again and mentally say "three," focusing on the number 3 and the inhalation. Hold your breath for three seconds. Exhale fully and completely, while mentally visualizing and saying 4. Inhale, counting 5; exhale, counting 6. Remember to visualize the number and focus on the inhalation. Inhale, counting 7, and exhale, counting 8. Repeat the entire sequence from 1 to 8. Slowly open your eyes.

Do you feel calmer?

Did you have any difficulty visualizing the numbers?

Were you able to focus on the inhalation?

Did you finish the exercise?

If you had any trouble focusing on the inhalation or visualizing the numbers, try to clear your mind of any distractions and try again. You might have been trying too hard if you didn't finish the exercise. Remember, trying too hard will only make you tenser. This exercise is not a race. Learn to be patient with yourself and the exercise; breathe slowly and pause between breaths. Do not try to force relaxation—this will only make it harder for you to relax, and you may find this very frustrating. Instead, find a way to give in to relaxation.

1-to-4 Count

Take a deep, full breath. Exhale fully and completely. Inhale again, and mentally count from 1 to 4. Hold your breath, and again count from 1 to 4. Slowly count from 1 to 8 while exhaling fully and completely. Repeat the sequence four times.

While exhaling, did you run out of breath before reaching number 8?

If you did, try again. On the second try, take a deeper breath and exhale more slowly. Be aware of full inhalation and full exhalation. If you had your eyes open and found it difficult to mentally count, close your eyes on the second try. This is a very powerful exercise if done correctly.

5-to-1 Count

Say the number 5 to yourself, and as you focus on the number, take a deep, full, slow breath. Exhale fully and completely, making sure to get the last bit of air out of your lungs. Mentally count 4 and inhale. As you begin the exhalation, tell yourself: "I am more relaxed now than I was at number 5." Be sure not to rush the thought. Inhale, mentally counting 3. Tell yourself: "I am more relaxed now than I was at number 4," as you exhale fully and completely. Count number 2 and then number 1, mentally repeating the phrase: "I am more relaxed

now than I was at number 2." Allow yourself to feel the deepening relaxation. As you approach number 1, you should feel calmer and more relaxed.

Three-Part Breathing

Take a deep, diaphragmatic breath. Imagine that your lungs are divided into three parts. Visualize the lowest part of your lungs filling with air. Use only your diaphragm; your chest should remain relatively still. Imagine the middle part of your lungs filling, and as you visualize the expansion, allow your rib cage to move slightly forward. Visualize the upper part filling with air and your lungs becoming completely full. Your shoulders will rise slightly and move backward. Exhale fully and completely. As you empty your upper lungs, drop your shoulders slightly. Visualize the air leaving the middle portion of your lungs, and feel your rib cage contract. Pull in your abdomen to force out the last bit of air from the bottom of your lungs. Repeat the exercise four times.

Did you have any trouble visualizing your lungs expanding and contracting?

Were you able to complete the inhaling visualization before you started to exhale?

If you had trouble visualizing, take a moment to put your thoughts out of mind. You can get back to them later when you are calm and relaxed. The visualization may seem more complex to you than it actually is; if you found yourself exhaling while still visualizing the inhalation, try and inhale more slowly. Be sure to exhale completely and push all of the carbon dioxide out of your lungs. This allows more room for life-giving oxygen to fill your lungs when you inhale.

— From *Guide to Stress Reduction*

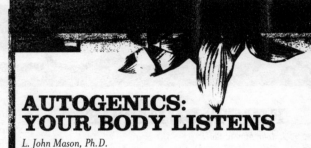

AUTOGENICS: YOUR BODY LISTENS

L. John Mason, Ph.D.

Sometimes you feel that you are a victim of your body, with its physiological processes beyond your control. When you feel well, you probably don't have this sense of helplessness. But when you are tense or anxious, you may suddenly feel out of control. Your hands and feet are icy; you jump at the slightest sound; trying to maintain an even keel consumes all your energy. You wish that you could tell yourself to calm down—and have your body listen. Though you may not be able to eradicate the stress-provoking incidents, with autogenic training you will be able to exert some control over your physiological processes and not feel so helpless. You will learn to recognize the signs and symptoms of tension and be able to reduce their effect on your life. *You do not have to be a victim of your own stress response.*

Once you have mastered deep breathing, autogenics can be the next step in your relaxation program. This method is easily learned and success usually increases with practice; the more you practice the exercises, the sooner you will effect a change in your tension level. You can use autogenics whenever you start to feel tense: for a few minutes at your desk, on the bus or in the subway, before going to sleep at night, or at any time you set aside during the day.

Continued ➡

In autogenic training you attempt to induce specific physical sensations that are associated with relaxation. By inducing any of the characteristics of the relaxation response, such as warmth and heaviness, you can break into the chain of physiological changes that occur when you are relaxed. Imagine that these changes are a row of dominoes, carefully stood on end and regularly spaced so that slightly pushing one domino causes all the others to topple over, one after the other. The warmth that you strive for is your perception of increased blood flow throughout the body, especially to the extremities (unlike the stress response, which constricts blood flow to these areas). The heaviness is your perception of the skeletal muscles relaxing (unlike the tensing of the stress response). If you can teach yourself to elicit warmth and heaviness at your command, then the other physiological changes that occur when you relax will follow, as in the domino analogy.

Johannes H. Schultz developed the autogenic method from his experiments with hypnosis. Schultz observed that hypnotized subjects, who had been commanded to relax and were in a state of deep relaxation, experienced two powerful and pleasurable sensations—warmth throughout the body and a feeling of heaviness in the limbs. Schultz developed the autogenic program for people wishing to achieve profound relaxation through self-suggestion, without the help of a hypnotist. Simple, yet effective, word phrases suggest relaxation to the unconscious mind, which then manifests the desired responses in the body.

Some people who practice the autogenic method have learned how to exercise considerable control over their automatic functions and can induce a variety of physical sensations as well as block out the feelings of pain. *Your body can listen, but you must abandon the will, rather than exercise it.* If you try to consciously control your body, you will fail. Passive concentration is the key—you focus on your body while in a state of deep relaxation. The effort necessary for mastering the autogenic technique is not in trying to do it; letting go and giving in to relaxation is the hardest part. Trying too hard will always create more excess tension and make it more difficult for you to learn to relax.

Autogenics produces a state of relaxation that is physiologically identical to that induced by meditation and other Eastern techniques. Unlike Eastern methods, autogenics focuses on physical sensations rather than abstract mental states; the Westerner may be able to understand and achieve deep relaxation more readily by utilizing methods deeply seated in Western culture. Autogenics gives you something concrete to do and experience. *The feedback is fairly immediate—you know if it is working.*

In some people autogenics can work quickly. A registered nurse, who had experienced true migraine headaches for over twenty years, came to me for help. Her headaches occurred three or four times a week, usually while she was working. Aware of the problem of drug addiction in chronic pain sufferers, she did not want to take pain pills; yet she worried that due to her intense discomfort she might make a mistake that would endanger someone's life. If she had a migraine and was dispensing medication, she often found herself checking and rechecking to make sure that the dosages and recipients were correct. She was a highly motivated person and very much wanted relief from her headache problem.

At the initial session I taught her the basic autogenic training phrases, and directed her to practice the exercises by herself at home at least twice a day. When she walked into my office for the second session, she had a big grin on her face. I was surprised because I had not seen her smile during the entire first session, and asked her what had brought about such a radical change in her behavior. She had not had a migraine all week and felt that she finally had control over her headaches and her life. She was absolutely elated.

Twice a day, and when possible, three times a day, the nurse had practiced autogenic training. It worked the very first day. We discussed her rapid progress and what seemed to be, at this time, her cure. She returned for three more sessions, and to her relief, there had been no recurrence of her migraines. The exercises had also taken on a new meaning for her; she found them so relaxing and rejuvenating that she continued practicing and discovered that they were also positively affecting her spiritual growth.

Of course not all people respond so dramatically, but I have found autogenics particularly effective with migraine sufferers; the success rate is about 85 percent. It has also been highly successful in treating high blood pressure, abdominal pain, anxiety, and nervousness.

In Basic Autogenic Training, some phrases imply heaviness, others warmth, others overall relaxation. Suggestions of heaviness are designed to relax skeletal muscles, and when they work, the arms and legs should feel very heavy, as they do when you are deeply relaxed. For those of you who hold tension in the muscles, releasing this tension may dramatically generalize to an overall relaxation. Phrases of warmth suggest increased blood flow allowed by the relaxation of the smooth muscles surrounding the arteries of the vascular system. If you constrict these arteries unconsciously and respond to tension with cold hands and feet, then these phrases will be especially helpful.

Autogenic Positions

Begin the exercises in the sitting or lying position with your eyes closed. Before assuming a position, make yourself as comfortable as possible: loosen your clothing, remove any jewelry or glasses, take off your shoes. These are the basic positions for many of the relaxation exercises included in this book, and I will often refer you to these positions. Learn them now, as correct posturing will facilitate deep relaxation.

Sitting Position

Sit near the front edge of a straight-back chair. Find the spot and position most comfortable for you. Your knees should be bent so that the angle between the calf and thigh is slightly more than 90 degrees. Sit up, as if a string were pulling you straight up through the crown of your head. Let your arms hang down freely at your sides. Now, crumple straight down with your neck bent forward. When you crumple, do it straight down, not forward or backward. Gently pick up your arms and lay them on top of your legs, about an inch above the knees. Spread your fingers. If you feel yourself pulling backward, move your hands slightly forward; if you are pulled forward, move your hands slightly back. There may be a pulling in your neck or shoulders, but as you become accustomed to this position, you will gradually stretch out and become comfortable. This sitting position creates the least amount of muscular tension.

Lying Position

Lie flat on a bed or on the floor. You may support your neck and knees by placing a pillow under them. Some people even prefer to place pillows under each arm. Spread your legs slightly and move your arms away from your torso, keeping your palms down and your elbows out. Separate your fingers so that they are not touching each other. If you are cold, cover yourself with a light blanket. Personally, I prefer the lying position, but if you find yourself inappropriately drifting into sleep, use the sitting position to remain awake.

Autogenic Exercises

I recommend exercising in the afternoon, before dinner, or in the morning before breakfast. It is always best to practice before meals rather than after eating. When you first attempt autogenics, try to reduce all outside distractions. Once you have become adept, you may be able to practice in an ordinary setting without preparation. Autogenics can be practiced for a few minutes at work; instead of grabbing a cup of coffee between phone calls, take ten minutes, request that someone take messages, and relax. Before attempting to practice in your office, you should have practiced at home and be familiar with the progression. There is no right way to experience these exercises; everyone's experience is unique. *Remember not to try too hard—it will only make it more difficult for you to relax.* Passive concentration is the key. Let any extraneous thoughts flow through you and out of you.

These phrases are easily read into a tape recorder; if you wish to use this method, see the section on using tapes in the first chapter.

This can be a vastly effective method of learning how to use autogenic training, though often people stop using tapes after they are familiar with the progression. The Autogenics and Deepening Visualization, which follows the Basic Autogenic Training, is most effective if read onto a tape or if someone reads it to you.

Basic Autogenic Training

Get into a comfortable position, either sitting or lying, and close your eyes. Take a deep breath, and exhale fully and completely. Remember to breathe properly throughout the exercise. Let the day's experiences and thoughts pass through you and out of you. Do not hold onto your thoughts; allow them to go. Watch them flow by as if on a movie screen or like billboards passed on the highway.

Repeat this mood phrase to yourself three times: **"I am at peace with myself and fully relaxed."** Remember to breathe properly, and on the exhalation, breathe away any tension.

Concentrate on feeling heaviness in your arms and legs. Right-handed people begin with the right arm; left-handed people with the left. Right-handed people begin: **"My right arm is heavy. My right arm is heavy. My right arm is heavy."** Left-handed people begin: **"My left arm is heavy. My left arm is heavy. My left arm is heavy."** Pause between each phrase—this is not a race. Take your time, and let any worries or thoughts that may enter your consciousness flow through you and out of you. Feel the heaviness in your arm. Proceed to the opposite arm and repeat the phrase to yourself three times: **"My left arm is heavy,"** or **"My right arm is heavy."** Feel the heaviness in your arm.

Then proceed to the legs, saying to yourself: "My right leg is heavy. **My right leg is heavy. My right leg is heavy.**" Feel the heaviness in your leg. Remember to breathe naturally, and take your time, pausing between each phrase. Then the other leg: **"My left leg is heavy. My left leg is heavy. My left leg is heavy."** Feel the heaviness in your legs.

Then say to yourself: **"My neck and shoulders are heavy. My neck and shoulders are heavy. My**

Continued ➔

neck and shoulders are heavy." Feel the heaviness in your neck and shoulders. Take a deep, calm breath, and exhale fully and completely.

Concentrate on feeling warmth as you relax the smooth muscles in the walls of the arteries. Right-handed people begin: **"My right arm is warm. My right arm is warm. My right arm is warm."** Left-handed people begin: **"My left arm is warm. My left arm is warm. My left arm is warm."** Feel the warmth in your arms; be aware of the pulse and the flow of blood through your entire body. Go on to the other arm.

Then let go of the tension in your legs, saying to yourself: **"My right leg is warm. My right leg is warm. My right leg is warm."** Feel the warmth in your right leg. Continue with the other leg and repeat the phrase to yourself three times. Feel the heaviness in your legs. Remember to breathe slowly and naturally, and let any thoughts flow out of you.

Move on to your neck and shoulders and say to yourself: **"My neck and shoulders are warm. My neck and shoulders are warm. My neck and shoulders are warm."** Feel the warmth in your neck and shoulders, and feel the warm blood flowing through your body. Just allow yourself to remain relaxed, don't try to force the feeling, and be aware of any sensation of blood flow or temperature change. Remember to breathe naturally and calmly.

Slow and calm your heart by saying to yourself: **"My heartbeat is calm and regular. My heartbeat is calm and regular. My heartbeat is calm and regular."** Some people may experience discomfort when they turn their attention to their own heartbeat. If you feel nauseated or light-headed, or notice any other disturbing sensation, change the phrase to: **"I feel calm. I feel calm. I feel calm."**

To slow your breathing, say to yourself: **"My breathing is calm and regular. My breathing is calm and regular. My breathing is calm and regular."** Feel the air completely filling your lungs when you inhale, and on the exhalation feel the warm air leaving your lungs. Pause between each phrase, and say the phrases to yourself slowly and calmly.

Concentrate on warmth in your abdomen, saying to yourself: **"My abdomen is warm and calm. My abdomen is warm and calm. My abdomen is warm and calm."** If you have serious abdominal problems, bleeding ulcers, or diabetes, or are in the last trimester of pregnancy, change the phrase to: **"I am calm and relaxed. I am calm and relaxed. I am calm and relaxed."**

Move on to your forehead, repeating to yourself: **"My forehead is cool and calm. My forehead is cool and calm. My forehead is cool and calm."** Feel the excess blood flowing out of your head. Remember to breathe the calm, full breath; allow any extraneous thoughts to flow through you and out of you.

When you have completed the last phrase, rest for a moment. To bring yourself back to a normal state of alertness, repeat the phrase to yourself: **"I am refreshed and completely alert. I am refreshed and completely alert. I am refreshed and completely alert."** Take a deep, full breath, flex your arms and legs, and stretch. You may wish to repeat the last phrase several more times. Slowly open your eyes.

Were you able to feel heaviness?

Was the technique more successful for one part of your body than another?

Did you experience any sensation other than heaviness?

Were you able to feel warmth?

Any sensation of blood flow?

Did you find the exercise pleasant or disturbing?

Did you feel any resistance to letting go?

If you were unable to feel heaviness in your limbs you may be trying too hard. Remember not to hold on to your thoughts—let them flow through you and out of you. You may have found it easier to feel warmth or heaviness in your arms or abdomen; this is not unusual and the rest will come with practice. Feeling warmth, especially in the legs and feet, may take some time. It took me almost two months of daily practice to feel warmth in my legs, so don't be discouraged if you are having difficulty with this part of the exercise. The feeling of increased blood flow will also be easier to recognize after more practice. The phrase used for the forehead suggests cooling and calming to relax the muscles of the head and face. A warming suggestion would increase blood flow to the brain and scalp, possibly causing a headache for migraine sufferers. Remember that this is the first time you've done the exercise—be patient. If you were able to let go and flow with the phrases, then you are on your way to being a relaxed person.

Practice the entire sequence at least once a day, twice or more if you want to learn more quickly. After you have followed the routine for several weeks, you may find that you can decrease the number of phrase repetitions because your body will be reprogramming itself and responding more readily to the suggestions. Also, after a few weeks reread the questions, and see if your responses are different. You may even wish to keep a journal; but don't use the journal to push yourself too much. This may just make you tenser and make it more difficult for you to let go. Try these techniques for at least a month; it takes that long to learn the phrases and to become comfortable with the exercise. You may wish to add a visualization to your exercise after two to three more weeks. If the combined autogenics and visualization doesn't work after ten to fourteen weeks, you might consider trying a different relaxation exercise.

Autogenics and Deepening Visualization

The author's taped version of this exercise is available at www.dstress.com. Look for Tape #102.

Get yourself into a comfortable position, either sitting or lying, and close your eyes. Take a deep, slow breath, and pause for a moment after you inhale. Exhale fully and completely. Allow yourself to continue to breathe slowly and naturally. Repeat the autogenic phrases to yourself slowly, and allow yourself to feel the heaviness and the warmth.

The first phrase is: **"I am at peace with myself and fully relaxed. I am at peace with myself and fully relaxed. I am at peace with myself and fully relaxed."** Breathe naturally and slowly, remembering to exhale completely. Try feeling the heaviness in your arms, as you say to yourself: **"My right arm is heavy. My right arm is heavy. My right arm is heavy."** Allow yourself to let go of the muscles in your arms as you say to yourself: **"My left arm is heavy. My left arm is heavy. My left arm is heavy."**

Continue to breathe slowly and naturally, and say to yourself: **"My right leg is heavy. My right leg is heavy. My right leg is heavy."** Let go of the tension in your legs as you say to yourself: **"My left leg is heavy. My left leg is heavy. My left leg is heavy."** Now say: **"My neck and shoulders are heavy. My neck and shoulders are heavy. My neck and shoulders are heavy."** Let your shoulders drop; allow the muscles to relax fully and completely.

As you continue to breathe slowly and naturally, say to yourself: **"My right arm is warm. My right arm is warm. My right arm is warm."** Feel the

blood flow through your arm and into your hand, and say to yourself: **"My left arm is warm. My left arm is warm. My left arm is warm."** Allow yourself to let go even more, and say to yourself: **"My right leg is warm. My right leg is warm. My right leg is warm."** Feel the blood flow through your leg and into your foot, as you say to yourself: **"My left leg is warm. My left leg is warm. My right leg is warm."** Now say to yourself **"My neck and shoulders are warm. My neck and shoulders are warm. My neck and shoulders are warm."**

Continue to breathe naturally and completely, while saying to yourself: **"My heartbeat is calm and regular. My heartbeat is calm and regular. My heartbeat is calm and regular."** Feel your strong, even heartbeat. Say to yourself: **"My breathing is calm and regular. My breathing is calm and regular. My breathing is calm and regular."** Feel your deep, full breaths and your complete, slow exhalations.

Continue on, saying to yourself: **"My abdominal region is warm and calm. My abdominal region is warm and calm. My abdominal region is warm and calm."** Then turn your attention to your forehead, and say to yourself: **"My forehead is cool and smooth. My forehead is cool and smooth. My forehead is cool and smooth."**

Breathe slowly and naturally, allowing yourself to breathe away tension with each and every exhalation. Imagine that any thought or experience running through your mind appears to you as a bubble, and just let the bubble float up and out of your consciousness. Just as if you were watching a glass of carbonated water, see the bubbles rise to the surface and burst. Let your thoughts or experiences rise up and out of your consciousness. Don't hold on to any of them—just watch them as they drift by. And just like in the glass of carbonated water, the bubbles gradually decrease in frequency, slowing and finally stopping, leaving the water clear and calm. As you continue to breathe slowly and calmly, your mind gradually becomes calm and clear as you let go of distractions and drift deeper into relaxation and peaceful calmness.

Imagine that you are at the top of a slow-moving escalator, and as you step on, you find yourself gradually riding down, deeper and deeper into relaxation. As you slowly ride down, you can feel yourself becoming more and more relaxed, deeper and deeper into relaxation. Gradually you can feel your muscles becoming heavier and more relaxed, as you allow yourself to drift deeper into a dream-like state of calmness and relaxation. As you near the bottom of this slow-moving escalator, you can see yourself surrounded by your favorite outdoor landscape. It is a calm and beautiful day, and as you step off the escalator, look around at this peaceful, calm scene.

Drift slowly over to the most comfortable spot, and allow yourself to lie down, just sinking into the warm earth. Gradually any excess tension melts away and is replaced by calmness and deep relaxation. Feel the warmth of the sunlight as it gently shines down and warms your hands and arms. Imagine that the sun and warm breezes warm your legs and feet.

Let the warmth of the sun spread to every cell of your body, melting the tension and allowing you to become more calm and relaxed. As the sunlight and warmth flow freely and easily through your body, simply let go of tension and allow yourself to drift deeper into a peaceful, calm state. See yourself completely relaxed, feel the increasing heaviness of your arms and legs as you melt into the earth. Feel the deep state of calmness and relaxation and register it in your mind, so that you can remember it in a fully waking state. Let yourself drift in this state of calmness for just a few moments.

Continued ➡

Every time you practice this exercise you will get better and better at it, being able to relax more deeply and more completely. Every time you practice, the will to control tension increases, and you can relax more quickly. The effects of the calmness and relaxation will carry over with you throughout your day. You will feel calm and relaxed and be aware of tension or excess energy whenever it manifests itself.

Now, gently bring yourself up and out of deep relaxation to a more alert state, gradually letting yourself become more aware of your surroundings, remaining calm and relaxed. Say to yourself: **"I am refreshed and alert. I am refreshed and alert. I am refreshed and alert."** Take a deep, full breath and stretch, letting the feelings of calmness and relaxation carry over with you into a fully alert state. You may wish to take another deep breath and stretch, and then gradually open your eyes.

Did you find this exercise more difficult than the basic exercise?

Did you have any trouble visualizing the bubbles?

Was it easier to feel warmth or heaviness?

Did you want to come out of the deep relaxation state?

Visualization can be extremely difficult for some people, so if this form of autogenics was more difficult for you than the basic exercise, don't feel that you have failed miserably. Once again, letting go and clearing your mind of distractions will make this exercise easier. If you had more difficult visualizing the bubbles in the carbonated water than visualizing yourself outside, you were probably more receptive by the time you reached the second stage of the visualization. Visualization is a skill that improves with practice. Warmth and heaviness, for some people, are easier to feel when the suggestions are accompanied by a visualization. If you found this to be true, then try to make it a practice to always accompany your autogenic sessions with a visualization. Not wanting to come out of a state of deep relaxation is normal, especially if you have trouble relaxing most of the time. Just remember that once you have achieved this state, you can recall that peaceful, calm feeling throughout the rest of your day.

—From *Guide to Stress Reduction*

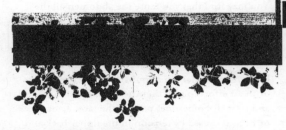

PROGRESSIVE RELAXATION: FROM HEAD TO TOE

L. John Mason, Ph. D

In autogenics words are used to trigger relaxation, focusing on the concrete sensations of warmth and heaviness. In active progressive relaxation specific muscles are contracted and released. Both autogenic and progressive relaxation techniques teach you how to focus on bodily sensations and how relaxation feels. Just as the act of inducing warmth and heaviness generalizes to an overall relaxation response, relaxing localized muscle tension generalizes to an overall relaxation response.

If you feel cut off from your body and find it hard to manifest warmth or heaviness through the autogenics technique, progressive relaxation may be

a good method for you. If your tension expresses itself as a backache, muscle spasm, tight jaw, stiff shoulders, or a tension headache—all forms of skeletal muscle tension—this may be the method that works best for you.

Progressive relaxation teaches you to be more aware of daily tension. Imagine that it is 2:45 on a Friday afternoon. You are waiting in a long line at the bank hoping to cash your paycheck and thinking about all the taxes deducted from your weekly salary. Your neck is stiff, and your shoulders are hunched up around your ears. Because you have practiced progressive relaxation, you are aware of the tension and know how to release it. This tension, in the past, has often developed into a full-fledged backache; now you know how to prevent this tension from manifesting itself later as pain. You zero in on the tension and feel it in your neck and shoulders. After tightening the muscles even further, you take a deep, full breath. As you exhale, you release the muscle tension and feel it leaving your body with the warm breath. Two more full, deep breaths, accompanied by a tension-releasing exhalation, and you are a new person, free of tension and neck pain.

Edmund Jacobsen said, "An anxious mind cannot exist within a relaxed body." Fifty years ago he developed a series of over two hundred exercises designed to relax the muscles by teaching muscle awareness and relaxation through tensing individual muscles. These exercises progress through the musculature—thus the term "progressive relaxation." Jacobsen used the exercises to treat a wide variety of physical complaints, and his research forms the foundation for our understanding of the mind/body awareness processes, and the use of relaxation in healing.

Two kinds of progressive relaxation have been developed from Jacobsen's original exercises: active progressive and passive progressive. In the active mode you tense your muscles and then relax them; passive progressive takes the process one step further and teaches you how to relax your muscles without first tightening them. *I personally find passive progressive relaxation more effective than the active form.* Active progressive can aggravate tension for some people. If you wish, you may go on to the passive form.

Active Progressive

Muscle tensing, followed by a conscious effort to relax the muscles, allows you to recognize clearly the difference between tension and relaxation. Once you feel your muscles tensed and then relaxed, it may be easier for you to induce relaxation. *These exercises are extremely beneficial for people who find it easier to concentrate while physically active.* I have not included Jacobsen's original exercise as it is too lengthy for most people, and it is not generally used for this reason. The first exercise follows his basic structure and incorporates the major muscles. The second, abbreviated version should only be practiced after you have used the first form.

These exercises work well on tape, and if you wish to tape them, follow the instructions in the first section. Many people are able to remember the sequence after practicing only three or four times and find tapes unnecessary. The sequence may be done quickly, but a slow initial session is most beneficial; you can speed up after you learn the basics of muscular relaxation.

Active Progressive Relaxation

Begin by sitting in a comfortable chair in a quiet room, or use the sitting or lying autogenic posi-

tions. Close your eyes gently and take a deep, diaphragmatic breath. Exhale fully and completely, letting the tension melt from your body. Pay attention to your slow breathing and let go of the days tensions and uncomfortable experiences. Relax as much as possible. Remember not to strain to relax as this only creates excess tension.

ARMS AND HANDS

Make a fist with your right hand, and concentrate on the tension as you gradually tighten your fist. Hold your fist tight for a few moments and notice the tension. After a few seconds release your fist and relax your hand. Take a deep, full breath, feel the relaxation, and let the tension flow from you as you exhale. Take a few moments to relax even further. Be aware of all the sensations in your hand and lower arm. Tense your right hand again, and repeat the process.

Do not forget to breathe naturally and let go completely when relaxing. Study the difference between tensed and completely relaxed muscles; become aware of the subtle degrees of tension. Repeat the exercise a third time and focus on any tension you may be holding in your fingers. Feel the tension in each finger, and feel the relaxation. Feel the warmth as the blood flows freely into your hand and each finger. Recognize increased circulation. Breathe deeply and fully, allowing the tension to flow from you.

Make a fist with your left hand. Remember to tense completely and relax fully. Notice any difference in the sensations between the left hand and the right. After clenching your left hand for the third time, take a moment and relax completely. Feel the relaxation in both hands and your lower arms. Now move up your arms to your biceps.

Contract your right bicep as tightly as possible. Concentrate on the tension for a few moments. After a few seconds release your bicep, and relax your entire upper arm. Take a deep, full breath, feel the relaxation, and allow the tension to flow from your body as you exhale fully and completely. Do the exercise two more times, while remembering to breathe naturally. When you have tensed and relaxed your bicep three times, focus on the relaxation in your right arm as it rests limply by your side.

Turn your attention to your left arm. Tense your bicep, and then release it, just as you did with your right arm. Do the exercise three times, remembering to exhale completely after each full breath and to release all the tension. Feel the relaxation in both arms.

Refocus your attention on your right hand and wrist. Spread your fingers apart and bend your hand towards you at the wrist as far back as you can. Feel the tension between your fingers, in your palm, in your wrist, and in your lower arm. Hold this position for a few moments, then relax, letting your hand go limp and releasing any tension in your hand and arm. Breathe away any remaining tightness and relax fully. Do the exercise two more times, remembering to breathe naturally. Feel the deep relaxation in your right arm and hand. Become aware of the increased blood circulation and notice how heavy your right arm and hand have become.

Practice the same exercise with your left arm and hand. Be aware of the difference between tension and letting go into relaxation. Remember to do the hand-spreading, wrist-bending movement three times. Be conscious of the different degrees of relaxation and how total relaxation feels.

Return awareness to your right arm. Stretch the arm out straight at a right angle to your body, pointing your fingers out straight so that you feel tension and a pulling in your arm. Tighten your

Continued ➜

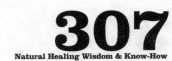

triceps and your whole arm and hand as much as possible. Remember to breathe naturally. Hold your arm in this taut position for a few moments, and then relax your arm completely and let it hang limp and relaxed at your side. Breathe fully and feel the relaxation. Straighten your right arm again; examine the tension and then relax. Repeat one more time and then take a few moments to relax completely, being aware of your right arm and hand. Repeat the entire sequence with your left arm and hand.

Do you feel any unique sensations in your arms?

Do your arms feel longer?

Do you feel tingling or warmth in your arms?

How about heaviness?

Your arms will feel different after doing this exercise. Most people report a sense of added length in their arms; your arms are actually longer because your muscles have relaxed and let go. The feelings of tingling and warmth are the result of increased blood flow, heaviness is experienced because you are more relaxed. This experience may make you more aware of the tension you always hold in your arms. After you practice this exercise for several days, you should notice progressively deeper relaxation and greater sensitivity to subtle levels of tension. If you practice twice a day for several weeks, you should be able to release the tension in your arms and hands completely, and have this relaxation generalize to your shoulders, neck, back, and chest. After two weeks of practice, try tensing and releasing both arms simultaneously.

LEGS AND FEET

Take a deep breath and relax. Follow your breathing, allowing it to slow and deepen naturally. Remember to exhale fully and completely, releasing any tension with the warm air. Turn your attention to your right foot. Curl your toes, and feel the tension as you progressively tighten them. Hold the tension as tightly as possible for a few moments. Be aware of all the sensations in your toes, foot, and ankle. Release the tension and take a deep, full breath, feeling the difference between tension and relaxation. Exhale, letting go of any remaining tightness. Let your breath become calm and regular. Do this sequence two more times, feeling the deep relaxation in your right foot.

Turn your attention to your left foot. Repeat the exercise three times. Remember to tense completely and relax fully, noticing any difference in the sensations between the left foot and the right. After curling the toes on your left foot for the third time, take a moment and relax even further. Feel the relaxation in both feet.

Now, back to your right foot. Bend your foot backward, toes reaching for the top of the ankle and lower leg. Feel the tension; bend it back even farther, stretching as far as you can. Hold for a few moments, and then relax your foot, letting it go limp. Take a deep, full breath, exhaling fully and completely. As you exhale, let go of even more tension; feel the difference between tension and relaxation. Let your breath become calm and regular. Repeat the exercise two more times, allowing your right foot to relax even more with each sequence.

Move on to your left foot. Tighten, and then relax, feeling the tension in your toes, arch, ankle, calf, and knee. Remember to breathe naturally throughout the exercise. Repeat two more times, and then let go for a moment, focusing on the complete relaxation in both feet.

Be aware of your right foot and lower leg. Arch your foot, point your toes, and tighten your lower right leg. Study the tension; tighten even further

and then hold for a few moments. Let go of the tension in your leg and foot, and relax even more by breathing away the tension. Let your breath become calm, and release even more tension with each exhalation. Practice the exercise three times. After also practicing the exercise three times with the left foot, feel the relaxation deepening in both feet and lower legs.

Remember to breathe properly, inhaling deeply and exhaling fully and completely. Tense your upper right leg; feel the tightness in the back of your knee and thigh. Tighten it further for a few moments and study the tension. Let go of all the tightness, and notice the difference between tension and relaxation. As your breath becomes even calmer, let your right leg sink deeper into relaxation. Repeat the exercise two more times, each time letting more of the tension fall away. Turn your attention to your upper left leg and repeat the sequence three times.

Next, turn your attention to your buttocks, becoming aware of the feelings there. Pull them in, tightening these muscles as much as you can. Tense the muscles of your buttocks tighter and tighter. Remember to breathe deeply. Pull your buttocks inward and feel the tension in your hips, thighs, and up and down your legs. Contract even further, hold a few moments at the point of complete tension, then relax. Take a deep, full breath, then exhale, breathing away every bit of remaining tension. Repeat two more times, allowing yourself to slip deeper into relaxation with each sequence.

Are you having trouble releasing all the tension?

Are your feet warmer than usual?

Are you more aware of how much tension you ordinarily hold in your legs?

Letting go is always the hardest part. If you are having a lot of difficulty in releasing the tension, perhaps you should use the passive progressive series. Some people tend to go into muscle spasm when they tense too hard or for too long. If your feet feel warmer, or if you are beginning to notice that they are always colder than the rest of your body, this exercise may be very beneficial for you. The feeling of warmth is the sensation of increased circulation to the extremities. The real benefit of these exercises is in making you more aware of the subtle levels of tension you tend to hold in various parts of your body. Perhaps now you will be more able to notice this tension and release it before it causes you pain. Even if you have not become instantly aware of all the places you hold tension, do not despair; such awareness is often cumulative or occurs suddenly after several weeks of performing the progressive series. After two weeks of practice, you will be able to tense and relax both legs at once and be more sensitive to relaxation and increased circulation in the legs and feet.

BACK AND TRUNK

Arch your lower back and consider the tension. Do not strain too hard, especially if you have a weakness in your back. Tighten slightly, hold for a few moments, feel the tension, and then relax. Take a deep breath, exhale fully and completely, allowing your lower back to relax. Tense your back again, being careful not to strain, and being aware of the tension in your spine, shoulders, and buttocks. You may even feel tension in your neck, chin, and legs. Study the tension, and realize how back tension affects you and how far this tension can generalize throughout your body. Remember to breathe properly and release any tension on the exhalation. Do not hold this position for too long, as you do not want to create too much tension in your back. Repeat once more.

Tighten your abdomen. Hold the tension and study it. Pull your muscles in even further, and then relax. Feel all the organs move comfortably back into position. Breathe calmly and release more tension as you exhale, allowing your breath to be calm and regular. Take a deep breath and release even more tension with the exhalation. When your breath is calm, repeat the exercise two more times.

Next, tighten your upper back and shoulders. Push back your shoulders, as if you were trying to get them to touch behind your back. Once again, do not strain too hard, especially if you have back problems. Hold; study the tension in your upper back, neck, shoulders, and up and down your spinal column. You may even feel it in your head or face. After holding for a few moments, release the tension and relax. Sink into the chair or bed, and relax completely as you exhale away any tension with the warm air. Consider the difference between tension and relaxation. Let your shoulders drop completely. Allow your breath to become calm and natural and repeat the exercise twice more; with each attempt, allow more tension to flow from your body.

Take a deep, natural breath and exhale fully and completely. Feel your rib cage relax as you exhale, forcing every bit of air from your lungs. Recognize the quietest part of the breath when you are wholly relaxed and free from tension, just before the next inhalation. Stay in this quiet space, and force out even more breath. Repeat twice, relaxing your rib cage more with each attempt.

In tensing your back, did you notice any special weak spots where you feel pain or disproportionate tension?

In tightening the abdomen, did you have a sense of the tension you ordinarily hold there?

Where did you feel the strain when you tightened your upper back and shoulders?

Often, people report feeling more tension in some particular area of their back—often the same spot where their backaches originate. This may also be the spot hardest to rid of tension during the relaxation exercises. The abdomen is another place where many people hold tension all the time. Tension is held not only in the muscles that can be consciously contracted and released, but also in the smooth muscles that regulate digestive movements. You may find that you tense the abdomen all the time, as if you were waiting for a blow, or that when you feel threatened, your arms immediately go to cover your abdomen as if to protect an especially vulnerable area. People sometimes hunch the upper back and shoulders in a similarly protective gesture or in an effort to pull their heads in from the world and retreat. Sometimes pain in the face, arms, neck, or head is caused by tension in the upper back and shoulders, even though you do not feel the pain there. Try to remember the discomfort of total contraction and the pleasure of complete relaxation. The next time you are standing in line at the bank, or hunched over your desk, or hiding in a corner at a party, ask yourself which of these two sensations you are closer to feeling. Perhaps after doing the progressive sequence for trunk and back, you will learn how to go along with tension for a moment, focus on the place where it is centered, contract as tightly as you can, and then really let go of it.

FACE AND HEAD

Open your eyes and mouth as widely as possible, as if you were a fish. Hold this position and study the tension in your forehead and jaw and around your mouth. You may feel tension up the sides of your neck as well. Hold this position for a few moments, and then relax your eyes and mouth, remembering

Continued ➡

to breathe naturally. Try the position again, this time opening your eyes and mouth even further. Relax and allow the tension to flow out of your whole face. Remember to unclench your jaw and relax completely, letting every bit of tension and any sign of emotion leave your face. Repeat again, relaxing even more.

Close your eyes and focus on your slow, calm breathing. Then, keeping your eyes closed, tense your face by tightening up around the nose as if you were trying to wriggle your nose. Purse your lips, tighten your jaws, and then tense your entire face just a little more. Hold the position for a few moments and then relax, letting all the tension flow from your face. Breathe away any tension with your calm, even, slow breath. Repeat twice more, remembering to keep your eyes closed throughout the exercise.

Be aware of your forehead; as it relaxes, let it feel smooth and calm. Take a deep, full breath and with the exhalation let your jaw drop, letting all the tension flow out of your mouth, along with the warm air. Feel your face soften into a state of total relaxation. Your eyes are loosely closed, your forehead unwrinkled, your skin smooth. Breathe calmly, slowly, and naturally.

Did you find it harder to relax your face than the other parts of your body?

How often is your face totally relaxed?

Many people find it harder to relax their faces than any other part of their body. This is because the many muscles of the face are in a constant state of tension, expressing emotion and moving when we speak. Even the act of hiding emotion creates tension. You may not know how many muscles you have in your face until you do this exercise. Most people are never without tension in their face except while sleeping. If you often get headaches, you may find that they magically disappear once you learned how to relax your facial muscles.

Abbreviated Active Progressive

After you have practiced Active Progressive Relaxation for three weeks and you can relax profoundly, you may be ready for the abbreviated form. Begin by getting into the autogenic sitting or lying position. Be sure that your back and head are supported. Close your eyes gently, and take a few diaphragmatic breaths and begin to relax. Exhale fully and completely, letting all the day's problems leave your consciousness, and allow yourself a moment of peace at that quiet time of the breath, just after exhalation.

Turn your attention to your right foot and any sensations you might be feeling there. Curl your toes. Tighten them even further and be aware of all the tension in your toes, foot, and ankle. Study this tension, and then relax. Be aware of the difference between tension and relaxation. Take a deep, slow breath, and with the exhalation, breathe away any tension you may still be holding in your right foot. Go on to the left foot, repeating the exercise. Be conscious of any difference in tension level between your left and right foot. Let yourself feel the increased blood flow moving through your toes, your feet, and into your legs.

Move back to the right foot and the lower right leg. Arch your foot, point your toes out, and then stretch to point them out even further. Feel the tension, and then relax, letting go of all the tension. Take a deep breath, and as you exhale, allow all the tension in your foot to leave your body with the warm air.

Tighten your upper right leg. Feel the tension in the back of your knee and thigh, and tense your leg even more. Hold the tension for a few moments, and then relax completely. Feel yourself slipping deeper into relaxation as you take a slow, easy diaphragmatic breath. Exhale fully and completely, allowing the exhalation to take every remaining bit of tension with it. Repeat the sequence with your left leg.

Now, direct your attention to your buttocks. Tighten them, pulling the muscles inward. Hold the constriction for a moment and focus all your attention there; then relax. As you relax, notice the pleasure in letting go of tension, the pleasure of just feeling your calm, relaxed body. Take a deep breath and then exhale, relaxing even more. Feel the relaxation deepen in your feet, legs, and buttocks, and spread to the rest of your body.

Tighten your abdominal region. Pull your stomach in, as if your abdomen could touch your back. Tighten it even further, hold this tension for a moment, and then relax. Realize the difference between tension and relaxation in your abdomen. Breathe deeply and then exhale, allowing all the tightness in your abdomen to flow from your body with the warm air. At the end of the exhalation, pause just a moment to appreciate the total peace of this quiet time of the breath.

Tense your shoulders and back. Study the tension, and then relax. Take a deep, full breath, and relax even more deeply, letting all the tension from your back and shoulders move out of your body with the warm exhalation. Sink into whatever surface you are sitting or lying upon. With the next exhalation, become aware of letting go of even more tension.

Contract your arm muscles and make fists with both hands. Concentrate on the tension and squeeze your arms and hands even tighter. Study the tension and then relax, letting your fingers unfold slowly, as you become aware of the tension gradually leaving your hands. Take a deep, full breath and with the exhalation, let go of any tension remaining in your hands and arms. Be aware of the blood flow returning to your hands; feel the warmth and the tingling. Focus on the heaviness in your arms, and allow your arms to sink into the chair or floor. Take another deep breath and exhale, becoming more and more deeply relaxed.

Squeeze your face tightly around your nose. Purse your lips, clench your jaws, and tighten up your entire face. Study the tension in your jaw and forehead, and then relax. Take a deep, slow, full breath and relax even more with the exhalation. Let your jaw drop slightly. Be quiet and still for a few moments, enjoying the feeling of total calmness and relaxation. Realize how good this state of total relaxation feels.

Did you find the abbreviated form as effective as the longer version?

If you had difficulty feeling relaxed with the abbreviated form, return to the longer form. More practice will make you more comfortable with the progression, which will make it easier for you to relax. Releasing all the induced tension is difficult for many people, and you might want to try the passive progressive exercises that follow.

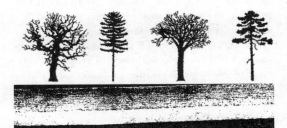

Passive (Gentle) Progressive

The first relaxation exercise I ever tried was a passive progressive sequence. Passive exercises start with the toes and progress to the head, based on the assumption that you first relax those parts of the body that are easiest to relax. I was in a class with a group of other novices, and because it was a warm, early fall day, we moved outdoors. I remember lying in the grass and listening to the voice of the teacher. I experienced a new sense of integration. It was a wonderful sensation to sink into the grass and to feel each set of muscles give up its tension and become part of the balanced wholeness of my body. I hope that the exercises which follow will allow you to have the same sort of deep relaxation.

In the passive form of progressive relaxation, proper breathing and a focus of awareness are combined to induce deep relaxation. The muscles are never intentionally tensed and remain totally unstressed. All tension leaves the body on the exhalation with the warm air. The most important factors in this exercise are the slow progression from one part of the body to another, pausing to focus on the various body parts while in a state of passive rather than agitated attention, and deep breathing to induce relaxation and as the focus of visualization.

Passive Progressive Relaxation

This exercise is available at www.dstress.com. Look for Tape #101.

Begin by sitting or lying in an autogenic position. Try to be very comfortable. To begin, take a few diaphragmatic breaths, exhale completely, allowing yourself to relax. Allow all the tension to leave your body with the exhalation. Let all the daily thoughts, events, and concerns pass through your mind. When you are ready to let go of them, take another very deep breath, and exhale completely, allowing the thoughts to pass out of your mind.

Turn your attention to your feet, for just a moment, and become aware of how your feet feel. Consider the way the skin of your feet feels against the surface of the floor or the bed. Notice the air around you. Is there a slight breeze or does the air feel still? Take a deep, full breath, and then focus completely on your feet. As you exhale, let any tension that you are holding in your feet be released with the exhalation. Then, just appreciate, for a moment, how good this state of relaxation feels.

Shift your focus of attention to your lower legs, and become aware of how your legs feel. If you notice any tension, focus on it. Breathe in, concentrating all your energy on your lower legs, and as you breathe out, let all the tension you are holding be released with the exhalation. If you still notice any tension, take another very deep, very pleasurable breath, and with the exhalation, blow all the tightness away.

Consider your knees and upper legs. Focus on any stress you notice there, any discomfort or tension. Inhale, focusing on the tension in your knees and upper legs, and as you exhale, allow this tension to flow from you, leaving your knees and legs totally relaxed. If you perceive any remaining tension, inhale again, releasing that last bit of tension with the warm air.

Feel your hips and buttocks resting against the floor, bed, or chair. As you take a deep, diaphragmatic breath, be aware of any tension in these areas. Focus on this tension and how it feels. Take a full, cleansing breath, and as you exhale, release the tension with the warm air. If any tension still remains, take another relaxing breath, and just imagine all the stress being carried from your hips and your buttocks by the exhalation.

Continued ➡

Gently consider your legs, from your hips down to your feet. They are probably beginning to feel heavy and relaxed. If there is any remaining tension, focus on it, inhale, and then let go of it completely as you exhale. You may wish to repeat this if you still feel any tension.

Move your focus to your lower back and any tension you may be holding there. Focus on the tension, and as you exhale, release this excess energy with the exhalation. Allow your back to become completely relaxed; let any burden you have been carrying there be lifted with the next exhalation. Focus on your shoulders and upper arms. Breathe in and consider any excess energy or tension that you may be storing there. Realize that you can let go of it, and with the next exhalation, let this tension flow out of your body with your breath.

Turn your attention to your lower arms and hands. Inhale fully and completely. With the exhalation, let all the tension from your lower arms and your hands be fully released. Let your arms sink into the surface upon which you are sitting or lying. If you perceive any residual tension, take another very deep, very satisfying breath and let every bit of stress in your arms or your hands be carried away with it.

Consider your back, your neck, and your head. Be aware of any excess energy, any stored tension, any stress, you are holding there. Focus on this tension, and then take a natural, diaphragmatic breath. As you exhale, send all the tension away and out of you. Now, focus on the top and sides of your head. If you feel any tightness, just inhale, and with the exhalation, allow the top and sides of your head to relax fully. Feel your head sinking into the surface upon which you are lying. Consider your forehead and the upper part of your face. Become conscious of any excess energy or discomfort there. Take a deep, full breath, and as you exhale, allow this tension to flow through you and out of your body. Pause for just a moment at the end of the exhalation to enjoy the peaceful feeling at the quiet time of the breath. Then, take another deep breath, and as you exhale, let go of every last bit of tension in your forehead and upper face.

Gently consider your mouth and jaw. Become aware of any clenching, any stored emotion you are holding. Allow yourself to breathe it away with the next deep breath. Focus your attention on this tension, and then, with the exhalation, let yourself release all this stored tension with the warm air. Breathe again, and as you exhale, let go of every last bit of tension. And with the next breath, be aware of any remaining tension in your neck, head, or face. Notice how it feels, and then with the exhalation, let it all go.

Move your attention to your chest and your diaphragm. If you are holding any tension there, and you sense yourself holding back just a little when you breathe, allow those areas to completely relax. Take another, very deep, very satisfying breath, and allow every last bit of tension to be carried away with the exhalation.

Become aware of how your abdomen feels. If there is any tension you are saving in your abdomen, where you are not allowing the breath to reach, then take a very deep breath, and focus on that held tension. Exhale and allow the tension to flow freely from your body, and allow your abdomen to relax completely. Take another very deep breath, letting the breath flow freely throughout your abdomen, and if there is any residual tension, let it flow from your body with your exhalation.

Consider your pelvis and your genitals. Focus on any excess energy or tension you may be holding there, and as you take a deep breath, really feel this

tension. As you exhale, let go of all the tension. Inhale again, and exhale slowly and peacefully, sending any remaining tension away and out of your body.

Take a very deep, very pleasurable breath, and appreciate the relaxation in your entire body. Feel the heaviness and the warmth. If you can identify any tension anywhere in your body, turn your awareness there and take another deep breath. As you exhale, allow this last bit of residual tension to flow from you and leave you completely at peace. Imagine yourself in this beautiful state of relaxation; your body is heavy and warm. Retain this mental picture, and whenever you start to feel tense, remember it. Focus on it and realize that you can relax completely any time you wish. Take a deep, full breath, stretch, and begin to return to a fully alert state. Inhale again, and become more alert on the exhalation.

Did you find the passive progressive technique as effective as the active?

Did you find it harder to relax some parts of your body than others?

Your relaxation and stress responses are uniquely your own. Some people find the active sequence more effective, others the passive. With either, remember that stress is a habituated response, one that you learned long ago and have been repeating unconsciously, probably for years. To reprogram your body to relaxation also takes time. For a while, it may seem that you are only going through the motions. If you continue, you will notice results. The part of your body that is most resistant to relaxation may be the place where you hold the most tension. For many people, the back, neck, and head are key areas. For others, the pelvis and abdomen are the most difficult to relax. Even if you cannot relax a particular area completely, the passive progressive sequence will make you more aware of how and where you hold tension and how tension feels. This is the first and most important step.

10-to-1 Passive Progressive Relaxation

This exercise is available at www.dstress.com. Look for Tape #103.

This exercise combines counting, breathing, and focusing on parts of the body. Counting provides a rhythm for the exercise and provides the suggestion for relaxation to deepen during the course of the countdown. The exercise lends itself well to taping. If you cannot tape it, you might ask a friend to read it to you for the first few times. Remember to speak slowly and to pause a moment for the first few times. Remember to speak slowly and to pause a moment after each sentence.

Get into a very comfortable position; use either the sitting or lying autogenic position. Allow yourself to begin to relax. Calm and quiet yourself, letting the day's worries leave your mind; you can cope with them later, but for now, just let them go. Gently close your eyes. If you wish, you may open them any time during the course of this exercise.

Begin by taking a deep, slow breath, pausing for just a moment after you inhale, and then exhaling completely. Allow yourself to continue to breathe slowly and naturally. As you sink into this slow, calm pattern of deep, diaphragmatic breathing, imagine that with every exhalation you can release excess energy or tension. You can just breathe it out and away; the warm air that you exhale carries with it all your tension, discomfort, and excess energy. The warm air carries with it anything that is holding you back from complete calmness. Throughout this exercise, continue to breathe slowly and naturally, breathing away tension from every part of your body. As you do this, you will experience a sense of heaviness and increased warmth.

Now, begin to count backward from 10 to 1. Picture the number 10 in your mind, or mentally say the word "ten" to yourself. Continue to just breathe very slowly and calmly, and focus on your entire being. As you become aware of any tension or discomfort, gently shift your attention to it, realizing that you can gradually begin to breathe it away. Just let go of all the tension, and allow yourself to drift deeper into a state of calmness and total relaxation.

Notice that the muscles throughout your body are just letting go of their tension, becoming calm, smooth, and perfectly relaxed. Now, as you picture the number 9 in your mind, or mentally say the word "nine," gently turn your consciousness to your arms and to your hands, letting any tension there be released. If there is any stress, any pain, any excess energy in your muscles, just let go of it, and let the exhalation carry it away. Focus on your upper arms, and as you breathe deeply, let the muscles in your arms go loose and limp. Let the exhalation take the tension with it. Feel the increased heaviness in your arms, spreading down into your elbows, causing all the muscles of your lower arms and of your wrists to become heavy and relaxed. Feel the heaviness gently spreading down into your hands and to your fingers, all the way into each fingertip. As you continue to breathe easily, inhaling deeply and fully, exhaling slowly and completely, just let the tension go with each exhalation. Allow every last bit of tension to leave your arms and hands so that they are absolutely, perfectly relaxed. Pause for just a moment after the exhalation and become even more aware of how heavy and warm they feel.

Now picture the number 8 in your mind, or mentally say the word "eight." Gently turn your awareness to your feet and then your toes. Let go of any tension in your toes and in the balls of your feet; slowly let go of it with your next exhalation. Then be aware of the relaxation spreading to your arches and to your heels, as all the muscles in your feet begin to let go. Now feel the relaxation spread to your ankles and then your lower legs. Take a deep, full breath and imagine any residual tension being carried away as you exhale. Breathe away the tightness in your knees, and let the relaxation freely pass into your upper legs. Continue to breathe slowly and calmly, inhaling fully, and exhaling slowly and completely. Notice any tension in your thighs and just let go of it; allow it to easily leave with the next exhalation. Become aware of the pleasant heaviness in your arms and your legs. Feel them sink into whatever surface you're sitting or lying upon. Just let go, and with each breath, allow yourself to relax further, more and more deeply. As you inhale fully and naturally, drift deeper into a state of calmness and peaceful relaxation.

As you continue to let yourself float, picture the number 7 in your mind, or mentally say the word "seven." Gently carry your awareness to the muscles of your back. Focus on any tension you may be holding there, and with the next exhalation, let them relax. Just let go of any tension or discomfort. Consider the muscles in your shoulders, and focus on any discomfort or rigidity there. Let your shoulders drop and relax, becoming loose and limp. Imagine the muscles on either side of your spine. Let them relax, and let the relaxation spread and follow your spine down into your lower back. Very slowly and calmly, drift deeper into a state of complete peace. Let go of every last bit of tension, and feel yourself sinking deeply into whatever surface you are sitting or lying upon. With each and every exhalation, feel the relaxation spread throughout your body and the feeling of complete peace deepen.

Continued ➡

As you picture the number 6 in your mind, or mentally say the word "six," turn your attention to your chest. Allow the muscles around your rib cage to relax, so that your breathing becomes even more relaxed and easy. Feel your calm, regular heartbeat, and the calm, regular pattern of your breaths. Become aware of the sense of calmness and relaxation spreading down into your abdominal region, increasing with every breath. Your abdomen feels completely calm and relaxed. Pause for just a moment, and let the very next breath take away any excess energy or tension still remaining in your abdominal region. With the exhalation, allow all the tension to leave, so that the energy flows freely, slowly, perfectly throughout your body. Let yourself drift deeper into a dreamlike state of calmness and total relaxation.

As you continue to drift deeper, become aware of the number 5 in your mind, or mentally say the word "five." Turn your awareness to your pelvis and the region between your lower back and the top of your legs. Just let those muscles relax completely, slowly and calmly letting go of any tightness, discomfort, or constriction. Allow the relaxation you are feeling to spread into these muscles as well. As you continue to breathe, realize that you continue to sink deeper into whatever you're lying upon. Feel the calmness spread to every part of your body. Take a deep, full breath and realize that you can control your own tension, that you can gently and slowly breathe it away. You need only allow yourself to calm and slow your breath, and then focus on the tension and let go of it with the exhalation.

Now, picture the number 4 in your mind, or mentally say the word "four," and gently consider the muscles in the back of your head and the sides and top of your head. Just as with the rest of your body, allow yourself to slowly and gently breathe away the tension as these muscles go loose and limp. Let your forehead relax, becoming calm and smooth, and let the muscles around your eyes relax even further. Just let go. Peacefully drift into a dreamlike state of calmness and relaxation. Allow this peaceful feeling to spread down into your face, around your mouth, within your jaw and your tongue. Continue to breathe slowly, very slowly and calmly, releasing every last bit of tension or discomfort. Just drift into deeper relaxation, letting go of all your tension, breathing it away with each slow and gentle breath, letting it go with each exhalation.

As the number 3 appears in your consciousness, or you hear the word "three" in your mind, gently turn your awareness to your neck. Let your head just sink into the pillow or chair or whatever surface it's resting on. As you continue to breathe, deeply and fully, exhaling slowly and completely, all muscles of your neck become loose and limp, and your neck becomes calm and comfortable. This pleasant feeling spreads gently downward into your shoulders.

As you picture the number 2, or mentally say the word "two," your shoulders relax completely and just let go, dropping into an easy, natural position and feeling loose and limp. As your shoulders relax, slowly breathe away any excess energy or tension and allow yourself to drift even deeper, into a deep, perfect state of peaceful relaxation.

Finally, picture the number 1, or mentally say the word "one," and enlarge your focus to your entire being, feeling total calmness and relaxation. Let yourself float further and further, deeper and deeper into relaxation, realizing that you can control your tension any time you wish, just by letting yourself breathe slowly and calmly, and breathing the tension away. This calmness and relaxation will carry over with you throughout the day, the week, and into the future. Pause for a moment, and just

appreciate the calmness. Your energies are flowing freely and easily, and the calmness is spreading to every cell of your body. Just feel the slow, easy calmness easing you deeper into a dreamlike state of complete relaxation. Realize that every time you practice this exercise, you will get better and better at it, and relaxation will come more and more easily. This total relaxation is very good for your mind and your body. It restores every cell of your body completely.

When you wish to complete the exercise and return to your normal alert state, take a deep, full breath and stretch. Allow yourself to feel completely rested and alert. Take another deep, pleasurable breath and stretch. Realize once more before returning to your activities, that you can experience this state of deep relaxation whenever you wish. You do not have to be a slave to your stress response, and whenever you need to, you have the right to relax.

Basic Guided Relaxation: Advanced Technique

This is a sophisticated progressive relaxation that many people prefer. It is best when someone reads this to you or you have taped this exercise for regular use. (This exercise is available at www.dstress.com. It can be found on one side of Tape #202, #203, #204.)

When you are ready to begin, start by getting into a comfortable position in a space where you will not be unnecessarily disturbed for at least twenty minutes. As you sit back or lie back, check to see if your arms and legs are in a relaxed and uncrossed position. Let your shoulders release tension and let your neck begin to relax by letting your head just sink back comfortably into the pillow or chair. Check the muscles of your head and face, especially the muscles around your eyes, even your eyebrows, and the muscles around your mouth, including your jaw and tongue.

Before we begin, let me remind you that I do not want you to try to relax too quickly. In fact, I do not want you to try to relax at all! Because, without any effort, you will be able to drift as deeply into relaxation as you wish by just letting go of stress, thoughts, and physical tensions.

To begin, start by taking three deep, slow diaphragmatic breaths, pausing after you inhale; then exhale fully and completely. You might even imagine that as you exhale you begin to release thoughts, tensions, even discomforts with the warm breath that you breathe out and away. (Pause.)

After these first three slow breaths, continue to breathe slowly, but naturally. As you breathe, please turn your attention to the relaxation that is beginning in your arms and down into your hands. You may feel that one of your arms is just a bit more relaxed than the other. It may be just a subtle difference in which one arm feels slightly heavier, as if the muscles in that arm are more loose or flexible. Or perhaps, one arm feels slightly warmer, as if blood and energy are flowing more freely and easily all the way down that arm into the hand and fingers. (Pause.) Or perhaps, both of your arms are equally relaxed. The only thing that matters is that you continue to breathe slowly and naturally, and perhaps you can begin to feel yourself drifting deeper into a dreamlike state where you feel greater calmness and comfort, and where you begin to develop even greater awareness and control.

As you continue to breathe slowly and gently, become aware of the relaxation that is starting down into your legs and feet. You may feel that one of your legs is a bit more relaxed than the other—slightly heavier, as if the muscles in that leg were more loose or flexible. Or perhaps, you may find that one leg feels slightly warmer, as if the blood

and energy is flowing more freely and easily all the way down that leg into your foot and toes. (Pause.) Or perhaps, your legs feel equally relaxed. What matters is that you continue to breathe slowly and gently, and allow yourself to drift deeper into this dreamlike state of calmness, comfort, and control.

Perhaps you can feel the control growing stronger as you feel yourself begin to sink back into whatever you are sitting or lying upon. Let the tensions begin to melt away.

The muscles of your back begin to relax even deeper. You feel the muscles there soften or loosen as you slowly breathe away any unwanted tension. The relaxation spreads to the other muscles of your back, even up into your upper back and your shoulders. Let your shoulders drop down into a more comfortable position. Feel the control grow stronger as your head sinks back, completely supported by the pillow or the chair; now your neck begins to relax even more. Even the muscles of your head and face can relax more.

Perhaps you imagine yourself outdoors on a warm and pleasant day. Perhaps you are standing near a pond of water; the water is calm and clear, and the surface is smooth. You feel the warmth of the sunlight and the warm breezes. If you were to drop a rock or a stone into the water, you could watch as the waves or the ripples spread across the surface of the pond in every direction. In much the same way, you imagine that you send soothing and cleansing waves of relaxation down from the top of your head, in every direction, to soothe, heal, and cleanse every muscle and cell of your body. These waves begin to drift down to relax the muscles at the top and sides of your head. Feel the waves drift down to deeply relax your forehead, letting it go calm and smooth. The waves wash down to relax the muscles around your mouth; even your jaw can loosen a bit better. The waves now slowly spread down to soothe and relax the muscles of your neck and shoulders, and now they drift down through your arms, slowly all the way down into your hands and fingers. (Pause.) Now the waves slowly drift down through your back and your chest. Your breathing is more calm and regular. Your heartbeat is more calm and regular. As you breathe slowly and freely, you may even be able to feel your stomach and abdomen begin to let go and relax more freely. Your lower back and pelvic area now relax further. The waves of relaxation begin to spread down your legs, slowly drifting all the way down and out through the bottom of your feet and into your toes.

Now you watch the pond of water once again become calm and still. The water begins to settle and become clear. Even the surface becomes calm and smooth again. You may wish to turn away from the pond and follow a pathway that takes you to perfect place. . .a place where you can be yourself and feel calm and comfortable. Once you arrive there, you look around to find the most comfortable place to lay down. As you drift over to that spot, you just sink back into whatever you would be sitting or lying upon. As you settle back, you feel the warmth of the sunlight gently shining down on you. You begin to soak up the warmth as the tensions just melt away. You may even be able to hear the sounds that surround you. Like the sounds of running water, birds, or warm breezes. Perhaps you even smell the fragrance of salt air, flowers, grass, or of the woods that may surround you.

Imagine that you soak up the warmth of the sun. You begin to breathe in the sunlight. As you fill with this warming, healing light and energy, remember that as you relax, there will be an increase of blood flowing more freely and easily to every cell of your body. Each cell is bathed in an increased supply of oxygen and nutrients to help

Continued ➡

heal and recharge itself. As the cells begin to fill with health and happiness, you can continue to drift in this peaceful state of calmness and relaxation. Though you remain calm and comfortable, you begin to see yourself healing fully and completely. You may even be able to see yourself in perfect health, smiling and celebrating in the sunshine on this warm and beautiful day. You see yourself active, smiling, playing, celebrating, dancing. . . . Remember that every time you practice this exercise you will get better at it. You will be able to relax more deeply and more completely. You will be able to let go more quickly. And the effects of the calmness and comfort will last longer, carrying over throughout your day, enabling you to be more calm and efficient with your available time and energy.

If you are using this exercise at bedtime, or if you wish to drift off to sleep now, then you can begin to do so. Continue to breathe slowly and gently. Focus on the relaxation in your arms and your legs, and drift off into a deep sleep where you are able to rest completely. When you awaken, you will be fully rested and alert.

If, on the other hand, you wish to awaken from this deep relaxation now, then begin to see yourself returning to this room, bringing the feelings of calmness and comfort back with you to a more fully waking state. You may wish to feel the bed or the chair beneath and slowly awaken, letting the feelings of calmness, comfort, health, and joy return with you to a fully waking state. Take a deep breath and slowly release it. You may wish to take another deep breath and stretch, becoming wide awake, feeling refreshed and alert.

—From *Guide to Stress Reduction*

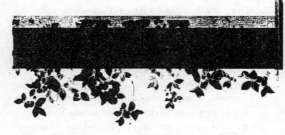

VISUALIZATION: IMAGINE

L. John Mason, Ph D.

During the course of this chapter, I have often asked you to imagine a hypothetical situation. You have even tried to envision impossible occurrences. In the Three-Part Breathing exercise, you visualized your lungs filling with air; when you did the Autogenics and Deepening Visualization, you pictured your thoughts as bubbles just floating away and later imagined yourself on a slow-moving escalator. Visualization is the use of positive suggestion through visual imagery to change a mental and/or physiological state. When you create a mental picture, your body can actually respond to the visualization as if it were a real experience. This technique can aid in relaxation and healing, or in changing destructive habits; used preventively, it can maintain your good health. It is often used as an adjunct to other relaxation techniques.

With visualization you attempt to affect unconscious processes (the stress response, immunological defenses, conditioned responses) with a conscious suggestion—a mental picture of the desired change. Although it is not understood exactly how a mental image can affect a physiological process, research shows that visualization can change your body's functioning. *Especially dramatic in the treatment of illness, visualization has successfully helped people suffering from terminal diseases.* Carl and Stephanie

Simonton are leading researchers on the effect of positive visualization on cancer. Dr. Carl Simonton discovered that tumor visualization (in a relaxed state of mind) in conjunction with traditional therapies, such as radiation, seems to have a much greater success rate than traditional therapies alone. The Simontons have had remarkable success in treating cancer patients with visualization.

Others have used their techniques with great success. A colleague worked with a six-year-old boy whose cancer had metastasized throughout his body. His parents were undergoing a lot of marital problems, and the boy felt responsible. He was always trying to reconcile his parents; when his efforts failed, he felt helpless and guilty. He was undergoing chemotherapy which had painful side effects; naturally he was resistant to the therapy. The chemotherapy was only moderately successful; his life expectancy was estimated to be about one year. The child began visualization therapy in conjunction with his chemotherapy. He imagined his cancer as a monster and his natural defenses as white knights. This was his own imagery; the therapist helped him to develop this imagery into a systematic visualization program. At the same time, the child and his parents began family counseling. This helped him to feel less responsible for his parents' problems and less helpless to control his own life.

The child's disease began to show signs of remission. In his visualization sessions, he reported seeing the monster weakening and the knights growing stronger. He told his visualization therapist that the monster would be conquered by the white knights by his next birthday. His objections to medication grew more vehement and the chemotherapy was discontinued. By the time of his birthday, he informed his therapist that the cancer wasn't there anymore—the monster was dead. His perceptions were accurate: the remission was complete and he showed no signs of cancer.

A sense of helplessness and the fear of losing his parents' love preceded the boy's disease. This is not at all uncommon, as helplessness and the loss of a loved one often seem to generate cancer—cancer often occurs six to eighteen months after the death of a loved one. Any significant emotional trauma that seriously impairs one's will to live can prefigure cancer. Visualization can rally the natural defenses and raise the spirit and positive energies.

Certain factors contribute to the success of visualization therapy. You should:

· Want to get better, or remain healthy. Ambivalent feelings or attachment to secondary gains may interfere.

· Be relaxed. Tensions seem to block the success of the visual suggestion.

· Use a positive visualization. A negative visualization will achieve negative results. Think in terms of becoming completely healthy, not in terms of becoming less sick.

· Visualize immediate results. The visualization must be phrased in the present tense.

First mentally picture your ailment. In the case of the little boy, his picture was not an accurate representation of the disease, but since the image of the white knights was real for him, it was very effective. *If you have a very powerful sense of the configuration of your illness, you should use that in your visualization.* You may wish to consult a medical text or your doctor. Some therapists feel that the more medically accurate your visualization, the more successful you will be. But if it is easier for you to imagine your disease as a weed eventually removed by a beneficent gardener than as a diseased cell being attacked by antibodies, then trust the stronger image. Don't use visualization as the only method of healing. If something is seri-

ously wrong, do not ignore it, or put off getting professional advice. Use visualization as an adjunct.

Visualization can be used to maintain health. See yourself in perfect health, exactly as you wish to be. See yourself doing something active, smiling and celebrating feelings of perfect health. You may know people who get a cold every four months; three and one half months go by, and they begin to wonder when the next cold will strike. They are programmed for the next cold. By programming continual positive health, you can reprogram yourself from the sickness model and prevent illness.

Just as visualization is effective in the control of disease, it can be useful in removing tension and stress from your daily life. *The same factors which influence the success of healing apply to relaxation visualization therapy.* You might want to imagine the tension in your body and the release of that tension, just as you would picture your disease and its cure. By visualizing relaxation, you are programming future relaxation and giving up the image of yourself as a tense person.

Habits and fears can be changed or reversed if you visualize the desired behavior. If you want to lose weight, picture yourself enjoying healthful, nonfattening foods. See yourself as a thin, attractive person wearing a particular garment in a smaller size than you now wear. If you have had negative sexual experiences, picture yourself having a joyous, mutually satisfying sexual relationship. If you are attempting to learn a new skill, picture yourself proficient.

Visualization Exercises

Tape the following exercises, or have someone read them to you. This will facilitate your involvement and make your visualization easier. You can change the visualization to fit your needs. Mentally phrase your objective in a positive way, leading to the desired response. If you wish to control your eating habits, do not think, "I will not eat junk food." Instead think, "I feel full and satisfied eating natural, healthful foods." Be sure you state the suggestion in the present tense. Remember, you are reprogramming your unconscious mind to achieve what you would like; you need to demand action now. Let the unconscious find a way to make it happen. People with inflammations should use cool colors (blue and green) instead of warm colors (yellow, gold, and red) in the following exercises.

Visualization for Relaxation

This exercise is available at www.dstress.com. Look for Tape #104.

Use the sitting or lying autogenic position. Gently close your eyes. Take one deep, slow breath. After you inhale, hold for a moment, and then exhale fully and completely. Allow yourself to continue to breathe slowly and naturally. Imagine that with each and every breath, you can breathe away tension or anxiety and allow yourself to relax more and more. As you continue to breathe slowly and naturally, imagine that any thoughts or memories that are running through your consciousness appear as bubbles, about to float up and out of your consciousness. Be aware of these thoughts, but do not hold onto any of them. Just watch them as they float by.

Imagine that you are watching a glass of carbonated water and all the bubbles are rising to the surface. See these bubbles float up to the surface, and as they burst, let go of any thoughts still in your consciousness. Watch the glass of carbonated water, and see the bubbles gradually decrease in frequency, slowly, slowly, until the water is clear and calm. Watch as your thoughts flow through your con-

Continued ➡

sciousness and gradually slow, as your mind becomes calm and clear, as it peacefully rests in quiet serenity. Let yourself drift even deeper into calm relaxation. Remember to breathe slowly and naturally.

As your mind calms and clears completely, thoughts or distractions leave you and you can focus on the various parts of your body. Allow your muscles to relax fully and completely, and as you become more and more deeply relaxed, your muscles just let go. Your muscles become heavy, flexible, and calm. With each and every exhalation, you breathe away more and more tension from your muscles.

Picture yourself at the top of a very slow-moving escalator. As you step onto the long escalator, begin to slowly ride down. Hold on to the side, and slowly drift down, down, down. Deeper and deeper you drift into a calm and relaxed state of mind and body. As you ride the escalator down, count backwards from 5 to 1. Imagine the number 5 in your mind, and say the number to yourself. Breathe slowly and calmly, and allow the tensions to flow out and away from you. Let yourself drift deeper into relaxation. Focus on relaxing your arms and your hands, letting the muscles go completely loose and limp. Relax your upper arms, and then your elbows, your lower arms, your wrists, your hands, down to the tips of your fingers. Feel the heaviness gradually increase in your arms and in your hands, as your muscles just let go and relax. Breathe calmly and naturally, exhaling fully and completely, while you slowly ride down the escalator. Feel the increased blood flow and warmth spreading down your arms and into your hands.

Visualize the number 4 in your mind, and say it to yourself. Gently turn your awareness to your legs and your feet, allowing your legs to relax fully and completely. Allow all the muscles to just let go, and the tension to melt away from your body. Feel your ankles and your feet relax, and allow this relaxation to spread to your knees and to your thighs. Feel your legs sinking into whatever you are sitting or lying upon, as the muscles let go and relax even further.

Continue to breathe slowly and naturally, as you see the number 3 in your mind. Say the number "three" to yourself, and realize that you are more relaxed now than you were at number 4. Allow your abdomen to relax, feeling all the muscles just let go. Your abdomen is relaxed, as you gently loosen all the muscles in your chest, and just breathe away any excess muscle tension. The muscles in your back relax, going loose and limp, as you just sink back, deeper and deeper into relaxation.

You are slowly nearing the bottom of the escalator. Visualize the number 2 in your mind and say it to yourself. Continue to let go of any remaining tension, and realize that you are more relaxed than you were at number 3. Relax the muscles of your shoulders and your neck, while breathing slowly and naturally. Exhale fully and completely, and feel the tension leave your body with each and every exhalation. Let the relaxation spread to your head and your face, letting your forehead become calm and smooth. The muscles in the back and the sides of your head and neck become loose, flexible, and free of tension. As you breathe slowly and calmly, the muscles around your eyes relax, and you simply let go of the tension in your jaw, your mouth, and your tongue. Let yourself drift deeper into a dreamlike state of calm relaxation. Just let go of as much tension as you wish to, by just breathing it away with each and every exhalation.

Become aware of the number 1, and say it to yourself while visualizing it in your mind. As you continue to breathe slowly and calmly, turn your awareness to your neck and your shoulders, letting your head sink into the pillow or chair. Just let go completely, and let your shoulders drop. Allow your entire body to relax, loose and limp.

As you continue to ride down the escalator, deeper and deeper into relaxation, let go and allow yourself to drift even further into calmness. Picture yourself getting to the bottom of the escalator, and as you step off you are surrounded by your favorite outdoor scene. You are in your favorite outdoor place on a calm and peaceful day. You are there all by yourself, noticing the beauty of the blue sky, the green grass, and the golden sunlight brightening to white light. Pick a very comfortable place, and go and lie down. Picture yourself just letting go, sinking into the ground, and letting the tension melt away, being replaced by calmness and relaxation. Continue to breathe slowly and naturally, and with each inhalation breathe in the warmth of the sunlight. Feel the calmness and serenity of this peaceful, beautiful scene.

Feel the warmth of the sunlight on your arms and hands and the warm breezes blowing on your legs and feet, warming you deep within. This gentle, golden sunlight is peaceful and healing. As you inhale, feel the golden sunlight fill you completely with brilliant golden-white light, warming your body. Your heartbeat carries this energy freely and easily to every cell of your body. Imagine every cell of your body bathed in golden-white light, nourished with oxygen and nutrients. As you continue to breathe in the golden light slowly and peacefully, every cell is able to absorb the healing light and energy, the oxygen, and the nutrients. Every cell becomes strong and vibrantly alive. You can see each cell grow healthy and strong. See each cell as a garden plant, slightly parched, growing robust and strong, healthy and revived, as you water it with golden light.

Health and energy, joy and happiness, well up within you. You feel full of health and happiness, and deeply at peace with yourself and the universe. Any time you wish to relieve yourself of tension and anxiety, and wish to replace these feelings with happiness, calmness, and health, all you need to do is breathe slowly and calmly, allowing yourself to relax. Any time that you wish, you can enjoy this beautiful, healing scene once again, restoring yourself with calmness and relaxation. You have control over the tension. You choose to breathe it away. You may let go of it at any time you wish.

Deep within you, there will remain a core of calmness and light, a being of light that dwells within your heart. It is your soul, your spirit. This being of love and light knows many parts of you. It sees and accepts your strengths and your weaknesses and realizes that they are tools that you can use to learn all of the lessons in life. This golden-white light and being grows brighter every time you practice your relaxation. It allows you to accept yourself even more, because you take the time to do really positive things for yourself, through calmness and relaxation, happiness and health, will carry over with you throughout your day, and throughout your week. Every time you practice this exercise, you will get better and better at it and be able to relax more deeply and more completely, more easily and more quickly. Remember that you have the choice to let go of tension by breathing it away and the freedom to feel calmness and relaxation.

Now gradually allow yourself to become more alert, bringing yourself back to the room you are in. Gently make yourself more and more alert, bringing with you into your completely alert state the feelings of calmness, relaxation, happiness, health, and joy. See yourself coming back to the room, and feel the chair or bed beneath you. Say to yourself: **"I am refreshed and alert. I am refreshed and alert. I am refreshed and alert."** Count to yourself from 1 to 5. At 1, feel yourself coming back to the room. At 2, you are becoming more alive and conscious, feeling your calm heartbeat. At 3, you are more alert. At 4, you begin to open your eyes. At 5, you are fully and completely alert. Take a deep, full breath and stretch. Let the feelings of calmness and relaxation carry over with you to your fully alert state. If you wish, take another deep breath and stretch, letting yourself become fully and completely alert. Remember that you have the choice to let go of tension by slowing and calming your breath.

Did you have any difficulty visualizing the carbonated water?

Did you find the image of yourself on the escalator pleasing?

Did you have to search for an outdoor place, or did one immediately come to mind?

When you ordinarily relax, do certain visual images usually come to mind?

Visualization is more difficult for some people than others. If you had a great deal of difficulty visualizing the carbonated water, you might try doing a breathing exercise first. This will put you in a more relaxed state and may make visualization a bit easier. Some people have difficulty controlling the imagery; for others distracting images may constantly crop up in their mind. If this happens, you might want to give yourself the freedom to explore those images. Perhaps you found that the escalator ride elicited a sinking or falling feeling. If this is the case, eliminated some of the escalator phrases from the visualization. A fantasy of the perfect garden may replace the recollection of a real locale; some people think of a childhood scene that has become idealized in their memories. Sometimes when you are not doing this kind of exercise but are using some other mode of relaxation, you will find that particular images may seem to be associated with the relaxed state. You may wish to incorporate these images into a visualization, or use them to become more aware of your inner life.

Relaxation and Self-Healing Visualization

One of the potentially best uses for visualization is to promote healing or for health maintenance. After initial relaxation is achieved, positive images and sensations can be used to reprogram the unconscious mind to optimum health. Remember that the autonomic functions, which are generated by the unconscious part of the mind, are responsible for maintaining proper metabolic equilibrium and for the not yet fully understood process of healing. The most important part of this exercise is to see yourself in perfect health, not in the future, but right now in the present.

Make yourself comfortable, and assume one of the autogenic positions. Take a deep, slow breath, and gently close your eyes. Exhale fully and completely. Inhale again, and see the number 1 in your mind. Hold your breath for a moment, and then exhale, visualizing the number 2. Be sure to exhale fully and completely, breathing away tension with the warm air. Inhale, visualizing number 3, hold for a moment, and then exhale visualizing number 4. Repeat the exercise until you have established your own natural, slow, calm rhythm. With each exhalation, let go of as much tension as you can, while passively allowing yourself to scan your body for excess tension. Without becoming alarmed, be aware of any place you are holding tension.

Imagine that with each exhalation your tension is being carried out with the warm air. Let your everyday thoughts and annoyances drift through

Continued ➡

you and out of your consciousness, as if they were credits at the end of a movie. Watch them gradually pass by and leave the screen blank. See yourself on the screen, lying in a meadow on a calm, beautiful, warm day. Gradually shift your perspective, slowly, slowly, so that you are looking down on your body. Watch your body become smooth and quiet, releasing any held tension and conforming to the contours of the meadow. You are completely alone, protected from any intrusion or distraction. Feel the warm sunlight shining gently upon you and spreading to your arms and hands, your legs and feet, your abdomen and your back. Sink deeper into the warm, soft meadow.

Feel the warm breezes blow against you, warming you to the very core of your being. See the beautiful, natural colors, the green of the grass, the soft, rich brown of the earth, and the deep, beautiful blue of the sky. Listen to the wind blowing and rustling the leaves and branches of the trees, and hear the birds' faint melody against the sweet running waters of the stream. See yourself relaxing more and more, drifting deeper into relaxation. Drift deeper into a beautifully relaxed state, becoming calmer and more peaceful. Feel yourself melting into the warm, receptive earth, becoming totally relaxed and at peace.

Become aware of your heart beating, and focus on its regular, even rhythm, pumping blood throughout the body, sending it anywhere that still feels tense or cool. See the lungs expanding with each breath and directing oxygen to each and every cell. Scan your body lightly, looking for any place where you may still hold tension, and gently breathe away the tension. See and feel the blood flowing easily and freely throughout your body, unrestricted to every cell. As the blood flows throughout your body, it carries rejuvenating oxygen and nutrients to each and every cell. The cells become vibrantly alive and healthy with each full and complete breath. Picture increased blood flow to your hands and your feet.

Send increased blood flow to any organ in your body that needs extra support or healing, gradually and slowly increasing the blood flow. See that organ becoming fully responsive and healthy, as the blood carries away the toxins. The organ begins to function perfectly, exactly as it is supposed to, as you help it return to its normal state with your own deep breathing. Visualize yourself in perfect health, smiling and celebrating, doing something active, dancing or walking, or sunning in the beautiful golden sunlight. See and feel yourself in perfect health, completely relaxed and free of any tension or anxiety.

Call upon this feeling of relaxation and health even throughout your day, and feel calm and relaxed once again. Every time you practice this exercise, you will get better and better at it. It will become easier and easier for you to relax, and the deep relaxation will happen more quickly each time. You will relax more deeply each time you practice. Allow this feeling of calmness and relaxation to be with you throughout your day. If you have any illness, each and every breath you take is gently healing you.

Take a deep, full breath, and exhale fully and completely. Gradually become aware of the surface you are sitting or lying upon, while maintaining a feeling of calmness and perfect health. Allow yourself to become fully alert, stretching and getting ready to return to your normal activities.

Was it difficult to watch yourself on a movie screen while feeling bodily sensations?

Did you feel in two places at one time?

If you have an illness, do you feel anxiety when you start to think about that part of your body?

In your dreams you may often observe your behavior from a distance, while also experiencing the feelings and actions associated with the behavior you observe. If you had difficulty with this part of the visualization, try to experience the sensation of being in two places at one time without subjecting it to rational thought. If you have an illness, it is natural for you to feel upset when you focus on that part of your body; but try to maintain the same easy, passive attention that you accepted in the rest of the exercise. After a while you will be able to experience a calm state of mind even when you turn your focus to your illness....

Magic Carpet Ride

This exercise enables you to use the creative centers of the mind to create the sensation and scene of flying off for a few moments of vacation from daily pressures and activities. As you use this technique, learn to develop an appreciation for detail and let your mind gently absorb all the beautiful, natural scenes that you may explore. You may treat this as a game, but it can help you to curb the unnecessary buildup of stress.

Get into a comfortable position, and close your eyes. Begin by taking a deep, full breath and exhaling fully and completely, allowing the last bit of air to leave your lungs. Do the breathing exercise with which you are most comfortable, until you are in a state of deep relaxation. Feel the relaxation spreading throughout your body. With each and every breath, feel any excess tension leaving your body with the warm air. Gently scan your body and locate any spot where you may still hold tension, and then breathe it away with an exhalation.

Picture yourself outdoors on a calm, beautiful spring day. The sun shines down and warms your arms and hands, your feet and your legs, your abdomen, your back, and your face. You become as calm and as comfortable as you would like to be.

Imagine that you are lying on a magic carpet, free to travel anywhere without effort. You are in complete control, safe and peaceful. No one is there to distract you or make any demands on you. Drift more deeply into relaxation, just enjoying the sensation of total calm and serenity. Flow freely with the drifting sensation as if you were gently floating on a raft on a warm and beautiful summer day, on a calm, warm, shallow lake. Feel yourself floating gently, deeper and deeper into relaxation. As you sense the feeling of floating, remain calm and sense the magic carpet beginning to float up off the ground. You feel very safe and at ease with your surroundings. The magic carpet rises a few inches above the ground, allowing you to enjoy the floating sensation even more. It is so peaceful that you relax even more and drift deeper into deep relaxation.

You can float as high as you wish to go and control both the speed and altitude of the magic carpet. You can look down and around and see all that surrounds you, as you remain totally calm and relaxed. You are free to fly anywhere you can imagine. If you wish, experiment with flying faster and then slower, higher and then lower. Perhaps you would like to visit some exotic locale or just get a different perspective on your daily environment. Feel the warm air currents blowing gently against your body and the warm sun shining down upon your magic carpet. Travel this way for a few minutes, noticing any detail that attracts you. Leave all your worries and thoughts behind you, and enjoy this brief vacation from your daily life. When you are ready, slowly return to the point of departure. Touch down gently, sinking into relaxation.

Calm and relax yourself, savoring any special moment you may have experienced in your ride.

Remember as much of your trip as you wish to and bring this feeling of calm relaxation to mind whenever you feel tension or anxiety. Gradually bring yourself to a state of alertness; take a deep, full breath and stretch. Take another breath and become fully alert.

Do you associate the floating sensation of the magic carpet ride with relaxation?

Do you ever have dreams or fantasies about flying or swimming in air?

Some people find it natural to associate deep relaxation with the sensation of floating or flying. Others feel more comfortable with the sensation of sinking or descent. If you found the ride anxiety-provoking, try increasing the size of your rug or imagine yourself floating on a soft, billowy cloud. If you often dream or fantasize about flying, this visualization may be easy for you to imagine; if you are always earthbound, consider what the freedom of flight might represent for you. You can use this exercise for a few moments during a break in your workday and actually feel as if you had taken a short vacation.

Wiseperson Guide Visualization

Some people have important questions and do not seem to have anyone to help them get answers. This exercise enables you to consult with your own innermost self (intuition, if you want to see it that way). You may wish to just enjoy this exercise to see what questions come up. People sometimes become conscious of problems they had not realized were causing mental or emotional distress. You may use this for personal growth, rather than for problem solving. Whatever you choose to explore, let this be a pleasant way to relax and learn to make better connections with the subtle, but powerful parts of your unconscious mind.

Get into a comfortable position and begin to relax. Inhale deeply, filling your lungs completely with air. Exhale, forcing every last bit of air out of your lungs. Picture your lungs as being divided into three parts. Take another deep breath and visualize the lowest part of your lungs filling with air. Then, imagine the middle part of your lungs filling, and finally the upper part. Your lungs are completely expanded, your shoulders back, your abdomen slightly pushed forward. Begin the exhalation. Visualize the air leaving your upper lungs as your shoulders drop slightly. Feel your rib cage contract as the air leaves the middle portion of your lungs. Pull in your abdomen to force out the last bit of air from the bottom of your lungs. Repeat the lung visualization twice. Continue to breathe calmly, at your own natural pace.

As you relax more deeply, picture yourself outdoors on a calm, gentle day. You are all alone, feeling very relaxed and at peace with yourself and the universe. Feel the warmth from the sun, healing your hands and your feet, penetrating to the very core of your being. You are relaxing more and more and slipping into deep relaxation.

You are in a clearing in a wooded area. Begin to become aware of your environment. Notice the colors, the smells, and the sounds. You are totally safe and comfortable in this special place. You are safe from outside distractions or interruptions. You belong here and can come back to this place any time you need to feel deeply relaxed.

A path appears leading up and away from your resting space. Slowly and gently get up and follow this path upward, until you come to a very sheltered, protected, peaceful clearing. A warm, bright fire burns in the center of the clearing. Gently become aware of your wiseperson sitting on the

Continued ➡

other side of the fire. The wiseperson sits calmly and peacefully, receptively awaiting your arrival. You are calm and relaxed as you approach to place another log on the fire.

Greet your wiseperson guide warmly, and sit together for a few moments. Look at your guide's face and gently become aware of the wiseperson's all-knowing presence. Breathe slowly and naturally and with each breath become more conscious of the safeness of your surroundings. When you feel totally relaxed, ask the wiseperson the question that you have brought with you. Listen carefully to the answer, letting it become clear and meaningful.

Rest for a few moments and absorb the wisdom that has come to you. Thank your guide, who embraces you gently and lovingly and gives you a special gift in remembrance of this occasion. Remember that any time you wish you may return to meet with your guide. You walk back down the path to your original resting place, feeling calm and satisfied. You are relaxed and happy, and your heart is full of joy and love.

Sit down in your resting place and focus again on your natural, slow breathing. Take a deep, full breath, exhale, and then stretch. Take another breath and begin to bring yourself back to a fully alert state. Carry with you the memory of this experience and the feelings of calmness and relaxation.

Did your wiseperson guide look as you expected?

Did your wiseperson guide undergo any transformation as you sat together?

Did a question come to mind immediately? Did you understand the answer?

When I first did this exercise, I expected my guide to be a wise, old, bearded fatherly figure. To my surprise, although the guide was a man, he was middle-aged, clean shaven, balding, and appeared to be wearing a pharmacist's smock. Because my expectations had been so different, it took me a moment or two to accept this guide. Don't be stunned by, or try to repress, the nature of your wiseperson guide. This visualization is not to reinforce what you already know, but to provide insight into your life. For some people, the wiseperson guide appears in one form and then undergoes a transformation right before their eyes. A man may become a woman, a woman may become a man, or the guide may become a person who has been important in your life. If a question did not come readily to mind, don't worry. Sometimes there is one crucial question which you must ask and other times the question is of less importance. The answer you received may be ambiguous, or it may not have directly addressed the question you posed. Each time you do this visualization, the appearance of the wiseperson may become more definite and the answer more coherent.

Deepening Relaxation

These abbreviated visualizations can be used to induce relaxation or to deepen relaxation when combined with another technique. Used alone, they will be most effective once you have become adept at the longer exercises and your body is accustomed to relaxing on cue.

10-to-1, 5-to-1 Count

The most basic and probably the most widely used deepening technique is counting backward slowly from 10 to 1. As you count, visualize each number, release more tension, and relax more deeply with each exhalation. You may combine counting with a short progressive relaxation, viewing and feeling the major muscle groups with each descending number, relaxing them more and more. Start at your neck and shoulders and work down to your toes; then go back to your face. You may also abbreviate this technique by counting backward from 5 to 1. Remember to focus on the number, seeing it in your mind and relaxing more deeply with each descending number.

50-to-1 Count

Another counting technique that works well for most people is counting backward from 50 to 1. As you count each number, insert the sequence 1, 2, 3, between each number. For example: 50, 1, 2, 3, 49, 1, 2, 3, 48, 1, 2, 3, and so on. If you actually visualize each number and let yourself be totally occupied with the exercise while you count backwards, your mind will take a nice vacation from extraneous thoughts or problems. Remember to let all the tension melt out of your body with each and every exhalation. This breathing technique is great for getting to sleep!

Escalator Ride

This exercise is often combined with autogenics or a longer visualization, but you can use it alone or combine it with any other relaxation technique. Imagine yourself riding an escalator that is slowly moving downward, deeper and deeper into relaxation. See and feel yourself slipping more deeply into relaxation as you ride gently downward. Combining this visualization with counting backward is particularly effective. Hold onto the moving escalator rail so that you feel secure. You may also imagine that you are riding down in an elevator, watching the floors descend and relaxing more deeply as you pass each floor. Walking down stairs can be used in a similar manner.

Melting Relaxation

Imagine yourself lying in a calm and comfortable place. Watch as the various parts of your body relax more and more. Feel them relax more than they ever have before, melting into whatever you are lying upon. Let your body melt completely into relaxation.

Watching the Clock

Imagine a clock with one hand moving backward. As it moves counterclockwise, relax more and more as it passes each number. When it gets to 11, you are more relaxed than you were at 12. When it reaches 10, you are more relaxed than you were at 11. When the hand eventually reaches 12 again, you are deeply relaxed and at peace with yourself. The clock hand should move very, very slowly. An alternative to watching a clock is to watch a pressure valve. Imagine that as the valve moves counterclockwise, the pressure is released and with it, your own tension.

Bubble Visualization

If you are having trouble with mental distractions, imagine that all your thoughts or problems are bubbles, floating up to the surface of a glass of carbonated water. As the bubbles reach the surface they burst and all your worries are released into the air. See and feel the word "calm," as you watch the bubbles slowly rise to the surface. Watch the bubbles until the water is completely clear and your mind is no longer distracted. This exercise can be inserted in any other technique if you are having trouble maintaining passive concentration.

—From *Guide to Stress Reduction*

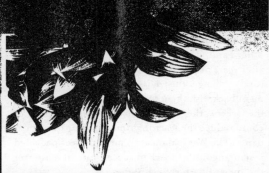

MEDITATION: EAST MEETS WEST

L. John Moson, Ph.D.

While meditating once, I saw myself as a drop of water in a stream. The stream was flowing from the mountains to the sea. I experienced the stream as a symbol of life; all the other drops of water were people and objects moving through life. I felt that I was everywhere in the stream at once. I saw the fast currents, the slow currents, and the eddies of the stream, as stream grew into river and swirled toward the ocean. I was one with all the drops of water in the stream; I was one with all the people and things in the world. I felt great joy. All of this happened in an instant, and yet I can recall this powerful experience, see it again, and describe it at any time. The impact of the symbols etched the vision indelibly into my mind.

Most of the relaxation techniques covered in this book originated in Europe or North America and grew out of a Western scientific and philosophical tradition. Meditation, which is thousands of years old, developed in Eastern cultures which pre-date Western civilization. I emphasize Western approaches because I find that readers can more easily relate to their philosophical bases. *For our purposes, meditation will be viewed as a relaxation technique outside of the various religious and ideological contexts in which it developed.* For many, meditation is only one part of a life philosophy.

Proponents of the diverse schools of meditation believe that different states of mind can be achieved with different meditative practices. Some forms of meditation seek to free "energy flows" throughout the body. These energy flows have not been recognized by Western medicine or scientific measurement. Inconclusive evidence does not mean that energy flows do not exist; it only means that a way to measure or explain them in Western scientific terms has not yet been found. In the same way, Western science may not be able to quantify subtle changes in state of mind that occur with different meditation practices.

The beneficial effects of meditation which can be measured are those associated with deep relaxation. These effects resemble the benefits of sound sleep, but in meditative states the mind remains awake and alert. (Most teachers of meditation warn against falling asleep during practice.) Meditation has been shown to relieve stress-related disease. Meditators show a substantial reduction in the frequency of such stress-related complaints as headache, gastritis, and insomnia. In blood pressure studies, it has been found that meditation significantly reduces blood pressure during the practice and enables the subjects to maintain lower blood pressures.

Skilled meditators develop a heightened awareness of their own autonomic functions and a heightened capacity for self-regulation. Elmer and Alyce Green studied yogis who were famed for their ability to control their own bodies and withstand extreme stress—such as pain—without manifesting a stress response. The results of the study are amazing. These holy men could slow their own heart rates to three or four beats a minute and warm one

Continued ➡

hand to a temperature 10 degrees higher than the other hand. This sort of control is only achieved after years of practice. In an interesting cross-cultural exchange, the yogis took biofeedback equipment back with them to India. In their work with the Greens, they realized that such equipment could reduce the learning times of their own students. The Western measurement devices provided instantaneous feedback of success rate in mastering the ancient Eastern techniques.

In *The Relaxation Response*, Herbert Benson reports on his exploration of the physiological effects of meditation. Benson began his research by investigating Transcendental Meditation (TM). TM was brought to the United States in the 1960s by Maharishi Mahesh Yogi, as a readily accessible meditation for uninitiated Westerners. In TM, an instructor selects a mantra, a particular Sanskrit word or sound, for each student. This sound is then repeated mentally while sitting still in a quiet place. The initiate is instructed to concentrate completely on the mantra, letting distractions simply pass over and through the consciousness. Subjects report that after repeated practice "the mantra seems to disappear from mind," they "fall into a space of rich darkness," and "the mind becomes blissfully quiet." They often report a loss of the sense of time passing while remaining fully awake.

In studying TM meditators, Benson found that the subjects were in a state of deep relaxation while repeating the mantra. Their oxygen consumption was markedly lowered; heart rates were slowed; galvanic skin resistance was raised; and blood pressure was lowered. *Benson went on to discover that these positive effects were not exclusive to TM and that individually selected mantras were unnecessary.* He devised his own modified mantra-repeating meditation and achieved similar physiological readings. Certain crucial factors, isolated by Benson, induce relaxation during meditation. They are:

- A quiet environment. At least when beginning to practice, the fewer external distractions the better. More advanced meditators may be able to shut out distractions despite the environment.

- An object to focus attention on. This can be a word, sound, physical object, an area on the floor or a wall, or a physiological function which can be monitored, such as breathing. It is important to concentrate on one thing only and cut down on the usual mental noise.

- A passive attitude. A willingness to let go of all distractions and troubling thoughts and an avoidance of ordinary linear thinking are most important. Refrain from considering the meditation as a performance.

These factors are usually stressed by most schools of meditation for those just beginning practice. They can be taken as guidelines for the meditations included later in this chapter.

All meditations direct attention and alter states of awareness. In our usual thinking, we progress quickly from thought to thought— the mind races and attention is scattered. We usually think in words and then become inundated by our own continuous string of verbalizations. We seldom attend to only one thing at a time or concentrate wholly on the action we're performing while performing it. *In meditation, attention is focused and we become wholly engaged in a single behavior.* Attention is cleansed of preconceptions, abstract beliefs, and distracting input so that phenomena are perceived more directly. Most practiced meditators speak of getting in touch with a self outside of thought, outside of social definition and cultural role. In my drop-of-water vision, I experienced a sense of being at-one-with-the-all

and of losing my self. This experience is common in meditation. Although meditations work by narrowing the focus of attention, the results are to enlarge the sense of being and eliminate the subjective distinction between self and environment.

The meditations provided here, with the exception of the Candle Meditation, are all twenty minutes long. They can be used once or twice a day, preferably before breakfast and before dinner. Always meditate on an empty stomach and do not meditate when you are likely to fall asleep. Consistency and discipline are important. Allow three to eight weeks to see results. Begin with the basic Yogic Mantra-Repeating meditation, Zen Breath-Counting, or Shavasana. You can use the Candle Meditation concurrently to help develop your powers of concentration.

Your first experience with meditation may not be entirely positive. A friend of mine, an attorney, went to a meditation class because he was suffering from recurrent bouts of anxiety. He had recently joined his uncle's law firm and was under a lot of pressure from the senior partners. Many of the clients had known him since childhood and didn't accept him in his new more authoritative role. The class was held in the local YMCA gymnasium. His classmates were already sitting in the middle of the room as he walked in and across the floor and then realized that everyone else was barefooted, their shoes in a neat line by the door. His every step echoed as he walked back to the door to take off his shoes and pick up a mat to sit on. The teacher explained the breath-counting meditation and then advised the class to "just sit" and count their breaths.

It had been a long time since my friend had just sat still anywhere. He began to feel nervous and a little rebellious. Most of his days were spent pacing, either before his uncles desk or in his own office, talking into a dictaphone. What good could just sitting still do him? Then the real distractions began. With each breath, the tip of his nose itched. He felt the urge to sneeze but denied it since the room was so quiet. No one else so much as squirmed. Then his back started to itch as well, and the sensation jumped all over his body. The backs of his knees throbbed. The mental distractions were as prevalent as the physical ones. He thought: " 1 (inhale) Did I leave my keys in the car? Someone is probably driving it away right now. 2 (exhale) Why did my uncle make that snide remark this afternoon? If he finds out I'm here, he'll think I can't take the pressure. 3 (inhale) What do I get for dinner if I make it through this ordeal?" At that thought his stomach growled. He repeatedly lost count of his breaths and one thought led to another, and some to whole narratives. But eventually, for only a moment, the rhythm of his own breathing carried him.

Zen Meditation

The meditation which my friend experienced is the most basic form of Zen meditation. In the more advanced forms of Zen, you do not narrow your focus of attention, but open your awareness to all the phenomena around you. You attempt to perceive everything with a clean, unappraising mind. This requires a high degree of discipline and self-regulation. Zen Breath-Counting develops discipline and self-awareness. It is performed while sitting still in one place, as sitting still in one place is an integral part of confronting yourself and shutting down noise. But Zen does not always require that you sit in one place; some Zen meditations are done while walking or even running. I have slipped into a meditative state of consciousness during a long, slow run, when my rhythm was regular and

effortless and my mind became calm. After running for several minutes in this state of mind, I came back to ordinary consciousness with a curious, but pleasant blankness.

Zen Breath-Counting

Begin by sitting in a comfortable position. The autogenic sitting position is fine, or if you prefer, use the traditional Zen cross-legged, half- or full-lotus. If you are sitting on the floor, you might want to use a small pillow to help support your buttocks and align and balance your body. Your spine should be erect, your torso perpendicular to the chair or floor, your head straight on your neck. You should feel comfortable, and your body weight should be balanced. Half-close your eyes so that they are unfocused and turned downward. Take a few deep, diaphragmatic breaths and begin to clear your mind. Let go of all the worries and concerns of the day. Allow your mind to slow down.

Focus your attention on the area of your lower abdomen. Imagine that there is a balloon in your abdomen and that with each inhalation the balloon is inflated. As you exhale, the balloon is deflated. Keep your focus of attention on your abdomen and see the balloon being inflated and deflated, filling and emptying. Feel the air move into the balloon. Feel the walls of the balloon expand. See the balloon inflate completely and then slowly deflate until the walls collapse on each other. As your breathing becomes more comfortable and begins to regulate itself, turn your attention from your abdomen to the air coming in and leaving your nostrils.

Begin to count your breaths, beginning with the next exhalation as 1. Count the next inhalation as 2, the next exhalation as 3, and so on, up to 10. Then go back to 1. If any thoughts come to mind, just let them pass over and through you. Do not hold on to them but do not reject them too vigorously either. Just allow them to come and go. Do not evaluate them, and do not judge yourself for having them. If you lose your focus of attention, relax your breathing and go back to 1. If you start to lose count for any reason, do not try to pick up where you left off; just go back to the number 1.

If you begin to carry on long internal monologues or fantasies, just relax and begin to count again. You can always return to the easy rhythm of your own breath, the sound of air entering and leaving your body, the feeling of air at your nostrils. Let your breath carry you and breathe itself. If you begin to breathe unnaturally, to hyperventilate, or to hold your breath, just attempt to relax all the muscles in your chest and abdomen. Return briefly to the image of the balloon to restore the easy pattern of your breaths. Then go back to your counting. Continue for twenty minutes.

What sort of distractions did you experience?

Was there any turning point at which the exercise became easier?

Distractions are the rule, not the exception. The body will resist sitting still and the mind will resist being quieted. Especially since you ordinarily program your body to keep moving and your mind to keep thinking, reversal of this process will not be immediate. In your normal workday you may be in a state of emotional arousal that you are unaware of, until you try to sit still and calm down. Distractions range from the usual string of mental verbalizations to visual fantasies. Thoughts are going to appear in your mind. The important thing is not to hold on to them and not to evaluate them. If a particular thought or image recurs, you might want to take a look at it when you are not meditating. Distractions can be illuminating—sometimes the meditative state can provide insight into what's really bothering you.

Continued ➡

Often people speak of a turning point at which the exercise becomes easier. This may not occur for weeks. It is similar to the turning point in acquiring any new skill; the gains in competence may be cumulative but are perceived as sudden. Sometimes you must get through the same hurdles and obstacles each time you sit down to meditate. Don't worry, they will probably fall away after the first few minutes of the meditation.

Shavasana

Shavasana (Sanskrit for "corpse pose") is another breathing exercise. It comes from the yogic tradition. Unlike the other meditations provided, it is performed in a reclining position. In research on this meditation and hypertension, subjects could lower their blood pressure an average of eleven points during the exercise, after a period of regular practice.

Basic Shavasana

Lie on your back with your legs slightly spread. Your arms should be separated from your torso, your palms open and upward. Make your body as straight as possible; your spine erect; your neck in a straight line up from your shoulders; your head erect on your neck. You should be comfortable and feel no undue strain anywhere in your body. Your breathing should be unrestricted.

Begin by taking a few deep breaths, and allow all the worries and concerns of the day to leave you. Allow your mind to begin to run down. Continue to breathe deeply and allow your breathing to establish its own easy rhythm. Focus your attention upon your breath. Become aware of the cool flow of air into your nostrils as you inhale, the warm flow of air out of your nostrils as you exhale. Focus on the point of your nostrils at which the air enters and exits your body. Let your body breathe itself. Do not force your breath; do not hyperventilate.

Feel the coolness at the tip of your nostrils, and pause for just a moment after the inhalation. Then exhale, fully and completely, feeling the warmth at the tip of your nostrils as the air passes out of your body. Pause again for just a moment after the exhalation. These pauses are the quietest times of the breath.

If any distractions come into your mind, let them go; you want to be aware of only your breath, of that pleasant flow of air into and out of your nostrils. Watch the thoughts just roll through your mind, remembering that you can choose to return to them at the end of the meditation, but letting go of them for now. Feel the warm air leaving your nostrils, the cool air coming in. After twenty minutes of focusing only on your breath, take another deep breath and stretch. Clench your fists for just a moment, and return to your normal consciousness, saying to yourself: **"I am refreshed and alert."**

How did this experience compare to the Zen meditation?

Did you find yourself getting sleepy in the reclining position?

You will find this experience somewhat different from the Zen meditation. Some people find counting easier but cannot detect the difference in temperature between air inhaled and exhaled. For many people, lying down is associated with sleep and makes them automatically sleepy. If this is true for you, stick with other meditations until you are more acquainted with meditative states. ...

Mantra-Repeating Meditations

Mantra-repeating meditations, like TM and Benson's variation, are common in the yogic tradition. Another form is the chant in which a mantra is sung, sometimes with musical accompaniment. In this case, the sound may be varied with each repetition, by variations in the rhythm or the inflection. This same sort of variation will probably occur in your mind; you may hear the sound stretched out or repeated at varying intervals. The mantra will probably start to sound "different" to you after you have repeated it a number of times.

Yogic Mantra-Repeating

Sit comfortably in a chair or on the floor as in the Zen Breath-Counting meditation. Your breathing should be unconstricted. Begin by taking a few deep, cleansing breaths, and allow all of the day's activities and concerns to wash over you. Just let them pass without allowing them to bother you. Do not hold on to any of them. Begin to focus upon your breath, breathing slowly and naturally. Let your body breathe itself, calmly and slowly. Do not force your breath or hyperventilate. Breathe away any experience of the day that may be distracting or disturbing you. As your mind begins to clear and your breathing begins to take care of itself, sense a greater calmness and relaxation coming over you.

Take a moment to scan your body and become aware of any held tension. Turn your attention to your feet and your legs, up to your abdomen, then to your chest, your arms and hands, shoulders, neck, and head. Let go of any tension remaining anywhere in your body. Just breathe it away and allow everything to go loose and limp. Sink into whatever surface you are sitting on. Continue to breathe slowly, releasing any tension in your back. Your jaw and tongue are relaxed; your face is calm and smooth.

Shift your attention back to your breath, which has established its own regular and even pattern. Begin to focus on a word or sound. Choose a word that does not have a lot of specific associations for you. Benson suggests the word "one." You may use a perfectly meaningless sound if you find the sound pleasant. Concentrate on the mantra, hearing, seeing, thinking, feeling nothing else. Whenever your consciousness wanders from the word, gently bring it back. See it for an instant written before you, or isolated on an otherwise blank movie screen. Continue to focus on this mantra, hearing it over and over again. After twenty minutes of this meditation, picture yourself coming completely out of this state. Make a fist with each of your hands and take a deep breath. Exhale fully and completely and open your eyes. Say to yourself: **"I am refreshed and alert."**

Did you have trouble concentrating on your mantra?

How did this meditation compare to Zen Breath-Counting or Shavasana?

Distractions are the most common occurrence during this or any meditation. Sometimes adding the visual sense, in mentally seeing the word on a screen, helps to clear the mind. Make note of how this meditation differs from Zen Breath-Counting or Shavasana. The overall feeling of relaxation should begin to be familiar.

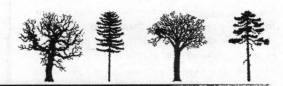

Visual Focal Point Meditations

The next two meditations utilize a visual focal point for focusing attention. They come from the yogic tradition. The visual focal point replaces a repeated mantra or your breathing as the center for awareness. When you look at an object this way, you may start to feel as if your eyes have become your hands and have touched the object. You may also feel a strange sense of unity with the object, as it fills your consciousness and you seem to merge with it.

Candle Meditation

This meditation is only five minutes long. You may repeat it twice in one sitting. It is designed to help you see more clearly and to develop your powers of awareness, attention, and concentration. It may also help you develop your ability to visualize.

Sit in a comfortable position so your breathing is unobstructed and your spine straight. There should be no undue pressure on any part of your body. Take a few deep breaths to begin to relax and clear your mind. Take just a moment to let the day's worries and distractions wash over you, as your breathing establishes itself in a fine, comfortable rhythm.

Place a lighted candle three feet from you. The room should be semidarkened so that you can see the candle well, but not so dark that there is a lot of glare when you look at the candle. Gaze directly at the flame for several minutes. Try to focus completely on the flame and not on a visual distortion. Then, close your eyes and press your palms against the lids.

See the flame again in your mind's eye. Concentrate on keeping this mental image of the flame as vivid as the sight of the real flame. Examine the image of the flame in your mind. Do not let it fade, become distorted, or disappear. Hold your palms against your eyelids for a few minutes. If the image starts to fade, look at the candle again for just a moment, and then shut your eyes and attempt to hold the image in mind. After a few minutes, move your hands away from your eyes and down onto your knees. Relax completely. Take a few deep breaths, and let the image go.

Did you have trouble holding the image of the flame?

The afterimage of the flame appears on your retina after you close your eyes. Holding onto this image and keeping it bright can be difficult, but the more you repeat this exercise the easier it will become. The image of the flame can be a model for you when you try to visualize brilliant light in the visualization and meditation exercises.

Spot-Staring Exercise

Sit in a comfortable position. Use either the autogenic sitting position or any other position you have found comfortable for the sitting meditations. Your back should be straight and your breathing unconstricted. Keep your eyes half-open, gazing upon a fixed object or a space. Either use a lighted candle's flame, a small object like a stone or shell, or a spot on the floor or wall. Avoid intricately detailed or patterned objects. Your focal point should be about three feet in front of you.

Take a few deep breaths and cleanse your consciousness of all distractions. Release any held tension anywhere in your body and let your breathing begin to carry you. Fix your gaze on your visual focal point and continue to breathe slowly and naturally. Do not force your breath and do not hyperventilate. Just continue to breathe, while focusing your entire consciousness on the point that you are gazing at. There is no room in your mind for any-

Continued ➜

thing but that point. If any thoughts or experiences from the day crop up, just let them roll through your consciousness. Watch them as if they are on a movie screen, just drifting by. Remember that you can always choose to return to any thoughts, memories, or impressions that are important.

Breathing slowly and naturally, become aware of any tension in your arms, hands, shoulders, or back. Let all the muscles of your arms, hands, shoulders, and back just let go. All of these muscles become loose and limp, as you continue to breathe. For just a few moments, consider your feet and legs, and if there is any tension there, allow it to just melt away. Allow your entire body to relax completely. Continue to gaze at your point, breathing slowly and calmly. Relax all the muscles of your head and face, allowing your jaw to relax and then your tongue. You face becomes calm and smooth. Let all the muscles of your neck relax, and then your chest and abdomen. Feel the breath coming freely into your chest and then into your abdomen. Then, allow the warm air to leave your body, leaving your abdomen and then your chest. If there is any tension remaining anywhere in your body, just breathe it away as you exhale.

Your body is just breathing itself. Your eyes are on your point, and you begin to lose yourself in it. You can relax deeper and deeper, allowing yourself to find the most comfortable position, settling yourself, stilling yourself, slowing your heart, and breathing in your calm, easy, natural pattern of breaths. Your whole being becomes centered in the point you're gazing at. The only other thing in your consciousness is the sound of your easy, natural breathing, the feeling of cool air entering your body at your nostrils, and the feeling of warm air leaving your body at your nostrils. You are drifting into an ever deeper state of relaxation, becoming more and more centered in that point. You drift into an even deeper state of relaxation, imagining that you can drift to the calmest, most peaceful spot, safe and absolutely peaceful. (Continue to gaze at your visual focal point for about five minutes.)

If you have drifted away from your point, gradually draw yourself back, becoming aware of your slow, deep, natural breathing. Fix your eyes again upon that point and allow yourself to really see it without anything else clouding or distorting your sight. See it as if you were touching it with your hands. Let that point be the center of your being. Remember now that all of the memories and experiences of this meditation can carry over with you, up and out of this meditative state, bringing them with you to a state of full awareness. Let the calmness and the relaxation carry over with you throughout your day and throughout the coming week. Feel the slow, deep relaxation. You can recall this feeling of serenity whenever you wish to for relaxation. Each time you practice this meditation, you will get better and better at it, more able to relax and more able to concentrate your attention on one point. Your meditative state will grow deeper.

Now tighten your fists. Take a very deep breath and stretch, letting yourself return to a state of normal consciousness. You may wish to write down any of the important thoughts or travels that you have experienced in your meditation. Take another deep breath, stretch, and become fully alert.

How do you find concentrating on a visual focal point as compared to focusing on a mantra or your own breathing?

Some people find it easier to focus on a visual object than on a mentally repeated mantra. The mantra is verbal and may stimulate you to produce other internal verbalizations. It may be easier for you to center yourself on a visual point. By all means try both forms of meditation.

Symbolic meditation comes from the yogic school. Instead of concentrating upon a meaningless mantra, you choose a word, scene, or object that holds some higher, symbolic meaning for you. It was during this meditation that I had the experience with which I opened this chapter. I cannot really explain why I feel so strongly about this experience or why it has had such a profound effect upon my life. But I do know that meditation provides for consciousness growth in a way that other relaxation techniques do not—and I find this particular meditation especially powerful.

The meditation is divided into three parts. In the first part, focus your attention fully upon the object or word you have chosen. This might be a word like "love," "peace," "calm," a specific landscape, or a star, cross, or other symbol that holds some meaning for you. In the second part of the meditation, allow your mind to go blank. Concentrate on keeping your mind as blank as an empty movie screen. In the third part of the meditation, close your hands and visualize pure white light surrounding you and filling your being.

Symbolic Meditation Exercise

Begin by sitting in a comfortable position. Use any of the sitting positions that you have found comfortable for the other meditations. Get into this position, and spend a few moments clearing your mind. Allow any disturbing or distracting thoughts or emotions to wash over you. Just let them pass through your consciousness. If you focus on any of them, just become aware and then let them go. You can always return to them later. As these ideas just float through and away from you, begin to breathe slowly and naturally. Take a few deep, diaphragmatic breaths, and with each exhalation, allow any worries or tension to be exhaled with the warm air. Your mind begins to calm and clear, and you begin to relax. The various parts of your body gradually become heavier and more relaxed. Continue to breathe slowly and calmly, letting your breath breathe itself and carry you.

Now place your hands together, palm to palm, and begin to focus on the word or symbol you have chosen. Hold this symbol in your mind. For the first ten minutes of this exercise you will just concentrate on your symbol, seeing it clearly in your mind. Avoid all distractions, internal verbalizations, or other thoughts. Be aware only of the symbol you have chosen and concentrate all your energies on it. (Allow ten minutes for this contemplation.)

If your mind has drifted, bring it gently back to your symbol. Try to see it clearly and become aware of its essence. Experience it with all your senses. Your breathing should remain calm, slow, and natural. Repeat the symbol over and over again in your mind. If it is a scene, explore it completely. When your mind wanders, just gently bring it back to center on the symbol. Now take a few more minutes to continue to concentrate, focusing all your energy upon the essence and feeling of the symbol you are contemplating. (Allow five minutes for further contemplation.)

Continue to concentrate on your symbol, while becoming aware of your breathing. Focus now on breathing very slowly, very calmly, very deeply. Open your hands and lay them on your lap, palms up. Put your mind into neutral gear so that it is perfectly blank. Imagine that you are staring at a perfectly blank movie screen. Whatever images crop up, whatever pictures come from your consciousness, sit back and watch them float by, as if you were seated in a

theater and they were moving by on the screen. Be aware of them but do not hold onto them.

Also be aware of the feelings of calmness and relaxation throughout your body. Start with your legs and work your way up through your torso, to your arms and legs, and up into your head. Gently and slowly make a survey of your body, feeling the total calmness and relaxation spreading. The tension is just melting away. Now just focus on the blank screen, not letting any distractions or interferences get in the way. (Allow five minutes for this contemplation of blankness.)

Clench each of your fists tightly, and then take a very deep breath, and stretch. Picture yourself surrounded by a white, absolutely pure light. Picture yourself standing in an all-white room. Imagine that you are outside in the snow on a beautiful, sunny day and all you can see for miles around you is white snow. You are jumping into a pool filled with milk. You are totally surrounded by white light; it absolutely fills you; you can see nothing but pure, white, brilliant light. Take another deep breath and stretch, becoming fully alert.

How did you find this symbolic meditation as opposed to the other meditations in the chapter?

Symbolic meditation offers individualized experiences. Each time I practice the meditation, my experience is different. Experiment with different mantras, and be receptive to the different experiences you may have. This is a good meditation to practice from time to time as a way of gauging your personal growth and exploring the changes in your psyche.

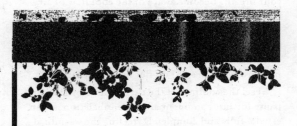

BIOFEEDBACK: CONVERSATIONS WITH A MACHINE

L. John Mason, Ph. D.

Imagine that you are a child again, absorbed in a game of "Hot and Cold" with a friend. You cover your eyes while your playmate hides a piece of candy. When you open your eyes and begin the search, your friend provides clues by calling out the words "hot" and "cold." The object itself is considered hot and the distance from it, cold. You dance around the room, peering over surfaces, scanning the shelves beyond your reach. When you approach the hidden candy, your friend screams, "Warm, warmer, getting hot," and as you take a wrong turn she chides, "Cooling off . . . brrr, it's the North Pole." Through a series of trial and error moves, always adjusting your behavior according to clues, you narrow down the territory. Taking smaller and smaller steps, making infinitely tinier moves, you finally discover the candy. At that moment your friend yells out, "Burning, burning up . . . you're on fire!"

"Hot and Cold" is a feedback system in which a measure of temperature provides a reading of proximity. Without consciously thinking about each move, the child alters his or her movements in order to stay "hot" and find the candy. Biofeedback works the same way. Monitoring devices provide a

Continued ➡

measure (a line on a graph, a blinking light, a buzzer, a tone) of autonomic physiological functions. Through a series of trial and error alterations in behavior, you strive to maintain the desired reading (a fork in the graph line, a blinking rather than a lit light, a sounding buzzer, a sounding tone). When you control the reading, you are also controlling the automatic process being monitored. The way in which you learn to control these processes is more complex than simply changing your location to find a hidden piece of candy.

Biofeedback training was first used clinically in the 1970s. It has quickly become important to the study of stress and is a popular technique for stress reduction and relaxation training. Biofeedback is the use of any instrument or technique to monitor physiological processes and feed back a measure of their function to the individual being monitored. *The beauty of biofeedback is that it allows systems to be monitored that could not otherwise be measured.* Once given information about these functions, we can learn how to consciously alter their functioning. Learning that we can control processes formerly considered beyond conscious intervention has revolutionized our understanding of the autonomic nervous system and all our beliefs about the nature of the control we can exert over our bodies.

Biofeedback has opened up research into the mind and body relationship and the interactions that produce psychosomatic illnesses. There is still much to learn about the control we can achieve outside of the biofeedback laboratory; relaxation techniques are an excellent way of becoming aware of our own physiological processes and beginning to achieve control over them.

Two separate studies led the way for the new science of biofeedback. Both proved that people can learn to control the electrical activity on the surface of their brains and change their brain waves. Researcher Joseph Kamiya amplified signals from the surfaces of his subjects' brains and fed them back to the subjects as auditory tones. Kamiya found that subjects could learn how to slow their own brain waves to produce the tones associated with slower waves. Barbara Brown translated her subjects' alpha brain waves into blue light. The subjects were able to control their brain activity and produce alpha waves in order to keep the blue light lit. These experiments have been readily duplicated. They proved, for the first time, that feedback provided in a usable, continuous, immediate form can teach physiological skills which had been considered beyond human capacity by Western science and medicine. Eastern yogis have been able to control many of the processes for centuries.

From brain waves, researchers went on to study other autonomic functions. These functions include the movements of smooth muscles (muscles which line the blood vessels and digestive tract, for example), the heartbeat, blood pressure, and enzyme and hormone secretion. The researchers found that not only can brain waves be controlled, but so too can the contractions of smooth muscles, heart rate, digestive functions, enzyme secretion, and perhaps every function of the body, down to the minute secretion of a chemical in the brain. Biofeedback researchers are presently directing their attention to perfecting feedback techniques for brain chemical secretion, blood cell manufacture, and other processes.

How do individuals learn to control their autonomic functions? What sort of effort is involved? How does the control acquired in the laboratory carry over into everyday life? In their first session with biofeedback equipment, most people spend some time just getting used to and playing with the equipment. Heart rate is easily monitored, and heart rate feedback often provides the first biofeedback experience. The subject is usually amazed to see what his or her own heartbeat looks like on a graph. Most people are surprised at how variable heart rate is and soon realize that it is sensitive to even minor changes in posture and very slight movements. Breathing has dramatic effects on heart rate, as it does on other physiological systems; since breathing is easily controlled, subjects soon discover its effects. Further experimentation reveals that mental states have definite effects on the measurements. Thinking about anxiety-provoking incidents increases heart rate; imagining restful scenes slows the heart. A particular sort of thinking—visualizing a special scene, or even a shape or color—may facilitate a particular physiological change.

Even the most adept biofeedback subjects may not be able to describe exactly "how" they control their own physiology. Just because they can affect their autonomic processes does not mean that they can "feel" them; they do not feel the blood coursing through their veins or the moment-by-moment movement of their digestion. But they do come to identify a complex of behaviors that elicits the desired results. Once they have learned how to control an autonomic process, people usually can duplicate the results outside of the laboratory.

The mental attitude most conducive to successful feedback work is not determined concentration, but passive attention. It is the same state of mind that we strive to achieve in any of the stress-reduction techniques.

Skeletal Muscle Tension

Skeletal muscle tension can be measured and monitored in the biofeedback laboratory by the electromyograph (EMG) machine. This instrument registers the very sensitive electrical discharge at the junction between nerves and muscles. In order for a muscle to contract or move, the nerve must electrically stimulate it. The impulse for movement is transferred through the nerve to the muscle, which then contracts in order for movement to occur. Muscles usually contract in groups and move the bones to which they are connected.

The EMG senses the nerve impulses that trigger muscular contraction, amplifies them, and converts the amplified impulses into a form usable by the biofeedback subject. The EMG can take a millionth of a volt discharge, amplify it, and use it to flash a light, sound a tone, or move a meter; such a signal indicates increase or decrease in electrical activity, depending on how the machine is set. The EMG measures changes in electrical activity level. The sensory signal gives the subject an accurate measure of excess tension in resting muscles; this level of tension would be required for movement, but is not normal in resting muscles.

EMG sensors can be placed in proximity to any skeletal muscles so that the subject can learn how to relax tight, tense muscles anywhere in the body. For a tension headache sufferer, the sensors can be placed above the eyes to measure the tension in the forehead. The sensory signal provides instantaneous, continuous feedback of any excess tension building in the muscles. The EMG makes the subject aware of held tension which may not have previously been recognized as tension at all. When using the EMG machine, subjects discover the combination of behaviors that are effective at reducing their muscle tension. Trying to relax the forehead is often ineffective, while deep breathing and daydreaming may produce the desired effect. Only the EMG can measure very low levels of tension and give a direct reading of reductions in those levels, but the following exercises will give you feedback on your muscle tension levels.

EMG Exercise

Other people can be a wonderful source of feedback. In the Eastern tradition, the guru gives the novice student of meditation continuous feedback as to his or her progress. In my stress-reduction classes, students often help one another pinpoint and describe each other's individual stress responses. In this exercise one person acts as the subject and the other as the "EMG machine." At the end of the exercise, reverse roles so you will both have an understanding of how muscle tension feels, subjectively and objectively.

In this exercise, verbal feedback can be provided in short appraisals and directives: "Relax the wrist. Relax the elbow." Or: "Let go of this tension here in your neck. Just let me move your leg." Feedback is most effective when it is short, factual, and fairly impersonal. Do not ask questions for which verbal responses must be made; do not comment on the personality of the subject or overall tension levels. Address all feedback to the area under focus and try to determine where the tension is centered. Is it more in the upper or lower arm? Does it come and go? Is it more present with some movements than others? Are there some movements that frighten the subject and cause a reflex tensing? You might also want to try the exercise without talking, communicating only nonverbally.

Begin by being the subject and have your friend be the EMG machine. Stand, facing one another. Have your friend gently, but securely, support your arm. Attempt to relax your arm completely, employing whatever relaxation technique seems most effective. Remember that relaxation is associated with heaviness and warmth, and strive to feel these two sensations. Your friend, the EMG machine, should consider how heavy your arm feels and how much resistance is encountered when the arm is moved. A relaxed arm will feel heavy, limp, and easily manipulated.

Sit in a chair. Be sure that your body is well supported and that no undue stress is placed on your legs. Allow your friend to hold your leg just above the back of the knee and at the calf. It is usually best to work with one leg at a time, since relaxed legs are very heavy. Have the machine move your leg slowly and gently. The leg should not be pulled or jerked suddenly. Be particularly careful in bending the knee. Tension is often pronounced in the calf and some people automatically tense when the knee is flexed.

Lie on the floor or on a couch or bed, with the EMG machine behind you, cradling your head. Have the machine cup his or her hand under your head and use the other hand to support your neck. Your friend should begin to slowly rotate your neck, moving in an even motion. Movements should be gradual, with the machine slowly rotating the neck in an even motion. The EMG machine should be especially sensitive to any resistance or strain. Be aware of any tension that you feel in the head, neck, forehead, jaw, mouth, or ears. When fully relaxed, the neck will rotate freely and to a degree not possible before relaxation. The machine should be aware of any differences in flexibility from one side to the other and any knots or areas of resistance. The head will feel very heavy, almost as heavy as a bowling ball.

Now switch roles. After you have both been the EMG machine and subject, ask yourselves the following questions. Discuss them together.

Continued ➜

Did the EMG's perception of my tension correspond to my own perception?

What resistance to complete relaxation did I encounter?

Did feeling another person's tension help me to become aware of how I carry tension in my musculature?

How did my ability to relax my arms, head, and legs in this exercise compare to my success with

   other stress-reduction techniques?

If there's a marked difference, does it have something to do with my relationships with other people?

Do I feel particular resistance about letting go of tension in the presence of another person?

Often your perception of tension is much different than feedback provided by another person. Another person's input may be very helpful in pinpointing areas where you hold tension. Feeling another person's tense muscles can bring you insight into your own tension. For some people, this exercise is much more effective than exercises performed alone. For others, an added resistance is associated with entrusting their arms, legs, and head to another person. If you encounter such resistance, begin to examine the connection between your stress response and various social situations. Let your reaction to this exercise provide some clues into your unique response to stress.

Skin Temperature

Skin temperature is affected by blood flow. The fight-or-flight response has a dramatic effect on blood flow, sending blood away from the extremities. The smooth muscles in the walls of the arteries which supply blood to the hands and feet constrict, and the hands and feet become colder than the rest of the body. Some people have cold hands and feet all the time. With relaxation, the arteries to the hands and feet dilate and the increased flow of blood warms them; most people, when relaxed, have a skin temperature reading of at least 90 degrees Fahrenheit in their hands. Those whose habituated stress response includes constricting the smooth muscles of the arterial walls can be greatly helped by temperature training.

The temperature trainer machine senses slight changes in the circumference of the arteries which supply blood to the hands and feet. It lets the subject know when the arteries begin to constrict so that he or she can relax them, and maintain warmth in the extremities. Temperature training is especially effective for people who hold tension in the vascular system and have conditions such as migraine headache, hypertension, and Raynaud's syndrome. We are accustomed to relaxing and tensing the skeletal muscles at will, but learning to control the smooth muscles is very different. You can become aware of differences in temperature, but you probably will not be able to directly perceive the constriction or dilation of the muscles lining the arteries.

Temperature Trainer Exercise

Temperature training at home is not as precise as in the laboratory, since vascular constriction and dilation cannot be measured at home. Hand temperature can be measured by loosely holding an aquarium or photo thermometer. Make certain that the thermometer you use has a wide calibration so you can clearly read each degree; it should go to at least 95 degrees Fahrenheit. Allow a few minutes for

the reading to stabilize. If the temperature is under 90 degrees Fahrenheit, then practice temperature control by attempting to raise it. You might want to employ one of the stress-reduction techniques, particularly autogenics, to warm your extremities. A reading of 93 to 95 degrees Fahrenheit feels very warm to most people and indicates deep relaxation.

If you have vascular problems, it can be very useful to take your hand temperature several times during the day under different circumstances. This can help you to identify the situations that cause tension. Once you know what makes you tense, you can begin to perfect a technique for alleviating the manifestation of that tension in your vascular system.

Galvanic Skin Response

Your skin responds to thoughts, emotions, and changes in the environment. Whenever you hear a noise, take a deep breath, think an emotion-charged thought, or react to phenomena around you, your skin responds. When you are tense or stimulated, you sweat more heavily; when you are relaxing or resting, you sweat less and your skin dries. *Becoming conscious of your skin's response to stress and controlling it can be useful in conquering anxiety.*

Galvanic skin response (GSR) is a measure of the skin's resistance to an electrical current. Moisture on the skin increases the electrical conductance between any two points on the skin. When conductance is increased, there is less resistance to an electrical current. A low GSR reading indicates tension: the skin is wet, conductance is high, and resistance is low. A high GSR indicates relaxation: the skin is dry, conductance is low, and resistance to the electrical current is high.

Skin response is an immediate and direct gauge of your emotional state and unconscious feelings. Your skin reacts before you are even aware of feeling the emotion which triggers it. Galvanic skin response is often used in polygraph (lie detector) tests in the belief that lying creates emotional tension. A low GSR might indicate the emotional stress of lying. In biofeedback, GSR is very useful in identifying stress-inducing situations and in helping people become more aware of their emotional responses. Even without using a machine, you can become more aware of your skin's responses to your emotions. What social situations make you perspire more? Do you ever notice that your hands are damp and sticky? When? What other symptoms accompany this response?

Stomach Acid

The digestive tract responds to stress immediately, just like the skin. Stomach acid feedback can allow you to focus on the specific stress response that is making you ill. Acid secretion in the stomach may be increased with tension, and overproduction of stomach acid can lead to ulcers. Subjects have been able to consciously prevent oversecretion of stomach acid and heal their own ulcerated stomach linings. In stomach acid feedback, a special acid-monitoring sensor is used. You swallow the sensor and it gives instantaneous electronic signals when the acid level in your stomach changes. You can become aware of shifts in acid secretion too subtle to be sensed otherwise.

Most people do not become aware of stomach acid production until it manifests as pain or discomfort. With biofeedback you can recognize and reverse this overproduction before its symptoms are manifested. Factors that contribute to increased

acid secretion can be easily recognized. You can identify the mental states and the tension-provoking situations that precipitate an attack and the particular state of mind that wards off attacks. As with all biofeedback training, the object is to take the information out of the laboratory and apply it to your daily life. In this instance, you would attempt to maintain the state of mind associated with decreased acid production and avoid the situations that lead to increased production. Although you probably will not learn to "feel" the acid secretion itself, you will identify the whole complex of feelings associated with it.

Abdominal Movement

Peristalsis is a progressive wavelike movement of the smooth muscles lining the intestine. It pushes the intestinal contents along. The contractions may be regular and even or spastic and irregular. Rate of movement and regularity of each contraction have a direct bearing on the functioning of the intestine. Slow movement may be associated with constipation and rapid movement with diarrhea. Spastic, irregular movement may cause discomfort and other digestive problems.

Abdominal movement can be monitored with a stethoscope or other amplifier so that you can hear your own bowel sounds. Once you become tuned in to your own peristalsis, you can learn how to regulate it and prevent spasms. You may be able to buy a stethoscope and listen to your peristalsis outside of the biofeedback laboratory, but it would be best to begin training with a physician or biofeedback therapist who can explain what you are hearing. Sometimes just placing your hands over the area where you sense spasm allows you to focus on the contraction and alleviate the irregular movement.

Heart Rate

Heart rate can be quite easily monitored today and often is as a matter of course in the emergency room. Usually the monitor is turned away from the subject's line of vision; many doctors believe that the subject doesn't know how to interpret the reading and will just become more agitated. *Research in the biofeedback laboratory has shown that subjects can learn to regulate their own heart rates.* This is significant for people who suffer from tachycardia (irregular heartbeats). Many people experience palpitations in conjunction with anxiety; heart rate biofeedback can help you control palpitations and curtail the entire anxiety response. You can buy a stethoscope for home use; but unfortunately, hearing your own heartbeat can be disturbing and more difficult to work with than a visual display. If you are using a heartbeat monitor of any kind, always remember to slow your heart by slowing your breath and quieting yourself.

Direct Blood Pressure

Several methods of direct blood pressure feedback are being researched. The sphygmomanometer, an indirect method, is the standard instrument used in most doctor's offices; it may distract or even alarm the subject. Researchers would like to develop a method that does not require the cuff and provides continuous, immediate feedback. If you are suffering with hypertension and would like to be involved in biofeedback study, check with your doctor or the closest medical training institution.

Continued ➜

Blood Chemistry

Blood chemistry may be directly monitored in the future. The potential of this feedback is very exciting. We may be able to control the metabolic secretion of hormones and antibodies and stimulate our own blood cell production. This would be useful in correcting hormonal or chemical imbalances, as well as in stimulating production of the antibodies needed to fight particular diseases. Biofeedback information could greatly augment self-healing visualization. We would then have immediate feedback as to the effectiveness of healing visualization in releasing the appropriate immunological agents.

Brain Activity

The first application of biofeedback and probably the most well known is brain wave feedback. The electroencephalograph machine (EEG) senses electrical activity on the surface of the cortex. This activity is amplified and translated into a pictorial representation or a set of auditory tones. Given feedback on their own brain activity, subjects are able to alter their brain wave patterns.

The electrical activity of the brain is characterized by general wave patterns which reflect different electrical frequencies. The four major wave frequency patterns are associated with four different states of consciousness. In the course of any day, brain waves fluctuate, and all four patterns probably appear intermittently. The association between particular wave frequency patterns and states of mind is general. Certain patterns do seem to predominate during the mental activities with which they are identified, although other kinds of mental activity occur. Brain waves are measured in Hertz, units of frequency equal to one cycle per second. Beta (13–30 Hz) are usually associated with wide awake, alert, problem-solving modes of thought; theta (5–7 Hz) are associated with dreaming or creative activities; delta (.5–4 Hz) are associated with dreamless sleep. Alpha (8–12 Hz) are the most celebrated and correspond to relaxation and contemplative, meditative states.

Early brain wave researchers were interested in the association between state of mind and wave frequency. They were especially intrigued by the correspondence between pleasurable, meditative states and alpha waves. "Alpha training" came into vogue in the 1960s but had fallen out of favor by the early 1970s. Proponents of alpha training believed that alpha states were beneficial and that by inducing such waves, total relaxation was guaranteed. It is true that for most people, alpha waves are associated with deep relaxation and peaceful contemplation, but alpha waves do not always indicate generalized physiological relaxation. Some people experience alpha in meditative states in which their minds are blissfully blank, though trying to make the mind a blank does not always lead to alpha wave production. The long-term benefits claimed by the alpha wave movement have not been proven. The brain is a very complex organ and does not lend itself to either generalization or complete understanding at this time. Brain wave biofeedback holds unlimited promise.

Feedback at Home

Of course you do not have to wait for the results of sophisticated research before you can take advantage of feedback techniques. The average household can become a feedback laboratory. You probably have a mirror, scale, thermometer, and other people at your disposal. A stethoscope and blood pressure cuff can be obtained at a medical supply store without a prescription. Used appropriately, these can provide a great deal of information about your stress levels and your unique stress response. The mirror is the most basic feedback device. It allows you to see your face where emotions and a good deal of whatever tension you are feeling are expressed. The following exercise should provide insights useful in performing every other exercise in this chapter.

Facing Yourself

Begin by taking a very close look at yourself. Try to forget the preconceptions you have about your own appearance. Look at yourself as if it were the first time you ever looked in a mirror. Where are the stress lines in your face? Are you holding your face in a rigid or strained position? Do your eyes look red, puffy, or tired? Are the pupils dilated or constricted? Is your jaw tight? Your mouth pinched or relaxed? How are you holding your neck and shoulders? Are you trying to burrow into your shoulders and hide? What emotion is expressed in your face? Anger? Fear? Sadness? Contentment? Boredom? Distress? Happiness?

Let your face fully express whatever you are feeling. Then let go of it. Release any tension held in your face, neck, or shoulders. Let your expression reveal relaxation. Use the mirror whenever you feel the need to verify your feelings. Be aware of how your self-image affects the way you hold your head and use your face to express emotions.

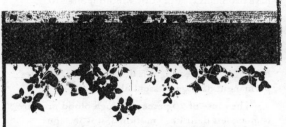

SPECIFIC AILMENTS AND STRESS REDUCTION: HELPING YOURSELF

L. John Mason, Ph. D.

Eighty to 90 percent of all disease is directly or indirectly related to stress. Stress reduction, practiced on a regular basis, can help prevent, modify, or eliminate the sources and symptoms of your physical complaints. Certain factors influence the rate of success: motivation, practice, and the willingness to "let go."

Dr. Carl Simonton's results, in his treatment of cancer patients, revealed that success rates were partially determined by the patient's attitude. Simonton found that a patient with a positive attitude toward the treatment, and an overall positive attitude toward life, had a better chance of positive results. People with negative feelings about the treatment, and life in general, had a lower rate of success.

In my own experience, I have found that people are not always motivated to continue a stress-reduction program, even when they know that the program works. A young woman, who was already an acquaintance, came to see me. Mutual friends had encouraged her to try stress reduction for her migraine headaches, but she was skeptical from the beginning. Migraines had plagued her for fifteen years; they were debilitating and often accompanied by nausea. I was determined to help her because I had had so much success with migraine patients, but I knew that motivation and willingness to give in, to go along with the technique, were all-important. Her lack of such willingness was a definite obstacle.

In our first session I taught her the basic autogenic training, and she went home to practice on her own. In our second session she reported a reduction in the frequency of her headaches, even though she had been inconsistent and resistant to her practice. The two headaches she did experience were shorter in duration and less intense than usual.

At our next session, I reiterated the importance of regular practice, and because she was a friend, spoke strongly to her of the need to perform the sequence regularly. She heeded my advice and, at our fourth and final session, reported relief and control over all her migraine symptoms, after instituting a daily program of autogenics. I reminded her to keep up the practice; she reassured me of her great pleasure at being relieved of her symptoms and left.

Several months later, I learned from mutual friends that her motivation had dropped. She had become negligent in her practice, and the headaches had recurred. For whatever reason, she had not been able to maintain a program, even when the alternative was pain.

My friend's success with autogenics was immediate, but this isn't always the case. *Relaxation is not a magic cure and is not a drug that can be taken for instant results.* It must be utilized on a daily basis and incorporated into your life. The body has disease and pain habits; stress-reduction techniques are helping you to reprogram the body. It is easy for you and your body to slip back into old habits.

Practicing once or twice a day, every day, is absolutely necessary for results. Relaxation and self-regulation come with practice, and for most, the changes are subtle; allow eight to ten weeks for the results to become noticeable. This doesn't mean that for some people the results won't be more immediate, but it is important to persevere even if you don't notice drastic changes right away. Remember again that trying too hard just creates more tension. You have to learn to "let go," and as difficult as that may be, "letting go" is the key.

WARNING: If you are suffering from any of the stress-related symptoms discussed here, it is advised that you seek the diagnosis of your physician to rule out serious physical symptoms which may be disguised as less dangerous stress-related disorders. If you are currently taking regular medication, please discuss your use of the following behavioral techniques with your doctor. Revisions to your medication regimen may be needed when using these powerful techniques. This caution is designed not to scare you, but is offered to allow for the very best treatment to help minimize if not eliminate your symptoms of stress and anxiety.

Migraine Headaches

Migraine headache is a severe and often debilitating vascular complaint that is relatively common. The cause of a "true migraine" is the constriction of the carotid arteries in the neck which supply blood to the head, followed by a dilation of these arteries. During the constriction, the prodrome characteristic of a true migraine occurs, followed by the severe, usually one-sided, pain of the dilation.

Most migraine patients know when a headache is coming on by the prodrome. Prodromes (presymptoms) range from flushing, dizziness, and

Continued ➡

visual aberrations to just a queer but unmistakable feeling. When you pick up the prodrome signal and respond quickly with the appropriate relaxation technique, you can often prevent the migraine.

In my practice, I have found that a regular regimen of relaxation can prevent migraine, even in people who have suffered for years. But you must set up a regular program, regardless of your symptoms; if you practice only when you already feel a headache coming on, you will find the technique less successful.

Migraine headache can be devastating, but it can also be controlled. *Eighty-five percent of the migraine patients I work with respond positively to stress-reduction practice.* The people who do not get better usually are not practicing consistently, because, for their own reasons, they are not quite ready to give up their migraines and discover a headache-free existence. I strongly recommend that migraine sufferers study the secondary gains they get from migraines and evaluate their lives to determine what needs are not being met appropriately.

Keys to Controlling Migraines:

- Learn slow breathing techniques to minimize stress.
- Know what conditions trigger your migraines and avoid them (if possible).
- Learn what presymptoms you experience and use these to prevent or minimize your headaches.
- Avoid being perfectionistic.
- Use biofeedback temperature monitoring for deep relaxation regularly.
- Use a relaxation tape regularly (like *Stress Management for High Blood Pressure*).
- Learn to warm your hands and feet to prevent headaches.

USING BREATHING TECHNIQUES REGULARLY WILL PREVENT STRESSES FROM BUILDING.

Breathing techniques that relax you and reduce stress in your circulatory system often can help to minimize headache activity when you catch the process early, in the prodromal stage. These techniques can also help to reduce the intensity of your headaches if they cannot be prevented.

KNOW YOUR MIGRAINE TRIGGERS.

Most migraines are triggered by specific conditions such as bright lights, noise, allergic responses, certain emotions, etc. If you experience these triggers, minimize your exposure by removing yourself or shorten your stay in these environments. If you experience any prodromal symptoms, remove yourself and begin to practice your relaxation strategies and your hand/foot warming techniques (including visualizations and physically warming your hands and feet while cooling your neck and head). If you can catch your headaches early or before they start, your chances of preventing them or minimizing them are greatly improved.

LEARN WHAT YOUR PRESYMPTOMS ("PRODROMES") ARE.

Many people experience certain "feelings" that are commonly perceived before the onset of their migraine headaches. These might be visual cues, certain "odd" feelings, or even pressures in their head or face. If you have identified these patterns (not every migraine sufferer has these), you can use them to stop or to minimize your headache pattern from developing. Stop when you feel these symptoms occurring and take preventive measures like relaxation and hand/foot warming to reduce possible headaches from occurring or becoming worse. .

Hypertension (High Blood Pressure)

Hypertension is not just a disease of aging. Young men and women can suffer from its damaging, sometimes deadly, effects. Please do not take this condition lightly. Get it treated as soon as possible before it creates lasting damage and adversely affects your life as you age.

Standard medical procedures today are being accompanied by relatively new behavioral approaches for treating conditions such as chronic pain and essential hypertension. These problems frustrate traditional medical practices and are expensive in both money and time lost from work.

High blood pressure, also called hypertension, is potentially fatal. Every year high blood pressure kills 60,000 people. It can lead to other serious health problems such as heart disease, stroke, kidney and liver disease, and arteriosclerosis.

High blood pressure is a dangerous, widespread disease affecting at least 15 percent of the adult population in the United States. *It is rarely caused by any single organic condition and is more often attributable to a whole complex of emotional and physical factors.* Hypertension is not to be treated lightly; medical attention and opinion cannot be replaced. Chronic hypertension can be asymptomatic and still damage the heart, liver, kidneys, and other organs. Untreated, it can precipitate stroke and heart attack. Consult your doctor; even get second and third opinions about your health. Whatever you do, don't drag your feet.

The need for treatment of this condition is an absolute necessity, and, unfortunately, physicians have problems treating this symptom effectively. Only about 30 percent of hypertension is caused by permanent physical factors such as hardening of the arteries (arteriosclerosis) or kidney damage. Because such physical problems offer little possibility of reversal, treating this disease before it creates permanent damage is essential.

The cause of 70 percent of high blood pressure is much less definite. Emotional, unconscious responses usually cause elevations in blood pressure. To understand the mechanism that occurs to elevate blood pressure because of emotional responses requires that the fight or flight response be understood. When excited by a stressor, the body will do several things which can raise the blood pressure. First, certain hormones are released, such as epinephrine and norepinephrine, which causes an elevation of heart rate and the constriction of many blood vessels. The sympathetic nervous system which controls the fight or flight response is responsible for the release of these hormones, and also will elevate the heart rate, therefore elevating blood pressure itself through direct nervous stimulation.

Seventy percent of all hypertension is diagnosed as "essential" hypertension, meaning that the doctor cannot find any organic cause. Some patients say, "I'm not worried. My blood pressure only goes up in the doctor's office." The situation, particularly that of the doctor's office, and your fear and apprehension can raise your blood pressure. It has been estimated that blood pressure rises as much as thirty points in the doctor's office, but it is unlikely that visiting the doctor is the only event that merits that response. The elevation in blood pressure you experience while trembling in the pressure cuff indicates that you respond to stress with an elevation in blood pressure. It also indicates that you hold tension in your vascular system. Holding tension in any physiological system on a regular basis can only weaken it.

It is important to remember that the blood flow patterns of the body are changed when responding to stress. For many people, the blood is redirected away from the extremities and abdomen into major muscle groups and to the central nervous system. As this redirection occurs, the vasoconstriction to the extremities can be monitored and can have direct bearing on the elevation of blood pressure. For this reason, tranquilizers, muscle relaxants, diuretics (to reduce blood volume), and a new series of chemical agents called beta blockers are often prescribed for treating and reducing hypertension. (Beta blockers are drugs that act to reduce the heart's output or to reduce resistance in blood vessels of the extremities. This is chemically induced stress reduction for the cardiovascular system.)

The problem with any of these medications is that they can create negative side effects, and these can be so unpleasant that the patient may stop taking the medication altogether and let the high blood pressure go unchecked. This is dangerous!

Another treatment for high blood pressure is the patient-responsibility approach that encourages change in lifestyle and change in personal response to emotional situations. Proper diet and physical exercise are key factors in conquering heart disease and have long been recognized as the best long-term remedies for treating hypertension. The use of stress management strategies to control the stress response is a technique gaining wide support. Awareness, relaxation, and response management are parts of a good stress control program.

People under a doctor's care for high blood pressure should inform their doctors that they are following a relaxation program. Since doctors often prescribe medication for this type of dysfunction, they must be informed so that medication levels can be periodically checked.

Hypertension Control Program

Since hypertension is a vascular problem, autogenics is a good technique. Progressive relaxation is also valuable; tension in your musculature probably contributes to your vascular dysfunction. Many people have had remarkable success using meditation. Zen-like active meditation combined with a long walk may be helpful; begin with short distances and increase your distance over time. While performing the combined autogenic and visualization exercise, focus on the blood flowing freely and easily throughout your body. Picture your blood vessels dilated and unobstructed. Generating warmth in your extremities will help, as will imagining yourself totally calm, peaceful, and relaxed.

Hypertension often responds to deep breathing exercises. Try to slow your rhythm of respiration. Do not starve yourself of oxygen or hold your breath; just slow and deepen your normal breathing rhythm. The 1-to-4 Count exercise in the section on breathing will slow your breath to four or five complete breaths per minute. Five to twenty minutes of this type of breathing can reduce your heart rate, and quite possibly, significantly lower your blood pressure.

If your high blood pressure is linked to particular situations that are unavoidable, then desensitization to the experience may be worthwhile. Read the chapter on desensitization and try following the program, changing it to meet your specific needs.

A relatively recent additional therapy has also been given much credence in the fight against hypertension. This is the use of biofeedback along with regular blood pressure checks, in the home, and the practice of relaxation techniques on a regular daily basis. Biofeedback is the use of instruments or techniques to monitor the changes within

Continued ➡

the body that are usually related to the stress response pattern. After these responses are monitored, the information is then offered to the individual, who learns to control these responses in a more positive way.

Temperature training, which is used to measure the changes of temperature of the skin of the hands and feet, is a simple but powerful tool to combat hypertension. When relaxed physically and emotionally a person should have a hand temperature above 90 degrees Fahrenheit. When you are completely relaxed, this can go up to 93 to 95 degrees in the hands and 90 degrees measured at the feet below the big toe.

If this can be done consistently by practicing relaxation techniques, then chances are excellent that blood pressure can be controlled. Remember that this control indicates that blood flow is not restricted by the stress response, so the blood pressure will drop and medication can be reduced—and often eliminated—under the care of a physician.

The difference between this new technique and the ones discussed earlier in the book is that specific criteria for both hand and foot warming are requested for true vascular control. Additionally, the regular daily monitoring of blood pressure and modification to lifestyle such as reducing time consciousness (self-pressuring) helps to increase awareness and control.

It sounds very simple, but it can take twelve to fifteen weeks to master the skill of relaxation so that the hands and the feet indicate a relaxed state of even blood flow. The patient learns to control the sympathetic nervous system's response to stress. Relaxation then can generalize to control of the internal mechanism that creates the high blood pressure.

As an example of this technique, Bob was referred to me by his slightly skeptical physician. The idea of biofeedback and behavioral changes controlling his blood pressure problem were not entirely the doctor's idea. Bob had pressured his doctor because of poor results with medication and its negative side effects.

Bob's high motivation to get off the medication definitely worked in his favor. He began regular relaxation practice on a daily basis, as well as self blood pressure checks and home temperature biofeedback. After experimenting for several weeks to determine the best relaxation format, he settled in to consistent practice. Bob discovered that he did not have to get so uptight at work or at home about the little things that had plagued him. He noticed that his blood pressure readings began to drop and his hand and foot temperatures began to climb during the relaxation practice.

In eight weeks he returned to his physician to show his progress of homework forms reflecting reduced blood pressure. Even his blood pressure taken in the doctor's office had dropped significantly. So he discussed reducing his medication needs with his doctor, and together they decided on a gradual highly monitored plan for withdrawal from medication. With the help of his doctor and continued daily relaxation and home monitoring, he worked his way off all medication.

Bob called me some months later to tell me of his pleasure with living medication and side effect free. This is not a random case, for with the additional parameters of specific training criteria the success rate reaches close to 90 percent with the motivated person.

Keys to Controlling High Blood Pressure:

- Breathe slowly.
- Use biofeedback temperature monitoring for deep relaxation regularly.
- Use a relaxation tape regularly (like *Stress Management for High Blood Pressure*).
- Learn to warm your hands and feet.
- Exercise aerobically and regularly.
- Avoid caffeine and other stimulants.
- Remain in the present, in your body, and in a positive frame of mind.
- Taper your high blood pressure medication after you have mastered the relaxation-biofeedback under your physician's care.

LEARN TO BREATHE DIAPHRAGMATICALLY. Place a hand over your upper abdomen. Push your abdomen out as you inhale. Let your abdomen move in as you exhale. Let your chest, shoulders, neck, and back relax as you breathe. Only on a very deep breath should these parts move in the breath. This may be the most important hypertension technique you can learn!

By linking one deep breath to a reoccurring work event like a telephone ringing or checking the time, you remember to take these slow deep breaths throughout your work schedule to avoid letting tensions build to painful or distracting levels. The secret is to check in with your body in the present moment, relax your major muscles, and slow and deepen your breath. This simple exercise can have miraculous results.

Other breathing techniques involve a short series of deep slow breaths, where you count as you breathe. Try counting slowly 1 to 4 as you inhale, pause and hold your breath as you count 1 to 4 again, and then release slowly, but completely, as you count 1 to 8. After four of these breaths you will be breathing easier and better able to control your body's pattern of holding tension. This process can in turn help you to control your hypertension. . . .

LIVE IN THE PRESENT. Many people with high blood pressure have trouble maintaining their thoughts in present time for focusing on their bodies in positive ways. Fears or angers from the past or apprehensions about the future seem to take up too much of their consciousness. Living in the present, letting go of negative emotions, and letting life's daily dramas roll off you are all important skills to develop.

TAPER YOUR HIGH BLOOD PRESSURE MEDICATION AFTER YOU HAVE MASTERED THE RELAXATION-BIOFEEDBACK, UNDER YOUR PHYSICIAN'S CARE. After you have learned to let go through relaxation and biofeedback training, you can monitor your blood pressure at home. When you have developed the skills of hand and foot warming, you will find that your blood pressure drops down to more normal ranges. Write these home blood pressure measurements down regularly to show to your doctor. In the doctor's office your blood pressure may still be higher than you like. Many people have "white coat syndrome" where their blood pressure will be ten to fifteen points higher in the doctor's office than it is at home. With your doctor's agreement and assistance you may be able to begin reducing your high blood pressure medication(s). Any changes to your normal medication may elevate your blood pressure, so reduce these medications slowly, in gradual steps.

Insomnia or problems with sleeping may affect your high blood pressure as well. If this is an issue for you, you may want to read the section on sleeping disorders and use the special tape at bedtime to help you get to sleep and so rest better.

You may also want to read the section on meditation from this book. The exercise entitled Shavasana, taken from yoga, has been researched and proven helpful in reducing blood pressure over twelve to twenty weeks. . . .

Tension Headache

Turn on your television set, and you will be besieged by commercials extolling the benefits of over-the-counter medications. One will combat the effects of fatigue; one will stop the "heartbreak of psoriasis"; and yet another will stamp out acid indigestion. Yet, far more patent headache medications are advertised than any other nonprescription drug.

Tension headache is the most common symptom of stress in our society. Muscle tension in the neck and shoulders, around the eyes, and in the jaw, often results in a throbbing tension headache. Tension may begin affecting you subtly; most people are not even aware that an energy-robbing headache is in the making. People start holding tension in their musculature as soon as they get out of bed in the morning, and by the beginning of the afternoon they have a worrisome, nagging, creeping headache. By evening they are holding their heads and looking for relief.

I usually buy my office supplies at the same store and often from the same salesperson. One day I noticed that he seemed irritable and asked if there was some way that I could help. He then told me that he had been getting excruciating tension headaches almost every day. Since I happened to have a tape of the 10-to-1 Passive Progressive Relaxation exercise with me, I suggested that he practice it daily and explained that it was important to become aware of the tension and learn to let go of it. Two weeks later, I returned to buy more office supplies. He was very pleased with the tape; control of tension headache had become possible for him. Any time he felt a headache coming on, he would take a few moments to relax. If possible, he would put on the tape and listen to it, even if he only had a few minutes. Awareness, letting go, and practice had worked for him.

Tension Headache Control Program

Knowledge of what triggers your stress response and where it manifests itself, and the realization that you can control muscle tension, is half the battle for stress reduction. The other 50 percent is learning to reduce or release the tension. Prevention is the best remedy. If you practice stress reduction for about twenty minutes a day on a regular basis, the number of headaches you get should decrease radically. For some people, this is enough to wipe out any tension headache problem. This may also be sufficient to alleviate other muscle tension complaints, such as back pain, muscle spasms, or tics.

Progressive relaxation deals directly with your muscles; some form of this exercise is recommended if you are commonly afflicted by muscle tension pain. Autogenic training phrases are also powerful control tools, and in combination with progressive relaxation and visualization, can be the most beneficial exercise of all. Breathing exercises will make you more aware of building tension levels, while continually releasing excess stress. The gentle movement exercises can be practiced just about anywhere and are excellent for reducing excess muscle tension. Just remember that stress-reduction practice will not only help you prevent or control your headaches; it will positively affect your emotional state as well.

Continued ➡

Keys to Controlling Tension Headaches:

- Learn slow breathing techniques to minimize stress.
- Use EMG biofeedback monitoring for deep relaxation of your muscles regularly.
- Use a relaxation tape regularly (like *Stress Management for Chronic Pain* or *10-to-1 Countdown*).
- Learn to relax your jaw, forehead, and neck/shoulders.
- Regular exercise can help prevent these complaints.
- Reduce your emotional triggers if these are a factor in your symptom activity.

USING BREATHING TECHNIQUES REGULARLY WILL PREVENT STRESSES FROM BUILDING.

Breathing techniques can relax you and reduce stress in your muscles. These techniques can also help to reduce the intensity of your symptoms if they cannot be prevented. . . .

REDUCE YOUR EMOTIONAL TRIGGERS IF THESE ARE A FACTOR IN YOUR SYMPTOM ACTIVITY.

Perfectionism (or needing to control most situations), repressed anger, and anxiety can all be potential triggers that either create tension headaches or make them worse. Get help in identifying these issues and seek out support as you work through them to find more appropriate ways to respond when these emotional states are triggered. Look for the issues that cause you to be "uptight" and can lead to you holding tension in your jaw or neck/shoulders.

Back Pain

After tension headache, back pain is the most common form of tension pain in this country. Lack of exercise, or underexercise, can be a contributing factor in persistent back pain, and a combination of stress-reduction techniques and appropriate exercise can be most beneficial. Often specific muscle groups may not be strong enough to support your body weight; the addition of environmental and emotional stress which tenses these weak muscles results in pain. A stiff neck, pain between your shoulder blades, lower back pain, and even a tension headache can result from stiff and weakened back muscles. Weakness in other parts of your musculature can also be a contributing factor. If your abdominal muscles are weak, which often occurs after pregnancy, you may suffer lower back pain. Compounded by the tension of taking care of an infant, this back pain may become excruciating.

I once treated a bank executive for persistent lower back pain. His doctor had checked him thoroughly, and after ruling out a disc problem, sent him to me for relaxation therapy. As the pain was located only on his right side, I questioned him about his work habits and discovered that he always kept the phone on his right side; he was right-handed and always answered the phone with his right hand. I suggested that he switch the phone to his left side and always pick up the phone in his left hand, for the time being. I also requested that he take one deep, full breath before answering the phone. The physician had recommended a specific exercise program, and I combined this program with autogenics and progressive relaxation. I instructed him to start switching his telephone from side to side after one week of keeping it on his left. He religiously followed the program and, after one month of practice, was rarely experiencing any lower back pain. Then, he had a setback. Since he had been doing so well and was obviously practicing

the exercises, neither his doctor nor I could understand what had triggered his relapse. Upon questioning, it all became quite clear.

Before he had started having trouble with his back, he had played tennis three or four times a week. Under a lot of pressure at work, he had played tennis for relaxation. After his back pain subsided, he started playing again; it was after only three days of tennis that his back started to hurt again. We talked about his tennis partners, when he played, and for how long. Flabbergasted, he realized that the tennis was adding to his tension, not reducing it as he had originally thought. His partners were all co-workers, and they often discussed work after they played; he often had a match on days when the tension at work was the worst. He was not a young man, but prided himself on consistently beating younger men who had been playing for longer than he had. I asked him if he stopped when he was tired or continued playing to the point of exhaustion. He laughed and said he played until the game was over, tired or not. I recommend that he stop playing tennis for three months and continue with his exercise program and relaxation techniques. Once again, the pain subsided. After three months he started playing tennis again; now, he played with his wife or children and stopped when he became tired. The back pain only rarely occurred, and only when he was under extreme pressure.

Back Pain Control Program

If you are suffering back pain, always make certain that you check with your physician before instituting any physical exercise program. Not all kinds of exercise may be beneficial. Some sports, such as football or golf, which may add stress to your life, may actually be harmful. Read the section on physical exercise for more information. *Backache, Stress and Tension*, by Dr. Hans Kraus, outlines a complete exercise program for people who suffer back pain. Included is the Kraus-Weber self-test, which will help you determine if any part of your muscle system is too weak to support your body weight. Specific exercise plans are keyed to specific problems and will help you develop or exercise any weak area.

Practice autogenic training, combined with progressive relaxation in conjunction with physical exercise. Concentrate on heaviness in your limbs and muscles while doing autogenics. Use passive progressive, since active progressive may tighten your muscles even more. Once again, motivation is a key factor in your success at eliminating back pain. Backaches are controllable, but it's up to you to exercise that control.

Keys to Controlling Back Pain:

- Learn slow breathing techniques to minimize stress.
- Use EMG biofeedback monitoring for deep relaxation of your muscles regularly.
- Use a relaxation tape regularly (like *Stress Management for Chronic Pain* or *10-to-1 Countdown*).
- Learn to relax your lower back and neck/shoulders.
- Regular exercise can help prevent these complaints.
- Reduce your emotional triggers if these are a factor in your symptom activity.

USING BREATHING TECHNIQUES REGULARLY WILL PREVENT STRESSES FROM BUILDING.

Breathing techniques can relax you and reduce stress in your muscles. These techniques can also help to reduce the intensity of your symptoms if they cannot be prevented.

REDUCE YOUR EMOTIONAL TRIGGERS IF THESE ARE A FACTOR IN YOUR SYMPTOM ACTIVITY.

Perfectionism (or needing to control most situations), repressed anger, and anxiety can all be potential triggers that either create back pain or make it worse. Get help in identifying these issues and seek out support as you work through them to find more appropriate ways to respond when these emotional states are triggered. Look for the issues that cause you to be "uptight" and can lead to you holding tension in your lower back or neck/shoulders.

DEVELOP A SENSE THAT YOU DO HAVE CONTROL OF YOUR BACK PAIN.

This is not easy in the beginning, but the behavioral techniques can help you to minimize the intensity of your back pain, if not eliminate it. Many people feel "out of control" when their pain becomes chronic. This can make the intensity of the pain worse because you have fear and anxiety regarding these ongoing challenges. Temperature training biofeedback can help you to learn to relax and to "let go" of the anxiety that can intensify your complaints.

Chronic Pain

Chronic pain ailments are very expensive and difficult to treat. The expense is both in quality of life and interference with productivity. The difficulties arise from the frustrations of dealing with a physical problem that does not seem to go away and the medical/insurance system that does not deal in a positive, productive way with a lot of chronic pain problems. In most cases, chronic pain has real physical origins that do not show up as clearly as some other physical complaints in typical medical testing. Broken bones can be discovered by X rays, MRIs, or CAT scans and treated by physical medicine including surgeries. But soft-tissue injuries that often comprise chronic pain complaints are frustrating for doctors and patients alike. They do not heal well or quickly for reasons to be discussed. And the frustration experienced by patients, doctors, and the insurance companies creates stress that can actually perpetuate chronic problems rather than help solve them.

Chronic muscle-contraction headaches, neck/shoulder pain, low back pain, and pain/tightness of the jaw are the most common, devastating, and expensive of these problems. There are others that certainly fit in here such as peripheral pain in the arms and legs, intercostal-muscular chest pain, and pelvic pain; however, these are not as common.

The most common reason that these problems do not heal easily relates to the nature of the injury and the healing process. If you were to cut yourself, what would you do? You would clean the wound and bandage it. The bandage helps to protect this location from added abuse and it helps to hold the wounded skin in place so that it may heal by a knitting together of the skin cells. However, in many low back or neck/shoulder injuries, after an accident that pulls or strains these muscles, tendons, or ligaments, it is unlikely that you have the luxury of just lying down and waiting for these injuries to heal. By moving in normal daily activities, you use these important muscle groups, and using these muscles groups is similar to pulling at either side of a cut. Movement and unconscious muscle tension keeps the deeper muscle or soft tissue injuries from healing. The catch-22 is that immobility will produce physical therapy problems as well. A "frozen shoulder," for example, can be a nightmare for people who avoid movement in that joint for a long

Continued ➡

period of time while trying to protect it from further injury.

The frustration experienced by chronic pain sufferers can also exacerbate their symptoms. The lack of progress and the sense of loss of control of their bodies and their lives often leads to an emotional state of tension that can intensify pain and slow the healing process. All of the muscles involved in these pain complaints are subject to unconscious tension from the major survival mechanism known as the fight or flight response. This automatic response prepares the body to defend itself from a perceived life-threatening situation by preparing to fight or to flee. When the muscle groups tighten to get ready for the action of fighting or fleeing the pain or emotional upsets, these muscle groups, if injured, can increase their own fatigue and go into the spasms that create pain or make existing pain or injuries worse.

I treated a construction worker whose leg had been grazed by a falling I beam. Though the accident had happened five years earlier, the man was still suffering severe pain. The original pain was a direct result of the accident, but the subsequent chronic pain was aggravated by several emotional problems. Since he could not work, he was deeply depressed and his self-esteem was low. His relationship with his family had deteriorated, and his wife was asking for a divorce. For the first session he limped into my office and gingerly sat down. All his complaints were neuromuscular: tension headache, low back pain, and leg pain. We worked on breathing techniques and autogenic training.

The second session I guided him through a pain visualization, in which he left his problems beneath a tree next to a fast-running brook. We also worked with progressive relaxation. After only one month of practice he informed me that his wife had agreed to try again with their marriage; his rapid and radical personality change had renewed her hope. He eventually learned how to control his neuromuscular tension; the backaches and headaches completely disappeared. After I worked with him for nearly three months and taught him how to take control of his life by practicing relaxation, he finally walked into my office without limping. Eventually he began vocational retraining and made significant progress in the relationship with his wife. He led a normal, pain-free life.

Though not all people who experience chronic pain have such emotional problems, many will find that their pain is intensified by anxiety and stress. Some people who suffer chronic pain and discomfort could find some, if not total, relief through mind control and stress reduction. Many doctors have become interested in pain management, and entire programs have been established to help people combat pain. Not all pain clinics are the same, but most are based on a combination of relaxation training, physical therapy, exercise, psychotherapy, and personality adjustment. Some clinics stress one type of therapy more than another, yet the basic philosophy is always the same: to help people find relief from pain. Check with your physician or hospital for the location of the center nearest you. Pain clinics may not be as plentiful as local drugstores, but they are located all over the United States.

Chronic Pain Control Program

Pain is a warning signal—a signal that something is wrong. Don't mask or medicate the pain before finding the source: is it caused by tension, anxiety, or even a psychological need? Secondary gains can be met by illness or pain; pain originally generated by an organic dysfunction can continue long after healing is completed. If you have this type of pain, you must ask yourself some questions which are often difficult to answer.

· Am I using my illness to get care and attention that I wouldn't normally receive?

· Do I enjoy not having to deal with people and situations I dislike?

· Am I extending my illness for this reason?

· If other people have high expectations for me, am I using my sickness to avoid dealing with failure? Or even success?

· Am I using my illness to avoid dealing with my own expectations?

· Do I feel like a victim?

If your answer to these questions is yes, then you need to make a decision. You need to decide to get better. Relaxation techniques which teach self-control, such as autogenic training, can help you get out of the pattern of being a victim, can help you take control of your life, and teach you how to take a more active role in your own healing.

Practice relaxation techniques daily, preferably twice a day. Use progressive relaxation or autogenic training to reach deep relaxation, or when the pain is severe. Use a long visualization with a deepening technique, stressing a pain-free existence. Such positive programming can be very beneficial. To increase circulation to the painful spot, use colored light in the visualization; warm colors like yellow, orange, red, and gold encourage warmth and increased blood flow. Blues and greens are cooling, soothing, relaxing, and comforting. Do not use warm colors if you have an inflammation.

When working with people referred for chronic pain, I often recommend that they start with gentle passive progressive relaxation to help control their stress and pain. The 10-to-1 Passive Progressive Relaxation is very effective when practiced regularly. This exercise not only helps to increase awareness and reduce muscle tension, but it can help to give much needed rest and sleep. When a person lacks sleep, a much lower threshold to pain and depression exists.

It is not surprising that chronic pain can lead to drug dependency problems. To treat these effectively, a program of supervised lifestyle adjustment is often needed. Inpatient and local outpatient facilities are springing up around the country to aid sufferers. Proper motivation of the patient is critical for this new pain clinic approach. Treatment is designed to help create awareness and positive alternatives to minimize the pain but cannot work without the positive desire of the patient.

Biofeedback and stress management are important parts of this work. The ability to control anxiety can give individuals more control over their energies and indeed over their lives. This sense of control is often missing from the sufferer of chronic pain, and this in turn can lead to more anxiety and depression. Breaking old patterns and substituting new control really help turn things around.

Many other unconscious factors can contribute to the creation or intensification of pain. Headaches, jaw pain, neck/shoulder pain, and back pain can all be made worse by habits such as poor posture and poor breathing. A potential factor in all of these chronic pains can be head position. We are unconsciously taught to be aggressive and many of us keep our heads or chins stuck out in front of us, as if to "lead" with our jaws/chins. This aggressive, attacking posture can put a major postural strain on the neck, shoulders, jaw, and lower back. Improper breathing can put an unnecessary, inappropriate workload on your shoulders and upper back. Diaphragmatic breathing should be learned to avoid headache, neck/shoulder pain, and back pain.

Motivation and the help of your family are the most important ingredients for conquering debilitating chronic pain. People who do not really want to get well have less success with these techniques. I have seen motivated individuals use stress-reduction techniques to overcome severe back pain and spasms, and return to a normal working life. Many people can successfully use stress reduction to eliminate, or at least reduce, discomfort and pain.

Offering any control over stress and pain gives the chronic pain sufferer a new lease on hope and future control by reducing symptoms even further with practice. This does not always work to reduce pain completely, but can help to get the person back to a more normal lifestyle and often back to work.

Marsha is a chronic low back pain patient who was referred to the pain clinic where I consult. Her depression and anxiety were very close to the surface. She had been suffering for a year with pain that had not responded to any medication or physical therapy. Her doctor did not believe that surgery was an appropriate option. Marsha did not realize how much her injury and lifestyle changes had influenced her level of stress, anxiety, and tension.

We discussed this and introduced her to biofeedback, so she could see for herself how tension was being held in her musculature when she waited for her sharp pains to recur. In fact, her anticipation at an unconscious level was bringing on a large measure of her tiredness, then spasms and pain.

Relaxation training was initiated, and Marsha was able to increase her awareness and control over the pain. She understood that her posture needed to change. Her patterns of communication were examined and slightly changed so that she did not withhold emotional stress as much, finding more appropriate outlets.

As her pain lessened, her activity increased. When last seen, she had begun taking classes to retrain herself for a more productive and physically easier job. Marsha's mood had changed dramatically from depression to optimism. And although she still needed to be careful and not overdo things, she was living a normal lifestyle.

Keys to Controlling the Stress That Creates or Intensifies Your Pain:

· Breathe slowly.

· Use relaxation techniques regularly.

— Use a relaxation tape regularly.

— Learn to relax your jaw and neck/shoulders.

· Exercise aerobically and regularly.

· Avoid caffeine and other stimulants.

· Vent your emotions.

LEARN TO BREATHE DIAPHRAGMATICALLY.

Place a hand over your upper abdomen. Push your abdomen out as you inhale. Let your abdomen move in as you exhale. Let your chest, shoulders, neck, and back relax as you breathe. Only on a very deep breath should these parts move in the breath.

Diaphragmatic breathing throughout your day should make relaxing at bedtime easier. By linking one deep breath to a reoccurring work event like a telephone ringing or checking the time, you remember to take these slow deep breaths throughout your work schedule to avoid letting tensions build to painful or distracting levels. The secret is to check in with your body in the present moment, relax your major muscles, and slow and deepen your breath. This simple exercise can have miraculous results.

Continued ➔

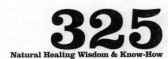

Other techniques involve counting as you breathe through a short series of deep, slow breaths. Try counting slowly 1 to 4 as you inhale, pause and hold your breath as you count 1 to 4 again, and then release slowly, but completely, as you count 1 to 8. After four of these breaths, you will be breathing better and more in control of your body's pattern of holding tension. This simple technique, if done regularly, can help teach you how to control your chronic pain.

PRACTICE RELAXATION TECHNIQUES.

Relaxation of the major muscle groups is very helpful for rest and sleep enhancement. And good sleep is necessary to manage pain.

Remember, the jaw and neck/shoulders are often the areas of the body that are tight and can distract you from falling asleep. These are also the most difficult parts of the body for most people to learn to relax.

Relaxation is easier in a quiet, comfortable space. You may want to be warm, but not too warm for restful sleep. If you have a lot on your mind, write out a list and prioritize it so you can begin to work on these items in the morning.

RELAXATION TECHNIQUES FOR SPECIFIC SYMPTOMS

Headache: Muscle contraction headaches can develop from muscle tension in the jaw, spreading to the sides of the head or to the forehead. Headaches can also develop from tension coming up from the neck and shoulders. This can create headaches at the back of head or at the base of the skull. This neck/shoulder tension can be related to improper head position (posture) or inappropriate shoulder breathing. Biofeedback monitoring of this muscle tension can help create awareness and can help you to develop the skills to relax these specific muscle groups.

Jaw Tension/Pain: Tension held in the muscles of the jaw around the temporomandibular joint (TMJ) is the cause of headaches and dental pain. Jaw and head position can affect this pain. Relaxation of this tension is essential and yet can take a surprising amount of time and practice. Use your regular breathing check-ins to reduce tension in the jaw and save lots of pain later in your day.

Neck/Shoulder Pain: Neck pain or tightness is very common. We have expressions like "pain in the neck" when we describe a difficult person or activity because this is where we habitually store our tension. The neck is a relatively poorly designed structure so it can be injured fairly easily over time. People will psychologically guard themselves in stressful situations by tightening their neck and shoulders to brace against trauma or stressors. Being aware and learning to let go of such guarding is very helpful for controlling pain.

As with headaches, neck/shoulder tension can be related to improper head position (posture) or inappropriate shoulder breathing. Biofeedback monitoring can help to create awareness and help you develop the skills to relax these specific muscle groups.

Low Back Pain: Back problems are very common and extremely painful. The low back is not a well-designed structure and so can be injured easily. Soft-tissue injuries in this area of the body are often overlooked but can contribute to the cause or increased intensity of low back pain. Look for muscle tension in back of the upper legs to create tension and pain in the lower back. Lower back pain can be related to improper head position (posture) or even inappropriate shoulder breathing. Biofeed-

back monitoring of this muscle tension can help to create awareness and can help you develop the skills to relax these specific muscle groups.

VENT YOUR EMOTIONS.

Frustration, anger, resentment, anxiety, and depression are normal by-products of coping with injury and pain. An appropriate and supportive way of discharging this potentially damaging emotional energy can be very helpful. Your church, pain clinic, psychological counselor/therapist, even your physical therapist may be able to help you vent your frustration. Getting this support from family and friends can be useful but may wear thin over time. You may need to search out the appropriate groups or professionals who are equipped to help you handle your frustrations.

Communication tools can help you vent your emotions safely and can save you wear and tear on your injured systems. Make a point of finding the best, most therapeutic method for you—this will be an extremely important key to managing your chronic pain.

Rheumatoid Arthritis

Though no one really knows the cause of rheumatoid arthritis, one thing is certain: stress and tension play a major role in the onset and recurrence of this disease. Young adults, at an average age of thirty-five and three times as many women as men, are stricken with this form of arthritis, the most widespread form in our country.

A severe emotional or physical shock often precipitates the onset of this disease. A death in the family, a business calamity, or a difficult operation may precede the first symptoms. Prolonged physical or mental stress may also be a factor. Heredity plays a role, as at least 50 percent of rheumatoid sufferers have the rheumatoid factor in their blood; often this factor is also found in their close relatives. Having this factor does not necessarily mean that you will get rheumatoid arthritis, but it does increase your vulnerability. Certain personality traits are associated with this dysfunction, and psychiatrists have compiled a list of traits culled from studies of rheumatoid sufferers. The following are typical: shy, inhibited, masochistic, self-sacrificing, anxious, depressed, resentful, and repressed anger. People who possess these characteristics along with the rheumatoid factor are the most likely candidates for this disease; *people who have a healthy psychological balance and the factor rarely suffer from the disease.*

Rheumatoid arthritis is an autoimmune illness. The body turns against itself and destroys healthy and unhealthy tissue indiscriminately. For example, if you had an infection in your joints, the antibodies would attack the infection, and under normal conditions, destroy the unhealthy tissue. In rheumatoid arthritis the antibodies cannot distinguish between healthy and unhealthy cells, and destroy both. Healthy cells, in an attempt to heal the system, begin to divide rapidly and more tissue is created than is necessary. This tissue creeps in between the joints, causing the swelling endemic to this form of arthritis.

Though this disease responds well, at first, to chemical treatment, often this treatment does not effect a cure. If the patient is subject to stress, the symptoms often flare up. Complete rest, with some form of exercise, is often prescribed; for many people this is financially infeasible, and the strain of an additional financial burden may create more excess tension. Climate also seems to have some effect, and in some cases a change from

the northern part of the temperate zone to a hotter climate brings about a remission or slows down the progression. But once again, this treatment is not possible for most sufferers and doesn't always work.

Rheumatoid arthritis commonly affects the joints of the body: the shoulders, elbows, hips, wrists, fingers, knees, ankles, and feet. In some people the disease may progress rapidly, while in others there may be flare-ups every few years, with little pain for years at a time. *Some cases have a complete remission, others are stabilized, and others progress over the years to severe debilitation.* Interestingly, the people who respond the best to stress-reduction therapy are those who have chronic, severe cases. People with sporadic, unprolonged attacks often lack the motivation necessary to follow the exercise program.

The onset of this dysfunction may be sudden, but usually it is gradual. The first sign is swelling and pain in the joints; the symptoms are often migratory, moving from joint to joint. Often the symptoms will abruptly disappear. After an indeterminate period of time, the pain and swelling reappear. Certain prodromal symptoms may be noticed, such as weakness and fatigue, loss of weight, anemia, and a tingling sensation in the hands and feet. The collagen fibers of the connective tissue are the most affected parts of the body; the cartilage may eventually be destroyed, and in severe cases, the bones themselves destroyed. Scar tissue forms and the joints become immobilized and deformed.

A woman who had tried just about every possible treatment for rheumatoid arthritis was referred to me for stress-reduction therapy. Her doctors had prescribed cortisone treatments, gold injections, and a combination of codeine and aspirin for pain. Though she had been temporarily relieved, the symptoms had always reappeared. Her parents had been missionaries, and she had had a very strict and structured upbringing. She was very guilty about not practicing Christianity, tended to be self-sacrificing to assuage her guilt, and had difficulty in recognizing and expressing anger. As she lived out of town, it was necessary for me to see her for an intensive two-week session. We worked on autogenics and visualization, and then she returned to her home and continued to practice on her own. After one month she had dramatically reduced her medication needs, which surprised her physician very much; but more importantly, she began to notice a reduction in the stiffness of her fingers. There was a noticeable difference in the amount of discomfort and pain, and the woman felt more positive about her condition and its effect on her life.

Rheumatoid Arthritis Control Program

I recommend autogenics and visualization for rheumatoid sufferers. Though you may not have a complete remission of the disease, the progression can be slowed down, and at the very least, your attacks can be reduced. Autogenics will work well because the suggestion of increased blood flow to the extremities eases pain and promotes healing. Visualizations which picture increased blood flow are also beneficial for the same reason, and visualization of the joints healing themselves can be valuable when used after a deep relaxation state is achieved. A warm bath stimulates the circulation and reduces severe pain.

If you plan to institute a stress-reduction program for rheumatoid arthritis, please check with your physician. Your medication needs may radically change as a result of stress management, and

Continued ➡

your doctor should monitor your progress. Do not expect any magic cure, but a positive, stress-free existence can only help your condition.

Keys to Controlling Rheumatoid Arthritis:

- Learn slow breathing techniques to minimize stress.
- Use biofeedback temperature monitoring for deep relaxation regularly.
- – Use a relaxation tape regularly (like *Stress Management for High Blood Pressure*).
- – Learn to warm your hands and feet to lessen your stress.
- Regular exercise can help prevent these complaints.
- Reduce your emotional triggers if these are a factor in your symptom activity.

USING BREATHING TECHNIQUES REGULARLY WILL PREVENT STRESSES FROM BUILDING.

Breathing techniques can relax you and reduce stress in your circulatory system. These techniques can also help to reduce the intensity of your symptoms if they cannot be prevented. . .

REDUCE YOUR EMOTIONAL TRIGGERS IF THESE ARE A FACTOR IN YOUR SYMPTOM ACTIVITY.

Perfectionism, repressed anger, and anxiety can all be potential triggers that either create rheumatoid arthritis or make it worse. Get help in identifying these issues and seek out support as you work through them to find more appropriate ways to respond when these emotional states are triggered.

DEVELOP A SENSE THAT YOU DO HAVE CONTROL OF YOUR RHEUMATOID ARTHRITIS.

This is not easy in the beginning, but the behavioral techniques can help you to minimize the intensity of your pain, if not eliminate it. Many people feel "out of control" when their pain becomes chronic. This can make the intensity of the pain worse because you have fear and anxiety regarding these ongoing challenges. Temperature training biofeedback can help you to learn to relax and to "let go" of the anxiety that can intensify your complaints.

Allergies and Stress-Related Respiratory Problems

One of the main manifestations of the stress response's range of physical symptoms is the effect upon normal respiration patterns. Asthma, chronic bronchitis, chronic respiratory infections, and even some allergic respiratory response can be irritated or prolonged by your response to life's changes. These conditions are not always created by stress, but can be made worse in stressful situations. People inherit characteristics both physically and emotionally that increase the possibilities of these types of symptoms. However, this does not mean that you are predestined to suffer from these complaints. You may need to change your lifestyle with behavioral techniques that can help you to get back in control of the way your body responds to stress and major life changes. (Respiratory symptoms that are created or made worse by stress can be confused with serious, sometimes life-threatening physical disorders. Please consult your physician to determine the source of your symptoms.)

Not all allergies are directly caused by stress, but stress and allergies are intrinsically related. Stress heightens your sensitivity to allergens because the immunological system is unbalanced when you are stressed. When you have an allergic reaction, your entire body is thrown into a stress response as strong as the fight-or-flight response; every time you have an allergic reaction, more stress is put on your system. This continued state of stress response makes you more susceptible to future attacks. Also, since allergic reactions perpetuate immunological disequilibrium, you become more susceptible to stress. During prolonged stress you are more prone to infection, which in turn may trigger an allergic response. This vicious cycle eventually weakens your entire system. Though drug therapy can help modify the allergic response, drugs also place stress on your system; though in many cases drugs are necessary, a stress-reduction program can help you reduce your need for medication.

When you have an allergy, your body overreacts to a foreign substance, an allergen, and responds as if that substance were a toxin. Allergies are usually characterized by an inflammation of the mucous membranes in the eyes, nose, and throat. You can be born with an allergy, it can disappear during adolescence, or an allergy can first occur during adulthood. There is no hard and fast rule about allergic responses. Some people respond immediately to an allergen, and others have a delayed reaction which may not occur for as long as twenty-four hours. Contact with an allergen may give you a slight reaction; the next contact may cause a severe attack. If you are constantly undergoing an allergic response, you may become more sensitive to other substances because you are placing added stress on your immunological system.

One manifestation of allergy is asthma, a reaction in which the bronchial tubes constrict, the breathing becomes labored, and a characteristic wheezing sound accompanies the exhalation. Emotional stress is a contributing factor and can often precipitate an asthma attack. Asthmatics not allergic to a particular substance often have an attack solely as a reaction to stress. If you have asthma, you can see how much of a role emotional stress plays in asthma; when you get more upset your attack often becomes more severe. Try to correlate your attacks with life events to discover what triggers them. You may notice a pattern of attacks occurring during certain kinds of emotionally upsetting situations.

Allergy and Respiratory Complaint Control Program

Meditation, biofeedback, progressive relaxation, and autogenics can be helpful in combating allergic reactions and asthma. Progressive relaxation and autogenics can be used for a long-term program for reducing the amount of excess stress in your life. Deep breathing and Zen Breath-Counting will help you move the focus of breathing from your chest to the abdominal region. Concentrating on releasing muscle tension in progressive relaxation will help you release muscle tension from your chest when you are experiencing an asthma attack. Visualizing blue and green colors, or cool blue water, will help reduce the inflammation of the mucous membranes associated with these dysfunctions.

A lifetime asthma sufferer that I worked with found that visualization gave him the most relief. He was not able to completely cure himself, but he was able to minimize the attacks. He was in his late twenties, and his barrel-chested, round-shouldered physique was typical of asthmatics. Though he was definitely allergic to smoke and specific chemical substances, his attacks were often triggered by visits to his dying mother. His job as a counselor of the emotionally disturbed also placed him in upsetting situations. We worked with a visualization of the complete dilation of his respiratory system, first picturing his bronchial tubes expanding and allowing for free air flow. Then he pictured himself as completely calm and relaxed, breathing easily and fully. He used this visualization as soon as he started wheezing and found that he was able to reduce the severity of the attack.

Keys to Controlling Stress-Related Respiratory Complaints:

- Breathe slowly.
- Remain in the present, in your body, and in a positive frame of mind.
- Avoid being perfectionistic and controlling.
- Use positive self-talk; avoid negative expectations.
- Use biofeedback temperature monitoring for deep relaxation regularly.
- – Use a relaxation tape regularly.
- – Learn to warm your hands and feet.
- Exercise aerobically and regularly.
- Avoid caffeine and other stimulants.
- Get support or professional counsel in confronting and then desensitizing yourself to fears/phobias related to your symptoms.

LEARN TO BREATHE DIAPHRAGMATICALLY.

Place a hand over your upper abdomen. Push your abdomen out as you inhale. Let your abdomen move in as you exhale. Let your chest, shoulders, neck, and back relax as you breathe. Only on a very deep breath should these parts move in the breath. (Use the other exercises from the chapter on relaxation through breathing.). . .

DEVELOP SKILLS OF CONTROL THROUGH POSITIVE EXPECTATIONS.

Do not let your fears escalate into losing control of your body and mind. By breathing slowly and staying in your body, in present time, you avoid falling into the negative pattern of fear and panic which can intensify if not create breathing symptoms.

The more you practice these relaxation techniques and practice the preventive lifestyle suggestions, the better your results will be in the near future. The key will be preventing the breathing difficulties. Early detection and positive actions during a respiratory flare-up will be the next best step. This will work most effectively after you have mastered diaphragmatic breathing and relaxation, and have the confidence to use these techniques even in the panic situation that accompanies breathing difficulties.

Remember that just as with other stress symptoms, respiratory difficulties are warnings to pay attention to our lives. We are being given an opportunity to examine our stresses and alleviate if not eliminate them.

Good luck! Remember to give this program enough time and practice so that you may gain the control you need to have for better breathing. . . .

Insomnia and Sleeping Disorders

Sleep dysfunctions are as common in our society as headaches. Difficulty getting to sleep, staying asleep, and resting during sleep are all forms of insomnia. Sleep remedies have become big business for the drug industry; they do not cure the problem. Drugs may induce a dreamless sleep that leaves you groggy in the morning, and regular use creates dependency.

Nearly everyone, at some point in their lives, is affected by sleeping difficulties—getting to sleep, staying asleep, or getting true rest while sleeping. For many people, these problems are inherited or learned in childhood. For others, they may be related to trauma or habit changes that have happened later in life. For still others, they may be

Continued ➤

related to physical changes that interrupt normal restful patterns of sleep. Such problems can become chronic unless you take action and develop the appropriate strategies to regain control.

To begin, insomnia is often related to the body's distraction and unconscious preoccupation with hypervigilance or hyperarousal. This often takes the form of unnecessary and inappropriately high levels of muscle tension, especially in the muscles of your jaw, face, neck/shoulders, back, and legs. With this habitual muscle tension as a distraction, it is difficult to relax and drift off into a restful state of sleep.

Usually insomnia has no organic cause, beyond protracted and chronic tension, though your diet may influence your sleeping patterns. Worrying about not being able to sleep well creates more tension, and it is not unusual for the condition to perpetuate in a snowball fashion. Ordinary daily tension can create enough anxiety, pain, and discomfort to keep you awake at night. If you have insomnia, institute a daily stress-reduction program. Stress-reduction techniques should be practiced before bed; you should also practice earlier in the day, since your anxiety about going to sleep will make it more difficult for you to relax at night.

Insomnia Control Program

Books have been written that are entirely devoted to sleeping disorders. This section is designed to get you started on a behavioral program for controlling the stresses that contribute to, if not cause, your sleeping problems.

Start your program with progressive relaxation, or the Visualization for Relaxation found in the chapter on visualization. Any autogenics, meditation, visualization, or breathing exercise may also be useful. Even if practicing relaxation does not completely stop insomnia attacks, relaxation can prevent the fatigue which often accompanies sleeplessness. *Twenty minutes of relaxation a day can take the place of two hours of sleep at night.* Your need for sleep may drop from nine to ten hours a night to six or seven hours. Mine did when I began to practice daily. This radical change is not at all unusual, and I recommend that people keep a diary of their sleeping habits so that they can become aware of any changes.

If relaxation cannot control the thoughts keeping you from sleep, maybe you should give in to them completely. Get up and take out your tape recorder. Speak all your thoughts, fears, worries, and irrational concerns into it. If some of your problems require action, record plans as to when, where, and how to act. Chronic worries or problems that you cannot immediately solve may obsess you; accept that you cannot resolve them. Close the book on these thoughts, return to bed, and try a relaxation technique.

Sometimes your body may just not be ready to go to sleep. Muscle tension may need to be released through physical movement, and a plan of daily physical activity combined with relaxation techniques can be the best "sleeping pill" of all. Check the section on physical movement; your activity doesn't need to be aggressive and extremely athletic to be effective. Gentle physical exercise can be even more appropriate and helpful than a set of tennis or handball.

I devised the following exercise to induce sleep, and my insomniac clients have found it very helpful. One client, a middle manager in a large corporation, spent every night awake, thinking about work-related issues. He worried about everything he had left unfinished on his desk; he worried about his relationship with his employees; he wor-

ried that he would be phased out by new "talent" in the firm. Because he did not get enough sleep, his work suffered: more and more work was left undone, and relationships with his co-workers deteriorated. His worries became self-perpetuating, and fear of replacement became more of a reality than an unfounded obsession.

He started to practice Relaxation for Sleep using my tape that is based on the progressive relaxation technique. After gaining some perspective on how his state of continual tension affected his health, he began to make definite associations between work events and sleepless nights. Once he consciously understood that he could control his sleeping habits and often positively affect difficult work situations, his behavior became less self-destructive. In a matter of months, his sleeping patterns had altered radically; he was sleeping peacefully every night of the week.

Relaxation for Sleep

An insomnia control exercise is available at www.dstress.com. Look for Tape #204.

This exercise works best if it is taped. Begin by getting into a comfortable position. Allow yourself to begin to calm and relax. Take one, deep, full breath, pause for a moment, and then exhale, fully and completely. Now, allow yourself to breathe slowly and naturally. Imagine that with each and every breath, you can exhale away excess energy or tension.

As you continue to breathe slowly and naturally, your muscles will gradually get heavier, and as you let go of more and more tension, your muscles will go loose and limp. As you continue to allow yourself to relax, focus your attention on your arms and hands. Imagine that the muscles of your upper arms are getting loose and limp as you let go of tension. Allow your upper arms to relax more fully and completely. Imagine that you can breathe away the tension, just exhaling it away with every full and complete exhalation. Remember that you can control tension and gradually you can let your muscles become even more relaxed.

Now, relax the muscles around your elbows, letting them go limp and relaxed. Let the relaxation spread down into your lower arms, while you slowly breathe away the tension, even from your wrists. Just release the tension, and feel it flowing through your hands, and then into your fingers, and out of your body through your fingertips. Let your muscles go loose and limp, and just allow the tension to flow from you, while you drift slightly deeper into calmness and relaxation.

Continue to breathe slowly and naturally, while considering your feet and your legs. Allow them to relax fully and completely, slowly breathing away the tension from the muscles in your toes and feet. Gently release the tension from your arches and your heels, letting the tension spread out of your ankles, and breathe away the excess energy slowly and completely. Allow yourself to relax your lower legs, just letting go of tension. Let the muscles go loose and limp. Relax the muscles around your knees, and in your upper legs, slowly allow the tension to melt away, as you sink deeper into whatever you are sitting upon or lying upon. Slowly allow yourself to drift deeper into a state of complete calmness and relaxation.

Gently turn your awareness to your back, and let the muscles around your shoulder blades relax. Just let go and allow these muscles to go loose and limp, allowing yourself to sink further into the bed or chair. Let the muscles on both sides of your spine relax, all the way down, down into your lower back. Allow the relaxation to spread slowly to all of

your muscles, and feel them totally relaxing as all the tension melts away. Remember to breathe calmly and naturally, exhaling fully and completely.

Let the relaxation spread down into your pelvic area, down into your lower back, and down into your legs. Just let go of the tension, and allow yourself to drift as deeply as you wish to, into a state of calmness and deep relaxation. As you continue to breathe slowly and calmly, gently become aware of the muscles in your chest and in your abdomen, and allow these muscles to relax. Your heartbeat is calm and regular, and your breathing is calm and regular. Feel the calmness in your abdominal region, and allow yourself to relax, letting yourself drift deeper into a dreamlike state of complete calmness and relaxation.

Now, become aware of the muscles in the back of your head, on the sides, and on the top of your head. Let these muscles go loose and limp, while breathing away the tensions slowly and naturally and allowing your forehead to go calm and smooth. Relax the muscles around your eyes and throughout your face. Relax your mouth, your tongue, and your jaw. Gently breathe away the tension, letting yourself flow into a peaceful state of calmness and deep relaxation.

Become aware of the muscles in your neck, and just let your head sink into a pillow or the chair, as your neck muscles go loose and limp. Relax your shoulders and your neck more completely now, letting your shoulders drop, letting go of the tension in these muscles, and peacefully easing yourself into a dreamlike state of calmness and deep relaxation. As you continue to breathe slowly and naturally, be aware that your arms and legs begin to feel heavier and more relaxed, and that the blood flow and energy flow is free and easy to every part of your body. You can control tension by breathing it away slowly and naturally, letting yourself drift deeper into a state of deep relaxation.

Imagine that you are outdoors on a very calm and peaceful day, in your favorite place, in a beautiful locale where you will not be disturbed by any distractions. Imagine that you can see yourself moving over to a very comfortable spot, and you lie down, just melting into the ground. Golden sunlight and its warmth gently shine down upon you. Feel the warmth on your arms and your hands, and feel the warm sunlight and breezes create pulsating, warming sensations in your feet and your legs. Just allow this feeling of warmth and relaxation to spread to every part of your body. Let your mind drift in a dreamlike state, as you continue to let go and drift peacefully along, deeper and deeper, into a sleepy, calm state of deep relaxation.

Feel yourself slowing and calming, just letting go more and more. Count backward from 5 down to 1, picturing each number, and slowing and relaxing even more, as each number fades from your peaceful, calm mind. As you picture the number 5, remember to breathe slowly and calmly, letting go and sinking deeper and deeper into relaxation. At 4, you are more relaxed than you were at 5, taking a step deeper into relaxation. At 3, you are more relaxed than you were at 4, relaxing and letting go, gently drifting down into deep relaxation. At 2, you can feel your slow, natural heartbeat gently pulsating to every cell in your body. And at 1 you are more relaxed than you were at 2, gently letting yourself drift even deeper into relaxation.

Drift into a dreamlike state of pleasant, relaxing slumber. As you let yourself drift off peacefully and comfortably, remember whenever you wish you can awake, feeling calm and relaxed. When you finally awake, you will feel refreshed and alert, and realize how much control you have over your tension and

Continued ➡

excess energy. By breathing it away slowly and calmly, you can let go even further, peacefully drifting into calmness and restful relaxation. Just continue to let yourself drift peacefully deeper into calmness and deep relaxation.

Keys to Controlling Insomnia:

- Breathe slowly.
- Maintain a regular schedule.
- Use relaxation techniques regularly.
  - Use a relaxation tape regularly.
  - Learn to relax your jaw and neck/shoulders.
- Exercise aerobically and regularly.
- Avoid caffeine and other stimulants.

LEARN TO BREATHE DIAPHRAGMATICALLY. Place a hand over your upper abdomen. Push your abdomen out as you inhale. Let your abdomen move in as you exhale. Let your chest, shoulders, neck, and back relax as you breathe. Only on a very deep breath should these parts move in the breath. (Use the other exercises from the chapter on relaxation through breathing.)

Relaxing/breathing throughout your day may make relaxing at bedtime easier. By linking one deep breath to a reoccurring work event like a telephone ringing or checking the time, you remember to take these slow deep breaths throughout your work schedule to avoid letting tensions build to painful or distracting levels. The secret is to check in with your body in the present moment, relax your major muscles, and slow and deepen your breath. This simple exercise can have miraculous results.

Other breathing techniques involve a short series of deep slow breaths, where you count as you breathe. Try counting slowly 1 to 4 as you inhale, pause and hold your breath as you count 1 to 4 again, and then release slowly, but completely, as you count 1 to 8. After four of these breaths, you will be breathing easier and better able to control your body's pattern of holding tension. This can help teach you how to control your insomnia.

Another breathing/counting exercise that works very well for many people is a technique of counting backward from 50 down to 1. The unique addition to this countdown is to add counting 1, 2, 3 to every number in your countdown. Example: 50, 1, 2, 3, 49, 1, 2, 3, 48, 1, 2, 3, 47, 1, 2, 3, 46, and so on. By focusing on these numbers, you will relax enough to drift off into relaxation and sleep.

MAINTAIN A REGULAR SCHEDULE. Make sure that you keep a regular bedtime, if possible. Changes in a regular routine can upset one's normal balance. This may even relate to the place and bed that you sleep in. Eventually you will not be so bound by time and environment, but to get a handle on this problem, it is best not to have too many variables. It is not recommended to schedule vigorous exercise or high-energy activities right before bedtime. A quiet, settling time would be best. Action books, arguments, movies, or even the news on TV may not be conducive to proper relaxation at bedtime. Eating too close to sleep may be another problem. Many people find that eating a heavy meal (with lots of protein or sauces) or spicy foods may interfere with getting sleep.

A warm bath or shower, a massage, or some other peaceful relaxation technique before sleep may encourage better sleeping patterns.

PRACTICE RELAXATION TECHNIQUES. Relaxation of the major muscle groups is very helpful for rest and sleep enhancement. You are encouraged to use the *Stress Management for Sleep* audiotape available from the Stress Education Cen-

ter (see the contact information in the back of this book) at bedtime to help you relax and fall asleep. You may need to practice with this tape for four to twelve weeks to develop the skill necessary to help you relax and drift off into a restful state of sleep.

Remember, the jaw, the neck, and the shoulders are often the areas of the body that are tight and can distract you from falling asleep. These are also the most difficult parts of the body for most people to learn to relax. It takes time!

Relaxation is easier in a quiet comfortable space. You may want to be warm, but not too warm for a restful sleep. If you have a lot on your mind, write out a list and prioritize it so you can begin to work on these items in the morning. . . .

Panic/Anxiety

Anxiety is the most prevalent type of neurosis in the United States and is the direct result of stress; its increase is in direct proportion to the increase of environmental and social problems such as noise pollution, air pollution, urbanization, inflation, crime, decay of the nuclear family, and divorce.

Everyone experiences anxiety. It is the normal reaction to a threat to your body, values, lifestyle, or a loved one. A certain amount is normal and even stimulating; it may provoke you to resolve conflicts and unhealthy situations. An excess amount of anxiety can be debilitating and, at the very least, interfere with your normal functioning. Healthy, normal anxiety usually decreases over a period of time as you become gradually desensitized by repeated exposure to the anxiety-producing situation. Neurotic anxiety increases with repeated exposure to the situation and eventually leads to avoidance or withdrawal from the dreaded circumstances.

Major transitions, trauma, and stress can lead to feelings of little or no control over one's life. As a result, a feeling of panic may ensue. A panic episode can come on suddenly or can awaken you from sleep with an overwhelming feeling of apprehension. Some people believe that they are having a heart attack because often there is chest pain, a shortness of breath, neck or arm pain, major stomach upset, an adrenaline rush, lightheadedness, dizziness, and other unpleasant feelings of fear and apprehension. These feelings can be triggered by specific events such as: driving (getting stuck in traffic); shopping; waiting in lines (at stores, banks, post offices, and so on); feeling trapped (in church, movie theaters, classes, and so on); traveling distances from home (especially by airplane); making a presentation in front of a group of people (or something else which draws attention toward oneself); doing new or unfamiliar things; meeting new people. Anything new or seemingly stressful where you fear losing control can bring on a panic episode.

Loss of control is the main feature of panic attacks. The anticipation of the attacks can be very frightening, and of course the attacks themselves give the feeling of no control. We may not know a panic sufferer by looking at him or her unless we look very carefully to notice the nervousness below the surface.

Fear may be out of proportion to the real threat in an anxiety attack. Some people may know what precipitates an attack, and others may not recognize the cause. The fear itself is always conscious, though the cause may not be. A client of mine exhibited fear and anxiety about going to work on the weekends, but was unable to determine exactly what was causing his attacks of rapid heartbeat and nausea. He felt fearful and always recognized his feeling as

fear; he did not know what was directly responsible for the fear.

His work as a lab technician in a hospital was rewarding and enjoyable. Life with his wife was stimulating, and they did not have any serious marital problems. At first he only disliked going to work; eventually his dislike became dread, and he refused to get out of bed and go to work on the weekend. I taught him autogenics combined with passive progressive relaxation. This helped him to partially control his anxiety and tension, and after two weeks of practice he realized what had generated his fear.

During the week he worked with other people and was not solely responsible for interpreting test results. He worked alone on Saturday. The strain of not being able to discuss and compare test results with other technicians made him feel inadequate and on edge. He realized that it had become almost impossible for him to analyze the tests when he worked alone. After eight weeks of intensive practice he no longer had attacks of nausea; going to work on Saturday was still anxiety-producing. He decided that the best thing he could do for himself would be to find another hospital job where he always worked with other people and was not personally responsible for analyzing findings.

Intense emotional reactions to ordinary events may indicate anxiety. Common tasks such as preparing a meal or socializing with friends may create an unnatural fear or dread. A feeling of inadequacy at meeting obligations, despondency, pessimism, and lack of concentration are indicators of an anxiety state. Decision-making becomes difficult and tolerance for frustration is decreased. Inability to determine the relationship between life events and unnatural feelings of fear can cause humiliation; you may view your fears and anxieties as a childish inability to control the functioning of your own mind.

A person suffering from an anxiety neurosis may exhibit certain physical symptoms: palpitations, chest pain, cold and sweaty extremities, bandlike pressure around the head, constriction of the throat, fatigue, lack of appetite, vomiting, and diarrhea. Not all of the symptoms will be present, but all acute anxiety attacks will manifest in some physical dysfunction. Often people suffering from severe anxiety believe that they have a serious illness; symptoms of panic and anxiety can be confused with life-threatening physical disorders. Please consult your physician to determine the source of your symptoms.

Heart problems, chest pain, and respiratory difficulties (hyperventilation and dizziness are common symptoms of panic/anxiety attacks) should be carefully examined by your physician. If no heart-related problem exists, but you are still in great fear of these occurrences of panic, then the following behavioral program, with practice, will greatly aid you in preventing or at least minimizing the episodes of panic. Also, remember that exciting/positive actions or events can raise your heart rate as well. This excitement is not bad or life threatening, and the fear of the physical symptoms of excitement can really hamper your enjoyment of life.

Panic/Anxiety Control Program

Any of the forms of relaxation you use and feel comfortable with can be of aid to you in a time of anxiety. I particularly recommend autogenics, visualization, progressive relaxation, desensitization, and meditation. Practice two to three times daily, and keep a first-aid tape on hand, such as a 10-to-1 Passive Progressive Relaxation tape. Use this tape if things get out of control; listening to and following the instructions will calm you.

Continued →

A therapist or doctor can help you regain your emotional equilibrium. Empathy, compassion, and the support of your family and friends are very important; it will be more difficult for you to help yourself if your family and friends are constantly reinforcing negative and destructive tendencies. Also, be aware of your diet, and any effect that it might have on your emotional stability. If you find yourself knocked off balance soon after you eat, evaluate what was in your food. Some people are radically affected by hidden chemicals and sugars.

Practiced on a regular basis, relaxation can give you more control over your mind and body, and help you take control of your own life. During deep relaxation, when the mind is calmed and quieted, you may be able to come to terms with what is really bothering you. Relaxation can be a safety valve for releasing excess tension and can keep you on an even keel in the sea of life.

Keys to Controlling Panic And Anxiety:

- Breathe slowly.
- Remain in the present, in your body, and in a positive frame of mind.
- Use positive self-talk; avoid negative expectations.
- Use biofeedback temperature monitoring for deep relaxation regularly.
  - Use a relaxation tape regularly.
  - Learn to warm your hands and feet.
- Exercise aerobically and regularly.
- Avoid caffeine and other stimulants.
- Get support in confronting and then desensitizing yourself to your fears/phobias.
- Taper your antianxiety medication after you have mastered the relaxation-biofeedback.

LEARN TO BREATHE DIAPHRAGMATICALLY.

Place a hand over your upper abdomen. Push your abdomen out as you inhale. Let your abdomen move in as you exhale. Let your chest, shoulders, neck, and back relax as you breathe. Only on a very deep breath should these parts move in the breath. (Use the other exercises from the chapter on relaxation through breathing.) This may be the most important panic control technique you can learn!. . .

PRACTICE POSITIVE SELF-TALK.

Do not let your fears escalate into losing control of your body and mind. By breathing slowly and staying in your body, in present time, you avoid falling into the negative pattern of fear and panic.

GET SUPPORT FROM YOUR FRIENDS, DOCTOR, AND A THERAPIST, IF NECESSARY.

Check your area for panic/anxiety support or treatment groups. Regular use of antianxiety medications may be better than taking your prescription only after the panic has begun. Reduce your medication in a supervised way after you have mastered the relaxation-biofeedback control techniques.

REMEMBER YOU CAN GET BACK IN CONTROL OF YOUR BODY AND YOUR LIFE!

You must make this a priority so you can avoid being a victim to this set of scary symptoms. Panic/anxiety is not always your enemy. This reaction is designed to protect you and may teach you something about the stresses and transitions you are going through. Denial of these challenges only creates a more stubborn set of symptoms that can be more debilitating. . . .

Terminal and Severe Disorders

If you have a severe or terminal illness you should be under a doctor's care. This does not mean that you should abdicate full responsibility for your cure, as you may be the best healer of your own body. In *Anatomy of an Illness as Perceived by the Patient*, Norman Cousins describes his "miracle cure." Diagnosed as having an incurable collagen ailment, he took an active role as partner with his physician in the healing process. He believes that positive emotions and behaviors, such as joy and laughter, can activate the immunological system's defenses; he maintained a positive attitude despite the prognosis.

Death of a family member or an acute trauma often precedes the onset of cancer or another serious illness by six to eighteen months. *Emotional upset seems to predispose human beings to severe illnesses.* If, like Norman Cousins, you can dwell upon positive emotions, your chances of getting well again are much better. When you are in a state of emotional upset, your immunological defenses are weakened; you are more susceptible to illness. People often use this information to blame themselves for having an incurable disease. This creates guilt, which is just one more negative emotion. Nor should you feel bad if you can't instantly mobilize all your positive feelings; it is natural to be angry, desperate, and afraid. It is better to accept these feelings rather than repress them, which just places more stress upon your system.

Carl and Stephanie Simonton have done extensive research with cancer patients. They have discovered that there is a definite correlation between attitude and cure rate. In their program, used as an adjunct to conventional medical treatment, cancer patients use visualization and also explore their attitudes toward their illness. Life drive is examined and patients are helped to determine if secondary gains play a large role in their disease.

A woman in her mid-forties was suffering from ulcerative colitis. Preliminary X rays indicated that about two feet of intestinal damage had occurred. She had severe emotional and family problems and a history of asthma, allergies, and migraine. She constantly worried about everything; even if the mail carrier was late, she worried that something had happened to him or that she would never get the mail. All her anger was repressed, and she never directly confronted anyone who had upset or inconvenienced her. Fifteen years before the onset of the disease, her husband had deserted her, leaving her with a three-year-old daughter. The child had always been overly dependent on her mother and for the two years prior to her mother's hospitalization had been undergoing psychotherapy twice a week. Her biggest fear upon entering the hospital was that her eighteen-year-old daughter wouldn't be able to feed and care for herself.

After her first hospitalization, when the physicians had diagnosed her illness, she returned home to recuperate before the surgery. She still experienced severe pain in her abdominal area; though she was very skeptical, she started attending a pain clinic two nights a week. She practiced a healing visualization twice a day until she returned to the hospital two months later. The doctors informed her that they had only removed a six-inch section of her intestines, as the original damage appeared to be partially healed. She believes that the healing visualization had a great deal to do with the improvement. Realizing that any added stress will possibly cause a recurrence of the disease, she is practicing stress reduction to control her anxiety.

Terminal and Severe Disorder Control Program

A combined program of relaxation therapy and self-healing visualization should be discussed with your doctor. If you are severely ill, I would recommend three relaxation sessions a day. After you have learned to relax, add a self-healing visualization to the exercise. Taping a relaxation-visualization exercise, rather than trying to memorize, would be ideal. In visualizing your ailment, picture your defenses defeating the infection or aberrant cells; use an image that seems most accurate to you. Your medical therapy is a positive agent, helping you to rally your natural defenses and destroy the disease. Use images for your disease that are weak and easily overwhelmed by your natural defenses.

Many people start this therapy with skepticism, and if you feel this way it doesn't mean you shouldn't try. Motivation does play a part in the healing process, but your unconscious is also involved. Listening to the tape over and over again can activate unconscious healing. You may need to revise your visualization as your health changes. If you are going to have surgery, visualize the entire procedure and its positive results. After surgery visualize complete healing of the area.

You may feel as if you have no control over what is happening in your body. To give yourself some hope, read Norman Cousins and the Simontons. Find a doctor or a clinic that will understand and cooperate with a relaxation and visualization program. More and more doctors are beginning to recognize the significance of the patient's attitude. Disease is complicated by many factors, but there are some factors you can control.

Keys to Controlling Terminal and/or Severe Disorders:

- Learn slow breathing techniques to minimize stress.
- Use of biofeedback temperature monitoring for deep relaxation regularly.
  - Use a relaxation tape regularly (like *Stress Management for High Blood Pressure*).
  - Learn to warm your hands and feet to lessen your stress.
- Regular exercise can help minimize or prevent these complaints.
- Reduce your emotional triggers if these are a factor in your symptom activity.

USING BREATHING TECHNIQUES REGULARLY WILL PREVENT STRESSES FROM BUILDING.

Breathing techniques can relax you and reduce stress in your circulatory system. These techniques can also help to reduce the intensity of your symptoms if they cannot be prevented. . .

REDUCE YOUR EMOTIONAL TRIGGERS IF THESE ARE A FACTOR IN YOUR SYMPTOM ACTIVITY.

Perfectionism, repressed anger, and anxiety can all be potential triggers that either create symptoms or make them worse. Get help in identifying these issues and seek out support as you work through them to find more appropriate ways to respond when these emotional states are triggered.

DEVELOP A SENSE THAT YOU DO HAVE CONTROL OF YOUR SYMPTOMS.

This is not easy in the beginning, but the behavioral techniques can help you to minimize the intensity of your pain, if not eliminate it. Many people feel "out of control" when their pain becomes chronic. This can make the intensity of the pain worse because you have fear and anxiety regarding these ongoing challenges. Temperature training biofeedback can help you to learn to relax and to "let go" of the anxiety that can intensify your complaints. Eventually, acceptance of your symptoms or illness may prove useful to minimize the anxiety and fears that can make pain worse. Lessening your physical and emotional pains will allow a better quality of life.

—From *Guide to Stress Reduction*

Continued ➡

SELF-HYPNOSIS

Adam Burke, Ph. D.

Self-hypnosis is a simple, practical tool for transforming beliefs. Why is that important? The beliefs we hold about self, others, and the world influence every single experience we have. If we believe we are not smart enough or that we are unattractive, that the world is not safe, or that we are not loved by other people, then our life becomes very limited, very constricted. On the other hand, if we believe that we are worthy, that the world is good, and that we are loved by others, then our life expands. It is really quite simple.

Beyond Limits

Our positive beliefs inspire us. They allow us to embrace dreams, to harness healing energy, to have hope and confidence, and to take empowered action. Positive beliefs strengthen and encourage us; perhaps we can say they liberate us. Certainly both types of beliefs, positive and negative, are within us. The thing to remember is that we always have a choice about which beliefs will constitute the core of our reality. If we want to be happy, if we hope to live a powerful life, the appropriate choice becomes clear. To experience deep healing and high happiness it is imperative that we act to reduce our limiting beliefs and to replace them with powerful new positive beliefs. We all possess the potential for an incredible life journey. Such a life begins and ends with empowered beliefs. If we can learn to work more intentionally with our beliefs then we will possess a key to achieving the greatest life possible.

The Healing Journey

When we heal our beliefs, those transformed beliefs can begin to heal us. The task of belief transformation, however, is not necessarily an easy one. It is challenging because of a number of internal mechanisms that are designed to protect our past beliefs and to resist the introduction of new information that might alter them. To succeed in the process of transforming and empowering new beliefs we need to strategically address those protective mechanisms.

One approach is to cultivate new beliefs through self-hypnosis. How does that work? It is a process by which we take in ideas, in the form of specifically structured visual or verbal information, and plant them at a deep level within our mind and body. When we work at this deep mind-body level we experience the information as its own reality, just as dreams are experienced as a reality. Self-hypnosis helps us to sink below the tangle of voices that say our dream is too big, that we will not succeed, that no one has ever done that before. It helps us to sink below those internal vigilance mechanisms that are designed to hold us in place by reducing receptivity to new information and new possibilities. Here we can explore new possibilities. With self-hypnosis we can enter a place of hope. The gates are open. Here our true vision can awaken, and we can wisely craft the life of our dreams.

Self-hypnosis gives us more access to life's potential. It can be used for working on relationship issues, body and health concerns, addictions, athletic performance, self-image, anxiety, public speaking, earning more money, improving one's sex life, experiencing greater courage, getting better grades, passing exams, finding a career; the list is endless. If your beliefs affect an issue, beliefs about yourself, the world, or life, then self-hypnosis can help. Self-hypnosis goes to the root level of our perceptions about life providing the requisite nourishment and vital energy necessary for deep change to occur. It is a simple tool that gives us a way to become the person we were born to be. . . .

The Goal

Having a clear sense of your desired outcomes is important. A vague goal will generate less insight, less commitment, and less motivation than a refined one. Water becomes a powerful force when it is focused and directed through a channel. Give direction to your dream, and it too will become empowering. You can also use hypnosis to arrive at a clearer vision if your issues are still muddy. Finding clarity can become your goal. Decide on the most important goal or goals that you want to begin manifesting.

Preparing Your Suggestions

Think of the suggestions you will want to use during your session. Make them appropriate, sufficient, positive, and varied. You will need a clear set of suggestions before you can do effective self-hypnosis. Work on the phrasing for your verbal suggestions, the imagery for your visual suggestions, and your choice of metaphors. Create a set of specific verbal, visual, and metaphoric suggestions to work with.

The Setting

Ideally you want to do your sessions in a setting that is conducive to relaxation, comfortable, reasonably quiet, and free from disturbances. If the lights can be lowered and some relaxing music turned on that is great. Reduce external input as much as possible, so there is less stimuli to pull your mind back out into the world. You want to create a sense of safety, relaxation, and comfort whenever possible.

Induction

Choose your induction method. The Fused Eyelids method is a good one to start with if you have not selected another one already. It is simple and very effective for most people. Whichever induction method you choose, remember that this is not about trying or struggling; it's about being and letting it flow.

Relaxation and Deepening

You can do self-hypnosis anywhere, but ideally you should find a good chair or couch to lie on. Make sure you stay warm too; use a blanket if you need it. Be comfortable. The magic words for relaxation are "warm, heavy, and relaxed." Tell yourself over and over, "I feel warm, heavy, and relaxed." That formula is simple and effective. For deepening you can use visual imagery, counting down, direct suggestion, and hypnotic phenomena. They can be used individually or in creative combinations. Counting down is a very effective approach.

Transformation

During your session, give your hypnotic suggestions—verbal, visual, and metaphoric. Alternate your suggestions with relaxation and other deepening methods. Continue to weave these elements to stay in the learning state while giving yourself your suggestions. See your outcome, feel it, tell yourself that you will achieve your goal, believe it. This is how old belief structures begin to dissolve and new powerful beliefs take root. Open the powerful mind-body matrix and drop in transforming images and ideas.

Conclusion

Come back. Tell yourself, I am returning now feeling refreshed, relaxed, and ready for the day. Come back slowly, noticing your breathing and your relaxation. Undo all hypnotic phenomena. Give yourself the posthypnotic suggestion that each session will be even more effective, and that during the day the positive effects of the session will become more and more evident. You can also give a posthypnotic trigger that will help you to reactivate the desired thought or behavior you are seeking to manifest.

Summary of Steps

- Vision your priority goals for greatest success and happiness
- Focus with your breath and induction
- Deepen with relaxation and other deepening methods
- Transform with verbal, visual, and metaphoric suggestions
- Cycle—for as long as you have time, cycle through your relaxation deepening methods and suggestions over and over to help you stay in a suitable state for deep transformation to occur
- Conclude the process, coming back slowly, ready for the day

Sample Script

The following script is offered both as an example and also as a useful framework for doing your own self-hypnosis sessions. It can be a good starting point, and as you become more familiar and comfortable with the material in the book you can bring in other methods and modify the script. If you choose to use this sample framework then read it to yourself several times to get a sense of the integrated process. As soon as possible, put the script down and just paraphrase the concepts in your mind. If you like you can also make a tape for yourself. It is easy to do, and it can be a useful way to work with your goals. You can write a short script, incorporating some of the ideas on specific issues from the next chapter, fine-tune the message, and then record it. The whole process will probably take an hour or two. You will then have a tailored product for your transformational process. If you do record your script then it can be a good idea to change the words "I and my" to "You and your." In this way the recording has the quality of someone speaking to you, which has a more engaging effect.

So give it a go. The core script provided here includes the following elements to work with:

- **Focusing**.
- **Fused Eyelids induction.**
- **Relaxation and Deepening,** including direct suggestions, counting down, floating leaf imagery, the hypnotic phenomena of catalepsy (immovable legs), and special workplace imagery.

Continued ➜

- **Suggestions** focusing on the specific topic of self-confidence for its verbal, visual, and metaphoric suggestion content. (As you create your own scripts it always useful to include core themes of self-confidence, the capacity to love, and a sense of having a deeply meaningful life.)
- **Concluding** with the posthypnotic suggestion of confidence during day before we undo the hypnotic phenomena.

So let us begin. Find a quiet, relaxing spot. Put on some peaceful music. Turn the lights down. Loosen any tight clothes, take off glasses and shoes. If you have to be finished by a certain time or if you are concerned that you might fall asleep, set a quiet alarm. Sit or lie down. Cover yourself with a blanket if desired. Get comfortable and gently gaze into the space in front of you.

Focusing

I will now take three deep breaths. [Take three slow, deep breaths.] Each breath allows me to let go and to begin relaxing. Three deep, relaxing breaths. Each breath out allows my muscles to soften, to become more comfortable. It feels so good to take this time for myself, time to manifest my vision, my life dreams. I know my dreams will come true. I know that everything I experience, every sound, every thought, every feeling and sensation will help me to go even deeper inside, into a place of safety, a place of comfort, a place of deep transformation. I continue to notice my body and mind relaxing. My breath is quieting. Every exhale helps me to relax even more deeply, more completely. I feel the chair/couch/bed beneath me, totally supporting me, completely supporting my body. It lets me relax completely. Letting go of every muscle now. Completely relaxing. My face, shoulders, arms, legs, breath, mind are so comfortably relaxed. I let go of every muscle now.

Fused Eyelids Induction

As I continue to relax I notice that my eyelids are becoming heavier and heavier. They are wonderfully heavy, just wanting to close. I know that when they do close I will go even deeper inside. My eyelids are getting heavier and heavier, so heavy, so relaxed. They just want to close to take me deep inside, into that place where dreams become real. My entire body is getting more heavy, more relaxed. Warm currents of comforting energy are flowing through me, just flowing through me. The colors are so beautiful. It is a perfect temperature. My eyelids are getting so heavy, taking me deeper and deeper inside. When they close I will not be able to open them. They will be so incredibly heavy. They will not open until my session is done, or until I am ready to open them. They are getting incredibly heavy, incredibly relaxed. Taking me deeper and deeper inside. [Repeat until eyes close.]

Relaxation and Deepening

My legs and arms are warm, heavy, and relaxed. I am floating in warm water, just floating. It feels so wonderful. [Repeat these phrases several times.] Slowly I begin sinking down, sinking down into a warm ocean of energy. With each exhalation I am going deeper and deeper inside. It is a very comforting feeling, very relaxing. Twenty. I am floating down now. Nineteen. Like a leaf floating down toward the earth. Feeling more and more wonderfully relaxed, more and more comfortable. Eighteen. My mind and body are going deeper, floating down. Seventeen. With every exhale I go deeper and deeper inside. The forest is quiet, peaceful. Sixteen. Everything is letting go. Floating slowly down

toward the earth, just letting go and floating. Fifteen. As I float down I am aware of a sense of deep peace. Fourteen. My body and mind are floating down deeper and deeper. The earth gently pulls me with its vast healing energy. Thirteen. My legs feel immovable; they are becoming so heavy and relaxed. My legs feel immovable; they are becoming so heavy and relaxed. Twelve. I am floating down. Eleven. I feel incredibly heavy, wonderfully heavy. Such an amazing feeling. Floating down toward the earth. Ten. Sinking deeper and deeper into the energy beneath me. Nine. Body and mind are melting into this peaceful space, very peaceful, very spacious. Beautiful colors, feeling so comfortable. Eight. It feels so relaxing. Deeper. Like an ocean, underwater canyons, deep. Seven. Deeper and deeper inside. Six. My legs are immovable. They are so heavy. The heavier they become the deeper inside I go. Five. Slowly floating in a vast spiral of energy, deeper and deeper, on warm currents of light. They are so heavy. The heavier they become the deeper I go inside. Deeper down, floating. Four. Floating deeper and deeper. Three. The colors are calming, so soothing, calming, so soothing. It is so peaceful here. Two. I am sinking deeper and deeper toward a beautiful light. One. I enter that light deep beneath me. Floating down into the light. Dissolving, just dissolving into that peaceful light.

Workplace Imagery

I am in a most amazing place now, an incredible grotto. There is a small waterfall and a crystal pool of sparkling water. There is a perfect place for me to lie down on the smooth, warm rocks, like nature's reclining chair. It fits my body perfectly. It is so comfortable, completely supporting my body. It is incredibly comfortable. As I sit there a leopard comes and lies down in front of me. I feel its weight pressing against my feet. I recognize this to be a guardian animal of this place, here to protect me. Floating on the surface of the pond is a beautiful pulsing light, an orb like a small radiant star. Directly beyond that is the waterfall. As I look at the waterfall its warm, translucent waters appear to display images. I can see images of my life. My body and mind are transfixed, immovable, so deeply relaxed. The air is fresh with the scent of pine and some incredible energy. It fills my body, and I can feel a healing energy, a purifying light, going into every cell. It fills every thought, every memory, every dream. The grotto is surrounded by ancient trees that rise up endlessly to the blue sky above. The rock wall surfaces are smooth and rounded. Moist ferns cover one wall. I watch the waters flowing and listen to the sounds.

Verbal Suggestion

I feel power running through my body and mind. I feel incredible. My energy is pure light. I remember who I am, where I am from, why I am here, how precious this adventure of life truly is. I have a wonderful sense that I can do anything at all, whatever I set my mind to. I believe in myself. I know what I can do, how many things are possible once I make my commitment to change, to grow, to heal, to succeed. I am committed now. The world needs me to be my fullest self. The world needs me to be my fullest self. The world needs me. I am alive now. I feel incredible. [Insert specific personalized suggestions.]

_____

_____

Visual Suggestion

I can see colors from behind the waterfall, like large shining gems. I see the color red, like some amazing ruby light. It is pure, extremely beautiful, very powerful, very intense. This light is flowing in a beam toward me, filling me with power like the morning sun. I am standing on a beautiful beach watching the sun rising up over the pure ocean. I see myself looking grateful, arms stretching up toward the sky. I am floating. I am powerful, so relaxed, so comfortable. It has been a most incredible year. I have done more, felt better, been stronger, kinder, more patient and persistent than at any time in my life. I look amazed and delighted. I see myself filled with confidence, the power of believing that I can. As I turn around I see down the beach my wiser, older self, twenty years into the future. A wiser, older self who has lived a powerful, self-respecting, confident life. I see a self that is capable, kind, courageous, powerful, very alive. That self sends a message that I feel deep inside. [Visualize any specific desired outcomes as completely as possible. Bring in positive emotion.]

Metaphoric Suggestion

As I sit here I sense the energy of my leopard guardian. I sense the leopard within me, the courage, the intensity, the sheer power. I feel the freedom of life, the power of life deep within my own roots. I am alive now. [Select appropriate metaphoric symbol.]

Relaxation, Deepening, and Suggestions

[Repeat this cycle until finished.] I hear a voice from the light star floating on the pool. It tells me to close my eyes. I continue to go deeper and deeper inside. I feel so incredibly comfortable and relaxed. My mind and body are so comfortable, such a beautiful color, such a comfortable feeling. Like floating down toward the earth. The more relaxed I become the deeper inside I go, deeper into confidence, deeper into power, deeper into self-respect. I see myself waking up in the morning with an inspiration. I am empowered by an incredible energy throughout the day that helps me to accomplish everything I need to do to move closer to my dreams. I feel incredible, warm, comfortable, relaxed. I am going deeper and deeper inside with each exhale. Like a leaf floating down deeper toward the power, deeper into an ocean of energy. Dissolving. Each exhale takes me deeper into this comfort, into this relaxation, deeper into confident peace. I can see my leopard body. I am stretching, claws digging into the side of a tree. My body is strong, supple, energetic, powerful. I sit quietly, watching, unstirred, powerful. I feel incredibly confident. I know I can do whatever I need to do to reach my dreams. I believe. Every exhalation takes me deeper and deeper into relaxation. During the week, every day at noon I will remember the sun in the sky above, and I will feel a surge of confidence. I will feel the ruby red energy of life filling me with confidence. I am filled with light and energy. I feel incredible. When I see the red color of a stop sign, I will stop. I will feel the power. I will be filled with a sense of pure confidence and joy, grateful to be alive. I love my life. I love life. I believe in life. I believe in myself. Life helps me in so many ways. Life is great. People are wonderful. I love my life.

Concluding

My dreams will come to me. I can see my goal totally, clearly. I will take a moment to let this experience integrate into my understanding deeply. I take a deep breath and let the images and ideas of

Continued ➡

success go deep inside me. Taking a breath I inhale these images, feelings, insights deep into myself. I see myself looking very accomplished, very happy. I know that whatever is perfect and best for me will come to pass. I notice my body now, my breathing. My eyelids feel normal, comfortable and refreshed. My eyelids feel perfect. My legs feel perfect, strong and relaxed. My legs feel wonderful. I am coming back feeling refreshed, relaxed, and ready for life. Each of my sessions will be more and more effective. This is going to be the most amazing week of my life. I feel incredible, and I anticipate positive success all week long. I come back slowly now, feeling great. Whenever I am ready, I slowly open my eyes to a most amazing day.

Short Version

Close your eyes, take several deep breaths, relax. Count down from twenty to one. During the counting down, tell yourself that you are feeling warm, heavy, and relaxed and that you are going deeper and deeper inside. You can imagine walking down a set of beautiful stairs or down a path. When you reach the number one, see yourself in a very beautiful, safe place, such as under a palm tree on a perfect beach.

Relax there for a moment.

Introduce suggestion: tell yourself about your success; see your outcome imagery; bring in a metaphoric symbol that supports your outcome vision. Give yourself a posthypnotic suggestion to reactivate positive expectation during the day.

Come back feeling refreshed, relaxed, and peaceful.

Priming

One other very useful quick strategy is an approach I call priming. This method can be used as a simple method to prepare for each day. Done early in the morning it sets the tone for everything you will do. It can also be done right before specific important events to give an increased sense of power and positive expectancy of achieving desired outcomes. The following version is used to prime the entire day. It is done in the morning before the day begins. To do priming just follow these eight simple steps:

1. Close your eyes and relax.
2. See yourself at the end of the day. You are sitting in a comfortable chair in your home. You look very happy, like you have had one of the most incredible days of your life so far.
3. Tell yourself mentally why it has been such an incredible day. Tell yourself that you successfully met your objectives for the specific things that you had to do for the day. For example, in my priming I might tell myself that I had an incredible day at work, extremely productive, that I was positive and supportive of people I met, that I worked out and my body feels great, that I ate healthy food. Pick a few of the key things for the day, your top daily or general life goals.
4. As you describe these things visualize them to the extent possible.
5. Bring positive feeling into the visual images (on certain days this may require a bit of effort).
6. Tell yourself that you feel incredible, that it has been one of the most amazing days of your life so far.

7. When you feel complete, inhale this energy deep into the center of your being, and then exhale it out into the universe.
8. Slowly open your eyes and begin your most amazing day.

To prime specific events, use the basic eight step process. Instead of seeing yourself at the end of the day, however, see yourself at the end of the specific event. See yourself as successful, happy, enthused, and specify that you are happy because of the positive nature of the event. Priming can be done for microevents, such as preparing to make an important phone call, all the way to macroevents, such as priming the day, month, or year.

Specific Applications

Now that all the elements are in place you can begin working with issues of personal interest. This section presents a broad range of issues and provides useful ideas for beginning your own self-hypnosis practice. If your particular goal area is not found here then select a related topic and work with the ideas provided.

Each topic in this section is approached comprehensively with the intention of providing ideas to begin creating an effective self-hypnosis transformation process. Under each one you will find three subsections: Action Layers, Hypnotic Suggestions, and Personal Plans. In the Action Layers, ideas are given for addressing the personal, behavioral, or environmental aspects of the issue. The Person layer focuses on a balanced body, calm and positive emotions, and a focused mind. The Behavior layer gives ideas for constructive, empowered action. The Environment layer examines how to make the external world support your success. The Hypnotic Suggestions include ideas for creating purposeful and effective verbal, visual, and metaphoric suggestions. Verbal suggestions should be positive and personal and have present and future perspectives. They should state clearly and strongly exactly what you want to hear so you will feel encouraged and capable. Visual suggestions should present as clear a picture as possible of what you truly want your life to look like. Metaphoric suggestions are best if they are strong, clear iconic images that empower you to succeed. Each topic concludes with a Personal Plans section where you can develop specific steps for beginning to make your own transformational process a reality. Take some time now to work with the following topics. Find your topic, work with the action layers and suggestions, add additional ideas from other resources such as issue-relevant books or Web sites, and create a tailored package for your success.

Addiction and Habit Control

ACTION LAYERS

Person

Dealing effectively with addiction involves working with emotional obstacles, challenging thoughts, and physical discomfort. Underlying emotional issues can be difficult to isolate, understand, and modify. They may be experienced as fear, unworthiness, helplessness, survival concerns, or a desire to die. You will need to develop a stronger sense of self-worth, positiveness, and a belief in your own abilities. You will also want to develop your ability to relax deeply and let go of tension, learning to use relaxation to work with physical discomfort and uneasiness. The key is to get your body and mind

balanced again and to activate the power stay in balance. Be patient, love yourself, and be proud of yourself for doing the work. Do not give up. Know that you can do it.

Behavior

Addiction and habits can relate to drugs, alcohol, tobacco, food, gambling, nail biting, shopping, and other behaviors. A key to changing any of them is to pay attention to the addictive pattern—when, where, why, and how much. When you start self-monitoring your pattern in this way you make it more conscious. So pay close attention to the pattern. This helps awaken the change process. Once you recognize the pattern you can start to do it differently, to break up the automatic behaviors. For example, you can change the time when you do it; you can do the steps of the pattern in a different order or change the speed, the location, or who you do them with; or do whatever you can think of to break up the habitual pattern. This helps some people change behaviors. Find new ways to make life work.

Environment

You may need to change elements of your environment to succeed in becoming independent. If you associate with other people who are struggling with their own addiction, they will challenge your success. Most likely, you will need to make new friends. That can be hard, but we are talking about your life. You will also need to regulate your environment to keep away from the thing that you are addicted to. Keep it out of your home, and avoid people and places where you can easily obtain it. Ask for help. Join a support group. There are many 12-step programs and other resources around that can be useful.

HYPNOTIC SUGGESTIONS

Verbal

I know I will survive. I know I am safe. I love myself and seek out others who respect themselves and who respect me. I am capable, and I am learning new ways to make my life work better and better. I deserve to live. I deal with any urges easily and effectively because I am strong. I enjoy my life free of _____. I am balanced and healthy, and I only do those things that bring me true happiness, strength, peace, and balance. I associate with people who are healthy and strong. I go to places that are life supportive and avoid those that are not. The old habit was about not loving myself. I love myself now, and that is why the habit is gone. I love who I am.

Visual Imagery

See yourself as addiction free. See yourself as dealing with urges very effectively now and being free of any urges. Imagine a relaxed, happy, confident you. You look great. See yourself one year and five years out in the future being independent, healthy, and very happy.

Metaphoric

Find an image that triggers a specific feeling that helps you deal with this change. For example, if you need to feel strong you could use an image of a brick wall (immovable in your commitment to finally loving yourself.) Maybe the word love is written on that wall. If you need courage you could use an image of a lion. Become the powerful lion. Feel the natural power within yourself. You could imagine a wise person who can offer you counsel. Ask them what they think you should do.

Continued ➡

_____

_____

_____

_____

_____

_____

_____

_____

_____

_____

Anxiety, Phobia, Fear, and Stress

ACTION LAYERS

Person

Relaxation is very, very helpful. Get your body vibrating at a lower, quieter level. Practice some relaxation method before a stressful event, such as right before an exam starts or right before a performance. Try a one minute method or priming. Banish any fearful thoughts, just banish them. Make them leave. You can also turn the fear into a small brother or sister. Take it by the hand and walk with it, but do not let it run and drag you. Talk to that small frightened child and reassure him or her. Remember, it is the vulnerable aspect of self that is afraid. Also focus on your goal and feel your passion. This makes obstacles smaller or invisible. Go with your passion. You have a purpose to fulfill. Focus on your goal, where you are going. Also, very important, remember to breathe deeply and slowly when you are anxious. Inhale through your nostrils. Breathe down into your abdomen. Exhale slowly.

Behavior

Reduce behaviors that increase your anxiety, such as procrastination and being late, alienating people because of your social fear, or drinking caffeinated beverages. Manage time, say no, get clear on your goals, and be responsible. You will succeed. Laugh, smile, do fun things, learn to be more at ease with things, get out of your head, go for walks at the beach, listen to quieting music, reduce your use of drugs and alcohol and stimulants such as coffee, keep your life in order, make more positive friends. Learn to meditate.

Environment

Reduce the number of things in your environment that increase your stress, such as angry people, stressful work, excess noise, clutter, and other imbalancing stimuli. Create a peaceful space. It can be helpful to use resources in the environment that can soothe the energy body, such as homeopathy and herbal products.

HYPNOTIC SUGGESTIONS

Verbal

I am calm and relaxed. My body is warm, heavy, and relaxed. I move toward my goals steadily. My mind is peaceful. Fear and negative thoughts flow out of me with each exhale. I am left clear and filled with happiness. I feel more and more relaxed every day. I am strong and confident; I manage my time and space. My life is organized and balanced. I make choices in my life that increase my sense of calm and peace. Relaxation is one of my main goals. I look forward to each day and to the opportunity to learn from life. I am flexible, happy, resourceful, and strong. I feel fantastic.

Visual Imagery

See yourself as being very calm and relaxed. Imagine being in a hot tub, in a cabin in the woods, or sitting on a sandy beach. When stress-inducing images come to mind during the day, modify them, make the images small and insignificant. Banish them; you are powerful. You have incredible power over them and with practice that power will grow. Take the reigns, change negative patterns, and substitute positive images for every negative one. Whatever your fear image is, during self-hypnosis see the opposite.

Metaphoric

Be a mighty warrior or champion fighter. Experience yourself interacting with all things with confidence. Use this as a metaphor of immense power. Or be like a child learning, playing, and having fun with life. Or be like a wise person who knows a great deal about life and is quite capable at dealing with events as they flow by. The old sage sits by the river of life and wisely observes the flow of life. All things come to that wise being in time. Be that sage.

Other Ideas

With phobia we often find a clear interrelationship between: person (negative imagery, internal feelings of fear, and physical discomfort); behavior (avoidance); and environment (fear-evoking stimuli). One of the easiest ways to work with this trinity is to disrupt it at one of its three points. A very effective method is to experience a deep state of relaxation (opposite of body discomfort) when you encounter the anxiety-provoking item. To do this, work on creating very deep relaxation. Give yourself the suggestion that you will feel relaxing energy whenever you come across the evocative stimuli. This will begin to create a new pattern, disrupting the old pattern of stimuli, fear, and avoidance. Be patient with the fear and with yourself, and you will transform.

PERSONAL PLANS

_____

_____

_____

_____

_____

_____

_____

_____

_____

_____

_____

Childbirth

ACTION LAYERS

Person

Keep your body healthy. Learn to relax very deeply. Banish fear and create positive expectations. Anticipate a wonderful, enjoyable experience. Be positive. Be calm. Relax your body. Relax your mind. Relax your emotions. Use self-hypnosis to promote a healthy pregnancy, delivery, and baby. Create powerful positive expectancy on all levels.

Behavior

Work regularly with relaxation, learning how to relax the muscles of your body, how to calm your mind. Practice the deep breathing methods taught in birthing classes. Practice those methods and associate that breathing with very positive, happy feelings. Join a birthing class to learn such useful skills. Stay healthy, take your vitamins, get your exercise, enjoy the process, and think of what a truly amazing event you are participating in.

Self-Hypnosis: A One-Minute Method

Adam Burke, Ph.D.

If you are like me, you do not want to read an entire book to find out how to do something. You want to start using a new skill now. This book is full of principles, techniques, and applications that will help you to become quite skillful in working with self-hypnosis over time. For those of you eager to begin now, however, the essence of all of those skills can be condensed to this simple formula:

- Induce and deepen a quietly focused mind-body learning state.
- Send transformative suggestions to that deep mind-body state.
- Come back refreshed and ready for life at a new level.

So, for those of you in a hurry, here is a one-minute method to get things started.

1. Sit or lie comfortably.
2. Close your eyes.
3. Take three deep breaths and release all tension.
4. Do the following:
   - Imagine you are holding a two-inch energy ball in your hand.
   - Squeeze it, physically squeeze it.
   - Pretend that the harder you squeeze the more it resists, that your forces match equally; you cannot modify the shape of the ball.
   - Tell yourself, "The harder I squeeze, the deeper I go inside."
   - Continue to squeeze for a minute; then absolutely, totally, completely release everything.
   - Feel yourself dropping down deep inside.
   - Give yourself your suggestion, "I feel incredibly energetic, confident, strong, loving, or..."
   - See the desired outcome; see a future image of that outcome.
   - Feel the positive feelings associated with that outcome.
   - After a few minutes, tell yourself that you are, "Coming back feeling refreshed, relaxed, and ready for an amazing day."
   - Then slowly open your eyes.

That's it. Now here we go!

—From *Self-Hypnosis*

Continued ➡

Environment

Keep your environment positive and healthy during your pregnancy. Eat well, rest, and be positive. Avoid tobacco, drugs, and alcohol. Get assistance if this is an issue. Pregnancy is an excellent time for healing old patterns and becoming a new person. Have your coach, partner, or other supportive people with you during delivery. Prepare the nest. Create a healthy, safe, loving space for your new family member.

HYPNOTIC SUGGESTIONS

You will ideally want to work on these practices for several months before the birth. Try to do some relaxation and imagery work every day.

Verbal

This is going to be a very smooth and wonderful birth. My baby is going to be healthy and happy. I will relax and breathe my baby into the world. My body feels strong and healthy during this pregnancy, and I feel very relaxed and calm during the delivery. My baby comes into this world easily, calm and incredibly healthy. I feel deep happiness during the entire process. Time passes quickly. It all goes so easily, so smoothly. I am warm, heavy, and relaxed. Once the baby arrives safe and healthy, my body will heal incredibly quickly.

Visual Imagery

See yourself having your baby easily and effortlessly. Your baby just flows out of you like light or an ocean wave, very healthy and happy. See yourself and everyone who loves you filled with joy. You are holding your baby and telling the baby how easy the birth was, how healthy, loved, and special he or she is.

Metaphoric

Here is a metaphor that is useful for delivery. Let it be spring, a nice time to hike down to the river. The waters are full. You can feel the joyful vibrations of the springtime river flowing. The waters are warm and easy, flowing effortlessly from the mountaintop to the vast blue ocean. The river feels its happiness and your happiness. It is a warm and joyful water moving down the mountain slope. Be joyful too.

PERSONAL PLANS

_____
_____
_____
_____
_____
_____
_____
_____
_____
_____

Energy

ACTION LAYERS

Person

Develop a positive mental attitude. Give yourself inspirational talks. Imagine that people are applauding you, like you are crossing the finish line, a winner. Energize yourself mentally. In the morning sing yourself an "I feel great" song to build your positive energy for the day. Remember that you are a learner. You are learning what you need to know to be happy. Remind yourself over and over that you will succeed, that you can do it. Self-love is also very energizing. Remove the garbage about yourself and your world from your mind. Just throw it out.

Behavior

Eat right. Enjoy the foods that make you feel light, happy, clear minded and able to work. Avoid excess in eating; it is hard on the digestive system. Stop smoking completely. Reduce use of unnecessary drugs. Also reduce alcohol consumption as it is a mild depressant. Exercise will increase general well-being and energy. Keep your life balanced. Discipline yourself, in a positive way. Place your goals out where you can see them to remind you of what you want in life. Track them and reward yourself for every success. The clearer and more committed and more enthusiastic you are about your dream, the more energy you will possess. Read about passionate people like Thomas Edison or John Muir. Passion is very energizing, and your dream is a strong connection to your passion. Live a life of no regrets. Go for your dream. Create your own joyful, energizing song and sing it in the shower each morning.

Environment

Get the junk food out of your house. Make it easy to exercise—buy a jump rope, move closer to the park, whatever will help. Keep images around the house, such as magazines that display active, energetic people.

HYPNOTIC SUGGESTIONS

Verbal

I am powerful, alive, and dynamic. Energy flows through me. I feel great. I feel incredible. I love my life. I am powerful, productive, organized, energetic, and totally effective. I can feel the power of life flowing through me. I feel the power of the earth, the sky, the wind, the water, the sun. The goodness of the world is in my heart and mind, and that power lifts me higher. I am strong and healthy. The radiant power of the sun is warming me. The surging power of the ocean is moving me. I am a warrior.

Visual

See yourself looking completely excited about life. You look very happy and enthusiastic. Perhaps you are jumping up and down with your arms up in the air shouting, "Yes." See yourself energized and feeling the power of life. See yourself doing something that totally energizes you—something physical, making a great deal, completing a major project. Get into a memory of personal power.

Metaphoric

Become an animal that represents full personal energy for you. You could become a galloping wild horse or a lion. Become something powerful and feel that power within you.

PERSONAL PLANS

_____
_____
_____
_____
_____
_____
_____
_____
_____
_____
_____

Health and Healing

ACTION LAYERS

Person

A positive attitude and a positive belief are very important. Hold strongly in your mind that you will be healthy and whole. Allow your mind to work constantly on bringing more strength to your body. Every thought, negative or positive, produces some effect. Seek to increase the number of positive thoughts moving through you and reducing the number of negative thoughts. Regulate your emotions, keep them smooth. Be positive and optimistic; deal with depression, anger, and other emotions that may burden you. If your emotions become imbalanced use creative measures, such as brief self-hypnosis, to return to center. Keep your body energy balanced.

Behavior

Do things that make you happy, bring you energy, help you remain optimistic, heal you. Eat right. Food is the first medicine in many ancient systems. One of the simplest ways to eat well is to eat for nutrients rather than caloric content. If you eat for nutrients you will be eating food that provides energy. Also, a light diet, one that is easy to digest, is good for healing. In ancient China they would cook rice soups for many, many hours to make them easy to assimilate for people who were ill. Eat foods that nourish deeply. Eat local, organic, and natural. Avoid pesticides and genetically modified foods. Eat what nature intended, not what the corporations mandate. Do what you need to do to get well. Be positive and proactive. Exercise appropriately if possible. Movement is good medicine. Walk, swim, ride a bike, stretch gently, whatever you can manage. Get fresh air when possible. Drink clean water.

Environment

Associate with positive people. Stay in healing energy places. Bring healing energy into your environment, such as plants, positive pictures and books, light, and fresh air. Get outside. Be in nature. Reduce the pollutants, energy emissions, toxic chemicals, and molds in your home and workplace if possible. Avoid toxic places, people, and things.

HYPNOTIC SUGGESTIONS

Verbal

I am getting stronger and healthier. Healing energy is flowing into my body from a very powerful place in the universe. I feel strong and whole. The universal life force is moving through me. Healing

Continued ➡

energy is flowing into me now. That energy is filling me with light, with freshness, with vitality. All toxic, stagnant energy is being removed from me. I am filled with light. Each cell of my body is glowing. I feel great. My body is a powerhouse. I am like a new plant. My leaves are catching the rays of the sun, and my body is creating energy. I am totally alive and feel powerful. I rest so deeply when I close my eyes. Each breath heals me. I am rested, healed, happy, alive.

Visual

See yourself as energetic, whole, and happy. Send healing energy (pick a powerful healing color) to any part of your mind and body that needs healing. Send healing sounds, words, or phrases to those areas; make them up, let them come from your deep mind. Let your deep mind guide you to take right action. Feel healing energy flowing through you, like an energy stream. Imagine that there is a powerful being, like a healing angel, working on you. Receive the healing. See yourself breathing in good, healing chi or energy and exhaling toxic, stagnant, putrid energy. Each breath heals you, energizes you.

Metaphoric

When you toss a stone into a pond it sinks, disappearing from sight, and the surface soon becomes calm again. Let your illness be that stone making momentary ripples, then sinking and disappearing. Let your entire energy field become balanced and harmonious again. Let your energy become smooth and calm. Imagine yourself as a radiant being, having a body of pure light.

Personal Plans

_____

_____

_____

_____

_____

_____

_____

_____

_____

_____

Insomnia

Action Layers

Person

Learn to relax. Do a lot of relaxation practice—feel warm, heavy, and relaxed. When in bed focus on your body instead of on your thoughts and feelings. When your mind starts rolling away on some idea, bring it back into your body, focusing on warm, heavy, and relaxed body feelings. Relax your body from your toes to your ears. When you are ready to sleep, then stop thinking about things. Successful people leave their work at work. Sleep is your time. Use it to heal. A good night's sleep will help you deal better with everything when you wake up. Let it go.

Behavior

Try the counting down method with the words warm, heavy, and relaxed. Count down from one

hundred to one, telling yourself that you feel more comfortable with each number down. Before bed do not exercise, study, or do other activities that stimulate the mind or body or emotions. Do not work too late at night. Avoid stimulants and spicy or stimulating food at night. Warm milk before bed can be relaxing, as can melatonin. You can also try chamomile tea, or tea with valerian in it. A warm, relaxing bath before bed is also a nice idea. People who get more sleep than they need will not fall asleep quickly at night. Avoid excess sleep or daytime naps.

Environment

Have a peaceful sleeping environment. A bit of fresh air in the room is nice if possible. Control the sound. Wear earplugs if you have to. Have clean, comfortable sheets. Use the right pillow for you. Make your sleeping space as conducive as possible to deep, healing sleep.

Hypnotic Suggestions

Verbal

I sleep deeply and soundly. I focus on my body when I go to sleep, noticing the feelings of heaviness and relaxation. My body is comfortable and heavy; my mind is quiet. I sleep deeply, feeling refreshed and relaxed when I awaken. I am going to awaken in the morning feeling great, I slept so deeply. I can see myself falling deeply asleep. My mind is quiet now. Nothing is important now. Peace is all that I feel. Everything in my life is going to work out perfectly. I trust in the perfection of life. I know that life is sometimes a mystery. I have no need to know all the answers to my questions now. I am at peace, knowing that everything that I need will come to me in time. I am at peace. I am falling into a deeply peaceful sleep.

Visual

See yourself being very heavy like a rock, sinking down into your bed. You are falling asleep, having a very hard time keeping your eyes open. Imagine that it is the next morning and the sun is coming in through the windows. You are waking up looking very, very happy and feeling refreshed, relaxed, and peaceful. You are smiling, stretching. You start to sing and laugh. You are happy to be alive. You are confident. You know that everything is going to be fine. You see yourself looking confident and more powerful than ever before. You look very happy and completely rested.

Metaphoric

Be a heavy rock sinking down in warm, soft sand. Be butter melting of top of hot oatmeal. Become the hibernating bear.

Personal Plans

_____

_____

_____

_____

_____

_____

_____

_____

_____

_____

Pain

Action Layers

Person

Chronic physical pain can create emotional issues—anger, frustration, and depression. These will have to be addressed. Then of course there is the physical pain sensation. Hypnotic analgesia can help with this. You will also want to work with relaxation. When the body has chronic pain, it can often create muscular tightening in the painful area in an effort to limit movement and discomfort. That tightening becomes a secondary source of pain, and it reduces flexibility causing other problems. Stay relaxed and upbeat as much as you can.

Behavior

Pain can produce secondary gain behaviors. This means that people's pain can be reinforcing because it gains the sufferer extra attention, access to drugs that can create dependence, and other dubious benefits. Secondary gains such as drugs and attention will reinforce the pain and make it harder to remove it. Any such secondary benefits will need to be examined and dealt with. Denial and false logic may present real challenges. The goal is to be as healthy and strong—physically, emotionally, and socially—as possible.

Environment

Use the resources in your environment that can help you, such as physical therapy, acupuncture and herbs, or massage. Be mindful when practitioners want you to get frequent X-rays, come back endlessly for treatment, or eagerly advise surgery or other expensive treatments. That often benefits them much more than it benefits you. Be a conscious consumer. Getting a second opinion in such cases can be very prudent. Seek reputable care. Become knowledgeable and more responsible for your own healing. Also, associate with positive, fun people.

Hypnotic Suggestions

Verbal

For pain: I am calm and relaxed. I feel the healing energy flowing through my body and through my pain. I love my body, and I work with it creatively and positively. My body feels great. My pain dissolves, and my body feels wonderful.

For secondary gains: I am free of artificial aids. I love myself and feel loved by the universe. I help myself. I take care of my needs, and I let others help me as needed. I am very independent and capable.

Visual

See yourself looking healthy, taking proactive steps to healing, being positive and strong. See yourself as happy and energetic.

Metaphoric

Become a tree. Trees are both strong and flexible. Work with metaphoric opposites. If the pain is cold, send it warm energy. If it is warm, send it cool energy. Ask your mind, "If the pain had a color, what color would it be?" Then ask your inner mind what the opposite, healing color would be. Send that healing color to the painful area over and over again. Speak to the pain and find out what it needs. When it answers through your inner mind, seek to give it the positive, healing things it needs.

Other Ideas

For specific pain, like headaches, menstrual cramps, or dental pain, relax and send cool or warm (depending on your need or preference) healing energy and a wonderful healing color to the area. Create hypnotic analgesia in your hand (so

Continued ➡

your hand becomes increasingly numb, chapter 8) and then place your hand on the area to transfer the analgesia to the pain directly. If you had dental work or some other type of surgery, you can suggest reduced swelling, rapid healing, healing energy flowing in the area, minimal pain, and good feelings. Pain can also be a signal of other things, such as more serious underlying issues or unresolved emotional concerns. If the pain persists see a medical professional to get an assessment. If the pain is a reflection of emotional issues, you may need to deal with the issue at the emotional (person) level for the problem to really heal. In that case, you may benefit from receiving professional counseling services.

PERSONAL PLANS

_____
_____
_____
_____
_____
_____
_____
_____
_____
_____

Sexual Health

ACTION LAYERS

Person

Relaxation is very helpful in improving sexual health. Your body has to learn to associate sexuality with pleasure, fun, and comfort. Relaxation is a good way to start. Banish negative thoughts about your body or your sexual ability. Just banish such useless garbage. Remove any comparisons with others; you are you. Patience and a noncritical attitude are essential. There is a good deal of confusion in our culture around sex because it has been made into such a commodity. Sex is really a simple thing. Let it be simple. Let it be pleasurable, fun, relaxing, and energizing. Let it be positive. It is about relationships with self, with other, and with spirit. Let it heal you.

Behavior

If your concern has more to do with sexual addictions then you should refer to the section on addictions. If you are troubled by some of your sexual behaviors or thoughts, it can be helpful to seek professional help. Our feelings and behaviors about sex are sometimes more common than we think, but they can still cause a lot of pain. There is no need for you to suffer. Regarding sexual performance, or function, trying to make things happen sexually is not the best strategy. Emphasize fun, not work. There is no need to hurry; why rush something pleasurable? Take your time. Make it enjoyable. Seek to make love, to generate more love. Ultimately that heals. Sexual healing is done through the mutual creation of love. Making love means to make love. Work with that concept. Explore it. This might include the need to improve relationships. Other things that greatly aid sexual healing are a high-quality diet, supplements, tonic herbs, regular exercise, limited use of alcohol, and abstinence from cigarettes and marijuana.

Environment

It takes two to tango. Sexual issues can be the result of incompatibility, unresolved emotional issues, or a million other things. The cause needs to be examined. It can be beneficial to work with a therapist who deals with couples or sexual issues. Ultimately the goal is to create a sexual experience that is mutually fun and is an evolving loving experience. Get the information you need to help you understand your issue, such as books on sex therapy or tantra. There are lots of good resources out there. Tantric approaches allow you to work with sexuality on an energetic level that can be very helpful.

HYPNOTIC SUGGESTIONS

Verbal

I enjoy making love. Sexual energy is healing my body and spirit. It is wonderful to connect with another human heart in a deeply loving way. I love my body. I love who I am. My sexual energy flows easily. The energy heals me and the one I love. I love making love. I am having fun. I can feel my energy in every part of my body. Vitality is filling every part of my body. I feel incredible. It is so great to be alive. I love people. My heart is healing, and I can feel love more and more. I want my love to heal others. I want love to heal me. I feel more and more at peace. I know that healing is happening now.

Visual

See yourself being sexual in a healthy, fun, loving way. See yourself and your partner having fun. See your body looking fit, energetic, vital. See yourself as playful and healthy, turned on, happy to be alive. Imagine that you are a body of pure energy. Feel the energy coursing through you. Feel the energy building and flowing. Recognize the vast power of life flowing through you.

Metaphoric

For functional issues, be a drawbridge going up or a garden gate opening. For sexual play, be an animal. Otters have fun, lions are sexually intense. Be a volcano or an ocean wave.

Other Ideas

Although it is not common knowledge in our culture, there is an ancient art of lovemaking called tantra. In the East this body of knowledge has been used for centuries. Although the bulk of tantric work in the East is more typically energy work of a nonsexual nature, there is a sexual branch to the practice. Tantric sex work is gaining popularity in the West. You can find many good books on the subject written by Westerners. These books contain helpful ideas regarding working with sexual energy. It is a very powerful energy, which can be used for high spiritual purposes.

PERSONAL PLANS

_____
_____
_____
_____
_____
_____
_____
_____
_____
_____

Skin Conditions

ACTION LAYERS

Person

Relaxation is very helpful in aiding skin conditions. Releasing anger and other negative emotions may also prove helpful in some cases. In Chinese medicine we often associate skin conditions with internal heat. Strong emotion can stagnate energy and generate such internal heat. Keep your emotions in balance, let go of your anger, and increase your gratitude. If physical anxiety or negative emotions cause you to eat poorly, then it is important to work on addressing those levels of the issue. Keep your body, mind, and spirit harmonious, positive, and happy.

Behavior

Determine whether any particular behaviors are related to your condition—such as inappropriate diet, stress, or not bathing every day—and work on that pattern. Try to pay attention to behavioral patterns that appear to be related to skin changes. Play with these patterns. Diet is very important. Watch what you eat. Oily foods, spicy foods, colas, and chocolate will often create acne and make other skin conditions worse. Try to eat greens and more vegetables; see what happens. Eat healthy, fresh foods. Avoid junk food. You deserve good things. Also, clip the stressors in your life. Relax more.

Environment

Determine what environmental factors may be stimulating or increasing your reaction. Many substances in the environment can be highly irritating and allergenic. This can include makeup, chemicals in body products, ingredients in foods, or materials in the workplace. Reduce your contact with these agents if you begin to recognize reactivity. See if it improves with reduced contact. Also, toxic social environments can stress the body-mind. See if you can mitigate their influence. Let the world work for you, not against you.

HYPNOTIC SUGGESTIONS

Verbal

I am very happy and take responsibility for my attitudes. They are very positive. My skin is smooth and soft. It is becoming healthier and healthier. My skin looks and feels very healthy. I feel great. I love how I look. I eat the right foods that balance my body chemistry and my skin. I take care of my health, and my energy is strong. My mind is calm, and my body is clean. I feel great.

Visual

See your skin becoming more and more balanced and nonreactive. Your skin appears smooth, your eyes are clear and bright, other signs of balance are evident. See yourself looking happy and healthy. Use counter imagery: if the condition is hot and dry then imagine cool, softening energy flowing through the specific affected area. If a skin patch is red, hot, and itchy then select an ideal antidote temperature, color, and feeling, and visualize that energy in the problem location. It can be a very simple and helpful strategy.

Metaphoric

Be the smooth surface of still, cool water. Be the water. Become the clear blue sky. Become a cooling, cleansing summer rain. Be smooth like satin. Be a baby again, with baby soft skin.

Continued ➡

_____
_____
_____
_____
_____
_____
_____
_____
_____
_____

Weight Management

ACTION LAYERS

Person

Have a positive attitude about your body and your ability to manage your weight. Know you will succeed in your goals. Give up on becoming some perfect weight. Get in shape and your natural ideal will become apparent. Love yourself. Have an upbeat outlook. Deal with depression, anger, and other burdensome emotions. Keep your emotions calm and steady. Stay positive as much as possible. Become a problem solver. Know that you have a great power within yourself to succeed. Allow yourself to be a success. Weight is often not the only issue, self-love is often a problem too. Work on both, and you will be exponentially healthy. Believe in yourself, love yourself, be yourself.

Behavior

Eat healthy—lower in fat, higher in protein and complex carbohydrates. Avoid fad diets. Exercise is also a key ingredient to successful weight management. Make exercise something fun, part of an enjoyable way to be healthy. Think of your health, with weight management being just one part of a bigger picture. Make the process pleasurable. Eat for nutrients, not for caloric content. Eat green, natural, and organic. Avoid pesticides, genetically altered foods, additives, sweeteners, artificial substances, and processed foods. Learn how to cook. Make that a fun thing. Make that a positive social experience.

Environment

Avoid eating at places that serve unhealthy foods. Keep your house free of inappropriate foods. Join a club or find other fun places to exercise. Find a place to exercise. Find an exercise partner. Make a plan and implement it. If it is helpful, join a group that assists people with eating and weight management. Get the books that you need or other resources. Take positive action. Associate with positive, affirming people.

HYPNOTIC SUGGESTIONS

Verbal

I love my body. I am healthy, energetic, and happy. I am at the ideal weight for my body. I feel great. I am so happy to be alive. I take such good care of myself. I eat right, exercise, drink fresh water, associate with loving people, read inspirational materials. I love my life. I have a strong desire to only eat healthy foods, to eat moderately, and to move my body. I have a tremendous capacity to accomplish my goals. I am excited about life. I look forward to getting up every morning and starting my day. My life is incredible. I feel great. My body is strong, flexible, vital, and alive. I love my body. I love myself. I love this life.

Visual

See yourself as fit, healthy, and energetic. You are doing active exercise and having fun. You are eating healthy food and loving the energy it gives you. See a radiant body of energy. You are like the sun. Warm, radiant light is coming from you. You feel that energy. It fills you with joy and peace. It is melting away sluggish, sticky energy. See yourself running with the wind. You are light and free. You feel fresh air on your face. The fragrance is uplifting. You have angel wings, and you are being carried up by the warm drafts of a summer breeze. You are light, soaring. You can see beautiful hills below. You fly to a special garden. There you are met by great healers. You sit in the garden with them. You feel their healing energy flowing into you. You are strong, peaceful, healthy; you feel wonderful, and you look great.

Metaphoric

Be powerful and physical, toned like a jaguar. You are a hillside covered with snow. The warm spring sun is melting away the layers of snow. Vital new life is rising up. The winter has ended. Spring is here.

PERSONAL PLANS

_____
_____
_____
_____
_____
_____
_____
_____
_____
_____

—From *Self-Hypnosis*

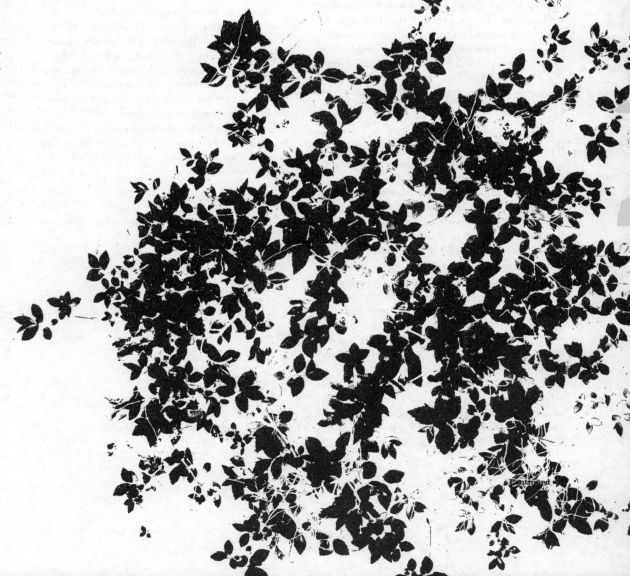

Healing with Foods, Nutrition, Diet, and Supplements

GOOD NUTRITION

Ellen Tart-Jensen

Let food be thy medicine and medicine be thy food.

—Hippocrates

It is sad that our foods have become so processed and denatured. Many people have lost their innate ability to know what their bodies need to eat in order to be nourished. Our taste buds have become dull from eating too many sweet and salty foods. Some people are hungry all the time and never feel satisfied after a meal. Thousands of American citizens eat enormous amounts of food, yet are overweight and undernourished!

The Laws of Nature

We are creatures of nature, just as all animals are. However, we have lost our understanding of the laws of nature. Animals know what to consume in order to be healthy. They know how to feed their young to ensure their strength and vitality. Many animals know how to store food for the winter. They avoid crops that have been heavily sprayed with chemicals—crops that humans eat. When insects get into our cupboards, they will go after the natural organic foods over their processed and highly preserved counterparts—whole grain over refined white flour,

for example, or real sugar over artificial sweeteners—though they have never read a book on nutrition!

I believe in an overall divine plan, and I believe that if people had always followed the laws of nature, health would be our birthright today. Early peoples once lived very close to nature. They knew how to hunt and fish and gather the herbs, nuts, and seeds of the land. Some planted crops and knew how to rotate them so the soil's minerals were preserved. They knew how to use healing herbs, whether in teas, salves, ointments, or poultices, and they drank pure water. They moved and worked in harmony, with the seasons and with nature.

When I was teaching in the Philippines a few years ago, I found that a large number of the people there were suffering from diabetes and decaying teeth due to the introduction of soda pop in their country. Everywhere I looked, people were drinking soft drinks!

It might have seemed wonderful at first, in the United States in the early 1900s, to have soda fountains and soft drinks. It might have seemed marvelous and wonderfully convenient when TV dinners became readily available and fast-food restaurants opened everywhere, but we need to wake up and take a close look at what we have created. We have more cancer and heart disease than ever before. Our children are suffering from obesity and attention-deficit/hyperactivity disorder (ADHD), both of which are exacerbated by foods high in sugar and

empty calories. We need to become responsible consumers and follow the laws of nature.

After my surgery as a child of twelve, I began to crave those easily available sweets. I had not cared much for sweets before the operation. In retrospect, I realize the tremendous stress that surgery caused my adrenal glands and therefore my pancreas. If my mother made a cake, I was unable to concentrate on my homework for thinking about that cake sitting in the cupboard. What was worse, the more I ate, the more I wanted! I never felt satisfied. As a teenager in high school, I was twenty pounds overweight. This disturbed me terribly. I couldn't understand why my willpower was weak in regard to foods when it seemed so strong in every other area of my life. I tried to eat less, but soon the hunger or craving for sweets took over and I would find myself eating more than I should. It took many years for me to learn about hypoglycemia and the types of foods I needed to eat to remain healthy and balanced.

In my practice, I have seen hundreds of people try to follow some sort of diet. Some of these diets are extreme. There are all-fruit diets, high-protein diets, low-carb diets, low-fat diets, low-cholesterol diets, low-sodium diets, starvation diets, and low-calorie diets to name just a few. People, in general, are confused by all the diets touted in the bookstores. I tried them all. I tried with all my might to stick to whatever diet I was on. If it wasn't on my diet, I ignored my instinct whispering that my body

Continued ➡

needed a specific food. When I was on the fruitarian diet, I started losing hair and feeling lethargic. When I was on the all-protein diet, I was constipated and tired. When I was on the low-fat diet, my skin and scalp became very dry and I felt hungry and wanted to eat something every hour. Now, after reading hundreds of books on nutrition, studying nutrition formally, and working with thousands of clients, I deeply believe that maintaining a balanced diet of fresh, natural foods is the key to good nutrition. I love Richard Simmons's philosophy that we should let go of the word *diet* because it has the word *die* in it! We want to eat nutritious, whole, beautifully prepared foods that promote life, health, and joy.

If you are rigidly following an extreme diet and you feel healthy, happy, and balanced and are truly listening to your inner instincts, it may be tight for you; just be open to change if you begin to feel out of balance. I respect whatever works for each individual. Raw foods and fruits may be eaten for a time in order to cleanse the body, but the body may require more variety after a while. Diets may vary regionally. People living in hot climates, such as India, are more suited to fruit and vegetable diets since their bodies don't have to shield them from freezing temperatures. People from colder climates, such as Norway and Switzerland, usually require more protein and some warm, cooked grains.

The nutritional plan I offer here has helped hundreds of people drop excess pounds, maintain their normal weight, feel energetic, and heal a majority of the health problems they were experiencing. Thin people have gained weight, and specific programs have helped people heal specific problems.

We want to adopt a way of eating that we can follow throughout life. We need some initial discipline to train ourselves to eat foods that are pure, fresh, and whole. However, we don't want to feel cheated out of the foods we like. I had a client recently who said she likes to plan a cheat day. She is very strict with her diet during the week, and on Saturday she eats whatever and as much as she wants—including ice cream, soda, pie, and candy. I asked her if this plan had accomplished what she wanted, which was weight loss, and she said no.

For years, I pondered how to maintain my weight through balanced eating. One night in the middle of the winter when I was studying natural therapies in Switzerland, I awoke in the early morning hours while it was still dark. I looked outside and saw snow falling gently on the Alps. At that moment, I heard a clear statement in my mind, "Eat and enjoy whatever you want, but pay attention to what your body truly wants. Eat only when you're hungry, and stop when you're full." Those words were very powerful for me. I wrote them down and worked with them for over a year in order to change my indulging-and-then-starving pattern. It took lots of practice to pay attention to what my body really wanted.

People who are on diets may think they want coffee and doughnuts all the time, but they really don't. My late father-in-law, Dr. Bernard Jensen, used to tell this story: A woman came to him as a patient and told him she could live on coffee and doughnuts as long as she said a prayer to bless them before she ate them. Dr. Jensen told her he would like for her to consume only coffee and doughnuts for one week and then call him. After a day and a half of coffee and doughnuts, the lady called Dr. Jensen and told him she was very sick to her stomach and felt severe nausea. He then asked her what she would like to eat and she replied, "Homemade vegetable soup!" We need to trust that our bodies will let us know exactly what they need. The great

thing is that when you do choose only nutritious foods, you start feeling better and lose the desire for junk foods.

Humbert "Smokey" Santillo, ND, writes in *Intuitive Eating: Everybody's Natural Guide to Total Health and Lifegiving Vitality through Food*:

Imagine being so sensitized to your body's genuine needs that you naturally gravitate towards the foods and the eating style that will work best for your system. This is no fantasy, however. It is a very real possibility for you, and one that I have lived and shared with thousands of people.

Making Healthy Food Choices Based on the Laws of Nature

Eat foods that are pure, whole, fresh, and natural (not processed). Choose foods that are organic and unsprayed. Chemicals used on crops to kill insects are harmful to our bodies. In 1962, Rachel L. Carson's book *Silent Spring* shocked many slumbering citizens and awakened them to the vast threat that the toxic chemicals on our foods pose. The book was dedicated to Albert Schweitzer, who wrote, "Man has lost the capacity to foresee and to forestall. He will end by destroying the earth." The title, *Silent Spring*, vividly conjures the possibility of a spring without the beautiful songs of birds. She wrote about toxic chemicals such as DDT that are sprayed on crops to rid them of insects but infect and kill birds as well. DDT has been found in the livers of ocean fish thousands of miles from where the chemical was used. The United States has since banned DDT, but it is still sold to Third World countries, from which we buy food. Half a million chemicals are now in use, and pesticide use has more than doubled since 1962.

Artificial chemical fertilizers are manufactured from petrochemicals and have very few of the trace minerals vital to our health. Soil exposed to artificial fertilizers produces poor plants, which therefore attract lots of insects, causing the farmers to use more chemical sprays, resulting in a vicious cycle. Organic foods are grown without pesticides and harmful artificial fertilizers. I know a wonderful Amish farmer named Jacob Miller who grows beautiful, large healthy crops of vegetables and herbs. He said to me, "The plants are healthy and free from bugs because the soil is healthy. The human body is much the same and will be able to resist disease and be free from 'bugs' [germs, viruses, or parasites] when it is healthy." He tests his soil each year to see which nutrients are deficient, then replenishes those nutrients with organic compost and minerals. We need to give our bodies whole foods rich in vitamins and minerals to keep them strong. We are literally made from the dust of the earth.

It is also important to choose foods that have not been preserved with artificial chemicals or dyed with food colorings. Read labels! If the words on a label are too long to understand, leave the product on the shelf. Chemicals are not natural and can harm our bodies. Dr. Ben Feingold researched children with ADHD and found that artificial preservatives and food colorings had definite detrimental effects on their behavior. He has written a very informative book called *Why Your Child Is Hyperactive*.

Choose foods that have not been irradiated. Irradiation is sometimes used as an alternative to chemical preservatives. Sadly, food irradiation is done with gamma fays from cobalt, which can cause genetic mutation, just like radioactive elements.

Don't choose foods that were cooked in a microwave oven. Research now shows that microwaved food is dangerous to our health. For example, according to a 1993 study by Dr. Bernard H. Blanc,

Swiss Federal Institute of Technology and University, and Dr. Hans U. Hertel, Environmental-Biological Research and Consultation,

Eight test persons—all on a macrobiotic diet—volunteered for this study. They committed themselves to a very strict regimen. All food, Which Was heated, defrosted or cooked in the microwave oven, caused significant changes in the blood of the test persons. These changes included: Decrease of all hemoglobin values, increase of the hematocrit, leukocytes and cholesterol values. Lymphocytes showed a more distinct short-term decrease after the intake of food from the microwave oven than after the intake of other variants.

The measured effects of microwave-irradiated food—as opposed to nonirradiated food—showed changes in the blood of test persons, indicative of an early pathogenic process, similar to the actual start of cancer.

According to Hertel, interviewed by Tom Valentine, "Common scientific belief states that cholesterol values usually alter slowly over longer periods of time. In this study the markers increased rapidly after the consumption of the microwaved vegetables." Also, the lymphocytes, which are a major part of our immune system, were decreased, and there were anemic tendencies in the subjects. In addition, blood changes were shown similar to those in the beginning stages of cancer.

According to a 1992 study by Richard Quan, MD, of Dallas, Texas, and John A. Kerner, MD, of Stanford University, microwaving breast milk is also unhealthy:

Women who work outside the home can express and store breast milk for feedings when they are away. But parents and caregivers should be careful how they warm this milk. A new study shows that microwaving human milk—even at a low setting—can destroy some of its important disease-fighting capabilities and "compared to heated breast milk, microwaved milk lost lysozyme activity, lost antibodies and fostered the growth of more potentially pathogenic bacteria.

Don't choose foods that have been packaged in aluminum cans, and don't cook your food in aluminum cookware or wrap it in aluminum foil. Also avoid baking powder that contains alum or aluminum. Many studies have shown that people with Alzheimer's disease have high amounts of aluminum in their brains. While the aluminum/Alzheimer's link remains unproven, lots of reports show that high levels of aluminum can be toxic to the body. According to the Agency for Toxic Substances and Disease Registry, people may have respiratory problems and coughing when exposed to high levels of aluminum in the air. They have also found that children and adults who have received aluminum in certain medical treatments developed bone diseases. Others that have used deodorants containing aluminum have developed serious skin rashes. The international science journal, *Neurotoxicology*, reported in April 1995 on a critical study that was conducted in Sydney, Australia, showing a direct pathway from tap water carrying aluminum through the intestinal tract, into the bloodstream and to the brain. Rats were given water treated with alum. Two weeks later, aluminum was found in their brains. Judy Walton, the scientist that performed the study, noted the worldwide increase in Alzheimer's over the past seventy years and stated, "We really should look seriously at revisiting this possibility that aluminum addition to foods and drinking water is a health hazard." I believe that waiting for definitive proof that aluminum can cause Alzheimer's before taking some measures of

Continued ➡

precaution is unwise. Foods should be cooked in stainless steel or glass cookware; clay pots and stainless steel waterless cookware are also wonderful choices.

When cooking your food, do not cook it to death with large amounts of water. Steam your vegetables in a stainless-steel steamer and keep them up out of the water or use waterless cookware. Do not fry foods in deep grease; saute them in a small amount of olive oil, grape seed oil, or coconut oil instead.

Tool Kit for Making Healthy Food Choices

Choose foods and substances that are pure, whole, fresh, and natural. Avoid denatured, preserved, processed foods; these can be harmful to our bodies. It is much easier to let go of foods that do not abide by the laws of nature if we have delicious foods to replace them with. This tool kit offers wonderful choices for eating healthfully.

Beans

Avoid:

Canned, salted pork and beans

Replace with:

Dried beans that have been grown organically and have been soaked before cooking so they are easier to digest, or bean sprouts

Dairy Products

Avoid:

Pasteurized milk

Ice cream that is high in preservatives and sugar or artificial sweeteners

Yogurt that is high in sugar and lacks friendly bacteria

Cheese that is made from pasteurized milk contains dyes, preservatives, and hormones Margarine

Eggs that have been fried in grease or overcooked

Eggs that have been salted and pickled

Replace with:

Certified raw goat's milk that is organic and hormone free

Certified raw cow's milk that is organic and hormone free

Almond milk that is organic and hormone free

Rice milk that is organic and hormone free

Oat milk that is organic and hormone free

Ice cream that is made from certified raw cow's or goat's milk, frozen bananas, or rice milk and is sweetened with maple syrup, raw honey, or stevia (a sweet, noncaloric herb)

Yogurt that is made from organic goat's or cow's milk and has live bacteria Cheese made from certified raw cow's or goat's milk, almonds, or seeds

Unsalted butter, preferably organic ghee (clarified butter)

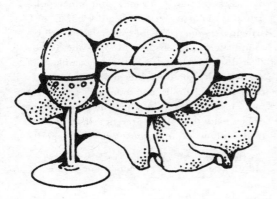

Organic coconut oil

Organic olive oil

Eggs that are organic, hormone free, and fertile

Fried Foods

Avoid:

Foods fried in deep grease

Replace with:

Foods sautéed in a small amount of organic olive oil, grape seed oil. or coconut oil

Fruits and Vegetables

Avoid:

Canned fruits with sugar and preservatives

Canned vegetables with salt and preservatives

Iceburg lettuce

Replace with:

Fresh fruits

Fresh vegetables

Romaine, butter, endive, green leaf and red leaf lettuces

Grains

Avoid:

Flour-based bread, especially white-flour bread

Crackers made from white flour

White-flour pasta

Cream of wheat and packaged cereals with sugar, salt, and preservatives

Replace with:

Breads made from sprouted whole grains

If sprouted-grain breads are not available, breads made from whole-grain flour such as barley, kamut, millet, quinoa, rice, or spelt

Crackers made from rice flour or rye flour

Rice cakes

Rice, corn, or quinoa pasta

Spaghetti squash (cooks up much like spaghetti)

Whole-grain cereals made from amaranth, brown rice, buckwheat, millet, quinoa, rolled oats, rye, or wild rice

Packaged cereals that are wheat-free and made from organic-grain without added sugar, salt, or preservatives

I usually recommend that people who are ill avoid all wheat. If you are not ill and are not suffering from sinus congestion, gas and bloating, or celiac disease (an inability to absorb gluten), you may eat whole wheat in moderation. More than a couple slices of whole wheat bread per day may cause weight gain or lead to gluten intolerance. Grinding your own wheat and making flour is of course the healthiest of all.

A NOTE ABOUT GRAINS AND ALLERGIES

Dr. Dan Kalish has done some research at his health clinic, The Natural Path. He has found, as I have, that many people have a subclinical, or hidden, gluten intolerance. Symptoms may include suffering from sinus congestion, gas and bloating after a meal, chronic fatigue, environmental illness, and lowered immunity. A highly specialized salivary test for subclinical gluten intolerance has accurately tested thousands of people with this disorder, making it easier to discover and treat the problem. Dr. Kalish explains:

Sub-clinical gluten intolerance refers to exposure to the gliadin molecule and to a specific inflammatory reaction, taking place in the small

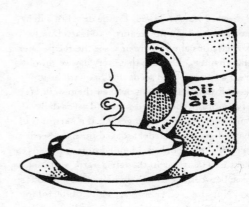

intestine of afflicted individuals. . . . To clarify, gliadin, the molecule that causes the problem, is present in some, but not all gluten containing foods. People with this problem must avoid glutens from the grains of wheat, rye, barley, oats, kamut, spelt, quinoa, amaranth, teff and couscous. Rice, corn, buckwheat and millet have glutens, but the glutens in these foods do not contain the gliadin molecule that can provoke the inflammatory reaction, therefore they are usually safe. In some cases people are allergic to rice, corn, buckwheat or millet, independent of the reaction to glutenlgliadin.

If you suspect you have a gluten intolerance, avoid wheat for a week. If you don't feel better, additionally avoid all grains containing gliadin including rye, barley, oats, kamut, spelt, quinoa, amaranth, teff, soy, and couscous for a second week and thereafter. It may take up to nine months to reduce inflammation in the small intestine and heal irritated tissue. Many who are gliadin intolerant also have corn allergies. If you don't feel well after two weeks of avoiding gliadin, omit corn for a week. If you have a corn allergy, you should feel better soon. Soaking grains overnight and cooking in a Crock-Pot is the best way to prepare grains. Hawthorne berry tea and flax seed tea may soothe the inflamed intestinal lining. Colon and tissue cleansing . . . is a remarkable way to help heal this disorder more quickly.

Meats

Avoid:

Pork, especially sausage and bacon

Processed meats, especially lunch meat and hot dogs containing nitrates, and nitrites in general

Replace with:

Veggie burgers

Veggie sausage

Turkey sausage and turkey bacon (60 percent less fat than regular pork bacon)

Lunch meats that have been sliced from freshly cooked chicken, turkey, and roast beef that contain no nitrates

Nut and Seed Butters

Avoid:

Peanut butter that is high in sugar and canola oil

Roasted nut and seed butters

Replace with:

Aflatoxin-free peanut butter (such as peanut butter made from sun-dried organic peanuts)

Raw. organic almond, sesame, or sunflower seed butter, which are much healthier than peanut butter

Soaked, blended nuts and seeds

Nuts and seeds can be soaked while they are sprouting, making them easier to digest. Soaking nuts and seeds also reduces the quantity of fat by

Continued ➡

half. Soaked nuts and seeds can be dried in a dehydrator or blended into creams. (To learn how to make delicious almond creams, see the recipe later in this chapter.) I believe that every day we should also eat a few nuts and seeds that have not been soaked. Either grind them or chew them well. We can eat more of the soaked nuts and seeds daily because they are so easily digested. If a person is ill or has a digestive disorder, soaked nuts and seeds are better for them. Soaked, blended nuts and seeds can be kept in a quart jar in the refrigerator and used as a snack between meals to help balance the blood sugar. Nut and seed creams are also wonderful for nursing mothers to help keep their milk from drying up.

Nuts and Seeds

Avoid:

Roasted, salted nuts and seeds

Peanuts

Peanuts are not really a nut, but a legume. Most people think of them as nuts, so they are listed here. Peanuts are high in calcium, magnesium, phosphorus, potassium, and protein. However, nonorganic peanuts are saturated with pesticides, and organic peanuts often contain a mold called anatoxin, which is carcinogenic.

Replace with:

A wide variety of raw, unsalted nuts and seeds

Raw nuts and seeds are high in beneficial oils (high-density lipoproteins), which help keep our arteries clean and skin glowing. Nuts and seeds contain lignans, which are believed to protect against hormone-sensitive cancers, such as those of the breast and prostate. Dr. Bernard Jensen used to say, "Think of the nuts and seeds as the 'glands' of the plants that can help to feed and nourish the glands of the body." The healthiest nut choices are almonds, Brazil nuts, and walnuts, which are very high in protein, calcium, magnesium, phosphorus, potassium, iron, selenium, zinc, and vitamin E. Calcium, magnesium, and potassium help prevent muscle cramping. Young people, who are growing rapidly and using their muscles a great deal, are often deficient in these three minerals and get leg cramps. These three minerals are also important in calming the nervous system. Iron is necessary for preventing anemia, and the bones need calcium and phosphorus to be strong. The heart is a muscle and needs potassium to be healthy. Selenium, zinc, and vitamin E help to strengthen the immune system and fight free radicals in the body, and they are well-known for helping prevent cancer. Black walnuts are high in all the minerals mentioned with the exception of selenium. Black walnuts also contain manganese, which is excellent for the memory.

Sesame, sunflower, and pumpkin seeds contain high amounts of calcium, magnesium, iron, phosphorus, potassium, and zinc. Pumpkin seeds are among the highest in zinc of all the nuts and seeds, and they are excellent for the prostate gland. Pumpkin seeds also kill parasites in the body. Ground flaxseeds are so beneficial everyone should include them in their daily nutritional plan. Flaxseeds are high in fiber and help keep the colon working smoothly. You must grind the flaxseeds, however, in order to receive their healthy benefits. The oil in the flaxseeds is high in lignans, which protect against several types of cancer. Many people take flaxseed oil, which, when fresh, is very good but lacks the soluble fiber so beneficial to the colon. According to research from Tufts University, even refrigerated flaxseed oil has a shelf life of only six weeks before it becomes rancid.

Oils

Avoid:

Canola oil

Cottonseed oil, which comes from heavily sprayed cotton crops

Foods containing partially hydrogenated oils, such as nondairy creamers or packaged baked goods and crackers

Oils that have been extracted by heat and processed to preserve them

Partially hydrogenated oils or fats, including margarine and shortening

Canola oil comes from rapeseed, a food we do not eat because it is highly toxic. According to John Thomas in *Young Again: How to Reverse the Aging Process*, "Rape is the MOST toxic of all food plants. Insects will not eat rape. It is deadly poisonous." He goes on to say that "canola oil . . . forms latex-like substances that form agglutination of the red corpuscles. . . . Rape oil (canola oil) antagonizes the central and peripheral nervous systems. Deterioration may take years to manifest." *Canola* is not the name of a natural plant. It is called canola because it was developed in Canada and it is short for *Canada oil*. Some documents state that it was developed by the genetic engineering of the rapeseed plant. Other authorities say it was developed by hybrid propagation techniques. It's confusing and it's controversial, and it comes down to this: Not enough long-term research has been done on this oil to consider it safe for consumption.

The hydrogen used to harden margarine also can harden bodily tissues. Trans-fatty acids occur when polyunsaturated oils are hardened into margarine through hydrogenation. According to James Balch, MD, and Phyllis Balch, CNC, in *Prescription for Nutritional Healing*, "One recent study found that trans-monounsaturated fatty acids raise LDL (bad) cholesterol levels. Simultaneously, the trans-fatty acids reduced the HDL (good) cholesterol readings." Some people think that eating margarine will help lower their cholesterol, but they are misinformed. Michael T. Murray, ND, and Jade Beutler, RRT, RCP, stated in *Understanding Fats and Oils: Your Guide to Healing with Essential Fatty Acids*, "Trans-fatty acids and hydrogenated oils have been linked to low birth weight in infants, low quality and volume of breast milk, abnormal sperm production and decreased testosterone in men, heart disease, increased levels of harmful cholesterol in humans, prostate disease, obesity, suppression of the immune system and essential fatty acid deficiency."

Replace with:

Organic, cold-pressed oils such as extra-virgin olive oil or grape seed, sesame, avocado, coconut, and sunflower oils

Olive oil is a wonderful oil because it helps balance the body's pH. If your pH is too acidic, it can damage the central and peripheral nervous systems. You may cook with grape seed, olive, or coconut oil because they can withstand high temperatures and retain their nutritional value. Never heat other oils to high temperatures; they will become rancid and toxic to the body. Keep all oils in the refrigerator.

Even a little real organic butter occasionally is better for you than margarine. Butter is high in vitamins A and D, which are very good for the eyes. Be sure to use organic, hormone-free butter, though. The hormones in dairy and beef products create all sorts of problems with women's menstrual cycles, including premenstrual syndrome (PMS) and menopausal imbalances.

Salt

Avoid:

Table salt and salted foods

Using too much salt has become a problem in our country. According to *The Supermarket Handbook*, by Nikki and David Goldbeck, "The most common form of salt on the supermarket shelf is a product referred to as 'table salt.' In [its] purifying process, iodine is added, plus dextrose to stabilize it, sodium bicarbonate to keep it white and chemical anticaking agents to keep it free flowing." Avoid using table salt and use caution when purchasing sea salt. When buying sea salt, look for unrefined sea salt; it will be light gray in color. Most sea salt is heated to extreme temperatures, thereby changing its molecular structure and robbing it of all essential minerals, then other chemicals are often added to iodize it, whiten it, and make it easy to pour. Unrefined sea salt is much better for us because it contains ninety-two essential minerals and trace minerals, while refined sea salt may contain only sodium and chloride. Almost all packaged foods contain an excessive amount of salt. Most people's taste buds have become so accustomed to added salt, they have lost the ability to taste the delightful flavors of foods. Each cell of our body contains a sodium-potassium pump that helps move fluids in and out of the cells. Eating too much salt upsets this system, causing our cells to retain too much sodium. When that happens, water is held within the cells, swelling occurs, and our heart has to pump harder, often causing high blood pressure. Our kidneys become overworked and do not release the fluids they should. High blood pressure is directly related to stress, poor kidney functioning, and/or an imbalance in the body's fluids and minerals. Avoid using table salt as much as possible. If you are ill, avoid using it altogether.

Replace with:

Salt-free powdered vegetable broths and seasonings

Liquid amino acids

Granular seaweed, such as dulse and kelp

Unrefined sea salt, in small amounts

If you have ever tasted your tears, you noticed they were salty. Lymph fluid needs natural sodium to lubricate the cellular membranes and hold calcium in solution. Sodium chloride in table salt has been isolated and refined from other nutrients that might help the body utilize it. When we take minerals into the body in plant form, we utilize the whole food. The body easily assimilates sodium from vegetables. Look for vegetable seasonings that are salt free. Add dried, organic herbal seasonings such as thyme, oregano, basil, rosemary, dill, garlic, onion, or sage to your food. Dr. Jensen called natural sodium the youth element because of its ability to keep the joints limber. The stomach also needs natural sodium for proper digestion. Under stress, sodium is depleted rapidly, causing digestive disorders, gout, and arthritic conditions. Organic sodium is found in celery, green leafy vegetables, okra, strawberries, goat's milk, and mineral whey drink. If you have digestive disorders, gout, or arthritis, try the recipe for mineral whey drink found later in this chapter. Mineral whey is the clear fluid that comes from the goat's milk while separating it from the solids in order to make cheese. It is naturally high in minerals and organic sodium. The juice from celery and green leafy vegetables helps to heal and prevent arthritis because the i sodium aids in dissolving calcium deposits.

Seaweed is a wonderful source of natural sodium, calcium, trace minerals, and iodine.

Continued ➡

Dulse, kelp, and kombu can be purchased in powdered form and used to season salads, soups, and vegetables; nori's the ideal "sushi" wrap for brown rice and vegetables; and hijiki, which looks like noodles when soaked, is crunchy and delicious in salads. Seaweed is a delicious way to fortify the body with minerals and to strengthen the thyroid gland with iodine. People in Japan do not often get goiter (an enlargement of the thyroid gland) because they eat lots of fish and seaweed, which are high in natural iodine. People in Switzerland have a tendency for goiter because they live in the Alps and do not get enough iodine in their diets. Salt from the sea that has been allowed to dry in the wind and the sun and is not highly treated or refined is rich in native minerals and may be used in small amounts.

Sugar and Sweeteners

A Note about Sugar

Glazed doughnuts, rich chocolates, chunky ice cream, creamy puddings, cakes, candies, pies, cookies: Many people think of these sweets with joy and anticipation. They may remind us of happy times from childhood such as birthday parties or holidays. Many people have been rewarded for a job well done with a sweet treat. In the old days sweets were truly a treat and were few and far between. They were often made with real maple syrup taken from a tree or honey pulled from a beehive. It took time to churn a freezer of ice cream by hand or make a cake from scratch. Today, ready-made sweet foods are everywhere. In addition to the myriad desserts available in the United States, as well as in a rapidly growing number of other countries, sugar is now in virtually every packaged food on the shelf. One 12-ounce soft drink contains the equivalent of thirteen teaspoons of sugar! Soft drinks were once sweetened with sugar derived from sugarcane or sugar beets, but now they are sweetened with high fructose corn syrup which is sweeter than sugar and costs the soft drink industry less. However, according to Sharon Elliott and other researchers in an article published by the *American Journal of Clinical Nutrition* (November 2002), high fructose corn syrup is metabolized differently in our bodies than sugar or glucose. While glucose can be metabolized by every cell of the body, all fructose must be metabolized by the liver. *Washington Post* writer Sally Squires reported on March 11, 2003, some very important information presented by George A. Bray, former director of Louisiana State University's Pennington Biomedical Research Center. Bray explained that when eating glucose, the body increases insulin production, which enables sugar to be carried into the cells to be used as energy. It also causes the body to produce a hormone called leptin that helps store fat and regulate the appetite. It suppresses production of another hormone the stomach makes that helps regulate food uptake, called ghrelin. She goes on to say that according to Peter Havel, associate professor of nutrition at University of California–Davis, that "Fructose doesn't stimulate insulin secretion. It doesn't increase leptin production or suppress production of ghrelin. That suggests that consuming a lot of fructose, like consuming too much fat, could contribute to weight gain." Meanwhile, a team of researchers led by Dr. Meira Fields of the U.S. Department of Agriculture found that when fructose was given to rats that were deficient in copper, they developed high cholesterol, enlarged thymus hearts, and anemia. Their livers were cirrhotic and filled with fat. Rats that were fed glucose were unaffected. (Fields, M. *Proceedings of the Society of Experimental Biology and Medicine*, 1984, 175:530–537.) Even peanut butter and ketchup are 30 to 40 percent sugar, mostly

in the form of high fructose corn syrup! High fructose corn syrup has replaced sugar in almost every food product on the market. It can be found in yogurt, bread, applesauce, fruit juices, cookies, crackers, and many other things. Read labels and avoid anything that contains it.

What has this sugar craze done to our bodies? Growing numbers of people throughout the United States and worldwide are suffering from diabetes, obesity, hypoglycemia, gum infections, yeast infections, tooth decay, and hyperactivity—all traced to the ingestion of excessive amounts of sugar.

When sugar enters the body, it feeds harmful bacteria that dwell in the mouth. Within minutes after eating a sugary dessert, tooth decay begins. Extensive ingestion of sugar without brushing the teeth creates gum diseases such as gingivitis and periodontitis.

Refined white sugar contains no nutrients, so the body has to draw from its storehouse of enzymes and nutrients to digest it. All of the B vitamins, which are vital to nerve health, and vitamin C, which is important to keeping the immune system active and to repairing connective tissue, are required. Excessive amounts of sugar can even leach calcium and other minerals from the bones to help process it. Place a chicken bone in a cup of pop for one week and watch how soft it becomes! Nor does white sugar give any nutrition back to the body. When one eats an apple, the apple contains sugar, but it also contains enzymes, vitamins, and minerals that help the body process the sugar.

A Note about Aspartame

Artificial sweeteners containing aspartame are two hundred times sweeter than sugar. Because it contains very few calories, aspartame has been tremendously popular with dieters and diabetics. It is in soft drinks, instant coffees and teas, sugar-free gum, breath mints, juice drinks, puddings, yogurt, laxatives, and even multivitamins. It is served in packets along with the sugar on tables in restaurants.

H. J. Roberts, in *Aspartame (NutraSweet): Is It Safe?*, writes about a significant number of people who used aspartame and reported having nausea and diarrhea, headaches, trouble with memory, problems sleeping, changes in their vision, moodiness, and confusion. Some even reported having convulsions.

There are three components in aspartame: phenylalanine and aspartic acid, which are both amino acids; and methanol, known as methyl alcohol or wood alcohol. Aspartame should not be used by persons with PKU (phenylketonuria). These people lack the enzyme necessary to digest phenylalanine, and if taken into their bodies, it can cause brain damage. A warning for phenylketonurics is found on aspartame products. Methanol can be poisonous and toxic in anyone. It can cause inflammation, swelling, and even blindness.

A Note about Splenda

Another artificial sweetener that has become most popular is sucralose, a synthetic compound known by its trade name, Splenda. It is four times sweeter than aspartame, twice as sweet as saccharin, and five to six hundred times sweeter than sugar. It is a chlorocarbon manufactured by the selective chlorination of sucrose. Short-term studies done by the manufacturer on rats revealed that sucralose caused shrunken thymus glands and swelling of the kidneys and liver. The FDA decided that because the studies were not done on humans they were not substantial and inconclusive. However, many people have given testimonials that report rashes, intestinal cramping, diarrhea, headaches, weight gain, disruption of

sleep patterns, numbness, and dizziness. In Dr. Janet Hull's new book, *Splenda: Is It Safe Or Not?*, she gives scientific evidence that suggests that sucralose may be dangerous for human consumption. I suggest avoiding it completely!

A Note about Saccharin

Saccharin has mostly been replaced by better-tasting products that contain aspartame. While aspartame is more toxic than saccharin, research has shown that saccharin caused bladder cancer in rats. Many researchers believe that it could be carcinogenic in humans when taken in sufficient dosages.

All artificial sweeteners are chemicals and are potentially toxic to the body. They are not food so they don't give the body the boost of energy it is calling for when one craves sweets. Therefore, when the body doesn't feel energized, it craves the carbohydrates. Often those who eat artificial sweeteners end up gaining more weight than those who eat sweeteners from natural sources. These natural sweeteners give the body the energy it craves so the person doesn't keep going back to the refrigerator for more food.

Avoid:

All products containing aspartame

Splenda and all products containing Splenda

Saccharin

Refined white sugar

Desserts made from white flour and white sugar

Replace with:

Stevia, a natural herb with few calories that can balance the pancreas and reduce cravings for sweets

Agave

Blackstrap molasses, which is high in minerals and B vitamins

Certified raw organic honey (except for children under two, who have not developed the ability to digest it)

Pure Grade B maple syrup which is less refined and contains more nutrients than Grade A syrup

Rice bran syrup, which is high in minerals including silicon as well as B vitamins

Unrefined cane sugar, for special occasions only

Carob candy, a nutritious substitute for chocolate

Organic chocolate, preferably raw, in small quantities for special occasions

Stevia is the best sweetener for someone who is watching his weight or has diabetes or hypoglycemia. Stevia is a sweet, noncaloric herb native to Paraguay that has been used to sweeten foods and beverages for centuries. It is two to three hundred times sweeter than sugar but has very little effect on blood glucose and does not cause cavities. It is sold in health food stores as a dietary supplement and comes in powdered or liquid form.

Organic blue agave nectar is a delicious and nutritious sweetener to use. The best, most natural agave nectar comes from the pineapple-shaped core of the blue agave plant, which is a desert succulent that grows in the mineral rich volcanic soil of Mexico. The nectar, or syrup, is light in color and thinner than honey. Research done by the Glycemic Research Institute in Washington DC has shown that the blue agave nectar is safe for non-insulin-dependent (type 2) diabetics because it has a low glycemic level. It is also great for hypoglycemics, those trying to lose weight, or anyone watching their carbohydrate intake. In recipes, three-fourths cup of agave nectar will equal one cup of table sugar. When purchasing agave nectar, make sure it

Continued ➡

has the Glycemic Research Institute (GRI) seal of approval on it.

Xylitol is a safe natural sweetener that comes from the bark of the birch tree, fibrous vegetables, and fruits and corncobs. It is also produced naturally in normally metabolising bodies. Xylitol looks and tastes almost exactly like sugar, but while sugar causes havoc in the body, xylitol helps heal and repair. Xylitol also helps prevent tooth decay and fights bacteria. It has 75 percent fewer carbohydrates than sugar, 40 percent less calories, and causes very little change in insulin levels. Xylitol is available in crystalline form and can be used in place of sugar to sweeten beverages, or in baking. Make sure xylitol is from the bark of the birch tree or other natural plant source before purchasing.

For healthy desserts, look for delicious cookies made from rice flour rather than wheat flour and sweetened with maple syrup, stevia, agave nectar, xylitol, or fruit juice. Practice making your own cookies with oat flour, spelt flour, or rice flour, and use maple syrup, stevia, or agave to sweeten them. Carob brownies and cakes can be made with rice, spelt, or whole wheat flour and maple syrup. Shop at health food stores for wonderful ice creams made from rice milk and Popsicles made from fruit juice. You can make your own tapioca pudding with rice milk.

Addictive Substances

Avoid:

Tobacco, nicotine, and social drugs

Organic tobacco is available, as are organic cigarettes free from pesticides and chemicals. However, tobacco smoke is very irritating to the lungs and arteries. It disturbs the blood sugar balance. In addition, nicotine is very hard on the adrenal glands and heart. If you are a smoker, ask yourself why you smoke. Is it for emotional reasons? Follow therapeutic remedies that will help you stop smoking. Any type of addiction enslaves us and keeps us from being free.

Avoid Free Radicals

Free radicals are highly reactive molecules or fragments of molecules that wreak havoc in our bodies. They have electrons that are unpaired in their outer orbits. Because of this imbalance, they are unstable and very aggressive with other molecules.

When a cell has been damaged by free radicals, the cell is less able to import oxygen and nutrients or excrete cellular wastes. Cells then begin to rupture and spill their damaging contents into the surrounding tissues. Free radicals can even alter genetic codes by damaging nucleic acids (RNA and DNA), causing abnormal cell growth. This destruction leads to rapid aging, the growth of malignancies, impaired immune function, arteriosclerosis, and damage to joint linings, which leads to arthritis and many other major health problems.

Air pollution, tobacco smoke, polyunsaturated fats, rancid fats, and processed foods are sources of free radicals. By avoiding these harmful substances and replacing them with wholesome, life-giving foods and juices, you will effectively decrease free-radical damage in your body. Antioxidants bind to and neutralize free radicals in the body. They are abundant in fresh fruits and vegetables. Several vitamins and minerals act as antioxidants as well. These include vitamin A, beta-carotene, vitamin E, and vitamin C. Selenium, zinc, copper, and manganese combine with enzymes and help fight free radicals.

Combine Foods Properly

Food combinations have many wonderful benefits that help improve health, though some restrictions do apply. Some people have become so paranoid about food combinations that they eat only one food at each meal. Also, I have had clients who were so concerned about proper food combining that they were afraid to eat and enjoy their meals, and they became malnourished. These responses are unnecessarily extreme. However, if you are extremely ill or have severe allergies, strict food combining is very important for optimal digestion and absorption.

It's best to eat fruits alone. Fruits digest very rapidly, and if they are eaten with grains, for example, they begin to ferment while the grains are still digesting. This causes gas. Too much gas over long periods of time can cause hiatal hernias because of the continuous pressure imposed on the cardiac sphincter muscle. So if you like fruit in the morning, have it at least ten to twenty minutes before your meal. Fruits can be combined with vegetables more easily than with grains because vegetables digest quickly. Our ancestors often ate vegetables from the earth and fruit from trees at the same time. Avocados combine well with all foods. Melons should definitely be eaten alone.

We should also separate starches from proteins. However, the body can tolerate the combination if the starch is a natural whole grain and not a white-flour product. Try the meal plans provided in the following tool kit, and notice whether you are having gas or burping. If so, you should eat fruits alone and even separate whole grains and natural starches, such as potatoes, from proteins. For example, have vegetables and a grain at a meal or vegetables and a protein at a meal.

Soaked nuts and seeds combine well with all foods except melons because they are digested and absorbed quite easily. It is important to soak all grains or beans for twelve to twenty-four hours before cooking them. They will digest easier and cause less gas. Beans contain enzyme inhibitors that are removed through soaking. You may want to take an enzyme supplement with your meal to aid digestion. Most Americans over the age of forty are deficient in natural digestive enzymes and should supplement them with their meals.

Eat a Variety of Foods

Nature has provided us with a multitude of beautiful, delicious foods of all colors to choose from. Different foods contain different nutrients. We should eat a variety of foods each day in order to provide our bodies with the vitamins and minerals they need to be well. Remember, our bodies are made up of the earth's elements. Our bones need calcium, our skin needs silicon, and our thyroid gland needs iodine to function properly. Each part of our body requires specific nutrients. If you are accustomed to living on sodas and chips, coffee and doughnuts, TV dinners, or all fruit or all meat, you are not getting the wide variety of nutrients your body requires on a daily basis. Deficient organs become sick organs and will not function properly. Follow the menu plans in this book to get a variety of foods in your diet each day.

Add Fiber to Your Nutritional Program

• Constipation, colon cancer, Crohn's disease, colitis, and diverticulitis have become too common in our modern world. The intestinal tract needs fiber to keep it clean and healthy. Fiber also promotes good peristalsis (healthy muscle contractions that keep food and waste matter moving through the

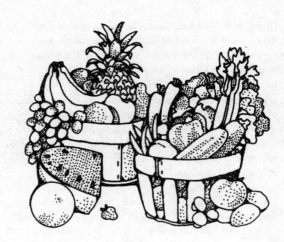

body), and it helps lower high levels of cholesterol. According to a study published in the *Journal of the American Medical Association*, oat bran was shown to lower blood cholesterol levels. Choose foods high in fiber from: fruits; vegetables; legumes; nuts; seeds, including ground flaxseeds; and whole grains such as brown rice, barley, millet, rye, quinoa, amaranth, and oats. A diet that is high in fiber can greatly regulate blood sugar levels and help manage both hypoglycemia and diabetes.

Eat Raw Vegetables with Your Meals

When we eat raw vegetables, we are eating foods as Mother Nature provided them. Raw vegetables are so good for us because they provide living enzymes, electrolytes, vitamins, minerals, and phytonutrients. Phytonutrients, also called phytochemicals, are the elements in most fruits and vegetables that help give them their color. Scientists have found that these valuable nutrients are potent antioxidants that help neutralize free radical damage and help the body fight disease by mobilizing natural killer cells and helper T-cells. They help to fight cancer and protect the heart. While some phytonutrients remain intact during cooking, such as those in broccoli, many are destroyed when exposed to high heat. Raw vegetables are also high in fiber. The enzymes help digest our meals better. If you have difficulty digesting raw vegetables, use a food processor or blender to chop and grind the vegetables, making them easier to chew and digest. Finely grind cabbage for coleslaw and carrots for carrot salad. Grind beets, zucchini, yellow squash, carrots, cucumbers, and jicama, and place them on a bed of lettuce. (See salad recipes later in this chapter.) Blended vegetables make good salads and cold soups.

Be sure to wash all raw vegetables well to remove any eggs, worms, or parasites. Soak them in raw apple cider vinegar and water for five minutes. Then scrub them with a good vegetable brush.

Choose 80 Percent Alkaline-Forming Foods and 20 Percent Acid-Forming Foods

Ripe fruits, including organic lemons and limes, that were ripened on the vine, raw apple cider vinegar, vegetables, and soaked sprouted grains, nuts, seeds, and beans are alkaline-forming foods. Meats, cheeses, eggs, beans that have not been soaked, white flour, soft drinks, coffee, and black tea are acid-forming foods. Oranges and grapefruits that were not ripened on the vine produce acids in the body.

Dr. Bernard Jensen recommended eating two fruits and six vegetables per day to achieve the 80 percent of alkaline-forming foods. He recommended 10 percent protein and 10 percent starch per day to make up the 20 percent of acid-forming foods.

Continued ➡

Fruits are alkaline-forming; however, they are high in fruit sugar, so I recommend no more than two fruits per day. If a person is ill, I recommend avoiding fruits altogether for a while. People with arthritis may have increased pain from eating too many fruits. People who want to lose weight should have no more than one fruit a day because the fruit sugar can turn to body fat. Of course, if it comes down to fruit or chocolate cake, fruit would be a nice substitute!

Vegetables are excellent for us, and we should eat a wide variety each day. Eating six different kinds of vegetables each day would be great. Consider having this many varieties in a salad.

We do need some protein. A large part of out body is made up of proteins, including our cell walls, digestive enzymes, and hair. Our brain and nervous system cannot function without protein. However, most Americans eat far too much meat. Dr. Samuel West, in *The Golden Seven Plus One*, shows how proteins can become trapped within the blood, causing pain, swelling, or inflammation in the body. The important thing is that protein come from natural organic sources and that it be digested well and absorbed. The balanced nutritional plans provided in this book improve health and well-being.

Understand Your pH Balance

Biochemist Carey Reams did a great deal of research on the importance of pH, which stands for "potential of hydrogen," a measure of the acid and alkaline balance in our bodies. We cannot be healthy if our bodies are too acidic or too alkaline. This balance is almost as important as breathing or the heart beating. When the pH within our bodies is balanced, it maintains healthy metabolism and allows the body to function optimally.

Dr. Robert Young has done extensive research on the pH of urine and saliva, and in his comprehensive book *The pH Miracle* he suggests the following normal pH ranges.

Saliva: 6.8 to 7.2 throughout the entire day. 6.8 to 8.4 right after meals

Urine: 6.8 to 7 before meals, 6.8 to 8.4 right after meals

ACIDOSIS, OR OVERACIDITY

Most Americans are overacidic because their diet includes processed foods and too much meat, sugar, salt, caffeine, and alcohol. According to Richard Anderson, ND, NMD, in *Cleanse and Purify Thyself*.

The further we deplete our minerals and move towards greater acidity, the more our bodies lose control over pH, and the more the liver and all organs are impaired. From this depletion of minerals and development of acidity, our immune systems become depressed. We also can lose the ability to create hydrochloric acid, the bile turns acid, our normal friendly bacteria mutates and we then become susceptible to infiltration of "germs"—various bacteria, viruses, fungus, Yest and perhaps protozoa. Both minerals and harmonious feelings are essential in maintaining this delicate pH and metabolic balance.

An overacid environment can lead to serious health conditions. Some of these include kidney stones, plaque in the arteries, osteoporosis, arthritis, cardiovascular deficiency, lowered immune function, free-radical damage, fatigue, weight gain, water retention, dry hard stools, burning tongue, and bad breath. We must have sufficient alkaline reserves to buffer the acids in our body. Calcium cannot stay in our bones if the body is overacidic. Stress, as well as acidic foods, causes acidity in the body. We can stay healthy by living a balanced life and consuming plenty of alkaline foods that are pure, whole, fresh, and natural.

ALKALOSIS, OR HIGH ALKALINITY

A less common condition in which the body is too alkaline can result from the long-term use of alkaline drugs, such as those used for ulcers in the stomach or intestinal tract. It can also result from excessive vomiting, diarrhea, and poor diet.

People suffering from alkalosis often have an intense, overexcitable nervous system. They may even have anxiety or seizures. They may feel cold or have sore muscles, cramps, allergies, sluggish digestion, constipation, immune deficiency, and urinary tract weakness. They may also have calcium deposits, such as bone spurs.

Test Your pH

If you sense that your body is overalkaline or overacidic, test your pH for six days by following the pH test provided below, based on Dr. Robert Young's research. You will need some pHydrion paper (pH paper strips), which can be purchased at most pharmacies. You will need one strip for each time you check your saliva and one strip for each time you check your urine.

Test Start Date:_____

Upon waking, test your saliva with pHydrion paper. Wet the end of a pHydrion test strip with your saliva before brushing your teeth, drinking, or eating. Note the color change and record the pH number. Optimally, the pH should be between 6.8 and 7.2.

First Saliva Test:

Day 1 _____ Day 2 _____ Day 3 _____
Day 4 _____ Day 5 _____ Day 6 _____

Now test your first urine of the morning. This is urine that has been stored in your bladder during the night and is ready to be eliminated when you get up. Urinate on a strip of pHydrion paper, note the color change, and record the pH number. Optimally, the pH should be between 6.8 and 7.2.

First Urine Test:

Day 1 _____ Day 2 _____ Day 3 _____
Day 4 _____ Day 5 _____ Day 6 _____

Next, test your morning urine a second time before eating any food. You will have eliminated the acid load from the day before, and optimally your second urine pH should be around 6.8 to 7.2.

Second Urine Test:

Day 1 _____ Day 2 _____ Day 3 _____
Day 4 _____ Day 5 _____ Day 6 _____

Eat breakfast. Wait five minutes, then check both your urine and saliva again. Record your results.

Second Saliva Test:

Day 1 _____ Day 2 _____ Day 3 _____
Day 4 _____ Day 5 _____ Day 6 _____

Third Urine Test:

Day 1 _____ Day 2 _____ Day 3 _____
Day 4 _____ Day 5 _____ Day 6 _____

Now wait a couple of hours after breakfast and check your saliva and urine again and record your results below.

Third Saliva Test:

Day 1 _____ Day 2 _____ Day 3 _____
Day 4 _____ Day 5 _____ Day 6 _____

Fourth Urine Test:

Day 1 _____ Day 2 _____ Day 3 _____
Day 4 _____ Day 5 _____ Day 6 _____

Two to three hours after lunch, check your saliva and urine again and record your results below.

Fourth Saliva Test:

Day 1 _____ Day 2 _____ Day 3 _____
Day 4 _____ Day 5 _____ Day 6 _____

Fifth Urine Test:

Day 1 _____ Day 2 _____ Day 3 _____
Day 4 _____ Day 5 _____ Day 6 _____

If you have sufficient alkaline reserves to buffer the acids in your system, the pH numbers will go up (greater alkalinity) from the first to the second urine and saliva tests. If you do not have enough alkalinity, then the pH numbers will show very little change or even go down from the first to the second and third morning pH tests. Our pH should always be between 6.8 and 8.4 right after meals and between 6.8 and 7.2 a couple of hours after meals. I like for my clients to test for six days in order to see a pattern, but really one can test their saliva and urine on a daily basis or (after the six days) periodically at various times throughout the week. Continue testing until your pH falls within a healthy range on a regular basis. Then you may want to check once a week to make sure you are maintaining a good pH.

IF YOUR BODY IS OVERACIDIC

- Eat lots of raw vegetables, salads, and steamed vegetables.
- Eat Avocado Pudding (see page 350) daily until your pH comes into normal range, then as often as you desire. It makes a great healthy morning breakfast or even dessert.
- Drink several glasses of raw organic vegetable juice throughout the day until your pH tests within range. Then continue with one glass of raw vegetable juice on a daily basis for maintenance and good health.
- Drink six to eight glasses of distilled water with ten drops of ionic liquid trace minerals added daily until proper pH is maintained.
- Take plant enzymes before each meal.
- Drink one to three liters of purified water with powdered green vegetables added. These green powders usually include a variety of all sorts of alkalinizing green vegetables such as celery, parsley, spinach, kale, collards, green kamut or wheat grass, alfalfa leaf, dandelion leaf, and barley grass. You may search for these in your local health store or call Bernard Jensen International.
- Eat seaweeds such as dulse, kelp, kombu, wakame, nori, and/or hijiki on a daily basis until pH comes into balance, then several times a week for maintenance.
- Take a liquid calcium-magnesium supplement daily until your pH comes into balance, then check with your health practitioner to see if you should continue.
- Drink potato peelings broth one to two times per day until your pH comes into balance, then once a week for maintenance; see the recipe later in this chapter.
- Drink mineral whey drink one to three times per day until your pH comes into balance, then

Continued ➔

- daily or at least several times a week for maintenance; see the recipe later in this chapter.
- Drink one tablespoon of Dr. Jensen's Whole Life Food Blend in eight ounces of water, one to three times daily until your pH comes into balance, then take it once daily for maintenance.
- Practice deep breathing and meditation.

IF YOUR BODY IS TOO ALKALINE

- Eat more acid-forming foods that are whole, fresh, and natural, such as whole-grain cereals, brown rice, beans, eggs, fish, chicken and turkey.
- Take enzymes with each meal daily until your pH comes into balance, then check with your health practitioner to determine if you should continue. If you see whole bits of food in your stools it is likely that you need them.
- Include liquid calcium citrate and methylsulfonylmethane (MSM) in your diet daily until your pH comes into balance.
- Take vitamin B complex and vitamin C daily until your pH comes into balance.
- Use acidophilus and bifidus daily until your pH comes into balance.
- Add essential fatty acids to your nutritional program.
- Cook foods with a minimum of water. A steamer, Crock-Pot, or waterless cookware is preferable. Never fry foods in deep grease. Pan fry with a little olive oil, coconut oil, grapeseed oil, ghee, or butter. Bake or broil rather than frying whenever possible.

Eat Essential Fatty Acids, the "Good" Fats

Not to be confused with trans-fatty acids, essential fatty acids (EFAs) are just that—essential. Christiane Northrup, MD, in her newsletter, *Health Wisdom for Women*, has reported that the following symptoms occur when people are deficient in essential fatty acids, the "good" fats:

- Dry "alligator" skin, cracked fingertips or cracked heels
- Bumpy "chicken" skin on backs of arms
- Brittle or soft nails
- Dry, unmanageable hair or dandruff
- Depression or moodiness
- Allergies, eczema, or psoriasis
- Hyperactivity
- Learning or memory problems
- Lowered immunity, frequent infections or poor wound healing
- Fatigue or weakness
- Excessive thirst or frequent urination

The good fats are terribly deficient in the American diet. These fats are the omega-3s and the omega-6s. Recent studies have shown that DHA, docosahexaenoic acid, an omega-3 fatty acid, is necessary for brain and nerve function, and is sorely lacking in the diets of those who are depressed, have learning disabilities, or have ADHD. Dr. Northrup states:

A deficiency in DHA is one of the main reasons individuals who've been on extremely low-fat diets for long periods of time become depressed. Several studies have shown a link between suicide or depression and following a very low-fat or fat-free diet. It's no wonder that the rise in the number of people on selective serotonin re-uptake inhibitor (SSRI) drugs such as Prozac and Zoloft seems to reflect the profusion of fat-free foods on the market.

She goes on to say:

The right kinds of fats are also important for the heart and cardiovascular system. Cardiovascular disease is the leading cause of premature death in the United States—for both men and women. . . In fact, research also suggests that deficiency of omega-3 fats is a factor in both Alzheimer's and Parkinson's disease.

Good fats are essential for our brain and nervous system, skin and nails, eyes, heart, and cardiovascular system, as well as the rest of our bodies. EFAs also are necessary to the development of a fetus's brain, nervous systems, and retinas, and they help to promote milk flow in nursing mothers. EFAs are an aid in losing weight since they help the body feel satisfied and keep it from feeling hungry for long periods of time. Plus EFAs help the body to release stored fat.

In people who have multiple sclerosis (MS), the myelin sheath that covers the nerves is destroyed. Michael T. Murray, ND, and Jade Beutler, RRT, RCP, in *Understanding Fats and Oils*, found that people with MS appear to have a defect in fatty acid absorption and transport, which would be a significant factor in their myelin deficiencies.

Essential fatty acids have been referred to as vitamin F, and they are the building blocks of oils and fats. Though they are vital to good health, the body cannot make them. Some of the best sources of DHA (an omega-3) are dark green leafy vegetables, organic eggs, and cold-water fish such as salmon, mackerel, rainbow trout, and sardines. Fish and fish oil can help heal psoriasis and dry skin disorders, high blood pressure, and arthritic inflammation. Good sources of other omega-3 EFAs, including linolenic and gamma-linolenic acids, are: eggs; free-range meat from animals that have consumed grass high in omega-3s; green leafy vegetables such as broccoli, collards, dandelion greens, and kale; legumes, raw nuts; seeds including ground flaxseeds; and oils such as fish oil, salmon, borage oil, primrose oil, sesame oil, and grape seed oil.

Good sources of omega-6 EFAs, which include alpha-linolenic and eicosapentaenoic acid (EPAs), are fresh deepwater fish, fish oil, walnut oil, and flaxseed oil. Essential fatty acids must be refrigerated and never heated in order to retain their beneficial properties. Heating oils to high temperatures changes the chemical bonds and creates dangerous free radicals.

Incorporate Lecithin, Another Good Fat, into Your Diet

Every living cell in the human body needs lecithin in order to be healthy. Lecithin is a type of lipid that is partly soluble in water and acts as an emulsifying agent, enabling cholesterol and other fats to be dispersed in water and carried out of the body. This helps to cleanse fat from the arteries and protect the vital organs from fatty buildup.

The sheath covering the brain, nerve cells, muscles, and cell membranes that are responsible for nutrient absorption are composed of lecithin. Lecithin contains B vitamins, choline, inositol, and linolenic acid. It is found in grains, brewer's yeast, eggs, fish, legumes, and wheat germ. Most lecithin in the market is made from soybeans. James Balch, MD, and Phyllis Balch, CNC, in *Prescription for Nutritional Healing*, explain about lecithin derived from egg yolks:

Recently egg lecithin has become popular. This type of lecithin is extracted from the yolks of fresh eggs. Egg lecithin may hold promise for those suffering from AIDS, herpes, chronic

fatigue syndrome and immune disorders associated with aging. Studies have shown that it works better for people with these disorders than soy lecithin does.

Respect Your Meals

Mealtimes should be pleasant, peaceful times during each day in which we sit down, relax, and enjoy our food. Observe your life. Are you allowing time and space to eat slowly and chew your food well? Or are you rushing through lunch, eating while driving and perhaps talking on a cell phone at the same time? Ask yourself if you are eating consciously, paying attention to the smell, taste, and texture of your food, or do you eat unconsciously without discernment about whether you are truly hungry or not? After you learn to make healthy food choices, it's just as important to learn when and how to eat the foods you have chosen. A bit of common sense can go a long way toward creating a healthy lifestyle. Read the following section and decide if you have healthy or unhealthy habits around eating. Write down the habits you have now and if they are not in alignment with creating good health, then write a new plan for change. Learn to make healthy food choices and also practice Wholesome eating habits. Treat yourself well during meals.

EAT ONLY WHEN YOU'RE HUNGRY, AND STOP WHEN YOU'RE FULL

People eat for various reasons, many of which have little to do with hunger. Some people eat because they are sad, others eat because they are happy. Some people eat to satisfy deep-seated emotional needs. Adults who were rewarded with foods when they were children—often with sweets—may still look for love from these foods.

Nature intended us to feel hunger so we would nourish ourselves and feel satiated so we would stop eating. We need to discern between food hunger and emotional hunger. We also need to learn to stop eating when we feel full. Practice eating in moderation and noticing when you feel comfortably full (not stuffed!). This may take practice if you are used to overeating. The more you eat nutritious foods, the less you will feel the need to overeat. Studies have shown that those who practice eating moderately live longer, healthier lives.

If you eat for emotional reasons, practice bringing more joy into your life by doing the things you love, and you will find yourself to be less hungry.

EAT IN PEACE

When you are hungry and it's time to eat, place your food on your plate. Sit at a table in a relaxed position (not on the couch in front of the TV). Pause before you eat, and place your hands in your lap. Take a few deep breaths in and out through your nose and relax. Your body needs to be in a relaxed mode, governed by the parasympathetic nervous system, while you are eating in order to digest well. The parasympathetic nervous system is responsible for all internal responses including the digestion of food. It functions when we are in a relaxed state. The sympathetic nervous system is associated with fight-or-flight responses and functions during emergency situations. It inhibits digestion and accelerates breathing and heartbeat. Therefore, we don't want to be watching a scary movie while eating because it could actually put us into a sympathetic mode which can stop digestion. So calm yourself before going to the dinner table. Bless your food before you eat in whatever way is comfortable for you, and eat it with an attitude of gratitude. You might light a candle or put a flower in a pretty vase on your table. Eat peacefully with good company or alone. Soft, relaxing music in

Continued ➜

the background can help facilitate proper digestion, or you may choose to eat in silence. Eating in peace can help you get rid of annoying food allergies too. According to Phyllis and James Balch in *Prescription for Nutritional Healing*, "particles of undigested food manage to enter the bloodstream and cause a reaction. Leaky gut syndrome is a term used to describe a condition in which the lining of the intestinal tract becomes perforated and irritated, and tiny particles of partially digested food enter the bloodstream, causing an allergic reaction." And Dr. Jeffrey Bland states in *Optimal Digestion*, "If food is poorly digested, it can produce ammonia, alcohol, and other chemicals in the body as a result of increased putrefaction. . . . The buildup of these toxins in the body can result in general toxicity. . . . Metabolic toxins may account for some cases of food sensitivity." Therefore, being in a relaxed state to allow the body to digest properly is crucial to the prevention of food allergies and poor health.

Food that is eaten in a hurry cannot be digested properly. Eating while you are walking around and talking on the phone severely compromises good digestion. Eating while driving through a fast-food restaurant or talking on a cell phone disturbs digestion. Too often, families watch the news while eating. It is no wonder people are suffering heartburn, gas, and ulcers!

I was very impressed when I was living in a small village in the Swiss Alps where, at noon each day, all the shops and businesses closed and everyone went home for lunch. Even the schoolchildren rode their bicycle home for lunch. Families spent time together between 12:00 and 2:00 each day. Eating food consciously is a step toward living lives consciously and with love.

Chew Your Food Well

Chew, chew, chew your food! Chew each bite of food at least twenty-five times. Digestion begins in the mouth. Food swallowed whole cannot be digested properly in the stomach. When we don't digest our food, we don't receive the vitamins and minerals it has to offer us. Undigested food can ferment and become food for parasites to live on and can create free radicals.

Never Consume Foods or Beverages that Are Too Hot or Too Cold

Ice-cold beverages and food or boiling-hot beverages and food can damage the delicate tissues in the mouth, esophagus, and stomach lining. Ice-cold or boiling-hot beverages taken with a meal can greatly impair digestion by paralyzing enzyme activity in the mouth and stomach. If you are accustomed to drinking really hot or cold beverages, try drinks that are a bit less extreme in temperature. Over time, you will prefer them and feel much better for drinking them!

Eat Your Evening Meal before 7:00 p.m.

It is important to eat your last meal of the day before 7:00 p.m. so your food will be fairly well digested when you go to bed. If you eat a heavy meal and then go to bed, your body will be digesting rather than relaxing. You may fall into a restless sleep, have bad dreams, and feel tired the next day. Quite often, people who eat late wake up between 1:00 and 3:00 a.m. because this is when the liver starts to cleanse. Eating late places a heavy burden on the liver, causing it to have to work harder. If you are hungry before going to bed, have a glass of raw vegetable juice, such as celery, parsley, cucumber, or carrot. The juice will help hold your blood sugar steady through the night and let you sleep.

Eating in Restaurants

Going out to eat can be relaxing and enjoyable. It allows you to spend time with friends and loved ones and have a night off from cooking. Others will serve you and wash the dishes afterward. However, many Americans have started eating out for breakfast, lunch, and dinner. This might be okay if they were eating at places that used organic foods and healthy recipes. But most of the time, this is not the case. People are eating in fast-food restaurants where food is prepared in deep grease that is saved and used again and again for days. Lots of white flour, white sugar, pasteurized milk, salt, and processed foods are used. I once saw a vial of blood that had been taken from a man who had just consumed a cheeseburger on a white-flour bun, french fries, and a milkshake. The vial was half full of creamy, thick fat thanks to that one meal! Fat clogs our arteries and veins, which causes our hearts to have to pump harder. This results in an enlarged heart, which is a tired heart and one that is much more likely to suffer a heart attack. Americans are among the most obese people in the world because of the types of foods they are eating coupled with a lack of exercise.

When you go out to eat, choose a restaurant that has a clean kitchen and prepares foods from scratch rather than using canned and packaged goods. Choose places that will cater to the customer and prepare foods with less salt and fat. Order seafood or chicken, and add salads made with Romaine lettuce, green or red leaf lettuce or butter lettuce (you may have to make a special request for these, but it's worth it because they are more nutritious and contain more chlorophyll than iceberg lettuce), vegetables, baked potatoes, or brown rice. Try to avoid fried foods and foods with heavy sauces and creams. If you are normally healthy and want to have a dessert once in awhile, do so and enjoy it. Just don't make desserts and sweets a daily habit. Eat your meal in peace and joy. This can be more healing than eating a healthy meal in anger or sadness.

Tool Kit for Creating Healthy Meal Plans

Make a list of the foods you are accustomed to eating on the following meal plan work sheet. Then look at each food and, following the guide presented in the preceding tool kit on foods to avoid and foods to replace them with, create a new healthy meal plan work sheet with foods you will enjoy. I have provided an example for you of how to change average American meals into healthy ones, followed by more great ideas for delicious, healthy meal plans.

Current Meal Plan Work Sheet

List what you eat now. You may want to keep a journal for a week.

Breakfast:

Snack:

Lunch:

Snack:

Dinner:

Do you snack in the evening? If so, what do you eat? Write it down. A lot of people are in the habit of eating at night and then skipping breakfast, even lunch. This is a sure way to gain weight! If you go to sleep with a heavy meal in your stomach, it will most certainly turn to body fat. Start eating breakfast, and you will not be as hungry at night.

Healthy Meal Plan Work Sheet

List healthy replacements for what you normally eat:

Breakfast:

Snack:

Lunch:

Snack:

Dinner:

Sample Meal Plans Based on the Average American Diet

Breakfast

Average: Coffee and a bagel with margarine and jelly

Replace with: Herbal coffee such as Teecino, which can be purchased in all health food stores, seven-grain sprouted bagel with organic butter and jelly sweetened with fruit juice

Average: Orange juice, toast made of white-flour bread, and instant oatmeal with one or two teaspoons of sugar and milk

Replace with: Fresh-squeezed orange juice from organic oranges or apple juice (have this about twenty minutes before meal), seven-grain sprouted toast, and cooked whole rolled oats sweetened with six drops of liquid stevia and rice milk. If you use vanilla rice or almond milk, you may not need the stevia

Average: Coffee and sugar-coated dry cereal with milk

Replace with: Herbal coffee and millet or rice flakes sweetened with six drops of stevia and vanilla rice milk

Average: Black tea with sugar, white-flour toast with margarine and jelly. scrambled eggs, and bacon or sausage

Replace with: Herbal tea of your choice, seven-grain sprouted toast with butter, fruit-sweetened jelly, poached eggs or soft boiled eggs and turkey bacon or turkey sausage

Midmorning Snack

Average: Coffee and a doughnut

Replace with: Herbal coffee and two cookies made of rice flour—such as buttered pecan, carob hazelnut, or macaroons—or a slice of raisin pecan bread made from rice and millet flour, toasted, with a little organic butter

Lunch

Average: Iced tea, french fries, and a hamburger or sandwich

Replace with: Cold herbal tea (no ice); baked "fries" (see the recipe later in this chapter); and a veggie burger, turkey burger, or organic hamburger, without a roll (or on a seven-grain sprouted roll), with healthy* mayonnaise, natural catsup, and mustard from your health food store, and with raw vegetables such as romaine lettuce, carrots, or celery

Average: Iced tea and a chicken sandwich on white-flour bread

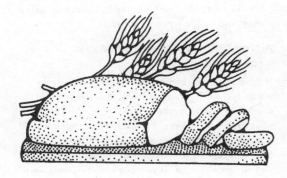

Continued ➡

Replace with: Cold herbal tea (no ice) and a sandwich made of chicken or turkey prepared from hormone-free fowl served on seven-grain sprouted bread with healthy* mayonnaise and/or mustard, and with raw vegetables such as romaine lettuce, butter lettuce, sliced tomatoes, carrots, celery, and coleslaw

Average: Iced tea and a hot dog

Replace with: Cold herbal tea (no ice) and a veggie, turkey, or chicken hot-dog with no bread (or on a seven-grain sprouted roll), with healthy* mayonnaise, mustard and catsup, and with raw vegetables such as carrot sticks or celery sticks

*Note on mayonnaise: It should be made without sugar, corn syrup, artifical preservatives, or canola oil.

Afternoon Snack

Average: Soft drink and a pack of peanuts or peanut butter and crackers

Replace with: Sparkling mineral water with lemon and stevia and rye crackers with organic almond, walnut, pecan or peanut butter

Dinner

Average: Spaghetti with white cream mushroom sauce and a salad made with iceberg lettuce and dressing

Replace with: Rice spaghetti or spaghetti squash with marinara sauce (vegetarian, made with grated zucchini, mushrooms, bell peppers, onions, and fresh basil or made with a little ground turkey or a little ground organic red meat); salad made from romaine lettuce and other raw vegetables such as grated carrots, jicama, and red bell pepper; dressing of olive oil and lemon juice or olive oil and raw organic apple cider vinegar with herbs such as basil, garlic, and thyme

Average: Pork chops, macaroni and cheese, and canned spinach

Replace with: Veggie burgers, lamb chops, or beef tenderloin; quinoa or rice macaroni with just a little raw organic grated cheese or almond cheese; steamed broccoli; and spinach salad with spinach, tomato, cucumber, and mushrooms, with olive oil and lemon juice or raw organic apple cider vinegar dressing

Average: Pork sausage, potato salad, and canned string beans

Replace with: Turkey sausage or grain sausage; potatoes dressed with healthy mayonnaise, mustard, and pickles; steamed string beans; and carrot sticks or celery sticks

Average: Fried chicken, mashed potatoes made from potato buds, and frozen broccoli

Replace with: Chicken tossed in cornmeal with herbs such as basil, sage, thyme, and paprika; baked tempeh seasoned with liquid aminos, basil, thyme, and sage; baked, mashed potatoes made from organic freshly steamed potatoes; fresh broccoli, steamed; followed an hour later by apple pie made with spelt flour and sweetened with apple juice and organic ice cream; or, better, a cored apple baked with cinnamon, nutmeg, walnuts, and maple syrup or stevia

A NOTE ON CANNED AND FROZEN VEGETABLES

It is best to use organic fresh foods, but in areas where it is difficult to get these, you might try canned or frozen organic fruits or vegetables in your health food store. Foods that have been picked at the height of ripeness and quickly frozen or canned properly will retain lots of nutrients necessary for good health. If you buy canned foods, look for cans that have an inner protective coating that protects the foods from the aluminum in the can. Read labels on both canned and frozen foods and make sure they are not filled with dyes, preservatives, sugar, high fructose corn syrup and salt. If you can foods yourself, make sure you put them in sterile glass jars with a tight seal to prevent spoilage. Also can with as little cooking time as possible and without salt and sugar. For excellent information on proper freezing and canning techniques, have a look at the Food pages linked from the Ohio State University Web site, www.ohioline.osu.edu. Here you'll find freezing and canning fact sheets prepared by OSU's Human Nutrition Department.

More Healthy Meal Plans

Breakfast

Natural rice, millet, quinoa. amaranth, buckwheat, or oat cereal sweetened with rice or almond milk and topped with half a banana or a quarter cup of blueberries or a few raisins you poured boiling water over. Cereal can be crispy from the health store or cooked whole. Whole cereal that has been cooked on low heat in a Crock-Pot overnight or soaked overnight and then cooked is much better for you than processed crispy cereals out of the package. If you have any problems with gas, do not combine fruit with grains. Eat your fruit first, then have the cereal fifteen minutes to a half hour later.

Cereal, as above, topped with one to two tablespoons of a mixture of ground almonds, flaxseeds, pumpkin seeds, and sunflower seeds

Fruit salad made with noncitrus fruits, such as apple, banana, blueberries, mango, papaya, peaches, pears, or pineapple, topped with almond cream and a ground nut or seed mixture

One fruit followed by one or two poached, soft-boiled, or over-easy eggs with seven-grain sprouted toast or rye toast (may have grits, millet, or quinoa instead of toast with a half teaspoon organic unsalted butter or ghee).

One fruit followed by one or two poached, soft-boiled, or over-easy eggs with grits, millet, or quinoa with a half teaspoon organic unsalted butter

Avocado Pudding (see page 350). This recipe tastes like vanilla or coconut cream and will not cause blood sugar imbalance.

Cornmeal pancakes, blue cornmeal pancakes, buckwheat pancakes, or whole-grain pancakes with blueberries, strawberries, or applesauce, a little butter or ghee, and a little pure, Grade B maple syrup. Wheat-free waffles are available in your health food store. If you have trouble with digestion, eat the fruit separately.

French toast made with organic eggs mixed with rice milk, cinnamon, and vanilla. Soak the sprouted bread in the egg mixture and cook in a little Olive, grapeseed, or coconut oil on top of the stove until golden on each side. Serve with almond cream and pure, Grade B maple syrup, ghee, or organic butter.

Lunch

Rainbow salad made with romaine, endive, red and/or green leaf lettuces and lots of colorful vegetables. Add a natural dressing. Use lemon juice or apple cider vinegar and olive oil as a dressing or use a sesame and sunflower seed dressing. Top with soaked sunflower seeds (soaking the nuts and seeds removes half the fat).

Turkey, chicken, or tuna sandwich on rye bread, with healthy mayonnaise, lettuce, tomato, and buckwheat sprouts. Serve with carrots and celery.

Two rice cakes slightly toasted. Top with raw sesame butter, a slice of tomato, and lettuce. Serve with raw vegetables.

Tuna salad on lettuce with raw vegetables

Vegetable soup and raw vegetables and rice or rye crackers or cornbread

Egg salad on lettuce with raw vegetables

Tabouleh salad made with quinoa or millet rather than cracked wheat

Cold "soup" made with blended romaine lettuce, avocado, cucumber, sprouts, tomato, carrots, garlic, and water. Season with vegetable seasoning, basil, and thyme. Serve in a bowl with pine nuts on top.

Dr. Bieler's potassium soup. (See the recipe later in this chapter.)

Dinner

Salad and stir-fry vegetables over brown rice or quinoa

Salad, baked potato, and broccoli

Steamed vegetable plate with beans and cornbread

Corn tacos with beans, ground turkey, or lean ground beef filling mixed with natural taco seasoning, chopped lettuce, tomatoes, onions, and celery

Baked or broiled chicken and string beans with salad

Broiled salmon patties, slaw, steamed vegetable, and cornbread

Spaghetti squash with vegetarian marinara sauce and salad

Steamed vegetable plate with string beans, beets, potatoes, black-eyed peas, and grated carrot salad. Top with ground sunflower, sesame and flaxseeds and a little olive oil.

Salad or coleslaw; baked or broiled organic fish, chicken, turkey, or lean organic red meat; and vegetables (steamed or baked)

Baked eggplant or zucchini "pizzas" topped with marinara vegetable sauce and a small amount of grated organic cheese or almond cheese

Salad, steamed vegetables, and veggie or ground turkey burgers

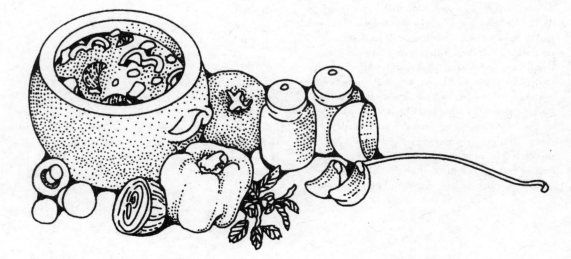

Vegetable or split pea soup and salad

Salad and stir-fry vegetables over brown rice or quinoa

Salad and rice or amaranth pasta with marinara sauce

A Note on Drinks

It is better to drink before or after your meal than with it. If you feel like drinking a beverage with your meal, take small sips of a beverage that is not too hot or too cold. When you first get up in the morning, drink hot water with fresh squeezed lemon, an herbal coffee substitute—such as Teecino—green tea, or other herbal teas such as peppermint, apple/cinnamon, or oat-straw tea.

Tool Kit for Choosing Healthy Snacks

Choose foods for snacks from a wide variety of pure, whole, and natural foods. If you eat snacks that are high in sugar and caffeine, such as a soft drink and chocolate bar, you may feel satisfied and energetic for a short time, but it won't be long before your blood sugar levels will crash and you will be hungrier than ever. Whole foods, as nature provides them for us, will balance your blood sugar and keep up your energy levels for hours. A healthy snack can improve your metabolism, keep your weight balanced, and help you think more clearly. Some snack suggestions follow.

Daytime Snacks

Snacks should be eaten between meals when you are hungry. If you are only slightly hungry, you may still have a small snack; this will keep your blood sugar balanced and even keep you from overeating when mealtime comes. Then, when mealtime comes, you won't feel so starved that you need to overeat.

Raw vegetables and hummus

Celery stuffed with raw nut butter, such as almond or sesame butter

One or two rice cakes, slightly toasted and spread with almond or sesame butter

Toasted sprouted bread with organic goat, cow, or almond cheese

Raw vegetables with feta cheese, goat or cow cheese, sesame sauce, or sesame butter (see the recipe for sesame sauce later in this chapter) Raw organic cottage cheese with carrots

One apple with twelve soaked almonds (soaked almonds are sprouted inside and will combine with fruit fairly well)

One-half papaya with a scoop of almond cream in the center (see the recipe for almond cream later in this chapter)

Sesame sauce dip with raw vegetables

A piece of fruit (if you do not have any problems with blood sugar)

Two-thirds cup of vegetable soup

One cup of organic yogurt

One glass of kefir (a beverage made of fermented cow's milk)

One-third cup of almond cream

Evening Snacks

If you are hungry in the evenings, have a light snack. You should never eat a lot of heavy food and then go to bed. The food won't digest properly, will probably keep you awake, and will likely turn to fat. The best food to have in the evening is a glass of raw vegetable juice. Here are some other choices:

Rice pudding

Glass of rice milk or almond milk

4 to 6 ounces goat's milk yogurt (organic)

4 to 6 ounces cow's milk yogurt (organic), if you are not allergic to it

One papaya or banana

One-half cup almond cream

8 ounces raw vegetable juice

Make Wise Food Choices

Many people are not aware that there is a connection between their health and the choices they make about eating. When we understand that some foods are life-giving and healing while others are actually harmful to our health, we can make more conscious choices about what we put into our mouths. The following list of foods are those used often and those most important to one's health. They are arranged starting with alkaline foods, including fruits and vegetables that we should eat often, and progress into more dense acidic foods such as bean, grains, and nuts, which we should eat less of.

Fruits

Eat one to three fruits per day, preferably not with other foods. When you are craving sweets, choose dates or figs stuffed with nuts, frozen banana ice cream (see the recipe later in this chapter), or other dessert choices in this book; when eating fruit as a dessert, have it at least a half hour after the meal.

Vegetables

Eat six different kinds of vegetables daily, raw, baked or steamed.

Potatoes

Potatoes can be eaten one to two times per week. Potatoes are best eaten baked or steamed with their skins on since most of the nutrients, especially potassium, is located there. Never boil or fry potatoes; these cooking methods destroy the nutrients. Cut out any eyes on the potatoes since they are toxic.

Beans

Lentils are probably the easiest bean to digest, but other beans are also good for you. Soak them overnight and then cook them. Eat beans several times per week with vegetables and salad. Beans are difficult for some people to digest. If this is the case for you, try the smaller beans such as adzuki, black, or navy beans.

Nuts

Nut butters and almonds are the best nut choices. However, walnuts, pecans, and Brazil nuts are also high in nutrients and good for us. Eat nuts in small portions, as they are high in fats. Soak almonds overnight. This starts the sprouting action inside the nut and reduces the fat content by half. Soaked almonds are delicious light snacks and much easier to digest than almonds that have not been soaked. Nuts are high in calcium, magnesium, and manganese.

Seeds

Seed butters, sesame seeds, and sunflower seeds or butter are best. Pumpkin seeds are also very nutritious because they are high in zinc and build the male and female reproductive systems. They kill parasites, which we should always watch out for. Grinding seeds in a coffee or spice grinder ensures better digestion. Soaked seeds are also very good for you and are easier to digest and absorb than seeds that have not been soaked. They contain half the fat content of unsoaked seeds. See recipes for seed sauce, salad dressings, and dips later in this chapter.

Breakfast Cereals

Cooked cereals are best or cereals prepared with the thermos method. Amaranth, buckwheat, cornmeal mush, millet, quinoa, and whole rolled oats are all good choices. You may eat packaged cereals at times but make sure they are wheat free and sugar free. Also check that they are free from additives and preservatives and are low in salt.

Whole Grains

Whole grains may be used in soups, breads, and pancakes. Consider amaranth, barley, basmati rice, brown rice, buckwheat, millet, quinoa, rye, wild rice, or yellow cornmeal.

Bread and Crackers

Have one to two servings of bread or crackers per day. You can make your own bread with any of the whole grains listed above. Eat wheat-free crackers such as rice crackers or rice cakes.

Wheat has been overused in our country to the point that most people have allergies to it. Wheat is high in gluten, which makes it very gluey and hard to digest. It can cause sinus congestion, lung congestion, and constipation.

Buy the following types of bread: eleven-grain sprouted, kamut, pumpernickel rye, rice, rye, seven-grain sprouted, or spelt. Be sure to toast all bread; toasted bread is less gluey and easier to digest. If you are sensitive to gluten, stick to rice, millet, buckwheat, and corn breads. Buckwheat is actually a flower and not a grain.

Milk and Milk Substitutes

Cow's milk is very difficult for some people to digest. Clean, certified, raw cow's milk is better for us because it is high in enzymes and friendly bacteria that make it more digestible. Many people have allergies to cow's milk that cause sinus congestion and/or gas and bloating. Some people fear that if they don't drink milk, they will not get enough calcium, but there are many other sources of calcium. A glass of raw carrot or green juice made with beet

Continued ➡

tops, parsley, and kale contains the same amount of calcium as a glass of cow's milk, and it is easier to digest and absorb. Almonds, sesame seeds, and green leafy vegetables are also wonderful sources of calcium. The following are great substitutes for cow's milk: almond milk, oat milk, raw organic goat's milk, rice milk (try vanilla), and rice milk ice cream. Have one to three servings of nut, oat, rice, or goat's milk daily.

EGGS

Choose fertilized eggs from free-range hens. Most eggs come from chickens that live in cages their entire lives and never see the sun. They are fed chemical foods. Their egg yolks will be very pale yellow and taste very bland compared to the rich yellow yolks of healthy range-fed chickens that live outside in the fresh air and sunshine, eating bugs and grass. I recommend eating only range-fed eggs, which are fertilized. Fertilization makes the eggs more nutritious and better tasting. Eggs fertilized by a rooster have lecithin, which naturally lowers cholesterol. Shelton Farms and Alta Dena are two companies that carry fertilized eggs from healthy chickens grown outdoors. The color of an egg's shell does not make a difference in how healthy the egg is for you. The color is determined by the type of chicken that lays the egg.

A recent egg scare made people afraid to eat eggs for fear they would increase their cholesterol, but this has now been proved to be untrue. Also, real eggs provide much more nutritional value than egg substitutes. An egg contains all the amino acids necessary for human life. Soft-boiled eggs ate best for you because the lecithin is still intact; cooking eggs at high temperatures for a long period of time destroys the lecithin. Lecithin helps to lower elevated cholesterol. And if you eat eggs from healthy chickens and gently wash the shells with soap and warm water right before use, you won't have to worry about salmonella.

MEAT

If you are not vegetarian, you should only eat organic meat such as veal, lamb, beef, or venison once or twice a week; chicken, turkey, or duck two to three times a week; and fish two to three times a week. These must be baked or broiled, never fried, and eaten in small amounts. Remember, you need protein every day, but you do not need animal protein every day. Avoid pork sausage and bacon which are very high in saturated fat.

BUTTER

A little butter is okay to eat. Butter is preferable to margarine that contains hydrogenated oils. Butter is also high in vitamins A and D, which are beneficial to the eyes, immune system, and nervous system. Butter should be organic and unsalted. Use small amounts for cooking and on foods.

GHEE

Ghee is clarified butter and is easier to digest than tegular butter. Look for ghee in the refrigerated section of your health food store.

OLIVE OIL

This is one of the few oils, in addition to grape seed and coconut oil, to be used in cooking (it is safe at high temperatures). It also can be used on salads. Olive oil helps to balance the body's pH, neutralizes acids, helps to cleanse the liver, and may dissolve gallstones and kidney stones. Combine olive oil and lemon juice to make a great salad dressing.

A NOTE ABOUT ACID/ALKALINE BALANCE IN OUR DAILY FOODS

Eighty percent of our daily food intake should be alkaline and 20 percent acidic. It's easy to reach these percentages if we remember to eat six vegetables and two fruits per day to provide the 80 percent alkaline foods that we need. By eating two different fruits per day and six different vegetables per day, we will get a variety of vitamins, minerals, and phytonutrients so important to our health. The rest of the foods below are more acid forming in the body, except for almonds which are more alkaline forming. Soaked nuts of any kind become alkaline and can be included as part of the 80 percent alkaline foods per day. It doesn't work out exactly to eat just one grain and one protein, for the 20 percent, but remember that we should only eat 20 percent acid-forming foods per day. So one might have two small servings of grains (one-fourth to one-third cup each), one small serving of beans (one-fourth to one-third cup), and one to two servings of fish or chicken in a day. One should only have one to two servings of red meat per week. If you are vegetarian, use fish, eggs, cheese, beans, nuts, and seeds for proteins. Soaked, blended nuts and seeds are excellent proteins and very easy to absorb.

Tool Kit for Preparing Healthy Recipes

Many people believe that eating healthfully means eating foods that taste bad. I have taught many classes in nutrition and showed people how to prepare nutritious foods in very delicious ways. The following recipes are both healthy and tasty. Enjoy!

* Denotes recipes by Kelly Worrall.

Drinks

ALMOND CREAM

1 cup almonds, raw

vanilla or stevia to taste

dates, soaked (optional)

1½ cups purified water

Soak one cup of raw almonds in purified water for twenty-four hours. Remove the almonds, and give the water to your plants or discard it. Place the almonds in boiling water for thirty seconds to loosen the peelings. Remove the peelings. Place the almonds in a blender. Cover them with one and a half cups of purified water, and blend until thick and creamy. Add vanilla, stevia, or soaked dates with soak water (adjust with water in the recipe) to taste. This nut cream can be combined with fruit because the nuts have been soaked. Serve over berries, mango, papaya, or peaches. Enjoy! Yields three cups.

ALMOND MILK

1 cup almonds, raw

3 cups purified water

Make almond milk the same way almond cream is made, only with more water to make it thinner. If you are making this drink for young children, strain it well through cheesecloth. It's very high in calcium, magnesium, and other minerals, which is great for building bones and teeth. Yields one quart.

FLAXSEED TEA

4 teaspoons flaxseeds

Bring one quart of water to a rolling boil. Add four teaspoons of flaxseeds. Turn the burner off, and let the mixture sit overnight. Strain the tea before using it. Yields four cups of brewed tea.

HOLIDAY ALMOND NOG

1 cup almonds, raw

8 dates, soaked, and date water

cinnamon, to taste

vanilla, to taste

nutmeg, to taste

Instead of eggnog, try almond nog! Prepare as almond milk, with soaked dates and date water, then add cinnamon, vanilla, and nutmeg. Delicious! Yields about one quart.

MINERAL WHEY DRINK

1 teaspoon mineral whey (goat milk whey)

1 teaspoon lecithin granules

1 teaspoon vegetable seasoning

Place all the ingredients in a large cup, and add one cup of hot but not boiling water. Let the mixture steep for five minutes and then drink. Yields one cup.

Mineral or goat milk whey is high in minerals and natural sodium, which help hold calcium in the bones and dissolve spurs and stones. The whey is the liquid part of the milk that separates from the solids when making goat cheese. It is very similar in consistency to our own clear lymph fluid that lines our eyes, sinuses, lungs, stomach, and joints. Lecithin helps keep arteries clean and lowers cholesterol. Lecithin also feeds the brain and nervous system. Vegetable seasonings may contain a variety of nourishing dried vegetables, including alfalfa, carrots, celery, parsley, pimento, spinach, or watercress; Bernard Jensen's Vegetable Seasoning has a wonderful consistency and flavor.

AVOCADO PUDDING

1 cup almond milk

½ cucumber

½ avocado

2 tablespoons soaked, peeled almonds

1 teaspoon vanilla or juice of ½ fresh lemon or 1 tablespoon shredded unsweetened coconut flakes

4 to 6 drops stevia

Blend all ingredients together. Yields about twelve ounces.

This shake is delicious and completely sugar free. I recommend it for diabetics, hypoglycemics, or people with Candida. It's great for everyone!

Grains

MILLET BREAKFAST CEREAL

½ cup organic millet, uncooked

1 cup distilled water

1 additional cup distilled water to soak millet

Soak the millet in one cup of distilled water overnight to soften the grains. Place the soaked millet in a saucepan with the water from soaking and one additional cup of distilled water. Bring the cereal to a boil, reduce the heat, and simmer for twenty to thirty minutes, stirring occasionally, until the cereal has thickened. Serve the hot cereal with almond cream if desired. Makes two six-ounce portions of cooked cereal.

Continued ➡

Soups

Soups provide a delicious soothing meal that's easy to digest and warming during cold months. Soups can be made ahead of time and frozen in strong rigid plastic containers or special jars made for freezing and canning. When ready to prepare, let soup thaw for about four hours, warm it up on the stove, and your meal is ready. Enjoy soups!

Vegetable Cleansing Solution

2 tablespoons raw apple cider vinegar

1 quart of water

To prepare vegetables for any recipe, combine them with the vinegar and water and soak for five minutes. This recipe can be multiplied as necessary for larger quantities of vegetables. This solution helps wash any harmful bacteria and chemical sprays from the vegetables without changing their flavor.

Dr. Bieler's Potassium Soup

⅓ cup chopped string beans

½ cup chopped celery

⅓ cup chopped zucchini

1 to 2 teaspoons chopped parsley

1 teaspoon vegetable seasoning (optional)

1 teaspoon liquid aminos (optional)

basil (optional)

garlic (optional)

onion (optional)

thyme (optional)

virgin olive oil (optional)

organic butter or ghee (optional)

In a steamer, steam the string beans for five minutes. Add the celery and steam for five more minutes. Then add the zucchini. Put the mixture in a blender with two cups of the water that the vegetables steamed over, and add the parsley. You may also add one teaspoon of broth powder or one teaspoon of liquid aminos and/or basil, garlic, onion, and thyme, to taste. Blend everything together, and serve the soup warm. Some natural virgin olive oil, organic butter, or ghee may be added after blending. Yields three cups.

Raw Vegetable Juice Soup

2 large carrots, cleaned and sliced

1 small beet, cleaned and sliced

3 stalks celery, cleaned and sliced

1 bunch parsley

1 small cucumber, sliced

1 tomato, quartered

1 tablespoon pumpkin seeds, soaked

1 tablespoon sunflower seeds, soaked

Juice all the vegetables, and pour them into a bowl. Sprinkle soaked pumpkin and sunflower seeds on top. Eat the soup slowly, and chew the seeds well; even though they've been soaked, they are still crunchy and should be chewed well for optimum digestion and absorption.

Other great toppings for raw vegetable juice soup are sesame and sunflower seed sauce (see the recipe under "Dressings and Sauces"). Put a dollop of each on top. So delicious and good for you too!

Raw vegetable juice soup is great for anyone, but it is particularly good for people with chronic illness or digestive disorders. The juice is loaded with nutrients, and the seed sauce is high in minerals and protein. Both are high in enzymes. The juice and seed sauces are easy to digest and absorb. Enjoy! Yields about one cup.

Lentil Soup

2 teaspoons olive oil

1 leek, chopped

2 cloves garlic, minced

7 cups water

3 tablespoons vegetable seasoning

2 large stalks celery, thinly sliced

1 cup sweet potato, cubed

1 cup carrots, diced

1 cup green lentils, rinsed

1 teaspoon dried thyme

1 teaspoon dried basil

1 large bay leaf

Warm the oil in a large saucepan or Dutch oven over medium heat. Add the leek, garlic, and three tablespoons of the water. Cook, stirring over medium heat for five minutes or until the leek and garlic are tender. (If necessary, add more water.)

Add the vegetable seasoning. Add the vegetables, lentils, thyme, basil, bay leaf, and remaining water. Bring everything to a boil, then reduce the heat. Cover and simmer for twenty minutes or until the lentils are tender. This is a delicious soup for lunch or dinner. Serve it with cornbread or rice crackers. Makes six servings.

Split Pea Soup (Vegetarian)

2 quarts water

2 cups green split peas

2 large carrots, scrubbed and chopped 6 stalks celery, chopped

1 large yellow onion, chopped

3 large potatoes, chopped

4 tablespoons vegetable seasoning

1 tablespoon olive oil

fresh parsley, chopped, for garnish

Place the water in a large pot, add the peas, and bring it to a boil. Reduce the heat, cover, and simmer for one-half hour. Add the carrots, celery, onion, potatoes, and vegetable seasoning. Simmer for an hour. Stir in the olive oil. Garnish with parsley. Yields about two and a half quarts.

Split Pea Soup

2 quarts water

4 small soup bones with a bit of lean beef on them

2 cups green split peas

2 large carrots, scrubbed and chopped 6 stalks celery, chopped

1 large onion, chopped (optional)

3 large potatoes, chopped

½ to 1 teaspoon unrefined sea salt

Place the water in a large pot and add the soup bones. Bring the contents to a boil. Reduce the heat and simmer for forty minutes. Add the peas and simmer for one-half hour. Add the vegetables and simmer for one hour. Add sea salt to taste and serve. Yields about two and a half quarts.

Potato Peelings Broth

2 cups scrubbed raw potato peelings, chopped (inner potato discarded)

2 cups celery and tops, chopped

2 cups carrots and tops, chopped

1 yellow onion, chopped

2 quarts water

Place the chopped vegetables and the water in a large stainless-steel pot. Bring the contents to a boil. As soon as the water boils, reduce the heat, and simmer the contents for one hour. Strain the mixture, and drink one to two cups per day. Yields about three quarts.

This broth is high in potassium, which helps relieve muscle cramps and restore calcium balance in the bones. This broth is wonderful for anyone with arthritis, muscular pain, or stress.

Hearty Vegetable Soup

2 quarts tomato juice

½ cup baby butter beans

½ cup yellow corn

½ cup string beans, broken

½ cup okra, chopped

1 cup broccoli, chopped

¼ cup yellow onion, chopped

½ cup ground lean beef or turkey (optional)

2 teaspoons dried basil

1 teaspoon dried thyme

½ cup kidney beans, cooked

½ cup barley, cooked

1 teaspoon sea salt

1 tablespoon olive oil

Put all the ingredients in a large pot except the cooked kidney beans, cooked barley, sea salt, and olive oil. Bring the mixture to a boil. Reduce the heat to simmer. Simmer the mixture for one hour, then add the cooked kidney beans and barley. Simmer for twenty minutes. Add the sea salt and olive oil. Stir and serve. Yields about three quarts.

Okra is mucilaginous and very soothing to the entire digestive tract. It's a wonderful food for people with colitis or ulcers. If you have ulcers or colitis, do not add meat to the soup.

Butternut Squash Soup

1 cup onion, finely chopped

1 tablespoon garlic, minced

1 tablespoon coconut, olive, or grape seed oil

4 cups butternut squash, cubed

4 cups vegetable broth

2 cups small white beans, cooked

5 tablespoons red bell pepper, chopped

unrefined sea salt, to taste (optional)

cayenne pepper, to taste (optional)

Sauté the onion and garlic in one tablespoon of oil. Add the squash and chicken or vegetable broth. Bring the mixture to a boil. Reduce the heat. Simmer the squash and onion mixture for one hour. Place the mixture in a blender; blend to a thick puree. Place the pureed mixture back in the pan. Add the small white beans and red pepper. Cook everything over low heat for another twenty to thirty minutes. When it is done, add a pinch of sea salt and a little cayenne pepper if desired. Yields about two and a half quarts.

Veggies

Baked Fries

2 baking potatoes, sliced very thin or cut in oblong shapes

olive oil or butter

seasoning mix

Slice two baking potatoes very thin or cut them into oblong shapes to look like french fries. Lay the pieces on a cookie sheet that has been greased with olive oil, ghee, or butter. Bake the "fries" at 450°F for one-half hour. Sprinkle them with seasoning mix. Bake them for fifteen more minutes or until crisp. Yields about two and a half cups.

Continued ➡

Baked Fries Seasoning Mix

⅓ stick of butter, or 2 tablespoons ghee

⅛ teaspoon sea salt

⅓ teaspoon thyme

1 teaspoon basil

Place the butter or ghee in a saucepan and melt it. Add the sea salt, thyme, and basil. Stir the mixture. Spread the seasoning mix over baked fries.

Borscht*

4 large golden beets, quartered

1 tablespoon olive oil

1 cup leeks, diced

¼ teaspoon caraway seed

¼ cup celery, chopped

½ cup carrot, chopped

½ cup tomato, chopped

2 cups green cabbage, chopped

4 cups vegetable stock

1 cup russet potato, mashed

½ teaspoon dried dill

2 teaspoons lemon juice

⅛ teaspoon cayenne pepper

2 tablespoons fresh parsley, chopped

sea salt, to taste

Heat the oven to 400°F. Place all the ingredients in an oiled, covered casserole dish. Bake for one hour. You may add unrefined sea salt to taste when the borscht is done. Makes six cups.

Onion Gravy*

½ cup onion, chopped

2 teaspoons ghee

⅛ teaspoon dried thyme

1 teaspoon fresh garlic, minced

2 tablespoons liquid aminos

1 cup flaxseed tea, vegetable broth, or water

1 teaspoon arrowroot powder

Sauté the onion in the ghee until translucent, about five minutes. Add the thyme and garlic, and let cook for another minute to release the flavors. Add the liquid aminos and flaxseed tea (or stock or water), and bring to a simmer. Make a slurry with the arrowroot powder and one tablespoon of cold water. Add the slurry to the onions in the pan. Cook the mixture until the arrowroot clears, adding additional tea, stock, or water as necessary to achieve the desired consistency. Serve with mashed potatoes. Makes one cup. Gravy should be creamy.

Tabouleh Salad

2 cups millet or quinoa, cooked

2 ripe tomatoes, chopped

1 large cucumber, chopped

1 small leek, chopped

1 red bell pepper, chopped

3 tablespoons lemon juice

1 tablespoon olive oil

1 clove garlic, minced

⅓ teaspoon sea salt

¼ cup fresh mint, chopped

⅓ cup fresh parsley, chopped

8 leaves of romaine or butter lettuce

sprig of mint

Place the millet in a large bowl. Add the tomatoes, cucumbers, leeks, and bell pepper. Toss them together. In a small bowl, whisk together the lemon juice, olive oil, garlic, and sea salt. Stir in the mint

and parsley. Pour over the millet mixture. With a fork, gently stir all the ingredients together Cover the salad, and let it stand at room temperature for half an hour to bring out the flavors. Serve on a bed of fresh romaine or butter lettuce with a sprig of mint on top. Yields about three cups.

Tabouleh is a Middle Eastern grain salad that can be made with bulghur (cracked wheat), millet, or quinoa. If you are allergic to gluten, try tabouleh made with millet or quinoa. These are delicious grains, high in protein. Tabouleh is a great salad for lunch and wonderful to take on a picnic. Enjoy!

Hummus

2 cups chickpeas (garbanzo beans)

5 cups water, distilled

2 cups raw sesame butter

2 tablespoons liquid aminos

3 Cloves garlic, pressed

juice of 2 large lemons

½ cup fresh parsley, finely chopped

Pinch of cayenne or paprika

sprig of parsley

Soak the chickpeas in five cups of distilled water for two hours. Place the chickpeas and water into a stainless steel pot, and bring them to a boil. Reduce the heat, and simmer for two hours. Strain the mixture, and keep one cup of the broth. Place a half cup of the broth, the sesame butter, liquid aminos, garlic, and lemon juice in a blender. Blend the mixture until creamy. Pour it into a bowl and set it aside. Pour the chickpeas and another half cup of the broth into the blender, and blend until smooth. Pour this mixture into the bowl with the sesame mixture. Stir. Add the parsley and a pinch of cayenne or paprika. Stir well, and serve with a sprig of parsley on top. Yields about five cups.

Hummus can be used as a delicious dip for vegetables, a topping for baked potatoes, or a spread for a sandwich. It is easy to digest and high in protein and minerals.

Dressings and Sauces

Sesame Seed or Sunflower Seed Sauce, Dip, or Salad Dressing

½ cup sesame or sunflower seeds

1 cup purified water

basil, to taste (optional)

thyme, to taste (optional)

dill, to taste (optional)

garlic, to taste (optional)

onion, to taste (optional)

Soak the seeds for twenty-four hours in one cup purified water. Discard the water. Rinse the seeds and strain them. Place them in a blender with the second cup of water and blend them. This sauce is great over salads and steamed vegetables. You may add basil, thyme, dill, garlic, or onion and serve it as a dressing or dip. Yields one and a half cups.

This topping is an excellent source of protein, calcium, and magnesium.

Sandwiches

Sandwiches are easy, convenient, and great for picnics. They can be made with all sorts of delicious, healthy ingredients. It is best to use whole-grain bread. If you have allergies to gluten, choose bread made from rice flour or use seven-grain sprouted bread. Sprouted wheat is less "gluey," and easier for the body to tolerate than bread made from wheat flour.

Veggie Sandwiches

2 slices whole-grain or sprouted whole-grain bread

mayonnaise made with cold-pressed oils

butter lettuce, green leaf lettuce, red leaf lettuce, or romaine

buckwheat sprouts

avocado slices

feta cheese, goat cheese, raw cheese, or seed cheese

fresh turkey or chicken slices, optional

Be creative with a variety of fixings to suit your taste. Have fun!

Fish and Poultry

Baked Halibut with Basil*

2 halibut or salmon filets

1 tablespoon lemon juice

1 teaspoon dried ground basil

⅛ teaspoon cayenne pepper

⅓ teaspoon unrefined sea salt

Heat the oven to 350°F. Place the halibut filets in a small baking dish. Pour the lemon juice over the fish. Sprinkle it with basil and cayenne pepper. Bake for about twenty minutes, until the fish is opaque throughout the thickest part. Sprinkle it with sea salt. Makes two servings.

Pan-Fried Fish

4 red snapper or flounder filets

1 cup cornmeal, stone ground

½ teaspoon basil

¼ teaspoon thyme

⅓ teaspoon dill

⅓ teaspoon unrefined sea salt

3 tablespoons olive, grape seed, or coconut oil

Place one cup of stone-ground cornmeal in a plate, and mix in the basil, thyme, dill, and a little sea salt. Roll the fish into the mixture. Put three tablespoons of olive, grape seed, or coconut oil in a stainless steel pan, and heat it on medium high. Add the fish when the oil starts to bubble. Watch the fish carefully and turn it regularly until golden brown. Serve with coleslaw, steamed broccoli, and yellow squash. Serves four.

Baked "Fried" Chicken

1 cup cornmeal, stone ground

⅓ teaspoon basil

¼ teaspoon rosemary

½ teaspoon sage

¼ teaspoon cayenne pepper

pinch of sea salt or vegetable seasoning

4 chicken breasts, thighs, or legs, skinless

1 tablespoon olive oil

Place one cup of stone-ground cornmeal on a plate, and mix in the basil, rosemary, sage, cayenne pepper, and sea salt or Jensen's vegetable seasoning. Roll the chicken into the mixture. Place the coated chicken in a stainless steel or glass dish that has been oiled well with olive oil and bake at 375°F for forty-five minutes or until done. The chicken should be crispy and golden brown.

If you use animal products, make sure they are organic (so they're not full of steroids or hormones). Salmon should be wild and not farm raised.

Continued ➡

Desserts

BANANA ICE CREAM

4 ripe bananas, chopped

1 cup rice milk or almond milk

1 teaspoon vanilla

Freeze the chopped bananas in a plastic bag. Place the bananas in a blender, cover with rice or almond milk, and add the vanilla. Blend the mixture until it is thick and creamy. Makes two and a half cups.

CAROB WALNUT SYRUP

4 to 5 tablespoons water

4 tablespoons maple syrup

½ cup carob powder

⅓ cup walnuts, chopped

Place the water and maple syrup in a pan. Warm them on low. Add the carob powder. Stir the mixture until it's free from lumps and creamy, adding water if needed. Simmer the mixture for three to five minutes. Add the chopped walnuts, and pour the syrup over banana ice cream. Makes one cup.

ALMOND CREAM PIE

1½ cups pecans and almonds, finely chopped

1 teaspoon cinnamon

2 cups almond cream

1 cup kiwis, mangoes, papayas, peaches, raspberries, or strawberries. sliced (noncitrus fruit in season)

⅓ cup dried coconut (optional)

Combine the chopped nuts and cinnamon. Spread them in a glass dish. Pour in half of the almond cream. Cover the mixture with sliced fruit. Top with another layer of almond cream. Decorate the pie with fruit on top. You may sprinkle it with dried coconut too. Enjoy! Serves six to eight.

SESAME COOKIES

1 cup butter, soft, or ⅓ cup olive oil

1 cup oat flour

1 cup rye or spelt flour

1 cup sesame seeds

2 cups dates, chopped

2 cups unsweetened coconut, shredded (may use 1 cup oatmeal instead)

1 cup pecans, chopped

2 cups almonds, chopped

1 egg, beaten, or 2 tablespoons flaxseed tea

¾ cup vanilla rice milk

1 tablespoon vanilla

4 tablespoons maple syrup

Mix together the butter, flour, and sesame seeds. Add the remaining ingredients, and mix to form a stiff dough. Shape the dough into flat circles, and place them onto a greased cookie sheet. Bake at 350°F for twenty to thirty minutes. Makes fifty cookies.

Other Suggestions for Healthy Desserts

Carob brownies

Pumpkin pie made with maple syrup

Apple pie made with spelt flour and sweetened with fruit juice

Pecan pie sweetened with maple syrup

Ice cream made with rice milk

Rice pudding

Cookies made with rice flour and sweetened with fruit juice

Cookies made with oats and rice flour and sweetened with maple syrup

Tapioca pudding made with rice milk

Dates stuffed with almonds or walnuts

Baked apples stuffed with cinnamon, maple syrup or stevia, almonds, walnuts, and pecans

Recipe Books

Here are several recipe books that offer great ideas for creating healthy meals.

A Cookbook for All Seasons, Elson Haas, MD

The Best Vegetarian Recipes, Martha Rose Shulman

Blending Magic, Dr. Bernard Jensen

The Cleanse Cookbook, Christiane Dreher, CCN, CCH

Back to the House of Health, Shelly Redford Young, LMT, and Robert O. Young, PhD

Fresh Vegetable and Fruit Juices, Norman Walker

Gaia's Kitchen, Julia Ponsonby

Gourmet Uncook Book, Elizabeth and Dr. Elton Baker

Intuitive Eating, Humbert "Smokey" Santillo, ND

The Quintessential Recipes for Vibrant Health, F. Naragali

Cooking for Health, Cheryl A. Matschek, PhD

Recipes for Better Health, Nenita Sarmiento and Leonard Mehlmauer

Ten Talents, Frank J. Hurd, DC, MD, and Rosalie Hurd, BS

Vibrant Health from Your Kitchen, Dr. Bernard Jensen

The Good Herb, Judith Benn Hurley

Organic Annie's Green Gourmet Cookbook, Ann Miller-Cohen

Nourishing Traditions, Sally Fallon

Living in the Raw, Rose Lee Calabro

The Raw Gourmet, Nomi Shannon

Summary of Practical Tools to Help You Eat Healthy Foods

You now have practical tools for making healthy food choices, creating healthy meal plans, choosing healthy snacks, and preparing healthy recipes. The following is a summary of these healthy food tools. A good way to use this list is to type it on a separate piece of paper and hang it somewhere in your kitchen. Slowly work toward following each item, on the list. When you have accomplished one of the items and are practicing it on a regular basis, check it off or put a gold star beside it. With each check or gold star you will be closer to practicing good food habits that will keep you nourished, healthy, happy, and wise. Take your time and move at your own pace, but be determined. Building good eating habits is a very important foundation for good health.

- Eat foods that are pure, whole, fresh, and natural.
- Avoid denatured, preserved, and processed foods. Replace them with natural whole foods.
- Cook foods with a minimum of water. Steam your foods or use a Crock-Pot or waterless cookware.
- Never deep-fry foods.
- Bake or broil foods rather than frying them.
- Practice combining foods.
- Choose from a variety of foods each day. Variety is the spice of life and our bodies need a variety of foods to get all the vitamins and minerals they need.
- Add fiber to your nutritional program each day.

- Eat some raw vegetables with your meals.
- Get 80 percent of your food intake from alkaline-forming foods and 20 percent from acid-forming foods.
- Add essential fatty acids to your nutritional program. Avoid hydrogenated oils.
- Avoid sugar, corn syrup, and artificial sweeteners and replace with stevi agave, pure maple syrup, or honey.
- Avoid salt and replace with vegetable seasoning or unrefined sea salt.
- Eat only when you are truly hungry, and stop eating when you are full. Learn to recognize when you are full. This may take practice at first if you are used to overeating. The more you eat nutritious foods, the less you will feel the need to overeat.
- Eat in peace.
- Chew your food well.
- Never consume beverages that are too hot or too cold.
- Eat your evening meal before 7:00 p.m. so you will have a restful sleep.

There are many drinks available on the market today. Many of them are loaded with refined white sugar, caffeine, aspartame, artificial color, preservatives, and chemicals. All of these additives are detrimental to the body. In order to build pure blood, vital organs, healthy muscles, and strong bones, we should enjoy delicious, refreshing drinks that are natural.

Tool Kit for Choosing Healthy Popular Beverages

Sodas, slushies, milkshakes, frappuccinos, cappuccinos, coffee, tea, beer, wine, lemonade, water—beverages are available everywhere, so which ones should we choose? In order to be healthy, we should make wise choices about the liquids we consume. Remember, we are organic creatures made from the natural elements of the earth. When we consume unnatural, synthetic substances in either our foods or our beverages, our bodies will rebel—sometimes immediately with an allergic reaction or sometimes slowly over time. Unnatural substances can weaken our immune systems, cause our adrenal glands, heart, and pancreas to overwork, and congest our arteries. Some good questions to ask when choosing what to drink are the following:

- Are the ingredients in this drink completely natural and without artificial colorings and preservatives? If so, this is a good drink to choose.
- Is this drink sweetened with natural sweeteners including stevia, xylitol, or agave? If so, this is a good drink to choose.
- Is this drink sweetened with natural sweeteners including raw organic honey, real maple syrup, or whole cane sugar? This drink is good for most people, but diabetics, hypoglycemics, people trying to lose weight, and people with Candida (yeast infections) should avoid these drinks.
- Is this drink sweetened with refined white sugar, aspartame, or Splenda? If so, this drink should be avoided by all for reasons previously mentioned.
- Does this drink contain refined white sugar, caffeine, or alcohol? If so. people with diabetes, hypoglycemia, and chronic fatigue should avoid these drinks. Even healthy people should proceed with caution.

Continued →

In this section, we will review various different drinks and popular beverages in order to help you make wise choices based on your current health conditions.

Water

The body is composed of approximately 60 to 70 percent water. Our digestive juices are 98 percent water. The human body excretes about one gallon of water every twenty-four hours. All of the body's cells need water to function. Clearly, water is an essential ingredient to good health.

F. Batmanghelidgj, MD, has written a fascinating book based on years of research called, *Your Body's Many Cries for Water*. In it he writes about water: "It is the solvent—the water content—that regulates all functions of the body . . . every function of the body is monitored and pegged to the efficient flow of water." He goes on to explain that a dry mouth is not the only indicator of thirst. He says: "When the neuro-transmitter histamine generation and its subordinate water regulators become excessively active, to the point of causing allergies, asthma, and chronic pains in different parts of the body, these pains should be translated as a thirst signal—one variety of the crisis signals of water shortage in the body." So we can see, based on this important research study, the vital importance of drinking water!

The healthiest water can be found in pristine regions of the world, where it is clean, pure, and vibrant. Its molecules, if viewed under a microscope, look a lot like snowflake crystals. All the water on our planet used to be this way until it became tainted and polluted with pesticides and chemicals. Tap water contains chlorine and often fluorine, both of which are toxic and place a burden on the liver. Chlorine not only kills harmful bacteria, it also kills good bacteria in the digestive tract, an important part of our immune system. Some water contains heavy inorganic minerals, the same ones that you see clogging up your iron, creating a ring in your teapot, and even staining your bathtub! It is impossible for the body to break down and digest inorganic minerals, and they can accumulate in the body's vessels and joints.

Steam-distilled water has had the heavy minerals, bacteria, and harmful chemicals removed. Steam-distilled water and water purified by reverse osmosis are two of the best water choices we can make. Distilled water is "empty" water because it does not contain minerals. Distilled water helps to cleanse the vessels and joints of mineral deposits. Herbal tea should be made with distilled water.

A small amount of minute minerals in our water is actually good for us. Thus, it's a good idea to add liquid ionic trace minerals to your distilled water. Ionic minerals are the smallest minerals and therefore more bioavailable and absorbable by the cells than the large inorganic minerals found in most water. Ionic trace minerals provide electrolytes that give us energy and neutralize the body's pH. Trace minerals nourish and strengthen the cells, giving them the life force necessary to throw off toxins and perform their jobs. Drink eight glasses of purified water daily; use about three drops of ionic trace minerals in each eight-ounce glass of water. It will help cleanse and build every organ of your body!

Soft Drinks

Soft drinks are addictive and very harmful to the body. One canned soft drink contains thirteen teaspoons of sugar. Some diet drinks are even more toxic because they contain aspartame—a serious poison! Beware of those sweetened with Splenda as well. Most soft drinks are high in caffeine and can cause heart palpitations. Many of our youth in high school and on college campuses are seriously addicted to soft drinks, and they are beginning to rot their teeth and destroy their pancreases at a young age!

If you are drinking soft drinks, you can replace them with delightful fruit juice drinks. Mix pure fruit juice with sparkling mineral water, half and half. Or mix sparkling mineral water with a dash of lemon or lime juice. Add some liquid stevia, agave, or xylitol as a sweetener. Drinks made with water and lemon or lime sweetened with stevia, agave, or xylitol actually nourish your body, balance the pancreas, add few or no calories, and place no burden on the liver. They don't cause blood sugar highs or lows. When people consume drinks sweetened with refined white sugar Of high fructose corn syrup, the pancreas must produce lots of insulin to manage the influx of concentrated sugar. They may feel energized for an hour, then weak when the sugar passes out of their systems. Stevia nourishes the body without making the pancreas have to work so hard. Blue agave nectar and xylitol also cause very little burden to the pancreas. If you are diabetic or hypoglycemic, use stevia, blue agave nectar, or xylitol for sweetening your drinks; or make drinks by mixing three-quarters sparkling mineral water and one-quarter fruit juice. Black cherry and apple juice are especially good with mineral water. Natural soft drinks, such as ginger ale are also available. These natural soft drinks contain good ingredients such as water, fruit juice, stevia, agave, xylitol, ginger, vanilla, or other natural flavorings. If you are diabetic or hypoglycemic consume drinks sweetened with fruit juice sparingly. Read labels when purchasing natural soft drinks. Some will say they are natural although they contain Splenda, artificial colorings, and preservatives.

Coffee

Most coffee on the market is highly processed and loaded with chemicals because crops are heavily sprayed. Organic coffees are better and even contain some antioxidants but still contain caffeine. Some decaffeinated coffees are also toxic because of the decaffeinating process, which uses chemicals such as methylene chloride to extract the caffeine. Methylene chloride is used by many industries for things such as metal cleaning and paint stripping. Methylene chloride is considered a potential carcinogen by Occupational and Safety Health Administration (OSHA). Water-decaffeinated coffees are better for you. Organic water-decaffeinated coffee is the best option, but remember that a bit of caffeine remains in it. A healthy person's liver can process caffeine better than an unhealthy person's. A new study has revealed that decaffeinated coffee is higher in fats and oils than regular coffee and more than two or three cups per day is not good for a person with high cholesterol. If you are a coffee drinker, and especially if you are ill, replace coffee with delicious substitutes such as Pero, Inka, Postum, and Caffix. These "coffees," made from chicory, are instant, so you only have to add water. If you like to drip or perk your coffee, try Teeccino. Delightful with a rich, full-bodied flavor, Teeccino is made from carob, barley, chicory, figs, almonds, and dates. It is high in potassium and gives you a boost of energy. It also contains inulin, a soluble fiber that enhances digestion and promotes regularity. Add a little rice milk and stevia if you ate accustomed to cream and sugar. Delicious! All of these coffee drinks may be purchased in health food stores.

The caffeine in coffee "kicks" the adrenals to produce an overabundance of adrenaline, which causes the heart to race and the pancreas to produce too much insulin. The insulin then drops the blood sugar and causes you to feel hungry or crave sweets an hour or two after drinking the coffee. Because of this, we often eat more and gain weight.

Some people think coffee keeps their bowels moving, because the caffeine kicks them into action. In reality caffeine increases acid production and may cause constipation.

If you are addicted to caffeine, wean yourself from it slowly. Start drinking half regular and half decaf coffee the first week, then change to one-third regular and two-thirds decaf coffee the second week. By the end of a month, you can be completely free from a caffeine addiction and able to switch to herbal teas or coffee substitutes.

Black Teas

Like coffee, black teas are high in caffeine and can be addictive. Replace black tea with any of the hundreds of herbal teas on the market. Try apple cinnamon, black cherry, peppermint, or whatever you prefer. Many herbal teas are already prepared for you in tea bags. Study the wide variety of herbal teas listed for you in this book. By learning what they do for you, you will be able to make wise choices about what your body needs at the moment. Green tea can be a great substitute for black tea, and it is a wonderful antioxidant.

Beer and Wine

In addition to containing alcohol, which can be harsh on the liver, beer is high in sugar and calories, which is why drinking lots of it over a long period of time can create a beer gut. Beer also contains yeast, which can promote the growth of *Candida albicans* and cause yeast infections. There are organic beers and alcohol-free beers, but they also contain sugar and yeast.

Red wine has been reported to be beneficial in cleaning the arteries and lowering cholesterol. Look for organic wines made from grapes that were not sprayed with pesticides. There are alcohol-free wines as well. Drinkers who are hypoglycemic often become alcoholics because their overproduction of insulin causes them to crave the sugar and alcohol in alcoholic beverages.

Hard liquor used daily can be extremely damaging to the liver, brain, and nervous system. It is best for those who are ill to avoid all alcoholic beverages.

Tool Kit for Choosing Healthy Juices

Raw vegetable and fruit juice is one of the finest foods we can take into our bodies. Because of its nourishing contents, raw juice can help heal all sorts of ailments, mend bones, reverse osteoporosis, cleanse and repair the cells, improve immune function, fight viruses and bacteria, oxygenate the cells, fight free radicals, energize, and invigorate. Raw juice can save the life of a person who cannot digest food, because it is so easily absorbed.

Raw juices build healthy red blood cells. For this reason you should take out your juicer, dust it off, and start juicing for your health! If you don't have a juicer, use your blender. A blender will not extract the fiber from the vegetables, so your drink will have more fiber and be more filling.

Enzymes

Enzymes are molecules that catalyze or initiate chemical reactions. Most enzymes are proteins that have special catalytic activity, but there are some RNA molecules that also have this property. Enzymes are responsible for the life force in our

Continued ➡

bodies with high levels of specificity. For example, the enzyme lactase catalyzes the breakdown or digestion of lactose. Raw juice is high in enzymes. These vital nutritional elements constitute the life principle in every atom and molecule of all living organisms. Enzymes are involved in all the body's activities and functions and are vital to healthy cellular activity. Thus, enzymes help our immune system function well by breaking down toxins that could cause illness. They help keep the arteries clean and are essential to our organs and metabolic pro-cesses. We would not be able to see, move our limbs, smell, taste, breathe, or think without enzymes!

Without enzymes, we become lethargic and exhausted. Edward Howell conducted extensive research on the effect that food enzymes have on our health. In *Enzyme Nutrition*, he says, "Enzymes offer an important means of calculating the vital energy of an organism. That which we call energy, vital force, nerve energy and strength, may be synonymous with enzyme activity."

Enzymes are destroyed at temperatures of 130°F or higher. People who live only on cooked foods deplete all their stores of enzymes and age more rapidly or become ill more often than people who eat plenty of raw foods. Undigested food ferments in the intestinal tract and becomes food for parasites and Candida. Eat raw vegetables with meals to provide enzymes for good digestion.

Raw juices are delicious and nutritional as well as medicinal. If you are healthy, drink twelve to sixteen ounces of vegetable juices daily to stay strong and well and prevent illness. Max Gerson, MD, helped hundreds of patients recover from otherwise "incurable" diseases. In *A Cancer Therapy*, he writes:

1. Juices consist of living matter with active ferments, fast-neutralizing oxidizing enzymes, which are most necessary for the sick body.
2. The body needs an equilibrium of active oxidizing enzymes supplied throughout the day. These cannot maintain active states except in freshly pressed juices, given at hourly intervals.

If you are ill, try to drink several eight-ounce glasses of raw vegetable juice each day.

Types of Juicers

The best juices are those that have been freshly extracted by a juicer. A juicer is one of the most important health-building appliances you can have in your kitchen. There are several types of juicers on the market. One is the centrifugal juicer, which works by grinding the fruits or vegetables and throwing the pulp against a round spinning screen. Another type of juicer has a round blade that grinds the fruit or vegetable, separates the juice through a screen, and expels the pulp into a bucket fitted in back. Then there is the heavy-screen juicer that presses the pulp through a stainless-steel screen and tosses it out the front while the juice falls through the screen into a bowl below. The wheatgrass juicer grinds very slowly and extracts juice from delicate wheatgrass or spinach leaves.

The latest juicer has twin gears and can be used to extract juice from both fruits and vegetables and from wheatgrass. This machine's gears run slowly, which eliminates oxidation caused by faster machines.

Preparing Fruits and Vegetables for Juicing

Use fruits and vegetables that are organic and free from pesticides. Wash your produce thoroughly, since it can contain certain parasites or their eggs. Prepare a solution with one tablespoon of raw apple cider vinegar to each quart of water. Soak your fruits and vegetables in this solution for five min-

utes. Then scrub them well with a natural-bristle vegetable brush. Make sure the vinegar you use is raw. Most vinegar is made from apple peelings that have been sprayed with pesticides and cooked at high temperatures, killing all living enzymes. Raw apple cider vinegar is high in enzymes and can kill parasites and streptococci germs.

Raw Fruit Juices

Fresh-squeezed fruit juices from organic fruits are best. A glass of freshly juiced fruit juice of any kind is delicious and much better for you than soft drinks. However, fruit juice is still high in sugar content and should be used sparingly. Sugar in fruit juice feeds Candida and parasites. You can dilute fruit juice with water and reduce the sugar content.

BLACK CHERRY JUICE

Black cherry juice is a very healthy juice and is high in organic iron. Organic black cherry concentrates are available. If you are tired or anemic, this is a great juice for you. It helps dissolve uric acid crystals in the body and may relieve the pain of gout and arthritis. Freshly juiced black cherry juice is even better for you when the cherries are in season. Black cherry juice diluted with distilled water is a good juice to give your baby when the baby is about four months old. By this time, the supply of iron in mother's milk becomes depleted, and the juice helps to supply iron.

CITRUS FRUIT JUICES

Citrus fruits should be ripened on the vine before they are picked or they will be very acidic in the body. Fresh-squeezed lemon, lime, and grapefruit juices cleanse the liver. Lemon, lime, grapefruit, and orange juice are high in vitamin C.

CRANBERRY JUICE

Cranberry juice can help heal a kidney or bladder infection. Cranberry juice has also been used in the treatment of asthma and kidney stones. It is very cleansing to the lymph system. Some of the key nutrients in cranberry juice are vitamin C, B vitamins, potassium, and beta-carotene. It also contains quercitin and ellagic acid, which are powerful antioxidants. The nutrients in cranberry juice keep bacteria from adhering to the cells of the bladder and thus flush it out of the body.

GRAPE JUICE

Use only organic grapes with the seeds in them. Never use seedless grapes. Juice the grapes, seeds and all. Grape seeds are a source of oligomeric proan-thocyanidins, or OPCs, which combat free radicals and improve immune function. They help to strengthen the capillaries in the eye and improve vision, including night blindness. OPCs also help repair connective tissue and thus heal varicose veins and hemorrhoids. Grape juice from the whole grape and seed can cleanse the veins and arteries, eliminate plaque, and promote cardiovascular health.

Dark purple grapes are high in iron. They help relieve gout and cleanse the liver. Grapes also fight some types of viruses, and bacteria. Johanna Brandt wrote a book titled *The Grape Cure*, in which she used grapes and their seeds to help heal cancer.

If you are hypoglycemic or diabetic, drink grape juice in small quantities or diluted.

LEMON AND LIME JUICE

The juice from fresh lemons and limes helps dissolve kidney stones and gallstones. Lemon pulp is high in bioflavanoids, which help strengthen the weakened tissue in those areas. Stanley Burroughs wrote about a "Master Cleanser" drink that was

made of lemon juice, organic maple syrup, and cayenne pepper. Here is a great way to prepare this drink:

Peel two lemons or three limes, cut them into quatters, and remove seeds. Place the chunks in a blender with twenty ounces of water, and add a half cup of pure organic maple syrup and one-eighth to one-fourth teaspoon of cayenne pepper or ginger powder. Blend for two to three minutes. Makes two servings.

Cayenne and ginger help to promote circulation and strengthen the heart. Cayenne also helps stop internal or external bleeding.

ORANGE JUICE

It's a good idea for nursing mothers to supplement breast milk with fresh-squeezed, strained orange juice. Breast milk is not high in vitamin C. Orange juice can be given to the baby by the third or fourth month. Oranges should be fresh, organic, and ripened on the vine. Dilute the juice to half-potency with distilled water. Fresh-squeezed OJ is good for people of all ages since it's high in vitamin C and calcium and also contains biofla-vanoids including rutin and hesperidin, which helps strengthen connective tissue in the body.

PAPAYA JUICE

Papaya juice is available in health food stores in concentrated form and helps facilitate digestion because it is high in enzymes. Papain is an enzyme that aids in protein digestion. Papain has proven valuable in the reduction of inflammation. Some important nutrients in papayas are vitamins C and A, pantothenic acid, and beta-carotene. These nutrients in combination with its soothing alkaline properties make papaya juice healing for ulcers and colitis. Papayas can be juiced or blended at home as well.

PINEAPPLE JUICE

Fresh-squeezed pineapple juice is high in bromelain, an enzyme that helps digestion and reduces inflammation. Studies have shown that bromelain prevents the aggregation of blood platelets and may be beneficial in the prevention of heart attacks and stroke. It also contains vitamin C, calcium, and potassium.

POMEGRANATE JUICE

Pomegranate juice is packed with wonderful nutrients that help clear up kidney infection, tighten the gums around the teeth, strengthen varicose veins and hemorrhoids, stop diarrhea, and improve bad breath. It contains vitamin C, riboflavin, and niacin. Its mineral content includes iron, potassium, calcium, and magnesium. The phytonutrients in pomegranate juice provide antioxidants and astringent properties; these include ellagic acid, beta-carotene, tannin, and pectin.

Watermelon Rind juice

When you juice watermelon, add the rind! Watermelon juice is delicious and great for the kidneys and bladder. It acts as a natural diuretic. The juice of the rind is high in sodium, which nourishes the lymph fluids and stomach lining. You will also receive chlorophyll from the rind, which builds the blood.

Raw Vegetable Juices

Raw vegetable juices are powerful antioxidants and slow the aging process. They provide highly absorbable vitamins and minerals of the finest quality. They both build and cleanse the body. Vegetable juices provide minerals including sodium and calcium in a balanced ratio that can assist the

Continued ➡

body in proper absorption so that calcium can be restored to the bones in cases of osteoporosis and arthritis. Bottled or canned juices have been heated or cooked, and all the living enzymes have been destroyed. Raw juices contain minerals that the body can absorb. On the other hand, the minerals in most water, such as lime, iron, and chalk, are hardened and not easily absorbed or utilized and can actually cause stones to form.

Blended salads and blended raw soups are very good for you, but not the same as juice because they still contain fiber. Fiber has its place and helps promote good peristalsis in the bowel and acts as little brooms to sweep the intestine clean. Juices contain more concentrated vitamins and minerals than blended salads and soups because the fiber is missing. Nutrients from the juice are more easily absorbed than when the fiber is included. I'm not suggesting you omit blended soups or blended salads. To use both in the diet is very beneficial. The only time juice alone is appropriate is during some types of cleanses or when a person is very ill and having trouble digesting fiber. Hypoglycemics and diabetics should stick with green vegetable juices in order to avoid the sugar content that is in carrot, beet, and fruit juices. To make raw vegetable juice in your blender, put the vegetables in the blender with water. Blend well, strain off the juice, and drink it. You will absorb more nutrients from the juice.

ALFALFA JUICE

Alfalfa juice is rich in nutrients including protein, vitamins E and K, beta-carotene, chlorophyll, calcium, magnesium, and potassium because the alfalfa plant's roots reach as far as 120 feet into the earth, absorbing vitamins and minerals from many different levels of soil. Alfalfa juice builds bones and blood, helps reverse arthritis, and promotes good bowel function.

ASPARAGUS JUICE

A wonderful diuretic, asparagus juice cleanses oxalic crystals from the kidneys and muscles and is a great blood builder. It's high in potassium, folic acid, thiamine, and vitamins C and A. It works best when combined with carrot and cucumber juice.

BEET JUICE

Beet juice is high in iron and helps build red corpuscles. It contains vitamin C, B vitamins, calcium, magnesium, and phosphorus. All of these nutrients along with beta-carotene and lutein work together synergistically to cleanse the liver and gallbladder, prevent jaundice, cleanse and soften hardened arteries, and strengthen varicose veins. It is high in organic sodium, which restores calcium to the bone, helps dissolve crystals in the joints, and may prevent or dissolve kidney and gallstones. It is also high in potassium, which strengthens the muscles, including the heart.

Do not drink more than one to three ounces of beet juice if you are not used to it. It is so cleansing to the liver and gallbladder, it can cause nausea. Combine beet juice with carrot and celery juice or carrot and cucumber juice to dilute its cleansing effects.

BEET GREENS JUICE

High in chlorophyll, potassium, calcium, magnesium, iodine, and iron, beet greens juice cleanses and builds the blood. It also strengthens the heart and thyroid gland, builds bones, and relaxes muscles.

BROCCOLI JUICE

Broccoli has tremendous cancer preventive properties. High in vitamin C, calcium, and phosphorus, it strengthens the immune system and builds bones. The American Cancer Society recommends eating broccoli several times a week to help prevent cancer. The best way to get the most benefit from broccoli is to juice it! A pound of broccoli makes three ounces of juice. Note: While broccoli juice can be very beneficial to those with hyperthyroidism, people with hypothyroidism should use in moderation.

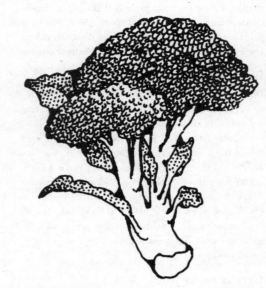

CABBAGE JUICE

More of a cabbage's beneficial nutrients are in its outer leaves, which most people discard. Why not juice them? A very important nutrient in cabbage juice is vitamin U or ascorbigen, which is one of the most effective cures for ulcers. The chlorophyll in cabbage juice provides iron and stimulates the flow of bile and cleanses the intestinal tract. Cabbage juice is high in vitamin C, which also boosts the immune system and helps protect the body from cancer. Cabbage is high in sulfur so it helps improve circulation and relieves arthritic pain as well as allergies. Other wonderful nutrients in cabbage are vitamin K, which helps the blood clot properly, and calcium, which strengthens the bones.

CARROT JUICE

High in beta-carotene, carrot juice has tremendous cancer-preventing properties. Beta-carotene is a powerful antioxidant and protects the body against free radicals. Carrots and carrot juice boost the immune function by enhancing the performance of white blood cells. Carrots are also high in calcium and strengthen the bones. People with osteoporosis or arthritis should drink lots of carrot juice! Carrot juice also cleanses the body and helps fight infection. The fiber in carrots can help lower serum cholesterol. And everyone knows carrots help improve sight. Our bodies convert beta-carotene to vitamin A, which helps keep the retina healthy. NOTE: Diabetics, hypoglycemics, and those with yeast or fungal infections should use sparingly becaue of the sugar content in carrot juice.

CELERY JUICE

Celery juice is high in chlorophyll, which cleanses the blood. It is also high in organic sodium, which nourishes the lymph fluid and helps hold calcium in solution. Celery juice thereby helps prevent, as well as to dissolve, the crystals that occur with arthritis, gout, kidney stones, and gallstones. The stomach is lined with natural sodium, and fluid in the eyes is high in sodium. Celery juice can be helpful in cases of dry eyes or stomach disorders, acting to neutralize acids in the stomach as well as

throughout the body. It contains coumarin which enhances blood flow and has antifungal and anti-tumor properties. It also contains pthalides, a phytochemical that can assist with lowering high blood pressure. Celery juice can calm the nerves, improve bowel function, help to lower cholesterol, and release excess fluids that cause swelling. It is high in potassium and can relieve muscle cramps. It is delicious mixed with carrot juice! NOTE: People taking blood thinners should use sparingly.

CUCUMBER JUICE

Cucumber juice is a delicious juice that is high in water content. It helps hydrate cells when you have a fever or are just "dry" and thirsty. A cucumber's precious naturally distilled water helps cool the body and calm the nerves. It acts as a natural diuretic and flushes the kidneys, and it assists in lowering high blood pressure. Please use only organic cucumbers, and juice the entire vegetable, including the skin. The peel is high in chlorophyll, which cleanses the blood, as well as silicon, a mineral that nourishes the nerves and connective tissue, helping prevent wrinkles, varicose veins, and hemorrhoids.

GARLIC JUICE

Garlic juice may sound terrible, but it can get rid of a cold or flu in a short period of time. Juice one clove of garlic with one apple. Drink two to three of these cocktails per day when ill, and you will heal rapidly. Garlic is high in a very potent antioxidant called allicin which helps fight many different types of bacteria and viruses. Garlic can also be juiced with carrots and celery or any other vegetables you prefer. If you are ill with salmonella, *Candida albicans*, or any bacterial infection, garlic is a must. According to research done by Steve Meyerowitz for his book, *Power Juices, Super Drinks*, "Garlic can even help in the war against AIDS." He found that "Garlic is also a powerful agent in the war against cancel." In addition to garlic's antibacterial properties, it is also high in sulfur, which can help with hardening of the arteries (atherosclerosis), high blood pressure, and cholesterol. NOTE: If you are taking any medications to dissolve blood clots or thin the blood, be careful with garlic, because it also acts as an anticoagulant in the blood.

GINGER JUICE

When combined with other juices, ginger juice is both delicious and good for us. I like to drink a combination of carrot, beet, celery, and ginger juice; or carrot, cucumber, apple, and ginger juice. Ginger warms the body and promotes circulation. It helps relieve nausea. Ginger juice can be added to hot water and honey for tea when you feel queasy or nauseous. Ginger helps people who are undergoing chemotherapy avoid nausea and pregnant women alleviate morning sickness. It can also help with motion sickness and vertigo. Ginger juice relieves inflammation associated with rheumatic pains, improves circulation, and loosens phlegm from the sinuses and lungs. The medicinal properties of ginger are in its volatile oils and pungent phenol compounds such as gingerols, shogaols, and zingibain. Important vitamins in ginger are vitamin C, vitamins B_1, B_2, niacin, and B_6. Its minerals include zinc, calcium, phosphorus, and postassium. Key phytonutrients are curcumin which is anti-inflammatory and quercitin, a powerful antioxidant. Note: Ginger also helps thin the blood so use with caution if taking anticoagulant drugs.

GREEN LEAFY VEGETABLE JUICE

Juice made from beet tops, turnip greens, celery tops, kale, broccoli, collards, chard, Chinese cabbage, or spinach will make you as strong as the car-

Continued ➡

toon character Popeye! These vegetables are loaded with minerals and chlorophyll that help improve red blood cell counts. All ate high in iron, and spinach is twice as high in iron as the rest, making them wonderful remedies for anemia. These juices are also very high in absorbable calcium and can help reverse osteoporosis! One cup of green juice from these vegetables contains more calcium than a glass of milk and is much easier for the body to absorb and utilize. Green leafy vegetable juices have phyto-chemicals, which can help prevent cancel and strengthen the eyes. If you don't like to drink these juices straight, combine them with carrot juice.

PARSLEY JUICE

Parsley juice is high in chlorophyll and helps oxygenate the blood and build red blood cells. Parsley juice is a natural digestive aid. It is also a natural diuretic and flushes the kidneys. It assists with healing kidney and bladder infections and with preventing kidney stones. It is also high in calcium, so it can help with tissue and bone repair. It is high in potassium and can prevent cramping. Carrot and parsley juice combined is delicious and great for you! Both contain beta-carotene, which is super for the eyes and immune system.

RADISH JUICE

Radish juice is a bit hot because it contains a potent oil, much like mustard oil, that's great for clearing the sinuses and lungs of excess mucus, relieving sore throat, and improving circulation. Radish juice contains salicylates (also in aspirin) that have been known to help relieve arthritis pain. Other important nutrients in radish juice are vitamin C, iodine, iron, calcium, and sulfur. Mix it with carrot and parsley juice, and you'll have a delicious drink!

RED BELL PEPPER JUICE

Red bell pepper juice is sweeter and better for you than green bell pepper juice. Red bell peppers are ripe, while green ones are not ripe and contain fewer nutrients. Red bell peppers are high in vitamin C and are great for the immune system. They are also high in silicon, which helps strengthen and repair connective tissue and prevent bruising.

TOMATO JUICE

Tomato juice should be made only from organic, vine-ripened tomatoes. Some of the tomatoes available in grocery stores in the winter are void of nutrients and hardly taste like tomatoes at all! Tomato juice is high in beta-carotene and vitamin C, which boost the immune system. They contain lycopene, a powerful antioxidant that helps prevent cancer and heart disease. Tomato juice is also rich in the amino acid lysine, which helps heal cold sores, and potassium, which is a great mineral for the muscles and heart. Some people worry that tomato juice contains too much sodium. This is because most people are drinking canned or bottled tomato juice that has added salt for flavor. Freshly juiced tomato juice contains some organic sodium, but this natural sodium is very helpful in dissolving crystals in the joints and holding calcium in the bone. Some tomatoes are a bit too acidic for some people and may cause indigestion. If this is the case, I suggest trying the more alkaline Roma tomatoes. Enjoy tomato juice! NOTE: If you have arthritis and are concerned that the foods from the nightshades including tomatoes, peppers, potatoes, and eggplants could be bothering you, leave out all nightshades for a week and introduce one at the time into your diet. If pain is worsened due to the nightshades, omit them from the foods you eat. It may be that after following a healthy nutritional plan for a year, your body will grow strong enough to tolerate the nightshades. If not, continue to avoid them completely.

WATERCRESS JUICE

Watercress juice has a bittersweet taste and is great juiced with carrot and cucumbers. It is a natural diuretic and helps prevent fluid retention. Drink watercress juice to strengthen your hair—it contains a lot of amino acids. It is also a good source of minerals, including sulfur, which helps arthritis and prevents cancer growth, and iodine, which is great for the thyroid gland. Watercress is also great for the immune system because its high in vitamins A and C.

WHEATGRASS JUICE

Wheatgrass juice cleanses the blood and acts just like a drain cleaner, killing bacteria and parasites as it goes through the system. If you don't have a wheatgrass juicer, the juice is often available in health food stores. It is also available in powder form. Barley grass and green kamut are similar because they are both good blood cleansers and detoxifiers and also come in powdered form. Ann Wigmore, who founded the Hippocrates Health Institute in Boston, is credited with discovering the benefits of wheatgrass juice. She had gangrene in her legs, and the doctors wanted to amputate. She started drinking wheatgrass juice and using poultices on her legs. Not only did her legs heal, but she went on to run the Boston marathon! Since then, many people with "incurable" diseases have gotten well using wheatgrass juice. I drink two ounces of wheatgrass juice often and feel energized! People with allergies to wheat will have no problem using wheatgrass juice, as wheat is a grain, while wheatgrass is a grass (not a grain). Wheatgrass juice is about 70 percent chlorophyll, which closely resembles hemoglobin in chemical composition. Chlorophyll has antiseptic cleansing properties. Wheatgrass juice is a wonderful source of protein, beta-carotene, B vitamins, and vitamins C, E, H, and K. It is said to contain a wide variety of minerals with more iron than spinach. Its nutrients nourish the body and give it a real boost.

Tool Kit for Choosing Therapeutic Herbal Teas

Herbal teas have been used for centuries both for healing and enjoyment. There is something wonderful about sitting with a cup of soothing tea in the midmorning, afternoon, or evening. You can curl up on a rainy afternoon on the couch with a blanket, a good book, and a delicious cup of warm tea or enjoy tea with a friend. When choosing a tea, make sure it is right for you. There are such a variety of teas with various benefits. For example, cramp bark tea is very useful to a woman with menstrual pains and may be helpful during pregnancy. When pregnant however, it would be wise to consult a knowledgeable herbalist or your physician before taking. Herbs are our friends and can comfort and delight. Some are medicinal and should be used with respect. To prepare a tea, it is best to use distilled or purified water. Never use tap water because in most places it is full of chlorine and other harmful chemicals.

Making Perfect Tea

Follow these rules when preparing your tea, and you will have wonderful tea each time.

- If the tea is leaves or blossoms, bring water to a boil, add the tea, turn off the burner, cover, and let it steep for about twenty minutes. Covering tea while it's steeping is most important in order to hold in the volatile healing properties.

- If the tea is seeds, bring the water to a boil, add the seeds, and reduce the heat to simmer. Simmer the tea for ten minutes, covered. Then turn off the heat, cover, and let it steep for twenty to thirty minutes.
- If the tea is roots, straw, or bark, bring the water to a boil, add the tea, cover it, then reduce the heat to simmer. Simmer the tea for twenty minutes. Then turn off the heat, and let it steep for thirty minutes.
- If the tea is a powder, pour boiling water over the powder, cover it, and let it steep for ten minutes.
- Use a teaspoon of each type of tea per cup unless directed otherwise.

Herbal Teas

Tea can make us more alert at work, help heal a sore throat, or help us to sleep at night. If you know the healing values in herbal teas, you can choose the best ones for your current needs. Herbs are rich in vitamins, minerals, and healing oils, and I have listed the most important of these for each tea. It is good to understand, however, that an herb's healing power lies within the synergistic interaction between all of the nutrients within it and not in one single element. Following is a list of various herbal teas and their medicinal benefits. These teas can be drunk with or without sweeteners. If you like your tea a bit sweet, add stevia, agave nectar, xylitol, pure maple syrup, or raw honey. Learn about the different teas and use them appropriately for yourself, your friends, and your family. Enjoy!

Note: If you do not want to drink these herbs as reas, but feel they would be beneficial to you, you may take them in capsule or tincture form. Check with a knowledgeable herbalist or physician to make sure they are right for you.

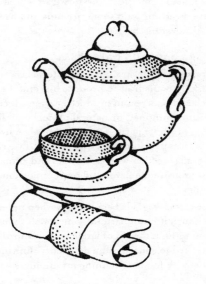

ALFALFA LEAF TEA

Alfalfa leaf tea is rich in minerals, including calcium, magnesium, iron, and potassium. It is also high in chlorophyll and vitamins A, B, C, D, K, and P. It contains all eight of the essential amino acids. Alfalfa leaf tea aids digestion, builds blood, and relieves inflammation. It can also be helpful with ulcers, urinary tract infections, and arthritis.

ANISE SEED TEA

Anise seed tea is a wonderful digestive aid. It relieves nausea, flatulence, and cramping. It can also be given to babies to relieve colic. Anethole, often referred to as the oil of anise seed, is aromatic and gives anise its licorice flavor. Anethole has carmitive properties, which help get rid of gas and settle the digestive system, and antispasmodic qualities, which soothe cramps. The anethole in

Continued ➡

anise is also an expectorant with antimicrobial abilities, which makes it excellent for releasing mucus and healing sore throats. Anise contains several phytonutrients including rutin, which helps tighten connective tissue in the gums. Key nutrients are vitamins A, B vitamins, C, and E. Its minerals include magnesium, calcium, iron, zinc, and potassium.

Burdock Root Tea

Burdock root tea purifies the blood, cleanses the liver, aids digestion, and balances blood sugar because it contains inulin, a plant starch that has been shown to have a favorable effect on the pancreas. Burdock root has been used as a diuretic and to help release uric acid from the kidneys and blood, thus relieving gout. It contains nutrients called polyacetylenes that have antibacterial and anti-inflammatory properties. Inulin, which helps to manage blood sugar in hypoglycemics and diabetics, makes up a large percentage of burdock root. Burdock is a fine blood purifier and has been used to heal arthritis and skin disorders. Burdock root is rich in vitamins A, B, C, E, P, as well as minerals chromium, phosphorus, selenium, iron, potassium, sulfur, iodine, silicon, zinc, magnesium, and calcium. Active compounds in burdock root are called sesquiterpene lactones (antimicrobial), volatile oils, and phytochemicals.

Cardamom Seed Tea

Cardamom seed tea relieves the gripping pain of stomach and intestinal cramps. It is both delicious and soothing. There are monoterpenes in the cardamom seeds that have antispasmotic, antiviral, antibacterial, and antifungal properties. The oil in cardamom contains limonene, terpineol, and terpenene, which have been found to relieve inflammation and pain. Cardamom seed oil also helps release mucus from the respiratory tract as well as improve digestion. Add some rice milk and have a cup in the evening.

Cascara Sagrada Bark Tea

Cascara sagrada bark tea is a safe, natural laxative that stimulates the liver to produce bile and the stomach and pancreas to produce enzymes. It contains anthraquinones, or natural phytochemicals, that help promote peristalsis in the bowel. A liver cleanser, it is useful in cases of jaundice. Take cascara sagrada together with cardamom and cinnamon to improve the flavor and prevent possible cramping.

Use cascara sagrada bark tea only when necessary. Though it is not harmful, our bowels should function without the aid of laxatives. Constipation is often related to a magnesium deficiency. Enhance your diet with foods containing magnesium.

Catnip Leaf Tea

Catnip leaf tea calms the nervous system and helps induce sleep. It also lowers fevers, eases symptoms of flatulence, stomach acids, intestinal spasms, and colic. This a wonderful tea to relieve colic in infants and promote rest. Catnip tea contains several minerals including calcium and magnesium that help calm the nerves and relax the body. It is rich in iron. Key vitamins are A, B_1, B_2, niacin, and B_6. B vitamins are very soothing to the nerves. It also contains a compound called valeric acid, a natural seditive also found in valerian root.

Chamomile Blossom Tea

Chamomile blossom tea soothes and relaxes the nervous system. It has a mild sedative effect, which can induce sleep. It also relieves digestive disorders, such as diarrhea, flatulence, and cramps. This tea can help relieve flulike symptoms such as aching muscles, inflammation, and coughing. Add four cups of chamomile blossom tea to the bath water to relieve muscular pain or sunburn. Chamomile contains the phytochemicals azulene (an anti-inflammatory), borneol (a digestive aide), salicylic acid (relieves pain), rutin (tightens tissues), and quercitin (an antioxidant). It's vitamins are B and C. Blondes can use this tea as a hair rinse to lighten their hair. NOTE: Those with an allergy to ragweed should drink chamomile tea with caution because it is very similar in nature to ragweed. Don't mix chamomile tea with alcohol or sleeping medications.

Chickweed Leaf and Stem "Tea

Chickweed makes a nice herbal tea with natural fatty acids that help with weight loss. It is also high in vitamin C, iron, and potassium and helps to cleanse the blood and reduce fevers. Add a little raw organic honey to the tea and it will soothe a sore throat.

Cinnamon Bark Tea

Cinnamon bark tea relieves symptoms of indigestion and helps stop diarrhea, stomach cramps, and nausea. The oils in cinnamon improve circulation and can encourage menstrual bleeding if a menstrual period is late. This tea has antifungal, antibacterial, and antiviral properties. Cinnamon contains beta-carotene—a form of vitamin A that boosts immunity and chromium that helps balance blood sugar in diabetics and hypoglycemics. NOTE: May take only small amounts during pregnancy, no more than one cup every few weeks.

Collinsonia Root Tea

Collinsonia root tea is wonderful for healing hemorrhoids and varicose veins because it strengthens the walls of the veins. The resin in it strengthens tissue and helps wounds to heal. The tannins in it are astringent and are beneficial in helping stop diarrhea. Tannins help fight bacteria and fungi. It also contains saponins which have cholesterol lowering abilities.

Cramp Bark Tea

Cramp bark is a wonderful tea for cramps of any kind, especially menstrual because it contains valerianic acid, the phytonutrient also found in valerian root that has relaxing properties. It can help regulate menstrual cycles and may be beneficial when there is potential for miscarriage. Cramp bark can also help ease heart palpitations because of its relaxing nervine properties. It contains the minerals calcium, magnesium, and potassium—also great muscle relaxants. It works wonderfully to relieve cramps when blended with false unicorn. NOTE: Consult an herbalist or knowledgeable physician before taking if you ate pregnant.

Dandelion Leaf and Root Tea

Tea dandelions are high in vitamins A, B, C, and D and the minerals calcium, iron, potassium, and sulfur. The tea is a wonderful spring tonic and blood and liver purifier. Dandelions are also high in inulin, which helps regulate the blood sugar and is a gentle laxative and natural diuretic. Dandelion leaf and root tea can alleviate anemia, jaundice, diabetes, gout, hepatitis, and constipation. It can also help reduce levels of uric acid and serum cholesterol. NOTE: Dandelion is a natural diuretic so do not drink this tea if you are taking medicinal diuretics. Also avoid this tea if you have gallstones.

Echinacea Root Tea

Echinacea root tea purifies the lymph and blood, thus helping fight off colds, bronchitis, sore throat, urinary tract infections, and flu. It contains the phytochemicals alpha-pinene, an antibacterial, and beta-carotene, a plant form of vitamin A that strengthens the eyes. It also contains the phytochemicals apgenin, a natural anti-inflammatory, and arabinogalactan, which boosts the immune system and protects against allergies. The tea stimulates white blood cells, which help attack germs, as well as interferon, which is a front-line component known to fight the development of cancer cells. It is antiviral and antibacterial. It is high in vitamin C, phosphorus, iron, and zinc. NOTE: This tea should not be taken for more than four to six weeks or it loses its potency in the body. Since this tea stimulates the immune system, it should be used with caution by those with autoimmune disorders. It should also be used with caution if you have an allergy to ragweed, daisies, chrysanthemums, or marigolds because echinacea has similar properties to these plants.

Eyebright Leaf Tea

Eyebright is high in beta-carotene and vitamin C. The tea is extremely beneficial in strengthening the eyes and maintaining good vision.

False Unicorn Root Tea

This wonderful tea helps regulate irregular menses and relieve cramping. False unicorn root tea relieves nausea that may come with menstruation or pregnancy. It has also been used successfully to help women become pregnant. Men who want to increase sperm count should drink false unicorn root tea. This tea helps rid the bowel of parasites as well. It contains the phytonutrients helonin, known to tone the female glands, and chamaelirin, known to strengthen both male and female systems, help impotence, and also act as a vermifuge.

Fennel Seed, Leaf, and Flower Tea

Fennel tea can be made from the seed, leaf, or flower. It is an excellent sore throat remedy. It also helps relieve coughs and colds and helps expel mucus. Fennel tea relieves colic, intestinal cramping, and flatulence. Fennel is very alkaline in nature so it's a great tea for an acid stomach or for those who have undergone chemotherapy. Its active constituents include terpenoid anethole, which has an estrogen-like activity that inhibits spasms in the smooth muscles due to coughing or abdominal cramping. It contains alpha-pinene, a phytonutrient which is antibacterial. Other key nutrients are beta-carotene, qurecitin, vitamin C, iron, and selenium.

Fenugreek Seed Tea

Fenugreek seed tea strengthens the liver. The seeds contain steroidal saponins, which have cholesterol lowering properties. These saponins also reduce the formation of secondary bile acids which are known to lead to colon cancer. Fenugreek contains the phytonutrient coumarin, which is antifungal, and kaempferol and quercetin, which are strong antioxidants and together have been known to reduce the proliferation of cancer cells. Oil of fenugreek helps soothe the throat and lungs and lubricate the intestines, and acts as a mild laxative. The oil may also reduce fevers and help asthma and sinus problems by clearing away mucus. Fenugreek contains amino acids, essential fatty acids, calcium, magnesium iron, phosphorus, zinc, potassium, B vitamins, and vitamin C. Because it is so nutritious, it strengthens the endocrine system and can help increase the flow of breast milk in nursing mothers.

Feverfew Bark, Leaves, and Flowers Tea

A wonderful anti-inflammatory, feverfew tea can relieve headaches, migraine headaches, and arthritic aches when used faithfully over a period of several

Continued ➡

months. It contains the phytonutrient parthenolide, which has been shown to be effective in relieving migraines and fighting leukemia. Parthenolide is anti-inflammatory. Key nutrients in feverfew are calcium, magnesium, potassium, selenium, zinc, iron, B vitamins, and vitamin C. Synergistically, its constituents help fight bacteria, yeasts, and fungi as well as inhibit the release of histamine in alletgic reactions. NOTE: People who take pain killers or medicines that thin the blood should not take feverfew without consulting a physician. Feverfew should not be taken during pregnancy.

FLAXSEED TEA

Flaxseed tea is mucilaginous and soothes the digestive tract, thereby helping relieve constipation. It is excellent for soothing and cleansing the urinary system as well. It contains the phytochemicals beta-sitosterol and campesterol, which are known to help in lowering cholesterol. Another phytochemical in flaxseed is apigenin, which is a natural anti-inflammatory and helps reduce cramping. Flaxseed are high in iron, potassium, sulfur, magnesium, zinc, B vitamins, and vitamin E.

GINGER ROOT TEA

Ginger root makes one of the finest teas to help relieve vertigo, nausea, and vomiting. It helps stop morning sickness in pregnant mothers and relieves menstrual cramps. It is also very helpful with colitis, stomach cramps, and flatulence. Ginger root tea increases circulation and warms the body, and it is wonderful for colds and flu.

NOTE: It's best to avoid ginger if you have gallstones or are taking a blood thinner. Pregnant women should take small amounts or consult their midwife or herbalist.

GINKGO BILOBA LEAF TEA

Gingko biloba leaf tea increases blood and oxygen circulation to all parts of the body, including the brain, thereby improving memory and easing the symptoms of Alzheimer's disease, headaches, and depression. It helps improve the transmission of information at a nerve cell level, thus improving mental performance. Ginkgo has been shown to improve the mental clarity of geriatric subjects and of people with attention deficit disorder. Ginkgo contains the flavonoids, ginkgolide, quercitin, and kaempferol. Flavonoids are compounds found in fruits, vegetables, and herbs that have powerful antioxidant, anti-inflammatory, antiviral, antifungal, and antitumor activities. Three important flavonoids in ginkgo are ginkgolide, quercetin, and kaempferol. Ginkgo has wonderful nutrients that are excellent for the brain, including manganese, phosphorus, potassium, and zinc. It contains vitamins A, B_1, B_2, niacin (helps circulation), and C.

NOTE: Children twelve years old and younger should not take gingko; nor should those using pain killers or blood thinning medicines.

PANAX GINSENG ROOT TEA

Panax ginseng root tea is a wonderful tonic for the immune system. It has been used in Asia since ancient times as a tonic, stimulant, and digestive aid. Panax ginseng is the only true ginseng and there are American, Chinese, and Korean panax ginsengs. Siberian ginseng, which is much less expensive, has similar properties, but it is important to note that it's not a true ginseng. There are two types of Panax ginseng, white and red. Red ginseng is made from the carmel-colored steamed root and is resistant to the invasion of worms and fungi. White ginseng has had the skin peeled off and is made from the dried underlying white part of the root. It is the red ginseng that is more commonly used in Oriental medicine. Panax ginseng contains phytochemicals called ginsenosides, saponins, panaxans, flavonoids, and volatol oils that work together as antioxidants, antiinflammatories, and immunity builders. They help to strengthen both male and female reproductive organs as well as the adrenal glands. Ginseng has been used to enhance physical endurance, increase energy levels, elevate mood, and improve memory. Ginseng root tea stimulates blood circulation and improves energy levels. Start slowly with ginseng; use small amounts at first. Studies have shown an absence of harmful effects, but some people may experience a feeling of hypertension. NOTE: Ginseng should not be used by anxious, nervous, or hyperactive people. People should avoid caffeine while using ginseng. Ginseng should not be taken if using aspirin or blood-thinning medications. Ginseng may exaggerate the effects of antipsychotic medication so they should not be taken together. It should not be taken if one is using an antidepressant. Ginseng may block the pain-reducing effects of morphine. It should not be used by children twelve years old and under. It should not be used by anyone with a heart problem, high blood pressure, insomnia, or asthma. Pregnant women and nursing mothers should avoid ginseng.

GOLDENSEAL ROOT TEA

Goldenseal boosts the immune system. It contains an alkaloid constituent called berberine that has been widely studied. According to research, berberine has powerful antibiotic, anti-inflammatory, and antibacterial properties. Goldenseal root tea soothes irritated mucous membranes and is helpful in healing gum diseases, yeast infections, colitis, colds, and flu. Note: Goldenseal also has been known to raise blood pressure. Do not use goldenseal for more than two to three weeks at a time, and do not use it at all in cases of high blood pressure. It should not be used in cases of insomnia or by pregnant women or nursing mothers. Since goldenseal is endangered, Oregon grape root is a good alternative.

GOTA KOLA NUT. LEAF, AND ROOT TEA

Gota Kola is native to India and has been used in Ayurvedic medicine for thousands of years. In China, it has been called a miracle elixir of life. Gota Kola is a great blood purifier and helps relieve high blood pressure. It decreases fatigue, increases sex drive, and helps with combating depression. Gota Kola contains several important sterols, including beta-sitosterol, campesterol, and stigmasterol. These natural lipids help lower cholesterol and nourish the brain and nervous system, enhancing memory. Important antibiotic properties are found in Gota Kola that support the immune system and promote wound healing. It is very alkaline in nature and may help reduce acidity in the body. Gota Kola contains beta-carotene, amino acids, vitamins B, C, and K as well as the minerals iron, calcium, magnesium, phosphorus, potassium, selenium, and zinc.

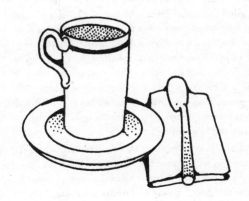

GRAVEL ROOT TEA

Gravel root tea is used to strengthen the urinary tract and dissolve stones. It can be very beneficial in slowing the frequency of excessive nighttime urination, as well as with enuresis (the involuntary discharge of urine). Gravel root contains the phytonutrients eupatorin and euparin, which work together as a urinary tract tonic. Gravel root helps strengthen the prostate and dissolve kidney stones.

GREEN LEAF TEA

Research shows that green tea is high in polyphenols, which are powerful antioxidants that help fight free radicals. Free radicals can cause disease and premature aging. Green tea has been shown to ptevent the growth of tumors, lower blood pressure, and prevent blood clots. Green tea also assists in fighting bacteria in the mouth that can produce cavities. It is antiviral and can aid in fighting influenza as well as the common cold. It is high in vitamin C and the bioflavonoids rutin and quercitin. It also contains B vitamins, potassium, zinc, and iron. Green tea does contain some caffeine, so drink it in the morning. It might help you kick the coffee habit. Decaffeinated green tea is also available.

HAWTHORNE BERRY TEA

Hawthorne berry tea is great for the heart. It is high in bioflavonoids, which build and repair connective tissue of arterial walls. It also helps reduce cholesterol levels and lower high blood pressure. Hawthorn contains amino acids, potassium, calcium, magnesium, and zinc as well as B vitamins and vitamin C.

HOREHOUND LEAF AND FLOWER TEA

Horehound is a must-have during times of coughs, respiratory infections, and colds. Horehound tea contains limonene, the same oil that is found in citrus and it helps clear the sinuses and lungs of mucus and helps the throat rid itself of thick phlegm. It soothes a sore throat and helps ease a cough. It contains tannins, which are antimicrobial and help the body to ward off infection. Horehound tea, made from leaves or flowers that also contain pectin, may help cleanse the liver, reduce indigestion, and rid the body of jaundice. Key nutrients in horehound are vitamins A, B, C, and E and potassium, and iron. NOTE: Use no more than one or two cups of horehound a day for no more than four to six weeks. Larger amounts may cause heartbeat irregularities. If you have heart concerns, consult your physician before taking.

HORSETAIL PLANT TEA

The horsetail plant, also called shavegrass, looks like a green horse's tail. Use only the plant, not the roots, for tea. When I hiked in the Swiss Alps in the summertime, we broke open the stem of a horsetail plant and used the white creamy milk inside to relieve rashes we got from the nettles that grew all around. High in silicon, zinc, phosphorus, calcium, and fluorine, horsetail taken internally helps repair weak or broken bones and strengthen the skin, hair, teeth, and fingernails. It is high in vitamin C, has been used to help stop bleeding, and can be very beneficial in treating ulcers.

JUNIPER BERRY TEA

Juniper berry tea is great for the bladder and helps heal bladder infections and prostate disorders. A natural diuretic, it releases fluids from the body when there is excessive swelling. It aids in relieving indigestion and gas. Its anti-inflammatory qualities help relieve arthritic and rheumatic pains. It is also useful in treating gout. Juniper berries are high in the antibacterial tannins, beta-carotene, and bioflavonoids. It contains chromium, which helps balance blood sugar, potassium, selenium, calcium,

Continued ➡

zinc, B vitamins, and vitamin C. NOTE: Large amounts of juniper berry tea—more than two cups per day over extended periods of more than four weeks—may intet-fere with iron absorption. Avoid juniper berry tea if you have a kidney disease until you have consulted with a knowledgeable health practitioner. Do not drink juniper berry tea during pregnancy.

Kava Kava Root Tea

Kava kava is a wonderful tea that contains the phytonutrients kavapyrones and kavalactones, which help to relax the nervous system thereby making it a natural sleep aid. Kava kava helps relax tight muscles and relieve pain. It's great for anyone with a pinched nerve, muscle spasms, muscle aches, or cramping. It could be very useful during moments of anxiety and panic. Kava kava also contains cinnamic acid, which is a natural antiseptic. NOTE: Should not be used with alcohol, sleep medications, or antidepressants. May cause drowsiness (if so, use only at night when you are ready for sleep). Not for those eighteen years old or younger. Pregnant women and nursing mothers should avoid.

Kombucha Tea

Kombucha tea is made from a mushroomlike fungus along with black or green tea, apple cider vinegar, and sugar. Some health food stores carry the brew ready-made. It has been reported to boost energy levels, strengthen immune function, normalize blood pressure, lower cholesterol, bring hair color back, ease arthritis pain, and fight AIDS and cancer. It has antiinflammatory and antimicrobial properties. It helps fight bacteria, fungi, and viruses. NOTE: Kombucha should not be taken by those with a weak liver. It is a powerful detoxifier and will pull toxins from the body and pass them through the liver. Because the tea is made with white sugar, people with blood-sugar imbalances and diabetics should use it with care. Pregnant or nursing women should not drink it at all because it contains some caffeine and alcohol and thereby may cause a toxic effect on the liver. Children twelve years and under should not take kombucha for the same reasons. Alcoholics in recovery should avoid kombucha because the small amount of alcohol contained in it could have a negative reaction in their bodies.

Lemon Balm Leaf Tea

Lemon balm leaf tea, also known as Melissa tea, contains balsamic oils and tannins that have antibacterial and antiviral properties that help fight colds, cold sores, and flu. It contains phytonutrients called terpines that help relax nerves and relieve feelings of anxiety or panic, relieve headaches (possibly migraines), and if taken at night, promote restful sleep. It contains another nutrient called eugenol which calms muscle spasms and aids with digestive disorders, such as cramping, flatulence, and nausea. Lemon balm has been effective with the relief symptoms associated with hyperthyroidism. Because of its special essential oils, it can help gently break a fever in children. NOTE: No toxic effects are known, but this herb should not be taken by pregnant women or nursing mothers. It also should not be taken with barbiturates or sleeping medicines, as it can enhance their sedative effects.

Lemongrass Leaf lea

Lemongrass leaves are high in lemongrass oil and the phytochemicals citral, geraniol, terpineol, limonene, spononin, and the bioflavonoids quercitin and rutin. The synergistic effects of these nutrients help reduce fevers, relieve headaches, soothe digestive disorders, and reduce flatulence. Its antispasmodic qualities may help relieve abdominal muscle cramps during menstruation. The oil

also has antifungal and antibacterial properties. It is high in potassium, calcium, magnesium, and zinc.

Lemon Verbena Leaf Tea

Lemon verbena leaf tea is an astringent herb with volatile oils that relieve cramping, including that which occurs during menstruation, and nausea, and it soothes the nervous system. It contains the phytonutrients limonene, geraniol, and terpineol, great antioxidants that help clear a stuffy nose or congested bronchial tubes. These phytonutrients have anti-inflammatory properties as well.

Licorice Root Tea

Licorice is a sweet, very nutritious root that helps to balance the adrenal gland, protect the liver, and dispel depression. The root can be chewed during hikes to help maintain energy levels. It also helps smokers kick the smoking habit and not gain weight. People who crave caffeine or sweets or are hypoglycemic can chew on the root as well to eliminate cravings and regulate blood sugar. The tea is delicious and can be added to other teas to sweeten them. Licorice root tea contains camphor, is antispasmotic, and reduces muscle spasms, soothes the digestive tract, helps heal ulcers, relieves nausea and gastritis, and helps ease colitis. Licorice root can also relieve sore throats, allergies, and asthma, help expel mucus, and fight colds, inflammation, and bronchitis. Licorice root contains a nutrient called glycyrrhizin that is known to be antiviral. Another one of its constituents is manitol, which helps scavenge free radicals and may act as a natural diuretic. Licorice root contains salicylic acid, the same ingredient in aspirin that relieves pain and fights inflammation. It also contains antioxidants including beta-carotene and quercitin. Another phytonutrient in licorice is geraniol, a natural antioxidant that may help prevent the growth of tumors. It is rich in nutrients including iron, calcium, magnesium, phosphorus, potassium, selenium, silicon, and zinc, as well as B vitamins and vitamin C. NOTE: Licorice root should not be used on a daily basis as it can raise the blood pressure. It should not be used by people with high blood pressure, glaucoma, diabetes, or heart disease. It should be avoided by people that have seizures or who have had a stroke. It should not be taken by pregnant women or nursing mothers.

Linden Flower Tea

Linden flower tea helps calm tension and relax the body because of its antispasmodic properties. It is high in flavonoids including quercetin and kaempferol, as well as p-coumaric acid, that act as diaphoretics that promote sweating. These nutrients work together to reduce fever and congestion during a cold or flu and soothe a sore throat.

Lobelia Leaf and Flower Tea

Lobelia tea, made from the leaves and flowers of the Lobelia plant, is excellent for healing coughing, wheezing, colds, bronchitis, sore throats, asthma, and pneumonia. It helps the bronchial muscles relax and liquefies thickened mucus that needs to be expelled from the sinuses or lungs. Lobelia tea can also help people addicted to nicotine let go of the habit with few withdrawal symptoms. Lobelia contains the active ingredient lobeline, which is similar to nicotine in its effect on the central nervous system. It stimulates the adrenal glands to release the hormone epinephrine, which relaxes and dilates the bronchioles (air passages in the lungs), thereby increasing respiration.

Lobelia is an herb to be respected and should be used in small amounts. Use no more than one-third teaspoon of dried lobelia to eight ounces of hot water. Sip it slowly and drink no more than

three cups per day. NOTE: Too much lobelia causes vomiting, dizziness, and nausea. Consult your healthcare practitioner before taking. Children should not take lobelia unless under the care of a qualified physician. Lobelia should not be taken by pregnant women or nursing mothers.

Ma Huang Stem Tea

Ma huang stem tea has been used as a bronchial dilator and decongestant to help reduce the symptoms of asthma, allergies, bronchitis, colds, and flu. It has also been used in weight reduction programs because of its ability to suppress the appetite and stimulate the metabolism. Ma huang contains two widely used alkaloids called ephedrine and pseudo-ephedrine. Ephedrine stimulates the thyroid gland and nervous system, thereby increasing the metabolic rate and suppressing the appetite. It can also alleviate feelings of fatigue and depression, and increase energy levels, alertness, and perception. Psuedo-ephedrine is a nasal decongestant and bronchodilator. It is a key ingredient in several over-the-counter cold and flu remedies.

NOTE: Ma huang should not be used by people with high blood pressure, heart disease, diabetes, prostate disorders, or thyroid problems. Nor should it be used by people on medications for hypertension or depression. Ma huang can cause insomnia and anxiety, so it should be used in small amounts and with respect. Consult your healthcare practitioner.

Malva Leaf Tea

Malva leaf tea is high in vitamin A, which helps to strengthen the eyes and the immune system. Malva contains flavonoids and demulcent qualities and is excellent for relieving inflammation in the mucous membranes. It is said to loosen phlegm in congested lungs. It soothes the digestive and urinary tract and acts as a mild diuretic. It has a mild laxative effect and works well as a laxative for children. When combined with eucalyptus in tea, it is an excellent remedy for coughs and other chest ailments.

Marigold Petal Tea (Calendula)

There are different varieties of marigolds (including African) which are often called American (*Tagetes erecta*) because they grow in North America, or French (*Tagetes patula*). The marigold that is used for tea and medicinal purposes is called the pot marigold or *Calendula officinalis*. Actually the pot marigold, though called marigold, is not a true marigold. It has beautiful orange and yellow flowers similar to the marigold family. The pot marigold petal tea contains calendula oil and vitamin E, which help soothe ulcers, lower or break fevers, and regulate the menstrual cycle. It also helps alleviate skin disorders, such as boils and shingles, and soften varicose veins and hemorrhoids. It has salicylic acid, which gives it antiseptic and antifungal properties that make it useful in reducing infections and treating gingivitis (gum disease), *Candida albicans*, yeast, acne, and athlete's foot. It also contains beta-carotene, which is an excellent antioxidant that fights the signs of aging and assists in healing wounds and eczema. The tea is mucilaginous and soothing to the digestive tract, especially in cases of colitis, diverticulitis, and ulcers. This soothing tea also makes a wonderful eyewash for dry burning eyes.

Marshmallow Flower, Leaf, and Root Tea

Marshmallow root tea soothes inflammation in the body. As marshmallow root is mucilagenous and slippery, it is great for relieving ulcers, diverticulitis, or colitis. It contains beta-carotene, quercitin,

Continued ➡

salicylic acid, and tannins, which make it an antioxidant and antimicrobial. It helps fight kidney and bladder infections, sore throat, and sinusitis, and helps the body release mucus from the lungs. Key nutrients in marshmallow flower are vitamin C, calcium, magnesium, potassium, selenium, and iron.

MOTHERWORT LEAF AND FLOWER TEA

Motherwort tea, made from leaves and flowers, is great for strengthening the heart because of its special oils and the antioxidants quercitin and vitamin C. It slows heart palpitations and a rapid heartbeat. It can also help lower blood pressure. It contains alkaloids, derivatives of amino acids, which may have a sedative effect. This tea calms muscle spasms, including leg cramps. It is great support for women's health, easing symptoms of PMS, menstrual cramping, and the hot flashes associated with menopause. It helps relax the nerves, calm anxiety, reduce stress, and ease depression. Motherwort may calm a hyperactive thyroid. The healing constituents of motherwort are rutin, which strengthens connective tissue and is especially helpful with hemorrhoids and varicosities, and alpha-pinene and tannins, which have wonderful antibacterial properties.

MULLEIN LEAF AND FLOWER TEA

Mullein is an exotic-looking plant, tall with soft velvety green leaves. It contains the phytonutrients hesperidin, which strengthens veins; coumarin, which has antifungal and blood vessel strengthening properties; beta-carotene, an antioxidant; and saponins, which have antibacterial and cholesterol lowering abilities. The mullein oil in mullein tea is a valuable destroyer of germs and viruses and has even been known to help get rid of warts. It is also high in mucilage. Because of these nutrients and its slippery consistency, mullein is a great decongestant and is very helpful in ridding mucus from the lungs and sinuses. It soothes the membranes in the throat and entire intestinal tract and may act as a mild laxative. It has been used for coughs, asthma, influenza, and urinary tract infections. Mullein has sedative properties and helps relax the body and relieve abdominal cramps.

To prepare the tea, use two heaping teaspoons in eight ounces of boiling water. Cover and let it steep for five minutes, strain, then drink.

NETTLE LEAF FLOWER. ROOT TEA

If you are going out to pick nettles, be sure to wear gloves. They are full of little stingers that are high in formic acid, which can cause a skin rash and itching. If you accidentally touch nettles, there are usually some horsetail plants growing nearby. Break open the stem of the horsetail, and use the creamy juice to coat the stinging area of your skin. This will greatly reduce the rash and promote healing.

Once nettles are dried or cooked for about eight minutes, they lose their stinging quality. Nettles, also called stinging nettles, ate high in vitamins C, K, pantothenic acid (B$_5$), and E, and minerals, including iron, calcium, magnesium, phosphorus, and potassium, and can be very beneficial in treating anemia. A cup of nettles tea may help prevent internal bleeding because the high dosage of calcium acts as a "knitter" to repair tissues (check with your physician). The tea helps purify and build the blood. Nettle tea can also be beneficial in calming allergic reactions. It can even help stop the itching and burning that often comes with allergies. Because of its rich nutritional content, which includes protein, natural lecithin, and essential fatty acids, nursing mothers will produce more milk while drinking this tea. Nettles tea has been know to stimulate hair growth. In cases of baldness, drink the tea and rub it into the hair follicles as well.

OATSTRAW TEA

A horse that eats oats has a shiny coat, silky mane, and great stamina. Oatstraw contains the minerals silicon, calcium, iron, copper, zinc, and magnesium, as well as the B complex vitamins. It strengthens and nourishes the skin, hair, fingernails, connective tissue, cartilage, and bones. It can also help people with hair loss or skin troubles such as acne, dandruff, eczema, and psoriasis. It can improve the sperm count in men. Oatstraw tea is a super nerve tonic that has a calming effect and strengthens the brain and nervous system. It has been known to decrease or stop bed-wetting. It is great for anyone who is trying to stop smoking, as it lessens withdrawal symptoms. Oatstraw tea is wonderful for athletes or anyone desiring more energy and stamina. This tea can be used as a delicious base for soups and broths.

ORANGE PEEL TEA

The inner portion of an orange peel is high in bioflavonoids, which build connective tissue, preventing bruising and promoting the healing of wounds and tissues. Orange peel tea can relieve flatulence and improve digestion. Be sure to use organic peelings that are free from chemicals.

OREGON GRAPE ROOT TEA

Oregon grape root is a powerful natural antibiotic with many of the same qualities as goldenseal. They are both high in berberine and Oregon grape root also contains tannins, which help strengthen the immune system and fight bacteria. Oregon grape root tea is a blood purifier and is remedial in treating skin disorders, including acne, cold sores, psoriasis, and eczema. It strengthens a weak liver and gallbladder and aids in digestion. NOTE: Pregnant women and nursing mothers, people with high blood pressure, insomnia, and people with an overactive liver should not drink this tea.

PARSLEY LEAF, STEM, AND ROOT TEA

Parsley leaf, stem, and root is a natural diuretic that is rich in chlorophyll. It helps cleanse the liver, kidneys, and bladder and fight urinary tract infections. It helps stop bed-wetting. The root is particularly helpful in dissolving stones. The entire parsley plant, including leaves, stems, and roots, is high in iron, phosphorus, calcium, manganese, B vitamins, and vitamins A, C, and K, making it great for building blood. The tea is also a wonderful digestive aid, helps relieve gas, and freshens the breath.

Note: Parsley tea can stop the flow of milk in nursing mothers. They should use the tea only after they have stopped nursing and are ready for their milk to dry up. Pregnant women should avoid using parsley tea completely because it can cause early labor.

PAN D'ARCO BARK TEA

Pau d'Arco bark tea has also been called La Pacho, Ipe Roxo, Taheebo, and Tecoma. It comes from the Pau d'Arco tree that grows in the forests of Brazil. This same tree grows in Argentina and is called La Pacho. Native tribes used it to treat cancers. Two primary active compounds in pau d'arco that have antifungal, antibacterial, antiparasitic, and anticancer properties are lapchol and beta-lapachone. Beta-sitosterol, a phytochemical in pau d'arco, helps lower cholesterol and is a natural anti-inflammatory. It has been reported to be beneficial in fighting Candidiasis in the intestines and vaginal tract. It has proved very helpful in treating diabetes, liver disorders, lung congestion, skin diseases, ulcers, immune dysfunction, infections, warts, smoker's cough, and allergies.

PEPPERMINT AND SPEAIMINT LEAF TEA

The menthol oil (called carvone) in these delightful teas helps them to soothe the digestive system, relieve heartburn, cramping, nausea, and flatulence. Peppermint and spearmint leaf teas are also great for relieving menstrual discomfort and morning sickness. They contain niacin, which is known to stimulate circulation and ease headaches. The oils and tannins in these teas give them antifungal, antiviral, antibacterial, and antiparasitic properties. Tannins are useful in soothing the digestive tract in cases of diarrhea, constipation, ulcers, and colitis. They can help heal colds, flu, and upper respiratory tract infections. Children tend to like spearmint tea because it's milder in taste. It can help them with the relief of stomachaches, coughing, and sinus congestion.

RED CLOVER TEA

Red clover is a natural blood purifier and tonic and contains salicylic acid, which has anti-inflammatory and antiseptic properties. It helps fight infection, cancers, and tumors. Red clover tea is great for helping heal skin conditions such as acne, eczema, and psoriasis. It is also wonderful for strengthening the immune system in both adults and children. Red clover has been used to treat asthma, bronchitis, pneumonia, arthritis, and gout. Its antispasmodic properties make it useful in treating coughs. Red clover tea can be beneficial to those who are trying to lose weight because it is a natural appetite suppressant. It is a good source of beta-carotene, calcium, chromium, magnesium, potassium, phosphorus, niacin, and vitamin C.

RED RASPBERRY LEAF TEA

Red raspberry leaf has often been called the herb for women because it helps stop frequent and excessive menstrual bleeding and relieves menstrual cramps. It can also relieve hot flashes. Red raspberry leaf strengthens and tones the uterus wall, helping to ease labor pains and facilitate childbirth. Pregnant women should not drink red raspberry leaf tea before their eighth month of pregnancy unless advised differently by their doctor or midwife. After pregnancy, because of its rich content of calcium, iron, phosphorus, the B vitamins, vitamin D, and vitamin E, red raspberry leaf enriches breast milk and helps the uterus return to its normal size and tone. Red raspberry leaf strengthens bones, skin, fingernails, and teeth, making it especially beneficial for children and elderly people. It is helpful in soothing urinary tract inflammations, treating colds, cold sores, flu, diarrhea, ulcers, bleeding gums, and colitis. NOTE: Herbalists may advise small amounts of raspberry leaf tea after the first trimester and increase the dosage during the last trimester depending on each individual, her history, and her needs.

ROSEHIPS TEA

Rosehips tea is higher in vitamin C and bioflavonoids than oranges. Bioflavonoids help build connective tissue. Rosehips tea is useful in preventing bruising, treating sore throats, colds, flu, and sinus infections.

SAGE LEAF TEA

The term sage describes someone old and wise. The herb sage is high in minerals, including manganese, phosphorus, and magnesium, that help improve mental clarity and memory. Sage contains the phytochemicals, saponins, rosmarinic acid, and tannins, which make it an antioxidant, an anti-inflammatory, and an antiseptic, and it helps with colds, cold sores, flu, and sore throats. Sage leaf tea can be used as a gargle to heal sore throats

Continued ➡

and as a mouthwash to heal gingivitis. It contains volatile oils that help improve digestion. Sage contains estrogenic substances that make it useful in relieving hot flashes during menopause, relieving menstrual cramps, and promoting blood flow if periods are delayed.

NOTE: Sage may be taken safely for a week or two, after which it should be used only periodically. Long-term regular use may inhibit the absorption of iron and other minerals. Pregnant women should not take sage because it stimulates the uterus. Nursing mothers should avoid sage leaf tea as it can dry up breast milk. Epileptics should avoid sage because it contains an antiseptic oil called thujone, which can trigger seizures.

Sarsaparilla Root Tea

Sarsaparilla is a blood purifier and tones the liver. It contains the phytochemicals stigmasterol, saponin, and beta-sitosterol, which work synergistically in the tea and help with skin conditions such as psoriasis, eczema, and acne. The tea also helps heal mouth sores and ulcers. Sarsaparilla may help the body utilize calcium efficiently, and it eases rheumatic pains. Sarsaparilla has been used throughout history to treat syphilis. It is rich in iron, phosphorus, zinc, selenium, and potassium. Boiling this tea causes it to lose its healing properties. Pour hot water over the tea and let it steep for one hour.

Saw Palmetto Berry Tea

Saw palmetto berry tea comes from a small palm tree and is very beneficial in healing the prostate gland, especially if it is swollen or enlarged. It contains the phytonutrients, sterols, beta-carotene, and ferulic acid, which are powerful antioxidants that help protect cells against the harmful effects of free radicals. It contains sterols and tannins, natural antiseptics which together help inhibit the action of testosterone on the prostate that contributes to swelling. It may act to relieve the need for frequent urination caused by an enlarged prostate gland pressing on the bladder. Saw palmetto is helpful in healing urinary tract infections and impotence. It has also been shown to help reduce unwanted hair growth in women.

Senna Leaf Tea

Senna leaf tea is used to relieve constipation. The active constituents in senna are sennosides, mucilage, volatile oil, and flavonoids. It is a powerful cathartic and stimulates peristalsis in the intestinal tract. However, it should be used seldom, if ever, and never on a regular basis to avoid laxative dependency. While using senna, some people have come to depend on it for bowel function without dealing with the true cause of the constipation. When they stop taking senna, they find their bowels have become dependent on the action of the senna rather than initiating peristalsis on their own. Senna may be used for occasional constipation but for no more than a week. If constipation has not diminished after a week, consult a knowledgeable health practitioner to determine what is causing the constipation. Senna is very harsh and should be combined with ginger and cinnamon to help prevent the abdominal cramping it can cause. Note: Pregnant women should never ingest senna because of the pressure it imposes on the intestinal tract. Senna is a stimulant, and it can keep sensitive people awake at night. Do not take if you have insomnia, inflammatory bowel disease, Crohn's disease, ulcerative colitis, abdominal pain, or nausea, or if you're experiencing vomiting. If you are nursing, consult your doctor before taking senna. Consult a physician before giving senna to children.

Shepherd's Purse Tea

Shepherd's purse tea, made from the whole plant, is high in vitamin K and acts as an astringent to help stop hemorrhaging, especially from menopausal disorders, endometriosis, or postpartum bleeding after childbirth. It can help stop the bleeding that often accompanies colitis as well. Shepherd's purse is high in chlorophyll, a natural anti-inflammatory and is a healing herb for urinary inflammations such as cystitis.

Skullcap Tea

Skullcap nourishes and soothes the nerves because of its large content of calcium and magnesium and vitamins B_1 and B_2. It can be used for treating convulsions, epilepsy, hysteria, anxiety attacks, stress, and insomnia. It is also very helpful in relieving headaches, muscle cramps, painful menstrual cramps, and nervous stomachs. Skullcap can relieve the withdrawal symptoms of alcohol and drugs.

To prepare skullcap tea, use one teaspoonful to twelve ounces of water. Never drink more than three half-cups per day because it can cause giddiness and an irregular pulse. Use only organic skullcap to ensure that it has not been combined with toxic herbs. NOTE: Skullcap should not be used by children eight years old and under.

Slippery Elm Inner Bark Tea

Slippery elm inner bark makes a slippery, mucilaginous tea that is wonderfully soothing to a sore, irritated throat and can help stop coughing. It is delicious with a little honey. Slippery elm inner bark tea contains mucilage and certain types of lipids, called campesterol, that soothe the entire digestive tract and can help heal ulcers, colitis, and hemorrhoids. Slippery elm inner bark tea is also very nourishing, and it can be given to anyone who is having trouble keeping down food. It also can be made into a porridge. Add cardamom and cinnamon for added flavor or to reduce nausea. This gentle herb can nourish tiny babies and the elderly. It is rich in nutrients including calcium, magnesium, phosphorus, potassium, manganese, iron, zinc, selenium, beta-carotene, and vitamin C.

Thyme Leaf Tea

Thyme leaf tea contains the oil thymol and the phytonutrients, tannin and caprylic acid, which are antiseptic and antifungal. It can help fight *Candida albicans* yeast infections and helps to relieve indigestion, gas, and diarrhea. It also helps clear the respiratory tract of mucus and infections. Thyme leaves have beta-carotene and vitamin C, which are wonderful antioxidants, as well as amino acids, essential fatty acids, calcium, magnesium, selenium, potassium, and zinc.

Turmeric Root Tea

Turmeric root tea contains the phytonutrient, curcumin, known for its anti-inflammatory properties that can help relieve the muscular pain associated with fibromyalgia. It also helps cleanse the liver and dissolves gallstones. Turmeric root tea regulates menstrual cycles, improves circulation, and can help alleviate arthritis. Other phytochemicals in tumeric are beta-carotene, an antioxidant; borneal, a digestive aide; alpha-pinene, an antibacterial agent; limone, an oil that helps cleanse the liver and lungs; and eugenol, which helps calm muscle spasms. It is a good source of vitamin C as well as iron, calcium, zinc, potassium, and phosphorus.

Uva Ursi Leaf Tea

Uva ursi leaf tea helps heal urinary tract infections, including nephritis and cystitis and prostate disorders. Uva ursi contains the phytochemicals ellagic acid, beta-carotene, and quercitin, which have powerful antioxidant properties and which protect the cells from free radical damage. Other phytochemicals are myricetin, which is an anti-inflammatory, and ursolic acid, which has antifungal, antiviral, and antibacterial properties. Uva ursi contains iron, phosphorus, potassium selenium, and calcium as well as vitamins C and B. NOTE: This tea is not recommended for pregnant women or nursing mothers. Children twelve or under should avoid it as well.

Valerian Root Tea

Valerian root tea is a wonderful relaxant. It contains the phytochemicals valerenone, valepotriates, and valerenic acid, which have a mild sedative effect and help promote peaceful sleep. Because of its calming abilities, it has been known to relieve cramps, coughs, high blood pressure, anxiety, and pain. Valerian root is very bitter and may be combined with cinnamon or ginger to make it more palatable. Valerian root contains fatty acids, calcium, magnesium, potassium, zinc, B vitamins, and vitamin C. NOTE: It should not be taken with sleep medications or alcohol.

Vervain Leaf Tea

Vervain leaf tea contains the phytochemicals verbenalin and verbenin, which help soothe and calm the nerves and relieve menstrual cramping. It contains the oils geraniol and limonene, which work to cleanse the liver and sinuses, promote menstruation, and the flow of mother's milk. Note: It may stimulate uterine contractions so should not be used during pregnancy.

Yarrow Leaf Tea

Yarrow leaf tea contains the volatile oils camphor and linalool, which promote sweating and can be used to reduce fevers associated wtih colds and flu. Yarrow is high in minerals including calcium, magnesium, and potassium that help stop cramping. It contains salicylic acid and tannins that are anti-inflammatoty and antibacterial and has been used to treat urinary infections. Yarrow also contains flavonoids that help tighten tissue and can be used topically as a styptic to help stop bleeding.

Yellow Dock Root Tea

Yellow dock root tea is high in iron and great for anemia. It is high in the antioxidants quercitin and beta-carotene and helps cleanse the liver and blood. It has rutin, which tightens tissues, and tannins that fight bacteria so it is helpful in healing skin problems such as eczema, psoriasis, acne, and herpes.

Yucca Root Tea

Yucca root tea is anti-inflammatory as well as antirheumatic, which makes it an excellent tea for healing arthritis and rheumatism. It can be a laxative, so combine it with cinnamon and ginger. It contains the antioxidant phytonutrients, beta-carotene, tannin, and sarsapogenin. It is rich in calcium, magnesium, potassium, phosphorus, iron, and zinc. It also has some B vitamins and vitamin C.

Watermelon Seed Tea

Watermelon seed tea is a natural dieuretic. It cleans and flushes out the kidneys and bladder. NOTE: To make, grind seeds and pour a pint of boiling water over one tablespoon. Steep for fifteen minutes, strain, and drink.

—From *Health Is Your Birthright*

Continued ➡

TARGETED NUTRITION

Ellen Tart-Jensen

Tool Kit for Choosing Healing Therapies

In this tool kit, you will find the tools you need to help heal the organs, nerves, muscles, and bones of the body. For each body part, you will be given a nutritional plan and specific physical exercises as well as emotional therapies to follow. Remember, the body works as one whole unit. While working with any one particular body part, you will be helping the rest of your body as well. For example, when we heal the adrenal glands, it helps improve the work of the heart and nervous system as well. Each part of the body needs the specific nutrients it requires to be strong. It needs exercise and movement to promote circulation and strengthening, it also needs for you to work with any emotions that may be keeping it from healing. We are physical, emotional, and spiritual beings, and we need to attend to all these areas in order to know health as our birthright.

Adrenal Glands

The two adrenal glands are small yellow masses of tissue that are triangular in shape and, true to their name (ad means near and renal means kidney), are situated on top of each kidney in the lower back. They are part of the endocrine system, which is made up of glands that secrete hormones directly into the bloodstream. Each adrenal gland is divided into two parts. The outer region is called the adrenal cortex. The inner core is known as the adrenal medulla. Although they are together anatomically, the cortex and the medulla are made of different types of tissue and function as distinct glands. Both help the body deal with stress and both help regulate metabolism.

The Adrenal Cortex: Vital to Life

The adrenal cortex's functions are vital. The adrenal cortex is divided into three zones which can be seen under a microscope. The outer zone secretes a hormone called aldosterone, which helps maintain blood pressure and blood volume by inhibiting the amount of sodium excreted in the urine. When there is a disturbance in the adrenal glands' functioning, too much sodium is excreted into the urine. This causes water to leave the body in large quantities, and the blood volume can become so low, a person could die of low blood pressure.

The middle and inner zones of the adrenal cortex work together and secrete several important hormones, including hydrocortisone, corticosterone, and androgen. Hydrocortisone, or cortisol, regulates metabolism and controls the way the body utilizes carbohydrates, proteins, and fats. Cortisol promotes production of glucose from amino acids and fats in the liver. This ensures adequate fuel supplies for the cells when the body is under stress. Hydrocortisone and corticosterone help suppress inflammatory reactions and regulate the immune system. They will act to suppress the immune system if it becomes overly reactive. Hydrocortisone counteracts inflammation, pain, and swelling of the joints due to arthritis and bursitis. Adrenocorticotropic

hormone, or Acth, produced by the pituitary gland in the brain, controls the secretion of hydrocortisone. Hydrocortisone is secreted in varying amounts throughout a twenty-four hour cycle. A minimal amount is secreted at midnight, rising to a peak at 6:00 A.M., then falling slowly throughout the day.

The adrenal cortex produces a small amount of female hormones in men and male hormones in women. A tumor in this gland can cause an excessive amount to be produced, causing feminine characteristics in males and masculine characteristics in females. Androgen hormones found in the adrenal cortex help stimulate the development of male sex characteristics. When the adrenal gland is unhealthy, it can produce an excessive amount of androgen, which can cause acne. In women, an excessive amount of androgen can also cause the growth of body hair on the face, arms, chest, or abdomen.

The Adrenal Medulla: Important for Fight or Flight

Within the inner core of each adrenal gland is an adrenal medulla. The adrenal medulla's tissue develops from nerve tissue and it is controlled by the sympathetic nervous system, the body's first line of defense against stress. The adrenal medulla secretes the hormones epinephrine, or adrenaline, and norepinephrine, or noradrenaline, in response to sympathetic nerve stimulation. Epinephrine is also released in response to hypoglycemia. These hormones are secreted when a person is physically injured, frightened, angry, or under stress. The adrenal medulla prepares a person physiologically to deal with threatening situations. Epinephrine and norepinephrine bring about all the responses necessary for fight or flight. People have been known to perform amazing feats, such as carrying a heavy piece of furniture out of a burning house or lifting a car to free a child trapped underneath.

The adrenal medullary hormones cause blood to be routed to those organs necessary for emergency action. Blood vessels to the skin become constricted, thus protecting the body from blood loss in case of lacerations. This explains why people often look pale when they are afraid or angry. Blood vessels to the brain and muscles are dilated; increased blood flow to the brain allows the person to become instantly alert, while more blood flow to the muscles causes a person to have more stamina. Glucose and fatty acid levels rise in the blood, assuring that we have the necessary fuel for energy. All the airways become enlarged so we can breathe effectively. Epinephrine and norepinephrine are secreted daily in small amounts.

Thus, we can see how important it is to care for our adrenal glands and keep them healthy. Our ancestors used adrenaline to fight wild animals to protect their families. In today's world, people produce adrenaline while sitting at stoplights when they are late for a meeting or preparing for an examination. However, they often are not exercising to use up the adrenaline. Some stressors, such as unhappy marriages or job situations, can go on for years. Prolonged chronic stress is harmful because there are negative side effects to long-term elevated levels of cortisol. Excessive amounts of cortisol can lead to ulcers, high blood pressure, arthritis, fibromyalgia, and atherosclerosis. Excessive amounts of epinephrine can lead to exhaustion.

Nutritional Suggestions

- Avoid stimulants such as caffeine, sugar, and nicotine.
- Take chlorella and spirulina, which are high in RNA and DNA, amino acids, and chlorophyll. They rejuvenate and cleanse the adrenal glands.

- Eat raw nuts and seeds. Soak the nuts and seeds for twenty-four hours; they will be easier to digest and the nutrients will be more fully available. Blend them to make dips and salad dressings.
- Eat licorice root, dulse, and kelp.
- Ingest ionic trace minerals.
- Take vitamin B complex, pantothenic acid, calcium, magnesium, and zinc keep the nervous system calm and support the adrenal glands.
- If you are suffering from exhaustion, take tablets of raw bovine adrenal.
- Herbs that calm and strengthen the adrenals are Chinese corticeps, ashwaganda, and schizandra.

Appendix

The appendix is a narrow tube attached to the cecum, or first part of the large intestine. It is located on the lower right side of the abdomen. N. W. Walker, DSC, writes in *Become Younger*, "The function of the appendix is to provide a secretion which prevents the feces from remaining stationary in the colon; at the same time its secretion neutralizes excessive putrefactive bacteria, in much the same way that the tonsils protect the throat." Appendicitis results when bacteria get into the appendix and it becomes swollen and inflamed. This is why it is so important to eat healthfully and keep our colons clean!

Nutritional Suggestions

- Eat cabbage and drink cabbage juice.
- Eat foods that are rich in sodium, such as celery, mineral whey, strawberries, and okra.
- Eat foods that are high in fiber, such as ground flaxseeds, oat bran, rice bran, whole grains, raw vegetables, alfalfa tablets, and chlorella.
- Include slippery foods, such as aloe vera juice, slippery elm tea, and flaxseed tea in your diet.
- Eat foods that are high in friendly bacteria, such as yogurt and raw sauerkraut.
- Include antiparasitic foods, such as garlic and onions, in your diet.
- Practice colon cleansing once or twice a year, and take parasite-fighting herbs, such as wormwood, cloves, black walnut, and garlic. The cecum is often called a "worm nest" because it's where parasites tend to lodge.
- Work on preventing constipation. When the colon becomes backed up with old fecal matter, it can become impacted and block the opening of the appendix into the cecum.

Blood

The blood is the stream of life that flows through the human body. Not a single part of the body can live without this red fluid. It picks up oxygen from the lungs, where it combines with iron molecules in the hemoglobin, and then carries the oxygen to every cell in the body. The blood also collects simple nutrients that have been broken down during digestion and distributes these within the cells, where they are used to build new tissue and produce energy. The blood also picks up waste products and carbon dioxide from the cells, and carries them away. The liver and kidneys remove most of the wastes, while the lungs remove carbon dioxide. In addition, the blood fights germs that cause disease when they enter the body. Blood has an amazing ability to clot and form a protective seal over a wound, keeping more blood from escaping the body. There are about ten pints of blood in a person who weighs 160 pounds.

Continued →

Red Blood Cells

A cubic millimeter of a person's blood contains about five million red blood cells! Red blood cells are manufactured in bone marrow. When fully grown, they leave the marrow. They circulate in the bloodstream for about four months, until they use up their supply of energy and are destroyed. To constantly replace these cells, the body must manufacture about two million new blood cells every second. When the body fails to make enough new blood cells or when the amount of hemoglobin falls too low, anemia results.

White Blood Cells

White blood cells are called leucocytes, and there are between five thousand and ten thousand in a cubic millimeter of blood. There are three main types of leucocytes: granulocytes, monocytes, and lymphocytes. Granulocytes are developed in bone marrow and devour bacteria that enter the body. Monocytes are produced in both bone marrow and the spleen, and they also destroy bacteria. Lymphocytes are formed in the lymph glands, and they produce antibodies that fight bacteria.

Nutritional Suggestions

- Eat foods that are high in chlorophyll, such as green leafy vegetables, green vegetable juices, and wheatgrass juice.
- Eat foods that are high in organic iron, such as green vegetables, red beets, black cherries, black berries, figs, and prunes.
- Take chlorella, blue-green algae, green kamut, and barley grass.
- Use red clover, chaparral, and Pau d'Arco teas to cleanse the blood.

Bones

Bones form the framework for our bodies, and they are tied together by ligaments that form the joints. About two-thirds of a person's bone weight is made of minerals, especially calcium and phosphorus. The rest comes mostly from collagen, a fibrous protein. When collagen is boiled, it yields gelatin. When bones are exposed to acidity, they begin to dissolve and eventually become so soft they can be bent or tied in a knot.

There are two types of tissue in bones. The hard, outer part of the bone is called compact tissue. The inner part is spongy and called cancellous tissue. Bone tissue is very active in the body. It cleanses the blood of harmful substances, including radioactive products. New blood cells are made in bone marrow. The bones store calcium, flouride, sodium, and phosphorus...

Nutritional Suggestions

- Include almonds, sesame seeds, kale, millet, celery, raw goat's milk, and raw vegetable juices in your diet.
- Take calcium, magnesium, sodium, sulfur, silicon, potassium, and phosphorus.
- Combine boneset, horsetail, and oatstraw into a mineral-boosting tea. You can also find them in capsule form if you prefer. Follow directions on the bottle.

Eyes

The eyes are our most important organs for learning about our world. They help us see our friends and family, our surroundings, and the beauty of nature. We can even view the stars, which are trillions of miles away!

The human eyeball is about an inch in diameter. It is seated in fat, inside a space, or orbit, in the skull, surrounded by bone. Each eyeball has six muscles attached, which move it and control the size of the pupil. The conjunctiva (a mucous membrane) covers the front of the eyeball, except for the cornea. Nerves within the conjunctiva warn us if a foreign object, like a particle of dust, enters the eye.

The cornea is a clear dome of tissue over the iris, the colored part of the eye. The iris is like a thin curtain of tissue in front of the lens. The crystalline lens is about the size of a small lima bean. The pupil, which looks like a black hole, is located in the center of the iris. Light passes through the cornea, the iris, and the pupil.

The center of the eyeball holds a clear jellylike substance called the vitreous humor. The retina is located in the inner layer of the eyeball. It contains light-sensitive cells called rods and cones. Cones help us see in daylight, and rods help us see at night. Nerve fibers come together in front of the rods and cones from all parts of the retina to form the optic nerve, which goes to the spinal cord.

Eye Color

Heredity determines iris color. For example, Asian, African, and some Hispanic babies are born with brown eyes. Their eyes remain brown, though they may darken. Caucasian babies and some Hispanic babies are born with blue eyes. Some of these babies begin to develop eye pigment soon after birth. The eyes usually become their true color between six months and seven years of age. Eye pigments may continue to develop throughout one's life.

Eye Defects

Hyperopia, or farsightedness, occurs when the eyeball is too short. Focus falls behind the retina, and the person has difficulty seeing close objects clearly.

Myopia, or nearsightedness, occurs when the eyeball is too long. Focus falls in front of the retina, and distant objects appear blurred.

With astigmatism, the shapes of the cornea and lens are abnormal. Light rays focus on, in front of, and in back of the retina. This results in blurry vision for both near and distant objects.

People who are color blind cannot distinguish between certain colors. This is an inherited trait.

Strabismus, or crossed eyes, mainly occurs in children. Imbalanced eye muscles cause one eye to turn out or in. Exercises may help strabismus. A patch over one eye may also help. Glasses or surgery may be required if all other techniques are unsuccessful.

Nutritional Suggestions

- Eat lots of green leafy vegetables, including spinach and raw juices from these vegetables, as well as carrots and carrot juice.
- Eat blueberries, celery and celery juice, cabbage, and egg yolks.
- Include soaked nuts and seeds and mineral whey in your diet.
- Take bilberry (320 milligrams per day to improve night vision) and eyebright.
- Take vitamins A, B complex, C, ionic trace minerals, and zinc.
- Eat whole grains, especially brown rice.
- Take latein.
- Eat egg yolks soft-boiled or raw in shakes.
- Eat plenty of fish, kale, raw goat's milk, and brewer's yeast.
- Do a liver cleanse once or twice a year...

Heart

The heart lies in the center of the chest between the lungs. The upper, wider portion of the heart points toward the right shoulder, while the lower part points toward the left side of the body. The heart beats in the lower section. This is why many people believe incorrectly that the heart is entirely on the left side of the body. The heart is a very busy pump linked by a hundred thousand miles of pipeline. It is about the size of a fist and weighs less than a pound. It beats seventy times each minute and pumps five quarts of blood through its chambers every sixty seconds. By the end of each day, the heart has pumped more than a hundred thousand times. The heart is essential to life. As long as it pumps blood, the body receives the oxygen it needs. When the heart stops, the oxygen supply is cut off and the body dies. A buildup of fatty deposits and calcium in the arteries causes a heart attack. We must keep the heart's pipeline clean and healthy.

Nutritional Suggestions

- Avoid foods fried in fat or hydrogenated oils.
- Cook only with olive, grape seed, or coconut oil.
- Eat only oils that have been cold-pressed.
- Include flaxseed oil in your nutritional program.
- Avoid heavily processed cheeses and creams.
- Avoid margarine, and eat organic butter sparingly.
- Eat lots of raw and steamed vegetables, raw nuts and seeds, and whole grains.
- If you eat meat, eat only lean meat sparingly, baked or broiled fish, chicken, and turkey.
- Eat foods high in potassium (see "Tool Kit for Selecting Healthy Minerals").
- Drink hawthorne berry tea.
- Take vitamin E, magnesium, A-flow (it chelates plaque from arteries), and policosanol (which lowers cholesterol). Also take CoQ10 or Co-enzyme Q10, which is found in every cell of the body and which acts as an enzyme and facilitates the activities of other enzymes. CoQ10 is a powerful antioxidant and acts as a catalyst to promote energy production in the cells. The heart and the liver contain and need the highest amounts of it...

Immune System

The immune system protects us from illness and is composed of highly specialized fighter cells called lymphocytes or white blood cells produced by a complex of lymphoid organs that contain lymph tissue. These organs include the bone marrow, lymph nodes (located near the joints), spleen (located in the upper left abdominal cavity), thymus (located just above the heart), tonsils, adenoids, and appendix. These fighter cells generate antibodies that defend and protect us from harmful invading viruses, bacteria, fungi, and even body cells that have gone astray such as cancer cells. Lymph vessels and lymph nodes carry a clear lymph fluid containing lymphocytes to every tissue of the body and eventually back into the blood. Two major classes of lymphocytes are the T-cells that grow to maturity in the thymus, and B-cells that mature in the bone marrow. T-cells alert B-cells to begin making antibodies. Other T-cells attack and destroy infected cells. B-cells secrete antibodies that neutralize bacteria, viruses, and fungi and prepare them for destruction by phagocytes (cells generated in the bone marrow that destroy foreign matter). A large part of our immune system is located in the intestinal tract. Peyer's patches are lymph tissue located in the walls of the small intestines that produce lymphocytes. We also have friendly bacteria called acidophilus and bifidus in our intestinal tract that

Continued ➡

fight harmful bacteria. Our immune system is vital to our health and most important to take care of.

Nutritional Suggestions

- Drink raw vegetable juices.
- Take vitamins A, B, C, E, zinc, and selenium.
- Take coenzyme Q10, a powerful antioxidant that fights free radicals.
- Take propolis.
- Take acidophilus and bifidus if you have had a round of antibiotics.
- Take colostrum.

If you feel a cold or flu coming on, the following may be taken until you are well:

- Goldenseal to fight infection.
- Echinacea to boost the immune system and cleanse the lymph.
- Grapefruit seed extract (in capsule form) to fight viruses, fungi, and bacteria.
- Colloidal silver, 10 parts per million, to fight viruses, fungi, and bacteria...

Kidneys

The kidneys resemble large purplish brown beans and lie above the small of the back on either side of the spine. The right kidney is slightly lower than the left to allow room for the liver. They are about four to five inches long and weigh about six ounces apiece. Blood moves into each kidney through the renal artery and returns to the heart through the renal vein. There are about a million tiny coiled tubes called nephrons in the kidneys. Nephrons filter out urea, uric acid, creatinine, and other wastes from the blood and pass them into the ureters. The ureters take the urine into the urinary bladder, below the pelvis, where it is expelled through the urethra. The body expels about a quart and a half of urine each day.

Kidney problems can cause elevated blood pressure. If there is a shortage of blood supply to the kidneys, they produce a chemical called angiotensin. This chemical constricts blood vessels throughout the body and raises blood pressure. Arteriosclerosis (hardened arteries) can decrease blood flow to the kidneys. Kidney and bladder infections can be extremely painful. Nephritis is an inflammation of the kidneys. When nephritis is severe, wastes accumulate in the blood, a situation that can result in death. Take care of your kidneys and bladder to prevent infections from occurring.

Nutritional Suggestions

- Drink lots of purified water with ionic trace minerals, at least eight glasses per day. If you are not used to drinking water, start with one or two glasses and build up.
- Drink eight ounces of water with a tablespoon of raw apple cider vinegar to cleanse the kidneys.
- Eat cucumbers, watermelon, carrots, green leafy vegetables, parsley, lemons, limes, grapefruits, apples, pears, and pomegranates.
- Avoid high-protein diets. Uric acid crystals build up in the kidneys from processed foods and high amounts of animal proteins.
- Avoid processed milk. The body is unable to absorb the calcium, and the calcium goes into the kidneys via the blood and creates stones.
- Drink raw vegetable juices such as carrot, celery, cucumber, and parsley.
- Drink herbal teas such as juniper berry, uva ursi, corn silk, alfalfa, and shavegrass.

- Avoid caffeine and alcohol. Caffeine pulls calcium out of the bone and causes it to pass through the kidneys.
- Eat foods high in magnesium, potassium, and natural sodium to keep the urine's pH alkaline and to hold calcium in the bone.

Liver and Gallbladder

The liver and gallbladder are miraculous organs indeed! They work together with the bile ducts as a team to perform the functions of the biliary system, which helps the body rid itself of wastes and processed fats. Weighing from two to three pounds, the liver is reddish brown and shaped like a cone. It occupies the upper-right abdominal cavity just beneath the diaphragm and has two main lobes. Its base touches the stomach, right kidney, and intestines. The gallbladder—a small sac, shaped like a pear—is tucked underneath and attached to the liver.

The remarkable liver has many vital functions. About one-quarter of the heart's output of oxygenated blood flows into the liver via the hepatic artery. In the liver, the artery divides into many branches to provide oxygen to all the liver cells. Blood, carrying such nutrients as fats and glucose from the intestines and spleen, enters the liver through the portal vein. Blood exits the liver through the hepatic vein, carrying away carbon dioxide and plasma proteins. Bile is produced in the liver and passed to the gallbladder where it is stored by means of a tube called a cystic duct.

The liver produces important proteins for blood plasma. One of these is albumin, which regulates the exchange of water between blood and tissues. Another is globin, which is a part of the oxygen-carrying pigment called hemoglobin. Others complement a group of proteins that play an important part in the body's defense system against infection. The liver also produces cholesterol and special proteins that help transport fats around the body. The liver regulates blood levels of amino acids, the building blocks of proteins. After a meal, some amino acids are converted to glucose, some to protein, and others to urea, which is passed out of the body through the kidneys and excreted in the urine. If not required immediately by the body's cells, the liver stores glucose (a form of sugar) as glycogen. When the body needs heat or energy, the liver converts glycogen back to sugar and releases it into the bloodstream.

Working together with the kidneys, the liver helps cleanse the blood of drugs, nicotine, caffeine, chemicals, and preservatives. A healthy liver absorbs these poisonous substances, changes their chemical structure so they are water-soluble, and excretes them into the bile. The bile carries waste products away from the liver and stores them in the gallbladder. The gallbladder contracts and expels bile into the duodenum (the first part of the small intestine) when the stomach sends food there.

The liver also processes estrogen. When estrogen is not processed properly, women may have an excess in their body. This can cause PMS symptoms, such as bloating, water retention, weight gain, irritability, headaches, anxiety, hypoglycemia (causing sugar cravings), an increase in prolaction (a hormone that can cause depression), an increase in inflammatory prostaglandins (which can cause pain), and cramping of the uterus's smooth muscles. Caffeine, alcohol, nicotine, sugar, fried foods, fast foods, and foods high in hormones, such as beef and milk, can hinder the liver in its job of processing estrogen and create premenstrual symptoms.

Nutritional Suggestions

- Eat lots of bitter greens such as kale, beet tops, cilantro, and arugula.
- Eat beets, raw or steamed, or take beet tablets.
- Drink raw juices such as wheatgrass, parsley, spinach, and beet.
- Take digestive enzymes with meals.
- Take chlorella.
- Use olive oil and lemon juice as a salad dressing.
- Take milk thistle, burdock, and yellow dock.
- Avoid heated oils, hydrogenated oils, rancid oils, and fried foods. . . .

Lungs

The lungs are organs of external respiration. Human beings have two lungs located in the chest cavity. These large spongy pyramid-shaped organs provide the blood with oxygen and remove carbon dioxide. The right lung has three lobes, and the left lung has two lobes. There are approximately six hundred million alveoli, or air sacs. If the walls of the air sacs were spread out flat and placed side by side, they would cover about six hundred square feet. Each air sac is lined with a network of tiny capillaries that carry blood. The blood is cleansed and purified of toxic carbon dioxide, brought in from all the cells to the lungs, and the toxins are released when we exhale. This is why proper deep breathing is vital to our health! All the cells in our bodies depend on the oxygen we breathe in. And if we did not breathe out, they would die from carbon dioxide poisoning. If we do not breathe deeply, we will become fatigued and exhausted.

Nutritional Suggestions

- Avoid dairy products, wheat, and sugar.
- Eat turnips, peppers, radishes, onions, and garlic to cleanse mucus from the lungs and promote blood circulation.
- Drink mullein tea to cleanse mucus from the lungs.
- Take echinacea, poke, and lobelia in small amounts and only when needed to relieve lung congestion.
- Avoid smoking. Tar and nicotine irritate the lungs and create congestion. . . .

Lymph Fluids and Lymph Nodes

The lymph, formed from blood plasma, is a colorless fluid. It contains much less protein than plasma and, unlike plasma, no red blood cells. Lymph fluid bathes and nourishes every cell of the body. Organic sodium carried within the lymph helps hold calcium in solution. An adult has about six pints of lymph fluid, which consists of water, white blood cells, digested foods, and wastes excreted by the cells. Lymph fluid moves through tiny vessels called capillaries and larger vessels called lymphatics. Muscle contractions keep the lymph fluid moving. Therefore, we must exercise in order to pump the lymph fluid.

Lymph nodes or glands are plentiful around the neck, under the arms, and in the groin. The nodes produce lymphocytes, which help defend the body against harmful bacteria and disease. They help regulate the amount of poisonous substances or microorganisms that enter the blood.

Nutritional Suggestions

- Avoid table salt.
- Eat foods high in natural sodium such as okra, green leafy vegetables, and mineral whey.
- Drink celery juice.

Continued ➤

- Drink potato peeling broth.
- Drink raw green vegetable juice, which is high in chlorophyll.
- Take mullein, blue violet, chaparral, and echinacea...

Muscles

There are more than six hundred muscles located throughout the body that make movement possible. Muscles are grouped into two types, the skeletal and the smooth. Skeletal muscles are attached to the bones and assist them in movement. They must be stimulated by nerves to operate. Therefore, injury to the nerves can result in paralysis. Smooth muscles are in the blood vessels and internal organs, including the digestive tract. They can be stimulated by nerves and hormones. The cardiac, or heart muscle has tissue that resembles both skeletal and smooth muscles.

Muscles, which depend on food for their energy, produce a waste product called lactic acid. When the muscles are overworked, lactic acid accumulates and causes muscle fatigue and pain. Rest allows the muscles to relax and the body to remove the wastes. Fear or anger can cause the release of epinephrine (adrenaline), which affects muscle movements of the autonomic nervous system.

NUTRITIONAL SUGGESTIONS

- Eat foods that are high in potassium, such as olives, bananas, green leafy vegetables, and potato peeling broth.
- Eat foods that are high in protein, such as soaked nuts and seeds, beans, eggs, goat's milk, goat cheese, fish, chicken, and turkey.
- Eat whole grains and root vegetables, both release carbohydrates that create energy for muscles.
- Include ionic trace minerals, calcium, magnesium, and potassium in your diet.

Nerves, Brain, and Spinal Cord

The nervous system is divided into two separate systems. The central nervous system is composed of the brain and spinal cord. The peripheral nervous system consists of the nerves of the autonomic nervous system as well as twelve pairs of cranial nerves that extend from the brain and thirty-one pairs of spinal nerves that extend from the spinal cord. Cranial nerves control sensations and actions, including sight, smell, taste, chewing, and swallowing. The thirty-one pairs of spinal nerves—including eight cervical, twelve thoracic, five lumbar, five sacral, and one pair of cocygeal—control the muscles. The autonomic nervous system acts independently of the central nervous system and regulates involuntary processes. It is made up of the sympathetic and parasympathetic nervous systems.

NUTRITIONAL SUGGESTIONS

- Eat whole grains, especially brown rice.
- Eat egg yolks soft-boiled or raw in shakes because they are high in lecithin.
- Eat soaked nuts and seeds because they are high in essential fatty acids necessary for nerve function.
- Eat plenty of fish, kale, raw goat's milk, and brewer's yeast.
- Take vitamin B complex.
- Herbs that soothe the nerves are kava-kava, valarian root, blue verrain, and lady's slipper...

Ovaries and Uterus

The uterus is a pear-shaped reproductive organ located in the lower-central abdominal area in women. An ovary (ovum-producing gland) is located on each side of the uterus and connected to it by fallopian tubes. Each ovary holds as many as four hundred thousand potential egg cells. Usually only one egg cell is produced each month, about eight or nine days after menstruation stops. The egg travels slowly to the uterus. If fertilization occurs, the egg-sperm combination attaches to the uterine lining, which becomes thick with blood vessels and fluids to nourish the embryo. If fertilization does not occur, the uterine lining sloughs off and results in menstrual bleeding.

The pituitary gland in the brain produces a follicle-stimulating hormone, which causes eggs to ripen each month. The ovaries produce estrogen and cause the uterine cells to divide and create a new lining each month. After an egg is released, the ovaries produce progesterone to continue building the uterine lining. For most women, menstruation begins around age twelve and ceases between the ages of fifty and fifty-five.

NUTRITIONAL SUGGESTIONS

- Eat soaked nuts and seeds, almond cream, and seed sauces.
- Use flaxseed, borage, and olive oils.
- Take vitamin E and evening primrose oil.
- Include magnesium, calcium, silicon, and trace minerals.
- Take black cohosh.
- Drink red raspberry leaf tea to reduce menstrual cramping and tone the uterus...

Pancreas

The pancreas is an elongated gland about six to eight inches long and one and a half inches wide. It is pinkish yellow. It lies in the back of the abdomen just behind the stomach. The duodenum, or first part of the small intestine that joins to the stomach, loops around it. The pancreas consists of both exocrine and endocrine tissue. The exocrine tissue secretes enzymes, including pancreatin, into the duodenum by way of a duct called the ampulla of Vater. These enzymes break down and digest proteins, carbohydrates, fats, and nucleic acids. The pancreas also secretes bicarbonate to neutralize the stomach acid entering the duodenum.

The endocrine tissue is composed of more than a million small clusters of cells known as the islets of Langerhans, scattered throughout the pancreas. About 70 percent of these cells are beta, or B-cells, which produce the hormone insulin. The remainder of the endocrine cells are alpha, or A-cells. They secrete the hormone glucagon. Both the alpha and the beta cells are regulated by the amount of glucose in the blood. If there is a low level of glucose, glucagon will be released to help increase blood glucose. High levels of glucose will stimulate the release of insulin to help decrease blood glucose. Together, these hormones regulate the blood's glucose levels.

When there is an abundance of sugar or glucose in the blood, B-cells secrete insulin directly into the bloodstream. The blood carries the insulin to cells throughout the body to help them utilize glucose, their main fuel. Insulin stimulates the liver, fat tissue, and muscle cells to take in glucose and metabolize it. It also stimulates the liver to store some glucose as glycogen, and it promotes the storage of fats and proteins to be used during leaner times.

When there is too little insulin, the cells cannot utilize glucose effectively. If glucose goes unused, it accumulates in the blood and tissues and is then carried out in the urine. Sugar in the urine is a major symptom of hyperglycemia or diabetes mellitus.

If the pancreas produces too much insulin, blood sugar is utilized too rapidly and can cause dizziness, frequent hunger, craving of sweets, and fatigue. These are the symptoms of low blood sugar or hypoglycemia. Hypoglycemia can be a precursor to diabetes because the pancreas is in the first stages of improper release of insulin.

A-cells secrete glucagon between meals when the blood sugar is low. Glucagon stimulates the liver to convert glycogen back to glucose, and it raises the blood sugar level. It causes the adipose tissue to release its stores of fatty acids into the blood. Adipose tissue is located just beneath the skin and helps provide insulation from the heat and cold. It is found around the internal organs and acts as a protective padding. In addition to providing protection and padding, its primary purpose is to reserve nutrients and store energy in the form of fat.

NUTRITIONAL SUGGESTIONS

- Avoid refined white sugar, high fructose corn syrup, and hydrogenated oils.
- Use natural sugars in moderation.
- Chew on licorice root if you don't have high blood pressure and drink blueberry or dandelion leaf teas.
- Eat whole grains and soaked nuts and seeds-foods that metabolize slowly.
- Eat raw honey, dates, molasses, and maple syrup in small amounts.
- Use stevia to sweeten herbal teas.
- Take chromium picolinate with trace minerals.
- Take gymnema sylvestre to regulate insulin and blood sugar levels.
- Other herbs that help the pancreas are bitter melon, agrimony, and cinnamon...

Prostate and Testes

The prostate gland is about the size of a walnut and is composed of muscular and glandular tissue. It is located below the urinary bladder and secretes a substance that transports sperm cells. The tube that empties the bladder, called the urethra, passes through the prostate. If the prostate becomes large and swollen due to disease or infection, it can press on the urethra and block the passage of urine. Cancer of the prostate gland is becoming more prevalent in the United States and is now the second leading cause of death among men in this country. The testes, the glands that produce sperm, are located near the prostate.

NUTRITIONAL SUGGESTIONS

- Eat soaked nuts and seeds whole or blended into creams, nut butters, and some nuts and seeds that have not been soaked. Grind unsoaked nuts and seeds or chew them really well in order to digest them properly. There are benefits to eating soaked nuts and seeds because soaking takes out about half the fat, makes them twice as nutritious because they have started sprouting a new plant inside, and makes them easier to digest. Nut butters and whole nuts and seeds are also nutritious because of the good essential oils they contain. We need smaller amounts of these than nuts and seeds that have been soaked.
- Take magnesium, calcium, silicon, zinc, vitamin E, lecithin, B complex, and B_6.

Continued ➡

- Use saw palmetto for the prostate, and damiana and ginseng for the testes.
- Use flaxseed and borage oil.
- Drink red raspberry leaf tea.
- Take pygeum, gravel root, and hydrangea.
- Drink herbal teas made from buchu, corn silk, and juniper berry…

Skin, Hair, Fingernails, and Connective Tissue

The skin is the body's largest organ and weighs about six pounds. If the skin of an adult were stretched out on a flat surface, it would cover nearly eighteen feet. The skin regulates body temperature and releases perspiration through the pores. Amazingly, a piece of skin about the size of a quarter contains four yards of nerves and twenty-five nerve endings, a yard of blood vessels, a hundred sweat glands, and over three million cells!

The skin is made up of two parts: the epidermis, or surface, and the dermis, or lower part. The epidermis contains nerves, but no blood vessels. Melanin pigment is located there and determines skin color. Epidermis cells are regularly pushed up to the skin's surface and sloughed off. The dermis, or lower portion, of the skin is made up of a closely woven connective tissue. Nerve glands, blood vessels, lymph vessels, and hair follicles are located in the dermis.

The skin also has two kinds of glands: one secretes perspiration and the other secretes oil. Two million sweat glands are distributed throughout the skin. They secrete liquid wastes and regulate body temperature. When sweat evaporates, the body is cooled. Sebaceous, or oil, glands open mostly into hair follicles. Oil from these glands keeps the skin moist and the hair shiny. Blackheads form when the oil becomes oxidized, or hardened, in the pores.

NUTRITIONAL SUGGESTIONS
- Eat foods that are high in silicon, such as oatstraw tea, horsetail herb, and bell peppers.
- Take bioflavonoids including rutin to build connective tissue and help heal varicose veins, hemorrhoids, and hernias.
- Include ionic trace minerals, calcium, and zinc in your diet.
- Include cabbage and cabbage juice and white pulp from grapefruits and oranges in your diet.
- Use oils rich in essential fatty acids, such as flaxseed and borage oil.
- Take juniper berry, parsley, and corn silk teas.
- Eat watermelon…

SPLEEN

The spleen is located to the left of and a little behind the stomach, below the diaphragm. It is about five inches long and three inches wide, and it weighs approximately seven ounces. The cells are similar to those in the lymph glands. The spleen filters and destroys foreign substances in the blood and destroys worn-out blood cells. It also stores blood cells and releases them during injury when the body requires extra blood.

NUTRITIONAL SUGGESTIONS
- Eat foods that are high in iron, such as green leafy vegetables and red beets.
- Eat foods that are high in chlorophyl, such as raw green juices.
- Eat foods that are high in sodium, such as mineral whey and celery juice…

Stomach and Intestinal Tract

The stomach is a large baglike organ shaped like a J, which lies between the esophagus and small intestine. It is positioned in the upper-left side of the abdomen. The top part of the stomach joins with the esophagus at the cardiac sphincter. The lower end of the stomach empties into the duodenum, or beginning of the small intestine, at the pyloric valve. Glands that secrete mucus to lubricate food and other glands that secrete hydrochloric acid and pepsin, which partially digest food, are found in the stomach wall.

Foods that are spicy, too hot, or too cold irritate the stomach. Unchewed foods irritate the stomach as well. Fear, anger, or constant tension can produce excessive secretions of stomach acids that burn the stomach or duodenum. This can cause ulcers. Poorly combined foods can cause fermentation in the stomach. Excessive gastric juice can be forced back up into the esophagus. When this happens on a regular basis, a hiatal hernia may develop.

The small intestine is a tube about twenty feet long and one inch wide, narrower than the large intestine. Most of the digestive processes take place here. Enzymes are secreted from the walls of the intestines as well as from the liver and pancreas. Digestion is completed in the small intestine, and the digested food is absorbed by fingerlike projections called villi. Blood and lymph fluid pick up the nutrients from the villi and distribute them to the cells.

The large intestine is about five to six feet long and two and a half inches wide. It consists of the ascending colon on the right side of the abdomen, the transverse colon that stretches across the top of the abdomen, and the descending colon that runs down the left side of the abdomen to the sigmoid colon and then the anus. The large intestine joins the small intestine at the cecum. The area where the colon bends from ascending to transverse is near the liver and is called the hepatic flexure. The point where the colon bends from transverse to descending is near the spleen and is called the spleenic flexure.

NUTRITIONAL SUGGESTIONS
- Eat cabbage and drink cabbage juice.
- Eat foods that are rich in sodium, such as celery, mineral whey, strawberries, and okra.
- Eat foods that are high in fiber, such as ground flaxseeds, oat bran, rice bran, whole grains, raw vegetables, alfalfa tablets, and chlorella.
- Include slippery foods that contain mucilage, such as aloe vera juice, slippery elm tea, and flaxseed tea in your diet.
- Eat foods that are high in friendly bacteria, such as yogurt and raw sauerkraut.
- Include antiparasitic foods, such as garlic and onions, in your diet…

Thymus

The thymus is located under the breastbone in the upper part of the chest. It is considered an endocrine gland because it has no ducts. The thymus plays a major roll in the processes of the immune system. Important fighter cells, called T-cells, grow to maturity in the thymus. The thymus selects the T-cells that are strong and sends them into the bloodstream to protect the body from invading germs. It also eliminates the weaker T-cells. The thymus is most active before puberty and begins to shrink in size, slowing its activity, when we grow older.

NUTRITIONAL SUGGESTIONS
- Eat carrots, cabbage, green vegetables, and seaweeds.
- Include red clover tea, vitamins A and E, zinc, and selenium in your diet. . . .

Thyroid

The thyroid gland is an endocrine, or ductless, gland located in the neck. It has two lobes, located on either side of the windpipe. The thyroid absorbs iodine from the blood. Iodine combines with other chemicals in the thyroid to form thyroxine. This hormone is released into the blood vessels located within the thyroid and distributed to the body's cells. As needed, thyroxin is then changed into several more hormones that regulate the rate at which oxygen and food are changed to heat and energy. This is why thyroid hormones are necessary for metabolism, body growth, and even mental development and function. Goiter, or enlargement of the thyroid gland, develops when the body doesn't have enough iodine. (See "Thyroid Disorders" in the next section.)

NUTRITIONAL SUGGESTIONS
- Eat plenty of green leafy vegetables.
- Eat seaweeds that are high in minerals and iodine, such as dulse (and dulse tablets), kelp capsules, and powder for seasoning.
- Include trace minerals in your diet.
- Include herbs such as Irish moss, watercress, and sarsparilla…

Tonsils and Adenoids

Tonsils and adenoids are both located in the back of the throat, with the adenoids positioned upward behind the nose. They are both made of lymphoid tissue. White blood cells called lymphocytes are formed in the lymphoid tissue. These germ fighters are the body's first line of defense, trapping poisons before they progress into the body. Do all that you can to avoid having them removed.

NUTRITIONAL SUGGESTIONS
- Avoid dairy products, wheat (gluten), and sugar.
- Follow the mucus cleanse program.
- Eat lots of fiber and vegetables to keep the bowels moving. When the bowels are constipated, the tonsils and adenoids must work harder to collect and filter poisons from the blood.
- Drink mullein tea. Take propolis and echinacea (only when you have a sore throat).

—From *Health Is Your Birthright*

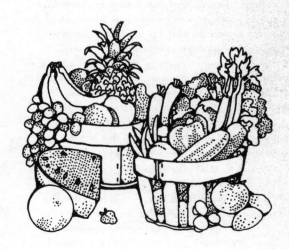

EASTERN NUTRITIONAL THEORY

Michael P. Milburn, Ph.D.

While the idea that how we live and eat can profoundly affect our health has come as a surprise in the West, the Chinese have explored the importance and power of nutrition and lifestyle for millennia.[1] Taoists obsessed with longevity searched for ways of eating that would prolong life; physicians searched for links between factors in their patients' lives, such as their eating habits, and the patterns of disharmony they observed; and farmers and tradespeople searched for foods that could offers sustenance and health. Over time, an approach to nutrition was developed that, while different in many respects from its Western counterpart, comes to conclusions about the foundation of a healthy diet with a striking resonance to those of the new biology.

Nutrition in the East

In Chinese medicine, who we are determines what is most beneficial for us to eat. And what we eat is considered to affect the expression of who we are.

—Beinfield and Korngold, *Between Heaven and Earth*[2]

Of Taoists and Ancient Physicians

Taoism is a religion that believes in, among other things, the importance of cultivating mental and physical health. Taoists practiced mental and physical hygiene, special breathing exercises, gymnastics and meditation, and maintained a strict dietary regimen that included many special herbs. They were strong in their belief that, with effort, people could greatly improve on their chances of living a long and healthy life.

Sun I-khuei, a renowned physician of the Ming dynasty and a contemporary of Li Shi-zhen, echoed this ancient belief in claiming that "One cannot entirely attribute events to fate; on the contrary, man can act in such a way as to conquer Nature." In his book *The Mysterious Pearl Recovered Near the Red River*, Sun discusses the importance of moderation in all things and the value of diet in preserving health. He laments that many people do not pay enough attention to their health at an early enough stage.[3]

Diet was an important topic in the earliest medical texts. The Lady of Tai was buried in an elaborate tomb in 166 B.C. along with her son and many artifacts of her time. Manuscripts written on silk and bamboo and found in an excavation of the tomb, deal with a wide range of topics from yin-yang theory to astronomy. Some of the texts addressed medical subjects, among them a book on eating for long life and another on the therapeutic and preventive use of exercise.[4] Several hundred years later, *Prescriptions for Acute Diseases*, a third-century medical text, claimed that good health is primarily to be found in food and that it is not possible to stay healthy without eating well.[5]

Sun Si-miao, the great Tang dynasty physician and Taoist who lived from 581 to 682, wrote the *Thousand Ounces of Gold Classic*. Sun argued that the superior physician looks for the root cause of ill health and tries first to change the condition with food. Only when food fails should she prescribe herbs.

Sun described dietary treatments for a number of diseases, including enlarged thyroid (goiter), night blindness, and beriberi, a deficiency disease common in Asia and characterized by numbness and tingling of the limbs and wasting of the muscles. He treated goiter with seaweed and pork thyroid, night blindness with beef, pork, and lamb liver, and beriberi with rice bran, all approaches congruent with modern Western nutrition. Goiter can be improved with a diet high in iodine, an element found in seaweed; night blindness is helped by vitamin A, of which liver is a good source; and beriberi is linked to thiamine (vitamin B_1) deficiency, a vitamin found in high concentrations in rice bran.[6] (Beriberi is associated with a preference for highly refined grains, such as white rice, which are polished to remove the outer bran, an excellent source of thiamine.)

The Basic Healthy Diet

The nutritional recommendations of ancient physicians like Sun Si-miao were developed from the perspective of Chinese medicine. Chinese nutrition differs markedly from its Western counterpart. Westerners know that oranges are good for them because they contain large amounts of vitamin C and milk is healthy because it is high in calcium. The Chinese people, in contrast, may choose bitter melon (a cucumber-looking vegetable considered the "king" of bitter foods) to balance the heat and humidity of a summer day, or might eat small red beans (adzuki beans) to improve a damp constitution. While Western nutrition focuses on the molecular components of food, Chinese nutrition considers its qualities and macroscopic actions.

Individual balance is the focus of Chinese nutrition. There is not a rigid, universal approach to eating suitable for everyone. Rather, there is a basic, healthy diet that must be adjusted to suit the person and environment, a flexible and evolving dietary regimen that will balance hot and cold, dryness and dampness, yin and yang. The basic healthy diet is built around generous helpings of whole grains and vegetables, with moderate amounts of legumes, fruits, and nuts and seeds. Animal products, if any, are eaten to supplement, not define, the meal. Food is usually lightly cooked, improving its digestibility without destroying its nutritive value.

According to Maoshing Ni, who practices and teaches Chinese medicine in California, the basic, healthy diet has equal portions of vegetables and whole grains, accounting for about 80 percent of food intake. Legumes, seeds, and nuts make up another 10 to 20 percent, with fruit comprising up to 10 percent. Animal products, if eaten, are to comprise no more than 10 percent of the diet. Ni also points to the usefulness of small quantities of sea vegetables such as nori, dulse, and kelp.[7]

The Five Flavors

In Chinese nutrition the basic, healthy diet must be adjusted to suit the individual and his or her environment and to accomplish this the Chinese describe foods in terms of their qualities and actions. Central to such a description are the five flavors of sour, salty, bitter, sweet, and spicy. The five flavors have five-phase correspondences linking each flavor with the various organ-meridian systems. The pungent or spicy flavor, corresponding to the metal phase, promotes the movement of qi and blood through its invigorating and dispersing nature. Many pungent foods, such as green onions and pepper, also warm the body. In contrast, salty foods, like seaweed and salt, tend to be cooling. Salty has a water phase correspondence and an affinity for the kidney. This flavor is softening and sedating.

Sour foods correspond to the wood phase and affect the liver channel. Sour foods like lemon and vinegar are obstructive and astringent. Bitter, the fire flavor, suggests both drying and heat clearing qualities. Bitter foods, like dandelion and bitter melon, are among the least popular of foods. The addictive sweet flavor has an affinity for the spleen and a correspondence to the earth phase. Sweet foods, like honey and yam, help to build blood and qi because of their tonifying and nurturing quality.

A healthy diet requires balance among the five flavors. The *Yellow Emperor's Classic* makes clear the benefits of a balanced diet: "[I]f people pay attention to the five flavors and mix them well, their bones will remain straight, their muscles will remain tender and young, their breath and blood will circulate freely, their pores will be fine in texture, and consequently, their breath and bones will be filled with the essence of life."[8]

Eating too much of any one flavor should be avoided. Too much sweet can damage the spleen, too much salt can injure the kidney, too much sour can stagnate the qi. According to the *Yellow Emperor's Classic*, sour in excess will cause the liver to produce too much saliva and will weaken the spleen; salt in excess will cause a decline in the health of the bones, weaken the muscles, and take away one's zest for life; sweet in excess will affect the balance of the kidney and produce fullness in the heart; bitter in excess will dry the spleen and affect the stomach; and pungent in excess will harm the muscles and spirit.

Many people are attracted to sweet foods, others are attracted to salty, sour, or spicy food—and most shun the bitter. These individual tendencies are a powerful diagnostic tool in Chinese medicine, offering an indication of the origin and location of disharmony. A patient with a sweet tooth bordering on addiction, for example, may be caught in an endless cycle of spleen disharmony. A malfunction-

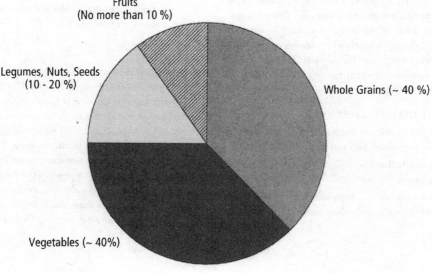

Fruits
(No more than 10 %)

Legumes, Nuts, Seeds
(10 - 20 %)

Whole Grains (~ 40 %)

Vegetables (~ 40%)

Continued ➡

ing spleen does a poor job of extracting qi from food, leading to lack of energy and a craving for sweet energy-giving foods. If the patient succumbs to his/her craving, the excessive consumption of sweet food will only aggravate the spleen disharmony.

Macroscopic Quality of Food

Flavor is one aspect of the macroscopic quality of food that helps describe its physiological impact. Another is temperature, a quality that has already been hinted at above. Some foods have a cooling quality, like salt and some salty foods; others are warming, including many pungent and spicy foods, like pepper and garlic. There is a continuum of temperature, from cold, cool, neutral, warm, and hot.

The quality of temperature ascribed to a food refers to its physiological effect. There are general signs and symptoms of heat in the body—including dark yellow urine, red face and eyes, affinity for cold, rapid pulse and red tongue—as well as indications of heat in particular organs. The same thing is true for cold, the presence of which is signaled by signs and symptoms like cold extremities, fear of cold, pale tongue, and slow pulse. Hot foods can be used to balance a cold environment, whether internal or external. A hearty beet soup with garlic, ginger, and a hint of chili can balance a cold, deficient constitution or buffer a cold Minnesota winter. Cool foods, in contrast, can balance heat. Mung bean soup with cucumber and lettuce salad provides a cooling repast appropriate for a scorching summer afternoon.

Chinese nutrition is also concerned with the physical temperature of food. Eating too many physically cold foods—such as ice cream straight from, the refrigerator— will weaken the digestive system and can lead to a deficient and damp spleen. Overconsumption of cold and raw foods—which also tend to be cooling—is a culinary faux pas of Chinese nutrition.

Food also has an effect on the moisture level of the body. Some people are constitutionally dry or yin deficient, with signs and symptoms of dryness like dry stool, dry skin, and thirst, together with signs of heat in the case of yin deficiency, while others are damp. Pathogenic dampness is indicated by a lack of thirst, digestive disturbance, a heavy feeling in the limbs, and a thick tongue fur. Drying foods can help improve a damp condition and moistening foods will counteract dryness, but generally moistening foods such as honey, millet, and milk should be balanced with drying foods such as adzuki bean and corn.

Some foods are very moistening and their overconsumption can disrupt the spleen, causing congestion and stagnation with symptoms of dampness—a problem commonly seen in the Chinese medicine clinic. Too many sweet foods, too many raw or cold foods, and too many greasy, fatty foods—common features of the typical Western diet—can precipitate a damp condition by weakening the spleen and impeding its function of transformation and transportation.

Method of preparation affects the properties of food. A carrot, for example, though cooling when raw becomes more strengthening and warming when boiled or steamed. And baking with a little honey and dried ginger fashions an even wanner and more tonifying carrot.

Healthy spleen and stomach are essential to good digestion. According to the *Yellow Emperor's Classic*: "Ingested fluids enter the stomach. Here, they are churned and their qi is strained off. The qi is then carried to the spleen and further distributed by the spleen qi." The spleen is thus the root of qi and blood production; the stomach manages the intake and breakdown of food, so its partner the spleen can transform and transport the purest essence.[9]

The spleen and stomach are a temperamental pair: the spleen fears dampness, the stomach hates dryness, requiring careful attention to the balance of moisture in the diet. The stomach is also susceptible to heat, which can engender dryness. The perfect diet supports the spleen and stomach, providing nourishment for the other yin and yang organs. On balance, it is not too cold or too hot, too damp or too dry. The five flavors are mixed delicately together without a hint of excess. It is, in the midst of extremes, just right.

From Cucumber to Black Bean

Many foods are traditional folk remedies. Cucumber, for example, is cool and sweet, and affects the spleen, stomach, and large intestine. It acts to clear heat, quench thirst, and promote urination. Cucumber consumption will improve acne, it can be applied externally for burns, and it can help relieve hot eye inflammations.[10]

Corn is neutral, sweet, and acts on the stomach and large intestine. Like cucumber it promotes urination. It is also considered to benefit the heart. Corn, particularly the corn silk consumed as a tea, is traditionally used to improve the function of the gallbladder. Radish is cool, pungent, and sweet, influencing the lungs and stomach. It has a downward action and is used in cases of indigestion with stagnant food. Radish is traditionally thought to improve lung function, help prevent cold and flu, and can be eaten in cases of cough with phlegm.

Fresh ginger root is warm and pungent, and associated with the lungs, stomach, and spleen. Ginger acts to promote sweating, improve nausea, and counteract the common cold. As these examples suggest, there is not a clear line between food and medicine. A few slices of fresh ginger are often added to Chinese herbal formula because of ginger's harmonizing effect on the digestive system and sometimes—because of ginger's ability to counteract toxins—to buffer the side effects of potentially toxic herbs.

Another herb-cum-food is job's tears, a barley-looking grain that can be eaten like rice and is used as a medicinal herb. Job's tears is sweet, bland, and neutral, and associated with the spleen, lungs, and kidneys. It clears dampness, strengthens the spleen, and helps to stop diarrhea.

Among the fruits, grape is neutral, sweet, and sour, and is considered a blood and energy-nourishing food. It influences the lungs, spleen, and kidney, and is thought to stimulate urination and improve the tendons and bones. Raisins are recommended as a folk cure for anemia.

Longevity Foods East

The Chinese, in their quest for long life and immortality, were not content with simply eating to avoid disease. They searched for special superfoods that would nourish the mind and body and take health to new heights. The sixth century Chinese scholar Yan Zhi-tui attributed his good health in old age to eating kidney-nourishing foods: "I have been in the habit of eating kidney tonics throughout my life which is why I could still read fine print when seventy years old with no gray hair on my head."[11]

In Chinese physiology, the health of the kidney is related to the strength of the *jing*-essence, a primary determinant of long life. With age, the yin aspect of the body wanes and the kidneys decline, a tendency that can be counteracted with appropriate supplements. Kidney-nourishing foods include walnuts and mussels. Walnuts are a tonic to the kidney, especially its yang aspect. They are used to boost sexual energy. Mussels strengthen the liver and kidney, and are particularly good for the lower back.

Ling zhi, the spiritual mushroom, is perhaps the quintessential longevity food. This woody bracket fungus, *Ganoderma lucidum*, or reishi in Japanese, was used for over a thousand years by the time Li Shizhen wrote about it in his encyclopedic work on natural history. He praised its ability to improve memory and benefit the qi of the chest. With regular consumption of the herb, claimed Li, one would stay agile and live a long time.

Another revered longevity food is the soybean, long a staple of Asian cuisine. The soybean has been grown in China since at least the eleventh century B.C., and its origins are the subject of numerous legends, all a testament to its high esteem in Oriental culture. The soybean is commonly eaten in derivative foods, like soymilk, tofu, tempeh, and okara, the leftover pulp from the milk-making process. The Japanese often call tofu and even okara "honorable" in everyday speech and fuss over soyfoods like tofu and miso as Westerners would fine wines.[12] Many long-lived Japanese attribute their good health to the regular consumption of miso.

Nutrition East and West: The Parallels

The best physician looks for the root cause of disease. Then he first attempts to cure it with food. Only if food fails should he use drugs.

—Sun Si-miao, *Thousand Ducat Prescriptions, Tang Dynasty*

In the past several decades major changes have t aken place in field of nutrition. Food is much more than a repository of various vitamin and mineral substances—it can be a primary cause of "Western" diseases and a veritable gold mine of potent phytochemicals useful in the prevention and treatment of disease. While nutrition is, in the old biology, largely irrelevant for medicine, it is, in the new biology, a foundation of health and healing.

The Basic Healthy Diet Revisited

With the rapid pace of research into the relationship between diet and health there is abundance of confusion. Many people sense that the standard American diet is unhealthy and are open to change. Yet with contradictory claims announced regularly in the popular press, it is hard to know what direction change should take. Part of the confusion lies in the emphasis on finding particular chemicals in food that represent the cause of disease. This molecular emphasis tends to obscure a perspective of the forest in the obsession with identifying trees.

Foods are composed of thousands of molecules, all with the potential to interact among themselves and with the thousands of molecules comprising the mind-body system. To make any sense, this molecular approach must be combined with a study of broader patterns in the relationship between food and health. And it is here, at the pattern level, that much less confusion reigns.

In their effort to study "Western" diseases, researchers like Cornell's Colin Campbell have noted a distinct dietary pattern associated with a high prevalence of Western diseases and another pattern where such diseases are much less common. As Campbell describes it, these diseases have "some very profound common causes." A rich diet containing a high proportion of animal foods, low in

Continued ➡

fiber and foods of plant origin, while high in fat and cholesterol, is this common cause. And the diet able to greatly reduce the risk of Western diseases is one that is low in animal products, fat, and cholesterol, while high in fiber and foods of plant origin.[14]

In light of the powerful evidence that food has a lot to do with health, governments have recently shifted their nutritional recommendations to favor a more plant-based eating pattern. In the United States, for example, the Department of Agriculture, which has issued "food guides" since 1916, now uses a food pyramid. Grains and complex carbohydrates, vegetables and fruits are the foundation of the pyramid, reflecting the fact that they are the foundation of a healthy diet. Dairy products and animal products are higher up on the pyramid, indicating that the quantity of these foods should be reduced in comparison to carbohydrates and vegetables. Fats, oils, and sweets are found at the top of the pyramid and should be used sparingly.

Government positions are inevitably subject to the fickle winds of politics and it is useful to turn to other sources of healthy eating wisdom. The Physicians Committee for Responsible Medicine (PCRM) points out that the government-issued Food Guide Pyramid suggests regular servings of meat and dairy products, reflecting a trade-off between health and agri-business interests. In response, the PCRM has developed its "New Four Food Groups": simply whole grains, vegetables, fruits, and legumes. In this recommended regimen, whole grains are given the most daily servings, legumes the least. The only known nutrient of concern in this entirely plant-based diet is vitamin B_{12}, which, although present in microorganism-transformed foods like miso and tempeh (B_{12} is produced by bacteria and other microorganisms), can be obtained with a supplement.[15]

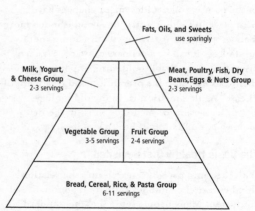

U.S. Department of Agriculture Food Pyramid

While this "new" way of eating—the standard fare of the world's agriculturalists for millennia—is a significant change in thinking from the nutrition of the old biology, it resonates strongly with the basic healthy diet of Chinese nutrition. In both systems, grains and vegetables form the bulk of the diet, supplemented by lesser amounts of legumes, fruits, nuts and seeds, and perhaps a small portion of animal-based food. The only minor difference is the recommendation in Chinese nutrition to eat an equal number of servings of vegetables as grains, while emerging Western guidelines suggest vegetable servings be less than grain servings. A minor point, but given the emerging recognition of the health benefits of vegetables, there may well be merit in this extra emphasis on vegetables.

The Complementary Nature of Nutrition East and West

There is considerable congruence between the basic healthy diet of new biology nutrition and that of Chinese nutrition, a confidence-generating fact in this time of often contradictory dietary claims. Yet a sticky point remains in the question of the extent to which animal products should be included in the diet. Some in the new Western nutrition, like the PCRM, suggest animal-based foods be completely shunned. The PCRM argues that a vegan diet—one that avoids meat, eggs, and dairy—can supply all known nutrients (except perhaps vitamin B_{12}). Dean Ornish, in his program for reversing heart disease, allows for a small amount of low-fat dairy and egg whites in an otherwise plant-based diet. In Chinese nutrition it is possible to find both an enthusiasm for the benefits of a plant-only diet and concern about possible deleterious effects of a diet completely devoid of animal products.

The Chinese tradition offers insight into the appropriateness of animal food in the diet through a system of constitutional typing emphasizing individual differences. For some people a complete abstinence from animal products can be beneficial; for others it may be useful to include supplementary foods of animal origin. This system combines an understanding of constitution with the proper ties of food to maintain individual balance.

There are a number of approaches used to categorize constitution. One approach is to work with three pairs of qualities: hot and cold, dry and damp, deficient and excessive. Symptoms of hot, cold, dry, and damp were discussed earlier in this chapter. Hot individuals counteract their constitutional tendency of overactivity by shifting the basic, healthy diet slightly in favor of cool and cold foods, reducing pungent and increasing bitter flavors. Cold constitutions, in contrast, need a wanner diet, with more sweet and pungent flavors, and less bitter. Dryness will benefit from a diet favoring moistening foods, while damp constitutional tendencies are moderated by increasing consumption of drying foods and avoiding foods with a dampening nature.

A deficient constitution is indicated by chronic tiredness, shortness of breath, passive personality, thin and pale appearance. The deficient constitution benefits from a greater quantity of strengthening foods, more sweet and less bitter flavors. The excessive constitution, with its non-stop energy, reddish complexion, loud voice, and boisterous personality, benefits from foods that promote the movement of blood and qi and a reduction in sweet and tonifying foods.[16]

By combining constitutional understanding with lifestyle and climate, a clearer picture of the role of animal products in the diet emerges. Strictly plant-based eating is widely considered beneficial for spiritual and intellectual pursuits, while the extra demands of a more physically strenuous lifestyle may be met with a small amount of animal food as a supplement to the basic, healthy diet. Damp constitutions—often with a tendency toward obesity—require a religious avoidance of excess fat and dairy products, foods that are dampness-generating. The richness of the Western diet is deleterious to those with damp constitutions and those with this pattern should eat few animal products.

A hot and dry constitution—deficient yin in the Chinese medical model—on the other hand, benefits from the moistening property of dairy products, as well as foods such as millet, clam, and barley. While deficient constitutions benefit from supplementary animal products, excess constitu-tions are poorly suited for the standard Western eating pattern and should strictly avoid a high-fat, low-fiber diet. A lighter vegetarian diet would even moderate their typically "Type A" personalities.

Food As Medicine

In the Chinese tradition, there is no clear line between food and medicine. Many foods/herbs can end up either in a herbal prescription or on the dinner plate. These foods have physiological effects that can be harnessed for the prevention or treatment of disease. Adzuki bean, a small deep-red legume with a hearty taste, for example, has the ability to remove heat from the body and promote urination. It is used in prescriptions for edema and topically as a paste for hemorrhoids. As a folk remedy, it is used to promote milk production in nursing mothers. Overconsumption of adzuki beans can lead to dryness, but regular consumption is ideal for those with a damp constitution.

Job's tears, a barleylike grain whose properties were discussed previously, is a dampness-clearing herb and a common food. There is some interest in its possible anti-cancer properties, and when lightly roasted it is used as a digestive tonic. Job's tears is also a folk remedy for warts.

Recently, new biology nutrition has rekindled an interest in food as medicine, paralleling the Eastern enthusiasm for the healing power of food. The simple soybean, for example, is now thought to be much more than a good source of protein for animals or people too poor to afford meat. Soy and its derivative foods are a nutritious addition to a vegetarian diet as well as a rich source of powerful phytochemicals, plant molecules with surprisingly powerful physiological effects. Phyto-estrogens, for example, can affect the hormonal system and are postulated to have a preventive effect against some forms of cancer.

While Chinese nutrition is focused on the qualities of food and its effects on the mind-body system, Western nutrition is focused on the molecular constituents of food and their biological effects. Despite these differences, Western ideas about food resonate with those of the East. The basic, healthy diet espoused by progressive Western organizations and Eastern nutrition are essentially one and the same. An awareness of the healing power of food, long part of Eastern culture, is now emerging from a scientific perspective in the West. It is possible to eat with confidence a diet that can help prevent and even reverse some of the common health problems of the modern world. As news reports chronicle newly discovered benefits of consuming various foods, it is interesting to reflect on this as a modern continuation of an ancient tradition.

Endnotes

1. There is a Western tradition of insight into the influence of diet and lifestyle on health. Some 2,500 years ago Hippocrates claimed that: 'Whoever gives these things (food) no consideration, and is ignorant of them, how can he understand the diseases of man?" For the most part these insights have been lost and ignored. Except for gross nutrient deficiencies, Western medicine has ignored the connection between diet and disease, a view demonstrated by the almost complete absence of nutritional training in Western medical schools.
2. Beinfield and Korngold, *Between Heaven and Earth*, 324.
3. Needham, J., *Science and Civilization*, Vol. 5, 46.
4. Ibid., pp. 136, 137.
5. Lu, *Chinese Foods for Longevity*, 32–33.
6. Lu, *Chinese System of Food Cures*, 5.
7. Ni, *The Tao of Nutrition*, 23–24.
8. Veith, trans., *The Yellow Emperor's Classic*, 109.
9. Wiseman et al., *Fundamentals of Chinese Medicine*, 76–79.
10. Information on foods adapted from Henry Lu's *Chinese System of Food Cures* and Maoshing Ni's *The Tao of Nutrition*.
11. Lu, *Chinese Foods for Longevity*, 32.
12. Shurtleff and Aoyagi, *The Book of Tofu*, 62.

Continued ➡

13. Ornish, *Dr. Dean Ornish's Program for Reversing Heart Disease*, 12–13.

14. Campbell, "The Dietary Causes of Degenerative Diseases," in *Western Diseases: Their Emergence and Prevention*, p. 69. In a description of his monumental China study, Campbell appeals to the need for synthesis and a broader view. As he puts it, "common causes cannot be fully understood by limiting investigations to the generalization of details of specific cause-effect relationships, a process that invites too much error, as has happened in this field too often in the past. Synthesis of detailed information into a larger picture is required."

15. The New Four Food Groups For Optimal Nutrition, PCRM, Washington, D.C. The PCRM works to debunk many of the nutritional myths that still linger. Protein, for example, immediately comes to many minds when the idea of a plant-based diet is considered. Yet it is actually difficult to get too little protein and most people eating a Western-type diet get more than enough. Iron is plentiful in a vegetarian diet and the excess of iron in a high-meat diet may actually be harmful. Calcium is plentiful in plant foods such as kale and sesame seeds, and evidence suggests that one factor responsible for calcium problems—like osteoporosis—is an excess of protein which increases calcium loss, rather than a deficiency of the nutrient in the diet. The World Health Organization RDA for calcium is about half that of Canada and the United States, which are deliberately set high to compensate for the loss of calcium in high-protein diets. Ironically, eating less meat and dairy products might help prevent the calcium problems epidemic in wealthy nations.

16. The Ayurvedic tradition also uses a diet-according-to-constitution approach. For further exploration of the Chinese nutrition system of diet-according-to-constitution see Beinfield and Korngold's *Between Heaven and Earth* and Henry Lu's *Chinese System of Food Cures*.

—From *The Future of Healing*

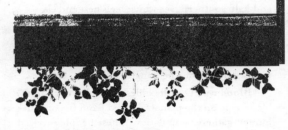

THE ENERGY OF FOOD

Lesley Tierra, L.Ac., Herbalist, A.H.G.

Most people are disconnected from the food they eat—they don't plant it, grow it, harvest it, or even cook it. In fact, many young children don't understand that the milk bought at a store actually comes from the cows they see in fields! The first medicine is always food; only after proper nutrition is established do herbs come next. If you want to heal, particularly from a complicated condition, it is necessary to treat your entire life, not just take a magic herbal bullet, and this starts with nutrition and diet.

Like herbs, every type of food has an inherent cool or warm energy. The cooling or warming energy of food affects the body by cooling it down, or heating it up. While in the West we create food groups, those in the East recognize the energy of food regardless of the group it is in.

Learning the energy of food is important in order to regain and maintain health. If you have Excess Heat and continue to eat warming and heating foods, then your body only becomes warmer inside, eventually creating disease. The same is true

if you have Coldness: eating a lot of cooling foods causes your body to get colder.

As a result, it is very important to choose foods according to their heating or cooling energies. If you are taking the right herbs to heal your condition but are eating foods with the wrong energy, then you will receive little or no benefit from the herbs: The herbal treatment will either be less effective, will take longer to heal, or will have no effect at all. For this reason, it is extremely important to learn about and understand the energy of food. Furthermore, eating appropriately for your body's energy helps prevent illness.

For example, Neil came to me with low energy and frequent colds. I gave him warming and building herbs and a balanced diet to eat, but he made little progress in two weeks time. When discussing his diet, Neil admitted he drank fruit juices, believing them healthy and important foods. Yet, these same foods continually caused his poor digestion, mucus, lowered immunity and tiredness. When Neil eliminated the fruit juices, within a week he felt stronger and had better digestion and more energy.

Rose had skin problems, frequently breaking out on her face, back and shoulders. Again I gave her an appropriate energetic diet along with Heat-clearing and detoxifying herbs. Within a few weeks, Rose felt better and her face cleared, but skin eruptions continued to appear on her back and shoulders. When questioned further I learned that she still ate a weekly dose of chocolate chip cookies, white sugar included. When she stopped these, Rose's skin fully cleared.

Every food we eat affects our bodies in some way. Food can add Warmth, Coldness, Dampness, Dryness, strength, weakness, maintain balance, create disease and so forth. Because most people eat two to three times a day, then two to three times a day the body's energy is affected by the energy of the food ingested. "You are what you eat" is not such a strange adage from this perspective.

The Energy of Food

A balanced diet is one that uses foods energetically, incorporating more foods with a neutral to cool and neutral to warm energy, less food with warm or cool energies and sparing use of hot and cold energy foods.

Consider this continuum as a child's seesaw and imagine a person sitting at each of the hot and cold ends, one in the air and the other on the ground. Now if the person on the ground suddenly gets off, the one in the air quickly slams to the ground. Likewise, if eating hot and cold foods at the extreme ends, the disease 'crash' is likely to be sudden, more intense and harder to cure.

Now imagine both people sitting a little distance away from the center point. If one gets off, the other only lightly taps the ground. Thus, eating closer to the balanced energy point creates less disease potential and only slight ailments may occur and are more easily healed. When eating according

to the energy of foods, include more foods close to the balance point and fewer foods away from it.

The more warm or hot foods you eat, the more potential there is for an excess-heat illness to manifest (such as high fever, thirst, constipation, craving for cold, blood in the nose, stool or urine, yellow mucus, stools or urine, red tongue body and rapid pulse). Likewise, the more cool to cold foods you eat, the more likely an excess-cold illness can manifest (such as feelings of coldness, diarrhea or loose stools, poor appetite, clear discharges, urine or mucus, no thirst, no sweating, a pale frigid appearance, frequent and copious urination pale tongue body, and slow, deep pulse).

You can determine yourself how food makes you feel by noticing how it affects you after eating it. Some effects are evident immediately, such as those from spicy hot peppers, or it may take three days or more for you to experience it, such as the effects of cold energy ice cream. Most foods affect you within three days. An excess amount of one type of food builds over time and within a month you can feel its effects.

Another way of looking at the warm-cool energy of food is in terms of acid-alkaline. The acid-alkaline determination is not the pH of food itself, but the residue ash that forms when food is oxidized. In general, foods that are cool or cold tend to make the body more alkaline. Foods that are warm or hot tend to make the body more acidic (of course there are exceptions). Most people eat too many acidic foods and not enough alkaline ones. Being either too acidic or too alkaline can imbalance your health (see page for specific acid and alkaline foods).

Sometimes just cutting back on acidic or alkaline foods quickly alters the body's condition. In fact, I know of one woman who healed herself of multiple illnesses simply by testing her pH balance frequently throughout the day and then altering her diet accordingly (you can purchase pH strips at your local drugstore and do this yourself).

The taste of each food also indicates its warming, cooling or neutral energy. Bitter foods, like endive or spinach, cool and eliminate toxins. Sour foods refresh and cool, like lemons, while small amounts aid digestion. Spicy foods stimulate and heat metabolism and move blood and Qi. Salty foods, like seaweed and miso, cool and soften because they retain Fluids in the body. Full sweet foods, like protein and complex carbohydrates, are hot to cool in energy and nourish bones, muscles, Qi and blood.

The energy of a food is inherent to it regardless of how the food is eaten or prepared, though the energy can be modified somewhat. Overall, adding heat, pressure, cooking time and spices makes a food less cooling and more warming. Adding water, refrigeration or freezing, eating raw and unspiced makes food less warming and more cooling. Yet, despite preparations, a cool food can never be warm and vice versa. For example, an apple, with a cool energy, can be baked with walnuts and cinnamon to make it less cool in energy instead. Likewise, eating warm shrimp in a raw state gives it a less warm energy since the shrimp isn't cooked.

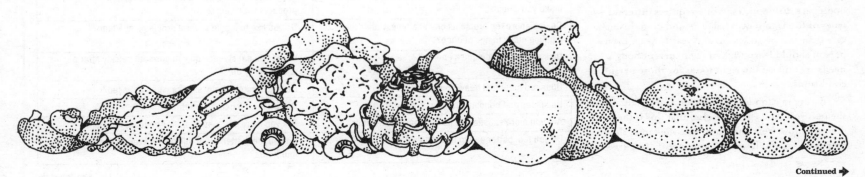

Continued ➡

Along with warming and cooling energies, foods are either empty or full. Empty and full refer to a food's building or eliminating effects on the body and not its nutritional contents. Like energy, empty-full is on a continuum; each food is not absolutely empty or full. Full foods are highly concentrated nutritionally, like animal protein. Empty foods lack protein, such as fruits and vegetables. Solid foods are building while simple foods are eliminating. Relative to each other, fruit and juices are empty, vegetables are neutral to somewhat empty, meat and dairy are full, grains and legumes are neutral, protein-rich foods are full and more water-containing foods are empty.

For instance, fruit and juices are empty foods, although they range from warm to cold in energy. They generally lower body temperature and metabolism by creating elimination. A little periodically eliminates toxins and moistens Dryness. Yet, if eaten too frequently or predominantly, they cause Coldness, poor digestion, gas, possible low-back pain. Dampness, lowered immunity and resistance and feelings of being ungrounded and unfocused.

On the other hand, prolonged eating of mostly full foods stagnate Energy, Blood, Fluids, Food or Heat, ultimately resulting in Excess conditions. Those who predominantly eat full foods often feel congested, stuck, explosive and hypertensive. For example, red meat and dairy are full foods, although they are neutral to warming in energy. They strengthen Blood and Qi, building strength and endurance. Yet, excess red meat or dairy ultimately creates too much congestion, resulting in a red neck and face, irritability, a loud voice, aggressive behavior, constipation and toxicity.

Putting empty-full together with warming and cooling energies helps us look at food in a different way. For instance, some foods may be warm in energy but also empty. The spice cayenne is hot, but it doesn't build or strengthen. Instead, it stimulates and disperses and, in excess, causes elimination. On the other hand, some foods may be cool in energy but also full, such as barley. It expands the intestines and eliminates Dampness, helping stop diarrhea. It also strengthens digestion.

Thus, along with the energy of a food, it is important to look at its empty-full effects. Overall, a balanced diet is comprised predominantly of foods with a neutral-warm and neutral-cool energy that are neutral-full to neutral-empty in quality. Eating large amounts of the more extreme foods, those that are hot, cold, full and/or empty, creates imbalance and disease.

Determining the Right Diet for You

I frequently hear this comment: "I've looked at every diet out there and they all say I should eat something different. I'm confused and don't know what to do. Which one is right?" Always I answer in return: there is no one specific diet for all people. This cannot be overstated. Because all people's bodies are different, everyone requires different types of foods to stay in balance, and even this may vary from season to season and year to year. Each person should learn what his/her current body's needs are and eat the right foods for those personal conditions.

Eating raw foods makes Karen feel so fantastic, she tells you (and everyone else) that this is the best diet to follow. Yet, when Suzie ate the same, she got diarrhea, gas and lowered immunity. Eating fre-

quent amounts of animal protein healed Ken of prolonged weakness and tiredness, and he scoffed at vegetarians. But it caused headaches, constipation and high blood pressure when Steve followed this diet. Thus, what benefits one person won't necessarily be healthy for your body, and could even make you sick over time.

Every one of us is born with unique traits based on ancestral heritage, blood type and inherited constitution. Further, your childhood dietary and lifestyle habits strongly influence your body type and food needs. The speed of your metabolism plus what you currently experience in life—stress, giving birth or having a specific ailment, for instance—also indicates what is best for you to eat. Therefore, diet must be individually tailored to your unique body needs. This is an extremely important point: never blindly follow a mass diet, no matter how good it sounds, or how much it has helped someone you know.

Most of us eat according to our minds or emotions, such as following a specific dietary regime for spiritual, cultural or peer group reasons, long-standing habits, according to ongoing emotional issues, or how we feel about food. Eating according to your mind or emotions rarely serves your body. Instead, choose to eat according to your individual body needs.

The following keys can help determine the appropriate diet for your individual needs.

Constitution: Each of us is born with a different constitution determined by the health of our parents at the time of conception, and inherited weaknesses and strengths. These help determine our immune strength, susceptibility to disease and, consequently, our food needs. Those with weaker constitutions must be much more careful with their diets, ensuring sufficient building foods are incorporated. Those with stronger constitutions do not need to be as strict.

Body Type: TCM categorizes body types according to the Five Phases—Fire, Earth, Metal, Water or Wood (refer to the Energy of Illness). Ayurvedic medicine recognizes the body types Vata (Air), Pitta (Fire) or Kapha (Earth). Other cultures identify further body types. For example, Western medicine used to categorize people according to sanguine, phlegmatic, choleric and melancholic. Each body type has its own dietary and lifestyle needs to stay in balance and eating accordingly maintains strength and immunity.

Metabolic Power: This is the ability to digest food normally. If metabolism is too slow, lethargy, sluggishness and easy weight gain result; if metabolism is faster than normal, foods burn too quickly, causing constant hunger, irritability and drastic energy drops (see table Slow Burner or Fast Burner? to determine which you are). People with slow metabolisms do better with lean proteins, little fat and some complex carbohydrates. Those with fast metabolisms need more concentrated proteins and healthy fats, both of which take much longer to metabolize than carbohydrates. Both types should avoid processed carbohydrates, the former because they'll experience severe blood sugar swings, the latter because they'll experience congestion and weight gain.

Ancestry and Genetic Heritage: People with unmixed heritages, like pure Japanese, Chinese, Indonesian, African, Indian, German, Italian, French, or Middle Eastern constitutions, for example, do better eating as their ancestors did and usually have stronger and healthier bodies. Most of us, however, have mixed heritages. To help determine your ancestral needs, consider whether most of your ancestors came from northern areas (cold climates) or southern areas (warm climates). Those from colder climates need concentrated diets with more protein and less carbohydrates. Those from warmer climates need lighter diets with less protein and more carbohydrates. If you are half-northern and half-southern, see which feels best and eat accordingly.

Blood Types: Much study has been done on how blood types affect us, not only on our nutritional needs, but also our personalities.

Blood type O is the oldest and most common blood type on the planet, derived from the original hunter-gatherer population. These people survived by eating lots of animal protein with some vegetables, fruits and wild grain supplementation (along with enormous amounts of exercise). Thus, O blood types need higher amounts of full proteins in their diets, especially from animal sources such as wild game. To offset the potential stagnating effects of this full diet, be sure to eat copious amounts of vegetables (part raw and part cooked), some fruit, plenty of water and get lots of exercise. Blood type O should especially avoid pork products and refined grains and flour products, since they don't as easily assimilate these domesticated products.

Blood type A generally does well with a vegetarian diet, needing protein from lean and carbohy-

---

Slow Burner or Fast Burner?

Answer questions that apply to you most of the time with a check. Add up every checked question. The column with the most checks determines which type you are.

Slow Burner	Fast Burner
Can you skip breakfast without losing energy or getting hungry?	Do you enjoy a hearty breakfast high in protein?
Do you prefer a "light" meal of salad to a "heavy" one of steak and potato?	Do you feel better eating steak and potatoes rather than leaner foods like chicken and vegetables?
Are you somewhat "laid back" and even-tempered?	Are you Type A, high strung or hyperactive?
Do foods like cheese, butter and avocados seem to make you sluggish?	Are cheese, butter, avocados and full-fat dairy products satisfying to you?
Do you approach problems one at a time, rather than juggling many things at once?	Do you like to juggle several problems at a time?
Do sweets give you quick energy?	When you eat sweets, do you burn out quickly after a short energy burst?
Does red meat feel heavy in your body?	Do you reach for salty snacks when stressed?
Do spices and condiments give an energy lift?	Do you have a hearty appetite?
Are you more satisfied by jam on toast than butter?	Are you more satisfied by butter on toast than jam?
Do you feel better eating two meals daily?	Do you feel better eating full meals every three to four hours?

Continued ➡

drate sources. They tolerate more grains, legumes and vegetables and should limit intake of red meat and dairy.

Blood type B appeared less than 10,000 years ago, after the introduction of grains into the diet. Thus, B blood types can handle a wide range of animal products, dairy and complex carbohydrates. This blood type should avoid chicken and sesame seeds/oil as they cause clumping in B type blood.

The most recent blood type on the planet and thus the rarest, **AB blood types** do very well on a vegetarian diet. They can easily digest dairy, grains and domesticated meat.

Environment/Climate Influences: This refers to the influences of where you live. Regardless of your heritage and blood type, for instance, if you live in a cold, northern climate, your body generally needs more protein and fewer carbohydrates. If you live in a warm, southern climate, your body needs a lighter diet of less protein and more complex carbohydrates.

Inherited Influences: What health issues exist in your family also determines your body needs or intolerances. If there's diabetes, it's generally safe to assume you may be sugar sensitive and thus need to ingest simple sugars (fruit, honey, etc.) and complex sugars (grains) in moderation. If there's asthma or allergies, dairy products should be limited. If there's alcoholism, there's generally a greater sensitivity to Liver heating and congesting foods such as nuts, nut butters, avocados, cheese, caffeine, alcohol, turkey, chocolate, and fried and fatty foods.

Putting It All Together: Taking all these keys into account, if you look at the current dietetic food pyramid guide you will be shocked to see that it is beneficial for only certain types of people (fast-burners, and A, AB and some B blood types living in warmer, southern climates). This guide is devastating for slow burners, O blood types and those living in colder, northern climates, and helps account for the rampant obesity, hypothyroidism, syndrome X, diabetes, and other health issues we see today. Thus, be sure to use these keys as clues so that when put together, they determine the right diet for you personally. The importance of one key over another varies individually. Experiment with these keys to help determine which are most important and influential for your unique dietary needs.

The Process of Digestion

Your digestion can be likened to a pot of soup bubbling at about 98–99 degrees F on the stove. In TCM, the pot of soup is the Spleen, the burner under the pot is the Stomach, and the pilot light of the stove is the Kidneys. Foods that digest easily in this soup pot are thoroughly cooked and warm in temperature.

When added to the soup pot, raw foods, cold foods eaten directly out of the refrigerator or freezer or cold energy foods all stop the soup from bubbling and slow the digestive process until they are heated up to match the body's temperature. If digestion is strong, this occurs fairly quickly, but over time the body has to turn up the burner underneath the pot to counteract the coolness obstructing digestion.

When the metabolic Stomach burner suddenly "turns up" symptoms often arise, such as forehead headaches, gum infections, bleeding gums, increased appetite, dry lips, mouth sores and/or bad breath. If the intake of cold foods continues, it also dampens the pilot light in the Kidneys, making

it difficult to stay lit. This is similar to putting wet wood on the fire—it creates smoke (Stomach Heat) and burns low, providing little heat (Deficient Spleen Qi and Yang).

Eventually, the burner cannot be turned up any further. Digestion becomes sluggish until, ultimately, food is not fully broken down and passes through the stools undigested, like wet wood dampening the fire so in time it goes out altogether (Deficient Kidney Yang). When digestion gets this Cold, other symptoms manifest, such as gas, bloating, sleepiness after eating, anemia, fatigue, weakness, lowered immunity, poor appetite, amenorrhea (lack of menstrual bleeding), loose stools or diarrhea, frequent copious urination, lowered sex drive, achy lower back and knees, and a variety of other complaints. Although these symptoms can occur at any time of year, they are generally aggravated in late summer (due to the excessive intake of cooling summer foods) or winter (the coldest season and Kidney time of year).

On the other hand, excessive amounts of hot foods, either from a high temperature or heating Energy, such as greasy or oily foods, excessive intake of hot spices or lamb, cause the soup pot to suddenly boil and splatter. This causes too much Heat in the body, leading to headaches, hypertension, irritability, restlessness, difficulty falling asleep, hyperacidity, hyperactivity, and thirst, among numerous other symptoms. Thus, you need the correct energied fuel to maintain healthy digestion and stoked fires.

Cooked Versus Raw Foods

Easily digested and assimilated foods build Blood and supplement your Essence trust fund with usable energy. When digestion is poor or sluggish, the body withdraws Essence in order to meet its daily demands. Ultimately, this causes Deficient Qi and Blood, aches and pains, anemia, gas, bloatedness, lethargy, weakness, lowered immunity, recurring infections and chronic ailments. This is why it is better to eat cooked foods rather than raw ones: they digest better and protect the digestive soup pot, thus providing more assimilated nutrients even if they do not contain live enzymes. Of course, healthy cooked food does not mean burnt or overcooked. It means properly soaked and cooked grains and legumes, slightly crunchy vegetables, and just-cooked meats.

At this point I am frequently told: "But raw foods are loaded with enzymes while cooked foods are dead! I need them to stay vital and well." Frankly, I have seen just as many sick raw vegetarians as I have meat eaters, and generally it is more difficult to bring them to health. While it is true raw foods have many "live" enzymes necessary for good digestion and health, if your digestion is sluggish, you won't fully metabolize or assimilate them and then the vitality of raw foods is totally lost. It is not only what you eat that is important, but also what you assimilate.

In addition, vegetable digestion takes little hydrochloric acid so that over time, your body produces a smaller amount. As digestive ability decreases, it becomes more difficult to digest other foods since they need more hydrochloric acid to metabolize. It is then that I hear, "I can't handle anything other than vegetables, fruit, and juices. Everything else is too heavy too digest." This is always a sign of impaired digestion. Now it takes time and focus, along with eating only cooked foods, slowly introducing more concentrated protein and taking digestive tonic herbs to restore good digestion.

This is why fermented foods and cultured products are so important throughout all cultures: they provide the valuable "live" enzymes so important for good digestion. As predigested foods, they are not only easily assimilated, but also provide the valuable nutrients and live enzymes our bodies need. Thus, fermented and cultured foods are the best substitutes for raw vegetables. Most traditional cultures have a native fermented or cultured food with every meal. Choose the ones that most closely match your ancestral heritage.

A Balanced Diet

The following basic balanced diet serves as a guideline for most people. It is broken into the Western categories, protein, carbohydrates and fats, with a look at specific food energies in each of them. To create your own personal dietary plan, vary the ratio of proteins, carbohydrates, and fats according to the keys given earlier in the section Determining the Right Diet for You. Then choose the appropriate energy foods within each category to match your body's needs.

PROTEIN

· Animal protein in amounts personally needed; eggs, grains and legumes together; cultured dairy in moderation; protein powders only as necessary; some fermented soy

CARBOHYDRATES

· Whole grains and legumes properly soaked and cooked
· Mostly cooked vegetables (still slightly crisp)—5 different ones per day of varying colors
· Dark leafy greens (collard, kale, mustard, bok choy, dandelion, chard, spinach)
· Fruit in season—mostly cooked and with spices (cinnamon, ginger, cardamom)
· Some salads in warmer seasons
· Fermented and cultured foods

FATS

· Small amounts of essential fatty acids, ghee, olive oil, sesame oil; small amounts of nuts and seeds as appropriate for your body's balance

Protein

Protein, the body's building block of life, creates Qi and Blood and from there, muscles, tissues and so on. It also gives strength, endurance, immunity, resistance and Heat. Excessive protein intake, however, taxes the kidneys and creates toxins, congestion, irritability and Excess Heat. Bear in mind that some proteins, such as red meat, are highly concentrated and only small amounts are needed, while other proteins, such as combined grains and beans, are less concentrated and so not as readily accessible to the body as are animal proteins.

Each person needs to determine his/her own protein level and needs. Don't go by an intellectual idea or theory but experiment with how you feel when you don't eat enough, or eat too much. Find what amount helps you feel good, strong, energetic and flexible. Bear in mind that your protein needs change from day to day and week to week according to what is going on in your life. In general, physical work requires more carbohydrates to sustain, while mental work demands more protein.

To determine how much and what type of protein you require refer to the keys under the section

Continued ➡

Determining the Right Diet for You. In general, those with O blood types, northern European or Northern Hemisphere ancestries and living in cold climates need substantial amounts of concentrated protein in their daily diets. Those with A or AB blood types, living in southern or hot climates and having Mediterranean, East Indian or tropical ancestries need less protein. B Blood types vary in protein needs; experimentation helps determine what is needed for each individual. Regardless of the quantity or type of protein eaten, everyone needs to include a complete protein with every meal, three times a day. It is the proper combination of protein, carbohydrates and fats that forms a complete nutritional meal.

Meat

Meat ranges from neutral-hot to neutral-cold in energy, yet it is full in quality. Meat, particularly red meat, is a very concentrated protein. If you have Excess Heat and need to eliminate, meat should be limited to white meats 2–3 times a week. If you need to build a Deficient condition, eat meat 1–2 times/day. In general, limit red meat and turkey to 1–2 servings per week (because they are quite congesting) and emphasize neutral-warm meats, such as fish and chicken.

A danger of eating meat is ingesting the drugs and chemicals injected into those animals. Thus, try to eat only organic meat because it is relatively pure and the animals are usually treated better. Avoid eating processed meats as they generally contain preservatives and carcinogens. Further, cook meat with spices, such as ginger, to help neutralize toxicity and aid quick metabolism and assimilation (see Recipes at the end of this chapter for how to detoxify meat).

The issue of whether to eat meat or not is a personal one. All foods are neither inherently "good" nor "bad" but subject to each individual's needs and preferences. I have seen people eliminate meat from their diets and feel much better. I have also seen ten-year vegetarians begin to eat a little meat and become healthier and stronger than ever before.

Excessive meat eating causes Heat, stagnation, toxicity and acidity, resulting in symptoms such as constipation, abdominal stuffiness, headaches, restless sleep, headaches, hypertension, heart attacks, arthritis, strokes, aggressiveness, irritability, red face and neck, rheumatism, stiff neck and shoulders, and gout. Also, as a food dense in protein and fat, excess amounts set up cravings for sugar (and vice versa), a substance high in carbohydrates and devoid of protein, minerals and fat.

On the other hand, vegetarians must eat more strictly to maintain health, eating only cooked food and a balanced protein at every meal. This does not allow for inclusion of many empty foods in the diet, such as fruit, salads, juices, and other raw uncooked foods. Be sure to include warming and building herbs to provide warmth, resistance and immunity. Ideally include some fish for a concentrated protein source.

In traditional medicine, meat is classified according to its therapeutic value (along with herbs and other foods): beef is neutral, sweet in taste and nourishes Qi and Blood and the Spleen-pancreas and Intestines, but its full energy easily leads to stagnation; lamb is hot in energy and nourishes Blood, the Heart, Spleen and Kidneys; pork is neutral, moistening and nourishes the Kidneys and Liver Yin; chicken is warming and tonifies Spleen, Stomach and Liver Qi; and duck is neutral, moistening and nourishing to the Lungs and Kidneys. Although a lean meat, keep turkey to a minimum because it is too Heating, Drying and stagnating to Liver Qi.

Consider adding small amounts of organ meats (liver, heart, kidney, gizzards, etc.) back into your weekly diet. Historically, organ meats have been an important part of most all culture's diets. They strengthen their associated organs and glands (heart strengthens the Heart, liver the Liver, and so on). The rampant hypothyroidism found today is often due to insufficient nutrition and poor glandular function, which organ meats support. Sausage was one of the best forms for eating organ meats as all edible parts of the animal were ground together to create this food. If you don't like organ meats, locate organic sausage made this old-fashioned way.

Dairy

The basic energy of dairy is neutral to warm and full/building. It adds valuable protein to the diet, especially for vegetarians, and moistens and builds, particularly for those who are underweight or have Dryness. In India, diary is widely used as a major source of protein. Yet, dairy is also Dampening and in excess, quite stagnating to Energy, creating mucus, cysts, fibroids, mood swings, cough, tight neck and shoulders, lung ailments, allergies and other conditions. Often children's asthma, coughs, runny noses, diarrhea or constipation disappear when dairy and juices are eliminated from the diet. This is even truer if the dairy is eaten cold directly out of the refrigerator.

Curtail dairy's dampening energy by drinking milk warm and eating yogurt or cottage cheese with cooked foods. Thus, be sure to heat dairy or bring it to room temperature before eating. Further, add a little cinnamon, cardamom, or ginger, plus take with some honey to counteract its mucus-producing effects.

Milk has different properties according to the animal from which it is taken. The cow has more fat content and its milk induces more mucus in the system. Yet, because the cow has a more peaceful disposition, its milk is "calmer." Goat's milk, on the other hand, is more alkaline and has a composition similar to that of human milk. Yet, goats tend to be more restless and aggressive, and this more "heating" characteristic of the goat makes its milk less mucus forming. Therefore, goat's milk is a better choice for people who can't tolerate cow's milk, get mucus easily, or have Coldness.

The best ways to ingest dairy products are in cultured forms (yogurt, cheese, clabber, curds, whey, kefir, koumiss, longfil, crème fráiche, sour cream, cottage cheese, yogurt cheese, kefir cheese, and buttermilk). This is because the fermentation (souring) process breaks down casein (milk protein), a very difficult protein to digest. Further, culturing restores many of the enzymes destroyed during pasteurization. Finally, cultured dairy products are much easier to digest and provide important friendly bacteria and lactic acid to the digestive tract. Often people who have dairy allergies do fine with cultured dairy.

Ideally, dairy products should be whole rather than low fat. Fats are needed with protein intake for mineral absorption and adequate protein utilization. Also, a lack of fat causes blood sugar dips, ultimately resulting in hunger and snacking (and weight gain rather than loss). Dairy should also ideally be purchased raw, non-homogenized and non-pasteurized. Homogenization makes fat more susceptible to rancidity and oxidation, while pasteurization destroys vital enzymes, making it less digestible and dairy allergies more likely. As well, be sure to eat only organic dairy to avoid drugs, hormones and antibiotics injected into cows (these substances concentrate in animal fat).

Eggs

Eggs, like meat, contain all amino acids and are high in protein and fat-soluble vitamins. They are neutral, full in energy and moistening. The idea that eggs increase cholesterol is a controversial one. In fact, eggs are high in lecithin, a cholesterol-lowering agent that also keeps cholesterol moving in the bloodstream. Eggs are best eaten in their whole, complete form, which contains both protein and fat together, an essential combination for protein metabolism and mineral assimilation. It is also best to purchase eggs from free-range chickens not given hormones or antibiotics.

Soy

When vegetarianism became popular in the late 1960s and '70s, many turned to tofu as their main source of protein. Fifteen to twenty years later, numerous of these same folks complained of fatigue, poor digestion, poor memory and hypothyroidism among many other symptoms. While several factors contributed to this, such as "poor vegetarianism" (i.e., insufficient protein and poor food combining), a main culprit was the heavy use of soy products. Children fed soy in school lunches react with vomiting, diarrhea, upper respiratory infections, rashes, fevers, extreme emotional behavior, immune problems, thyroid disorders and pituitary insufficiency. Infants fed soy-based formula have a higher incidence of learning disabilities and early-onset puberty.[1]

Clinically I have seen such issues over and over and experienced them personally with family and

Energy of Meat				
Hot	Warm	Neutral	Cool	Cold
Lamb	Chicken	Herring Pork	Mussel	Clam
Trout	Fresh ham	Oyster Beef		Crab
	Anchovy	Sardine Eggs		
	Shrimp	Duck Carp		
	Turkey	Goose Tuna		
		Whitefish Oyster		

Energy of Dairy				
Hot	Warm	Neutral	Cool	Cold
	Goat's milk	Cow's milk	Mussel	Clam
	Goat's cheese	Cow's cheese		Crab
	Butter	Cottage cheese		
	Ghee	Yogurt		

Continued ➡

friends. Since then, much important research brings the true nature of soy to light, despite the explosion of soy protein sources over the last decade from intense marketing strategies promoting its apparent health benefits.

Traditionally, the soy legume was used to fix nitrogen in the soil. Only when fermentation processes were applied around 2500 years ago was soy eaten as food—tempeh, miso, natto, and soy sauce. In recent times, it was processed into the common forms used today—soymilk, tofu, soy protein powders, texturized vegetable protein, soy protein isolate, and soy infant formulas.

In actuality, soy contains many antinutrients, or natural toxins. It is rich in potent enzyme inhibitors that block the action of trypsin and other enzymes needed for protein digestion, resulting in reduced protein digestion and amino acid deficiencies. Soy also contains hemagglutinin, a clot-promoting substance that causes red blood cells to clump. As well, both trypsin and hemagglutinin are growth inhibitors. Fortunately, these components are deactivated during the process of fermentation.

Soy also contains goitrogens—substances that depress thyroid function (babies fed soymilk formula have a higher incidence of thyroid issues). Hypothyroidism is now a rampant problem in the West, and excess intake of soy products is certainly a contributor. As well, soy is very high in phytic acid, a substance that interferes with protein absorption and blocks the uptake of essential minerals in the intestinal tract, particularly calcium, magnesium, copper, iron, iodine, and especially zinc. Such mineral deficiencies can lead to problems involving the bones, blood sugar, nerves, memory, and brain. Further, soy notably lacks important vitamins such as A, D, and B_{12}.

Energetically, soy is cold and dampening, depleting digestive fires (Spleen Yang) and slowing metabolism (Kidney Yang), setting the stage for hypothyroidism, Candida, chronic fatigue, cold hands and feet, gas, bloatedness, coldness, lowered immunity, anemia, and scanty menstruation, among many other conditions.

By now many of you are wondering about all the touted soy health benefits, such as lowering cholesterol, aiding menopause with estrogen-like compounds, and preventing cancer. Yet, how can soy help alleviate osteoporosis if it blocks calcium absorption? And all beans contain genistein, the cancer-reducing component of soy. Further, while Asians do have a lower incidence of breast, uterine and prostate cancer, they have much higher rates of other types of cancer, especially of the esophagus, stomach, pancreas and liver.

Thus, many of these health claims are premature and biased. While the Japanese do consume soy daily, it's mainly in fermented form and only as much as 1–2 tsp./day. Further, a mineral-rich fish broth and serving of fish or meat generally follow it.

Thus, if you eat soy, only eat fermented soy products, such as tempeh and miso. Limit intake of soymilk, tofu, soy isolate protein powders and all other soy forms if you are concerned about their cold, dampening energies, mineral-blocking effects, enzyme inhibitors, goitrogenicity, endocrine disruption and increased allergic reaction results.

Protein Powders

Protein powders, mostly made from whey or soy, are now readily available in pure form, or mixed with sugar (usually fructose) and vitamins/minerals. Like all supplements, these are concentrated substances separated from their whole food source. It is always better to eat a whole food rather than its parts, because the whole food contains added components that metabolize and balance its other elements. However, for those with Deficiency, or vegetarians who won't eat meat but need higher levels of protein than a typical vegetarian diet provides, protein powders can be useful, even essential.

I generally recommend undenatured whey protein powder rather than soy because it metabolizes better, doesn't have any added sugar and boosts immunity (some are even lactose free). Soy protein powders tend to be genetically manufactured, have added sugar, are difficult to digest and their processing leaches high levels of aluminum into the final product, not to mention the other negative effects of soy (read about soy above).

Because protein powders are mostly predigested, they quickly metabolize. Yet, a small part generally remains in the stomach unless the protein powder is taken with carbohydrates, such as whole grains, vegetables, or fruit. The bulk and fiber of carbohydrates help metabolize the residue protein, moving it through the stomach and intestines. If protein powders are taken alone, the undigested portion remaining in the stomach blocks digestion in time, causing food stagnation, stuffiness in the abdomen, constipation and headaches. Further, if the protein powder isn't natural, but partly artificial, the artificial part causes toxicity, as seen in resulting skin outbreaks.

Other Protein Sources

The combination of grains with legumes/seeds/nuts provides all the amino acids necessary to form a complete protein. For many people, particularly blood types A, AB, and some B's, this less-concentrated protein is adequate, especially if living in hot, southern climates. For blood type O and some B's, and for those living in cold, northern climates, grains and beans alone usually do not provide sufficient protein for all meals, and so some animal protein usually needs be included to maintain a healthy body. This is because grains and legumes are carbohydrates high in fiber, which must first be broken down in order to get to the protein. Thus, grains and beans are considered a "weak" or less concentrated protein.

Carbohydrates

Carbohydrates are comprised of starch and sugar. When broken down in the body, they form the primary sugar in the blood. There are three types of carbohydrates: complex, simple, and processed. Complex carbs include whole grains, legumes and starchy vegetables, such as potatoes, broccoli and asparagus. They digest slowly in the body.

Simple carbs include all sugars and sweeteners, such as sugar, honey, molasses, and the fructose found in fruit and fruit juices. Simple carbs enter the blood at various rates, though much more quickly than complex carbohydrates, raising blood sugar levels and increasing fat storage (fructose and agave are the slowest metabolizing of the sugars).

Processed carbs act just like simple carbs in their effect, whether from whole sources or not. They include all flour products, such as pasta, breads, pastries, pie crust, cakes, crackers, cookies, bagels, muffins, cold cereals, rice cakes, quick oats, pre-prepared and packaged foods, many desserts, pancakes, waffles, flour-coated fried foods, donuts, and all types of chips. Often people gasp when they see this list, for these foods usually comprise 70% or more of their diet! Further, junk food is generally made from vegetable oils, white flour and sugar. While it quickly satisfies taste buds and hunger, it just as quickly stores as fat and drops blood sugar levels.

Flour products acidify and strongly imbalance blood chemistry. Even those from recently ground, whole grain, organic flour are made from flour and water which together form—does this sound familiar?— glue, or paste. This is exactly what these foods turn into inside our intestines. In excess, they cause tremendous congestion, particularly if coupled with insufficient protein.

I frequently see people develop carbohydrate sensitivity leading to food allergies, hypoglycemia, Candida, leaky gut syndrome, Syndrome X, hypothyroidism, weakness, gas, bloatedness, anemia, diabetes, lowered immunity, food allergies, and/or chronic fatigue as a result. Folks usually eating diets high in carbohydrates and low in protein for ten to twenty years and developing these health issues are generally O blood types with northern European ancestries. When eating flour products in excess, even those made of organic whole grains, coupled with insufficient protein intake, these ailments (and many others) ultimately arise.

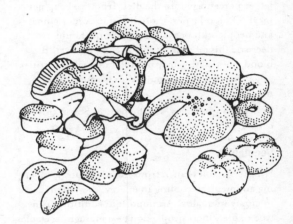

Grains and Legumes

Grains and legumes are predominantly neutral-warm and neutral-cool in energy and neutral in quality. A complex carbohydrate, grains are broken down slowly by the body, giving long-lasting energy and strength, particularly to AB, A, and some B blood types. Adding beans to grains provides a complete protein that should be regularly eaten by those who don't include meat, or as a periodic protein substitute for meat eaters. Further, beans are high in genistine, an anticancer agent. Bread and pasta are not substitutes for grains, even if organically grown and made from whole grains. Once ground into flour and mixed with water, you get a glue-like flour product that is dampening and congesting to digestion.

It is extremely important that all grains and legumes be soaked before they are eaten. As complex carbohydrates, their protein content is not readily available, but obtained only after the fiber is broken down. Soaking grains 12–24 hours and beans 12–36 hours catalyzes this process and, more importantly, neutralizes the phytic acid content. If not soaked, phytic acid actually interferes with protein absorption. When grains and beans are properly soaked, phytic acid is neutralized and protein availability shoots up sixfold. Fermented foods with phytic acid, like tempeh, are fine as the fermentation process neutralizes this acid.

After eating a high-grain diet for ten to twenty years, many Westerners today are experiencing low energy, depressed immunity, Candida and hypoglycemia (among other problems), especially those of O blood type and northern European ancestry. This occurred because the grains and legumes generally weren't soaked and were also used as the primary source of protein along with soy products. While eating lots of grain usually works fine for AB,

Continued ➡

Energy of Grains and Legumes

Hot	Warm	Neutral	Cool	Cold
	Sweet rice	Adzuki (azuki) bean	Barley	Soymilk
		Kidney bean	Wheat	
		String bean	Tofu	
		Rice	Mung bean	
		Yellow soybean	Soybean	
		Black soybean	Millet	
		Peas	Buckwheat	
		Corn	Wheat gluten	
		Rye		

A and some B blood types, over time it causes a myriad of problems for O blood types. Thus, the proper quantity of grains to include in your diet varies according to your blood type, ancestry, climate, and digestive strength.

In general, those with blood types AB and A, living in southern climates, or with strong digestions tolerate grains well and can incorporate a larger percentage into the diet, from ½–1 cup per meal. O blood types, those living in colder climates and people with weakened digestions should decrease this amount to ¼—⅓ cup per meal. B blood types may or may not tolerate high quantities of grains; determine your needs through experimentation.

For soy products, see the section Soy in this chapter.

Vegetables

While vegetables range from slightly neutral-warming and neutral-cooling in energy, they are neutral to empty in quality. An important addition to any type of diet, most people don't eat enough vegetables and they should comprise about 30–40 percent of each entire meal. Ideally, eat a minimum of five different vegetables a day and from all color groups (green, white, yellow, orange, and red), as the various colors supply the different nutrients our bodies need. Dark leafy greens, such as kale, collards, dandelion, mustard and bok choy, are one of the most important groups as they clear Heat, toxins and acidity from the Blood, decongest Liver Qi, aid in grain digestion and supply important vitamins and minerals. Their tremendous value cannot be overstated.

Most vegetables alkalinize the body, creating balance to acidifying meat, grains and flour products. They also supply nutrients and are a primary help in waste elimination. Since a wall of cellulose that is difficult to break down surrounds vegetables, cook them to facilitate assimilation of their vital nutrients. While raw vegetables supply vital "live" enzymes, they are extremely difficult to digest, so less nutrition is metabolized from them than from cooked vegetables (use fermented and cultured foods for the "live" enzymes). However, never overcook vegetables so they are mushy, as this destroys important nutrients. Cooked and still slightly crunchy, vegetables are less cold and digest and assimilate well. A little bit of raw food is beneficial for meat eaters, who can healthily include some salads, fruits and juices to help counteract their warmer diet.

Unfortunately, most vegetables today (even organic) are grown in soil depleted of nutrients, particularly minerals. Thus, it is extremely important to include sea vegetables in the daily diet, as they provide the essential minerals our bodies need. Some, such as arame and hiziki, are bland and make colorful additions to vegetable dishes. Others are stronger in taste, such as the more detoxifying kelps, and cooked best with legumes.

All sea vegetables are very cooling and Dampening in nature, particularly the kelps, yet therapeutically they soften lumps and masses in the body.

Energy of Vegetables

Hot	Warm	Neutral	Cool	Cold
	Onion	Carrot	Cucumber	Tomato
	Garlic	Shiitake mushroom	Eggplant	Seaweed
	Winter squash	Beet	Mettuce	
	Mustard leaf	Potato	Swiss chard	
	Kale	Sweet potato	Button mushroom	
	Chestnut	Yam	Watercress	
		Cabbage	Asparagus	
		Pumpkin	Summer squash	
		String bean	Celery	
			Lotus root	
			Spinach	
			Cauliflower	
			Broccoli	

Energy of Nut and Seeds

Hot	Warm	Neutral	Cool	Cold
	Walnut	Almond		
	Pinenut	Sesame seed		
	Chestnut	Peanut		
		Sunflower seed		

Nuts and Seeds

When combined with grains, nuts and seeds provide all needed amino acids to form a complete protein. However, and this is a BIG however, nuts and seeds are highly concentrated foods high in fat, which in excess easily stagnate Liver Qi, causing PMS, tight neck and shoulders, depression, moodiness, anger, irritability, stress, headaches, and gallbladder pains, just for starters. Because they are so rich, most should be eaten infrequently and even then in moderation, like a condiment.

The only exception I've seen is walnuts, since they tonify Kidney Yang, thus supporting Liver Qi. Walnuts, (and almonds), are also roborants (thus building the body and increasing weight). A couple tablespoons of walnuts each day can treat chronic weakness of the lower back and joints and lung weakness. Peanuts make delicious stir-fries and sauces, and help circulate Blood. In general, you can consume more seeds, such as sesame or sunflower, than nuts. Sesame seeds are a great tonic food that can be added to dishes as gomasio, a Japanese condiment.

Fruit

Rich in vitamins and minerals, but lacking in protein, fruit has a neutral-warm, neutral-cool or cold energy and an empty quality. Fruit is best eaten locally grown and in season, and better digested and assimilated when eaten baked, stewed, sauced, or cooked, with cinnamon, ginger, and/or cardamom and walnuts added to make it less cooling. Additionally, include a little protein on the side to balance its higher glycemic (blood sugar raising) effects.

Meat eaters should regularly include fruit (of different colors) in their diets to eliminate Heat toxins, acidity, and Excess. Young children (who naturally have more Internal Heat) also benefit from moderate fruit intake on a daily basis with occasional use of juices (be sure to add a dash of ginger, cinnamon, or cardamom and dilute it by half with water to lower its concentrated fruit sugar). Excessive intake of fruit juices, however, contributes to children's runny noses, coughs, and diarrhea.

Vegetarians should moderate fruit intake and only eat it cooked and with spices and protein. Excess fruit thins the Blood and creates Dampness, causing anemia, weakness, scanty menses, fatigue, poor digestion, weakness, lowered immunity, diarrhea, frequent and recurring colds and flu, mucus, chronic asthma and other lung problems, low back pain, sciatica, impotence, infertility, nasal drip or runny noses, and many other ailments. This is especially true of fruit juices, which are highly concentrated. Few people could eat the eight or more carrots or apples it takes to make a glass of juice, plus the important fiber is lost, which aids in the fruit's digestion. Thus, keep juices to a minimum, dilute them and add spices to aid in their digestion.

While eating fruit and protein together is generally considered poor food combining, many who experience gas, bloatedness, runny nose, diarrhea, and abdominal cramps after eating fruit alone do not experience these symptoms when intaking fruit with a protein (try cottage cheese). Further, these folks feel more satisfied, don't get blood sugar peaks and drops, or hypoglycemia, and their energy is sustained longer.

Continued ➡

Energy of Fruit				
Hot	**Warm**	**Neutral**	**Cool**	**Cold**
	Cherry	Fig	Apple	Banana
	Date	Grape	Lemon	Mango
	Peach	Loquat	Lime	Watermelon
	Coconut milk	Papaya	Pear	Cantaloupe
	Guava	Plum	Strawberry	Grapefruit
	Kumquat	Raspberry/blackberry	Tangerine	Star fruit
		Blueberry	Orange	Melons
		Olive	Mandarin orange	Persimmon
		Coconut meat		Mulberry
		Pineapple		
		Apricot		

Fats

Perhaps the most misunderstood food group is fats. Many people run from fats, fearing they cause weight gain, high cholesterol, and heart disease. Yet fats are not only unharmful to the body, they are essential to protein metabolism and mineral absorption, and are the primary fuel warming your body and providing energy to your muscles. They also slow carbohydrate release and keep your appetite satisfied for hours.

What is most important about fat is *quantity* and *quality*. Slow-burners, A, AB, and some B blood types, and those living in warmer climates need less fat. Fast-burners, O blood types and those living in colder climates need more fat. In terms of fat quality, be sure to consume only organic fats, as chemicals and pesticides are concentrated in fats. Further, there are three types of fats: saturated, unsaturated and transfats and not all of these act the same in the body.

Saturated fats, solid at room temperature, are found in meat, dairy, lard, beef tallow, and coconut and palm kernel oils. They provide good sources of stored energy for the body, insulate vital tissues against the cold, provide fat-soluble vitamins and enhance immunity. The problem related to saturated fats has more to do with their excess consumption rather than the fats themselves. Many saturated fats are hidden in restaurant foods, fast foods and highly processed and frozen foods.

There are two types of unsaturated fats: monounsaturated and polyunsaturated. Monounsaturated fats, solid at cold temperatures, include canola oil, olive oil, peanuts, almonds, cashews, and avocados. They metabolize quickly and can increase weight gain because the body mostly uses saturated fats for energy. (Olive oil, ghee, or clarified butter, and sesame oil are monounsaturated fats that don't go rancid.)

Polyunsaturated fats are found in fish (salmon, mackerel, halibut), vegetable oils (sunflower, safflower, sesame), and botanicals (borage, evening primrose). These fats rapidly go rancid from heat and light, and should be used quickly, or refrigerated in dark containers.

It is from the polyunsaturated fats that we obtain essential fatty acids (EFAs)—once known as vitamin F. There are two types of EFAs: omega 3's and omega 6s. Omega 3 oils come from flax, chia and pumpkin seeds, walnuts, canola oil, seaweeds and cold-water fatty fish such as salmon, sardines, butterfish, tuna and anchovies. Omega 6 oils come from plant sources such as unprocessed, unheated vegetable oils (safflower, sunflower, corn and sesame), botanicals (borage, evening primrose), and saturated animal fat (choose free-range organic meats because drugs concentrate in animal fat).

While omega 3s and 6s each have individual functions, both are necessary for health and should be taken in equal amounts rather than one over the other.

Trans fats, "modern" manufactured oils, are hands down the most harmful fats for your body. They include hydrogenated and partially hydrogenated vegetable oils shortening, margarine, and soybean oil. The manufacturing process of trans fats strips the original oils of their EFAs, creating a chemical makeup closer to plastic. Subsequently, these fats cannot be broken down in the body, but are stored in fat tissues (like the breasts), eventually leading to such diseases as cancer, obesity, diabetes, heart disease, depressed immunity, and the formation of free radicals (causing wrinkles, age spots and tumors for starters). Trans fats are commonly found in commercial as well as health foods, such as breads, crackers, chips, cookies, rolls, muffins, cakes, pies, donuts, preprepared packaged foods, and most restaurant foods. Read labels for hydrogenated oils and avoid margarine, whether from butter, vegetable, or soy sources.

In excess, most fats create Heat in the body, particularly in the Liver and Gallbladder, causing hypertension, PMS, depression, headaches, insomnia and a propensity toward anger and irritability. Those with Liver Heat or stagnant Liver Qi should only use small amounts of saturated fats. Nuts, nut butters, avocados and tahini all have a very high fat content and should be eaten infrequently and in small amounts. The best fats include olive oil, sesame oil, and ghee (clarified butter). These are natural sources of important vitamins and minerals. Not only do olive oil and ghee not go rancid, ghee has the added energetic quality of sparking metabolic fires without adding unwanted Heat.

Now before you shy away from fats altogether, remember the problem is not with fats themselves, but with the quantity and type. We do need fat with every meal, but most of us don't need more than ½–¼ teaspoon, depending on our dietary needs. In fact, fat is needed to lose fat! Those who lose body fat from reducing food fats in their diet usually do so because they were eating excess fats to begin with.

However, those who don't eat fat, or only low fat, may ultimately gain weight. If there is not enough fat in the diet, then protein can't be properly metabolized and the unsatisfied body tells the brain to keep eating. This is the reason most people cannot stay on low-fat diets and eventually develop other health problems, such as mineral deficiencies. Fat is essential for mobilizing stored fat out of the body; thus, some fat in the diet is necessary for reducing stored body fat.

Fermented and Cultured Foods

Fermented and cultured foods are extremely important, not only for digestion, but also for health and well-being. These foods are partially predigested, making them easily digested and assimilated. The fermentation or culturing process further adds invaluable enzymes back into the food, which provide nutrients and assist digestion. These foods also supply friendly bacteria to the digestive tract. Thus, fermented, cultured, pickled, leavened and sprouted foods are the best substitutes for raw, "live" vegetables and juices.

Most traditional cultures have a fermented or cultured food with every meal. For example, yogurt is traditionally eaten in India, sauerkraut in Germany, kimchi in Korea, cultured dairy products in Scandinavia, miso and umeboshi plums in Japan, and pickled fruits and vegetables in many countries. Choose the fermented or cultured products that most closely match your ancestral heritage.

An easy recipe is to chop enough vegetables to fill a mason jar ½ full. Place cut vegetables in a bowl and mix with 3 tsp. salt and 2 Tblsp. whey (make yourself by straining yogurt through cheesecloth overnight, catching the liquid—this is the whey—if you don't add whey, add 4 tsp. salt). Toss mixture well, stuff into mason jar and pack down. Screw on lid and let sit unrefrigerated for 3 days, turning once a day. Then refrigerate and eat small amounts with every meal.

Extreme Foods

There are several other foods worth discussing here since they frequently comprise a large percentage of most diets: sugar, salt, alcohol, and caffeine. Tobacco, although smoked and not eaten, is still ingested and, since its effects are severe and serious, it's also included here. Ingesting any of these extreme foods usually sets up a craving for the other and creates an endless cycle. For example, after eating sugar for awhile, the body craves salt and vice versa. Yet this type of "balance" is extreme, like the seesaw described in The Energy of Food.

Processed sugar causes Stomach Heat with accompanying forehead headaches, gum problems, dry lips, mouth sores and bad breath, among other health issues. As well, sugar overtonifies the Spleen, eventually leading to digestive problems, poor energy and a big stomach (sugar expands the abdomen).

Refined white sugar is an empty food that leaches important vitamins and minerals (such as calcium) from the body, depletes the immune sys-

Fermented and Cultured Products				
Fermented		**Cultured**		
Umeboshi plum	Sauerkraut	Yogurt	Sour cream	Cheese
Pickles	Kimchi	Cottage cheese	Clabber	Curds
Pickled vegetables	Pickled rinds	Yogurt cheese	Kefir cheese	Kefir
Chutney	Pickled fruit	Crème fraiche	Cream cheese	Whey
Pickled grape leaves	Relishes	Koumiss	Longfil	Buttermilk

Continued ➡

Energy of Extreme Foods				
Hot	**Warm**	**Neutral**	**Cool**	**Cold**
	Coffee	Honey	Green tea	Salt
	Tobacco	White sugar		Sugar cane
	Vinegar			
	Wine/alcohol			
	Brown sugar			
	Malt/maltose			
	Molasses			
	Chocolate/cocoa			
	Black tea			

tem by half and feeds infections. As well, white sugar causes muscle cramps and spasms and makes it difficult for the body to hold alignment (because it weakens the Kidneys). If that were not enough, it also gives an energy boost so you skip eating when food is actually what your body needs. Excessive sugar intake also causes salt cravings.

Many people are amazed at how good they feel simply by eliminating sugar from their diet. Those with strong sugar cravings generally eat insufficient amounts of protein. Rarely do I tell someone to stop eating sugar. Rather, when people increase protein, grains, and legumes in their diet, their sugar cravings quickly disappear.

Whole sugars, such as maple sugar, honey, barley and rice malts and raw unrefined sugar cane, are healthier choices, though they should be used sparingly since they are empty foods. Fructose metabolizes more slowly than other sugars and so is frequently used in health foods. Yet, fructose is bleached and so should be eaten more sparingly. Agave metabolizes slowly, too, perhaps even more so than fructose (Native Americans traditionally use cactus sweeteners like agave with no problems, but quickly develop diabetes on refined white sugar). Thus, agave is one of the best sweeteners to use.

Salt is cooling and softening in nature. A little salt tonifies the Kidneys, but in excess it causes water retention and subsequent edema, high blood pressure and other problems. Ideally, use unrefined sea or earth salts because they are high in minerals. Alternatively, use gomasio, a combination of sesame seeds and salt (see Recipes at the end of this chapter). When the seeds are ground, their oil coats the salt particles, thus metabolizing the salt directly into the cells and preventing water retention. Excessive eating of salty foods causes sugar cravings.

Alcohol, caffeine, and **tobacco** all cause Heat and irritation, particularly in meat eaters. In vegetarians, alcohol, caffeine, and tobacco can provide the Heat the body craves since it is usually fed a very cooling diet. This quite often makes it much more difficult, if not impossible, for vegetarians to quit smoking tobacco and drinking coffee without a diet change, even more so than meat eaters. In addition, because of its sugar content, alcohol creates the same sugar swings and addictions as sugar does (this is why it goes so well with a meat diet), and it is quite Heating to the Liver and depleting to the Kidneys. As well, alcoholic beverages cause stagnant Blood, which can be seen as a purplish discoloration on the nose and cheeks of alcoholics or heavy alcohol drinkers.

Caffeine drains energy reserves from the adrenals to create a temporary sense of well-being. Drinking coffee to push through tiredness ultimately leads to adrenal exhaustion, which is very difficult to replenish (bags under the eyes are one impending sign of this). It may take years for adrenal exhaustion to show up, and then suddenly take you by "surprise." Coffee is especially harmful this way and becomes a catch-22 of needing coffee to wake up while at the same time it makes you tired (the adrenal exhaustion). If you can drink coffee after 5 P.M. and it doesn't affect your sleep, worry about it! This means your adrenals aren't responding and well on their way to exhaustion. (See the chart, Caffeine Contents, for specific foods and how much caffeine they contain.)

While not containing caffeine, chocolate contains theobromine and mate contains mateine, both of which energetically act like caffeine by creating Liver Heat and depleting Kidney Qi, Yin and Yang. Further, when eaten excessively, chocolate causes toxins in the Liver, which generally show up as skin outbreaks. Perhaps the only caffeine exception is green tea, which is Cooling and Drying in energy rather than Heating and Dampening. It clears Heat from the Liver, is antitumor and anticancer and has the lowest caffeine content of all caffeinated substances.

To get off caffeine, drink a beneficial coffee substitute, such as dandelion/chicory "coffee" made from 1 part dandelion root with ½ part roasted chicory root (to prevent caffeine withdrawal headaches, slowly reduce the caffeine while proportionately increasing the dandelion/chicory coffee). Grind the herbs like coffee beans and put in a filter or percolator. The resulting tea is dark, full bodied, and bitter in flavor, satisfying all coffee needs but the taste. Yet, it does exactly the opposite of coffee: it clears Heat, Dampness, and toxins from the Liver and helps the Kidneys to filter fluids.

Alternatively, try drinking grain drinks, green tea or herb teas to eliminate coffee. The longest I've seen it take people to regain their true energy after quitting coffee is about a month. Until that time, you may experience more tiredness than before, but keep going, for the results are well worth it. Once caffeine is eliminated from the diet, you'll not only feel more energy, but also

Caffeine Contents*	
Substance	**Caffeine in Mg.**
Drip coffee (7 oz.)	115–175
Jolt (12 oz.)	100
Espresso (7 oz.)	100
Iced tea (12 oz.)	70
Instant coffee (7 oz.)	65–100
Tea, brewed, imported (7 oz.)	60
Mountain Dew (12 oz.)	58.8
Coca-Cola (12 oz.)	45.6
Tea, brewed, U.S. (7 oz.)	40
Diet Pepsi (12 oz.)	36
Cadbury Chocolate Bar (1 oz.)	15
Hot cocoa mix (one envelope)	5
Decaf coffee, brewed (7 oz.)	3-4
Jello Pudding Pop (47 g.)	2

* From seas.upenn.ed/~epage/caffeine/FAQmain, copyright 1994 by Alex Lopez-Ortiz.

notice that it is of better quality and clarity than you ever felt while on caffeine.

Tobacco injures the circulation because it constricts blood vessels. It also robs the cells of their much-needed oxygen supply, causing a weakening of cell functions throughout the body and injuring the Blood. Further, it causes wrinkles, lung mucus, and a husky voice, not to mention all sorts of cancers. To get off tobacco, smoke herbal cigarettes, gradually reducing the amount over time. As well, take 2–3 drops of lobelia tincture when cravings arise, ingest 2–4 caps 3 times daily of a lung decongesting formula (such as equal parts mullein, coltsfoot, chickweed, horehound, loquat, and grindelia or yerba santa) and eat a piece of honey-soaked ginseng (slice ginseng root very thinly and "marinate" in honey) periodically throughout the day.

Water is worth mentioning here because it, too, can cause disease when taken improperly. Often the brain is unable to distinguish between the need for water and the need for food. Most people are underhydrated rather than overhydrated and so need to drink more water. Most meat eaters crave iced water because it seemingly offsets their thirst, which is caused by the Internal Heat and acids created by excessive red meat eating. Yet iced water is one of the largest contributors to weakened digestion.

Imagine throwing iced water on a fire and the resulting steam and eventual extinguished fire. The same occurs in the stomach where digestive fires must be kept continually burning. If doused by iced water, the results are gas, bloatedness, lethargy, forehead headaches, drippy and stuffy nose, postnasal drip, ulcers, and poor digestion, among other ailments. Thus, drink water warm, or at room temperature.

The average meat eater should have a minimum of 6–8 glasses of pure water daily to dilute and flush meat toxins from the body and uric acid from the blood (it also relieves chronic pains in the joints and lower back). For those who eat little or no meat, less water is needed, from 4–6 glasses a day, because vegetable foods have higher water content. Excessive drinking of water causes frequent urination, while too much carbonated water creates gas, bloatedness, hiccuping, poor digestion, dizziness, spaciness, lethargy, and poor bone formation. Further, excess water intake in vegetarians can cause Dampness and overwork the Kidneys, thus weakening them.

Supplements

While herbs are whole food–like substances, supplements are concentrated components extracted from whole foods and synthesized in laboratories. Taking extensive amounts of vitamins, minerals, body-building substances, energy boosters, and other similar products have strong actions that, over time, can imbalance the body. While many people are familiar with excess vitamin C intake causing diarrhea, most do not know that prolonged excessive intake of supplements creates toxic Heat and stagnation in the body, in time causing many health issues. In fact, minerals are best absorbed by the body in their whole organic form, i.e., in food.

Taking a multivitamin or mineral supplement can be useful over a short period of time (several months), yet prolonged intake of these and/or other supplements is not a substitute for good food and proper nutrition. In time, health issues arise, not to mention digestive problems, such as gas, bloatedness, diarrhea or constipation, headaches, poor appetite, and low energy.

Supplements create a false environment—they are not the body's true energy. Only use them short term as an aid and support while getting your diet,

Continued ➡

rest, sleep, and general life back on track (unless, of course, you are dealing with serious health issues that need such supplementation). Using herbs to obtain your desired vitamins and minerals can also cause problems because herbs have many other uses that may not be appropriate for you. For instance, while nettle is high in iron, it's a diuretic, and while goldenseal contains vitamin C, it's drying to the Blood and very cooling, all of which actions may not be suitable for your particular body.

Food Therapy

Food can be used therapeutically to heal disease by following its inner warming or cooling nature. A body with Excess Heat can be balanced by eating more cooling foods and less heating ones. A body with Excess Coldness can be balanced by eating more warming foods and less cooling ones. Thus, it's important to tailor your diet according to any disease or imbalance you're experiencing, along with taking the proper herbs. Known as food therapy, this not only enhances the healing process, but usually speeds it up as well. In contrast, eating improper foods can actually drain your healing energies and prolong illness.

To use food therapeutically, first determine if your condition is one of Coldness, Heat, Dampness, Dryness, Excess, or Deficiency as outlined in The Energy of Illness. Then create your food plan accordingly. If the plan is to maintain existing good health, then follow the balanced diet outlined under the section A Balanced Diet, earlier in this chapter.

More specifically, when treating an illness of Heat (feeling irritable, thirsty, always hungry, sweating easily, and always feeling warm), it's important to eliminate foods with a hot energy, eat only a few with a warm energy, and focus more on neutral, cool and a small amount of cold energy foods. Eat mostly cooling foods until the illness is healed and the body is brought back to balance. Then a balanced diet should be adapted, for otherwise, the continued eating of cooling foods (salads, raw foods, fruit juices, etc.) over time creates the opposite energy in the body: Coldness.

It is not uncommon for someone with too much Heat from excessive meat eating to adapt a vegetarian or raw foods diet and feel great for a while. Yet, upon continued eating of these foods, Coldness is created several years later, eventually causing emaciation, lowered immunity, fatigue, and a feeling of coldness. Thus, it is very important to always come back to a balanced diet once the illness has healed.

When treating an illness of Coldness (frequent colds and flu, lowered immunity, runny nose, tiredness, weakness, diarrhea, poor appetite, and/or feelings of chill and cold), eliminate all cold foods, eat some cool foods, but only in cooked form, and focus more on balanced, warm, and some hot energy foods. This means eating only cooked foods and eliminating all raw foods, salads, fruit and vegetable juices, and anything directly out of the refrigerator or freezer. Along with the cooked foods, more concentrated protein and warm-natured foods should be ingested with every meal three times a day, including animal protein such as beef, fish, pork, or chicken. In time, adding more warming foods and meat into the diet makes vegetarians feel great again. When the illness is healed and the body brought back to balance, adapt a balanced diet, for if these foods are eaten to excess over a few years, then problems of Excess Heat and stagnation can eventually arise.

In general, vegetarians must eat much more strictly to regain and maintain balance in the body. This means ingesting only cooked foods, including sufficient protein with every meal, and cooking food with spices such as cumin, coriander, garlic, and onions to warm and spark digestion. Further, vegetarians with O type blood and/or northern European ancestry have even less leeway and absolutely need adequate protein 3 times/day to maintain health.

The following categorizes foods according to their energies and effects in the body.

DIGESTION-IMPAIRING FOODS
- Sugar
- Refrigerated/frozen foods and drinks (iced drinks, frozen yogurt, ice cream, Popsicles)
- Excessive intake of raw foods, including salads
- Excessive intake of flour products (breads, pasta, chips, cookies, crackers, pastries, etc.)
- Fruit; fruit and vegetable juices
- Potatoes (in excess)
- Excessive and prolonged intake of supplements
- Insufficient protein and nutrition

OVERLY HEATING FOODS
- Turkey
- Lamb
- Nuts and nut butters
- Alcohol
- Caffeine (coffee, black tea, cocoa, colas, mate, chocolate)
- Fried, fatty and greasy foods
- Hard cheeses
- Vinegar
- (Plus: tobacco smoking)

OVERLY COOLING FOODS
- Refrigerated/frozen foods and drinks (iced drinks, frozen yogurt, ice cream, Popsicles, etc.)
- Raw foods, including salads
- Most fruit and vegetable juices
- Melons
- Bananas
- Crabmeat and shellfish
- Soymilk, tofu

ACIDIC FOODS
- Flour products (breads, pasta, chips, cookies, crackers, pastries, etc.)
- Red meats
- Grains (except millet, barley, amaranth, and quinoa)
- Citrus (except lemons and limes)
- Tomatoes
- Green bell peppers
- Sugar

ALKALINIZING FOODS
- Umeboshi plums
- Lemons, limes, grapefruit, cranberries, blueberries
- Millet, quinoa, amaranth, barley, white rice

DAMPENING FOODS
- Flour products (breads, pasta, chips, cookies, crackers, pastries, etc.)
- Bananas, citrus, persimmon
- Cucumber, plantain, olives, seaweed
- Raw foods, including salads

- Wheat, wheat gluten, oats, potato
- Refrigerated or iced foods and drinks
- Dairy (cheese, milk, sour cream, cottage cheese, etc.)
- Honey
- Frozen foods, such as yogurt, ice cream, Popsicles
- Salt
- Potatoes
- Fruit and vegetable juices
- Excessive intake of fruit
- Soymilk, tofu, and other soy products
- Goose, oyster, clam, pork, duck

DRYING FOODS
- Adzuki, kidney, and mung beans
- Asparagus, celery, carrots, cabbage, lettuce, dark leafy greens
- Barley, rye, millet, quinoa, rice
- Tuna, chicken, lamb
- Berries

WIND-AGGRAVATING FOODS
Avoid if there's arthritis, rheumatism, asthma, or any other patterns with Wind:
- Shrimp
- Prawns
- Crab
- Lobster
- Spinach
- Rhubarb
- Mushrooms
- Caffeine
- Alcohol

Foods That Strengthen or Weaken Each Organ

Each food has a special affinity for a specific Organ. When eaten in moderation, it strengthens that Organ, but weakens it when eaten to excess. The charts on page 380 and 381 lists foods according to the Organs it strengthens or weakens.

Whole Foods

Regardless of the energies of food, there is a big difference between whole (healthy) foods and disease-causing foods. Whole foods are those that come directly from nature with the least possible interference. This means they are unrefined and preferably organic (and ideally from animals given free-range and humane treatment). As well, we should ideally consume foods that are locally grown, limiting those that come from far away. Brown rice, maple syrup, earth salt, and organic vegetables and meats are examples of whole foods.

On the other hand, disease-causing foods are highly refined with additives, preservatives, hormones, chemicals, and/or colorings added. Refined white rice, white sugar, table salt, flour products, and prepared packaged foods are examples of processed, disease-causing foods. The chart Whole Foods on page 381 suggests healthy foods to eat and unhealthy foods to avoid.

Unfortunately, many chemicals, additives and preservatives are hidden in food. For instance, MSG is a known irritant that causes skin rashes, headaches, nausea, palpitations, insomnia, hyperactivity, depression, panic attacks, migraines, and asthma, for starters. Yet, MSG is hidden in many

Continued ➡

forms, such as hydrolyzed vegetable protein, natural flavors and natural flavorings, autolyzed yeast, sodium or calcium caseinate, and more. Thus, get in the habit of reading labels and researching "foreign" names.

In today's mass-produced food market, most every stage of development is negatively affected in some way. Fruits and vegetables are hybridized to grow bigger and faster and are subjected to plant hormones, insecticides, and chemical fertilizers to increase production. Unfortunately, this sacrifices flavor and enhances the potential of disease. Animals are force-fed, given massive amounts of antibiotics, and subjected to extremely inhumane treatment, all to increase production. The result is toxicity and lowered immunity in those who eat these foods. Thus, get in the habit of reading labels and shopping selectively. There are plenty of healthy alternatives available. Eating whole foods according to a balanced energetic diet is eating to maintain strength, health, and disease prevention.

Further, more and more foods are genetically manufactured organism (GMO), completely mixing different food chemistries together in order to prolong shelf life, resist pests and enhance other commercial purposes. European countries, such as the UK, strictly forbid all GMO foods, while in the U.S. these foods are slipped past an unsuspecting public because no legal requirements exist for their labeling. In fact, most soy is now genetically manufactured, including that widely used in health foods.

How foods are cooked affects their quality as well. Never use aluminum pots and pans as aluminum is toxic, contaminates food, and causes disease, such as Alzheimer's. Glass, stainless-steel, and ceramic containers are best for cooking food. As well, use gas or wood heat, as electric heat is fine for strong bodies, but for those with lowered immunity and severe or degenerative disease, it can alter the food enough to interfere with the healing process. Microwaves should ideally never be used. They rearrange the molecular structure of the food, altering the electromagnetic field of its atoms and making the food something different than nature created. Microwaved food doesn't cook evenly and even tastes strange to some.

Ideally, eat foods within two days after being prepared. After 24 hours food quickly loses energy and nutrients, while molds start growing, even though they can't be seen. Thus, prepare food as freshly as possible. The best methods for food preservation include cold storage (refrigeration), drying, salting, fermenting, pickling, and smoking. Only freeze foods with low water content to prevent cellular deterioration caused by water's turning to ice. Eat canned foods only sparingly, as many nutrients are lost in the canning process (foods must be cooked at very high temperatures to create a vacuum and resulting hermetic seal, killing important nutrients).

Healthful Eating Routines

How food is eaten and prepared also contributes to health or disease. . . The most important thing to remember is no matter what or how you eat, be fully present with your food and give thanks for it. When you do this, you'll digest it better and become more aware of what and how you're eating.

Spleen–Strengthening Foods	Spleen–Weakening Foods
Protein (all proteins, especially beef)	Insufficient protein and nutrition
Cooked foods	Excessive intake of raw foods, including salads
Warm/room temperature drinks	Refrigerated foods and drinks
Root vegetables	Iced drinks
Winter squash	Frozen yogurt, ice cream, Popsicles
Rice, quinoa, barley, amaranth, buckwheat, millet; peanuts; tofu	Excessive intake of flour products (breads, pasta, chips, cookies, crackers, pastries, etc.)
Spices (garlic, cumin, ginger, black pepper, etc.)	Excessive hot, spicy foods (ex. Salsa)
Soups	Excessive intake of vegetable juices
Congees	Excessive intake of potatoes
Peach, apple, mango, papaya, loquat; cook fruit with spices	Excessive intake of fruit and fruit juices
Beets, cabbage, carrot, yam, sweet potato, potato, string beans, peas, winter squash, lotus root	Excessive intake of supplements
Small amounts of whole sugar, especially malt	Excessive intake of sugar, especially white, refined

Lung–Strengthening Foods	Lung–Weakening Foods
Black beans, tofu	Dampening foods
Rice	Digestion-impairing foods
Almonds, walnuts, peanuts	Citrus
Pear, loquat, tangerine, olive	Dairy
Garlic, onions, black pepper	Flour products
Duck, chicken	Raw foods
Warm foods and drinks	Cold refrigerated and/or iced foods and drinks
Water chestnuts, mustard greens, carrot, lotus root, asparagus, radish	Cigarette smoking

Kidney–Strengthening Foods	Kidney–Weakening Foods
Adzuki beans, kidney beans	Raw foods
Pork, duck, lamb, oyster	Alcohol
Asparagus, celery, sweet potato, string beans, parsley	Caffeine (coffee, black tea, cocoa, colas, chocolate)
Black sesame seeds	Refrigerated foods and drinks
Grapes, plums, raspberry, strawberry, black cherry, blueberry, tangerine	Excessive intake of fruit and fruit juices; sugar and sweets
Millet, wheat	Insufficient protein and nutrition
Seaweeds; salt	Excessive protein intake (prolonged high-protein diets)
Walnuts	Marijuana and similar recreational drugs
Sufficient protein	Iced drinks
	Frozen yogurt, ice cream, popsicles

Liver–Strengthening Foods	Liver–Weakening Foods
Mung beans, garbanzo beans	Alcohol
Beef liver, oysters, pork	Turkey
Vegetable juices	Fried, greasy and fatty foods
Carrots, beets, celery, tomato, seaweed	Avocados; nuts and nut butters
Dark leafy greens (collards, kale, bok'choy, dandelion, chard, spinach), burdock root	Caffeine and caffeine-like substances: coffee, black tea, cocoa, colas, chocolate, mate)
Lemons, loquat, plum, raspberry, strawberry, mulberry, watermelon	Cheese
Oats; black sesame seeds	Chips of all kinds
Shiitake mushrooms	Excessive intake of vinegar
Vinegar in small amounts	Excessive intake of oils
Essential fatty acids	Recreational drugs
	Cigarettes
	Mega doses of vitamins
	Environmental chemicals
	Synthetic drugs

Heart–Strengthening Foods	Heart–Weakening Foods
Mung beans, adzuki beans	Fried, greasy and fatty foods
Lamb	Excessive red meat intake
Amaranth, rye, wheat	Alcohol
Cherry, papaya, watermelon	Hard cheeses
Burdock root, lotus root, eggplant	Insufficient protein and nutrition
Dark leafy greens (collards, kale, bok choy, dandelion, chard, spinach)	Caffeine (coffee, black tea, cocoa, colas, chocolate)

Continued ➡

Whole Foods	
Healthy Foods	**Unhealthy Foods**
Whole, organic grains	White sugar
Organic legumes	White flour
Vegetables, especially organic	White bread and other flour products
Sea vegetables	"Junk foods"
Sea or earth salts	Refined (table) salt
Fermented foods	Additives; preservatives; artificial colorings
Organic fruit in season and cooked (if needed)	Chemicals in foods (MSG, etc.)
Small amounts of whole, organic dairy	Soda pop
Sufficient organic protein for your body's needs	White sugar
A little sea or earth salt	Tobacco
A little honey, maple, or grain syrups, or whole unrefined sugar cane	Caffeine (coffee, black tea, mate, cocoa, chocolate)
Very small amounts of red wine or beer	Larger amounts of alcohol
	Genetically manufactured food (GMOs); irradiated food

Kitchen Tips

Those with busy lifestyles (probably most of you!) may feel overwhelmed at first with this diet change. To heal disease, regain health and maintain wellness, however, an appropriate energetic diet is absolutely essential. Old habits die hard, yet new ones can actually be formed fairly quickly with attention and intention. Give yourself two to four weeks of focused energy on your dietary changes and needs. Afterward, it'll be much easier and slip into your lifestyle as new habits. Following are several tips to aid this process.

Plan Ahead

Always think of what must be done for the next three meals. For instance, put grains and legumes on to soak and marinate meats a day in advance. Prepare your evening meal in the morning (try a Crock-Pot) so it's ready after a busy afternoon. Plan meals several days ahead so you can shop for what you need only once or twice a week.

Crock-Pots

Although cooking with electricity is not ideal, Crock-Pots are so convenient and useful, I recommend them. It's an easy way to prepare meals, soups, stocks, beans, breakfast, and dinner with little time and effort. Ingredients are put into the pot at night for the next morning, or in the morning to be ready for dinner. Turn pot on high, medium, or low, depending on length of time available/needed to cook its contents.

Meal Ideas

Breakfast: Throw away all your whole-grain boxed cereals even if organic and start your day with oatmeal, multigrain cereal, soup, congee, kicharee, or even leftover dinner. Side proteins can include eggs, sausage, Canadian bacon, tempeh or cottage cheese, or if necessary, whey protein powder, for instance.

Lunch: Heat up leftover dinner, kicharee (see Recipes at end of this section) or soups. If traveling away from home, put in wide-mouthed thermos or warmth-holding food containers (pickled and fermented foods do not need refrigeration and can be kept in a drawer at work). Sandwiches also travel well.

Eating out: Ethnic restaurants usually offer the most nutritional and balanced meal choices, such as Chinese, Indian, Japanese, Korean, Indonesian, Middle Eastern, and Malaysian. Avoid fast-food restaurants.

Condiments

Add condiments to every meal to aid digestion and impart flavor and color. This is very important, not only to the taste of food, but its desirability. Try garlic powder, kelp powder or dulse flakes, miso paste, umeboshi plum paste (instead of salt), ginger powder, tamari, Bragg Liquid amino acids, yeast flakes, and varied spices.

Enzymes

Include a little fermented, cultured, or sprouted food with every meal. These aid digestion and provide invaluable nutrients, especially when eating mostly cooked foods. See Fermented and Cultured Foods listed earlier in this chapter. To make your own, refer to the Bibliography for a book with recipes.

Meat

Many cookbooks teach how to cook meat (see Bibliography). Roasting is also an excellent and simple method. Cook all meat with ginger to aid digestion of meat and prevent toxin buildup.

To detoxify chicken and other poultry before cooking: remove skin, rub salt (rock salt is best) over chicken for one minute, rinse, then cook with ginger.

To detoxify red meat before cooking: rub with salt (rock salt is best) one minute, then soak in water for ten minutes to remove the blood. Cook with ginger.

Recipes

Kicharee

This wonderfully balancing food detoxifies, yet supports. It makes a good fast for all body types, though it may be eaten as a meal any time. Vegetables may be added or eaten on the side. Vegetarians and O blood types benefit from cooking the rice and mung beans in meat stock, or adding meat on the side.

To make: Soak and cook I cup rice and ⅓ cup mung beans separately. Brown I tsp. turmeric powder, I tsp. cumin seed and ½ tsp. coriander powder in 2 Tbsp. ghee (or sesame oil). Mix all together. Add water to make soupier, if desired.

Congee

Congee, called *jook*, is a well-cooked soupy grain or fortified porridge. A very therapeutic food, it's perfect during convalescence from sickness, for treating acute diseases, strengthening digestion and assimilation and alleviating general debility and low vitality.

Congee gives strength and energy to the whole body and helps those who can't digest carbohydrates or keep food down. Traditional Chinese families serve congee to the whole family on a weekly basis, varying herbs according to weather and health needs to enhance immunity, strengthen digestion and prevent illness.

Congee is made with a grain, usually rice (or ½ part rice and ½ part barley or coix), water, and your chosen herbs. It is then cooked a long time over low heat, which slowly and thoroughly breaks down the grain so it's extremely easy to digest and assimilate. Thus, the body gets the most nutrients possible, perfect for weak digestion, those who are ill, convalescing, or needing strength and vitality. Ideally enamel, clay, glass, or good-quality stainless-steel pots are used in making congee. Don't use aluminum, iron, or water-soluble metal pots. A Crock-Pot may also be used. Vary herbs to satisfy your current health and healing needs. In a pinch you can use herbal tablets instead of fresh herbs.

BASIC MORNING CONGEE RECIPE

(Four servings)

6 cups water

I ounce herbs

I cup rice, or ½ cup rice and ½ cup coix or pearled barley

Combine all ingredients and cook in Crock-Pot for 8–10 hours, or in glass-covered dish in 250 degree oven for 4–6 hours. If congee consistency is too thick, add water to thin. Include honey, as desired.

Gomasio

Gomasio, or sesame salt, is a great way to include small amounts of salt in the diet. When made, the salt crystals are coated with sesame oil, aiding its quick assimilation into the body's cells while preventing water retention. Gomasio also provides a good source of calcium to the diet and is beneficial to the heart.

To make: Separately, dry toast sesame seeds and sea salt in pans. Then grind 20 parts sesame seeds with I part sea salt in a surabachi, nut and seed grinder, food processor, or blender. Bottle a small amount and leave on table; refrigerate the rest. Yellow sesame seeds are typically used; black sesame seeds are best for tonifying Yin.

Ghee

Ghee, or clarified butter, is the oil par excellence because it sparks digestive fires without creating Heat, as do most other oils. Further, it doesn't go rancid and so needn't be refrigerated.

To make: Melt I lb. unsalted butter in a pan over low heat. Periodically scrape foam off surface. When golden and clear, pour through sieve into container.

Dark, Leafy Greens

Include ½–I cup of dark, leafy greens (collards, kale, bok choy, mustard, dandelion) per day in your diet.

To cook: wash, chop and blanch (boil) greens in I–2" water for 5 minutes. Drain, set aside, and add miso to greens' water to create an additional nutritious drink or broth. Add lemon juice to greens to make the iron more available, top with a little olive oil or salad dressing, if desired, and make these vibrant greens your daily "salad" rather than raw foods.

Stocks

Stocks have been used worldwide for a very long time. They are extremely nutritious and easily

Continued ➜

assimilated. Use them for soups, grains, beans, stir-fries, and cereals and to flavor other meals. Stocks are excellent for vegetarians. They supply highly assimilated nutrients and protein not found in vegetarian food. Cook all beans and grains in stocks to increase flavor and nutrition. Stocks can be made in bulk (easily done in a Crock-Pot) and stored until needed. They keep several months in the freezer (pour into ice cube trays).

To make: Prepare stock by stuffing a large pot full of bones. Add any vegetable peelings and eggshells (saved in freezer). Add water, covering bones by 2-3 inches, and ¹/₂ cup vinegar to pull minerals out of bones. Add whole cut vegetables (such as onions, carrots and celery) and herbs (if desired). Cook in a Crock-Pot, or simmer on stove, for 12-72 hours, removing dirty foam for first two hours or so. Strain, then cool soup overnight. Skin off fat the next morning, then pour resulting stock into pint-size mason jars or ice cube trays. Refrigerate and/or freeze.

Bones to use: ribs, knuckle, meaty shanks, oxtail, lamb, beef, pork and/or chicken bones, wings, backs, breastbones, necks, whole fish carcasses and heads.

Cooking Beans

All beans need picking through for stones and washing before soaked and cooked. At cooking, add a strip of kombu or other seaweed for minerals and to aid digestion.

Hard beans, such as adzuki, black, and garbanzo beans, must be soaked 12-36 hours to neutralize phytic acid (and other antinutrients) and increase protein content substantially (or otherwise it prevents protein absorption). Beans also cook more evenly and prevent gas formation. Cook 2 hours.

Softer beans, such as lentils, split peas, and dhals, should be soaked 3 hours, then cooked 30–60 minutes.

Cooking Grains

Presoaking grains 12–48 hours increases protein content six-fold (a USDA-published fact). It also neutralizes their phytic acid content (and other antinutrients), which otherwise inhibits protein absorption, and they become more digestible and increase in protein content substantially. Try mixing various grains together. Below is a table of grains and their cooking specifics.

Endnotes

1 For further information and scientific studies, refer to the article "Newest Research On Why You Should Avoid Soy", by Sally Fallon and Dr. Mary G. Enig, extracted from *Nexus Magazine*, volume 7, number 3 (April–May 2000).
2 From seas.upenn.ed/~epage/caffeine/FAQmain, copyright 1994 by Alex Lopez-Ortiz.

—From *Healing with the Herbs of Life*

Grains			
1 cup grain	Cups water	Cooking time	Yield
Amaranth	3	45 min.	2½ cups
Barley, hulled	2½	1 hr.	3½ cups
Barley, pearled	2	30 min.	3 cups
Buckwheat groats	2	20 min.	2½ cups
Couscous	1	20 min.	1½ cups
Millet	2½	30 min.	2 cups
Oat groats	2	1–2 hr.	2½ cups
Polenta	4	20–25 min.	3½ cups
Quinoa	2	15 min.	2½ cups
Basmati white rice	2	15 min.	3 cups
Basmati brown rice	2	45 min.	3 cups
White rice	1	15 min.	3 cups
Brown rice	2	45 min.	3 cups
Wild rice	3	1 hr.	4 cups
Rye berries	2	45 min.	3 cups
Teff	4	15 min.	2½ cups
Wheatberries	2	1½ hr.	2 cup
Bulgur wheat	2	20 min.	2½ cups
Kamut and Spelt: follow directions on package			

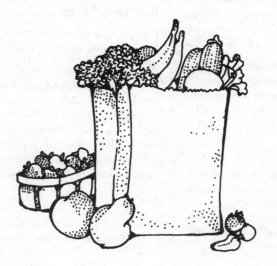

TRADITIONAL YOGIC DIET PRINCIPLES

Michele Picozzi

Overview

The ancients have known all along what science and health practitioners are rediscovering today: diet plays a significant role in sustaining and restoring good health and well-being and maintaining a smooth-functioning nervous system. Today, research continues to support a plant-based diet—one that is low in fat and rich in complex carbohydratesto prevent and treat heart disease; some types of cancer; digestion disorders, including gallbladder disease; diabetes; and hypoglycemia. Such a diet also allows for others to eat well and helps ensure the health and continuation of planet Earth.

The yoga of food is called *anna yoga*. According to yogic scriptures, food can affect us in three ways: it provides nourishment for energy, strength, and emotional equilibrium; it can be the source of illness and mental confusion; it can impede function, which leads to sickness and even death.

The yogic ideal encourages cultivation of the sattavic foods in the diet to encourage a state of mind that is lucid, alert, and capable of higher realizations. The most revered of the yogic scriptures, the Bhagavad Gita, offers specific dietary advice on how certain foods will cultivate a particular nature. While yogic scripture contains much dietary advice, the overriding guiding principles in a yogic diet are to eat minimally and to fast regularly.

Food Categories

Yogic philosophy divides foods into three categories—*tamasic, rajasic,* and *sattavic*. It recommends avoiding tamasic and rajasic foods as they can upset physical, mental, and emotional equilibrium. *Sattavic* foods, on the other hand, encourage energy, clarity, and creativity.

Tamasic Foods

- stale, over- or underripe foods
- meat, fish, mushrooms, and vinegar
- frozen and canned foods
- overcooked and reheated foods
- drugs and alcohol

Rajasic Foods

- sour, bitter, and acidic foods
- coffee, tea, onions, garlic, and eggs
- chocolate, white sugar, and flour
- strong spices and hot peppers

Sattavic Foods

- fresh fruits and vegetables
- milk, butter, beans, and honey
- cereals
- fresh fruit juices
- pure water

Continued ➡

In more modern times, the traditional yogic diet has been decidedly lacto-vegetarian, including dairy products with the exception of eggs. Eating eggs has largely been discouraged, as they possess a *rajasic*, or stimulating, quality while bean and grain combinations and soy food are favored, as they provide protein and do not cause negative effects on the mind and body. Milk and related products possess sattavic nature; dairy foods are reputed to be easily digested, easy on the system. However, milk is considered a food and should be consumed slowly.

Vegetarianism

The basic principles of the yogic diet are good health and common sense and hence, vegetarianism. This type of diet is thought to encourage compassion for all living things, a more refined mind, and a higher consciousness. Certain foods help the mind to become more refined, and others keep it at the consciousness level of an animal.

The basic yogic diet features:

- vegetables and herbs
- fruits
- nuts and seeds
- grains
- legumes
- specific dairy products such as yogurt and ghee (clarified butter)

Ideally, these foods are consumed raw or lightly cooked to preserve their life force or *prana*.

However, the decision to become a partial or total vegetarian should not be forced. It should be undertaken willingly and only if there is no risk to maintaining health. Not everyone is cut out to be a vegetarian. Your body may require the nutrients found only in meats or in more concentrated quantities. On the advice of his doctors, even the Dalai Lama does not practice vegetarianism, although many of his followers do. To a yogi, however, health reasons are secondary to the idea of nonviolence. The concept of nonviolence includes not only refraining from harming living creatures, but also from harming oneself. To start out on the road to vegetarianism by forcing yourself to eat differently before you are ready or doing it because you think you should is a form of violence. Eliminate meat from your diet gradually, and explore other sources of protein.

There are several types of vegetarian diets:

- lacto-ovo, where dairy products and eggs are permitted
- lacto-vegetarian, which allows dairy products but no eggs
- vegan, which refrains from all animal products
- fruitarian, where only "fallen fruits"—so no plants have been destroyed during harvesting are consumed
- macrobiotic diet, similar to vegan but with a heavy emphasis on consuming brown rice

A regular hatha yoga practice helps us become more aware of our eating habits and reduces cravings for junk food. As a result, many practitioners find it easier to maintain a healthy weight.

How to Eat Healthfully

During her many trips to India, its adopted daughter and revered yoga teacher Indra Devi acquired dietary advice that she has passed on to her students over the years:

- Do not overeat.
- Avoid dead foods—ones that have been robbed of their natural vitamins, minerals, amino acids, and enzymes by processing. This includes canned, preserved, pickled, bottled, bleached, polished, and refined foods.
- Eat plenty of fresh fruits, salads, and vegetables or fruit and vegetable juices every day.
- Drink lots of fresh water.
- Inhale a sufficient of quantity of fresh air.
- Eat foods that support the "rate of life," or metabolism. The best foods include vegetables, particularly the green variety, fruits, whole grains, honey, oils, nuts, milk, eggs, fish, and meat. These foods contain all the necessary vitamins, minerals, amino acids, and enzymes, the life-chemicals that control metabolism.

Serious yogis also avoid consuming alcohol, as it is in direct opposition to yoga's purpose. Alcohol lowers the vibrations of the astral body, while the purpose of yoga is to elevate these vibrations. Eating meat is also thought to have a detrimental effect on the astral body.

Water

Most of us don't drink enough water. By the time thirst sets in, so has mild dehydration. Eight-tenths of the body consists of water, and we eliminate about two quarts every day—even more in higher altitudes. Insufficient water intake is responsible for constipation, a congested colon, malfunction of the liver and kidneys, and clogged bowels. As a general rule of thumb, drink one glass of water each day for every fourteen pounds of body weight. For most of us, this translates to five to eight glasses of water daily.

As a rule, yogis never drink cold water or water with ice. This is particularly important during meals, as it impairs the flow and potency of the enzymes necessary for digestion. Ideally, water should be consumed at room temperature. A glass of fresh, pure water is recommended first thing in the morning and last thing at night. If constipated, drink water hot with some lemon. On hot days, try hot water or herb tea with honey or lemon, as it actually cools the body.

Fasting

In the yogic context, fasting goes beyond skipping meals or starving oneself as a form of discipline. Fasting, when done for spiritual and health purposes, should be approached with the same seriousness and dedication as practicing *asanas*, *pranayama*, or meditation.

Benefits of Fasting

- removes toxins and poisons from the body
- rejuvenates *prana*, or life energy
- purifies the mind
- furthers spiritual practice
- expedites the removal of waste materials from the bowels, kidneys, skin, and lungs
- engenders a feeling of lightness and freshness
- rests the digestive system

How to Fast

Fasting monthly for a period of twenty-four hours is considered the most practical and efficient method for busy Westerners. However, fasting is not appropriate for people with these health conditions: diabetes, kidney disease, bulimia, or anorexia. It is also not advised for those who have recently undergone a detox program for drug or alcohol dependency.

Drink only mineral water or diluted fruit juice and nothing else. Drink plenty of water. If fasting more than two days, use a small amount of fresh lemon juice. Lemon juice is a natural disinfectant for the stomach and cleanses the liver and kidneys.

Rest as much as possible, doing light yoga stretches, restorative poses, *pranayama*, meditation, and walking outdoors.

Eat lightly upon breaking the fast, slowly introducing solid foods.

Tongue and Nose Cleaning

Both these hygiene customs have been long practiced in India and Nepal, using special equipment to accomplish the task. A curved, stainless instrument is used to scrape away the coating of impurities that build up over time on the tongue. This cleaning is best done in the morning before drinking or eating to avoid washing the collected impurities into the digestive system. A spoon, used in an inverted position, can do the job nicely.

Irrigating and cleansing the nasal passages is done with a *neti* pot, a small ceramic pot with a bowl and spout for mixing the right amount of warm water with a pinch of salt. Besides aiding breathing, running water through the nose also helps to keep the sinus passages healthy.

—From *Pocket Guide to Hatha Yoga*

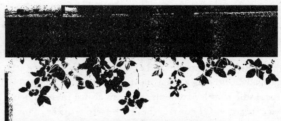

MACROBIOTICS
Carl Ferré

What is Macrobiotics?

Macrobiotics is the practical application of the natural laws of change. The term comes from the Greek; *macro* means "great," and *bios* means "life." It is a tool that allows one to learn to live within the natural order of life, the constantly changing nature of all things.

Macrobiotics as it is known today is the result of the tireless work and vision of George Ohsawa (1893–1966). Ohsawa developed tuberculosis at the age of fifteen. By the time he was eighteen, his mother, younger brother, and younger sister had all died of the same disease. His own illness had progressed to the point that the doctors had given up all hope for him. Determined to overcome his condition, Ohsawa began searching for alternative theories of health. He based his theory and practice of macrobiotics on Sagen Ishizuka's (1850–1910) theory of balancing mineral salts, the early heaven's sequence of the I-Ching, yin and yang, and other

Continued ➤

ancient Eastern concepts. He lived to the age of 73, devoting his life to teaching macrobiotic theory and writing on science, ethics, religion, and philosophy from a macrobiotic point of view.

While macrobiotic principles can be applied to all areas of life, this book emphasizes their application to diet and health. The macrobiotic approach to diet emphasizes whole grains and fresh vegetables. For the most part it avoids meat, dairy foods, and processed foods. The goal is to provide the body with essential nutrients so that it can function efficiently without loading it with toxins or excesses that must be eliminated or stored. And since the body is always adjusting to changes in the environment and in its own aging process, its needs will always change as well. The idea is to balance the effects of foods eaten with other influences on the body, largely through diet, and to adjust to changes in a controlled and peaceful manner.

A basic tenet of macrobiotic thinking is that all things—our bodies, foods, and everything else—are composed of yin and yang energies. Yin energies are outward moving, yang energies are inward. Every thing has both yin and yang energies, but with either yin or yang in excess. Most of the foods that make up the standard American diet have very strong yin or yang characters and also tend to be acid-forming. In contrast, macrobiotic practice emphasizes the two food groups—grains and vegetables—that have the least pronounced yin and yang qualities, making it easier to achieve a more balanced condition within the natural order of life. Living within the natural order means eating only what is necessary for one's condition and desires, and learning to adjust in a peaceful way to life's changes. Learning the effects of different foods allows one to consciously counteract other influences and maintain a dynamically balanced state. The resulting freedom from fear and the new sense of control are two of the most important benefits of a macrobiotic practice.

A macrobiotic practice encourages the body's natural ability to heal itself. If the body is not burdened by toxins and excesses, it can function better and thus heal any illness that does occur. Anybody who begins a macrobiotic diet goes through a period of healing, beginning with the elimination of accumulated toxins and excesses. Those who are already following a macrobiotic diet may also have periodic health problems, and can adjust their diet accordingly. Of course, there are factors other than diet that affect health; true macrobiotic practice emphasizes balancing extremes in all areas. Finally, the goal of macrobiotics is not to avoid death, which is part of the cycle of life. Rather, it seeks to ensure that each person's life is long, healthy, and enjoyable.

The conventional nutritional approach holds that each individual needs certain amounts of proteins, fats, carbohydrates, vitamins, and minerals each day, based on a statistical average of everybody's needs. This makes the recommended daily allowances easy to comprehend, but does not allow for the uniqueness of each individual's changing needs. It eventually leads to stagnant thinking. The macrobiotic approach maintains that what works for one person will not necessarily work for another, and that what works one day may not work the next. Therefore, using macrobiotic principles means to determine the foods best suited to us based on our current condition and what we want to become. In other words, a macrobiotic approach requires a change in thinking from a static view of life to a dynamic and flexible one. This leads to real freedom. The first and most important step is to change from a diet based on meat and sugar to one based on grains and vegetables.

Very few people can make such a radical shift overnight. Instead, most people learn macrobiotics in stages.

Beginning Stage

In my experience, the easiest way for relatively healthy people to start a macrobiotic practice is to follow a basic diet that emphasizes whole grains and fresh vegetables. The food we eat affects the way we feel, think, and act. Learning to use macrobiotic principles is much easier after a transitional time of using a basic macrobiotic dietary approach.

The main benefit of a standard macrobiotic diet is that the body becomes cleaner as toxins and old excesses are discharged. This alone can sometimes relieve minor aches and pains. As our bodies are cleansed, our minds become more clear and our natural good judgment begins to return. People who are in relatively good health may begin a macrobiotic diet after consulting books or relatives or friends who are more familiar with macrobiotic practice. The following pages provide all the information that is needed, but a good macrobiotic cookbook is also invaluable.

People with a serious illness should consult a health care advisor or a macrobiotic counselor who is familiar with the effects of dietary change before making big dietary changes. Most people need help learning to use macrobiotic principles effectively to remedy serious illness. A standard macrobiotic diet must be tailored to the individual's condition. Even two people with the same illness need different dietary adjustments.

Many people who are beginning a macrobiotic diet, or are considering doing so, are taken aback by the number of Japanese foods in a standard macrobiotic diet. Japanese foods are often emphasized simply because Ohsawa was Japanese. The expression of macrobiotics is becoming less Japanese as more Americans write and teach about macrobiotics.

A second source of confusion is that there are three primary expressions of macrobiotics: that of George and Lima Ohsawa, and those of Ohsawa's students Michio and Aveline Kushi, and Herman and Cornellia Aihara. This section unifies their three different expressions of the macrobiotic approach. Still, in consulting any source of macrobiotic information, readers may find seemingly conflicting advice.

Intermediate Stage

In the intermediate stage one begins to learn the principles of macrobiotics. Macrobiotics is based on the principle that there is a natural order to all of life. What a person does and eats determines who that person is and how that person feels. If one lives and eats in harmony with the natural order, the effect is the natural condition of health and happiness. If one lives and eats in disharmony with the natural order, the result is a condition of minor sickness and eventually major sickness. A return to living and eating in harmony with the natural order leads to an improved health condition and outlook on life.

The way to learn about the natural order is to study yin and yang. These Eastern concepts provide a view of life that allows us to live and eat in harmony with the natural order. The knowledge of yin and yang is used to change a weak condition to a strong one, sadness to joy, sickness to health. It is a working knowledge of yin and yang that leads to greater freedom and more control over our health. The second section of this book provides an introduction to yin and yang; learning how to apply these principles to life is the goal of the immediate stage. Of course, we can start this stage at any point, even from the first day. As our understanding increases so does our enjoyment of life; as our physical, mental, and emotional health improves so

does our judgment increase. We can better evaluate the appropriateness of advice from others. This increase in confidence leads in general to a more positive outlook toward life.

Advanced Stage

At the advanced stage, we have reached the dietary goal of macrobiotics: To be able to eat whatever we want whenever we want without fear. No food is forbidden. This stage is very different from the beginning stage. It is complete freedom rather than a set of rules. Judgment is so developed that we know what to do without having to stop and think about the principles involved. We know the effect of each food and how to counterbalance that effect.

People at the advanced stage realize the importance of sharing their knowledge with others, and they are searching for additional tools with which to better their lives. They understand that macrobiotics does not provide all the answers, but rather is a way of viewing life that can incorporate any and all other disciplines and methods of growth. People at this stage of practice can be recognized by their health, happiness, and honesty.

Benefits of Macrobiotics

In general, the more we know about macrobiotics and the more we practice it, the greater the benefit. However, since every individual is different and no two people have the exact same reaction to changes in diet and lifestyle, the exact benefits for each person differ. Here is a brief list of common benefits:

- Less or no fatigue.
- Better health: relief from all pains and sicknesses, including colds, the flu, and cancer.
- Better appetite, able to eat the simplest food with complete joy and deep gratitude.
- Better sexual appetite and more joyful satisfaction.
- Deep and good sleep every night without bad dreams.
- The ability to fall asleep within minutes of lying down.
- Improved memory, leading to better relationships.
- Greater freedom from anger, fear, and suffering.
- Ability to view difficulties as positive learning experiences.
- Better clarity in thinking and promptness in action.
- More generosity in our interactions.
- Greater control over personal destiny.
- The belief that nothing in life is too difficult.
- Greater honesty with oneself and others.
- Improved understanding of Oneness (God).

Many of these benefits are obviously related to health. In fact, in macrobiotic thought all of these benefits are the product of good health. The third section of this book outlines the macrobiotic view of sickness and healing, and provides some information on macrobiotic diagnosis, as well as natural home remedies that can be helpful during the healing process.

Macrobiotic Approach to Diet

A Beginning Macrobiotic Diet

The origin of the macrobiotic approach to diet is Ohsawa's relatively complex cosmology called the order of the universe. All life comes from oneness—the infinite, pure expansion. Oneness divides into yin and yang, and from these three all things are

Continued ➡

created. The inorganic world is created first. This is the world of magnetism, vibration, electricity, atoms, stars, planets, and so on. It is the origin of the organic world. In the organic world, the vegetal world (plants and vegetables) is created first and from it the animal world (animals and humans) is born.

The principal food of humans then should be vegetal foods such as whole grains, fresh vegetables, beans, and sea vegetables. Anything else is a supplement or a luxury. Thus, the macrobiotic dietary approach is to eat a diet largely composed of whole grains and fresh vegetables. This is a major readjustment for people who have been eating a diet based on animal products and canned or frozen vegetables.

Selection

This section outlines the foods that make up a basic macrobiotic diet, some of which can be found in supermarkets. However, a local health food store or co-op is usually the best source for natural foods, especially for whole grains. Such stores can often offer suggestions for dietary changes, or at least may know of people who follow a macrobiotic approach. Most of the nonperishable foods can be ordered through the mail.

The quality of food is extremely important. No matter what the food, the more natural—the less processed or refined—the better. Try to avoid foods that have been colored; preserved; sprayed with synthetic fertilizers, herbicides, or pesticides; irradiated; or treated in any way with chemicals. Foods grown with genetically engineered seeds should also be avoided. Organically grown or produced foods are preferable; organic foods taste great, reduce health risks, and are best for the health of the soil and water. Select locally grown and seasonal foods as often as possible, especially when buying fresh vegetables. Locally grown foods are most adapted to the local environment, and eating them helps aid the body to adapt to the local environment as well.

There are an increasing number of convenience foods, such as quick-cooking grains and miso soups, crackers, and snacks. Those without additives, preservatives, or other chemicals are suitable for occasional to moderate use.

A standard beginning macrobiotic diet consists of:	
grains	40 to 60 percent daily
vegetables	25 to 30 percent daily
beans	5 to 10 percent daily
soups	5 to 10 percent, 1 to 2 cups (bowls) daily
sea vegetables	3 to 5 percent daily
beverages	regularly according to thirst
condiments	several times a week to daily
garnishes/seasonings	small amounts daily, used to balance dishes
pickles	several times a week to daily
fish	0 to 3 times per week
fruit	2 to 3 times per week
desserts	2 to 3 times per week
nuts, seeds, snacks	several times a week to daily
sweeteners	0 to 3 times per week

Foods

These food groups are discussed below. Each category contains primary foods (at least 40 to 50 percent of the diet) that are used most often in the beginning of macrobiotic practice, secondary foods (at least 25 to 30 percent of the diet), occasional foods that are used in small amounts, and foods that should be avoided in the beginning. One should eat a wide variety of foods from each category to ensure a nutritious diet. However, one need not eat all of the foods. People generally base their diet primarily on the foods they like and can find easily.

In the charts that follow, foods are listed in more-or-less yin to yang order. *Those foods that should be avoided when you first begin a macrobiotic diet are in italic type.*

Note that the recommendations in this section are for those beginning macrobiotic practice. People at the intermediate level who have learned more about yin and yang select foods to suit their condition and surroundings. Those who are more advanced find that they understand the effect of each food and know how to counterbalance that effect.

Finally, people with major illnesses should read the section on Macrobiotic Healing before beginning a macrobiotic diet. Women who are pregnant or breastfeeding should read the subsection on macrobiotic eating for families.

Grains: In temperate climates in the spring and fall, whole grains comprise 40 to 60 percent by volume of daily food consumption. The percentage is increased to 50 to 70 percent in colder climates and seasons, and reduced to 30 to 50 percent in warmer climates and seasons. The grains should be whole and unrefined and may be prepared in a variety of ways.

Of the whole grains, brown rice is the most frequently used, primarily because of its nutritive value and favorable sodium-to-potassium ratio. Of the several varieties, short-grain brown rice is primarily chosen for daily use all year. While any whole grain may be eaten at any time as a primary grain, the heartier ones such as buckwheat, millet, rye, and whole wheat are chosen more in colder climates and seasons, while whole oats, corn, hulled or pot barley, and medium-grain rice are chosen more in warmer climates and seasons. A wide variety of whole grains should be eaten every day.

In practice, many whole grains are consumed in a partially processed form. Examples are cornmeal, rolled oats, bulghur, couscous, creamed cereals, noodles, and flour made from any whole grain. The general recommendation for a beginning macrobiotic approach is to eat mostly whole grains for daily consumption, and to eat products made from whole grains occasionally. Refined or "enriched"

Whole and Partially Processed Grains

less yin: ramen noodles, somen noodles, udon noodles, long-grain brown rice, whole wheat crackers, couscous, tortillas, chapatis, cornmeal, corn grits, corn, rolled oats (oatmeal), unsalted rice cakes

less yang: whole oats, pearl barley, wild rice, basmati rice, pot (hulled) barley, buckwheat noodles, medium-grain brown rice, mochi, rye flakes, wheat flakes, sweet brown rice, bulghur, brown rice cream, sourdough whole wheat or rye bread, unyeasted whole wheat or rye bread, rice kayu, cracked rye, lightly salted rice cakes, lightly salted cracked wheat

more yang: rye, whole wheat, quinoa, short-grain brown rice, amaranth, teff, millet, buckwheat

grains are avoided in the beginning stages of macrobiotic practice.

Vegetables: Fresh vegetables comprise 25 to 30 percent by volume of daily food consumption. Fresh means vegetables as they come out of the garden—not canned, frozen, or processed in any way. Organically grown vegetables are preferable, the more locally grown the better. Vegetables are prepared in a variety of ways, such as steamed, in a stew or soup, or served raw in salad. Root vegetables are used more in colder climates and seasons, and green leafy vegetables, including raw salads, are used more in warmer climates and seasons, and for balancing heavy meat consumption. A variety of vegetables is eaten daily all year.

In areas with long cold winters, locally grown vegetables, stored without the use of chemicals, are preferable. However, fresh vegetables from another climate are preferred over canned or frozen vegetables. Local farmers in any area should be able to say what foods can be grown and when they are normally available.

Vegetables

extremely yin: *potatoes, eggplant, tomatoes,* shiitake mushrooms, albi, *avocados, sweet potatoes,* mushrooms, *yams, zucchini,* yellow summer squash, patty pan squash, *bell peppers,* artichokes, bamboo shoots, *spinach, Swiss chard, asparagus,* alfalfa sprouts, okra, Jerusalem artichokes, chives, Brussels sprouts

more yin: Chinese cabbage, escarole, kohlrabi, snow peas, green peas, corn on the cob, radishes, string beans, yellow wax beans, purple cabbage, leaf lettuces, endive, cilantro, parsley, bok choy, mustard greens, scallions, collard greens, turnip greens, dandelion greens, beets, broccoli, cauliflower

less yin: kale, green cabbage, celery, butternut squash, buttercup squash, Hubbard squash, acorn squash, Hokkaido pumpkin (kabocha), turban squash, leeks, daikon, onions, watercress

less yang: turnips, rutabaga, salsify, parsnips, carrots, cress, lotus root, burdock

Some macrobiotic teachers suggest that some vegetables should be avoided, or used only occasionally. Eating too much of certain foods can be unhealthy, especially for those with certain health conditions. Many lists of macrobiotic foods are designed to be appropriate for everybody. A better approach—the complete macrobiotic approach—is for each person to learn the effect each food has on his or her body, so that each person can enjoy the widest possible selection of foods nature has to offer.

These are the vegetables that require you to be judicious in using them: the nightshade vegetables, such as potatoes, tomatoes, eggplant, and all peppers other than white and black pepper; those containing large amounts of oxalic acid, such as spinach and beet greens; and other vegetables such as asparagus, avocados, zucchini, sweet potatoes, and yams. They are all extremely yin as shown in the vegetable chart.

Beans, Soups, and Sea Vegetables: Beans, soups, and sea vegetables comprise anywhere from 10 to 25 percent by volume of daily food consumption. Beans are a good protein complement with whole grains, and 5 to 10 percent of the diet consists of bean dishes or soybean products (processed by natural methods without the addition of chemicals) such as miso, natural soy sauce, and tofu used in a variety of ways, including in soups. Soy milk and products made from it are luxury foods used on special occasions, or as transitional foods from a standard American diet to a macrobiotic dietary approach.

Continued →

A wide variety of soups and stews can be made using any combination of vegetables, grains, beans, sea vegetables, and fish. The most common daily soup in macrobiotic practice is miso soup with vegetables and sea vegetables. Of the many varieties of miso available, barley (mugi) miso is most commonly used daily.

Sea vegetables (seaweeds) grow in and are harvested from the sea. Their nutrient-rich composition and relatively clean growing environment make them an important addition to any vegetal-based diet. They can take time to get used to. Some sea vegetables seem to disappear in bean dishes, and small amounts in soups can be tolerated immediately. Interestingly, sea vegetables are used widely in processed foods, including ice cream, salad dressings, and bread.

Beans and Bean Products

extremely yin: soy milk, bean sprouts, soybeans, black soybeans, split peas, tofu, natto, blackeyed peas, lima beans, whole dried peas, white Northern beans

more yin: tempeh, pinto beans, kidney beans, black beans, black turtle beans, bolita beans, anasazi beans, chickpeas, broad beans, mung beans, red lentils

less yin: aduki beans

more yang: natural soy sauce, miso

Sea Vegetables

less yin: nori, agar agar (kanten), Irish moss, dulse, sea palm, arame, kelp, alaria, nekabu, mekabu

less yang: wakame, kombu, hijiki

Beverages: Beverages are consumed regularly according to thirst and need. Beverages for primary use include bancha twig tea (kukicha), teas made from roasted whole grains such as barley or brown rice, and spring, well, or filtered water. A good source of water is important for maintaining health, especially since most cooking is done with water. Filters that remove chlorine, lead, odors, volatile organic chemicals, and other contaminants from tap water are often a good solution.

Other beverages used in a basic macrobiotic dietary approach are teas and drinks made from vegetables, sea vegetables, grains, beans, or a combination of them. Most macrobiotic cookbooks contain recipes for a wide variety of natural beverages. Fruit juices, soy milk, and naturally fermented alcoholic beverages such as beer, wine, and saké are used for special occasions. Milk and dairy-based drinks, sugared drinks and sodas, coffee, and other stimulant drinks are avoided at first.

Beverages

extremely yin: *sugared drinks*, natural wine, natural beer, natural saké, fruit juice, soy milk, *coffee*

more yin: green tea, black tea, herb teas, amasaké

less yin: carbonated water, mineral water, spring water, well water, carrot juice, vegetable broth, brown rice milk, grain milk (kokkoh), bancha stem tea

less yang: bancha twig tea, mu tea, kombu tea, dandelion tea, roasted barley tea, roasted brown rice tea

yang: grain coffee (yannoh), ginseng tea, sho-ban tea, lotus root tea, burdock root tea, umeboshi tea

---

While each drink, juice, or tea has its own effect, beverages such as sugared drinks, fruit juices, and herb teas have been grouped for simplicity into their general yin (or yang) category. Some herb teas have a yang effect.

Condiments, Seasonings, Oils, and Pickles: Condiments are used as needed to add flavor to cooked dishes and to add nutrients. In addition, they help stimulate appetite and in many cases are an aid to the digestion of grains and vegetables. Gomashio, roasted ground sesame seeds and sea salt, is used for adding salt at the table. The oil from the sesame seeds coats the salt, making the salt easier to process in the body and less yang in effect. Some of the other more popular condiments are listed below. Macrobiotic cookbooks explain how to make or purchase and use these helpful foods.

Seasonings are another way to spice up an otherwise "bland" diet. They are especially helpful to those whose taste buds are adjusting from the highly stimulating standard American fare to a macrobiotic approach. Many seasonings may be used as garnishes for variety in serving or as a complement to help balance the effects of some dishes. For example, grated daikon or grated radish would be a good garnish for fish.

Cooking herbs, including basil, oregano, cinnamon, curry, cloves, and others are used in small amounts. Using natural sea salt is very important because it contains many minerals that are lost during the refining process of commercial salt.

Vegetable oils are used in cooking and occasionally for flavoring and in salad dressings.

Pickles are used as condiments. Many macrobiotic advisors recommend eating a small piece of pickle after each meal as an aid to digestion. Natural pickles may be purchased at natural food stores or from mail-order suppliers, but many macrobiotic practitioners make their own at home.

Condiments

more yin: natural mustard (for fish), toasted nori

less yin: powdered sea vegetable, roasted sesame seeds

less yang: ground shiso leaves, gomashio

more yang: scallion miso, tekka, umeboshi plum, shio kombu

Seasonings

more yin: lemon juice, orange juice, brown rice vinegar, umeboshi vinegar, green mustard paste, yellow mustard paste, red pepper, garlic and other herbs

less yin: ground black pepper, grated ginger root, grated daikon, grated radish, grated horseradish

more yang: sauerkraut brine, umeboshi paste, natural soy sauce, miso, umeboshi plums, sea salt

Oils

extreme yin: *coconut oil*

more yin: peanut oil, corn oil, olive oil, soybean oil

less yin: canola oil, mustard seed oil, sesame oil, safflower oil

Pickles

less yin: pressed salad, sauerkraut

yang: nuka (bran) pickles, takuan pickles, umeboshi pickles

more yang: soy sauce pickles, miso pickles, salt brine pickles, salt pickles

---

Supplemental Foods: Fruit, nuts, seeds, fish, and sweeteners are used as supplemental foods up to two to three times per week within a basic macrobiotic dietary approach. One of the major differences between a macrobiotic diet and other diets is the limited use of fruits, because they contain fructose, a simple carbohydrate that has a similar effect on the body as refined sugar. Still, for a relatively healthy person, eating freshly picked fruit can be one of life's pleasures. Organically grown fruits are preferred, the more locally grown the better. Dried fruits from temperate climates also may be used as part of the weekly amount. Avoid fruits that have been picked unripe or have been sprayed or coated with chemicals before or after picking. Tropical and semi-tropical fruits are avoided on a beginning macrobiotic dietary approach.

Nuts and seeds are used as supplemental foods because they are rich in fat and are somewhat harder to digest than whole grains. In general, smaller seeds and nuts contain less fat and are recommended most. As mentioned earlier, gomashio, a condiment made from sesame seeds and salt, is used daily, or as desired. Nuts and seeds are used primarily as snacks, in baking such as in cakes and cookies, as garnishes, or ground into nut or seed butter.

While the basic macrobiotic diet avoids meat, fish is used as a supplemental food, especially when needed for health; in colder climates and seasons; as extra protein for those active in sports; or as a transition to a grain-and-vegetable-based diet. Less fatty white meat fish is preferable for more regular use, and blue-skinned and red-meat varieties are used for special occasions.

Sweeteners are used in desserts and snacks. They are used sparingly (two to three times per week in small amounts) within a basic macrobiotic approach, especially in the beginning. People who

---

Fruit

extreme yin: *mango, papaya, pineapple, bananas, kiwis, dates, figs, grapefruit,* grapes, raisins, green olives, black olives, currants, lemons

more yin: peaches, apricots, plums, prunes, pears, tangerines, nectarines, oranges, honeydew melon, blueberries, watermelon, cantaloupe, mulberries

less yin: apples, cherries, blackberries, strawberries, raspberries

---

Nuts and Seeds

extreme yin: Brazil nuts, cashews

more yin: macadamia nuts, pistachios, filberts, hazelnuts, peanuts, pecans

yin: almonds, chestnuts, pine nuts, walnuts, poppy seeds

less yin: squash seeds, pumpkin seeds, sunflower seeds, white sesame seeds, black sesame seeds

---

Fish and Seafood

less yang: oysters, bluefish, clams, octopus, tuna, carp, scallops, mussels

yang: lobster, halibut, trout, flounder, mackerel, sole, pike, perch, haddock, cod, swordfish, smelt, scrod

more yang: salmon, shrimp, herring, sardine, red snapper, small dried fish (iriko), caviar

---

Continued ➡

are used to a diet high in refined sugar may need to use the listed sweeteners more often as a transition, but none of them replaces the immediate stimulation of refined sugar. (Eventually, naturally sweet vegetables satisfy the need for a sweet taste.) Grain-based sweeteners are preferred. Simple sugars, such as refined sugar, honey, and molasses, are best avoided.

Sweeteners

extreme yin: *mirin*, maple syrup, juice from fruits that grow in temperate climates (such as apples), cooked or dried fruit from a temperate climate

more yin: *amasaké*, barley malt, brown rice syrup

Preparation

Careful and varied food preparation is crucial in a macrobiotic approach. Foods should be tasty and appealing, retain their nutrients, and be appropriate for the people eating them. How a food is cooked changes its quality, and more importantly, its effect on whoever eats it. A more yang food can be made more yin, or a more yin food can be made more yang. One can balance the foods and preparations for a meal so that some are more yin and some more yang, or one can make the entire meal more yin or more yang depending on the season and the needs of whoever will eat the food. A good understanding of food preparation gives the macrobiotic cook flexibility and control over nutrition and health.

The following chart lists some common examples of food preparation methods. In addition, several factors are used to make any of these preparation styles more yin or more yang: the longer the food cooks, and the more pressure, heat, or salt used, the more yang the result; the more water or sweetener and the less time and heat, the more yin.

Among the best introductory macrobiotic cookbooks is *Basic Macrobiotic Cooking* by Julia Ferré. It provides a straightforward guide to preparing whole grains and fresh vegetables.

Food Preparation Methods

more yin: served raw, steaming

less yin: boiling, waterless cooking, sautéing with water

less yang: pressure cooking, sautéing with oil, stir-frying, roasting

more yang: baking, deep-frying, broiling, pressing with salt

extreme yang: pickling, drying

Consumption

How food is consumed is important. Chewing food well is most important—the more a food is broken down, the more nutrients will be absorbed by the intestines. Saliva aids in the digestion of complex carbohydrates. People who chew each mouthful fifty to one hundred times often experience at least a few of these benefits: a reduced tendency to overeat; reduced craving for sweets; reduced desire for excessive amounts of liquid after a meal; better control of salt intake and needs; and greater energy and less overall fatigue.

It is also important to control liquid intake according to thirst and the body's needs. Drinking too much or too little can overwork the heart and the kidneys. Even though grains and vegetables contain a greater percentage of water than animal foods, drinking a sufficient amount of water for proper electrolyte functioning is important.

Quantity also matters. Eating too much food—even good-quality, well-chosen, properly prepared fare—overburdens the body and can reduce the amount of nutrients the intestines can absorb. Too much of various nutrients can be harmful. For example, too many minerals, such as those from sea vegetables, can cause hardness or tightness in the body. Too much or too little salt can cause fatigue. In general, moderation is one of the keys to a happy and healthy life. One of the benefits of a macrobiotic dietary approach is that it helps people pay attention to what their bodies tell them, making it easy to determine the proper amounts of each food.

How often to eat is an individual decision. But whether one eats two, three, or four times a day, it is best to eat at the same times each day. Proper digestion of foods takes several hours, so eating just before going to bed is not recommended. Some macrobiotic counselors advise not eating for three hours before bedtime. Eating in a peaceful environment also aids in proper digestion and is beneficial to one's health and outlook on life.

Macrobiotic Eating for Families

Since each person is unique and has specific dietary needs, preparing macrobiotic meals for a family may seem very difficult. However, if everyone in the family is relatively healthy and wants to eat according to macrobiotic principles, it is not difficult to prepare meals that are appropriate for all family members by making a variety of dishes and by using condiments.

Meals for a large family, or for a small family with a great variety of needs, should include at least one dish that is more yang and at least one dish that is more yin. Those who need more yang cooking should simply eat more of the yang dish or dishes and those who need more yin cooking should eat more of the yin dish or dishes. Second, pickles, condiments, or seasonings that can be used by each family member to adjust the meal to their desire and need should always be served. Dishes should be prepared keeping in mind the person needing the least amount of salt. Those needing more salt can add gomashio or other salty condiments at the table. At least one dish each day should be high in protein. Those who need more protein can eat a higher proportion of that dish.

If someone in the family is sick or needs to avoid certain foods, there should always be a plain grain dish, such as pressure-cooked brown rice, and a cooked vegetable dish without extensive seasoning. Those who need to avoid certain foods such as sweeteners need to be aware that their condition is temporary and that others in the family may need these foods for their conditions. It is not a good idea to force everyone in the family to eat a restrictive diet because one person is sick.

Macrobiotic cooking in a family where one or more family members refuses to follow a macrobiotic approach is more challenging but still feasible. It is easier if the person who cooks wants to practice macrobiotics. It is possible for other family members to benefit from a macrobiotic approach if the person cooking is willing to prepare dishes at each meal that can be eaten both by those following a macrobiotic approach and those who are not. In practice this means that whole grain and fresh vegetable dishes are available every day. Those following a macrobiotic approach simply avoid the meat, sugar, and other dishes.

Changing to a macrobiotic approach may be difficult for children from the ages of three to sixteen. In general, the older the children the more difficult it can be. Talking openly and honestly is always a good approach; if they refuse, one can still substitute better quality food, such as natural cheese

from a natural food store rather then commercial cheese. Gradually introducing more vegetables and whole grain dishes will usually be accepted. If children start to feel better and have more energy and if they see a parent's improvement, they may decide for themselves to adopt macrobiotics. In any case, forcing a diet of grains and vegetables on kids who are used to eating meat and sugar may cause resentment and lead to greater family problems.

Another question that is sure to arise in families with kids is the question of candy. Children aged five and older may require some autonomy. When children are given sugary foods at Little League games, scout meetings, friend's houses, or on Halloween, it may be helpful to give them three choices: trade it for a better-quality snack at home, refuse it, or eat it. Refusing is hard. If the children choose to eat the candy, they should pay attention to the effects on their bodies.

A macrobiotic dietary approach is very appropriate during pregnancy and childbirth. If the expecting mother has been following a macrobiotic approach for some time, few adjustments need to be made. Working with a midwife or doctor who has had positive experiences working with macrobiotic families is best. Flexibility is the key to a positive birth experience. Cravings should be satisfied within reason. If a midwife or doctor is concerned about protein, calcium, iron, or any other nutrient, there are many excellent sources of each nutrient within a macrobiotic diet.

If the expecting mother has recently changed to a macrobiotic approach, it may be difficult to determine true cravings—something the mother or baby really needs—from cravings for foods the body is still discharging. In this case satisfying the craving is still recommended. If the food that is being craved is filled with chemicals, sugar, or preservatives, determine what the body is really craving, such as the sweet taste, and substitute something of more natural quality.

What should be avoided is profound changes in one's overall diet during pregnancy and while breastfeeding. The discharge process from an extensive dietary change can be so strong that caution is needed at this time. Major changes in the diet cause discharges of excess toxins; some of these may affect the unborn or breastfeeding baby. Small changes can be made such as finding better-quality foods. A complete change from a meat-and-sugar diet to a grain-and-vegetable diet is too drastic during pregnancy or while breastfeeding. Similarly, a major change from a macrobiotic approach to any other dietary approach should be avoided.

The best food for a baby is milk from its mother. The first milk, called colostrum, helps the baby's immune system and encourages the expulsion of meconium wastes that have collected during the time the baby spent in the womb. If for some reason breastfeeding is not possible, there are supplemental drinks that can be made from grains. Consult macrobiotic child care books for recipes, and consult a midwife or health care advisor.

Opinions vary on how long to breastfeed a baby, as well as when and how to introduce solid foods. Like each adult, each baby is unique and has its own needs and desires. Some want and need to breastfeed longer than others. Some want solid food sooner than others. When first introducing solid food, especially before the age of ten or eleven months, the mother should prechew the food so that it is mixed with her saliva because babies do not produce ptyalin, an enzyme helpful in the digestion of carbohydrates, before this time.

One concern expressed by doctors and other health professionals is the amount of fat, especially cholesterol, needed by small children for proper

Continued ➡

brain development. A well-rounded macrobiotic approach along with breastfeeding will supply plenty of the needed fat. However, if breastfeeding is not possible, if the child is developing too slowly, or if there is any other concern over the need for more fat, you should select the most natural quality food possible. Remember, there is no food that is absolutely prohibited in a macrobiotic approach. If dairy foods, meat, or even sugar are necessary for anyone's condition, the macrobiotic approach is to eat that food, buying the most natural product available and eating it only as long as it is necessary. The next section discusses the nutritional issues of eating meat, dairy, and other foods.

Nutrients

Each person has different needs. While a macrobiotic diet provides more than adequate amounts of all nutrients, how you feel is a better guide to what you should eat than any list of recommended daily allowances.

The macrobiotic diet contains 12 percent protein, little or none of it from animal sources. It is low in fat (15 percent, including only 2 to 3 percent saturated fat), low in simple carbohydrates (5 percent), and high in complex carbohydrates (68 percent). In contrast, nearly all of the 12 percent of protein in a standard American diet is from animal sources. It is also high in fat (42 percent, including 16 percent saturated fat), high in simple carbohydrates (26 percent) and low in complex carbohydrates (20 percent). (These figures reflect what most Americans eat, not the United States government's dietary guidelines. The diet recommended by the government, like a macrobiotic diet, emphasizes grains and produce.)

The differences between the standard American diet and a macrobiotic diet have important consequences, since what a person eats affects what she or he needs to eat. The body works most efficiently when the proper amounts of nutrients are available, but cannot do its work well when there is too little of a nutrient or when it must work hard to eliminate excesses.

For example, a person who eats a typical American diet high in animal foods and refined carbohydrates needs large amounts of minerals and vitamins such as calcium and vitamin C, very little added salt, and must be careful to get enough dietary fiber. A person who eats foods on a macrobiotic diet needs less calcium and vitamin C, more added salt in cooking, and gets plenty of dietary fiber from whole grains.

The recommended daily allowances (RDAs) are based on the average needs of people who eat a standard American diet. Changes in these daily allowances are based on the needs of those eating large amounts of animal foods. For example, in 1975, the RDAs for calcium and vitamin C were about half what they were in 1995. The recommended daily allowances suggested by the World Health Organization are closer to the needs of people who eat a diet based on grains and vegetables. For example, the United States recommends that a 154-pound male eat 52 grams of protein each day, while the World Health Organization recommends 37 grams. The recommended allowances for a 122-pound female are 44 grams and 29 grams respectively.

Since there is no one macrobiotic diet, it is not possible to perform double-blind studies to show that the macrobiotic diet works. The proof that a macrobiotic dietary approach works for any person is how she or he feels. Furthermore, each person's way of practicing a macrobiotic approach is valid only for that person, since each person is unique. Beware of any studies that show that a specific mac-

robiotic diet works; the very idea is counter to fundamental macrobiotic principles.

Protein: A majority of people throughout the world eat enough protein with little or no animal food. In fact, a macrobiotic diet contains about 12 percent protein, as does a typical American diet. The only real difference is the source.

Proteins are the building blocks of the body and are used for growth and repair of cells. They are the primary solid constituent of enzymes, hormones, blood, and cellular fluids. Amino acids are the components of protein. After a meal, the body breaks down protein into amino acids, and then reassembles them into the specific proteins it needs. Eight of the twenty-two amino acids are called essential because they can be obtained only from food. These eight amino acids must be eaten at the same meal in certain quantities. If one essential amino acid is lacking, the body can make only a limited amount of usable protein.

Since animal foods contain about the right proportion of all the essential amino acids, they may seem the best source of complete protein. However, they also contain large amounts of saturated fat, which can lead to heart disease and other problems. Also, foods that contain a high percentage of protein, such as animal foods, create many waste products during decomposition that take energy for the body to deal with, and, in excess, overburden the kidneys and liver. Excess protein from animal sources can create toxins from fermentation in the large intestine as well. Complex carbohydrates provide more energy and create less waste products as they are converted to energy, so they are a much better source of energy than animal protein.

A macrobiotic diet approach contains plenty of all the essential amino acids, especially if miso, soy sauce, sesame seeds (gomashio), or beans are eaten daily with whole grains. Grains are high in some essential amino acids and beans are high in others, so when they are eaten at the same meal the body gets all the protein it needs. Nuts, seeds, and fish, which are supplemental foods in a macrobiotic dietary approach, are also good sources of protein. For more about protein and amino acids, see *Basic Macrobiotics* by Herman Aihara, which discusses amino acids and protein requirements at length.

Fat: The body needs fat for a variety of reasons. However, the typical American diet contains about 42 percent fat, and more than one third of this is saturated fat. The health risks of such a diet are well known. Any diet in which fat consumption is more than 20 percent of total intake can lead to problems, including heart disease, cancer, and diabetes.

The macrobiotic diet contains about 13 percent unsaturated fat plus only 2 percent saturated fat. This is enough fat under normal circumstances and is easily obtained from vegetable oils, beans and soy products, whole grains, nuts, seeds, and fish.

Carbohydrates: Because fat provides more than twice as much energy per gram as protein or carbohydrates, many people think it must be the best source of energy. This is not so. First, there are the problems associated with too much fat. Second, animal foods, which are high in fat, are far from natural. They are full of chemicals, additives, hormones, etc. Third, dietary fat converts to body fat much easier than either protein or carbohydrates.

Carbohydrates are a much better source of energy than protein or fat. Complex carbohydrates, such as those in whole grains, beans, and vegetables, are a better source of prolonged energy than the simple carbohydrates in refined grains and processed sugar. Complex carbohydrates take longer to digest and therefore produce a longer-

lasting energy supply, whereas simple carbohydrates convert to fat in the body very easily and, in excess, can lead to conditions such as hypoglycemia or diabetes. While a typical American diet contains about 46 percent carbohydrates, over half are simple carbohydrates from refined grains and flour products and simple sugars. A macrobiotic diet contains about 68 percent complex carbohydrates, providing sustained energy over a longer period and producing less waste products than energy produced from protein or fat. Whole grains, vegetables, and beans are excellent sources of complex carbohydrates. Also, these foods are rich in fiber, which can be very helpful for people with constipation and other problems with the bowels.

Minerals: A macrobiotic diet provides ample minerals. Many people believe that dairy foods, which are rich in calcium, are necessary for a healthy life. Calcium is needed to help build strong bones and teeth. It also helps with blood coagulation, regulates the heartbeat, activates some enzymes, and normalizes the metabolism. A basic macrobiotic diet includes many excellent sources of calcium. Leafy green vegetables such as broccoli, collard greens, kale, and turnip greens are particularly high in calcium. Sea vegetables, soybeans, and soy products also are good sources. Sesame seeds are very high in calcium, making gomashio (ground sesame seeds and salt) an excellent source. Small dried fish (iriko) are a good choice for people who wish to get a large amount of calcium from one source.

Iron is needed by everyone but is of particular concern for women, especially during childbearing years when a significant amount of blood is lost through menstruation and during pregnancy. One of the main functions of iron in the body is carrying oxygen to the tissues. Iron also activates the formation of bone, brain, and muscle tissue. While a lack of iron is one cause of anemia, magnesium, calcium, copper, vitamin E, vitamin C, many of the B vitamins, and adequate levels of protein are also necessary for building blood. A basic macrobiotic diet includes plenty of sources rich in iron—a 3.5 ounce serving of hijiki (sea vegetable) alone contains almost five times the amount of iron in beef liver. In fact, millet, chickpeas, lentils, soybeans, pumpkin seeds, sesame seeds, and all sea vegetables contain more iron than a comparable amount of beef liver.

Sources of Minerals

sodium	natural sea salt; miso; sea vegetables, especially dulse; green leafy vegetables; sesame seeds
magnesium	sea vegetables, especially dulse; dried beans, especially soybeans and lentils; leafy greens; whole grains
iron	sea vegetables, especially hijiki; sesame seeds; pumpkin seeds; leafy green vegetables, especially radish tops; millet and other whole grains
iodine	sea vegetables, especially kelp; green leafy vegetables; fish; organically grown vegetables
potassium	sea vegetables, especially dulse and kelp; beans and soy products; vegetables, especially cabbage; nuts; dried fruit
calcium	sesame or other seeds; sea vegetables, especially dulse and hijiki; leafy green vegetables, especially kale and parsley; nuts; soy products
phosphorus	sunflower seeds; beans, especially lentils; grains; sea vegetables

Continued ➡

Some of the other minerals necessary for a healthy life are sodium, which aids in the formation of digestive juices and helps maintain water balance throughout the body's cells; magnesium, which activates enzymes in carbohydrate metabolism and helps strengthen nerves and muscles; iodine, which stimulates circulation and helps in the oxidation of fats; potassium, which helps regulate the heartbeat and aids in the formation of glycogen from glucose and fats from glycogen; and phosphorus, which helps with the transport of fatty acids, blood coagulation, and the building of strong bones and teeth. Minerals needed in small amounts are known as trace minerals. Sufficient amounts of all these minerals are available within a macrobiotic diet.

Minerals work together. If one is lacking or is too abundant, it affects the proper functioning of all the minerals. This is why it is best not to take megadoses of any one mineral. Any mineral supplement taken should contain a balanced amount of all the major minerals. However, people who eat whole foods and sea vegetables, as in a basic macrobiotic diet, should not need any supplements at all. Natural sea salt is used in a macrobiotic dietary approach because it contains a good supply of trace minerals.

Minerals help produce an alkaline condition in the blood and body fluids so that acidic metabolic by-products can be neutralized. If enough alkaline-forming minerals are not present in the diet, the body uses calcium and any other alkaline-forming minerals it can find, leading to deficiencies and later diseases like osteoporosis. See the section on acid and alkaline for more information.

Vitamins: Vitamins are co-enzymes or catalysts. They help the body use the energy in food. Since there are plenty of vitamins in whole foods, people who eat a wide variety of whole grains, fresh vegetables, sea vegetables, and beans do not need vitamin supplements under normal conditions. In fact, synthetic vitamins can be harmful: any vitamin supplements should be made from natural sources.

Large amounts of vitamins are not needed by those following a macrobiotic diet. For example, people who eat a lot of animal foods need large quantities of vitamins, including vitamin C, to help break down the protein and use it for energy, especially if the diet is low in complex carbohydrates so that protein is the body's main energy source.

Most food is cooked in a macrobiotic diet. Since cooking destroys some vitamins, some people worry that this approach does not provide sufficient vitamins. The macrobiotic view is that proper cooking minimizes the loss of vitamins and makes the nutrients more accessible to the body by breaking

---

Sources of Vitamins

vitamin A . . . . . .soybeans, carrots, winter squash, rutabagas, other yellow or orange vegetables, broccoli, kale, other green leafy vegetables, nori

vitamin B$_1$ . . . . .whole grains, soybeans and other beans, vegetables, seeds, nuts, sea vegetables, especially nori and wakame

vitamin B$_2$ . . . . .whole grains, beans and soy products, broccoli, lettuce, cabbage, turnips, sunflower seeds, nori, wakame

vitamin B$_3$ . . . . .whole grains, beans and soy products, peas, seeds, nuts, shiitake mushrooms, leafy greens, sea vegetables, especially nori and wakame

vitamin B$_6$ . . . . .whole grains, beans, cabbage, nuts

Sources of Vitamins

vitamin B$_{12}$ . . . . .sea foods, especially small dried fish (iriko); soy products such as miso, soy sauce, and tempeh; sea vegetables; bacteria bound to the skins of some organically grown vegetables

vitamin C . . . . . .broccoli, parsley, mustard greens, kale, other green leafy vegetables, parsnips, cabbage, carrots, daikon, horseradish, sprouted grains and beans, and fruits, especially strawberries and cantaloupe

vitamin D . . . . . .sunlight

vitamin E . . . . . .whole grains, beans, leafy greens, unrefined vegetable oils, nutsvitamin Kwhole grains, radish leaves and other green leafy vegetables, cauliflower, hijiki

---

down the tough cellulose walls of the plant cells and that the body has the natural ability to manufacture certain vitamins out of other substances not destroyed in cooking. However, people who have eaten large amounts of animal foods and refined sugar for years can lose this ability, and it may take some time of eating primarily grains and vegetables before it returns. If there are no major health concerns that would make raw foods inadvisable, such people should eat more raw foods such as fresh salads, especially in warmer climates and seasons.

Cooking food the proper way, especially over wood or gas heat, condenses the food, making it more yang, without losing the food's vitality. Energy is gained from the heat, from the greater accessibility of nutrients, and from the yangizing of the food. This is not intended to imply that yang is better as both yin and yang foods and preparations are needed for a healthy active life.

Vitamin C (ascorbic acid) receives much attention these days. One of its main functions is helping with protein metabolism, especially in the digestion of animal foods. Since vitamin C cannot be stored in the body, is destroyed by cooking, and is lost with cold, heat, fatigue, and stress, the recommended daily allowance is very high. Macrobiotic thinking is that large quantities of vitamin C are not needed if animal foods are avoided. A more questionable view is that humans should be able to produce their own vitamin C but that they may have lost this natural ability by eating too much of it in the past. In any case, a basic macrobiotic diet includes ample supplies of vitamin C. Good sources of vitamin C in a macrobiotic diet are vegetables, sprouts, pressed salad (with or without salt), and raw salad. Horseradish and daikon are high in vitamin C, which is why they are often served raw (grated) with fish.

All of the vitamins in the B complex work together. This group includes B$_1$ (thiamine), B$_2$ (riboflavin), B$_6$ (pyridoxine), B$_{12}$, B$_3$ (niacin), B$_{15}$, B$_{17}$, and biotin, choline, inosital, folic acid, pantothenic acid, paraminobenzoic acid, and Bt (carnitine). These vitamins are the only vitamins that help with carbohydrate metabolism, and they also help with protein and fat metabolism. The bran and germ of whole grains (the outer layers) contain all the B vitamins needed to metabolize the carbohydrates contained in the whole grains. Refined carbohydrates, such as refined flour and simple sugar, lack the necessary B vitamins, so that the body uses stored vitamins for metabolism. This results in a net vitamin loss. Vitamin B$_1$ (thiamine) is one of the most important vitamins. It is destroyed by cooking, especially pressure cooking. However, it can be reassembled in the intestines

---

and can be produced in the large intestines from the cellulose of vegetable foods. Deficiencies in any of the B vitamins are extremely rare in those following a macrobiotic approach.

A lack of vitamin B$_{12}$ can cause pernicious anemia, a serious disease in bone marrow that inhibits proper blood formation. Vitamin B12 is found mostly in animal sources. A study done in Europe, which concluded that macrobiotic children were not getting enough B$_{12}$, worried many macrobiotic followers, especially those eating no animal products. The non-seafood sources listed above contain small amounts of B$_{12}$—but then only small amounts are needed. People who think they need more B$_{12}$ should try seafood. If this is not adequate, then a natural supplement may be needed. A more extreme option is injections; once started they may always be needed. Studies have shown acceptable levels of B$_{12}$ in adults who had eaten no animal products at all for more than 17 years.

Vitamin A (retinol and beta-carotene) is in very good supply within a basic macrobiotic diet, and since excessive amounts can be stored in the liver, deficiencies are very rare. A deficiency of vitamin E has never been observed in humans. A deficiency in vitamin K is not likely because healthy people produce vitamin K in the intestines, except immediately after birth or after prolonged treatment with certain drugs.

Vitamin D is made by the cholesterol-related substances in skin when it is irradiated by the suns ultraviolet rays. Of the more than twenty different forms or analogs of vitamin D, only vitamin D$_3$, available from sunshine, is natural. Milk is fortified with vitamin D$_2$, a nonnatural analog. Some believe vitamin D$_2$, actually a steroid, is the root cause of many disorders, and that products containing it should be avoided. Plenty of sunshine, an average of about 15 to 20 minutes of facial exposure per day, is enough for the adequate production of vitamin D. Production is directly related to the surface area of skin exposed to the sun and the darkness of the skin (the lighter the skin the more produced). People who live or work in areas where the sun's ultraviolet rays are obscured much of the time should be careful to spend enough time in the sun when it does shine. If enough time in the sun is not possible, fish liver oil is the only dietary source of natural vitamin D.

In summary, whole foods give whole nourishment. There is no need to worry about the latest findings based on the needs of those who eat a diet based on animal and dairy foods, new drugs, or the newest miracle vitamin or supplement once the body has regained its natural healthy condition.

Acid and Alkaline

The theory of acid and alkaline is a very valuable contribution to macrobiotic thinking. This aspect of proper nutrition is rarely considered within the more conventional approach. It is based on maintaining the proper balance of acid and alkali in the blood. Solutions with a pH of less than 7.0 are acid (the lower the number the greater the acidity), and solutions with a pH of more than 7.0 are alkaline (the higher the number the greater the alkalinity). For a balanced health condition, the pH of the blood should be slightly alkaline—between 7.35 and 7.45—all the time. If the blood pH reaches 6.95 (slightly acid) or 7.8 (slightly more alkaline than normal), death is the result. The pH of the blood is so important that the body has several highly effective blood buffer mechanisms to maintain a constant pH. Thus, many people believe that eating a diet that balances acid and alkaline is not important.

In his book *Acid and Alkaline*, Herman Aihara challenged that view (as well as the idea that acid is always more yin and alkaline is always more yang).

Continued →

Using various scientific methods, Aihara determined which foods are more acid-forming and which are more alkaline-forming once metabolized by the body. The result is four categories of foods: yin acid-forming foods, yin alkaline-forming foods, yang acid-forming foods, and yang alkaline-forming foods.

Good health depends on eating a balanced amount of acid-forming and alkaline-forming foods (and yin and yang foods) each day. In fact, in my experience most people who have practiced macrobiotics for many years and still feel fatigued much of the time do not pay enough attention to acid and alkaline. They eat too many grains (acid-forming) and not enough vegetables (alkaline-forming), especially raw salads, and not enough sea salt (alkaline-forming).

The situation is more complicated for people who eat a typical American diet. The foods that make up a large part of the American diet, that are not included in a macrobiotic approach, tend to be overly yin and overly acid-forming, making it much more difficult to maintain the body's balance. These foods are also much more extreme both in their yin and yang natures and their acid-forming and alkaline-forming natures than the foods emphasized in a macrobiotic diet. Dairy foods act as buffers. They make acid-forming foods less acid-forming, and alkaline-forming foods less alkaline-forming. However, they do not completely neutralize the effects of strong acid-forming or alkaline-forming foods. Overall, dairy foods tend to be more acid-forming.

yin acid-forming foods	yin alkaline-forming food
grain sweeteners	beverages
oil	fruit
nuts	sea vegetables
beans	seeds
some grains	most vegetables
most grains	some root vegetables
fish	some sea vegetables
	salty soy products
	(miso, soy sauce)
	sea salt

Here, then, is a chart of the foods eaten mostly in a modern typical American diet.

yin acid-forming foods	yin alkaline-forming foods
most chemicals	coffee, honey, and
most medicinal drugs	spices
sugar and sugar products	fruit
psychedelic drugs	refined grains
vinegar and saccharin	raw salads, potatoes
whiskey and beer	heavily salted
most dairy products	processed foods
salted cheese	commercial salt
poultry	
red meat	
eggs	
some anti-depression	
drugs	

Whether a food is acid- or alkaline-forming is largely determined by its mineral content. The more acid-forming the diet, the more alkaline-forming minerals are needed to metabolize them.

The typical American diet does not contain enough alkaline-forming elements. Instead, animal foods that produce large amounts of sulfuric and phosphoric acid are consumed. In addition, people are consuming less salt (sodium), an alkaline-forming mineral. While salt in conjunction with large amounts of fat can lead to higher blood pressure and heart problems, the real problem is the fat and not the salt. Since salt is being reduced, the recom-

mended amount of calcium (alkaline-forming) keeps being increased. However, to get enough calcium, people eat dairy products, which produce more sulfuric and phosphoric acid. The cycle continues. The long-term health effects of such a diet are presented in the section on macrobiotic healing.

In contrast, a macrobiotic diet contains foods that break down easily in the body without the need for extra amounts of alkaline-forming elements. In addition, the foods themselves contain alkaline-forming elements in ample supply.

There is one more fact about the balance of acid and alkaline to mention: All active activities such as work, play, worry, and stress cause acid in the body. The opposite and more passive activities such as rest, relaxation, meditation, and breathing deeply help to balance the more active acid-forming activities. An excess of active activities, coupled with a diet of an excessive amount of acid-forming foods, can lead to fatigue and a dulled mental awareness, and then to greater sickness.

Macrobiotic Yin and Yang

At the root of macrobiotic thinking is the realization that there is a natural order to life: day turns to night and night to day; spring follows winter, followed by summer, autumn, and winter again; inhaling is followed by exhaling, the heart expands and contracts in the pumping of blood throughout the body. These changes take place whether or not we pay attention to them.

The words *yin* and *yang* help classify and categorize things within this natural order. They have meaning only when used to describe or compare things. Yang represents the inward or contracting force of life, and yin represents the outward or expanding force. The first step in learning to use yin and yang is to learn how to classify things as either more yin or more yang.

In terms of space, when the heart is expanding it is becoming more yin. When the heart is contracting it is becoming more yang. Similarly, when the lungs are expanding while inhaling they are becoming more yin, and when the lungs are contracting during exhaling they are becoming more yang. Yin always follows yang and yang always follows yin, in the same way we breathe in and then out. This is the natural order of all things.

Macrobiotic practice is to study and then intentionally live within this natural order. There is always change from yin to yang and yang to yin. The macrobiotic idea is to have calm change instead of violent change, orderly change instead of chaotic change, comfortable and healthy change instead of unpleasant change involving sickness. In fact, people begin to return to the natural order once they begin to eat more natural foods and less processed and chemicalized foods. The ability to comprehend yin and yang increases the more natural foods they eat and the more they study.

Any pair of opposites can be classified as more yin or more yang. Some of these classifications make sense immediately, while others require more thought.

Charting opposites is relatively easy because the difference between yin and yang characteristics is very great. For example, it is easy to say that 30 degrees Fahrenheit is cold and therefore more yin. Similarly, 100 degrees is hot and therefore more yang. But what about 65 degrees? Is it more yin or more yang? Compared to 30 degrees, 65 degrees is warmer, and therefore more yang. Compared to 100 degrees, however, 65 degrees is cooler, and therefore more yin. This is nothing more than what

more yang	more yin
contractive	expansive
inward	outward
fire	water
hot	cold
heaviness	lightness
inner	outer
active	passive
drier	wetter
summer	winter
day	night
brighter	darker
descending	ascending
time	space

one instinctively knows. If one is cold (more yin), she or he seeks warmth (more yang). If one is too hot (more yang), she or he seeks coolness (more yin). To put it another way, the natural order is to unify all opposites. Somebody who is too yin or too yang seeks the opposite quality in order to become more centered, calm, orderly, comfortable, or healthy.

Note that the macrobiotic usage of yin and yang is different from the way yin and yang are used in Chinese or Oriental medicine. Chinese medicine uses yin and yang as a curative technique. The macrobiotic way uses yin and yang as a way to restore natural order and gain freedom. Both systems work, and many macrobiotic followers and counselors have learned both usages in order to understand life more fully.

The Twelve Principles of Yin and Yang

Ohsawa wrote volumes on the natural order of the universe and yin and yang, which he called "the twelve theorems of the unifying principle." I have reworded and expanded on these principles here. Of course, there is much more to say about each one, and many more principles for further study. The first four principles have already been mentioned in various ways.

1. Yin and yang come from oneness, the infinite, and represent the two fundamental forces (outward and inward) or activities of oneness. For any thing or phenomenon to exist in this finite world, its opposite must also exist. (For example, we know what it is to feel cold only because we know warmth.) Yin and yang are produced infinitely and continuously from oneness.

2. An infinite variety of combinations and proportions of yin and yang produces energy and all other things, both visible and invisible. Without the fundamental forces of opposition (yin and yang), nothing, including life, would be possible.

3. Yin activity is the outward force and produces expansion, lightness, cold, and so on. Yang activity is the inward force and produces contraction, heaviness, heat, and so on.

4. Yin attracts yang and yang attracts yin. Someone who is more yin will be attracted to people and things that are more yang, and vice versa. The finite world only exists as long as opposites exist. By unifying opposites one reaches toward the infinite world of oneness where there is no separation. The ability to unify opposites is one key to a happy and healthy life.

5. The force of attraction between two things is directly proportional to the difference of yin and yang in them. For example, something that is extremely yin and something that is extremely yang will have a much greater affinity than something that is extremely yin and something that is less yin.

Continued ➡

6. Yin repels yin and yang repels yang. Someone who is more yang will be repelled by people and things that are more yang, and vice versa.

7. The more alike two things are, the more they will repel each other. The farther away or less alike they are, the weaker the repulsion. (Many troubled relationships could be helped with an understanding of this and the previous three theorems. Between any two people or things there is always a force of attraction and a force of repulsion. People or things with similar yin and yang qualities will repel each other more and attract each other less, while people or things with different yin and yang qualities will repel each other less and attract each other more.)

8. Every thing in this finite world is composed of both yin characteristics and yang characteristics. There is nothing that is all yin or all yang. In other words, yin and yang are not absolute qualities; they are relative qualities. This is one of the most important principles of yin and yang theory.

9. There is nothing that is neutral. Either yin or yang is in excess at any given time within every thing. If the yin characteristics dominate, then the thing is called "more yin." If the yang characteristics dominate, then the thing is called "more yang." If the yin or yang characteristics dominate, but just by a little, then the thing is called "less yin" or "less yang."

10. Every thing is constantly changing its yin and yang characteristics—every thing is restless. What is more yin one day can become more yang the next, and vice versa. In my experience this is the hardest principle to understand, but it is also the most rewarding. It allows one to change an overly yin condition of sickness to a more healthy balanced condition.

11. At the extremity of development, yin becomes yang and yang becomes yin. Because many of the charts in macrobiotic literature are two dimensional, people see yin and yang as opposites. But if one thinks of the seasons, it is easier to see how more yin (winter) can become more yang (summer), and vice versa.

12. The surface (periphery) of every thing is more yin and the center of the same thing is more yang, since yin is the representation of the outward force and yang is the representation of the inward force.

While everything in this finite world has yin and yang aspects, macrobiotic practice emphasizes the yin and yang of food and of the body. What one eats influences what one thinks and as such is an important determinant of health.

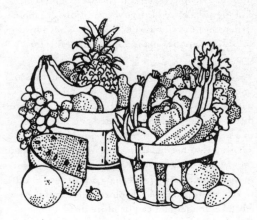

Yin and Yang of Food

Macrobiotic teachers have determined how yin or yang various foods are from theoretical understanding, practical experience, or a combination of both. All foods have many yin and yang qualities. These are some of the aspects of each food that must be considered:

Yin and Yang Qualities of Food

Composition	
more yang	**more yin**
rich in sodium	rich in potassium
more dry (less atery)	more watery (less dry)
high in complex carbohydrates	high in fat
Color and taste	
more yang	**more yin**
red, brown, orange, yellow	white, green, blue, violet
darker shades of color	lighter shades of color
bitter, salty	sweet, sour, spicy

Growth	
more yang	**more yin**
more downward or inward force	more upward or outward force
vertical below ground	vertical above ground
horizontal above ground	horizontal below ground
slower growth	faster growth
Season and Climate in the Northern Hemisphere	
more yang	**more yin**
grown more in winter months	grown more in summer months
grown in colder climates (grows bigger or more abundantly in the North)	grown in warmer climates (grows bigger or more abundantly in the South)
Manner of production or processing	
more yang	**more yin**
organically grown	grown with chemical fertilizers
needs longer cooking time	needs shorter cooking time
whole food	refined food
Size, weight, and hardness	
more yang	**more yin**
smaller, shorter	bigger, taller
heavier, harder	lighter, softer

To determine the placement of each food on a chart, all the factors or characteristics are taken into consideration. However, it is not an exact science. Adding up all the yin and yang characteristics of any food is very subjective. First, just how much more yin or more yang each food is for each aspect must be determined. Then, how much weight to give each aspect must be calculated in order to reach a sum total.

In practice, after the measurable theoretical considerations are noted, a final decision is made based on the observable effect of each food. Because every person is different and reacts differently to various foods, these decisions are somewhat subjective. Since the first yin-yang charts of foods were made by George Ohsawa, newer charts have been made that reflect the theoretical understanding and practical experience of more recent writers. In fact, different books list foods in slightly different yin to yang orders. All macrobiotic food charts are most useful as general guidelines. Ideally, everybody should create their own charts, based on how foods affect them.

Here is a detailed list of food categories from more yang to more yin.

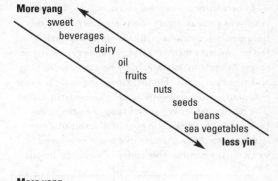

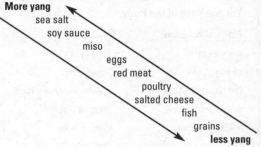

The yin or yang qualities of foods within one category may overlap the yin or yang qualities of foods in other categories. For example, an extremely yin vegetable such as a potato is more yin than a less yang sea vegetable such as kombu, even though sea vegetables as a category are more yin than vegetables.

This leads to some confusing terminology in the macrobiotic literature. For example, in the macrobiotic literature bananas are said to be more yin and strawberries are said to be more yang. But in fact, strawberries produce a yin effect and not a yang effect because the whole category of fruits is more yin. This is confusing. Therefore, the charts in this book more clearly reflect the actual yin and yang qualities of foods. The terms "extreme yin" and "extreme yang" and "less yin" and "less yang" are used to further differentiate among the various yin and yang qualities.

The food and preparation charts in the beginning macrobiotic diet chapter along with the understanding gained in this chapter may be used in deciding what to eat each day. They may be used to prepare balanced meals or to tilt the meal toward yin in the summer or toward yang in the winter. They may also be used to correct an overly yin or yang condition by preparing meals emphasizing the opposite quality. Since the principal foods used in a macrobiotic diet are those with the least pronounced yin or yang qualities and are more toward the center than those in a standard American diet, one can prepare healthy balanced meals with relative ease.

Yin and Yang of The Body

The condition of the body is continually changing as it reacts to foods eaten, the seasons, aging, situations in one's life, and all other aspects of one's daily environment. Macrobiotic practice emphasizes the role of food in both determining a person's condition, and changing it. A person's overall condition is determined by many different factors, such as whether the pulse is weak or strong, the person is more extroverted or introverted, thinks more about the past or the future, or prefers physical activities to mental activities. Some of these conditions, such as height, do not change much. Others, especially emotional conditions, can change in a

Continued ➡

moment. A mix of yin and yang conditions is needed for a balanced, healthy life. However, if any factor, or group of factors, becomes extreme enough to cause discomfort, this can lead to trouble, signaling a need to move that factor, or group of factors, toward the center area.

Every thing always seeks its opposite. If extreme yin foods such as sugary foods are eaten, the body becomes more yin. Seeking the opposite quality, the body craves meat or salt (more yang). Eating an excess of meat or salt, the body becomes more yang and seeks yin again. Furthermore, the body is never completely balanced—yin or yang is always in excess. The natural order is yin and yang changing into each other, forever. The goal of macrobiotic practice is to make the changes in a more comfortable way within a comfortable range of dynamic balance.

Yin and Yang of the Body	
Physical condition	
more yang	**more yin**
strong pulse	weak pulse
red face, pink face	yellow face, pale face
drier (less watery)	(less dry) wetter
smaller, shorter	bigger, taller
heavier, harder, stronger	lighter, softer, weaker
Emotional condition	
more yang	**more yin**
laughing, over joyous	sadness, crying
anger, complaining	worry, whining
overconfidence, arrogance	inferiority, doubt or fear
stubborn, screaming	complacency, silence

Psychological condition	
more yang	**more yin**
extrovert, aggressive	passive, introvert
optimist, positive thinker	negative thinker, pessimist
focused	spaciness
talker	listener
Mental condition	
more yang	**more yin**
specific thinker	universal thinker
dealing with the past	dealing with the future
materialistic	spiritual
Activity	
more yang	**more yin**
physical, social	mental, emotional
jogging, dancing	meditative, sleeping
disco, rock and roll music	blues, religious music
talking	writing

I have not placed male and female on the list, as macrobiotic literature does, because it leads to the wrong conclusion that females are, or should be, more yin and males are, or should be, more yang. Every person has both yin and yang characteristics and should determine the proper combination for their condition and desires. One can change an overly yin or an overly yang condition to a more balanced and healthy condition. First, one pays attention to the body's condition and how it changes each day. If any particular quality becomes overly yang or yin, and causes discomfort or gets one in trouble, one does the opposite to move oneself back to a more balanced condition. Someone who is too yang should eat more yin foods and

engage in more yin activities. Someone who is too yin should eat more yang foods and engage in more yang activities. For example, someone who drives to work gripping the steering wheel tightly and getting angry at other drivers needs to loosen up (become more yin). Someone who does not pay attention to how her or his driving is affecting others' needs to become more focused (more yang).

Ohsawa suggested checking one's daily eliminations. An overly yang condition of the stools implies that more yang food was consumed. Less salt and a greater proportion of yin foods would be the remedy. An overly yin condition implies that more yin food was consumed. More salt or a greater proportion of yang foods is suggested. Dark urination usually indicates an excess of salt (sodium) and light or clear urination often means too much liquid was consumed. The general guideline is for males to urinate three or four times in twenty-four hours, and for females to urinate two or three times per day. It is normal for those over fifty to urinate more often.

Yin and Yang of Daily Eliminations	
Stools	
more yang	**more yin**
darker in color	lighter or greenish in color
harder, constipated	softer, diarrhea
Urination	
more yang	**more yin**
darker in color	lighter in color
less frequent	more frequent

Many disorders can have both a yin cause or a yang cause as will be explained in the next section. The overall idea of macrobiotic diagnosis is that the part reflects the whole, so that any part gives a picture of the whole condition. For example, each part of the face corresponds to a different organ. Every aspect of the body can be more yin or more yang, and books on diagnosis study everything from the top of the head to the bottom of the foot, including voice, body odor, and conditions such as stiffness. Here are just a few examples of very specific indicators.

Some Specific Yin and Yang Indicators	
Eyes	
more yang	**more yin**
eyeball low (white showing above)	eyeball high (white showing below)
narrow distance apart	wide distance apart
smaller or slanting downward	larger or slanting upward
iris turned inward (toward the nose)	iris turned outward (toward the ears)
Nails	
more yang	**more yin**
convex, downward at end	concave, upward at end
short, wide	long, narrow
Shoe Wear	
more yang	**more yin**
front wears out first	heel wears out first
more wear on the inside	more wear on the outside
Baldness	
more yang	**more yin**
back of head	front of head, top of head

Macrobiotic Healing

In macrobiotic thinking, health is a condition of living in dynamic balance between yin and yang. In health, the movements between yin and yang are easy and smooth. Sickness is a condition of imbalance occurring when the changes between yin and yang are more difficult and rough, or when there is a blockage of movement between them. Healing is the process of going from an unbalanced condition to a more balanced one. It is most important to understand that there is no perfect balance—yin or yang is always in excess in every thing, in every person, and at every time. Thus, healing is an ongoing process and everyone is constantly healing. In times of health, the interplay between yin and yang is hardly noticed but it is there just the same. In times of sickness, one recognizes the need for change more readily.

Macrobiotic principles are used in an attempt to stay in the balanced area of health as much of the time as possible and to minimize both the time and severity of any imbalance. Changes in the season, climate, diet, environment, stress levels, and all of life requires adjustments in order to accomplish this goal. The macrobiotic way is to allow the body's own healing power to work by avoiding over-burdening the system with excesses or extreme foods. This is done by using a macrobiotic centering diet, by using the principles of yin and yang, or by using any of a number of natural home remedies. These methods are explained in detail in this chapter.

Macrobiotic healing is not medicine; it uses no medication or surgery. Macrobiotic healing methods may be used along with other therapies, including medical intervention, but this is beyond the scope of this book. Other holistic approaches such as homeopathy, naturopathy, Ayurvedic, and traditional Chinese medicine that take into account the whole person rather than just the disease symptoms work well with the macrobiotic approach. If a person chooses such a course of action, seeking the advice of a qualified macrobiotic counselor or care provider is recommended.

No matter how one lives and deals with life's changes, the body will wear out eventually. Macrobiotic practice strives to make the most of each person's constitution, giving them a longer and healthier life than they might enjoy otherwise. While death is inevitable, the manner in which one dies varies greatly. The possibility of dying in one's sleep of natural causes (the body simply wearing out) and not of a major disease is one of the objectives of macrobiotic living.

Looking more closely at health and sickness, just as there is a natural order to life and health, there is a natural order or progression to sickness. In order to maintain a healthy physical condition, most internal body conditions must remain fairly constant. Examples include the pH level of the blood, blood sugar levels, internal body temperature, oxygen and carbon dioxide levels, and so on. As long as balanced internal conditions are maintained, health is the result. When balanced internal conditions are not maintained, sickness is the result.

Sickness is the body's warning that there is an imbalance, and thus can be viewed as the body's natural attempt to maintain balanced internal conditions. If the warning is heeded and taken care of in a natural way, health returns quickly. If the warning is unheeded or taken care of in an unnatural way, the body must take more extreme measures to maintain balanced internal conditions. The sickness gets progressively more severe and the remedy takes longer and can be more difficult.

Continued ➡

This section contains an explanation of the stages of sickness from a macrobiotic viewpoint as developed by George Ohsawa and Herman Aihara. Within the stages, while there are usually immediate causes of any new difficulty, the underlying root cause is the same—an excess of yin or yang or both. Stage one and stage two sicknesses are transitory in nature, while stages three through five are chronic conditions that require greater care. The sooner any imbalance is remedied the better.

The section continues with a part on macrobiotic centering diets and diagnosis, showing that often a simple natural diet is the best approach to healing. The section on the process of macrobiotic healing explains what to expect if dietary changes are made. Natural home remedies that are supplemental and may be used for relief of symptoms are explained next. The section concludes with a part on some of the factors in health other than food, although examples both of nonfood causes and nonfood remedies can be found throughout this section on the stages of sickness.

Stages of Sickness

Stage 1: Fatigue. As with many disorders and sicknesses these days, fatigue is seen as a natural occurrence rather than as a sickness. However, from a macrobiotic perspective, fatigue is the first sign of sickness. If the fatigue is understood and dealt with in a natural way, more serious sickness can be avoided. There are many causes of fatigue and dulled mental awareness, including:

- Too much acidity in the body.
- Any reduction in the oxygen supply to the cells, such as too much fat in the blood, a low red blood cell count, or low blood sugar.
- Poor circulation from a lack of exercise. Too much strenuous exercise also causes fatigue.
- Elimination disorders, such as constipation or diarrhea.
- Overworking, overeating, or too much stress.

Any fatigue is a sign that the body, and especially the organs, are having to work too much. Sometimes a brief rest or a vacation is all that is needed. In other cases, more must be done. Here are some ways to counteract fatigue or dulled mental awareness.

- Breathe deeply and completely, concentrating on the exhalation. This helps increase the amount of oxygen and decrease the amount of carbon dioxide in the body. Put your hands on the front and back of your abdomen just below your belt. This area should move outward in both the front and the back when you breathe in. Learn to breathe so this area moves outward when inhaling.
- Chew your food well. Eat less if fatigue comes from overeating and your body can handle eating less.
- Improve blood circulation by taking hot foot baths, alternating hot and cold showers if your body can handle the shock, or by exercising. Do exercises that elevate the heart rate as your condition allows.
- Avoid strenuous exercise if that is the cause of your fatigue or if your condition does not allow it. Walking, gardening, Do-In self massage, and other mild circulation-enhancing exercises are helpful.
- Apply ginger compresses over the kidneys.
- Consume more alkaline-forming and less acid-forming foods and drinks. This is better than taking antacid pills.
- Take cool showers or baths. Hot baths are more acid-forming.

- Learn to control tension in your body. Any kind of meditation or muscle relaxing technique is helpful.
- Become more open and honest with your feelings. This helps by reducing stress.
- Live within your limits. Every child knows when to stop, but adults often do too much. Learn what you can and can't effectively influence and act accordingly.

Stage 2: Aches and pain. If fatigue or dulled mental awareness is not dealt with in a natural way, the next stage is pain, often in the form of headaches. Also, a state of fatigue makes one more vulnerable to injuries that result in various kinds of pain.

Pain is a warning that something is wrong and needs attention. In cases of injury such as a cut or a bruise, one deals with the pain and tries not to let the same thing happen again. However, most people suffer from little aches and pains that they have learned to live with. These are also warnings that something is wrong. The modern response is to stop the pain. The macrobiotic response is to determine the cause of the pain and then to deal with that cause. Both responses get rid of the pain; however, the modern response does nothing to remedy the cause of the pain, and the sickness progresses to the next stage.

Almost every injury or sickness has pain associated with it. According to Herman Aihara, the actual cause of the pain is a shortage of oxygen in the nerve cells. For example, a shortage of oxygen in the brain leads to a headache. Taking aspirin or other headache medication stops the pain by shutting down the warning system. It's similar to killing the messenger who brings bad news. Taking drugs is more dangerous than the pain—most painkillers also damage the nervous system and often lead to more severe illness. It is far better to learn how to deal with the pain in a more natural way.

The most lasting relief from recurring aches and pains—from headaches to stiff shoulders to back pain to foot pains—is a change to a macrobiotic approach to diet and lifestyle. Achieving such relief can take weeks to years, depending on the depth of the underlying sickness. Here are some common natural remedies for temporary relief of pain.

- A ginger compress applied to the affected area increases the circulation of blood to that area and gives temporary relief from pain. An albi plaster is often used immediately after a ginger compress.
- A tofu plaster is usually used on the head, and green plasters are useful for milder pains on either the head or the body.
- Massaging the painful area is helpful, especially for headaches.
- Various teas, including sho-ban tea and umesho bancha tea, are useful.

See the chapter on natural home remedies for instructions on making and applying many of the remedies listed here. Consult *Natural Healing from Head to Toe* by Cornellia and Herman Aihara or a similar book for additional useful home remedies.

Stage 3: Infections and infectious diseases. The next stage of sickness is infections and infectious diseases. Many microbes live within the body. These microbes aid in digestion and metabolism, and are necessary for a healthy life. When the natural order is not followed, unhealthy microbes can grow and cause inflammation, swelling, itching, and pain, damaging healthy cells. The most dangerous microbes can survive without oxygen and therefore are harder for the body's immune system to deal with. Problems occur most frequently when there are too many microbes in the body. The environ-

ment that causes microbes to grow excessively is produced by any or all of the following conditions.

- Too much simple sugar, such as from refined sugar or fruit.
- Excess water or liquid intake.
- Excessive amounts of protein.
- Too little sodium.
- A warm environment or season. (Unhealthy microbes have trouble living in too cold or too hot an environment).

These conditions all lead to an overly yin condition and a weakened immune system. Winter is the most yin season. An overly yin diet in the winter leads to a greater chance to develop a cold. The natural remedy for these conditions that encourage the growth of microbes is quite simple. Avoid simple sugars, excessive liquid or protein intake, and use enough sea salt in cooking to ensure an adequate amount of sodium in the body fluids. A macrobiotic diet meets all these requirements perfectly. In addition to the home remedies discussed in this book, the topical applications as discussed in *Natural Healing from Head to Toe* can bring natural relief from inflammation, swelling, itching, or other symptoms associated with infections.

The modern typical approach is to stop the symptoms; for example, taking aspirin for a fever. According to macrobiotic thinking, a fever is not only the body's warning that something is wrong, but also the body's natural attempt to deal with excessive unhealthy microbes or bacteria by creating an environment that is too hot for them. Stopping the fever only allows the microbes to get an even stronger hold, leading to deeper diseases. The macrobiotic approach is to let the fever run its course unless the temperature rises too high (over 103 degrees). In this case, natural remedies are used to reduce the fever to a manageable temperature and then to let it finish running its course.

Another modern typical approach to infections is antibiotics. Here again the response is to kill the messenger rather than dealing with the underlying cause. Antibiotics do stop the symptoms of infections and are often referred to as wonder drugs. The overall effect on the immune system is not positive however. With antibiotics many infectious diseases have been "cured" miraculously. As stronger and stronger infectious diseases have developed because the bacteria become resistant to the antibiotics, newer and stronger antibiotic drugs have followed. The reason for the stronger diseases in the first place is that the use of antibiotics weakens the body's immune system, contributing to the development of diseases such as candida, environmental sensitivities or illnesses, herpes, AIDS, and many more. Here again the response is to kill the messenger rather than dealing with the underlying cause.

Stage 4: Autonomic nervous system. Ignoring or destroying the body's warning signals and eating poorly eventually weaken the autonomic nervous system. The result is problems with hormone secretions and the proper functioning of the organs. This is another result of an overly acidic diet, which causes first nerve cell function and then hormone secretions to slow down. Problems with insulin, cortical hormone, and thyroid gland secretions are examples of the results of a long-term diet of too much fatty animal foods, sugary foods, processed foods, and foods containing chemicals.

Diabetes, one of the leading causes of death in the United States, is a good example of the fourth stage of sickness. There are two types of diabetes, insulin-dependent and non-insulin-dependent, but in both cases the problem is insufficient

Continued ➡

insulin. Frequent urination, constant thirst, weight loss despite eating a lot of food, cramps, blurred vision, and feeling tired and run-down all the time are some of the symptoms of insulin-dependent diabetes. According to macrobiotic thinking, the underlying cause is a diet that includes too much sweet food and drinks, including fruits and fruit juices. These foods cause the beta cells that produce insulin to be weakened so that not enough insulin is produced. Another underlying cause is too much fat in the diet. In this case, the body may be able to make insulin but neither insulin nor glucose can pass through the membranes of either blood vessels or cells because of the excess fat. The cells die from starvation. Non-insulin-dependent diabetes is similar, except that overconsumption of fatty foods is the major underlying cause.

The natural home remedies chapter and books such as *Natural Healing from Head to Toe* provide remedies for the symptoms associated with diabetes and other nervous system disorders, but only a change to a more natural way of eating such as a macrobiotic diet or macrobiotic centering diet allows the body to return to its natural healthy condition. Injections or stimulants and depressants used to control hormonal secretions are not the answer. They do nothing to remedy the underlying cause, and only serve to drive the sickness deeper into the cells and organs.

Stage 5a: Organ diseases. These are the life-threatening diseases such as heart disease and cancer. Here is a brief introduction to macrobiotic thinking regarding heart disease, as an example of organ diseases.

Even though the percentage of deaths from heart disease has decreased due to a greater understanding of the role of fats and cholesterol, heart disease is still the leading cause of death in the United States. Fats and cholesterol narrow the artery walls, restricting blood flow and limiting the amount of oxygen available to the heart. In the case of a heart attack, the lack of oxygen causes pain, and if action is not taken quickly enough, death is often the result. The modern response is to use drugs to control the amount of cholesterol and triglycerides, another type of blood fat. If this doesn't work, surgery to clear the blockage is often the next or only option.

According to macrobiotic thinking, the underlying causes and risk factors that contribute to heart attacks are:

- A diet high in fat and cholesterol from animal food sources.
- A diet high in simple sugars, including fruit sugar. Excess simple sugars easily turn to fat in the body.
- Too much or too little salt. Too little salt weakens the body's ability to make white blood cells and thus weakens the immune system. Too much salt can lead to kidney problems, and too much salt in conjunction with too much fat leads to high blood pressure.
- Smoking, stress, or obesity.
- Overwork, fatigue, or a sedentary lifestyle.

The macrobiotic approach is to deal with the underlying causes of heart disease. A macrobiotic diet—a balanced diet that is low in fat and protein from animal food sources and in simple sugars, and high in complex carbohydrates—is a good preventative for heart disease. Of course, people who have had a heart attack or who have any advanced heart disorder must deal with it quickly—a change in diet and lifestyle simply may take too much time. After medical intervention, however, a change in diet and lifestyle is definitely the best option.

Stage 5b: Cell diseases. Organs and cells work together closely. Organs, of course, are made up of cells. And one of the main functions of the organs is to maintain constant conditions for the body fluids, such as the blood and cellular fluids, that make cells healthy. If the body fluid is not healthy, the cells become sick and the organs become weaker. Weak organs cannot maintain constant conditions for the body fluids, so the cells become weaker, and so on. Here is a brief introduction to macrobiotic thinking regarding cancer, the worst-case example of cell sickness.

According to Herman Aihara, cancer (the malignant growth of cells) begins as a result of overly acidic body fluids. The blood needs to be slightly alkaline, with a pH from 7.35 to 7.45. The organs, and especially the kidneys, filter out acids to maintain such an alkaline condition. The overconsumption of acid-forming foods and fats leads to overworked and weakened kidneys.

The underlying cause of cancer is a diet or lifestyle that produces too much acid. A diet of animal foods (especially fatty meats), simple sugars and sugary foods, and synthetic chemicals such as flavorings, colorings, preservatives, and conditioners can cause cancer. The metabolism of fat creates large amounts of acid wastes, and fats slow blood circulation. The metabolism of simple sugar increases the level of carbon dioxide, leading to an acidic condition. Simple sugars also destroy red blood cells. Fruits are alkaline-forming; however, they are more yin and further weaken an already weakened immune system. And because fruit sugar readily changes to fat in the body, avoiding fruits is usually recommended by macrobiotic counselors for those with cancer.

Animal protein, animal fat, and simple sugars also help the cancer cells grow and thrive. The macrobiotic approach to cancer is to avoid these foods and follow a diet low in fat and simple sugars. Cancer cells cannot grow without excessive amounts of these nutrients; they eventually die without developing new cancer cells. Many other substances, such as known carcinogens, x-rays, atomic radiation, and asbestos, also contribute to the development of cancer. As in the case of heart disease, people who have an advanced cancer (for example, the cancer cells are strong and growing quickly) should consider medical or alternative intervention because the macrobiotic approach may take too much time.

The role of the kidneys is so very important in all fifth-stage disorders, and most people have weakened kidneys from the advice to drink as much as one can. Here are some ways to strengthen the kidneys—any one or all are helpful. See the section on natural home remedies for instructions.

- Follow a macrobiotic dietary approach, which does not require large amounts of excess liquid.
- Apply a ginger compress over the kidney area for twenty minutes each day for at least one month. Continue as needed.
- Walk barefoot on the grass in the early morning for five to ten minutes every day.
- Take two or three salt baths per week in a 1 percent salt solution (one pound of any kind of salt in twelve gallons of water) for about twenty minutes per bath.

Stage 6: Psychological sicknesses. Psychological sicknesses or imbalances are another warning signal that changes in diet and lifestyle need to be made. While physical sicknesses generally follow a pattern from stage 1 to stage 5, psychological imbalances can happen at any time and can trigger or greatly contribute to physical sickness. Conversely, a physi-

cal sickness can trigger or greatly contribute to psychological sickness. Psychological imbalances themselves follow a natural progression or order. For example, feelings can be positive or negative. Positive feelings are alkaline-forming, add to one's sense of strength, and lead to more energy. Negative feelings are acid-forming, use up energy, and lead to fatigue.

During each person's life there are times of loss, from the loss of friendships, to the loss of a job, to the death of a spouse or relative. Anxiety is the fear of hurt or loss. Hurt, loss, or anxiety over loss all lead to pain. If one grieves for the original loss near the time of the loss, a return to psychological balance is the result. Any pain left inside demands a response of energy that is directed outward and is usually expressed as anger. Anger held in leads to guilt, and unrelieved guilt leads to depression, a disruption of the flow of feelings that consumes all energy. In other words, the imbalance of emotions progresses until it is dealt with in a natural open and honest way or until it becomes so severe that it completely overwhelms you. Physical sickness or food imbalances make it more difficult to deal with any psychological imbalance. Physical sickness itself is a loss—the loss of health. Thus, physical sicknesses and psychological imbalances often feed on each other. Here are some warning signals that show psychological imbalance.

- Not wanting to get up in the morning or feeling that little can be done to change one's life. A healthy person is full of motivation to get up and work each day and knows all problems can be solved sooner or later.
- Blaming oneself for a long time for failures or disappointments. Everyone fails at times. A healthy person can deal with failures or disappointments quickly and honestly.
- Feeling that plans will turn out badly, that planned events will be canceled, or shying away from difficult tasks out of fear of failure. A healthy person is positive about the future and does not shy away from difficult tasks.
- Always looking to others for cures of even minor symptoms. A healthy person lets the body's own healing power remedy such symptoms. Always taking medications or always going to the doctor is a sign of imbalance. Doing whatever someone else says out of a fear of taking responsibility for one's decisions is a sign of deeper imbalance.
- Paranoia. A healthy person is instinctively afraid of crazy or threatening people, but a fear of everyone is a signal of imbalance.
- Often feeling alienated or separated from others, or having few close relationships. A healthy person fits in with others and has close friends with whom to share failures or temporary unhappiness.
- Difficulty showing anger. A healthy person is able to express anger appropriately in a non-threatening way when necessary.

Most of these conditions are a result of a diet that is too yin. For example, it may include too many simple sugars. A change in diet can be most helpful in restoring balance to one's emotional and psychological condition. Creating the space, time, privacy, and peace to get in touch with and to be open and honest about one's feelings daily is very helpful as well.

Stage 7: Spiritual sickness. A spiritually healthy person has faith in oneness, the natural order of life; takes responsibility for all his or her actions; is not exclusive; lives with infinite gratitude and appreciation for life. A lack of faith and a lack of

Continued →

appreciation for the oneness of life is spiritual sickness—the deepest sickness of all. This is the beginning of the dualistic dunking that sees enemies and leads to an unhappy life of fear. For example, modern medicine sees unhealthy microbes and cancer cells as enemies that must be killed before they kill us. The macrobiotic understanding is that all so-called "enemies" exist to help us understand the natural order of life. Thus, unhealthy microbes and cancer cells are part of us, and therefore are part of the world of oneness. They are necessary warning signals. A person who understands that unhealthy microbes and cancer cells are a blessing because they help show the cause of such a condition is well on the way to a natural healthy life.

Ohsawa outlined seven judging abilities to show people how to regain spiritual health. According to his theory, judgment develops in stages:

- Physical judgment begins almost immediately after birth and is characterized by instinct or unconscious reflexes guided by hunger and thirst.
- Sensory judgment begins some days after birth and develops into the ability to distinguish colors, sounds, smells, tastes, and textures, as well as the beginning of understanding what is agreeable and disagreeable.
- Sentimental or emotional judgment begins after some months. It includes the ability to discern like or dislike, love or hate, sadness or joy, and so on.
- Intellectual judgment begins around the age of four and develops with an interest in knowledge, asking questions, and the desire to find the causes of things.
- Social judgment develops about the age of six out of a desire to be the same as others (to have friends). Later, in the teen years, there is usually a different expression of social judgment in which the desire to be different develops.
- Ideological judgment usually begins around the age of twenty and is characterized by religious thinking and justice, and includes the ability to distinguish and understand good from bad and right from wrong from a philosophical perspective.
- Supreme judgment begins when an understanding of absolute and universal love that seeks to unify all apparent opposites is reached.

To reach supreme judgment, all the other judging abilities must be developed—all are necessary for life. Paying attention to physical and emotional warning signals is one step in this development. Here are some ways to develop each judging ability.

- Physical judgment can be increased by having more contact with nature or by creating movement anywhere there is stagnation, such as through a change in dietary approach or through physical exercise. The goal is greater adaptability.
- Sensory judgment can be increased by developing greater sensory awareness of one's surroundings or by developing a greater appreciation for art, music, or dance. The goal is greater sensitivity.
- Sentimental or emotional judgment can be increased by finding others to share in one's life and any changes one is attempting. The goal is greater stability and expressiveness.
- Intellectual judgment can be increased by challenging oneself more and by asking more questions. Ohsawa advised people not to believe others, to question everything, and to

find out about things for themselves. The goal is greater clarity and insight.
- Social judgment can be increased by having a family and by helping or serving others more. The goal is greater empathy.
- Ideological judgment can be increased by creating social challenges and learning from failures. Giving up a habit, such as watching television, can lead to greater spiritual awareness.
- Supreme judgment can be increased by studying yin and yang and the natural order of life, as well as developing each of the other judging abilities. The goal is oneness or freedom.

A person who reaches supreme judgment can unify all opposites. Hate changes to love, enemy changes to friend, sickness changes to health, unhappiness changes to happiness. Such a person has absolute faith, has no fear, and can maintain peace of mind, leading to eternal happiness. A person who truly understands and possesses supreme judgment can cure any sickness easily and naturally by allowing the body's healing power to remedy any disorder.

Macrobiotic Centering Diet and Diagnosis

Most diseases in civilized society come from excesses rather than from deficiencies. The macrobiotic way of expressing this is too much yin, too much yang, too much extreme yin and yang, or too much acid-forming food. (Cases involving too much alkaline-forming food are very rare.) In simple cases a dietary remedy is easy: simply eat more foods with the opposite qualities and less foods with the same quality.

However, many cases are more complex. Nothing in this world, including one's condition, is ever all yin or all yang. Just as with categorizing foods, all the yin characteristics and yang characteristics of a condition must be added up to determine if someone is overly yin or overly yang. There may be swelling (more yin) and redness (more yang) and so on. Adding up all the factors and deciding how much weight to give each one can be confusing.

Fortunately, simply eating a basic macrobiotic diet helps to restore the body's own healing power. One approach to healing is to eat a variety of foods when healthy and to use a beginning macrobiotic centering diet when sick or uncomfortable for any reason. This approach is used for short periods of time and is often all that is needed to restore health depending on the sickness (overly yin conditions respond best) and the strength of a person's natural healing power.

A macrobiotic centering diet is a restricted basic macrobiotic diet, eating and drinking only what is necessary for one's life, and toward the center of yin and yang balance. This means eating primarily whole grains, vegetables, beans, and sea vegetables. Sea salt either by itself or in miso, soy sauce, umeboshi, or gomashio, and liquid, usually bancha tea (kukicha), are also needed. Everything else is kept to a minimum or avoided altogether. This approach allows the body's natural healing power to heal from within.

For a macrobiotic centering diet, the percentage of whole grains is increased to 60 to 80 percent daily and pressure-cooked brown rice is usually the largest portion of this amount, although a variety of other whole grains may be used. If digestion of whole grains is a problem, or if a pressure cooker is not used, brown rice cream is recommended. This is whole brown rice roasted in a dry pan, ground, and then made into a porridge. Any of the less yang and less yin vegetables listed in the beginning mac-

robiotic diet chapter are eaten daily, totaling from 20 to 30 percent by volume. The extremely yin vegetables are avoided and of the more yin vegetables, leafy greens and broccoli are eaten most often.

Beans, primarily miso, natural soy sauce, aduki beans, chickpeas, and lentils, comprise from 3 to 10 percent daily. Of the sea vegetables, wakame, kombu, and hijiki are used most, from 3 to 5 percent of daily intake. One to two bowls of soup, usually miso soup, using the vegetables, grains, beans, and sea vegetables listed above are included in a centering diet. Bancha twig tea is used as one's primary beverage. Other teas found in the natural home remedy chapter are used for specific purposes.

Of the condiments, gomashio (ground roasted sesame seeds and sea salt) is used most. It, and any of the more yang condiments, are used as desired. Any of the more yang or less yin seasonings are used in small amounts for flavoring or to balance dishes. Of the oils, sesame oil is preferred, used sparingly. All of the supplemental foods, fruit, nuts, seeds, fish, and sweeteners, are avoided until one is better.

Quality becomes even more important with a macrobiotic centering diet. One should obtain the best water and the most organically grown foods possible. Chewing each mouthful of food at least one hundred times is recommended so that the body spends less energy breaking down food and more energy on the healing process. Overeating is avoided for the same reason.

This diet is to macrobiotic healing what a basic macrobiotic diet is to a macrobiotic dietary approach. It is a beginning simplified diet that can be used for general healing for ten days to two weeks or longer, as long as one is benefiting from it. A complete remedy may take longer, requiring the next step—the introduction of yin and yang principles. Once a person is well it is important to widen the diet to include a greater variety of foods.

Developing a working knowledge of yin and yang, which provides a greater understanding of the natural order of life, gives one greater control over the healing process. To begin, one adjusts the basic macrobiotic dietary approach, or the macrobiotic centering diet, based on the yin and yang qualities of foods eaten in the past and on one's present yin or yang condition of the body, emphasizing either yin or yang foods, as appropriate. Many of the guidelines needed for these adjustments are included in the section on macrobiotic yin and yang. If one makes a mistake and uses yin when yang is needed, the body keeps issuing warning signals, and the remedy can be changed. Nonetheless, to remedy a specific ailment using yin and yang, it may be necessary to consult a book or someone with more experience. Either increases one's understanding of yin and yang.

The rest of this section presents some of the conditions that signal that a change of diet is needed. Most of these warning signals rely on the principle that the condition outside reflects the condition inside. In addition, the chapter briefly mentions some of the disciplines studied by practitioners of macrobiotic diagnosis—a field that is far too detailed and complex to cover fully here.

Here are some useful diagnosis tools for each organ. They show an imbalance and an actual or impending sickness if corrective measures are not taken.

Lungs: An overall white or pale skin color indicates lung trouble, as does excessive yawning. Frequent headaches, melancholy, or depression may indicate insufficient oxygen in the brain due to poor lung functioning.

Continued ➡

Large intestine: Evacuating more or less frequently than once a day (or a person's normal amount) or bad odor in the feces may signal a problem with the large intestines. If the feces are shrunken and dry, it indicates too much salt. If the feces have no shape, it indicates too little salt plus as excess of milk, fruit, or simple sugars. An easy test is to walk barefoot on stones—pain indicates poor functioning of the digestive organs, including the large intestine and the kidneys.

Stomach: A blue line along the inside or at the base of the thumb, a white tongue, and chapped lips (except as a normal changing of the skin) are signals of possible stomach problems. A thick upper lip indicates overeating, especially sugary yin foods and refined foods. A cyst on the lips shows overacidity in the stomach and a possible ulcer.

Spleen/pancreas: Malfunctioning of the spleen/pancreas is shown by yellowish skin, cracked feet, excessive sleeping during the day, anemia, dull legs, or cravings for sweets. Forgetfulness and overworry indicate spleen trouble, which is usually the result of eating too much sweet foods.

Heart: The tip of the nose shows the condition of the heart. A purple color or puffiness indicates a weak overexpanded heart, usually from too much alcoholic drink or fruit juice. A red color shows an inflamed heart and possible high blood pressure. An oily or shiny condition shows an excess of animal protein. A red tongue or a large deep crack down the middle of the tongue is another indicator of possible heart problems.

Small intestine: An expanded lower lip indicates the overeating of fatty foods and problems with the intestines. Pimples and rashes indicate an excess of toxins in the body, usually from the overconsumption of animal foods. Stiff shoulders or trouble turning the head from side to side indicates possible small intestine problems.

Urinary bladder: Frequent urination that is dark or black indicates a contracted bladder. Other bladder problem indicators are sensitivity to cold and wind, itchy running eyes, and pain in the neck, backbone, kidney area, or ankles. If the vessels on the back of the hands are bulging or if there is pain when the back of one hand is slapped by the fingers of the other hand, the body has too much liquid. Watery eyes, a runny nose, or sneezing also signal too much liquid.

Kidneys: Bags or puffiness under the eyes indicate weak kidneys. Dark brown or black color under the eyes indicates overly yang kidneys, as does dark urine or a shrunken small toe with a very small nail. Athlete's foot comes from bad kidneys, as a result of too much animal protein. Other indicators of weak (overly yin) kidneys are light-colored urine or frequent urination that is like water, along with cold feet. The ears and skin also show the condition of the kidneys; any ear or skin problem indicates that the kidneys need help. In all cases, control liquid and salt intake and avoid animal foods.

Circulation/sex (heart governor): Dark lips or coldness in the hands or feet show poor blood circulation, usually from excess animal foods and strong yin foods such as simple sugar. A horizontal line between the mouth and the nose indicates a malfunction of the sexual organs. Swelling in the armpits, constant thirst, and rancid-smelling breath are further indicators of heart governor problems.

Pituitary/hormonal system (triple warmer): Trembling hands or fingers indicates a problem with the triple warmer, as does significantly different temperatures between the top and bottom parts of the body (such as constantly being cold from the waist up while warm from the waist down).

Gallbladder: Swelling around the upper eyelids shows the possibility of gallstones. Yellow palms on the hands indicates a problem with the gallbladder along with the spleen/pancreas and possibly the liver.

Liver: Lines between the eyebrows indicate liver problems and that a person is temperamental. Vertical lines show that the overworked liver is in a more yin condition, and reveal a tendency toward complaining. A horizontal line between the eyebrows shows a more yang liver, and reveals a tendency toward anger. A red color in the whites of the eyes indicates the overconsumption of food, especially fatty animal foods. Visible blue blood capillaries, dry throat, or the inability to bend forward or backward also indicate possible liver trouble.

Many of these indicators of organ trouble may be visible at the beginning of a person's macrobiotic practice. Others may develop as the body removes toxins and returns to health. The interrelationship between the organs and certain parts of the body comes from the theory of five elements, an ancient Chinese system reported to be over four thousand years old. In this system each of five fundamental elements are given a direction, season, yang organ, yin organ, emotion, grain, vegetable, and a host of other classifications. With study one can determine the best foods to strengthen each organ.

Just as there is a system of arteries and veins carrying blood throughout the body, there is also a system of meridians that carries energy through the body. This is the system used by acupuncturists to control and change one's condition using needles. The same system is used in Do-In self-massage for similar purposes. The meridians follow definite paths through the body and all pass through one of the fingers or one of the toes. Moving and massaging each finger and each toe every morning stimulates all of the organs. Moving all the joints from the fingers to the toes and tapping the bottom of each foot with the opposite fist every day is also beneficial to all the organs.

Here are some ideas on the yin and yang of organs. Again, the macrobiotic usage is different from traditional Chinese (Oriental) medicine. The organs are paired in terms of function so that one organ is more yin, and one is more yang. There are two "organs" that are used in traditional Chinese medicine, acupuncture, and Do-In that are not used in Western medicine. One is called the "heart governor" and is often referred to as "circulation/sex." The other is the "triple warmer" and is often referred to as "pituitary/hormonal system." Here are the yin and yang organ pairs and the corresponding fingers and toes where their meridians either begin or end.

Yin and Yang of Organs	
more yang	**more yin**
kidneys (little toe/bottom of foot)	urinary bladder (little toe)
liver (big toe)	gallbladder (fourth toe)
heart (little finger)	small intestines (little finger)
spleen/pancreas (big toe)	stomach (second and third toes)
lungs (thumb)	large intestines (index finger)
heart governor (second finger)	triple warmer (third finger)

While all the organs are important for a healthy body, the more yang organs are necessary for any life at all. In other words, a person can survive for longer without the more yin organs. The more yin organs work and then they rest, whereas the more yang organs are always working. It is important to let the yin organs rest. One of their functions is to protect the yang organs, a problem with a yang organ indicates a prior problem with the corresponding yin organ. For example, a person with a lung problem should look for ways to strengthen the large intestine as well as the lungs.

In using the meridian system, one learns that all the organ energies are connected. Sickness may be viewed as an imbalance in this energy system resulting from an excess or deficiency in one or more organs, often a blockage of the energy flow. Knowing where the meridians are can be useful in diagnosis of a condition. For example, a second toe that is longer than the big toe shows an overly expanded stomach, and thus a tendency toward a weak stomach. Redness or pain in a finger or toe would indicate a problem with the corresponding organ. Again, the basic principle is that the outside condition reflects the condition inside. Similarly, the face, eyes, ears, teeth, and feet are examples of more visible parts that reflect the condition of the inside.

The Process of Macrobiotic Healing

Just as there is a natural order to life and health and a natural order to or progression in sickness, there is also a natural order for turning an unhealthy body to a healthy one. This section explains how people who are using or changing to a macrobiotic approach move from sickness to health. Of course, every individual is different and will experience different results.

Healing always occurs in three stages. Any change to a more natural diet and lifestyle begins with a temporary worsening of the body's condition as it discharges toxins. This occurs as the body's natural healing power gets stronger from not having to deal with excesses or additional toxin-producing substances. The usual order is from yang to yin, or more specifically in the following order: meat, cheese, excessive fruit, dairy, alcohol, refined sugar, and drugs. It's clear what is being discharged because cravings, sometimes intense cravings, accompany the elimination. The discharge process may last for days, weeks, or longer. Discharges vary greatly from intense, dramatic events to slower, more tame affairs depending on the substances being discharged, the severity of the imbalance, and the length of time the body has been unbalanced. Still, one should expect some level of temporary discomfort. It almost always involves some pain, usually beginning in the neck and traveling downward through the body to the fingertips and toes and upward to the top of the head. Pain will be felt also in any weak or malfunctioning organs. A person undergoing a discharge may appear quite sick, but is often happy, especially if they understand the healing power.

The toxins may be expelled in any way possible, from the normal elimination channels of breathing, sweating, urinating, and defecating, to vomiting and discharges from the nose, ears, eyes, and reproductive organs. Green liquid bile and a colorless sticky substance from the intestines may come out. Black feces containing tiny stones are not uncommon. Massaging the naval area can help move old stagnant feces.

During the discharge process, white or yellow moles may appear at the back of the tongue that move toward the tip until they disappear, signaling

Continued ➡

a return to health. Black moles indicate the possibility of cancer. Redness on the body shows that the bloodstream is being cleansed. When the redness is only in the fingers and toes the discharge is about over. A headache often signals the end of a discharge and some people report seeing ghosts or visions at this time.

It is best to let the healing process finish naturally, but eating a small amount of the food being discharged will stop a discharge of toxins that is happening too rapidly and painfully. Medications and painkillers are not recommended; they can make the condition worse in the long run. Drinking less can hasten the discharge but will also increase the desire for foods and drinks that are being discharged. During a discharge, a simple diet of whole grains and fresh vegetables is best.

The second step in healing is to restore a healthy condition of the red blood cells. The red blood cells change completely every three months, becoming healthier very quickly. Most people who make a change to a macrobiotic dietary approach experience a marked improvement in health after the initial discharge period. Shortly after the change of red blood cells, the intercellular fluid (the fluid between cells) is changed. This time, usually the second to the fourth months, can be quite exhilarating. Many people feel that they have found the answer to healthy living.

The third step, however, is more gradual and can be much more difficult, and there may even be an occasional worsening of one's condition. This step is the healing of the rest of the body cells themselves. Nutritive substances from the improved intercellular fluid enter the cells and gradually make them healthier. However, most cells are not as adaptable to change as the red blood cells and the intercellular fluids. In other words, they do not easily adapt to the new intercellular fluid and while the benefits of new, more healthy body cells are on the horizon, another temporary weakening or worsening of condition is felt. This usually happens anywhere from the fourth month to several years after beginning a macrobiotic dietary approach. It is important to understand that this worsening of condition is a prelude to greater health.

Since the natural order is change, even after the first dramatic healing process has been completed, the body is continuously expelling toxins or excess materials or making adjustments and experiencing temporary worsenings of its condition. These are opportunities to increase one's understanding of the healing process. These are actually signs that one is in good health but must simply learn from experience and from solving new problems.

Natural Home Remedies

Simple home remedies made from foods can be helpful for people who have followed a macrobiotic approach to diet for a long time, as well as people just beginning a macrobiotic practice. Home remedies can bring relief from discomfort stemming from many causes, including: old toxins or undischarged excesses; toxic materials in houses, furniture, cosmetics, or polluted air; or too much stress.

The remedies in this section fit a macrobiotic approach because they are made of natural foods and contribute to the healing process. There are many other natural home remedies used within macrobiotic practice, and any natural food or drink, including medicinal herbs and herb teas from other holistic healing approaches, are used as needed or desired. However, the yin or yang effect of such remedies must be factored into the total healing process. In contrast, synthetic drugs, which tend to be extremely yin or extremely yang, fre-

quently stop or hinder the healing process. However, no home remedy cures a disease; it can simply relieve symptoms and encourage healing.

Many of the preparations use ginger. This yin spice acts as a stimulant, boosting circulation and helping internal cleansing of the body. The remedies listed here also make use of ginger's ability to increase respiration, digestion, and nervous-system function. The recommended readings include a few books that discuss more home remedies.

Ginger Sesame Oil

Ginger sesame oil may be used for massaging any area, and is useful for headaches, dandruff, pain in the spine or joints, skin problems, or numbness. To help heal a curved spine, put the ginger sesame oil on the index and second fingers and massage down the spine with one finger on either side of the spine. Do this for about 30 minutes each time. This massage is very relaxing for anybody.

To make the ginger sesame oil, grate 1 to 2 teaspoons of fresh ginger with a fine Japanese grater (available from Asian markets, some natural food stores, or mail-order suppliers). Squeeze the juice into a small bowl. Add an equal amount of sesame oil, and mix well. Any sesame oil will work, but pure dark sesame oil is best.

Ginger Bath

Freshly grated ginger juice added to your bath water is useful for improving blood circulation; relieving pain in the joints; itchiness, or other skin disorders; and for helping to remove old salts from the body. Ginger baths can be strong, and should be taken by adults only. Bring 20 cups of water to a boil and shut off the heat. For a medium-strength bath using fresh ginger, grate about 2/3 cup of ginger with a Japanese grater and put it in the middle of a square piece of cheesecloth. Bring the four corners together and tie them so that the ginger is inside. This is a "cheesecloth bag." Put the bag into the hot water. Do not boil the ginger, as this can reduce its effectiveness. After a few minutes, squeeze the bag with any utensil (such as a pair of chopsticks) so that all the ginger juice is expelled into the hot water. Place the ginger water in a bathtub and add enough warm water to cover the navel when lying down in the tub. Lie in this water for about 20 minutes. Use a greater proportion of ginger for a stronger bath or if the ginger is old. Decrease the proportion of ginger for a milder bath.

Ginger Footbath

This footbath is good for improving blood circulation in general and for kidney disorders and insomnia in particular. Prepare the ginger water as for a ginger bath and put it in a pan. Soak the feet for about 10 minutes at a time.

Ginger Compress

The ginger compress is useful for any kind of pain, and when applied over the kidney area on the lower back is most helpful for strengthening the kidneys. It is simple, inexpensive, and very strong. Caution is suggested for several disorders. Ginger compresses are not recommended for use on the breast in cases of breast cancer, on the head when there is high fever, or on the uterus area during pregnancy. It should not be used for appendicitis pain when there is fever, or on a baby. For an elderly person in a weakened condition, use a mild ginger compress (reduce the proportion of ginger juice) until the person's strength returns. Prepare ginger water as for a ginger bath, only using 10 cups of water and 1/3 cup of freshly grated ginger. The water may be reheated (do not bring to boil) and used again for up to 24 hours.

Dip a cotton or linen hand towel or other cotton cloth into the ginger water and squeeze out the excess water. (If your fingers are sensitive to the hot water, either wear rubber gloves or roll the towel lengthwise so you can put it in the ginger water without getting the ends wet.) Twist the towel by the ends, one end clockwise and the other counterclockwise, so that the excess water drips back into the pan. You need to keep the ginger water hot but not boiling, since each time the towel is dipped heat will be lost. Keep the pan covered when not dipping the towel, or heat it intermittently.

Apply the hot towel to the affected area. If it is too hot, let it cool in the air before applying it to the skin. A thin dry towel may be used between the skin and the hot towels until the hot towels can be applied directly to the skin without discomfort. Cover the hot towel with a dry bath towel to keep the area being treated warm. Use two towels, and apply newly dipped towels every few minutes for 10 to 25 minutes. When changing towels, lift the dry bath towel and the previously applied towel off the skin and replace with a newly dipped towel and the same dry bath towel. This keeps the area as warm as possible with the least amount of cooling between towels. Stop when the area has turned red, or when the pain is gone. Ginger compresses applied to the kidney area are very relaxing.

Albi (Taro Potato) Plaster

The albi plaster is often used following a ginger compress. It is useful for relieving pain and helping to remove excess toxins from the body. Like the ginger compress, an albi plaster is quite powerful and caution is needed in certain conditions. It may be used with confidence on the body if cancer or other serious illness is not present. Consult home remedy books or a trained macrobiotic counselor before using an albi plaster on a person with cancer or if you wish to use an albi plaster on a person's head. Albi (taro potato) may be found in Asian markets, some natural food stores, and some mail order catalogs. Powdered albi is available but fresh albi is preferred.

Choose a light-colored (more white) albi that is small and fresh. Peel the albi and discard the skin. Grate the albi using a Japanese grater. Grate enough fresh ginger to equal 10 percent of the amount of albi and mix together. (If the plaster causes itchiness, reduce the amount of ginger next time.) Add unbleached white flour until the mixture is the consistency of an earlobe, like thick dough or paste. Spread the mixture on a cotton cloth—flannel works well—to a depth of one-half inch, and apply the paste side directly on the area being treated. Secure with a gauze bandage if necessary. Leave the albi on for up to 4 hours. Discard after removing and do not reuse, as it will be full of toxins.

Tofu Plaster

The main uses of a tofu plaster are to relieve head pain; to reduce very high fevers; to provide cooling relief to overly heated areas (such as in inflammations) of the body or head; and in emergency cases of internal bleeding where medical help is unavailable. Any kind of tofu may be used. Squeeze the excess water out of a block of tofu and then mash well. Beat the tofu to remove lumps, and add 1 tablespoon peeled and grated ginger per 8 ounces of tofu. Next, add enough unbleached white flour to make the mixture sticky. Apply directly to the area being treated, about 3/4-inch thick, and secure with a bandage. Leave on for 2 to 3 hours or until the plaster turns yellow or becomes hot. In cases of fever, apply to the forehead. Change more often for high fevers or when used on the chest. Discard the plaster after using it.

Continued ➡

Salt Bath

Herman Aihara popularized the salt bath for improving the overall condition of the kidneys; correcting mineral imbalances in the body; and for relieving pain, insomnia, worry, or other stress. The optimum salt bath contains 1 to 2 percent salt. Less than 1 percent is not effective and more than 2 percent is too strong. Any kind of salt may be used; use the cheapest salt available. One pound of salt in 12 gallons of bath water makes a 1 percent salt solution. Fill a tub using an empty gallon container and mark the tub at the height of 12 gallons. (Next time, just fill the tub to the mark.) Any comfortable temperature of water may be used. Simply sit in the water for 20 minutes or longer. A person with a weak heart should avoid extremely hot water. He or she should stay in the tub only 5 to 10 minutes at the most and get out immediately if the heart starts beating faster or there is any discomfort in the chest area.

Daikon Hip Bath

The daikon hip, or sitz, bath is useful for bladder inflammation, menstrual cramps, ovarian and uterine problems, and many other female disorders, as well as for postpartum care of the mother. It also is useful for skin problems, for eliminating excess fat or oil from the body, and for anal pain.

Daikon root is sold in many stores, but often the greens are discarded. Ask the produce manager if you can have or buy the greens. Natural food stores leave the greens on the daikon. Some mail-order suppliers sell bags of dried daikon leaves ready for use. Hang fresh greens in the shade to dry until they are brown and somewhat brittle—about four to seven days. Put the dried greens from 7 daikons (about 8 cups) in a pan with 15 cups of water, bring to a boil, and simmer for 30 to 60 minutes. The water will turn dark brown in color. Add ¼ cup of any kind of salt and turn off the heat. Strain and let the water sit for 5 to 10 minutes. Pour the liquid into a small tub (big enough to sit in) and add enough hot water so that the bather's hip bones are covered. The feet and hands remain out of the daikon water. Cover the upper body and legs with a large towel or blanket to stay warm and to induce sweating. Stay in the bath for 15 to 20 minutes or until the hips become red or very hot, or the bather wishes to stop sweating. After drying off, keep the hip area warm. It is best to take the bath immediately before going to sleep. If it is taken during the day, wait at least one hour after eating and rest for at least 30 minutes after bathing before becoming active. Drink some sho-ban tea if overly tired.

Bancha Tea

Bancha tea is the basic macrobiotic beverage. It is useful as a daily beverage or for any disorder involving weakness or poor blood circulation. It also helps satisfy cravings for sweet foods after a meal. Bancha tea is made from twigs or stems (about 60 percent) and leaves (about 40 percent) of the tea plant. It is called kukicha twig beverage if made from 100 percent twigs or stems. Place ¼ cup bancha tea (twigs, or twigs and leaves) in 4 cups water and bring to a boil. Simmer for 20 minutes. Strain and serve hot.

Sho-ban Tea

Sho-ban tea is useful for fatigue, anemia, and any yin disorder, overly acidic condition, or weakness. It helps strengthen the blood and promotes good blood circulation. Place 1 teaspoon soy sauce in a cup and add ⅔ cup boiling bancha tea. Drink hot. Decrease the proportion of soy sauce to tea if a weaker tea is desired.

Umesho Bancha Tea

This tea is useful for digestive disorders, fatigue, and all cancers. It also helps improve blood circulation, regulate the heart rate, and strengthen the reproductive organs after the delivery of a baby. Umeboshi plums are plums pickled with salt and beefsteak leaves. They are available from natural food stores or mail order suppliers. Bring ½ umeboshi plum (pit removed) and ⅔ cup already prepared bancha tea to a boil and simmer for 5 minutes. Grate enough fresh ginger to yield ¼ teaspoon ginger juice after the ginger is squeezed. Place the ginger juice and ½ teaspoon soy sauce in a cup and add the umeboshi bancha tea. Drink hot.

Umesho Kuzu Tea—

This tea is useful for diarrhea, upset stomach, and a lack of appetite. Kuzu, a starch extracted from the root of a wild Japanese plant, has a strong contracting power. It is available from natural food stores and mail order suppliers. For adults, break an umeboshi plum into several pieces, add 1½ cups water, and bring to a boil. Dissolve 1 tablespoon kuzu in 3 tablespoons cold water and add to pot. Simmer, stirring constantly until the liquid becomes clear. Add 1 teaspoon soy sauce and bring to boil. As soon as it boils remove from heat and add about 7 drops of juice squeezed from freshly grated ginger. Drink immediately. For kids, increase the kuzu to 1½ tablespoons and decrease the soy sauce to ½ teaspoon.

Kuzu Bancha Tea

Kuzu bancha tea is another useful tea for the intestines. Dissolve 1 teaspoon kuzu in 1 tablespoon cold water in a cup. Add 1 cup boiling bancha tea and a pinch of sea salt. Drink as soon as the kuzu turns from a milky color to clear.

Lotus Root Tea

This is helpful for all respiratory problems, including congestion, coughs, and sinus problems. Fresh lotus root is best, but dried or powdered lotus root may be used if necessary. For adults, grate about ½ cup lotus root, place in cheesecloth, and squeeze out the juice. For 3 tablespoons of lotus root juice, add 1 teaspoon ginger juice, a pinch of sea salt, and 1 cup water. Boil slightly and drink hot or warm. For children, use 1 tablespoon lotus root juice, 2 to 3 drops ginger juice, a pinch of sea salt, and ½ cup water. To use dried or powdered lotus root, follow the directions on the package to make 1 cup or (½ cup for children) of tea. Then, add ginger and a pinch of sea salt as above.

Other Factors in Health

Eating well and wisely is only one of the factors that affect health. Indeed, everything we eat, breathe, see, hear, touch, smell, feel, think, and experience influences health. And since everything is connected and related, each factor affects all the others. For example, a stressful situation often affects your overall attitude and ability to get a good night's sleep, causing you to be cranky with loved ones or friends. Thus, learning to give proper emphasis to each area of your life helps you move toward a more balanced condition. Similarly, being unbalanced in any area tends to be unsettling in general. Different factors affect people differently, depending upon their condition and personality. This section discusses a few factors that tend to be most important for many people.

Attitude: People who are happy and positive about life tend to have an easier time with the healing process. People who are fearful or negative tend to have a harder time. There are two types of fear:

normal fear, when one is in danger, and abnormal fear, when one is fearful of life itself. Abnormal fear, especially the fear that one cannot heal, is the greatest destroyer of human health. It leads to negative thinking. Health is positive thinking. Healing is the process of going from negative thinking (I can't) to positive thinking (I can). Abnormal fear can affect the immune system. Strong abnormal fear leads to depressed T-cells, which leads to a weakened immune system, which leads to greater sickness, which in turn leads to yet greater fear. One of the greatest benefits of macrobiotic thinking is the belief that everything can and will change. One can reverse the cycle of abnormal fear, repair the immune system, and thus achieve greater health and less abnormal fear. Love is the greatest benefactor to health, and the greatest expression of love is to live within the natural order of life. One who can do this completely will be healthy and will be able to overcome all abnormal fear of life.

Adaptability: Being able to adapt to change is very important for a healthy life. Sickness can be viewed as stagnation or blockage, either physical or mental. The remedy is to create movement. Ohsawa suggested that people learn to be adaptable. His ideas were to learn to cook whole foods, to raise or be around kids, or to visit a totally different culture. Long-time macrobiotic people sometimes lose adaptability, especially if their practice of macrobiotics is to follow a rigid set of rules. Following lists and guidelines from others is needed at first, but at some point one must create one's own lists and guidelines.

Breathing: Breathing happens without any conscious effort, but it is so important to health that learning to breathe fully and deeply can be very beneficial. There are two main functions of breathing. Inhaling brings oxygen into the body. If the breathing is complete and full, the air is of good quality, and if there are no blockages in the body, the cells get the oxygen they need. Exhaling removes about 70 percent of the body's wastes and contributes greatly to well-being. If the quality of the air you breathe is poor, you might consider an air purifier for your home. Also, the more house plants you have, the better.

Sunshine: Sunshine lifts the spirits. Today, there are warnings about spending too much time in the sun without a sun block to protect the skin. However, if the body's healing power is reasonably strong, one can enjoy moderate time in the sun without needless worry. For longer times in the sun, some protection is needed. Natural sunblocks are available from natural food stores, and are better than other sunblocks. However, there are some indications that the active ingredients in all sunblocks may be harmful.

Environment: The quality of the surrounding environment is becoming more and more important. Breathing clean air and consuming pure water is particularly important. Natural unpolluted spring water is best, but is getting harder to find. Well water is another good source if not contaminated. Water filters also work well.

An increasing number of natural products are available, including natural foods, natural clothing, natural insect repellents, and natural cosmetics. One might first pay attention to the things closest to the body, such as clothing and cosmetics, and to the places one spends a substantial amount of time, such as the bed. Natural products are those substances that exist in nature and are as close to the way nature provides them as possible. For example, cotton, wool, and silk are natural fibers that promote health. Polyester is a manufactured product

Continued ➡

that is not natural and wearing it does not promote health.

In my experience, people who change to a macrobiotic approach first become more sensitive to environmental pollutants, and later gain strength for dealing with them. It is best to eliminate as many pollutants as possible. Houses and modern-day workplaces often do more to hinder health than promote it.

Social support: Health depends partly on friendship because a friend shares life's stresses and joys, and supports one's decisions. This reduces one's stress and improves one's self-esteem. The number of true friends a person has can be an indicator of her or his level of health. Friendships, like all relationships, require give and take, but some take more time and effort than others. Relationships that create excess stress can be damaging to health and may need some time and space. Sometimes improved health can lead to an improved friendship.

People who follow a macrobiotic approach need not lose their friends who do not follow such an approach; nor need they stop going to parties. If one cannot avoid sugary foods or meat, one can eat a small amount and chew it well. Or simply saying, "My condition does not allow me to eat these foods," is a response that should not make other people uncomfortable about what they are eating.

Making new friends who are making similar changes in their lives can be rewarding. A note on a message board at a local natural food store, announcing a macrobiotic potluck or merely stating one's interest in finding other macrobiotic people, is one way. There are also macrobiotic gatherings, such as the French Meadows summer camp.

Stress: Stress has become a large factor in most people's health. Stresses at work, financial concerns, and family matters can be energy drainers. Dealing with unusual stress such as the death of a loved one or the loss of a job only adds to the amount of energy it takes to deal with everyday stress. Being open and honest and dealing with as much pain as possible when the loss occurs is best. As overall health improves, one's ability to deal with everyday stress and unusual stress also increases. Stress is acid-forming, so more alkaline-forming food and activities can be helpful.

A relative of stress is overworry. Macrobiotic people often worry too much about whether or not to eat a certain food. The worry can be more detrimental than the food; eat it and be happy, or don't eat it and don't worry about it.

Electronics: Advances in technology make life more simple and enjoyable in some ways but the cost in terms of health is oftentimes high. For example, computers can speed work, but even moderate use can cause headaches and other symptoms, even if you have a good diet, frequent breaks, radiation shields, etc.

Television can consume too much time. People have reported that frequent headaches disappear when they stop watching television or sleeping near a clock radio. Microwaves "heat" food by making the molecules move in a chaotic and unnatural manner. The effect on a person's health may be negative and caution is advised.

While there is no reason to avoid all machines, a person who is sick—especially if the sickness is stubborn and hard to cure—should try to determine whether some machine may be a cause of or a contributor to the discomfort. Books on applied kinesiology and biofeedback can provide further information.

Religious values: All religions and religious practices fit well with a macrobiotic lifestyle. In other words, a macrobiotic approach can be used by members of any religion. The macrobiotic viewpoint is that everyone is a part of Oneness (God), and that a positive relationship with one's Creator, God, Oneness, Infinity (or whatever the name) is very important. Knowing who one is, where one comes from, and where one is going spiritually provides tremendous healing power.

Sleep: Good sleep is necessary for good health, and it is a sign of good health. Having trouble falling asleep or not sleeping deeply through the night is a signal something is wrong, such as a poor diet or strong emotional stress, and action must be taken. It is important that the bed be comfortable and made of natural products; then, after major excesses have been discharged, sleep will be good and deep.

The general macrobiotic recommendation is not to eat before going to bed—some say for up to three hours. The amount of sleep one needs will most likely vary as one's health changes. Too much sleep can be more tiring than too little sleep. In any event, it is normal to wake up refreshed and ready to meet the challenges of the day. If one doesn't, this is a signal that one's condition is not the best.

Sex: The macrobiotic view is that sex is a unification of opposites, yin and yang, and thus an expression of the natural order of life. Many macrobiotic people report better sex and an increased sexual appetite once their body's natural health is restored. I have heard of some couples who were previously unable to conceive who have conceived and delivered healthy babies after a switch to a macrobiotic dietary approach.

Movement: Activity is necessary to use food fully. In fact, a lack of exercise is one of the main reasons why some longtime macrobiotic followers feel fatigued. There are many forms of exercise, including weight lifting, jogging, hiking, calisthenics, gardening, yoga, aikido, and house cleaning. People with cancer or other serious illness should take milder forms of exercise, such as non-strenuous gardening and walking. A person who is at all uncertain about exercising should check with a health care advisor before beginning any exercise program, especially a strenuous one.

Toward Macrobiotic Living

There are as many ways to learn macrobiotics as there are people. In talking to people over the years, I have heard of many different approaches. Some want to change quickly, others take their time and ease into it more gradually. Some want to learn all they can about macrobiotic principles and increase their understanding and enjoyment of life as much as possible using those principles. Others are content to follow a macrobiotic dietary approach and enjoy more limited benefits. Some will be moved to begin a macrobiotic lifestyle the minute they read or hear a fair presentation of it. Others wait until they have cancer or some other major disease. Some people love the idea of being self-reliant. Others will never feel comfortable being in charge or control of their own destiny—they are happier paying for and accepting the advice of others, be they macrobiotic counselors, alternative health advisors, or medical doctors.

In my opinion, the biggest mistake in macrobiotic education is giving knowledge to people rather than teaching them how to think. From an early age, most people are taught to believe others rather than to trust in their own judgment. Giving knowledge in the form of lists of things to eat or do and things not to eat or do is fine for a beginning but in the long run creates slaves instead of free persons who can think for themselves. It is your life and it depends on your decisions. Thus, improving your judgment is most important.

This does not mean that you shouldn't accept the advice and help of others when it is needed. A macrobiotic lifestyle is learning from life. It includes doctors and other professionals, books and nature, family and friends, successes and failures, sickness and health, and on and on. Each person is a part of the totality of life and experiences only a part of life; life is bigger than any one person's perception of it. It is bigger than any theory of it, including macrobiotics.

Macrobiotics is a study of life—the natural laws of change. But like any expression of life, it is only a partial picture. Using a macrobiotic approach to life as a tool, you can begin to see more of the total picture—it becomes clearer, more focused. The whole picture is there all the time but your view of it changes as your ability to focus— your judgment—increases or decreases. More clarity comes from increasing your judgment, which comes from a greater understanding of the natural laws of change, which in turn comes from eating well and living in harmony with the natural order of life. Blindly following a prescribed set of rules is not the goal of macrobiotics. Instead, the goal is to live a happy and healthy life in which you freely make your own decisions and gladly accept the consequences of those decisions. You always will need books and other people to give you guidance and to answer your questions, but after a while you need to begin to rely more on your own judgment and to answer your own questions.

The suggestions offered here are based on my experience in talking with many people over many years about beginning a macrobiotic approach to life. There are many roads to the final destination, but the idea and willingness to begin must come from you. How to begin and how to travel is outlined here, but the decision to travel, the speed at which you go, and the direction are totally up to you.

- Be prepared to change. Macrobiotics is a philosophy of change that leads to the oneness or unification of all things. Many thinkers in many centuries have taught change. When you begin macrobiotic practice, you will change. You can control the rate of change by the rate at which you make dietary and lifestyle changes. If you are inspired to change all at once, go for it—just do it. If you prefer a slower transition, this is okay also. In either case, being prepared for and open to change will ease the transition. A healthy life includes both constancy and change.

- Gain a working knowledge of the concepts and principles behind macrobiotics. Reread and study the chapters on yin and yang and healing as you proceed. You will find that your understanding of the principles changes, even though they are constant.

- Be realistic about the results that can be reasonably expected. In order to gain a wider appeal for macrobiotics, some authors have made it sound very easy to gain fantastic results. This book attempts to provide enough information so that there are not many unexpected changes. Many people drop out of macrobiotic living because of unrealistic expectations.

Continued ➜

- Develop a plan. There are many books on how to develop a plan for changing different kinds of behavior. While these may be helpful, people often spend more time in planning than in doing. Still, there are several areas of plan development that are worth considering.

  — Breaking the large overall goal up into smaller ones can be useful to get started. Set attainable goals, a time limit for reaching the goal, and a reward that you will give yourself for making progress toward or reaching the goal.

  — Knowing yourself, your strengths, weaknesses, and present condition allows you to honestly evaluate your chances of success and helps you set reasonable goals.

  — Knowing the resources available to help you reach your goals is probably the most helpful. For example, in addition to your own personal resources, there are macrobiotic counselors, support persons, study centers, camps and conferences, books, magazines, directories, natural food stores, mail order suppliers, family, friends, and so on. Having a support person to whom you report your progress can be helpful. Knowing others who are working toward similar goals can be very valuable; you can share experiences and understandings.

- Establish helpful everyday habits. Here is a list of habits that can be valuable.

  — Exercise. At the very least, give yourself five to ten minutes a day of stretching and organized movement that includes breathing deeply.

  — Chew well. One of the best exercises is chewing food. If you feel sick, try to double the amount of chewing for each mouthful.

  — Reflect. Give yourself five to ten minutes time each day to reflect on the day, relationships, and yin and yang. And listen to nature each day as much as possible.

  — Eat sensibly. Eat a grain-centered diet without being overly rigid or fanatic (unless your condition demands it). Your daily diet is most important; an occasional deviation can be refreshing and easily tolerated.

  — Write. Write in a personal journal every day. Writing about what happened and your reactions to what happened is enough. Or write to family and friends about your experiences.

  — Read. Reading inspiring and supportive literature, even one page a day, is very helpful.

  — Check-up. Pay attention to your condition every day, especially after the initial discharge period, by checking your urine, feces, and body for warning signals of imbalance.

  — Create. Choose a hobby that allows you to express yourself, such as playing music, writing poetry or novels, painting, drawing, acting, and so on. Or, be creative in thinking of ways to help others or yourself.

  — Contemplate oneness. For at least one moment every day stop and view life from the perspective of oneness. From this view, no person is Better than any other person, or any other thing for that matter. Every one and every thing is connected. Most people spend too much time looking at what separates us rather than at what unites us.

These are some ideas for developing a macrobiotic approach to living. I sincerely hope that you

will find these suggestions useful and that you will develop your own lists and your own plan. You can and should be the director of your own life. Always ask questions and answer them yourself to gain a deeper understanding of oneness. This is the macrobiotic way.

As your natural judging ability and instinct increases, you will be able to live a more healthy and happy life. Then, you can go beyond beginning macrobiotics and become eternally peaceful and infinitely free. It is the understanding of the natural order of all things, the oneness of all things, and the changeability of all things that allows you to live a life that is truly happy, healthy, and free.

Exercises in Distinguishing Yin and Yang

Learning to use yin and yang is like learning a new language or musical instrument—it takes time and practice. In order to learn a new language you have to practice with that language. Any amount of working knowledge you obtain is useful and allows you to learn more. At some point, yin and yang, just like a new language, becomes instinctive and you no longer have to think about the elementary concepts in order to use them in your daily life.

Practicing every day, even though the time may be brief, is better than the same amount of total time spent all at once. It is helpful to work with yin and yang each day for at least 10 minutes. Many people who try to learn yin and yang too quickly and all at once become frustrated and confused. A working knowledge of yin and yang only comes with daily practice over a period of time. This time can be spent studying this or other books and magazine articles on yin and yang, or practicing discriminating between yin and yang among common objects or within your own body.

Any of the following exercises can increase your working knowledge of yin and yang. During the first year of macrobiotic practice reread these suggestions at least once a month. After the first year reread the chapter on macrobiotic yin and yang from time to time. You'll be surprised how your understanding deepens over time. As you practice with the ideas that follow, refer to the principles and charts as needed. These exercises can be used in any order.

- Go to the store and pick any vegetable or fruit to study. For example, pick up any two Red Delicious apples. In terms of size the smaller one is more yang (less yin) and the larger one is more yin. In terms of color the darker one is more yang (less yin) and the lighter one is more yin. After you have evaluated the apples for as many characteristics as possible, find the two most similar apples and the two furthest apart in yin and yang qualities. Each time you visit the store, follow the same process with another vegetable or fruit.

- While at the store, choose two different vegetables or two different fruits and evaluate their yin or yang characteristics. The first few times choose similar vegetables such as carrots and parsnips or kale and collards. Compare different varieties of the same fruit such as Red Delicious apples and Granny Smith apples. Later, compare carrots and kale or apples and oranges in terms of yin and yang.

- Using the procedures in exercise 1, buy an amount of carrots that are more yin and the same amount of carrots that are more yang (less yin). Using the same cutting and cooking method, and ideally the same kind of pan and heat, compare the yin carrots and the yang carrots in terms of their effect on you. Did they cook the same or differently? The more differences and similarities you can determine the better.

- Using the same manner of preparation and cooking method, compare the effects of similar vegetables such as carrots and parsnips and then very different vegetables such as carrots and leafy greens. People's reactions vary. One person may find that buckwheat has a more yin (cooling) effect, and another may feel a more yang (warming) effect. Both reactions are valid and demonstrate the variable nature of yin and yang. Similarly, you may not always notice a difference between similar vegetables.

- Compare organic vegetables and non-organic vegetables in terms of yin and yang characteristics, taste, and vitality; that is, the energy you get from eating each. The difference can be quite subtle or indistinguishable. For example, I cannot tell the difference in effect between different carrots, except that organic ones taste better and seem to have more vitality, giving me more energy once eaten.

- Study the effect different cooking preparations have on you. Is there a difference between vegetables cooked with salt and vegetables with sweetener added? Boiled carrots versus baked carrots are very different in their appearance and effect. Just by paying attention to the differences, you will become very familiar with yin and yang.

- If you are cooking on an electric stove or using a microwave, find a way to cook over gas or wood heat for at least a month and compare the difference in how you feel. If you are fatigued much of the time, a change to gas or wood heat can have a positive effect. If you have a sensitivity to natural gas, check your appliances for leaks and correct any found.

- Look in the mirror daily and honestly evaluate your condition. Pay most attention to the factors that change the most. Is your face more red (yang) or more pale (yin) in color? Do you have any puffiness or swelling (yin) anywhere? Evaluate the condition of your eliminations. Are they more yin or more yang? What does this tell you about the food you ate yesterday?

- Pay attention to how your emotions and mental conditions change, both due to seasonal changes and to daily dietary changes. Ask yourself how you feel every day. After some time these evaluations become automatic.

- Compare yourself with family members or friends. Decide who is most yin and most yang in terms of height, weight, and other physical conditions. Compare emotional and mental conditions also. If you know someone else learning yin and yang compare your evaluations. The store or the office is a good place to look at people in terms of yin or yang. It does not take long to tell the difference between meat eaters and vegetarians, for example. Another fun thing to do is to look at people in the store and what's in their shopping baskets. After a while you only have to look at one to know the other.

- Compare other books or magazine articles on yin and yang and diagnosis with this section. If your experience indicates a different yin or yang order, change the charts accordingly.

- Make up your own questions and find the answers yourself. This is most important for your continued development.

If you are making big changes in your diet, your body will be throwing out stored toxins. Evaluations of the effects of certain foods or cooking methods may need to wait until your body has rid itself of these toxins.

Continued ➡

Don't worry if yin and yang seems difficult to learn—a change in diet is more important at first. Taking your time and learning every step completely will give you a deeper understanding and greater working knowledge of yin and yang in particular and of life in general.

—From *Pocket Guide to Macrobiotics*

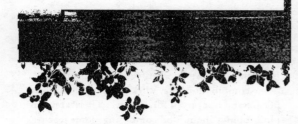

RAW FOODS DIETS

Jeremy Safron

What is Raw Food?

In the beginning, all creatures consumed their food in a raw form. Somewhere along the way, mankind left Eden and began to use fire on foods. Some people suggest that this was in order to help the food keep longer; others speculate that it was an accident that led to an addiction. Either way, man is now exporting this cooked consciousness to other civilizations and to domesticated animals. Fire is known as a destroyer; if we place an item in the flames, all that is left is ash. When we expose our flesh to fire, we usually get burned (fire-walkers and fire-eaters excluded). If our bodies reach extreme temperatures (above 112°F), we can die. Once man started using fire on food, pioneers and advocates who wished to protect the true diet of man researched, taught, and brought to light all the beauties and benefits of the raw food diet.

Raw food is often defined as anything edible that comes in its uncooked form, referring to anything that occurs naturally. Clearly, fresh fruits right off the tree are as raw as it gets. Fruit is love! To ensure survival, the trees want to have their fruits picked so the seeds can be carried off to be planted elsewhere. We are the parents of the next generation of fruit trees. Leaves and roots are also crucial parts of a balanced raw diet. Many tubers, herbs, greens, and roots that can be found in health food stores are edible wild. Flowers, berries, vine fruits, mushrooms, and sea vegetables are also raw. Most land creatures live primarily on all of these.

Sprouts are also raw. All seeds, nuts, beans, and grains are sproutable, and, in fact, many birds make their diet of sprouts. Fresh foods and sprouted foods are more common in nature, and that is why they represent a greater part of a raw food diet. Cultured foods represent another form of raw food. They are found in nature when the sprouting process is interrupted or when food starts to be eaten by good bacteria. Yet another segment in a raw diet is food that has been dried or dehydrated. Foods can be dried naturally outside where it is hot and dry after a fruiting season or grain harvest.

With human intervention, raw food is much more elaborate. We can create a delight of combinations and plan exquisite meals. One great aspect of a raw food diet is that it is easily prepared and can be radically transformed from its original form. Ultimately, by putting positive intentions into the preparation, beautiful and healthful meals can be created and enjoyed.

Benefits of Raw Food

Consuming a diet of primarily or solely raw organic vegan foods provides a large range of benefits. Eating raw food provides 100 percent of the nutrition available to us. The same food in cooked form can have up to 85 percent less nutritional value. Eating living foods also helps us obtain all the enzymes, catalysts that help us digest our food. Enzymes remain intact within living foods not exposed to temperatures above 116°F; otherwise, the enzymes are destroyed, and our bodies have to work harder to digest the foods we consume. Enzyme-rich foods help provide our body with a more realistic and efficient energy source. These foods can rapidly break down in our stomach and begin to provide energy and nutrition at a quick rate. When cooked food is consumed either alone or before raw food, it can cause a condition called leukocytosis, an increase in white blood cells. Our body may respond to cooked food as if it were a foreign bacteria or a diseased cell, which causes our immune system to waste energy on defending us. By eating only raw food or eating raw food before cooked food, you can prevent leukocytosis.

There are two primary conditions that affect the body: assimilation and elimination. These two functions represent the body's abilities to take in what it needs and get rid of what it doesn't want. All diseases can find their roots in these two conditions. Every ailment is a symptom of either poor elimination or lack of assimilation.

The foods many people have consumed earlier in life have often been less than healing for their bodies, and this can result in a clogged colon. The colon is where we get most of the nutrition out of our foods. At present, many people have their colons clogged with fecal mucoid matter. This debris can sometimes cover the majority of the surface area of the intestinal walls. The walls of the intestines are covered with many folds, curves, and fingerlike projections called villi, which are designed to take in nutrition. The more surface area we have, the more we can assimilate food. When the colon gets overly impacted with fecal mucoid matter, our ability to take in nutrition is degraded.

Many people eat a lot and yet are unable to get what their body needs. A contributing factor to effective assimilation is a healthy intestinal flora (see Live Cultured Foods). Eating correct combinations and chewing well allow for greater assimilation. Some of the best-fed people in the world suffer from malnutrition. Fresh raw juice and fruits are the easiest to assimilate. Greens and fibrous foods are wonderful for cleaning out the intestines of old debris. Eating raw food allows for maximum assimilation of what that food has to offer. Many of our true food cravings are nutritionally based. Our bodies know what they need and send word to our senses to seek out foods with these nutrients. In order to absorb the nutrients we seek, we need to have healthy assimilation. If not, we will eat much greater amounts of food in an attempt to get the nutrients we need. Raw food with all of its nutrients and enzymes intact is very easy to absorb and often helps cleanse the body and promote greater assimilation.

Elimination is the process of removing something from the body that is useless or toxic. Many people pick up bacteria or toxic food substances and get ill. This is because their bodies are not releasing the harmful substances. When a healthy body encounters toxic materials, it will quickly pass them out of the system. When toxic materials are encountered by a body suffering from poor elimination, they may get stuck in the system and cause

disease. Toxic debris can build up in the body for many years and eventually cause health issues. By eliminating potentially harmful substances, we protect our body and promote greater health and longevity.

There is a wide range of benefits from eating an ideal diet. One of the best forms of life enhancement through eating raw food is the abundant amount of energy that is present. Energy that is spent digesting cooked food can be made free for us to use for other things when eating raw. People eating raw foods find they need to sleep less to feel rested and often attest to achieving goals in their lives that on a cooked food diet seemed unfathomable. Many athletes have found that light raw meals give a more sustainable form of energy and allow them to surpass their previous records. Students also find that raw food gives them a more balanced blood sugar level and helps them think more clearly and stay more focused. Indigenous people throughout the world demonstrate the great life extension benefits that raw food has to offer. Many of these cultures eat a primarily raw diet and live much longer lives. People eating raw food also find it enhances their beauty. Most of all, people who eat well feel good. Feeling good is the essence of life. We enjoy our lives more when we feel good. The Hawaiians say that the most valuable thing a person can have is a positive attitude. By eating well and feeling good, we can be more positive and create a better life for ourselves and those we love.

Four Living Food Groups Chart

Eating 100 percent raw food is easy. It requires eating a balanced diet with certain understandings. Knowledge of nutrition is of great import in order for us to know what our bodies need and to make certain these requirements are met. The body takes in food and will use different parts of it in different ways. The chart pictured below gives a general guideline of what makes a well-balanced raw food diet. By increasing the amount of fresh foods in a cooked food diet, the cleansing process begins and helps flush out old toxins and the addictions that go with them. Greens and fresh fruits are especially helpful in pushing harmful debris out of the cells and the colon. These two primary raw food sources allow a person in transition to adjust his body to eating more and more raw food. As a person feels fuller and more nutrified from eating an increase in raw food, he may begin to experiment with letting go of cooked food. The cultured foods will really help initiate this by increasing the amount of assimilation through proper intestinal flora. The dried foods also assist a person transitioning by giving him a raw food way to satisfy a cooked food craving for something heavy. The chart shows an ideally balanced raw food diet that can be continued through life.

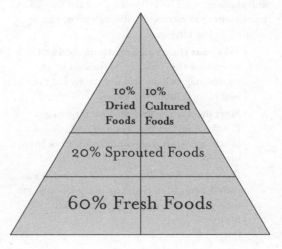

Continued ➤

Transitioning Strategies

Each person is unique, and so is her way of eating. In order to transition to a raw plant–based diet, some people may need to take a short amount of time, while others might take years to comfortably shift. People who were raised on a standard American starch-and-meat-based diet may take up to three years to properly transition to a 100 percent living foods diet. Through fasting and cleansing practices, the body can be rebuilt. The cleaner and healthier the body is, the quicker and easier the transition. The four living food groups chart can help structure a transition that is easy and healthy. It is helpful in moving toward healthier eating to work in conscious steps and to keep within your comfort zone. Senseless struggle and self-judgment only impede growth. Dried foods are the closest to cooked foods and can help people who are used to eating bread and pasta. Refer to the information below in order to see the proper percentages that can support transition.

Average American (Poor) Diet

80 percent cooked food

20 percent raw food
Of the 20 percent raw food, most is dried, and some is fresh

"Healthy" American Diet

60 percent cooked food

40 percent raw food
Of the 40 percent food
20 percent is fresh
10 percent is sprouted
10 percent is dried

A Sustaining Transitional Raw Diet

40 percent fresh food

20 percent sprouted food

20 percent cultured food

20 percent dried food

A Rejuvenating Transitional Raw Diet

20 percent fresh food

40 percent sprouted food

40 percent cultured food

A Balanced Raw Diet

60 percent fresh food

20 percent sprouted food

10 percent cultured food

10 percent dried food

Transitioning Tips

Change is the only constant. In our eternal growth, we often seek out new ways of thinking, living, and even eating. The transitory period between one way and another can be smooth and easy or quite rough and challenging. The following are a few tips on transitioning to raw food, although many can be applied almost anywhere.

· **Take your time and be patient.** Add and accentuate the positive. Be focused on the good things you ate and did today. Eat the raw and natural foods you enjoy.

· **Start the day raw and see how far you go.** Drink smoothies for breakfast, eat salad at lunch, and start your dinner with a raw soup or salad.

· **Have a raw food dinner party or potluck at your home.** It's a great way to try new dishes, turn people on, and support your new lifestyle.

· **Eat one new raw food each day.** Find out what foods you like and don't. Discover the variety of delicious flavors nature has to offer. If you know your foods, you can create any dish.

· **Go on local plant walks** and familiarize yourself with herbs, fruits, flowers, and greens that grow wild near your home.

· **Dine out at raw cafés** and then go home and re-create your favorite dishes. It is also fun to make old cooked favorites as raw dishes.

· **Always make the best choice**—eat the thing with the most lifeforce and the foods that you know will help your body.

· **Know yourself and educate yourself.** Knowledge is power.

Fresh Raw Foods

Fresh food is any type of raw food that is ready for use in its vibrant form. Examples of fresh food are: fruits, vegetables, herbs, and other harvested food. It is very important to consume large amounts of fresh food. These should make up 60 percent of your daily intake of food. Fresh food contains a high source of organically distilled water (up to 85 percent). Fresh food also contains many vital nutrients and is rich in vitamins. There is a wide variety of fresh foods and it is often best to eat fresh food grown in your own area. These foods represent the element of water, meaning that they are life giving.

Organically Distilled Water

Plants have the natural ability to distill water. A tree will draw inorganic minerals into its roots from stream runoff, rain, and underground springs and transform this into organically distilled water, which it will store in its leaves and fruits. This organically distilled water can be obtained by juicing or eating watery fruits or by drinking coconut water. Inorganic water contains toxic minerals in their inorganic elemental form. These minerals may cause kidney stones and could possibly clog the arteries. The human body does not have the ability to assimilate the metal found in most spring, tap, or rain water. Organic water is held inside the cells of organic matter. This intercellular water easily passes through living tissue carrying in nutrients and filtering out toxins.

Why Organic?

Organic foods are grown without any chemicals, pesticides, or fungicides. Nonorganic or conventionally grown foods may contain deadly poisons that can cause cell damage and toxic buildup and eventually lead to death. These synthetic poisons are completely foreign to humans and animals, and we are just now beginning to see their effects in civilization. Most farms grow sprayed foods because it keeps the pests away, thereby ensuring a larger crop even though the food is deadly. Organic foods are grown the way nature intended with only natural fertilizer that is compost of other organic foods or sea vegetables or plant matter. Plants grown only with these fertilizers are considered grown in a vegan manner (with no animal products). Other organic methods entail using manure and fish emulsion; these are considered organic only if the animals were fed organically.

Seasons of Fruits

Most fruits go from a fruiting season to a dormant stage, to a leaf and branch growing stage, into a flowering stage, and then back again to fruiting. Each variety of fruit has its own internal cycle; therefore, some trees may fruit in the summer, while others fruit in the spring or fall. Some trees may even fruit at different times based on the elevation at which they are grown. Many fruits do have definite seasons, though they vary by geography. For more information, contact your local farmers to verify what fruits are in season, where and when, and start keeping a local seasonal calendar.

Food Combining

Many varieties of foods are available—some that go together quite well, such as mango and papaya, and others that do not combine so well, such as onions and persimmons. For the most part, food combining is intuitive; we do what feels best for our body. Some combinations may work wonderfully for one person and not as well for another. There are many philosophies about food combining; some teachings suggest that it is best to eat fruits separate from vegetables. Some beliefs even advise eating each type of food alone. The main reasoning behind these ideas is that different foods take different amounts of time to digest and some can even impede the digestion of other foods.

Often foods are divided into groups such as acid, subacid, and sweet fruits, grains, greens, and other veggies. People who practice proper food combining try to eat only foods that are classified in the same group. It has been said that fruits if eaten alone take only thirty minutes to digest, whereas most other foods take up to seven hours to digest. For example, melons are best to eat alone. The reason behind this is that melons will be absorbed into the body in fifteen minutes if eaten alone, whereas if eaten in combination with other foods, melons may be forced to take as long as normally required for the other ingested foods to digest. The best message to look for is the quality of stool produced and the sensation the foods give to the body. When foods are eaten in a proper combination, they will feel good and produce no flatulence, and the stool will be solid and will not contain any undigested food particles. Creative digestion is the practice of eating what feels good because the body always knows best.

Juicing

Juicing is extracting the organic water and concentrating vitamins and minerals by removing the pulp and fiber. Juicing is a great way to stay hydrated and enjoy a wide range of nutrition. Juicing is extremely cleansing and healing.

From the Tree Right to Me

Fresh is best! There is a great beauty to consuming foods right under the tree they grew from. Much of the publicly available food is shipped all across the world and is also stored for extended amounts of time. Food when attached to the root or plant is still in the process of growing. When we harvest fruit or other types of fresh foods, they hold their life force for a short time, and then they begin to decompose. The closer you are to the source of harvest, the better the quality of food, and the more vital it is. There are a variety of ways to get closer to the source of growing. One way is to contact local farmers in your area. Another way of obtaining fresh foods is to go to a local farmers' market. Of course, the easiest way is to grow your own. Food that we coparent is of the greatest value because it becomes imbued with our own energy. Interaction with the plants we eat can heal us and help us grow. Remember, you are what you eat!

Cutting and Storing Fresh Foods

When we bite or cut into a fresh food, we rupture its auric field. We are essentially breaking the safety seal that the fruit has. This seal is made up of all the

Continued ➡

cells of the food, and, when we slice or puncture these cells, we open the fruit up and allow it to begin to oxidize. Oxidation is the process where oxygen combines with other available minerals and feeds bacteria so the fruit can go back to the soil and nourish the seeds within it. All of us have experienced biting into an apple, setting it down for a few moments, and seeing it turn brown; that's oxidation. The best method found for extracting juice from a fruit or vegetable is to press it. By pressing, we cause cells to rupture from within rather than by cutting or popping the cells from the outside. Pressed juice takes up to twenty-four hours to oxidize, while any masticated or centrifugally made juices oxidize in under an hour. Storing of foods is also important. The ancient Egyptians stored food in pyramids. This allows grains and seeds to be stored for considerably longer periods of time. The kamut found in King Tut's tomb thousands of years later was still viable and sprouted. Temperature and light play major roles in the storage of foods. Warmth and direct light make food break down more quickly. So keep your fruits dry. cool, and out of the sun.

Sprouted Foods

The Benefit of Sprouts

Sprouts are potential energy unleashed. All seeds, nuts, beans, and grains are sproutable. The sprout is the young growth of a seed or nut when the enzyme inhibitors have been released and the food has become enzyme rich. Sprouts are abundantly rich in chlorophyll and are quite diverse. Sprouts are a very high source of protein. Sprouts are a high-energy food providing a wide realm or nutrients. Plants know that their seeds or seed-laden fruits will be eaten—in fact, they plan for it. All seeds, nuts, beans, and grains are coated with an enzyme inhibitor. This inhibitor is designed to protect a seed from the digestive system of animals. The enzyme inhibitors are contained on the shell and skin of a seed, and, when eaten whole and raw, the seed can pass through the entire digestive system whole and be planted in a pile of fertilizer to grow a new plant. The best way to release the enzyme inhibitor is to sprout the seed or grind it into a powder. When we grind a seed, we are able to digest it mostly because we have created a greater surface area and broken through the enzyme inhibitor-coated skin. Chewing well is a great way to grind seeds. Sprouting completely releases the enzyme inhibitor and also activates the seeds. Soaking a seed for fifteen minutes releases up to 50 percent of the enzyme inhibitors. The recommended soaking time is for maximum enzyme inhibitor release. Sprouted seeds also have more nutrition than their dry predecessors. Some types of sprouts have as much as five times their original nutritional value. A sprout is the baby plant, so it puts an enormous amount of energy into getting those first few leaves out. The sprouting cycle of a plant's life is where it has the most concentrated nutrition. This is because the sprout wants to become a plant and it knows that it must get a root in the ground and a leaf up to the sky. Once rooted, survival will be much easier. Much like all creatures, sprouts go through their most rapid development at this early stage. The equivalent in humans would be learning to walk or talk; for a sprout, it is creating a wide range of enzymes and vitamins and minerals to get a good start in life. The young sprouts and grasses contain the highest amount of chlorophyll that the plant will ever attain. Sprouts are very nutritious and have many rejuvenating benefits.

Sprouting

Jeremy A. Safron

Sprouting is the easiest way to grow foods for yourself. All seeds are sproutable. The sprout is the young growth of a seed or nut when the enzyme inhibitors have been released and the food has become enzyme rich. Sprouts are abundantly rich in chlorophyll, quite diverse, and a very high source of protein and other nutrients.

To sprout, first select the type of seed you wish to grow and refer to the chart on page 44 to find out the optimal soaking time. You can sprout seeds in just about any container, though a large glass jar (½ to 1 gallon) with a screen cover is the most popular setup. As a general rule, for a yield of ½ gallon of sprouted seeds, use 2 to 3 tablespoons of small seeds such as alfalfa or clover; 1½ cups of medium seeds such as wheat, oat, and garbanzo; and 2 to 3 cups of nuts and rice. Soak the seeds using the time on the sprouting chart. Next, drain the sprouts. After that, rinse the sprouts with fresh water at least twice a day until the tails are at least three times the size of the seed in length. Next, expose your sprouts, still in the jar, to sunlight for about 15 minutes to activate the abundance of chlorophyll. Now, chow down!

Seed Soaking and Sprouting Times

Type of Seed	Amount	Soak Time	Sprout Time* (comments)
Adzuki	1½ cups	8 hours	3 days
Alfalfa	3 tablespoons	6 hours	3 days
Almond	3 cups	8 hours	1 to 2 days
Barley	2½ cups	7 hours	2 to 3 days (plant in soil for grass)
Buckwheat in hull	2 cups	6 hours	2 days (plant in soil for greens)
Buckwheat no hull	2 cups	10 hours	1 day
Cabbage	3 tablespoons	6 hours	3 days
Cashew	3 cups	5 hours	1 day
Chia	3 tablespoons	5 hours	2 to 3 days
Corn	2 cups	8 to 10 hours	3 days
Cumin	1 cup	7 to 9 hours	1 day
Dill	3 tablespoons	5 hours	2 days
Fenugreek	½ cup	7 hours	3 days
Flax	3 cups	6 hours	2 to 3 days (1 hour is okay)
Garbanzo	1½ cups	8 hours	2 to 3 days
Hazelnut	2 cups	8 hours	2 to 3 days
Kamut	2 cups	7 hours	2 to 3 days (plant in soil for grass)
Lentil	2 cups	7 hours	3 days
Macadamia	3 cups	5 to 7 hours	4 days
Millet	2 cups	8 hours	3 days
Mung bean	2 cups	8 hours	3 days
Mustard	3 tablespoons	6 hours	2 days
Oat groats	2½ cups	6 hours	2 days
Peanut	2 cups	8 hours	2 days
Peas	2 cups	7 hours	3 days
Pecan	2½ cups	4 hours	—
Quinoa	2 cups	6 hours	1 day
Radish	3 tablespoons	6 hours	3 days
Red clover	3 tablespoons	6 hours	3 days
Rye	2 cups	8 hours	3 days (plant in soil for grass)
Sesame	2 cups	6 hours	2 days
Soy	2 cups	8 hours	3 days (1 day for tofu)
Sunflower	3 cups	7 hours	2 days (plant in soil for grass)
Triticale	2 cups	6 hours	3 days
Walnut	2½ cups	4 hours	—
Wheat	2 cups	7 hours	2 to 3 days (plant in soil for grass)
Wild rice	3 cups	9 hours	3 to 5 days

* Sprout time is from drain time to time of consumption. The length of sprouting time may vary based on climate. These instructions are for a ½-gallon jar or bag.

—From *The Raw Truth*

Continued ➡

Chlorophyll

Chlorophyll is liquid life. All plant life is based upon it. Plants use chlorophyll to transform sunlight and CO_2 into sugar and oxygen. The chlorophyll cell and the human red blood cell are molecularly almost identical.

When ingested, chlorophyll is almost instantly absorbed into the body and feeds abundant amounts of oxygen to the blood, brain, organs, and all cells, allowing them to function at an optimal level. It creates an unfriendly environment for harmful bacteria, helping to protect the body from viruses and infections. Chlorophyll helps build the immune system, detoxifies the organs and cells of the body, cleanses the liver of accumulated toxic oils, and aids in healing wounds. Chlorophyll helps protect cells from the harmful effects of radiation from electricity substations, television, computers, X-rays, nuclear power plants, and nuclear waste. Chlorophyll can be found in all green plants, and specific plants such as wheatgrass contain as much as 70 percent chlorophyll and heal wounds extremely quickly. Sprouting seeds begin the production of chlorophyll using light and water to create life. Chlorophyll-rich food is high in vital enzymes and in B vitamins. Chlorophyll is a healer, protector, and revitalizer. It increases cell growth and thereby helps the body regenerate. Young grasses and sprouts contain some of the highest sources of chlorophyll. Chlorophyll is destroyed by heat. A temperature of greater than 108°F begins to break down the chlorophyll in plants. The greater the temperature, the more quickly the chlorophyll is destroyed. Therefore, food rich in chlorophyll should be eaten raw and not cooked.

Sprouting

Sprouting is the easiest way to grow foods for yourself. You can grow sprouts in any climate anywhere in the world. If you can live there, so can sprouts. You can even sprout in cities right on your windowsill. Sprouting can be accomplished in a variety of ways. You can use a jar method or you can soak your seeds in a cloth bag or even a wicker basket. To sprout, first select the type of seed you wish to grow and refer to the chart on page23 to find out how long to soak it. Soak the seed. Six to twelve hours later, drain the sprouts. Then rinse the sprouts at least twice a day until the tails are at least three times the size of the seed in length. Next, expose your sprouts to sunlight for about fifteen minutes to activate the abundance of chlorophyll. Now chow down!

SPROUTING TIPS

The length of sprouting time may vary based on climate.

- Sprout time is from drain time to time of consumption.
- Amounts are for half-gallon jar or two-quart sprout bag.
- If using the jar method, it is important to set the jar at a 45° angle. This promotes the maximum amount of drainage and an ideal amount of airflow.
- Make sure the sprouts can breathe—use wide-mouth jars whenever possible.
- Sprouts can drown! Be conscious of the soaking time.
- Buckwheat and sunflower are best when planted like wheatgrass in soil and grown into tasty greens.
- Always rinse with filtered water to promote clean sprouts.

How to Grow Wheatgrass

Wheatgrass is fun and easy to grow. Just follow the sprouting directions on the Sprout Chart for sprouting wheat and then spread a thick layer of wheat sprouts on the surface of a tray filled with soil or spread the sprouts on the ground. Then cover the sprouts with a thin layer of soil. Next, cover the tray with mesh or another tray. Water the wheatgrass every day, and after three days it will push up the top tray. Remove the tray and continue to water as needed. When the grass is about 5 inches tall, expose it to sunlight for a few hours to help enrich the chlorophyll. Wheatgrass is one of the highest sources of chlorophyll, containing as much as 70 percent chlorophyll.

There are many varieties of wheat, and all have different purposes. The winter wheat is better for wheatgrass, the soft spring is best for fermenting, and the summer is nice for dehydration and cereal. Wheat has been around for a long time as a staple grain.

It is said that the Essenes had known the abundant value of the benefits of the grass and grew it as a food and lived healthily. Dr. Ann Wigmore has helped enlighten the world to the benefits of wheatgrass. Dr. Ann helped many people overcome their disease and move into a more living foods lifestyle.

Live Cultured Foods

Cultured food is any type of food that has friendly bacteria in it. These cultures live on this food and digest it completely. Cultured foods are filled with enzymes and living bacteria that are extremely necessary for good assimilation. These bacteria, once inside our intestines, deconstruct food and hand us the vital parts. Higher concentration of good bacteria allows for maximum absorption and faster assimilation. A strong concentration of friendly bacteria will also maintain a healthy balance within the intestines and will not leave room for unfriendly bacteria to grow. Cultured food represents the element of fire and is energizing and protecting.

What Are Cultured Foods?

Cultured foods are a type of food that has been predigested by a helpful bacteria such as acidophilus, bifodus, or koji. These cultures are highly beneficial to the body. Live cultures reside on the villi, small fingerlike projections that extend from the intestinal walls. The greater the surface area of the villi, the more room for healthy cultures to live there. The helpful bacteria that now reside in our bodies originally got there through our mother's milk (if we were breast-fed). Cultured foods are live foods. Some cultured foods may have lived on a cooked product. These foods, such as miso, contain none of the original cooked food, only the live raw culture (unless they are pasteurized, in which case the culture is cooked). Many cultured foods live on raw food and are considered both raw and live. These are the most ideal. Some cultures are even grown on sprouts and are extremely excellent tasting and good for us.

What Do Cultured Foods Do for Us?

Cultured foods both protect us from foreign bacteria and energize us through proper assimilation. These helpful bacteria, such as acidophilus, allow for high rates of assimilation of nutrients from our food. Cultures such as acidophilus also act as a protective barrier against harmful cultures that may seek to invade the body. By eating cultured foods, we can increase the strength of our immune system as well

Type of Seed	Soak Time	Sprout Time
Aduki	8 hours	3 days
Alfalfa	6 hours	3 days
Almond	8 hours	1 to 2 days
Buckwheat	6 hours	2 days
Cabbage	6 hours	3 days
Cashew	6 hours	2 days
Chia	5 hours	2 to 3 days
Corn	8 to 10 hours	3 days
Dill	5 hours	2 days
Fenugreek	7 hours	3 days
Flax	6 hours	2 to 3 days
Garbanzo	8 hours	2 to 3 days
Lentil	7 hours	3 days
Macadamia	5 to 7 hours	4 days
Millet	8 hours	3 days
Mung bean	8 hours	3 days
Mustard	6 hours	2 days
Oat groats	6 hours	2 days
Peas	7 hours	3 days
Quinoa	7 hours	2 to 3 days
Radish	6 hours	3 days
Red clover	6 hours	3 days
Rye	8 hours	3 days
Sesame	6 hours	2 clays
Soy	8 hours	3 days
Sunflower	7 hours	2 days
Triticale	6 hours	3 days
Wheat	7 hours	2 to 3 days
Wild rice	9 hours	3 to 5 days

as the amount of nutrient absorption in the body. New cultures, both helpful and harmful, enter into the system through the foods we eat. When we create an ideal healthy environment for positive cultures, they grow and proliferate. The same is true for unhealthy cultures when we create an unhealthy environment in our colon. Healthy cultures protect us from disease by standing guard in the intestines and ushering harmful cultures on their way. Often, cleansing practices such as colonics or enemas can wash away health-giving bacteria along with the fecal mucoid matter impacted on the colon. It is important to continually reintroduce healthy bacteria into the system both orally and rectally when following a colon therapy program. Fasting can also deplete the active cultures living in our system, so it is important after long water or dry fasts to reintroduce cultures into the system.

How to Culture Food

Cultured foods can be created by obtaining a starter or by creating the ideal environment for healthy cultures to begin to grow. Often airborne cultures are present, and there is no need for a starter. The starter is a great method for being certain to obtain the correct flavor and is the preferred method. A starter is an already cultured food. Unpasteurized kim chee or miso can be your starter for making your own batch.

Continued ➡

STARTER METHOD

(example: kim chee)

Grind or chop 1 to 3 heads of cabbage.

Add ¼ cup of caraway seeds.

Add 3 crushed cloves of garlic.

Add the juice of 5 lemons.

Add 1 tablespoon of a previous batch of kim chee or 1 teaspoon live acidophilus culture.

Place in Harsch crock or in glass bowls 5 to 30 days (some kim chee is aged for months).

A Harsch crock is obtainable through Loving Foods or your local Asian distributor. It is an earthen crock that has a V-ring seal on the top. This means that the mouth of the crock is fluted and water sits in the ringed V-shape and the lid sits in the groove of the V, thereby sealing the crock and its contents. Air goes out but not in. For more cultured food recipes, see my book *The Raw Truth* (Ten Speed Press, 2003).

THE AIRBORNE JAR METHOD

(Example: Rejuvelak)

Soak 1 cup of quinoa in a half-gallon jar for eight hours.

Drain and rinse the seeds twice daily.

After 24 hours, grind seeds with 6 cups of fresh water and place in a half-gallon jar.

Let it sit for 12 hours. Drain off the rejuvelak and compost the seed pulp.

Refrigerate and enjoy. (Reminder: if it smells too pungent, don't eat it. It should smell lemony).

Where to Obtain Cultures

Cultures can be obtained through a variety of sources. Purchase a previously made cultured food product from your local retail store or contact a health product distributor. These cultured products contain the mother or starter and can be used to create your own cultured foods at home. Some common cultured products available are:

- Seed Cheez from Mount Shasta Rejuvenating Foods
- Kim Chee from Rejuvenative Foods
- Sauerkraut from Fermentations
- Live Apple Cider Vinegar from Braggs
- Sauerkraut from Cultured
- Kombucha mushrooms (get them from friends)

Cultures can also be purchased in their whole form (not on a substance). These are usually sold dry as a powder or as a liquid. Try to get cultures that are growing on something, because they are usually heartier and are specific to what you want to make. When buying a starter, make certain that it is refrigerated. Cultured foods are very temperature sensitive and will no longer be viable if exposed to extreme heat or cold. Here is a good source or live cultures through mail order:

Gold Mine Natural Foods
7805 Arjons Drive
San Diego, CA 92126
(800) 862-2347

Dehydrated Foods

Dehydrated food is any type of food that has had the water removed from it. These foods are very concentrated. Since the water has been removed and the mass of the food has been decreased, dehydrated food allows the intake of greater quantities of nutrients and leaves an intensified version of the food. Dried foods are considered alive only if they were dehydrated below 108°F (the point where enzymes begin to die and minerals and vitamins are denatured). Most dried foods have a longer nutrient retention time due to the lack of oxidation caused by water trapped in the cells. Dried foods can also be rehydrated. Dried food represents the element of earth and is very grounding and sustaining.

The Value of Dried Foods

Dried foods are concentrated nutrition. Most foods can be easily dehydrated by evaporating the water (which makes up anywhere from 30 to 85 percent of the fresh food). A fresh apple that might take us twenty bites to eat takes only three to seven bites to eat dried. Most nuts and seeds are sold dried to create longer stability of the oils. Sea vegetables, fruits, and vegetables are dried for storage. Oils are considered a dried food because they come from a dried seed or nut. Spirulina is also a dried food. In fact, many South American tribes would sun dry spirulina into patties in order to carry the nutrient-rich dried food with them on their long journey across the Andes Mountains.

Dried foods give us a wide range of concentrated minerals and vitamins and a concentrated amount of protein. Dried foods also slow down the metabolism in order to maximize assimilation. The body will rehydrate the dried food and take its time digesting it. Dried foods can be very grounding. Often people transitioning to a raw diet find that they constantly want food. Dried foods will easily fill this need by slowing the digestion and allowing for maximum absorption of both the dried food and other foods that are also in the body. Dried foods can be especially helpful to people who are transitioning to raw food and are used to eating a lot of starchy cooked food.

Methods of Dehydrating

Drying food can be accomplished in a number of ways. One of the most ancient and free ways is to place the food you want to dry in thin layers on a ceramic or glass tray in the sun. Another sun-drying method is to hang a hammock made of mesh or screen outside and put the food to be dried on it. It can be helpful when using these outdoor methods to cover the food with screen and put it in a hard-to-reach spot to prevent other appreciators of drying food from getting to it. Building a solar or home dehydrator is a great project and a simple way to dry food. Buying a commercial or home dehydration unit is often the easiest and most guaranteed way of drying food. The basics are: expose food to 108°F or less until the ideal texture and dryness are obtained. For suggested times, see drying chart.

Kissed by the Sun

The sun is the great provider of life. It is a powerful healer and giver of warmth. Most food enjoys its days basking in the sun, growing sweet and ripe and nutrient rich. The sun blesses us with both light and warmth, two very powerful forms of energy. Drying foods helps concentrate even more of this powerful manna. By drying food, we get to concentrate even more sunlight into an already sun-laden food and thereby enhance the food with more energy.

Dried Foods for Travel

Dried foods have always been the choice for travelers. In ancient times, people would dry part of their harvest for winter or for a long migration to warmer climates. Even today, people going to work or school will bring dried fruit or nuts because they are lightweight and stable. Dried foods can be kept for considerably longer than when in fresh form.

Dried foods are great for hiking because of the concentrated nutrition and energy. Dried foods are often dehydrating on the body, so be certain to drink lots of fluids or eat fresh foods to rehydrate the body.

How to Build Your Own Dehydrator

SOLAR

Step 1. Find a suitable cardboard or wooden box.

Step 2. Punch holes in the sides and bottom.

Step 3. Cover sides and bottom with dark-colored breathable screen or black cloth.

Step 4. Place a rack or hang a piece of breathable screen in the middle of the box.

Step 5. Put items to be dried on suspended screen.

Step 6. Cover box with glass or plastic.

Step 7. Place box in the sun.

Solar dehydration can be tricky. In some climates, the sun is too hot and it is best to use early morning sun. Other climates require all day drying. Be conscious of what you are drying the first few times, to get an accurate gauge on how your climate affects the drying time. A plastic strip thermometer can be purchased at a tropical fish or pet store to give you an accurate temperature in the box.

ELECTRIC

Step 1. Find a suitable box. A cardboard box will work, yet for extended durability use a wooden box. Either build it yourself or use an old wooden trunk. Some people even turn an entire closet into a dehydrator. Ventilation is important, so make sure the moist evaporated air has some exit point.

Step 2. Purchase a small space heater, ideally with a built-in fan, and set it in the back of the box. You will probably need to cut a hole for the cord, the temperature setting, and on/off switch.

Step 3. Glue or nail thin slats of wood or cardboard to the side of the box in order to slide trays in and out.

Step 4. Create trays by making square frames of wood and covering them with a mesh or by taking cardboard squares, cutting out the centers, and lining them with screen.

Step 5. Put items to be dried on trays and turn on space heater.

A plastic strip thermometer can be purchased at a tropical fish or pet store to give you an accurate temperature in the box. If drying in your closet, you may want to take temperature readings at a variety of heights to find the most suitable drying area.

Raw Survival Foods

A few foods that are eaten raw can sustain the human body and give maximum energy for minimal consumption. These foods are power packed with concentrated nutrition and provide an abundance of vital energy. Diversity is important when eating raw, so it is challenging to live solely on these foods, yet it could be done if you were in a survival situation. Otherwise, these foods of sustenance are some great staples for a raw/living food way of eating.

Sprouted buckwheat: Buckwheat is the highest source of protein in the seed kingdom. Buckwheat is the fruit of a small herb plant and is praised as a staple in many Eastern countries. Buckwheat is easy to digest and is a wild food.

Continued ➡

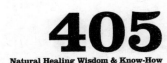

Drying Methods, Time, and Temperature

Food	Method	Drying Time	Temperature
Apple	Sliced	13 hours	108°F
Apple	Ground	10 hours	108°F
Banana	Whole	28 hours	108°F
Banana	Sliced	18 hours	108°F
Banana	Ground	14 hours	108°F
Carrot	Ground	8 hours	108°F
Coconut	Sliced	18 hours	108°F
Coconut	Ground	21 hours	108°F
Corn	Whole	18 hours	108°F
Corn	Ground	15 hours	108°F
Com	Ground sprouts	15 hours	108°F
Flowers	Whole	3 to 5 hours	98°F
Garlic	Whole	12 hours	108°F
Garlic	Ground	8 hours	108°F
Herbs	Whole	5 to 7 hours	100°F
Kiwi	Sliced	16 hours	108°F
Mango	Sliced	21 hours	108°F
Melon	Sliced	24 hours	108°F
Melon	Ground	21 hours	108°F
Oat sprouts	Whole	15 hours	108°F
Oat sprouts	Ground	24 hours	108°F
Onion	Sliced	13 hours	108°F
Onion	Ground	10 hours	108°F
Papaya	Sliced	20 hours	108°F
Papaya	Ground	16 hours	108°F
Peach	Sliced	24 hours	108°F
Peach	Ground	18 hours	108°F
Pear	Sliced	15 hours	108°F
Pear	Ground	13 hours	108°F
Persimmon	Whole	48 hours	108°F
Persimmon	Sliced	18 hours	108°F
Persimmon	Ground	15 hours	108°F
Pineapple	Sliced	21 hours	108°F
Potatoes	Sliced	16 hours	108°F
Sapodilla	Sliced	12 hours	108°F
Sea veggies	Whole	15 hours	100°F
Sprouts	Whole	13 hours	100°F
Sprouts	Ground	20 hours	100°F
Starfruit	Sliced	13 hours	:108°F
Sunchoke	Sliced	16 hours	108°F
Tomato	Sliced	18 hours	108°F

Chia seeds: Chia was one of the foods used by the Aztecs for hiking long distances. The chia seed, like flax, produces a saccharide gel around it that is an easily assimilatable starch. Chia is a power food.

Coconut water: This pure tree-filtered water is nearly identical to human blood plasma and has been used as a way to get intravenous medicine into the body instead of the IV liquid used in hospitals. Plasma makes up more than 55 percent of our blood content. Coconuts are more hydrating than water and more nutrient balanced for the human body.

Kelp: Seaweeds are the highest source of organic minerals available. Kelp is an excellent salt replacement and a great seasoning as well as a nutritional supplement. Kelp has more iron, magnesium, and trace minerals than any other substance known.

Spirulina: This single-celled alga is the sister plant to wheatgrass, providing a similar range of nutrients (all that are needed for survival), and spirulina is the highest source of protein on the planet (a whopping 89 percent). Spirulina has been used by the Aztecs as well for endurance.

Wheatgrass: The young shoots of the wheat plant are a great source of energy and nutrition. Wheatgrass is a power food and provides every vitamin and mineral necessary for human survival as well as helping to reduce radiation poisoning and remove other toxins from the body. Wheatgrass is protein packed, and one ounce of wheatgrass is equal nutritionally to four and a half pounds of vegetables.

Honey: The collected nectar of flowers is a potent and sustaining food. Honey gathered in the area you happen to be in grants a powerful immune booster and protects you from allergies. Honey is an ancient food and the honeybee, like the coconut, hasn't changed in over 20 million years. Honey comes from flowers and is gathered by bees in a completely natural and harmonious way. Just as the fruit that is sold in stores is gathered by workers, honey is collected by bees.

Raw Warnings

These warnings are designed to educate. We all make the best choices we can in each situation, and we grow as we go. Be patient, take your time, and vibrant health will follow behind.

Braggs Amino Acids: This product made only out of soybeans is still one of the most controversial "living food" products. At this point, no one knows how it is made. We do know that Paul Braggs was a health pioneer and that the other Braggs products are raw and living. There have been many questions about this product, and the answer is we still don't know. Braggs is non-GMO and supposedly "organic."

Nama shoyu: This is a fermented product made from soybeans, wheat, salt, and a starter. This product is cooked before being allowed to culture. This is a living food product as long as it is unpasteurized. The *Asperigillus oryzae* culture has proliferated so much by the time you purchase it that there are more culture and very few remnants of the soy-wheat soup that the culture lived in.

Nutritional yeast: This bacteria is superabundant in B vitamins, especially B_{12} (one often lacking in a vegetarian diet). Some companies freeze-dry their yeast, while most kiln-dry it at 375°F for three seconds. It is essentially cooked, yet there are a few companies that still do it the old freezer way. Also, there are some companies that add things to their yeast. They are always listed, so just read the label.

Spirulina: Most spirulina is freeze-dried. This breaks open the cell wall (due to water expansion), increases the digestibility, and makes spirulina more absorbable. This freeze-drying process does destroy the life force (the ability to grow and create more life). A few companies still solar-dry their algae. Freeze-drying is considered raw by most, and so is spirulina.

Nori: Most nori contains fish! In fact, nori can be up to 10 percent fish and remain labeled as only nori. When nori is harvested, it is caught as a big mass of sea lettuce in nets. This wet seaweed is then lightly rinsed, put in a big blender, and then spread out like paper to dry. A few companies provide a fish-free nori (Buddhist and kosher varieties).

Sea vegetables (hijiki, arame, and so on): Most of the sea vegetables sold in packages have been cooked. It says on the back of packages of arame and hijiki that they are cooked for several hours before sun drying. Just because it says sun dried doesn't mean it wasn't cooked first.

Nuts and nut butters: There is a huge question about how nuts and seeds are dried. Many seeds such as sesame are hulled using steam. Some places still machine hull. Nuts must be dried before selling, and many companies dry in kilns and ovens at well over 200°F. Nut butters that are made from "raw" nuts are sold as raw even if the nut butter-making equipment heated up to well over 200°F. Truly raw nuts are usually freeze-dried.

Young Thai coconuts: These raw coconuts imported fresh from Thailand are definitely not

Continued ➡

organic. These nuts have been treated with various chemicals, including formaldehyde and bleach, and are processed by machines.

Sea salt / Celtic sea salt: Watch out for iodized salts and kiln-dried mineral salts. Sun-dried salt is the best.

Apples and cucumbers: For the purpose of shelf life and aesthetic visual beauty, apples and cucumbers are often waxed with a synthetic or carnuba wax. These items are labeled organic and have been grown organically. Later, they are treated by the shipping or distribution company.

Anything organically grown: Organic doesn't mean consciously grown. Many organic farms are using conventional methods that are harmful to the environment and are farming for money rather than to produce good healthy natural food. Biodynamically grown foods are more conscious, yet only foods you get from farmers or grow yourself are truly consciously grown and sustainable. It is important to be able to eat locally year-round or store up local supplies in summer and fall for winter, because any food that must be transported by planes, trains, boats, trucks, and cars is not truly sustainable. The food comes from far away, and it has been said that 70 percent of the world's transportation is used for moving food. That is a lot of fuel and wasted time. Think globally. Eat locally.

Honey: Many beekeepers harm the bees when they collect the honey. Some smoke out the bees, or even fumigate the hive. Many commercial hives have all the honey removed and leave none for the bees during the winter. Tropical honey is usually the safest bet since there are always flowers and therefore always more honey nectar to collect. Some honey contains larvae (baby bees) and this is not vegan. Many beekeepers use separators to keep the queen out of the top layers so the eggs don't get laid in that honey. Be sure to get honey from a source you trust, and make sure they are using non-impregnated cells to claim their golden nectar.

Cacao: Cacao beans, or nibs, are becoming ever popular in the raw food scene. While cacao may have some helpful properties, such as amino acid compositions and high levels of antioxidants, it can also be toxic and cause mild hallucinations at dosages over 40 beans. Cacao is shunned by all animals in nature and domesticated animals that are fed cacao often contract cancer and can die of toxicity. Cacao contains a chemical very similar to caffeine that acts a stimulant on the central nervous system, causing extreme mood swings and aggressive tendencies.

Agave nectar: The nectar from the agave cactus is used by many people in the living food world as a sweetener. When harvested fresh, this sweet liquid is similar to maple water or coconut water. In order to stabilize it and concentrate the sugars, agave is heated to temperatures above 150°. This prevents it from fermenting and turning into alcohol. Commercially-available agave nectar is a cooked product. It can, however, be obtained in its pure, raw form.

Types of Raw Food Diets

Raw foods: This is a general term referring to those who consume a diet of foods prepared without any fire. A person following the raw foods diet may not be vegan, but is likely to be vegetarian. Raw foodists often attempt to properly combine their foods.

Live foods: People eating a live food diet eat all raw foods (often with the exception of nightshades) as well as live foods. Live foods may be cooked and then have a living culture introduced to them. This culture will then grow upon the cooked food, and as it breaks down it creates more cultures. Some examples are miso, tofu, and amazake. Live foods are not necessarily cooked. Some raw/live examples are rejuvelac, sprouts, and seed cheez.

Living foods: A living foods diet is a synthesis of raw foods and living foods. The teachings of living foods have been expounded by Dr. Ann Wigmore. Living food eaters will eat all raw foods as well as raw living. Living foodists often include wheatgrass as a major part of their diet as well as a range of cultured foods.

Essenes: The Essenes were a sect that lived over 2,000 years ago. They sun-dried their breads and sprouted their seeds. A large portion of their diet was made up of fruits. The Essenes also understood much about intentional eating and bodily cleansing for healing.

Breatharians: A breatharian is someone who consumes no food or drink. People following this path are very few because of the extreme nature of the discipline required. Most breatharians reside in areas where they do not have to interact with society. The few I know do not have jobs or cars or even go to towns. Many breatharians will sit and meditate with a piece of fruit in order to "absorb its essence"; other say they exist on *prana*, "air/energy."

Fruitarians: Fruitarians are those who ingest only fruit. Some fruitarians eat only one type of fruit at a time, while others will eat any fruit in any combination. This type of diet is better suited to those who live in warmer climates.

Sproutarians: People who consume only sprouts are known as sproutarians. Sprouts are the youngest stage of growth for a plant. They have the highest vitality and nutritional value at three to seven days' growth. There are two types of sprouts, hydroponic and soil based. Some young grasses are considered sprouts.

Hydrorians: Hydrorians, or liquidarians, are people who ingest foods only in a liquid form. Fresh juices make up the primary diet of these people. Some hydrorians do not drink water, while others make it a primary part of their diet.

Natural hygiene: Natural hygiene (NH) is a type of raw diet that involves the use of only completely natural substances. Natural hygienists do not use shampoo, soap, cleansers, or other "beauty products." The rest of the diet is varied. Many of the different NH groups disagree about general principles. NH is based upon the teachings of H. Shelton, T. C. Fry, and Viktoria Bidwell.

Instincto: This diet is all raw. The instinctos eat anything raw: plants, animals, insects, and so forth. They believe in eating one type of thing at a time (for example, only mangos or only spiders). Instinctos eat based on instinct, as the name suggests.

Vitarian: The vitarian diet is based on the teachings of Dr. Johnny Lovewisdom. Essentially, this is a raw, mostly fruit-based diet. One primary practice is the retention of sexual fluids in order to extend life.

Sun foods: Sun foods are foods that are blessed by the sun. This includes mostly fresh foods. The sun food system uses a food pyramid that balances sweet foods, fatty foods, and green foods to keep the body in its ideal state.

Life food nutrition: Life food nutrition is the use of food as medicine. This is a branch of raw food that is conscious of the glycolytic rate of foods (how their sugars are processed in the body and specifically how they affect the liver). Life foodists choose to not eat any starchy foods, such as carrots or bananas. Essential oils, such as flax or hemp, are an important part of this diet. Life food is also very big on nutritional fasting, which is fasting on blended foods. Life food is a part of whole brain functioning, which also includes other physical and psychological tools to aid in healing.

Loving foods: The philosophy of loving foods is that at every intention, from planting seeds to the point of ingestion, food affects us. Loving foods advocates the use of all vegan raw-living organic foods. The theory is that every hand, machine, and tool that touches our foods adds to the intention being put into the food. Anyone who has eaten food made by an angry chef knows the difference between that and food made by someone you love. Foods prepared with proper intention will nourish the body far more than foods that go through a range of harsh experiences and then sit in a supermarket only to be microwaved and eaten. Loving foods believes in acquiring foods as close to the source as possible. Grow your own or buy from your local farmer and always grow sprouts. A loving foods diet does not include any animals or animal-based products (eggs, dairy), heavily refined products (sugar, flour), or pesticides and chemicals. Loving foods advocates the use of the four living food groups to create a balanced raw food diet. Loving foods also sees the value of exercise and right livelihood to create true balance, health, and happiness.

—From *The Raw Foods Resource Guide*

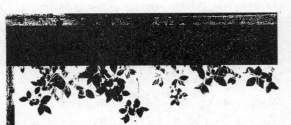

RAW FOODS AND RECIPES

Jeremy A. Safron

Finding pure food has become a challenge in the modern world. Foods that are labeled organic can still be mass-produced, possibly using "natural" pesticides which are still toxic. (Purely natural pesticides like bay leaves or marigolds are not harmful, but in my book, biodynamic farming—using living plants to deter bugs—is still the only way to go.) Even worse, companies may claim their food is organic when it's not just to get more money. On the flip side, there is also pure, truly natural food sold without labels and high price tags that is actually organic; it's just that the farmers who grow and sell them can't afford certification as organic farmers.

To be absolutely sure your produce is pure, grow it yourself or forage it in the wild. Planting trees, growing a garden, and especially growing sprouts are all excellent ways to obtain food. Foraged foods are most ideal since nature grew them on its own. Participating in local herb walks and interviewing docents can both provide a solid education about the habitats and seasonal availability of local foods.

Farmers' markets are usually the next best source of fresh produce. They're also a great place to learn about local produce that's available for foraging. In fact, many farmers' markets have a side selection of foods that grow wild in the area; look here for information and inspiration. Farmers also

Continued ➡

sell directly from their farms so check the phone book for local resources and stop at local farm stands. What the farmers don't sell themselves will go to the shelf of a local store or co-op; ask around and find local markets that buy produce directly from local farms.

For exotic and hard-to-find items, check Asian or Mexican markets as they usually carry a wide range of tropical produce and special items. There are also some companies that mail order exotic foods and fresh produce direct from farms, so no matter where you live, you should be able to find a nice array of produce.

Herbs

Herbs are the greens and flowers of annually blooming plants commonly used for seasoning and medicine. Used both fresh and dried.

Basil—A sweet, broad-leafed aromatic herb that grows rapidly. Some varieties are purple basil, French basil, Thai basil, and lemon basil. Basil is commonly used in Italian and Thai cooking.

Cilantro—A flat-leafed herb widely used in Latin American and Southeast Asian cooking. Sometimes called Mexican parsley, fresh coriander, or Chinese parsley. This plant's seeds are known as coriander.

Dill—A soft, wispy, refreshing herb.

Fennel—A wispy herb similar in appearance to dill, with a slightly sweet licorice taste and smell.

Lamb's-quarter—A common herb found throughout the Northeast and Northwest areas of the United States.

Lemongrass—A long, hearty, sharp-edged green grass with a lemonlike scent.

Lovage—A sweet, beautiful flowering herb with a strong scent

Malva—A slightly bitter, richly green herb.

Marjoram—A pungent and aromatic herb.

Mint—A refreshing and cool herb that's available in many varieties and grows almost anywhere.

Apple mint—A sweet mint with a slight apple taste and round leaves.

Chocolate mint—A superbly rich mint with tiny, dark leaves.

Lemon mint—A mild mint with a distinct lemon aroma.

Peppermint—A strong, darkly colored mint with smooth, long leaves.

Pineapple mint—A mild, sweet-tasting mint with a hint of pineapple to its taste.

Spearmint—A light-colored, mild, cooling mint with pointed leaves.

Oregano—A mildly sharp-flavored herb available broadleaf or creeping and often used in Italian recipes.

Parsley—A clean-tasting, refreshing herb available curly or flat and high in vitamin C.

Peppergrass—A thin grass with a mildly spicy pepper flavor.

Purslane—A common, round-leafed herb that is quite nice in salads.

Rosemary—A piney, minty herb resembling evergreen needles.

Sage—A robust, pungent, aromatic herb with long, whitish, fuzzy leaves.

Sheep sorrel—An herb with a tangy flavor and high in vitamin C and potassium.

Sourgrass—A wild type of sorrel with yellow flowers, a lemony flavor, and a slight bite.

Tarragon—A tart, mild herb that tastes of anise.

Thyme—An earthy-flavored herb that comes in over forty varieties.

Wintercress—An herb with a slightly spicy, slightly bitter taste, often found growing in moist areas.

Edible Flowers

There are many types of edible flowers found all over the world. They go wonderfully in salads or as a garnish on any dish. Make sure you use only unsprayed, organically raised blossoms in your food. Edible flowers have a very short shelf life so it is best to grow them yourself either in a garden outdoors or in a window box.

Arugula—A delicate, pale lavender or white blossom with a slightly spicy taste.

Borage—A blue, star-shaped flower with a mild, watery, cucumber flavor.

Calendula—A yellow-orange flower that is sweet and calming to the nervous system. It is also known as pot marigold.

Chrysanthemum—A silvery white flower with a slightly spicy taste.

Day lily—A yellow-orange flower. The petals of this plant are edible, while the young buds are not. Day lilies have a nutty, sweet taste.

Garlic—A white or purple flower from the garlic chive with a spicy, garlicky taste.

Geranium—A mild-tasting flower available in many varieties, such as rose, lemon, almond, and mint.

Hibiscus—A bright red, orange, or pink flower that makes wonderful sun tea.

Honeysuckle—A deliciously sweet, honey-flavored, yellow-white tiny flower.

Impatiens—A five-petaled, pastel-colored flower with a mildly sweet taste.

Lavender—A flower with a blue-purple blossom that tastes almost as strong as it smells.

Nasturtium—A very spicy flower available in a variety of colors, from yellow to bright red.

Pansy—A velvety-textured, mild-flavored flower available in many colors.

Red clover—A purple-and-white-topped flower that can be grown from clover seed or found in fields in the early summer. This herb contains high quantities of vitamin C.

Rose—A soft, sweet, aromatic flower.

Scotch broom—A sweet, honey-flavored, bright yellow flower.

Squash—A tender, huge, orange flower with a sweet and slightly starchy taste.

Tiger lily—An exquisite orange flower that tastes like sweet crispy lettuce.

Violet—A purple-pink flower with both sweet and spicy overtones. The flowers, stems, and leaves of the violet are all edible and contain vitamins A and C.

Sea Vegetables

Sea vegetables have an abundance of minerals and trace elements. They are an ideal source of organic salts. They are high in calcium, iodine, potassium, magnesium, phosphorous, iron, niacin, and vitamins A, B_1, B_2, B6, B_{12}, and C. Sea vegetables are very helpful in cleaning the prostate and the whole lymphatic system. Although eating fresh sea vegetables is ideal, sea vegetables can be purchased dried and then soaked to rehydrate.

Some companies boil their vegetables before drying them. Check the labels carefully; if they don't specify that the vegetables were or were nor boiled, find another brand or call the company's customer service number and ask. Always read the package and look for kosher certification to verify that it contains no animal or fish products. Purchase dried sea vegetables at Asian markets or directly from Gold Mine Natural Food Co. (www.goldminenaturalfood.com).

Agar-agar—A clear, gelatinous seaweed product available in flakes or bars. Agar-agar is used to gel liquids into a more solid form.

Arame—A dark brownish green, broad-leafed sea plant most commonly shredded into fine strands. This sweet, nutty sea vegetable is abundant in calcium, phosphorous, iodine, iron, potassium, and vitamins A and B. (Grows around Japan, the Pacific coasts, and South America.)

Dulse—A leafy, purple sea frond from cold northern Atlantic waters that can be eaten dried or rehydrated. Its flat, fan-shaped fronds have a chewy consistency. Dulse has a very high concentration of iron. It is an excellent source of magnesium and potassium and is quite rich in iodine, calcium, phosphorous, vitamins A, B_2, B_6, C, E, and many trace minerals. (Grows in cold waters worldwide.)

Hijiki—A stringy black seaweed that looks like twine. It is thicker and stronger-tasting than arame and is very high in calcium. It also has ample amounts of vitamins A, B_1, B_2, phosphorous, and iron. (Grows in waters around southern Japan, Hawaii, Taiwan, and the Indian Ocean.)

Kombu (kelp)—A green seaweed with chewy, sweetish blades that is dried and used as a condiment or flavor enhancer. Kombu is rich in potassium, sodium, and vitamins A and B. Monosodium glutamate (MSG) is derived from kombu. Dried kelp is available in strips, flakes, and in powdered form as well as vinegared and shredded, giving it a breadlike flavor. (Found in cold waters worldwide, including Japan, northern and mid-Pacific coast, and Atlantic coast.)

Nori—A bright, light purple when growing, this flat-bladed sea vegetable dries purple or black-green. Nori is most commonly found shredded and pressed into sheets and used in sushi. Nori is an excellent source of calcium, potassium, manganese, magnesium, and phosphorous and is especially rich in niacin and protein. Nori also contains large amounts of vitamins A and C. (Grows in the colder waters of the Atlantic and Pacific and along the coasts of Japan, California, Hawaii, the Philippines, and Europe.)

Sea palm—A sea frond that is gray-green with vertical ridges. It is quite firm and slightly jellylike.

Wakame—A dark green seaweed that is sweet and becomes a beautiful light green when rehydrated. It is quite slippery when wet. Wakame is an abundant source of calcium and niacin and is high in vitamins A, B_1, B_2, and C. (Grows in the cold waters of the northern Atlantic and Pacific including the coasts of northern Japan, the United States, and the British Isles.)

Continued ➡

Algae

An organism that transforms sunlight into chlorophyll, algae is a substance known for its blood-building and cleansing properties. Algae is abundant in trace minerals, and very digestible and easily assimilated because of its simplicity. Many people use algae supplements for their high amino acid content, naturally available protein, and high levels of trace minerals. The powder and liquid forms of single-celled algae are the only raw options; algae flakes contain soy lecithin, which in its preparation is steamed at temperatures 140°F and higher.

Chlorella—A powdered algae originally discovered by Christopher Hills and Hirashi Nakamura, renowned scientists whose research provided a lot of information about algae to the West.

Phytoplankton—A sea variety of algae that grows in deep waters and still produces chlorophyll from water-filtered sunlight. Phytoplankton is no longer commercially available.

Spirulina—A spiral-shaped algae known for its potency and easy digestibility. Dried spirulina powder is the highest source of protein known, containing almost 70 percent fully absorbable proteins.

Mushrooms

Not all mushrooms are fit for raw consumption. Use caution when harvesting any wild mushroom. Mushrooms can provide a rich and meaty texture that is satisfying to people transitioning to a vegetarian diet.

Chicken-of-the-woods—A thick, yellow-orange, many-layered tree fungus with a fibrous texture. Used fresh.

Enoki (enokidake)—A tiny, slim, white mushroom that often grows in clusters. Used fresh.

Hen-of-the-woods—A light gray tree fungus that grows in bunches similar to chicken-of-the-woods. Used fresh.

Kombucha—A flat fungus grown in a jar or tank of water with green tea and a sweetener. A well-cared-for kombucha colony will continuously divide and multiply, producing an endless supply of kombucha-infused tea if desired. Kombucha tea is known for its healing properties.

Morels—A spongy, wrinkly, brown-black wild mushroom with an elongated head. Used fresh and dried.

Maitake—A small-capped mushroom well known for its immune-building and cancer-fighting abilities. Used fresh and dried.

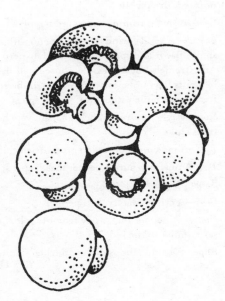

Portobello—A large, tender mushroom with a smooth, white-brown surface and white stem. Used fresh.

Shiitake—A small, butter-flavored mushroom used in Oriental recipes. Used fresh and dried.

Silver ear—A silver-white fungus that looks like a sponge or coral. Used fresh and dried.

Straw—A very fleshy mushroom. Used fresh (avoid canned).

Tree ear—A dark, round fungus. The smaller varieties are known to be the tastiest. Used fresh.

Truffles—A very rare (and therefore expensive), wild delicacy. A must for the mushroom connoisseur. Used fresh and dried.

Wood ear—A small, gold-brown fungus with a woody flavor. Used fresh.

Legumes

Also known as beans, legumes grow in pods, mostly on vines.

Adzuki beans—A red-skinned dried bean with a sweet flavor when sprouted.

Black beans—A dried black bean with a starchy flavor when sprouted.

Garbanzo beans (chickpeas)—A beige, dimpled dried bean, very good for sprouting.

Kidney beans—A variety of red-skinned legumes that are kidney shaped. These dried beans have a bland taste when sprouted.

Lentil—A traditional ingredient in Indian cuisine, the lentil is a small, flat, and round bean that is sold dried. Lentils come in many colors, are high in protein, and make for very sweet sprouts.

Green lentils—When sprouted, good in salads.

Red lentils—Use sprouted in soups and sauces.

Yellow lentils—Good for making sprout loaves and pâtés.

Lima bean—A large, green-yellow, kidney-shaped bean, with a sweet taste when fresh. Available both fresh and dried.

Mung bean—A fresh, yellow- or green-skinned bean whose sprouts are used frequently in Asian cuisine.

Navy bean—A white dried bean with a mild taste when sprouted.

Pea—A green, round legume with a deliciously sweet flavor when fresh. Dried varieties are also available. Also makes great sprouts.

Peanut—A legume often referred to as a nut, this fresh bean has a rich, nutty flavor.

Pole bean—A fresh, long, pod bean that is crisp and sweet.

Snap pea—A fresh, superbly sweet bean. These crunchy little bright green pods are delicious in salads.

Snow pea—A traditional Chinese pea pod that is sold fresh and is slightly blander than the snap pea.

Soybean—A powerhouse of protein, the soybean is extremely versatile. In either fresh or dried form, the soybean provides the basis for tofu, soy milk, miso, tamari, and many other products.

String bean—A fresh, long, thin, crispy, green pod with small beans inside.

Wax bean—A fresh, long, thin, yellow pod similar to the string bean.

Greens

Leafy green plants grow in heads in a huge array of colors, flavors, and textures. They are rich in chlorophyll, silica, and fiber.

Arugula—A peppery green with a slightly spicy flavor.

Bamboo shoots—The young shoots of certain types of bamboo are edible.

Beet greens—A plant with dark green leaves with a red vein. It tastes mildly bitter, with a woodsy flavor.

Bele (tree spinach)—A plant with large, broad leaves from the Philippines. This plant's tough gelatinous leaves are almost 30 percent silica and are great for rolling burritos.

Chard—A member of the beet family, chard has coarse leaves and a woodsy taste.

Chicory—A dark green plant (often found in the wild) with narrow, frilly leaves, a pale green center, and a bitter flavor.

Comfrey—A plant with broad, fuzzy leaves that can aid in cellular regeneration and the healing of wounds and muscle and bone injuries. Best for raw consumption when the leaves are young and tender.

Dandelion—A bitter green with small and narrow dark leaves. Look for dandelions growing in the wild.

Curly endive—A crisp, light green to white compact head with frilly leaves and a slightly bitter flavor.

Escarole—A broader, less bitter, and curlier green than endive. Escarole is part of the chicory family.

Fiddlehead fern—Often wild, this young sprouted fern has curly light fronds and a delectable nutty, asparagus flavor.

Frisée—A bitter, light yellow to white salad green with curly leaves.

Green butter lettuce—A crispy, large-headed lettuce with generous, wide leaves.

Green leaf lettuce—A loose-headed green with frilly edges and a mild taste.

Green oak lettuce—A loose-headed green with frilly, tapering finger leaves.

Katuk—An African tree whose leaves are more than 30 percent protein and taste like nuts.

Mâche—A mild and delicate green with small, round leaves.

Malabar spinach—A purple and green variety of garden spinach.

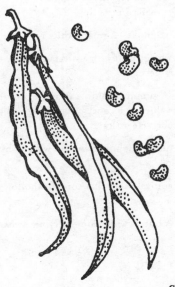

Continued ➡

Mizuna—A jagged-leafed, slightly spicy green often used in Asian foods.

Mustard—A very pungent, spicy, tart green abundant in vitamins A and B.

New Zealand spinach—A crispy vinelike spinach that grows wild.

Plantain—A long-leaved plant that is common in North America.

Radicchio—A type of red chicory, radicchio has a loose white head and tangy crimson leaves.

Red butter lettuce—A crispy, large-headed lettuce with a red tinge.

Red chard—A large, leafy green with a red vein running up its middle. A member of the beet family.

Red hibiscus—These burgundy-colored leaves have a lemony taste. Red hibiscus can often be found growing in the wild.

Red oak lettuce—A loose-headed green with frilly, red-tinged, tapering, fingerlike leaves.

Red orach—A blossoming, burgundy-colored green with mild flavor.

Savory—A distinctly peppery green with a spicy flavor.

Spinach—A deep green plant whose delicate leaves have a rich, earthy flavor.

Tango—A pungent and flavorful green with a rich flavor.

Tat soi—A round, crispy green with a sweet taste.

Travissio—A sweet and spicy green.

Watercress—A round-leafed, fast-growing green with a bitter aftertaste.

Roots

Roots are starchy, nourishing plants that grow underground. Most root greens are edible and highly nutritious. A root can be cut into a few pieces which, if put in the ground, will each grow new full roots (each piece must include some portion of the roots's external surface).

Beet—A large, bulbous root with red and green leaves.

Chioga—A red-and-white-ringed beet that looks tie-dyed inside.

Golden—A golden variety that makes a beautiful decoration.

Red—A common variety of beet quite high in iron.

Carrot—A long, orange root with a wispy green top.

Celery—A large root with multiple stalks that are high in water and organic sodium content and have small leafy greens on the tips.

Chinese artichoke—A small, white root.

Ginger—A beige root with a sweet and spicy flavor grown in riverbeds.

Ginseng—A gummy root in a variety of colors. Especially value for its energy-boosting and yang-tonifying characteristics.

Jicama—A large, light brown root with a white, crispy inside.

Lotus—A conical tuber that contains hollow tubes in a ring.

Parsnip—A bitter, white root—very nice when shredded.

Potato—A smooth-skinned, eye-covered root that grows prolifically.

Golden russet—A golden watery potato (very starchy raw).

Purple—A dark-skinned, purple-fleshed dry potato.

Red Romano—A red-skinned, white-fleshed, very starchy potato.

Radishes

Daikon—A long, large, white, crispy, spicy root.

Horseradish—A very spicy white root.

Red—A round, red-skinned, juicy radish.

White—A slightly spicier version of the red.

Rutabaga—A purple-and-white-skinned crispy root with a watery taste.

Salsify—A brown, long, skinny, slightly hairy root.

Sweet potato—An orange-fleshed, very sweet root.

Taro—A dense tuber that causes intense mouth and throat discomfort when eaten raw.

Turmeric—A pungent, bitter, orange root used often in Indian food.

Turnip—A spicy and bitter, large, round, white root.

Yakon—A sweet root related to potatoes, with an apple flavor.

Yam—A very similar root to the sweet potato in taste and appearance.

Yucca—A plant also known as cassava that is too dense and starchy to eat raw.

Raw Foods

Brassica

These hardy plants grow in cooler climates in clusters flanked by leaves. They are coated with layers of acidophilus, which helps increase intestinal flora.

Broccoli—A green, clustered, flowerlike plant with some purple overtones that is very high in calcium.

Brussels sprout—A plant that looks like miniature, tight cabbages growing on a stalk.

Cabbage—An acidophilus-rich plant that grows in cooler climates.

Bok choy (Chinese chard)—A cabbage with thick white stalks and broad, dark green leaves.

Choy sum—A cabbage similar to bok choy with a more slender appearance.

Miniature red—A smaller version of the normal red.

Napa (*Chinese cabbage*)—A plant with layers of dark green, purple-veined leaves.

Red—A cabbage with deep magenta leaves on a compact head.

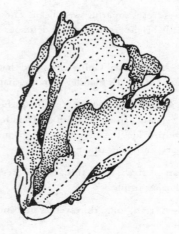

Savoy—A cabbage with crinkly, pale green leaves and a loose head.

White—A dense, firm head with smooth, yellow-green leaves.

Cauliflower—A white, flowerlike plant with a creamy taste.

Kale—A dark green to purple plant with overlapping leaves and red-purple veins.

Kohlrabi—A round and green plant with a purple stem.

Turnip—A plant with tart leaves and a spicy root.

Allium

Allium are pungent, bulblike plants that grow underground and produce green shoots. They are anthelmintic—they help remove intestinal parasites.

Asparagus—A plant with long branches that end in flowerlike tops with a robust taste.

Chive—A delicate, slender, mild-tasting plant with an onion flavor.

Garlic—A white-skinned bulb composed of cloves individually wrapped in a parchmentlike membrane and with a spicy, often strong flavor.

Leeks—A grasslike plant with a slight onion flavor.

Onions

Kula—An oblong, very sweet onion with a white interior and yellow skin.

Red—A spicy onion with purple-red skin.

Spanish—A yellow-skinned, slightly spicy round onion.

White—A crisp and sweet onion with a white skin.

Scallions—A long, green, grasslike shoot.

Shallots—A small brown bulb with a taste between garlic and onion.

Nightshades

Nightshade plants grow at night and produce a fruit with fine-lobed ears and edible flowers of various colors.

Artichoke—A flowerlike, green plant with sharp leaves.

Eggplant—A large, purple fruit with a light green, seeded interior.

Okra—A pointed, cylindrical green to purple fruit.

Peppers

Hot

Anaheim—A long, mild, thin, fresh green chile.

Cayenne—A long and winding orange to red, pointed, dried chile.

Chile—A small, round-tipped red pepper.

Chipotle—A smoked and dried jalapeño with a smoky flavor and spicy aftertaste. Habanero—An extremely hot fresh chile whose small size belies its fiery taste. Jalapeño—A medium-sized fresh green chile with a nice, gentle spice.

Scotch bonnet—An orange, bell-shaped, very hot fresh chile.

Tepín—A medium-hot, red to green dried chile.

Thai—A tiny, red-purple pepper that's super spicy.

Sweet

Green—A crispy, watery, bell pepper.

Orange—A pepper that, aside from its color, is very similar to the red.

Purple—A bland, almost bitter, purple-skinned

Continued ➡

bell pepper.

Red—A very sweet and crunchy bell pepper.

Yellow—A very sweet and quite juicy bell pepper.

Tomatoes

Beefsteak—A large, watery, light red to pink tomato.

Cherry—A tiny, round, very sweet and juicy tomato.

Pear—A pear-shaped, small tomato that grows in a variety of colors.

Plum—A medium-sized red tomato.

Roma—An oblong and light red tomato, great for slicing.

Curcubits (Vine Squash and Melons)

Circubits are fruits that grow on vines and contain many seeds. All flowers from curcubits are edible.

Acorn squash—A large green and brown squash resembling an acorn.

Melons

Cantaloupe—A commonly known melon, the cantaloupe has fairly dense orange to pink flesh with beige, scaly or bumpy skin.

Crenshaw—A lightly scaly-skinned, golden-fleshed melon that is the ultimate in juiciness.

French—A golden orange-fleshed melon that is a very sweet type of cantaloupe with smooth, beige skin.

Honeydew—A smooth, firm, green-yellow-skinned melon with pale green, ultrasweet flesh.

Honeyloupe—A cross between a cantaloupe and a honeydew, this fine treat has a smooth, firm skin and sweet, pale orange flesh.

Muskmelon—A melon with a scaly, netted skin and extremely sweet, yellow-orange to yellow-green flesh.

Sharlyn—A melon with skin like a cantaloupe, this ultrasweet melon has golden-orange flesh.

Sugar baby—A delectable, smaller, ultrasweet, seedless version of watermelon. Watermelon—A large melon with a smooth, green or dark yellow, mottled or striped skin and crisp, pink to red flesh composed of 96 percent water. A great kidney cleanser.

Yellow baby—A strain of watermelon that has a creamy yellow flesh.

Pumpkin—A large, rounded, orange squash with many seeds.

Yellow squash—A sweet and crunchy, yellow-skinned summer squash with a mild taste.

Zucchini—A long, green summer squash with an earthy flavor.

Seeds

A seed is defined by the fact that its hull can be removed, and that it produces two leaves upon sprouting. Seeds are the potential energy of plants-to-be and as such have highly increased nutritional value. Seeds can be used in a variety of forms. Store-bought seeds are a dried food and are concentrated. If seeds are soaked, their enzyme inhibitors release and they become more digestible. This can also be accomplished by grinding a seed into powder or by chewing very well. Sprouting seeds is a great way to get more bang for your buck: it increases the seeds' nutritional value as well as their size, thereby providing more food mass.

Alfalfa—A seed that sprouts quickly and provides many valuable nutrients.

Buckwheat—A black-hulled grain that produces sweet greens. Buckwheat is the highest in protein of any seed.

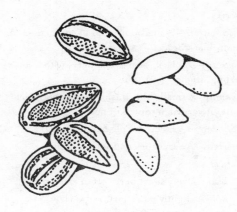

Celery—A seed that helps to inhibit molds and is useful to add to other seeds for sprouting.

Chia—A seed that produces a gelatinous coating before sprouting and is packed with energy.

Clover—A seed that provides a chlorophyll-rich sprout.

Coriander—A seed with a mildly spicy flavor.

Cumin—A robust-tasting seed that is quite earthy.

Fennel—A seed with a distinctive licorice flavor.

Fenugreek—This seed produces a rich and tasty sprout that is great in salads.

Flax—A seed that creates a gelatinous coating when soaked. Provides a good balance of omega oils and essential fatty acids and works well as an egg substitute.

Garlic—A very spicy seed with a reddish hue when sprouted.

Hemp—A rich, tangy seed, high in essential fatty acits

Mustard—A versatile seed that makes great sprouts and is used dry as a spice.

Onion—A sweet and spicy seed, great for sprouting.

Poppy—A round, blue seed with a delightfully crunchy texture.

Pumpkin—A very robust and sweet seed that provides a good balance of omega oils and essential fatty acids.

Radish—A spicy and bitter seed, good for sprouting.

Sesame—A very sweet, tiny, white seed.

Sunflower—A pointed, gray seed, great for making Essene bread and pates.

Wild rice—Black long-grain wild rice is the only rice that is a seed and not a grain. This seed also sprouts without any oxygen.

Grains

Grains are the kernel of a plant that produces only one shoot, a grass. Grains are permanently affixed to their hull and usually contain gluten. These close relatives of seeds are abundant in carbohydrates and most digestible when sprouted.

Amaranth—A grain native to the Americas and the second-smallest grain, amaranth plants grow soft red and white flowers. The seeds sprout easily.

Corn—A starchy, sweet, juicy grain that grows in a number of colors. Wonderful both raw and sprouted.

Millet—A small, yellow grain with a starchy taste when sprouted.

Oat—A very sweet grain to sprout. Lots of fiber.

Quinoa—A grain worshipped by the Aztecs, quinoa is the third-smallest grain and creates a spicy sprout.

Rice—The staple grain of China. Most rices are edible when sprouted, though not very tasty. Experiment with the length of sprout time for varied flavors.

Basmati—A translucent long grain.

Brown long grain—A long, round, brown grain.

Brown short grain—A short, stubby, brown grain.

Jasmine—A white, sweet rice with a delicate fragrance.

Spanish—A long, yellow rice.

Sushi—A white, round grain used in the making of sushi.

Sweet—A white, stubby grain.

Rye—A brown seed good for making Essene bread.

Teff—A very small grain, sweet and gray. High in protein.

Wheat—A grass rich in chlorophyll. The staple grain of America, it produces a tasty sprout.

Hard winter—A good variety for growing wheatgrass.

Soft winter—A wheat that is very good for making Essene bread.

Summer—A sweeter wheat variety. Good for making breads and salads.

Nuts

Nuts are the inner center of a fruit that is contained by a shell. Nuts are very sweet when harvested and get much more oily when dried.

Almond—A white, oblong nut, pointed on one end, that comes in a beige shell.

Brazil—A creamy, oily nut that is often an inch in length.

Cashew—A white, very sweet, crescent-shaped nut that is poisonous unless sun dried.

Chestnut—A brown-skinned, large, round, crunchy nut that is sometimes bitter.

Hazelnut—A dark brown-skinned, small, round nut with a rich flavor.

Macadamia—A sweet, white nut with a delightful crunch and a very hard shell.

Malabar chestnut—A light brown-skinned, sweet nut that is crispy when sprouted.

Pecan—An oblong-shelled nut with a wavy interior. This nut is very sweet. Pine—A golden, tiny, teardrop-shaped seed from a pine cone. It tastes quite rich.

Walnut—A round-shelled and warped-shaped nut.

Fruits

Fruit is a beautiful, colorful, delicious membrane made of cells filled with organic water and nutrients. Fruit is love since it is designed to feed the seed inside or feed a creature and with that creature's cooperation spread the seeds around the local area making more fruit trees and more fruit. Fruits come in every flavor and color.

Annona or moya family—Annonaceous fruits have scaly skins, black seeds, and creamy flesh.

Atemoya—A hybrid between the sweetsop and cherimoya.

Bullock's heart—A purple-skinned fruit consisting of an exterior with rounded scales and an interior flesh that is sweet and creamy.

Continued ➡

Cherimoya—A sweet and juicy version of the sweet-sop, with far fewer seeds.

Rollinia deliciosa—A black and gold, spiky fruit with the sweet flavor of lemon pudding.

Soursop—A spiky, green fruit also known as the guanabana, with a sour and sweet white flesh and many poisonous seeds that must be removed before consumption.

Sweetsop—A green, round, scaly fruit also known as the sugar apple, with a seed-filled interior and a sweet and creamy taste.

Apples

Discovery—A red apple that fruits late in the season.

Gala—A medium-sized, crisp, juicy apple, with skin that is mostly red with some yellow.

Golden Delicious—A golden, sun-filled apple with a sweet taste.

Granny Smith—A green, hard apple with a sweet-tart taste.

Jonagold—A golden apple with a mild flavor.

McIntosh—A small, red and white apple that is good when soft.

Pippin—A crispy and crunchy apple with red skin.

Red Delicious—A large, red apple with a sweet flavor and a hard crunch.

Spartan—A medium-sized, red and green apple with a mildly sour taste.

Starkling Delicious—A small, red and gold apple.

Asian pear—A beige-skinned, sweet fruit that has a taste and texture similar to pear but looks like an apple.

Avocados

Alligator pear—A watery, light-colored, small, slender avocado.

Bacon—A rich bacon-flavored avocado with dark green, smooth skin.

Cocktail avocado—A sweet avocado that is the smallest of its kind.

Common—A round, hard-skinned avocado with creamy insides.

Ettinger—A green, mildly rough-skinned avocado with creamy flesh.

Fuerte—A watery avocado with a sometimes purple, smooth skin.

Hass—A dark, rough-skinned avocado with a buttery taste. One of the most popular varieties.

Napal—A large and purple avocado whose flavor varies from tree to tree.

Reed—A round, green-skinned, sweet and creamy avocado.

Sharwil—A green-skinned, dry, buttery avocado.

Bananas

Apple—A small, starchy banana with a reddish interior.

Bluefield—This is the largest, fattest, and sweetest of its kind.

Chinese—A long and very sweet banana. Slightly thinner than the Bluefield.
variety.

Cuban red—A red, semistarchy, semisweet banana.

Dessert—A medium-sized, sweet and creamy banana.

Ice cream—A large, triangular banana with white flesh reminiscent of vanilla ice cream.

Lady finger—A tiny and supersweet banana.

Plantain—A dry and starchy banana.

Berries

Black raspberry—A medium-sized berry formed of many black beads.

Blackberry—A black, seed-filled berry with a very strong, slightly sour taste.

Blueberry—A small, blue bush berry with a sweet taste. A very high source of pectin.

Boysenberry—A sweet, purple berry.

Cranberry—A very tangy and sour red berry.

Currant

>*Black*—A very sweet berry often eaten dried.

>*Red*—A slightly more tart, red variety.

>*White*—A whitish yellow variety.

Dewberry—A sweet, tiny cousin of the raspberry.

Gooseberry—A green bush berry related to the blueberry.

Mulberry—A black, sweet berry that has a sweet and sour flavor and grows on trees.

Physalis fruits

>*Chinese lantern*—A tiny, yellow, sweet, tomato-like fruit coated with a papery skin.

>*Tomatillo*—A green-purple, very sweet, tomato-like fruit also covered with a papery husk.

Raspberry—A red, very sweet, oblong fruit from a bush that grows in cold climates.

Strawberry—A red, pointed berry that has a distinct taste and grows on low ground shrubs.

>*Alpine*—A white variety not as sweet as the traditional raspberry.

>*Hot boy*—A very crimson berry with a tart bite.

>*Red gauntlet*—A large, red variety with a high sugar content.

>*Scarlet*—A dark red, very sweet, medium-sized berry.

>*White*—A white to yellow, tiny berry.

>*Wild*—A miniature berry with little flavor that grows in small clusters in the shade.

Tayberry—A very sweet and mild berry also known as the thimbleberry.

Breadfruit—A round, scaly fruit that tastes like a bread pudding when eaten very ripe.

Cacao—Food of the gods. Cacao pods, ranging in color from yellow to purple and resembling a papaya in shape, contain both a sweet, white pulp and a number of small seeds. The seeds, when dried and roasted, are the source of chocolate.

Carob—Carob pods are nature's candy bar: they taste like chocolate-covered caramel. The seeds are as hard as rocks, so remove them before eating or navigate around them carefully.

Cherries

Barbados—A black, small cherry with a large seed.

Bing—A very tangy cherry.

Dukes—A large, black cherry with a rich taste.

Early rivers—A red cherry that is quite sweet.

Surinam—A small, light red, sour cherry shaped like a small pumpkin.

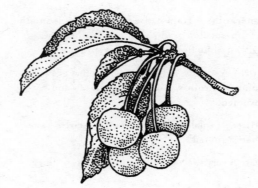

Citrus, sour

Calmondin—A tiny, very sour orange.

Citron—A medium-sized, yellow fruit with lemony flavor.

Kumquat—A small, orange fruit with a sweet and sour flavor.

Lemon—A sour fruit with golden juice and skin.

>*Ugli fruit*—A rough-skinned version of the lemon.

>*Meyer lemon*—A sweeter and juicier lemon.

Limes

>*Green*—A green-skinned fruit with sour flavor and sweet undertones.

>*Kaffir*—A small pear-shaped lime, whose leaves, which are uniquely shaped like two leaves joined end to end, are often used in Asian cuisines.

>*Tiny*—A round, yellow to green, small lime.

>*Yellow*—A yellow-orange variety.

Orangequat—A sour orange with mild flavor.

Citrus, sweet

Grapefruit

>*Pink grapefruit*—A slightly more sour version of the red.

>*Pomelo*—A very large and thick-skinned grapefruit.

>*Ruby red*—A red-fleshed, very sweet variety of grapefruit.

Oranges

>*Blood*—A red-and-orange-skinned, very sweet fruit.

>*Clementine*—A tangy and juicy orange.

>*Mandarin*—A tiny and tart orange.

>*Mineola*—A very juicy, sweet orange.

>*Navel*—A very round and mild orange.

>*Satsuma*—A small, Oriental variety with a tangy aftertaste.

>*Seville*—A sweet, golden-fleshed variety.

>*Sour*—A sour version of the navel orange.

>*Valencia*—A very common variety that is easy to cultivate.

>*Tangelo*—A cross between a tangerine and an orange.

>*Tangerine*—A very dark orange in color, with soft, sweet fruit. Resembles a squished orange.

>*Unique fruit*—A rough-skinned, sour fruit.

Coconut—A hard-shelled fruit of a palm tree that contains both water that is high in electrolytes and a white gelatinous meat that is very rich and protein packed.

Coconuts are the fruit of a palm that has been around since prehistoric times. This prolific plant has made it to the shore of every continent except Antarctia and is available in over 100 varieties. Coconuts can float for three months in the ocean and land on a sandy beach and still sprout up a tree that will bear up to ten thousand coconuts in its lifetime.

Coconuts can be used at almost any stage of ripeness. Baby or bitter coconuts are used for their water as they have not yet developed any meat. The water in these young nuts is slightly bitter and is considered medicinal in many island nations around the world as well as throughout Asia. As they develop slightly sweeter water and a small amount of clear jelly on the inside of their shell, baby coconuts are then called jelly nuts or spooners. Next, the coconut graduates to young or green coconuts, the most popular variety for use in food and for drinking. These young nuts have very sweet water and a coating of rich, creamy, soft meat a centimeter or more thick on their inside shell.

Continued ➡

Mature coconuts are the kind most people are used to seeing in a supermarket. These brown nuts have had most of the husk removed down to the shell layer. These nuts are old and the water is either bad or has fermented and tastes like coconut champagne. Mature coconuts are used for oil and cream made from the hard meat. If a mature nut falls to the ground and has a chance to germinate it becomes a coconut sprout—once considered the most powerful food in the Hawaiian Islands. Sprouted coconuts contain a spongelike heart that tastes like cotton candy. Its meat, known as copra, is very thin and crispy and has a thin layer of natural coconut oil. The oil can be obtained (for nutritional, medicinal, or cosmetic purposes) just by rubbing a finger on the inside of the copra. Coconuts are essential to the raw food diet so it is important to know how to find them at the desired ripeness and then, of course, how to open them. Since there are so many varieties of coconuts, it can be challenging to tell what stage of ripeness a coconut is at. Look for the the three nubs at the base of the nut; if they're close together, the coconut is most likely young (as the nut ages, the nubs spread farther apart). High moisture content in the coconut's husk can also help determine how young a nut is; the higher the moisture content, the younger the coconut since the husk dries out as it ages. Though most young nuts have a green stage, don't be thrown off by color: some nuts are always red, brown, gold, or green.

To open a coconut, using a machete or a heavy knife, shave one side of the coconut's outer layer at a 45° angle, until a hole providing access to the coconut water is created. Reserve or drink the water, then chop the coconut in half lengthwise with the grain. Some industrious people also open coconuts with power drills. At Chinese and Mexican markets, you may find young coconuts sold with their husks removed; typically these nuts don't keep as long or taste as fresh but they are much easier to open. The meat of mature nuts can be scooped out by using the back edge of a butter knife, carefully avoiding the hard shell which isn't fun to eat. To remove the meat from a young coconut, all that's needed is a spoon since the meat is thinner and softer.

Coffee—A small red bean of a tropical tree.

Date—The fruit of a palm that, when fruiting, produces up to three hundred pounds at a time. Dates are used as the primary sweetener in a raw-food diet. Dates range in color from green to golden brown to black depending on ripeness and variety. My favorite varieties are Bahari for its wonderful flavor and Medjool for its large size and nice texture. No matter the variety, choose soft dates, as they're more likely to be fresh and have a better flavor.

Bahari—A very sweet, soft, almost honeylike date.

Bread—A very dry, chewy date.

Deglet Noor—A large and creamy variety.

Halawi—A brown, soft, sweet date.

Honey—A sticky, honey, flavored, golden date.

Medjool—A very sweet date that is one of the largest.

Zahidi—A small, dark date with a taste that has hints of maple.

Durian—A yellow fruit that smells like sulfur but tastes like vanilla ice cream.

Fig—A very sweet, small, plump, pear-shaped fruit filled with many seeds and small fibers. This fruit is delicious fresh and also can be dried. Dried figs are even sweeter and often the fig sugars will crystallize on the outside.

Guavas

Common guava—A hard, yellow-skinned fruit with pinkish flesh and many seeds.

Pineapple guava—A guava also known as the feijoa, that tastes like pineapple.

Quince—A pear-shaped fruit also known as the guava pear.

Strawberry guava—A tiny, red guava filled with a tart, white membrane.

Jaboticaba—A small, black-skinned fruit that is very sweet and grows directly from the trunk of the tree.

Jackfruit—A large, spiky fruit weighing up to seventy pounds that has an edible membrane surrounding a seed that tastes like Juicy Fruit gum.

Kiwi—A small, brown, hairy fruit with distinctive bright green and black insides and a taste that is a cross between strawberry and banana. Peel before eating.

Longan—A fruit also known as the dragon's eye, with a hard, brown skin and a white membrane-covered seed that is quite juicy.

Lychee—A red, rough-skinned fruit similar to the longan although sweeter.

Mabolo—A fruit known as the velvet apple, with a velvety skin and a flavor like apples and bananas.

Mango—A sweet and juicy fruit that is grown in hundreds of varieties around the world and ranges greatly in shape, color, and flavor.

Alphonso—A juicy, orange mango with a honeylike taste.

Haden—A sticky, sweet, very orange mango with multicolored flesh.

Julie—A small, sweet mango with mild flavor.

Kent—A cold-climate mango with a creamy flavor.

Mangosteen—A fruit known as the queen of the fruits, that has a purple skin and a number of white, gelatinous, moon-shaped pods inside.

Miracle fruit—A red and tiny fruit that, when eaten before sour foods, makes them taste sweet for about thirty minutes.

Monstera—The large, tubular fruit of the Monstera deliciosa plant, with many green scales. It can only be eaten a little at a time to avoid stinging from the acids in the fruit. It tastes like pineapple and banana.

Papaya—A pear-shaped fruit that contains many black seeds and takes nine months to ripen.

Babaco—A giant, mountain papaya that is mild in flavor.

Common—A yellow-skinned and yellow-fleshed, very sweet papaya.

Strawberry papaya—A red-fleshed version that is much sweeter than other varieties.

Passion fruit

Common—A yellow-shell fruit filled with a sweet-sour, yellow membrane surrounding many edible seeds.

Purple—A purple-shelled variety with a slightly more acidic taste.

Velvet—A very sweet, orange, soft-skinned passion fruit with white membranes.

Peanut butter fruit—A small, red fruit also known as a ciruela, that tastes similar to peanut butter.

Pears

Anjou—A large green pear.

Bartlett—A red-skinned, very sweet pear.

Bosc—A beige-skinned pear best eaten soft.

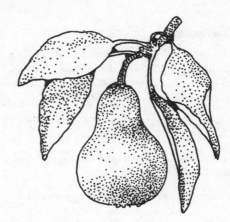

Persimmon—A sweet orange fruit commonly grown in Asia and California.

Fuyu—A round variety that is like an apple when eaten hard and like a Hachiya (below) when soft.

Hachiya—A pointed variety that is only eaten when soft. Hachiya are very gelatinous and sweet.

Pineapple—The very juicy and sweet fruit of a small ground bush with sharp leaves. It is known as the "King of the Fruits" because of its crown.

Common—A variety that grows rapidly and produces medium-sized fruits.

Sugarloaf—A sweet variety with a beautiful golden color.

White—A white-fleshed pineapple that has a lower acid content than most pineapples and tastes very creamy.

Prickly pear—A fruit from a variety of cactus, it has a very sweet and melonlike flavor and is filled with seeds. This fruit comes in purple and green and contains very simple sugars that can provide quick energy. If foraging this fruit, beware of its many miniscule barbed thorns. Clean very well before use.

Rambutan—A cousin of the lychee, oblong with red, hairy tendrils all over its exterior.

Sapote—A subtropical, round fruit with a sweet flesh and several seeds that should be removed before using. The eggfruit and sapodilla are both members of the sapote family, but the vanilla sapote (below) is not.

Chocolate pudding fruit—A fruit with a creamy brown inside and a green skin that tastes like very ripe bananas. It is also known as the chocolate persimmon or black sapote.

Eggfruit—A rich, orange fruit also called a canistel or yellow sapote, that has very cakelike meat.

Mamey—A caramel-flavored fruit with brown skin.

Orange sapote—An orange-fleshed, creamy, oblong fruit.

Sapodilla—A small, brown-skinned fruit, also called a chico, that tastes like cinnamon and sugar.

Vanilla sapote—A green-skinned fruit with a white, vanilla pudding-like interior.

Tamarillo—An oblong, red fruit that is also known as the tree tomato and tastes of basil and tomatoes.

Tamarind—A rich seed with a sweet-tart flavor.

Vine fruit

Black Grapes

Flame—A dark purple, sweet grape.

White Grapes

California seedless—A seedless variety of the white grape.

Italia—A strain from Italy often used for wines.

Muscat—A light green grape with a very sweet taste and small seed.

Sultanas—A variety of grape used often in desserts.

Thompson seedless—A darker, seedless variety.

Continued ➤

Raw Condiments

These foods are designed to season and flavor your dishes and recipes. Variety is the spice of life so use these to enliven and enhance other foods. These foods are available at local health food stores.

Beet powder—Red beets that have been dehydrated and powdered. Excellent for coloring food.

Bragg Liquid Aminos—An aged soy product used to replace salt.

Carob powder—A soft inner lining of the carob pod.

Cayenne pepper—Dried hot pepper available in a range of Btu's (British thermal units). The lower Btu's are for food and the higher ones are for medicinal usage.

Curry powder—A mixture of Indian spices: curry leaf, coriander, and tumeric.

Dried shredded coconut—Dehydrated coconut meat finely shredded.

Enzyme sprinkle—Dehydrated green papayas and lime juice.

Kelp powder—A dried and powdered form of kombu used as a salty seasoning.

Mirin—A sweet Asian rice wine.

Miso—An aged and cultured soy paste.

Nama shoyu—A fermented soy and wheat sauce.

Nigari—A dried form of sea water that coagulates tofu.

Nutritional yeast—A type of yeast grown on beet sugar that contains a wide range of B vitamins especially B12 which is considered challenging for vegetarians to find naturally.

Oil—Any dry nut or seed, olive, or oily fruit (such as coconuts) can be pressed for oil. Be certain to look for cold-pressed oils rather than oils that have been extracted using solvents. Also, be aware that "cold-pressed" is commonly used to describe oils that result from heating ground ingredients to 160°F before pressing. Omega Flow oils are truly cold pressed; ask at your local health food store for other brands if Omega Flow oils aren't available. Oils don't last very long separated from their whole food; store them in a dark container (light may cause spoilage) in the refrigerator. Stable oils (like olive oil) maintain their integrity when heated; unstable oils (like flax oil) become toxic when heated. The oils listed here can be found in the refrigerated or vitamin section of local health food stores.

Avocado oil—It is quite rare to find a cold-extracted avocado oil. However, avocados are often very oily on their own and can be used as a whole food replacement for other oils.

Coconut oil—Coconut oil is one of the best fats you can consume. It is delicious and creamy and can be used both in recipes and as a moisturizer.

Flax oil—Flax oil is high in essential fatty acids and is one of the healthiest oils to eat. Flax has a rich taste and is a delight in sweet and savory dishes.

Hemp seed oil—Hemp seed oil has a very nutty flavor and can be used in place of flax oil. This oil is unstable and should never be heated or used in recipes that are dehydrated.

Nut and seed oils—Dried seeds and nuts can be pressed for their oils. Many commercial nut and seed oils are heated during processing and are therefore not raw. Look for cold-pressed nut and seed oils in specialty stores.

Olive oil—Olive oil is the most stable oil; it can handle slight amounts of heat and is very tasty in recipes.

Other oils—There are a wide variety of oils sold in health food stores that may be far less than healthful. Fractionated or overheated oils become rancid quickly and some oils are even toxic for human consumption.

Stevia—A green herb that is one hundred times sweeter than sugar and is useful as a nonfruit sweetener.

Sun-dried sea salt—This salt looks gray and feels wet. That is because it is slow-dried sea water. Sun-dried sea salt contains far more minerals than table salt.

Vinegar—Always buy vinegar that says "with the mother" on the label because that is a sure sign that it is live and raw.

Apple cider vinegar—A fermented apple product with a tangy taste.

Red wine vinegar—A fermented grape vinegar.

Wasabi—A spicy, condiment made from horseradish roots and gardenia flowers. This bright green paste is served with Japanese food. Wasabi is also available in powdered form.

Recipes

Food can be art. The best chefs are artists of visual appeal as well as flavor and texture. Once you know how to use the tools and what foods work with each other, you can create dazzling dishes to delight the eyes and mouth. All it takes is a little self-expression. These recipes are some fantastic discoveries that I made along the way. Remember to use your head, act with your heart, and follow your tongue.

Fruit Dishes

TROPICAL FRUIT SALAD

Tropical fruits can provide delicious new realms of flavor as well as varied forms of nutrition to your diet. Many of the tropical fruits in this salad can be obtained in Asian markets. If you live in the tropics, remove the seeds from the papayas, persimmons, and cherimoya, and plant them. In time, you'll be able to harvest and enjoy your own fruit.

Serves 4

2 ripe papayas, peeled, seeded, and cut into ½-inch cubes

2 ripe mangoes, peeled, seeded, and cut into ½-inch cubes

1 ripe pineapple, peeled and cut into ½-inch cubes

3 ripe Hachiya persimmons, seeded and cut into ½-inch cubes

1 ripe cherimoya, peeled, seeded, and cut into ½-inch cubes

1 small bunch ripe bananas, peeled and thickly sliced crosswise

1 ripe star fruit, peeled and thinly sliced crosswise

1 ripe kiwi, peeled and thinly sliced

Freshly shredded coconut, for garnish

Place the papayas, mangos, pineapple, persimmons, cherimoya, and bananas in a large serving bowl. Alternate star fruit and kiwi slices in a spiral over the top. Garnish with the shredded coconut.

MIXED MELON BALL SALAD

This dish is entertaining due to its shapes and colors as well as its delicious flavors.

Serves 2 to 4

1 ripe cantaloupe, halved and seeded

1 ripe honeydew melon, halved and seeded

1 ripe watermelon, halved

Juice of 2 limes

Scoop out the flesh of the melons with a melon bailer and place in a large serving bowl. Mix gently. Splash with the lime juice and serve.

PAPAYA FUNDAE

These "fundaes" are a great party dish and have always been one of the most popular desserts at our restaurants.

Serve 2 to 4

Carob Sauce

6 dates, seeded

¾ cup filtered water

2 tablespoons olive oil or hemp-seed oil

¼ cup raw carob powder

Black Raspberry Kreme

5 dates, seeded

¾ cup filtered water

1 cup soaked cashews

⅓ cup black raspberries

8 ripe medium bananas, peeled and thickly sliced

2 ripe papayas, halved and seeded

Chopped walnuts, for garnish

To prepare the sauce, place the dates in a small bowl, cover with the water, and soak for about 1 hour, or until soft. Drain, reserving the liquid. In a food processor, combine the dates and the oil, slowly adding the reserved liquid as needed until the mixture is smooth. Add the carob powder and pulse until combined.

To make the raspberry kreme, place the dates in a small bowl and cover with the water, and soak for about 1 hour, or until soft. Drain, reserving the liquid. Place the dates, cashews, and black raspberries in a blender cup or blender, and while blending, add the reserved liquid as needed, until smooth.

Put the frozen bananas through a homogenizing juicer with a blank plate in place, or puree in a food processor until smooth. Fill the papaya halves with the pureed bananas, dividing equally. Top with 3 heaping tablespoons of the raspberry kreme. Drizzle the carob sauce over the papayas and raspberry kreme and garnish with the chopped walnuts.

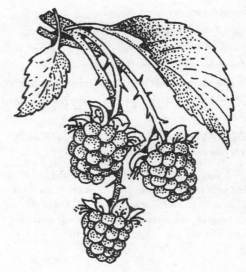

Continued ➡

Apples with Ginger Chutney

Serves 2 to 4

10 dates, seeded

¾ cup filtered water

1½-inch piece fresh ginger

¼ cup freshly squeezed orange juice

Pinch of ground cinnamon

4 crisp apples, thinly sliced

Apples are available year-round and make excellent "chips." By thinly slicing the apple lengthwise around the core, you can obtain an average of ten slices per apple.

Place the dates in a small bowl, cover with the water, and soak for about 1 hour, or until soft. Finely grate the ginger with a ginger grater or fine grater to extract its juice (you should have about 1 tablespoon). In a blender, combine the dates and their soaking water along with the ginger and orange juices and cinnamon. Blend until smooth. Arrange the apple slices on a plate and pour the date mixture over them, or serve the date mixture in a bowl with the apple slices around it.

Banana-Date Pudding

This dish was originally inspired by a banana-date-tofu pudding at an Asian vegetarian restaurant in New York City that made. I never did get the recipe for it, but this creation is an amazingly close raw version.

Serves 2 to 4

½ cup filtered water

Seeds from ¼ of a split vanilla bean

6 ripe bananas, peeled and halved crosswise

Chopped walnuts, for garnish

Place the dates in a small bowl, cover with the water, and soak for about 1 hour, or until soft. In a food processor, blend the dates, their soaking water, and the vanilla seeds until smooth. Add the bananas and process until smooth. Spoon the pudding into individual serving bowls. Cover and refrigerate for 2 hours, or until chilled. Garnish with the chopped walnuts and serve.

Persimmon Sunburst

Hachiya persimmons, also known as Japanese persimmons, are very high in tannic acid when under-ripe and taste like very bitter chalk. To avoid this, make certain that your persimmons are fully ripe and soft. The skin should peel off the fruit easily if totally ripe.

Serves 2 to 4

6 dates, seeded

½ cup filtered water

½ cup fresh blueberries

4 ripe Hachiya persimmons

Place the dates in a small bowl, cover with the water, and soak for about 1 hour, or until soft. In a food processor, combine the dates, their soaking water, and the blueberries and process until smooth.

Starting at the point of each persimmon, slice an X shape through the skin, cutting all the way down to the nub on top. Place the fruit, point up, on serving plates. Gently peel the skin away from each fruit, and leave it hanging like the petals of a flower. Using a melon bailer or a small spoon, scoop out a piece of each persimmon from the top of the open fruit. Spoon some of the blueberry sauce into the open persimmon points and drizzle more over the tops.

Applesauce

Applesauce is a great treat for kids and a quick and easy side dish. As a variation, add 1½ teaspoons of fresh ginger juice.

Serves 2 to 4

¼ cup raisins

¾ cup filtered water

Juice of ½ lemon

2 large, crisp apples, peeled and diced

Ground cinnamon, for garnish

Ground nutmeg, for garnish

Place the raisins in a small bowl, cover with the water, and soak for 1 hour. In a blender, combine the raisins, their soaking water, and the lemon juice and blend until smooth. Add the apples and blend until smooth. Sprinkle each serving with cinnamon and nutmeg.

Pineapple-Pepper Salad

Peppers give this recipe just the right crunch. Apple mint adds an especially nice flavor to this salad, hut if you can't find it, any sort of fresh mint will do.

Serves 2 to 4

1 large pineapple

2 red bell peppers, seeded and diced

4 kiwis, peeled and thinly sliced crosswise

¼ cup minced flat-leaf parsley

¼ cup minced apple mint leaves

Juice of ½ orange

With a sharp knife, carefully cut the pineapple in half lengthwise, remove and discard the core, and cut out the fruit, leaving 4 pineapple "boats." Remove the abrasive, brown eyes from the fruit. Dice the pineapple fruit.

In a large bowl mix together the diced pineapple, peppers, kiwis, and herbs. Stir in the orange juice. To serve, divide the salad among the empty pineapple halves.

Pineapple-Ginger Pudding

Pineapples are the highest source of bromelain, an enzyme that breaks down protein. They are so high in these enzymes that they can be used as a digestive stimulant that helps ease gastric issues and aids digestion.

Serves 2 to 4

10 dates, seeded

¾ cup filtered water

¾-inch piece fresh ginger

4 cups chopped, peeled pineapple

1 cup freshly squeezed lemon juice

Crated zest of 1 lemon

Coarsely ground almonds, for garnish

Place the dates in a small bowl, cover with the water, and soak for about 1 hour, or until soft. Drain, reserving the liquid. Finely grate the ginger with a ginger grater or fine grater to extract its juice (you should have 1½ teaspoons). Place the pineapple, lemon juice, zest, and ginger juice in a blender. Blend slowly, adding the reserved liquid as needed until smooth yet thick. Pour the padding into a decorative bowl, sprinkle grated almonds over top, and serve.

Mango Pudding

Mangoes are among the most popular fruits in the world, and there are over three hundred varieties. The fruit's avid fans have cultivated it all over the world, and people still breed new strains today.

Serves 2 to 4

4 dates, seeded

½ cup filtered water

4 ripe mangoes, peeled, seeded, and quartered

4 ripe bananas, peeled and halved crosswise

Freshly shredded coconut, for garnish

Place the dates in small bowl, cover with the water, and soak for about 1 hour, or until soft. Drain, reserving the liquid. In a blender, combine the mangoes, bananas, dates, and ½ cup of the reserved liquid and puree. If needed, add additional reserved liquid until the mixture is smooth yet thick. Transfer to a serving bowl and refrigerate 2 hours, or until well chilled. Garnish with the shredded coconut and serve.

Apple-Cinnamon Cup

This dish was inspired by harosset, a traditional dish made of apples, walnuts, and wine eaten at Passover. Whenever I go to a Passover seder, I bring this dish, and it's always a big hit.

Serves 2 to 4

6 seeded, soaked dates (see above), drained

Juice of ½ lemon

1 teaspoon ground cinnamon

1 teaspoon ground allspice

1 teaspoon freshly ground nutmeg

5 crisp apples (such as Fujis or Galas), shredded or cut into matchstick-sized pieces

¼ cup soaked raisins, drained

2 tablespoons chopped walnuts, for garnish

In a food processor, combine the dates, lemon juice, cinnamon, allspice, and nutmeg and process until smooth. Transfer to a large bowl and stir in the apples and the raisins. Spoon the apple mixture into individual bowls or ramekins, garnish with the chopped walnuts, and serve.

Fruit Soups

Ginger-Pear Soup

The pear makes this soup—so he sure to pick a good one. When selecting pears for this dish, it is best to use softer ones that are very ripe. I like to remove the skin before making this recipe as it yields a smoother consistency. To peel a ripe pear, just hold it under running water and rub the skin right off.

Serves 2 to 4

6 dates, seeded

2 cups filtered water

¼-inch piece fresh ginger

4 ripe pears (such as Bartlett), peeled

½ teaspoon cinnamon

2 fresh anise flowers, or ½ teaspoon anise seeds, or a few wisps of Florence fennel

2 mint leaves

Black and white sesame seeds, for garnish

Place the dates in a small bowl, cover with the water, and soak for about 1 hour, or until soft. Drain, reserving the liquid. Finely grate the ginger with a ginger grater or fine grater to extract its juice (you should have ½ teaspoon). Place the dates, pears, cinnamon, anise, mint, and ginger juice in a blender. Slowly add the reserved liquid as needed while blending, until smooth. Pour into bowls. Garnish with the black and white sesame seeds.

Continued ➡

Peach-Melon Soup

I had always been told that melons should either be eaten alone or left alone. In making melon soups, I've found that melons actually combine quite well with other foods—providing great taste and ease of digestion.

Serves 2

1 large cantaloupe, halved and seeded

2 peaches, pitted

1½ cups freshly squeezed orange juice

½ teaspoon ground nutmeg

Using a metal spoon, scoop out the cantaloupe flesh, reserving half of the fruit for another use. Set aside both cantaloupe bowls. Place the remaining half of the cataloupe flesh, peaches, orange juice, and nutmeg in a blender. Blend until smooth. Divide the soup between the reserved cantaloupe bowls and serve.

Fennel-Berry Soup

In Kula, on the island of Maui, the Kula black raspberry grows. Wherever the raspberry grows, wild fennel grows as well. I would often rub my fingers on the fennel flowers and then pick the berries. The taste was fabulous and that is how the flavor combination for this soup was created.

Serves 2 to 4

3 cups raspberries

3 cups blueberries

2 tablespoons chopped fresh fennel leaves

2 cups filtered water

1 ripe avocado, pitted and peeled

Fresh fennel leaves, for garnish

Place the berries in a blender with the fennel. Blend while slowly adding the water. Add the avocado and continue to blend until smooth. Pour into bowls, garnish with the fennel leaves, and serve.

Watermelon Soup

A few years ago someone taught me a new technique for testing the ripeness of a watermelon: Set the watermelon on a table as it would sit on the ground. Take a dry straw from a broom, or a piece of hay, and lay it across the watermelon crosswise. The piece of straw will turn on its own toward the length of the watermelon. The more it turns, the riper the watermelon.

Serves 2 to 4

8 cups peeled, chopped, and seeded watermelon, juices reserved

Juice of 1 lime

Filtered water, as needed

Place the watermelon in a sealable plastic container or plastic bag and freeze for about 3 hours, or until very cold but not frozen. Transfer the watermelon to a blender; add the lime juice and the reserved watermelon juice and blend until thin but still chunky. If needed, add the water, ¼ cup at a time, until the correct consistency is reached. Transfer to a pitcher and freeze until well chilled, about 1 hour. Pour into bowls and serve.

Nectarine-Cardmom Soup

With its cardamom and cashews, this summertime delight has an East Indian flair.

Serves 2 to 4

4 nectarines, pitted

2 teaspoons ground cardamom

½ cup soaked cashews, drained

1½ cups filtered water

Pinch of black sesame seeds

Place the nectarines, cardamom, cashews, and water in a blender. Blend until smooth. Pour into bowls, garnish with black sesame seeds, and serve.

Apple-Almond Soup

This is a classic combo. It tastes like apple pie in a bowl. If time allows, try sprouting the almonds as it makes for a less oily soup.

Serves 2 to 4

2 apples, cored

½ cup soaked or sprouted almonds, drained

1½ cups filtered water

1 teaspoon ground cinnamon

Place the apples and almonds in a blender. While slowly adding the water, blend until smooth. Pour into bowls and sprinkle each serving with cinnamon.

Drinks

Banana Mylk

In Hawaii, banana trees grow everywhere; from seed, it takes only nine months to get a hundred-pound stalk of bananas. Bananas are excellent for making mylk as they provide a creamy texture and a sweet yet subtle flavor. There are hundreds of varieties of banana, but Williams and Bluefield work the best. As a flavoring variation, try any of the following: blend in 2 tablespoons raw carob powder; blend in the seeds of half a vanilla bean; blend in the seeds of half a vanilla bean and 2 tablespoons raw cacao. You can also first freeze the bananas and enjoy a banana mylk shake with or without any of the above variations.

Serves 2 to 4

4 dates, seeded

1 cup filtered water, plus additional as needed

4 ripe bananas, peeled

Place the dates in a small bowl, cover with 1 cup of the water, and soak for about 1 hour, or until soft. Transfer the dates and their soaking water to a food processor and blend until smooth. Add the bananas and blend until creamy. The consistency should be creamy. If needed, add a little more water and pulse a few times until combined. Serve in a tall glass.

Banacado

One day while traveling the road to Hana, on Maui, I had the pleasure of harvesting both a ripe stalk of bananas and some ripe avocados. Being hungry after a long drive, I began munching on the bananas when I noticed that one of the avocados had gotten squished. I started eating the mashed avocado along with the banana and discovered a delicious new combination. Later I found out that the banana-avocado combination is a Hawaiian tradition.

Serves 1 to 2

2 dates, seeded

2 cups filtered water

4 ripe bananas, peeled and thickly sliced

½ ripe avocado, peeled and pitted

Place the dates in a small bowl, cover with the water, and soak for about 1 hour, or until soft. Drain, reserving the liquid. Place the bananas, avocado, and the reserved liquid in a blender and blend until combined. Add the dates and continue blending until a thick, smooth consistency is achieved. Serve in a tall glass.

Almond Mylk

I never really understood the concept of humans drinking milk from a cow. Cow's milk is designed to take an eighty-pound calf and turn it into a three-hundred-pound heifer in a few months. Almond Mylk has more nutrition than cow's milk and is far more absorbable into the human body. Sprouted almonds are also a great source of protein and amino acids.

Serves 1 to 2

3 dates, seeded

3 cups filtered water

½ cup sprouted almonds

Place the dates in a bowl, cover with the water, and soak for about 1 hour, or until soft. Transfer the dates and their soaking water to a blender, add the almonds, and blend until smooth. Strain through a wire-mesh strainer into a tall glass and serve. (The pulp can be blended again for a lighter batch or used for "rawies," or dehydrated cookies.)

Cashew Mylk

This sweet and rich nut mylk is one of the most delicious and filing treats. Cashews blend up better than any other nut, so if you are looking for a really creamy consistency, use cashews. As a variation, blend in the seeds of half a vanilla bean or 3 tablespoons of raw carob powder along with the dates and nuts.

Serves 1 to 2

2 dates, seeded

½ cup cashews

3 cups filtered water

Place the dates and cashews in a small bowl, cover with water, and soak for about 1 hour, or until soft. Drain. Place the dates, the nuts, and the water in a blender and blend until creamy. Pour into a tall glass and enjoy.

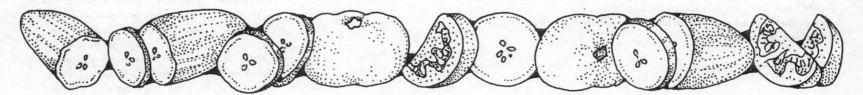

Continued ➡

Tropical Ambrosia

This pina colada–style smoothie is a delicious tropical drink. Pineapples are propagated by planting the top crown. A few years later, a new pineapple grows out the center of the crown of the old one.

Serves 1 to 2

1 pineapple, peeled and cored

1 cup fresh, finely chopped coconut meat

4 bananas, peeled, frozen, and thickly sliced

Place the pineapple in a juice press or juicer and juice. You should have about 2 cups of pineapple juice. Reserve the pineapple flesh for making Fruit Rawies. Place the pineapple juice, coconut, and bananas in a blender and blend until smooth. Serve in tall glasses.

Banabrry

This is your standard smoothie. All I can say is it is berry good.

Serves 1 to 2

½ cup raspberries

½ cup hulled strawberries

½ cup blueberries

2 bananas, peeled, frozen, and thickly sliced

1 to 2 cups fresh apple juice (2 to 4 apples) or filtered water

Place the raspberries, strawberries, blueberries, and bananas in a blender. While slowly adding at least 1 cup and up to 2 cups of the apple juice, as needed, blend until smooth.

Nature's Nectar

This smoothie tastes like coconut cream pie.

Serves 1 to 2

3 dates, seeded

2 cups filtered water

1 cup freshly shredded coconut

Place the dates in a small bowl, cover with the water, and soak for about 1 hour, or until soft. Transfer the dates and their soaking water to a blender, add the coconut, and blend until smooth. Pour into a glass and serve.

Coconut Milk

Coconuts have the bad reputation of being high in fat, but coconut water contains no fat and coconut meat, depending on its maturity, can contain lots of healthy, good fats. It is amazing how much misinformation is out there.

Makes 1½ cups

½ cup fresh coconut meat

1 cup coconut water

Place both ingredients in a blender and blend until smooth. Strain.

Storange Smooth

This is a vitamin C–packed smoothie. Many people think of oranges as a great source of vitamin C. Although oranges do contain a fair amount of the vitamin, the top honors go to acerola cherries, hot chile peppers, and strawberries.

Serves 1 to 2

½ cup hulled strawberries

2 cups freshly squeezed orange juice

2 bananas, peeled, frozen, and thickly sliced

Place all of the ingredients in blender and blend until smooth. Serve in a tall glass.

Fruit Root

Apples and carrots both are harvested in abundance in the fall. Combining the fruit of the tree and the root of the earth creates a tasty and well-balanced drink—the best of the earth and sky.

Serves 1 to 2

6 apples, seeded

6 carrots

Process both ingredients through a juicer into a bowl. Pour into glasses and serve.

Apple Zing

This zippy drink is a delight to the taste buds. It is nice to juice the rind of the lemon through the juicer for an added spark of flavor.

Serves 1 to 2

10 apples, seeded ½-inch piece fresh ginger

⅓ of a lemon with rind, or juice of 1 lemon

Process the apples and ginger through a juicer into a bowl. Juice the lemon with rind, or stir in the lemon juice once the apples and ginger have been juiced. Pour into glasses and enjoy.

Thin Mint

This smoothie was inspired by everyone's favorite Girl Scout cookie, and it's as tasty as its namesake. For a different treat you can dehydrate this smoothie into rawies.

Serves 1 to 2

6 dates, seeded

1½ cups filtered water

1 large sprig fresh mint

3 tablespoons raw carob powder

1 cup coconut milk

4 bananas, peeled, frozen, and thickly sliced

Place the dates in a small bowl, cover with the water, and soak for about 1 hour, or until soft. Place the dates and their soaking water in a blender, add the mint and carob powder, and blend until smooth. Blend in the coconut milk and the bananas until smooth. Serve in a tall glass.

Complementary

The look of this delicious smoothie determined its name. When blended up, the drink's orange color is perfectly set off by the flecks of blue scattered throughout.

Serves 2 to 4

1 ripe mango, peeled and seeded

2 ripe peaches, peeled and pitted

½ cup blueberries

4 bananas, peeled, frozen, and thickly sliced

2 cups freshly squeezed orange juice or coconut water

Place all of the ingredients in blender and blend until smooth. Pour into tall glasses and serve.

Nut Shake

When using frozen bananas, slice them up before putting them in the blender. This will ensure that all of the pieces blend up evenly, resulting in the most creamy "milk shake" imaginable.

Serves 1 to 2

5 dates, seeded

2¾ cups filtered water

Seeds from ½ vanilla bean

½ cup sprouted almonds

4 bananas, peeled, frozen, and thickly sliced

Place the dates in a small bowl, cover with _ cup of the water, and soak for about 1 hour, or until soft. In a blender, blend the dates, along with their soaking water, and the vanilla seeds until smooth. Add the almonds and the remaining 2 cups of water and blend until smooth. Add the bananas and continue blending until smooth. Pour into glasses and serve.

Ruby Cooler (Sun Tea)

Sun tea uses concentrated sunlight to extract flavor and essence from herbs, fruits, and flowers. The pH of the water determines how fast it will extract the tea. The more alkaline the water, the faster it will extract the tea.

Serves 2 to 4

⅓ cup dried hibiscus leaves

⅓ cup dried rose hips

6 cups filtered water

½ cup freshly squeezed lemon juice

1 cup freshly squeezed orange juice

½ cup pineapple juice (optional)

2 to 4 lemon or orange wedges, for garnish

Place hibiscus leaves and rose hips in a large glass jar and cover with the water. Cover the top and set the jar in direct sunlight for 3 to 6 hours. Stir in the lemon, orange, and pineapple juices, and refrigerate until chilled, about 2 hours. Serve in tall glasses, garnished with a wedge of lemon or orange.

Black Raspberry–Prickly Pear

Prickly pears grow prolifically in Hawaii and in the Southwestern United States. Many native tribes subsisted primarily on the fruit for almost one third of the year, while it was in season. The prickly pear is covered with hundreds of tiny thorns, so when dealing with it, be careful! The barbed thorns are as small as fiberglass. Make certain to wipe down all cutting areas after preparing this fruit.

Serves 2 to 4

7 large prickly pears

10 black raspberries

1 cup filtered water or coconut water (optional)

To peel the prickly pears, make a _ inch-deep, lengthwise cut through the skins. Cut off both ends of the prickly pears, and peel back the skins, removing the fruit. Discard the skins. Juice the prickly pears along with the raspberries in a juicer or puree in a blender and strain. Transfer to a pitcher, add the water if a thinner consistency is desired, stir to combine, and enjoy!

Ginger Blast

Ginger grows wild in riverbeds and the jungles throughout Maui. While hiking in the woods, the smell of fresh ginger is everywhere. Its wonderful scent and flavor enhance this bracing drink.

Serves 1 to 2

1 pineapple, peeled and cored

2- to 3-inch piece fresh ginger, peeled and minced (about ¼ cup)

½ cup filtered water

Juice of 2 lemons

Process the pineapple through a juicer into a large measuring cup (you should have about 2 cups). In a blender, thoroughly blend the ginger with the water. Strain through a sieve, discarding the ginger solids. In a pitcher, stir together the pineapple juice and lemon juice. Add the ginger water and stir to combine. Chili before serving.

Continued ➡

EVE-8

This flavorful drink combines eight vegetables and is power-packed with a wide range of nutrients that provide long-lasting energy.

Serves 1 to 2

2 tomatoes

1 carrot

1 beet, peeled

1 yellow bell pepper

1 cucumber, ends trimmed and rubbed (see recipe below)

2 stalks celery

½ cup loosely packed parsley leaves

1 to 2 cloves garlic

Shots of wheatgrass juice (optional)

Process the vegetables through a juicer into a bowl and stir to combine. Pour into glasses. Add a shot of wheatgrass to each glass for a lively kick!

COOLING GREEN

This light and juicy drink is satisfying and provides an abundance of minerals. Cucumbers contain much of their vital nutrients in their skin. Unfortunately, the flavor of a cucumber's skin is quite bitter. Remove this bitterness by following these simple instructions, and enjoy a far tastier cucumber—skin included: Cut the tips off of the cucumber. Take the tip from one end and rub its exposed flesh in small circles on the skin near the opposite end until a milky white sap comes out of the skin. Repeat, using the other tip on the skin of the opposite end. Cut off the new ends now coated in white sap and use your new, improved cucumber.

Serves 1 to 2

1 large cucumber

5 stalks celery

1 teaspoon powdered kelp

Process the cucumber and celery through a juicer into a bowl. Stir in the kelp. Pour into glasses and enjoy.

INTESTINAL CLEANSE

Every once in a while it is a good idea to help clear the intestines. Many people eat far more than needed or could have eaten better foods in their youth and are now ready to cleanse the unhealthy remains from their systems. This drink is a sweet and easy way toward better health.

Serves 1 to 2

10 apples, seeded

Juice of 1 lemon

1 tablespoon psyllium husks

Process the apples through a juicer into a bowl (you should have about 4 cups). Blend or stir in the lemon and psyllium. Pour into glasses and serve.

IRON LION

This earthy root drink is made with a classic vegetable combo: carrots and beets. It is nice to do this one with dark red beets for a really earthy taste. Golden beets provide a far lighter flavor but are very nice in this drink, too. Beets are an excellent source of iron.

Serves 1 to 2

6 carrots

1 beet, peeled

½ cup loosely packed parsley leaves

Process the carrots, beet, and parsley through a juicer into glasses and serve.

Salads

SHREDDED SALAD

Salads of shredded vegetables are a welcome side dish to any meal; they're quick to make and are highly filling.

Serves 2 to 4

3 carrots, shredded

2 purple potatoes, shredded and rinsed

2 beets, shredded

2 cups shredded cabbage (about ½ head)

2 cups Carrot-Cashew-Ginger Dressing

In a salad bowl, toss together the carrots, potatoes, beets, and cabbage. Drizzle the dressing on top, and serve.

GARDEN SALAD

This salad is standard fare in any restaurant. Nothing fancy, no frills, just your basic side salad. It's a quick and easy addition to a meal that just needs a little something extra. Make it with the freshest ingredients and it will be something special.

Serves 2 to 4

1 small head red leaf lettuce, torn into small pieces

1 small head green leaf lettuce, torn into small pieces

1 cup radish, clover, and sesame sprouts

1 cucumber, thinly sliced large tomatoes, cored and cut into wedges

2 cups Green Goddess Dressing

2 carrots, shredded Pansy flowers, for garnish

In a large bowl, make a bed of the lettuces and sprouts. Top with the cucumber and tomatoes and drizzle with the salad dressing. Garnish with the carrots and pansies.

ZUCCHINI-SQUASH SALAD

The curcurbits sometimes have a bitter taste to them. To improve their flavor considerably, soak the chopped zucchini and yellow squash in water with a pinch of salt and a dash of lemon juice, then rinse thoroughly.

Serves 2 to 4

2 zucchini, cubed

2 yellow squash, cubed

1 onion, diced

1½ cups Almond-Cumin Dressing

In a salad bowl, combine the zucchini, yellow squash, and onion. Drizzle the dressing on top, and serve.

WALDORF SALAD

The Waldorf salad was a popular dish originally created for the Waldorf Hotel in New York City. This raw evolution of the traditional salad is tastier than the original and offers a unique flavor combination.

Serves 2 to 4

1 small Belgian endive, separated into leaves

1 large head red leaf lettuce

¼ cup peeled, shredded jicama

3 stalks celery, diced

1 apple, diced

1 cup sunflower sprouts

½ cup walnuts, chopped

1 cup red or green grapes

2 cups Waldorf Dressing

Arrange the five nicest endive leaves into the shape of a star around the sides of a salad bowl. By hand, tear the lettuce leaves into small pieces, then slice the remaining endive leaves crosswise. Mix together the sliced endive leaves and the torn lettuce and add to the salad bowl. In another bowl, combine the jicama, celery, apple, and sprouts. Place the jicama mixture on top of the greens. Sprinkle the chopped walnuts on top of the jicama mixture and the greens, then arrange the grapes on top to form a ring. Finish by drizzling the salad with the dressing. Serve immediately.

CORN, CARROT, AND PEA SALAD

This salad evolved from a cooked dish using frozen corn, carrots, and peas that I remember eating at summer camp. When I finally got around to making it raw, I was amazed at how much better it was than the original. Machine-processed, frozen, thawed, and cooked vegetables just don't compare to their fresh, natural counterparts.

Serves 2 to 4

2 cups corn kernels (approximately 4 ears of corn)

4 carrots, shredded

1 cup peas removed from their pods (approximately 1 pound peas in their pods)

1 small onion, diced and rinsed

Combine all of the ingredients in a salad bowl. Toss and serve.

DELUXE SALAD

This was the standard salad at the Raw Experience. Many of the restaurant's recipes changed over the years hut this one stayed the same. If it ain't broke, don't fix it.

Serves 2 to 4

1 head romaine lettuce, torn into small pieces

1 head red oak lettuce, torn into small pieces

2 heaping tablespoons alfalfa sprouts

2 heaping tablespoons shredded carrot

2 heaping tablespoons shredded beet

½ avocado, peeled, pitted, and thinly sliced

2 tablespoons seeded, chopped bell pepper

2 cups Carrot-Cashew-Ginger Dressing

In a large salad bowl, make a bed of the lettuces and sprouts. Top with the carrot, beet, avocado, and bell pepper. Drizzle the dressing on top and serve.

CUCUMBER-JICAMA SALAD

This cool and crisp salad is a great option when you want a lively texture. It has a great crunch to it and is fun to make.

Serves 2 to 4

1 cucumber, diced

1 jicama, peeled and diced

1 apple, diced

2 stalks celery, diced

2 cups Creamy Herb Dressing or Cucumber-Dill Dressing

Combine the cucumber, jicama, apple, and celery in a salad bowl and gently toss. Drizzle the dressing on top, and serve.

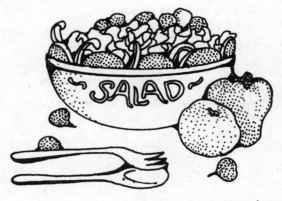

Continued ➡

LITTLE ITALY SALAD

This rich and aromatic salad—a classic from the Raw Experience kitchen—makes a hearty side dish you can also serve on a bed of greens and drizzle with Italian Dressing Marinated portobello mushrooms and sun-dried tomatoes lend a meaty flavor. The tomatoes and black olives also give a nice color contrast.

Serves 4

½ cup dry-packed sun-dried tomatoes (golden if available)

1 large portobello mushroom, stemmed and cut into ½-inch pieces

2 tablespoons Bragg Liquid Aminos

1 small clove garlic, pressed

2 to 5 basil leaves, coarsely chopped

2 oregano sprigs, coarsely chopped

Juice of ½ lemon

¼ cup olives, pitted and diced

2 tablespoons diced red bell pepper

2 tablespoons minced onions

2 tablespoons olive oil

Place the sun-dried tomatoes in a small bowl, cover with water, and soak for about 1 hour, or until soft. In another bowl, combine the portobello, Braggs, garlic, basil, oregano, and lemon juice. Cover and marinate for at least 1 hour. Drain the sun-dried tomatoes and slice them into small strips. In a separate, large bowl, combine the sun-dried tomatoes with the olives and bell pepper.

To keep their flavor from dominating, rinse the onions with water in a wire-mesh sieve. Drain the mushroom mixture, reserving the marinade for other uses. Add the onions and the mushrooms to the bowl containing the sun-dried tomatoes, add the olive oil, and stir to combine. If needed for additional flavor, add ¼ cup of the reserved marinade.

GREEN PAPAYA SALAD

Island people all across the South Pacific, including Hawaii, eat green papaya salad. There are two things referred to as the green papaya: One is a long large papaya that doesn't ripen well and is only used green; the other is just a regular papaya that is used before it is ripe. Either may be used in this recipe. Green papaya has a much higher papain content than ripe papaya and therefore is even better as a digestive stimulant. Seeds of the green papaya, when dried and ground, make an excellent replacement for black pepper.

Serves 4

2 green papayas, peeled and seeded

1 yellow bell pepper, seeded and diced

1 red bell pepper, seeded and diced

½ cup diced red onion, rinsed and drained

¼-inch piece fresh ginger

2 tablespoons minced fresh parsley

2 cloves garlic, pressed

1 esh jalapeño, minced

2 blespoons olive oil

2 tablespoons apple cider vinegar

3 tablespoons Bragg Liquid Aminos

Juice of 1 lemon

Juice of 1 lime

Shred the papaya using a hand shredder or the shredding blade of a food processor. In a large bowl, combine the papaya, yellow and red bell peppers, and onion. Finely grate the ginger on a ginger grate or fine grater to extract its juice (you should have about ½ teaspoon). Add to the papaya mixture

along with the parsley, garlic, and jalapeño. Season with the olive oil, vinegar, Braggs, lemon juice, and lime juice.

Serve as a side dish or on bed of mixed greens with Spicy Papaya-Lime Dressing

CREAMY COLESLAW

Coleslaw has always been one of the great American picnic foods. This version's creamy consistency—the result of a special balance between its acids and oils—and its flavor of vinegar, tahini, and dates together enhanced by the mustard seed, make it a slaw to remember.

Serves 4

Dressing

½ teaspoon dried mustard seeds

5 tablespoons raw tahini

2 teaspoons apple cider vinegar

1 teaspoon sun-dried sea salt

2 tablespoons nutritional yeast

2 seeded, soaked dates drained

1 large red cabbage, shredded

1 large savoy cabbage, shredded

3 carrots, shredded

To prepare the dressing, using a mortar and pestle, crush the mustard seeds into a fine powder. In a blender, combine the mustard seed powder, tahini, vinegar, salt, yeast, and dates. Blend well.

In a large serving bowl, toss together the red and savoy cabbages with the carrots. Drizzle the dressing over the top, toss well, and chill for 1 hour before serving.

ROOT SLAW

Shredded root vegetables of different colors make for a festive and bright salad. They also hold their color for a long time. Root vegetables are sturdy and can be carved and shaped in various ways to add flair and texture to a dish. Experiment with different styles of shredding and slicing to make this dish look unique. Look for the mirin in Japanese markets.

Serves 4

½ jicama, shredded

1 beet, shredded

2 carrots, shredded

4 sunchokes (if available), shredded

½ yakon (if available), shredded

2 tablespoons nama shoyu or Bragg Liquid Aminos

2 tablespoons mirin

2 tablespoons flax oil

Juice of ½ lemon

½ teaspoon cumin seeds

ground ½ teaspoon mustard seeds

ground ½ teaspoon kelp powder

In a large serving bowl, combine the jicama, beet, carrots, sunchokes, and yakon. In a blender, combine the shoyu, mirin, oil, lemon juice, cumin, mustard seeds, and kelp powder. Blend until smooth. Pour the shoyu mixture over the roots, toss well, and let sit for 1 hour, mixing once every 15 minutes or so. Serve.

TABOULI

I was introduced to this traditional Middle Eastern vegetarian dish by the little gyro shops of the Lower East Side in New York City. Traditionally, tabouli is made from bulgur or crushed wheat. Sprouted quinoa has almost the same taste and a very similar consistency. I originally made this with ground sprouted wheat but the whole sprouted quinoa has more life force (being whole) and is softer. The

quinoa only needs to soak overnight and sit out and sprout for part of a day, and then it's ready for use. Black quinoa can be used for this dish for an exotic look.

Serves 4

3 cups sprouted quinoa (see page 403)

¼ cup olive or flax oil

1 teaspoon sun-dried sea salt

2 tomatoes, finely diced

½ large red onion, minced and rinsed

1 green onion, thinly sliced

1 red bell pepper, seeded and finely diced

½ yellow bell pepper, seeded and finely diced

2 to 3 sprigs of mint, coarsely chopped

¼ cup minced parsley

¼ cup minced cilantro

Juice of 2 lemons

Mixed salad greens, for lining platter

In a bowl, mix the quinoa, oil, and sea salt. Stir well. Add in the tomatoes, onions, green onion, and bell peppers. Mix in the mint, parsley, cilantro, and lemon juice. Stir until the colors are mixed evenly throughout the dish. Serve on a bed of mixed salad greens.

Dressings

WALDORF SALAD DRESSING

This Waldorf-style dressing is a perfect replacement for the traditional mayonnaise dressing. This recipe has as its base a great raw, vegan mayo replacement. The raw mayo is further enhanced with orange juice, dill, and onion, making an easy and delicious dressing for a Waldorf salad.

Makes 2½ cups

Raw Mayonnaise

½ cup raw tahini

¼ cup freshly squeezed lemon juice

2 tablespoons apple cider vinegar

2 seeded, soaked dates, drained

2 tablespoons Bragg Liquid Aminos, or 1 teaspoon sun-dried sea salt

¼ cup freshly squeezed orange juice

2 tablespoons dried dill

2 tablespoons minced onion

1 cup filtered water

Combine the mayonnaise ingredients in a blender and blend until smooth. Add the remaining ingredients and blend until combined. The dressing can be covered and refrigerated for up to 2 days.

CREAMY HERB DRESSING

Avocados are the best thing to use to make a creamy dressing. It is important to choose a rich, fatty avocado, not a fruity, watery one. Sharwil and Haas avocados are both good choices. If you don't know the variety, it's often a challenge to tell what it will be like inside. Since there are over three hundred varieties of avocado, it's best to try every type you can find, and once you find one you like, use the same type in all of the avocado dishes you like.

Makes 2 cups

1 ripe, fatty avocado, peeled and pitted

2 tablespoons chopped fresh parsley

2 tablespoons chopped fresh cilantro

2 tablespoons chopped fresh basil

Dash of Bragg Liquid Aminos

1 cup filtered water

Continued ➡

Combine all of the ingredients in a blender and blend until smooth. The dressing can be covered and refrigerated for up to 1 day.

SPICY PAPAYA-LIME DRESSING

This traditional Hawaiian Island dressing has a fruity flavor with a real kick.

Makes 3 cups

1 ripe, medium to large papaya, peeled

Juice of 1 lime

1 tablespoon cayenne pepper

1 cup filtered water

2 to 3 tablespoons Bragg Liquid Aminos

Seed the papaya, reserving 2 teaspoons of the seeds. In a blender, blend the papaya, lime juice, cayenne, water, and reserved papaya seeds until smooth. Add the Braggs to taste. The dressing can be covered and refrigerated for up to 3 days.

GREEN GODDESS DRESSING

There are many dressings out there called "Green Goddess." This recipe was the Raw Experience version. I don't know what is in any of the other ones, but I do know that this was created out of my garden. It was composed from the gifts of the earth goddess, and since the dressing was green, I called it Green Goddess.

Makes 3 cups

1 cup sunflower sprouts (see page 403)

2 tablespoons chopped fresh parsley

2 tablespoons chopped fresh dill

2 tablespoons chopped fresh cilantro

Juice of 1 lemon

2 tablespoons Bragg Liquid Aminos

1 cup filtered water

Combine all of the ingredients in a blender and blend until smooth. The dressing can be covered and refrigerated for up to 1 day.

MANGO-GINGER VINAIGRETTE

This Asian-style dressing is sweet and tangy.

Makes 2 cups

1 ripe mango, peeled and seeded

3-inch piece fresh ginger, peeled

3 tablespoons apple cider vinegar

1 cup filtered water

Juice of 1 lemon

Place all of the ingredients in a blender and blend well. The dressing be covered and refrigerated for up to 4 days.

HERBED VINAIGRETTE

Centuries ago, Europeans began scenting their oils or vinegars with herbs by leaving herb sprigs to sit in glass jars of oils and vinegars for months, and even years, in the dark to slowly extract the essence of the plant. This vinaigrette is a tribute to that tradition. If you like, keep the herbs whole and place the ingredients in a covered glass jar, leave it to sit in a cool dark place for a month or so, and then blend.

Makes 3/4 cup

1/4 cup olive oil

1/4 cup red wine vinegar or apple cider vinegar

2 tablespoons Bragg Liquid Aminos

1 clove of garlic, crushed

3 sprigs fresh parsley, chopped

4 sprigs fresh dill, chopped

3 sprigs fresh cilantro, chopped

Combine all of the ingredients in a blender or food processor and puree until smooth. The dressing can be covered and refrigerated for up to 4 days.

CARROT-CASHEW-GINGER DRESSING

This Raw Experience classic is zingy and creamy. Some people even eat it as a soup.

Makes 2 1/2 cups

6 carrots

1-inch piece fresh ginger

2 tablespoons soaked cashews drained

2 tablespoons Bragg Liquid Aminos

Process the carrots through a juicer into a large measuring cup (you should have approximately 2 cups). Reserve _ cup of carrot pulp from juicing the carrots. Process the ginger through the juicer into the bowl of a food processor. Add the carrot juice and the cashews and process until smooth. Add the reserved carrot pulp and Braggs and pulse once or twice to combine. The dressing can be covered and refrigerated for up to 2 days.

AVOCADO-PARSLEY DRESSING

This creamy dressing has both strong and subtle flavors. The parsley gives the dressing an herbal and earthy tone, while the lemon's acidity cuts through the fat of the avocado and offers a light yet smooth texture.

Makes 2 cups

1 ripe avocado, peeled and pitted

1/2 cup loosely packed parsley leaves

1 tablespoon Bragg Liquid Aminos

1 teaspoon ground cumin

Juice of 1/2 lemon

1 cup filtered water

Combine all of the ingredients in a blender or food processor and blend or pulse until smooth. The dressing can be covered and refrigerated for up to 1 day.

ITALIAN DRESSING

The herbs used in this recipe are some of the easiest to grow at home. Fresh basil, oregano, cilantro, and parsley can all add true flavor to your meals. Each also produces a flower that makes a beautiful garnish and helps bring out the subtler flavors.

Makes 2 1/2 cups

2 tablespoons chopped basil

2 tablespoons chopped fresh oregano

2 tablespoons chopped fresh cilantro

2 tablespoons chopped fresh parsley

Juice of 1 lemon

4 teaspoons apple cider vinegar

1 tablespoon olive oil

1 tablespoon Bragg Liquid Aminos

1/2 cucumber, thickly sliced

1 tablespoon dried onion flakes

1 teaspoon paprika

1 cup filtered water

Combine all of the ingredients in a blender or food processor and blend or pulse until smooth. The dressing can be covered and refrigerated for up to 2 days.

CUCUMBER-DILL DRESSING

This is a nice light dressing that is perfect when you want the flavor of the salad to he stronger than that of the dressing. Its flavor is sweet and sour yet not overpowering.

Makes 2 cups

1 cucumber, thickly sliced

1/4 cup chopped fresh dill

1 tablespoon Bragg Liquid Aminos

Juice of 1/4 lemon

1 cup filtered water or cucumber juice (from about 2 cucumbers)

Combine all of the ingredients in a blender and blend until smooth. The dressing can be covered and refrigerated for up to 2 days.

ALMOND-CUMIN DRESSING

This simple dressing has a rich and robust flavor. Cumin seed is the dominant flavor, giving it an earthy taste.

Makes 1 1/2 cups

1/2 cup sprouted almonds (see page 403)

1 cup filtered water

2 teaspoons Bragg Liquid Aminos

1 teaspoon ground cumin

Combine all of the ingredients in a blender or food processor and blend or pulse until smooth. The dressing can be covered and refrigerated for up to 2 days.

Savory Soups

CREAMY CARROT-GINGER SOUP

This smooth and spicy soup was one of the most popular soups at the Raw Experience.

Serves 4

1/2-inch piece fresh ginger 6 large carrots

1 ripe avocado, peeled and pitted

2 tablespoons loosely packed cilantro leaves

1 tablespoon Bragg Liquid Aminos

1 1/2 cups White Sauce

Black sesame seeds, for garnish

Finely grate the ginger on a ginger grater or fine grater to extract its juice (you should have about 1 teaspoon). Using a homogenizing juicer, homogenize the carrots (you should have about 2 cups).

In a blender, blend the ginger and carrot juices, avocado, 2 tablespoons of the cilantro, and the Braggs until smooth. Pour the soup into individual serving bowls, top each with about 1/3 cup of the sauce, and garnish with the sesame seeds.

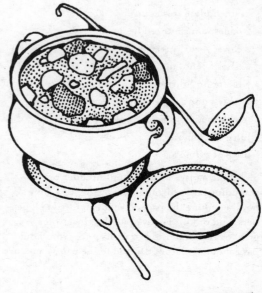

Continued ➡

TOM YUM

This traditional Thai-style soup is my personal favorite. I love coconuts and this soup is all about the coco. I like to use different ages of coconut meat to get varied textures. A more mature nut makes a chunky soup, while a younger one makes a creamy soup. I also like to use a variety of hot peppers: jalapeño, scrrano, and even the super spicy Thai chile, just to get a wide range of spiciness. Some peppers are hot as you eat them, others after you eat them; my favorite are hot only when you stop eating them.

Serves 2 to 4

- 1 coconut
- 7 leaves basil, plus additional for garnish
- 3 leaves oregano
- 5 sprigs cilantro, stemmed
- ½ Thai, jalapeño, or serrano chile, seeded and minced
- 2 tablespoons Bragg Liquid Aminos or nama shoyu

Open the coconut with a machete, cleaver, drill, or knife. Pour the coconut water into a blender. With a metal spoon scoop out the coconut meat and place in the blender with the coconut water. Add the 7 leaves of basil, the oregano, cilantro, chile, and Braggs, and blend until smooth. Pour the soup into individual serving bowls, and garnish each with a few basil leaves.

MAUI ONION GAZPACHO

The Maui onion is a special thing. It grows up at high elevations on the side of Haleakala crater. The onion is crisp and sweet, almost like an apple. In fact, there are people on Maui who eat them whole. Maui onions are what make this soup so good. If you don't have access to them, then find a suitable sweet onion to replace it with.

Serves 2 to 4

- 3 large tomatoes
- 1 Maui onion, diced (about ¾ cup) and rinsed
- 1 yellow or red bell pepper, seeded and coarsely chopped
- 1 clove garlic
- 1 ripe tomato, chopped
- 1 cucumber, peeled and chopped
- 2 tablespoons chopped fresh dill
- Juice of 1 lemon
- 1 to 2 cups filtered water
- Bragg Liquid Aminos or sun-dried sea salt

Using a homogenizing juicer, homogenize the tomatoes (you should have about 2 cups). Place the onion, pepper, and garlic in a food processor. Pulse a few times to blend slightly. Add the chopped tomato, cucumber, dill, lemon juice, tomato juice, and 1 cup of the water. Pulse a few more times, until thin but still chunky. If the soup is too thick, add up to 1 cup of the remaining water, and pulse just once or twice to combine. Do not blend until smooth. Add the Braggs to taste. Serve immediately.

GAZPACHO

Many people think of soups as something warm or hot. Yet in the heat of the summer, most people don't want a hot soup. Gazpacho is a delicious raw soup traditionally served chilled. The soup originated in the Andalusia region of southern Spain, and is the basis for this amazing creation.

Serves 2 to 4

- 2 large or 3 medium tomatoes
- 2 cups diced tomatoes (approximately 4 tomatoes)
- 1 small onion, minced and rinsed
- 1 cucumber, diced
- 2 green onions, chopped
- Juice of 1 orange
- Juice of 1 large lemon
- 1 clove garlic, crushed
- 2 tablespoons apple cider vinegar
- 2 tablespoons olive or flax oil (optional)
- ⅓ cup coarsely chopped fresh parsley
- 1 teaspoon coarsely chopped fresh tarragon
- 1 teaspoon ground cumin
- ⅓ cup coarsely chopped fresh basil
- ⅓ cup coarsely chopped fresh cilantro
- Pinch of ground cayenne pepper (optional)
- Bragg Liquid Aminos or sun-dried sea salt

Juice the tomatoes using a juicer or puree them in a blender and strain. Set aside.

In a food processor, pulse the diced tomatoes, onion, cucumber, and green onions only a few times to mix and chop the ingredients, not to grind them. In a blender, combine the reserved tomato juice, orange juice, lemon juice, garlic, vinegar, and oil. Add the parsley, tarragon, cumin, basil, cilantro, and cayenne pepper, and blend well. In a large bowl, combine the chopped vegetables with the blended soup. Add the Braggs to taste. Chill for about 2 hours before serving.

CREAMY RED PEPPER SOUP

This soup has a bright and sweet flavor that is well supported by the richness of the avocado.

Serves 2 to 4

- 1 red bell pepper, seeded and chopped
- 1 ripe avocado, peeled and pitted
- 2 cups filtered water
- Leaves from 1 sprig oregano
- 2 tablespoons chopped fresh cilantro
- 2 tablespoons chopped fresh parsley
- Bragg Liquid Aminos
- Black sesame seeds, for garnish

Place the bell pepper, avocado, water, oregano, cilantro, and parsley in a blender, and blend until smooth. Add the Braggs to taste. Pour into serving bowls and garnish with the sesame seeds.

CORN CHOWDER

On a visit to Georgia, a friend of mine turned me on to raw corn chowder. It was summer and corn was readily available, so each night we experimented with new evolutions of corn chowder. We decided this final version was the perfect chowder.

Serves 2 to 4

- ½ cup sprouted almonds (see page 403)
- 1 cup filtered water
- 1 clove garlic
- ¼ cup coarsely chopped fresh cilantro
- 2 large carrots, shredded
- 1 cup fresh corn kernels (approximately 2 ears corn)
- 2 tablespoons chopped onion, rinsed
- Pinch of nutritional yeast
- Bragg Liquid Aminos, for seasoning

Place the almond sprouts, water, garlic, and cilantro in a blender, and blend until creamy. Add the carrots, corn, onions, and yeast and blend until chunky. Add the Braggs to taste. Pour into bowls and serve.

BORSCHT

This classic cabbage and beet soup is known throughout Russia and the Slavic region of Europe. Borscht is hearty, healthy, and fun to say.

Serves 2 to 4

- 2 to 3 cups chopped red cabbage
- 1 beet, shredded
- 2 tablespoons red miso
- 1 clove garlic
- 1 cup filtered water

In a blender, blend the cabbage, beet, miso, garlic and water until smooth. Pour into bowls and serve.

CASCADILLA SOUP

Cascadilla means "cascade" or "waterfall" in Spanish, which is an accurate description of the outpouring of flavor from this sweet and tangy soup.

Serves 2 to 4

- 5 tomatoes
- 1 avocado, peeled and pitted
- 1 red bell pepper, seeded and chopped
- 1 cucumber, chopped
- 1 green onion, chopped
- 1 clove garlic, crushed
- 2 seeded, soaked dates, drained
- 1 teaspoon chopped fresh dill
- Bragg Liquid Aminos, for seasoning

In a blender, blend the cabbage, beet, miso, garlic, and water until smooth. Pour into bowls and serve.

Using a homogenizing juicer, homogenize the tomatoes (you should have about 4 cups of juice). In a blender, blend the tomato juice and avocado. Add the bell pepper, cucumber, green onion, garlic, dates, and dill, and blend well. Add the Braggs to taste. Pour into bowls and serve.

PEA SOUP

Fresh peas are a fun summertime treat. Peas still in the pod are always the sweetest—plus they're fun to shuck.

Serves 2 to 4

- 2 cups shelled fresh peas (approximately 2 pounds peas in their pods)
- ½ avocado, peeled and pitted
- ¼ cup loosely packed fresh cilantro leaves, plus additional for garnish
- 1 cup filtered water
- Bragg Liquid Aminos, for seasoning

Place the peas, avocado, the ¼ cup cilantro, and water in a blender and blend until smooth. Add the Braggs to taste. Serve in bowls, garnished with the additional cilantro.

PESTO SOUP

This Raw Experience creation has a robust flavor and chunky texture that make it "soupreme"

Serves 2 to 4

- 10 large fresh basil leaves
- 1 clove garlic
- ¼ cup pine nuts
- 1 tablespoon red miso
- 1 tablespoon nutritional yeast
- 2 cups filtered water
- 2 cups diced tomato (approximately 4 tomatoes)
- ¼ cup diced red bell pepper
- 2 tablespoons shredded carrots
- 2 tablespoons shredded beets
- 2 tablespoons minced onion, rinsed
- 1 tablespoon Bragg Liquid Aminos
- Basil flowers, for garnish

Continued ➡

Place the basil, garlic, pine nuts, miso, and yeast in a blender and blend while gradually adding the water. Add the tomatoes, bell pepper, carrots, beets, onion, and Braggs, and pulse until chunky. Serve in bowls, garnished with the basil flowers.

CREAM OF BROCCOLI SOUP

Broccoli and cauliflower are two of the most beautiful plants in nature. When flowering, these members of the Brassica genus have giant bulbous flower heads surrounded by olive green, cabbagelike leaves. Broccoli stems can be used as well as the flowering part—just peel and use.

Serves 2 to 4

　1 cup sprouted almonds
　3 cups filtered water
　1 small head broccoli, chopped (about 2 cups)
　½ cup chopped red onion
　¼ cup loosely packed fresh parsley leaves
　2 tablespoons nutritional yeast
　1 tablespoon Bragg Liquid Aminos
　2 tablespoons minced onion, for garnish
　2 tablespoons chopped cilantro, for garnish

In a blender, blend the almonds and the water until smooth. Stir in the broccoli, red onion, parsley, yeast, and Braggs. Spoon the soup into individual serving bowls. Top each with a little of the minced onion and cilantro and serve.

Appetizers

PESTO WRAPS

These delightful little treats were one of the many bite-sized creations that I came up with for a catering gig, and they became such a hit that people requested them forever after.

Serves 4 to 6

　3 large zucchini, peeled
　Pinch of sun-dried sea salt
　Juice of ½ lemon

Presto Pesto

　2 cups walnuts
　2 cups loosely packed fresh green and purple basil leaves
　3 cloves garlic
　1 heaping tablespoon red miso
　2 tomatoes, cubed
　Chopped green and purple basil, for garnish

Using a vegetable peeler or mandoline, cut thin, wide strips lengthwise down the zucchini. Place the zucchini strips in a bowl, cover with water, add the sea salt and lemon juice, and soak for 2 hours, or until they taste clean (not starchy). Drain, rinse, and drain again.

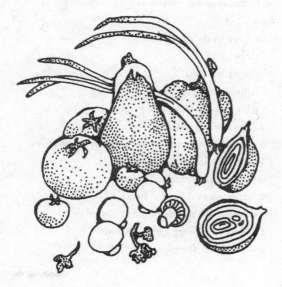

To prepare the pesto, place the walnuts, basil leaves, and garlic in a homogenizing juicer or food processor, and homogenize, creating an oily paste. Transfer the paste to a bowl and stir in the red miso.

To prepare each wrap, lay a zucchini strip flat on the workspace. Drop a teaspoon of pesto in the center of the zucchini strip. Press a small piece of tomato into the pesto. Fold or roll up the zucchini strip. Secure the wrap with a toothpick or place it seam side down on a serving plate. Serve garnished with the chopped green and purple basil.

FLAX-DULSE CHIPS

Flax crackers are possibly the simplest chip or cracker to make and are a crunchy delight. All you will want is "just the flax, ma'am."

Serves 2 to 4

　3 cups flax seeds
　4 cups filtered water
　¼ cup dulse

Place the flax seeds in a bowl, cover with the water, and soak for 15 minutes. Mix in the dulse flakes. Drain through a sieve. Using one of the methods described thinly spread the flax-seed mixture 1/4 inch thick on the appropriate drying surface for the chosen method. Dry for 18 hours, or until crispy.

VEGGIE KABOBS

This dish has a high entertainment value. There is something to he said for fun food. These display beautifully and are almost as enjoyable to make as they are to eat.

Serves 4

Marinade

　2 teaspoons olive oil
　¼ cup Bragg Liquid Aminos
　2 cups filtered water
　2 tablespoons apple cider vinegar
　1 clove garlic, pressed
　Juice of ½ lemon
　Pinch of paprika
　Pinch of chile powder
　Pinch of dried cilantro
　10 cherry tomatoes
　1 avocado, peeled, pitted, and cubed
　1 onion, cubed and separated into thin squares
　10 pitted olives
　1 large red bell pepper, seeded and cut into chunks
　1 small pineapple, peeled and cut into chunks

To prepare the marinade, in a large bowl, combine the olive oil, Braggs, water, vinegar, garlic, lemon juice, paprika, chile powder, and cilantro. Mix well.

To prepare the kabobs, spear the tomatoes, avocado, onion, olives, bell pepper, and pineapple onto 10-inch wooden skewers, alternating ingredients so that the tastes and colors mix.

Place the kabobs in a shallow bowl and pour the marinade over them. Marinate the kabobs for at least 1 hour and up to 10 hours before serving.

MINI PIZZAS

This may be one of the ultimate recipes in the world of raw-food cuisine. This mini-pizza recipe will convince anyone that raw food isn't just salads and nuts.

Serves 4

　Dough for 4 mini pizzas (recipe follows)

　2 cups Red Sauce
　2 cups White Sauce
　½ cup chopped fresh basil, for garnish

Beginning 1 day in advance, prepare the pizza crust.

To serve, place the pizza crusts on a tray. Spread ¼ cup of the red sauce on top of each crust, then ¼ cup of the white sauce. Garnish with the basil and serve.

PIZZA CRUST

Makes dough for 4 mini pizzas

　2 cups sprouted buckwheat or soft wheat, sprouted for 2 days
　3 large carrots
　2 tablespoons shredded carrot
　2 tablespoons shredded beet
　2 tablespoons minced onion
　¼ cup flax seeds
　2 tablespoons finely chopped fresh parsley
　2 tablespoons finely chopped fresh cilantro
　2 tablespoons finely chopped fresh basil
　2 tablespoons nutritional yeast
　2 tablespoons caraway seeds
　2 tablespoons sun-dried sea salt

Homogenize the sprouted buckwheat with the whole carrots in a homogenizing juicer. In a bowl, mix the wheat mixture with the shredded carrots, beet, and onion. In a coffee grinder or small food processor, grind the flax seeds into a powder. Add the ground flax seeds, parsley, cilantro, and basil to the wheat-carrot mixture. Stir in the yeast and caraway seeds, and add salt to taste. Mix well (you may need to sink your hands into this one).

Using wet hands, press the dough into 3-inch disks, ¼ to ½ inch thick. Using one of the methods described dehydrate the crusts for about 12 hours, or until dry. To decrease the drying time, occasionally flip the crusts.

RED SAUCE

Makes 3¹/₂ cups

　7 dry-packed sun-dried tomatoes, soaked in water until soft, and drained
　2 large tomatoes, chopped
　1 clove garlic
　4 fresh basil leaves, chopped
　2 tablespoons Bragg Liquid Aminos
　2 tablespoons olive oil
　1 tablespoon nutritional yeast

Place the sun-dried tomatoes in a blender. Add the chopped tomatoes, garlic, basil, Braggs, olive oil, and yeast. Blend well, until smooth. The sauce should be very thick.

WHITE SAUCE

Makes 3 cups

　½ cup macadamia nuts
　¼ cup pine nuts
　½ cup cashews
　2 tablespoons olive oil
　1 tablespoon Bragg Liquid Aminos
　2 teaspoons nutritional yeast
　Juice of 1 lemon
　1 cup filtered water, plus additional for thinning, if needed

Place the macadamia nuts, pine nuts, and cashews in a bowl, cover with water, and soak for 2 to 6 hours. Drain. Place all of the ingredients in a blender and blend until smooth, adding additional water, if needed, to obtain a creamy consistency.

Continued ➡

Potato Chips

This is the raw food solution to the potato chip. These easy-to-make chips are a crispy snack that tastes great with guacamole or salsa.

Serves 2 to 4

3 purple potatoes, sliced crosswise ⅛ inch thick

2 tablespoons Bragg Liquid

Aminos 2 tablespoons chile powder

I teaspoon red miso

Filtered water, for soaking

Place the potatoes in a bowl and add the Braggs, chile powder, red miso, and enough water to cover the potato slices. Mix well, then drain. Using one of the methods described dehydrate the potato slices on the appropriate surface for the chosen method for 21 hours, or until crispy.

Sides

Kim Chee

Kim chee is an Asian version of sauerkraut, or fermented cabbage. Much like durian, the malodorous Malaysian fruit, you just have to get past the smell and you will really enjoy yourself. Kim chee has a tangy and spicy flavor that will keep you coming back for more. It is also considered a healing food because it helps bring healthy balance back to the intestinal flora. To start the culture, you'll need a tablespoon of prepared kim chee. Using some of a previous batch is best, but you can also purchase kim chee—just make sure it's "live" (unpasteurized) kim chee and doesn't contain any sugar or chemicals.

Serves 4

½ head red cabbage

½ head napa cabbage

I-inch piece fresh ginger

I heaping tablespoon red miso

I jalapeño chile, seeded and diced

I tablespoon prepared kim chee

There are three different traditional styles of chopping the cabbage for this dish: (1) Thai style: shred the cabbage either using the shredding blade of a food processor or a hand shredder; (2) Korean style: slice the cabbage using the small slicing blade of a food processor or by hand using a sharp knife; (3) Hawaiian style: using a blender, a homogenizing juicer, or food processor, grind the cabbage until it becomes mash. Using one method or some combination of the three, prepare the red cabbage and the napa cabbage. Place both cabbages in a large ceramic bowl or a traditional kim chee or sauerkraut crock, and toss.

In a homogenizing juicer, juice the ginger and ¼ cup, firmly packed, of the prepared cabbage. Place the juiced cabbage and ginger in a bowl, add the miso, jalapeño, and prepared kim chee, and stir well. Add this mixture to the tossed cabbage in the bowl and toss well to combine. Cover with a piece of cheesecloth. Place a second bowl of the same size on top of the first. (This second bowl will act as a weight.) Leave in a warm (75 to 90°F), dark location for 2 days. When your kim chee is ready it will smell strong. It is good to know what kim chee should smell like when fully fermented; buy some in a store and get a good smell.

Traditional Guacamole

Avocados may be the most celebrated fruit in the world of raw foods. This traditional guacamole is a Mexican recipe handed down to me by my friend Josh.

Serves 4

2 very ripe avocados, peeled and pitted

I large tomato, diced

¼ onion, diced

½ teaspoon sun-dried sea salt

2 tablespoons chopped fresh cilantro

Juice of ½ lemon

Pinch of nutritional yeast

Pinch of cumin

Lettuce leaves or Flax-Dulse Chips and sliced veggies, for dipping

In a large bowl, mash the avocados. Add the remaining ingredients and stir well. Roll in lettuce leaves to make burritos, or serve with flax chips and sliced veggies for dipping.

Star Fruit Guacamole

A giant star fruit tree behind the Maui Raw Experience inspired this delicious guacamole.

Serves 4

2 avocados, peeled and pitted

2 small star fruits, ribs removed and diced

I tomatillo, diced

¼ cup diced shallot

I tablespoon Bragg Liquid Aminos

Juice of I lemon

2 tablespoons chopped fresh cilantro

Lettuce leaves or Flax-Dulse Chips and sliced veggies, for dipping

In a large bowl, mash the avocados. Add the remaining ingredients and stir well. Roll in lettuce leaves to make burritos, or serve with flax chips and sliced veggies for dipping.

Star Fruit Salsa

One winter while vacationing on Maui, I created this fabulous salsa. I had an abundance of star fruits and was going to a potluck gathering. I had had mango salsa and papaya salsa, both of which are Hawaiian specialties, so I decided to discover star fruit salsa. This sweet and tangy salsa was a huge hit and often appeared on the menu at the Raw Experience.

Serves 4

5 star fruits, ribs removed and diced

I cup pitted olives, diced

I small onion, minced and rinsed

1½-inch piece fresh ginger

2 tablespoons minced fresh cilantro

I tablespoon apple cider vinegar

I clove garlic, crushed

2 tablespoons Bragg Liquid Aminos

Juice of I lemon

Bottom half of a jalapeño chile, seeded and minced

Flax-Dulse Chips, for serving

In a large bowl, combine the star fruits, olives, and onion. Finely grate the ginger on a ginger grater or fine grater to extract its juice (you should have about I tablespoon). Add the ginger juice, cilantro, vinegar, garlic, Braggs, lemon juice, and jalapeño to the star fruit mixture; mix well. Cover and let sit in the refrigerator or at room temperature for I to 4 hours, until the flavors mingle. Serve with flax chips.

Tomatillo Salsa

Tomatillos have a high entertainment value because nature decided to make this fruit come complete with wrapping paper. A tomatillo is like a cross between a berry and a green tomato and has papery husk surrounding its fruit.

Serves 4

I pound tomatillos, husked and diced (about 3 cups)

I cup diced, pitted olives

½ cup diced yellow bell pepper

¼ cup diced tomato

½ cup diced onion

2 tablespoons minced fresh cilantro

2 tablespoons Bragg Liquid Aminos

Juice of I lime

I habanero chile, seeded and minced

Sliced veggies (such as sunchokes, carrots, or jicama), for dipping

In a large bowl, mix the tomatillos, olives, bell pepper, tomato, onions, and cilantro. Add the Braggs and lime juice and mix well. Add the habaneros to taste. Cover and let sit in the refrigerator or at room temperature for I to 4 hours, until the flavors mingle. Serve with sliced veggies for dipping.

Red Pepper–Chipotle Salsa

The chipotle chile (a dried and smoked jalapeño) has a robust and smoky flavor. Both black and red dried chipotles are sold; the red ones seem to have more flavor, but the black ones are far spicier. These chiles are available pickled and in adobo sauce, but only the dried chipotles are raw.

Serves 4

I chipotle chile

5 dry-packed sun-dried tomatoes

2 red bell peppers, seeded and diced

I large tomato, cubed

½ cup diced onion

2 tablespoons minced fresh cilantro

2 leaves fresh basil

I tablespoon olive oil

½ teaspoon sun-dried sea salt

Juice of ½ lemon

In a small bowl, soak the chipotle and sun-dried tomatoes in water to cover until soft. Drain. Mince the chipotle and sun-dried tomatoes. Set aside. In a large bowl, mix the bell peppers, fresh tomato, and onion. In a blender cup or blender, mix the cilantro, basil, chipotle, sun-dried tomatoes, and olive oil. Blend until the consistency is that of a chunky paste. Add to the large bowl and mix well. Add the sea salt and lemon juice. Mix well. Cover and refrigerate the salsa for I to 4 hours, until the flavors mingle.

Chile Mole

Many ingredients go into making a good mole. In Mexico, chocolate or cacao is traditionally used in the preparation of mole. This mole features a range of vegetables and offers many layers of flavor.

Serves 4

I large tomato, diced

½ red bell pepper, seeded and diced

½ purple or yellow bell pepper, seeded and diced

I medium avocado, peeled, pitted, and cubed

1½ cups corn kernels (approximately 3 ears corn)

¼ cup loosely packed fresh parsley leaves

¼ cup loosely packed fresh cilantro leaves

½ cup dry-packed sun-dried tomatoes, soaked until soft and drained

2 tablespoons Bragg Liquid Aminos

2 cloves garlic, pressed

Juice of ½ lemon

I teaspoon nutritional yeast

Pinch of cayenne pepper

Continued ➡

In a bowl, mix the tomato, bell peppers, avocado, and corn. In a blender, blend the parsley, cilantro, sun-dried tomatoes, Braggs, garlic, lemon juice, and yeast until creamy. Season with the cayenne. Add the blended mixture to the bowl containing diced vegetables. Stir until all of the ingredients are evenly combined and a thick consistency is achieved.

PEA MOLE

Sometimes avocados aren't available, yet we crave a good guacamole. This pea mole is a great substitute for these occasions. Fresh peas are less oily than avocados but are just as creamy.

Serves 4

    3 cups shelled fresh peas (approximately 3 pounds peas in their pods)
    ¼ cup loosely packed fresh cilantro leaves
    Juice of 1 lime
    Pinch of sun-dried sea salt
    Cucumber slices or corn chips for serving

Place the peas, cilantro, lime juice, and sea salt in a food processor and process until smooth. Serve in a bowl alongside the cucumber slices.

SPROUTED HUMMUS

Garbanzo beans, or chickpeas, sprout quickly and easily. When sprouting garbanzos, make certain not to overfill the jar. Garbanzos expand so rapidly that they can shatter a glass jar. The best flavor comes from using garbanzos that have been sprouted for one day.

Serves 4

    4 cups sprouted garbanzo beans
    ¼ cup chopped fresh parsley
    1 clove garlic
    ¼ cup raw tahini
    ¼ cup freshly squeezed lemon juice
    Sun-dried sea salt

In a homogenizing juicer with the blank plate in place, homogenize the garbanzo beans, parsley, and garlic into a bowl. In a blender, blend the tahini and lemon juice. Stir the lemon-tahini mixture into the bean mixture. Add sea salt to taste. Serve.

BABA GHANOUSH

This Middle Eastern dish is hearty and earthy. The longer you marinate the eggplant, the better it gets. Serve the baba ghanoush with Hummus, Falafel, or Tabouli.

Serves 4

    1 large eggplant, peeled and thinly sliced
    Generous pinch of sun-dried sea salt
    Juice of 1 lemon
    1 clove garlic, crushed
    1 teaspoon sprouted cumin seeds
    ¼ cup raw tahini
    1 medium onion, minced and rinsed
    ¼ cup minced fresh parsley
    Bragg Liquid Aminos

Put the eggplant in a large bowl, cover with water, add the sea salt and lemon juice, and soak for 4 to 10 hours. (This will help cure the eggplant and improve its flavor.) Drain. In a homogenizing juicer with the blank plate in place, homogenize the eggplant with the garlic and cumin sprouts into a large bowl. Add the tahini, onion, and parsley and mix well. Mix in the Braggs to taste.

Entrées

FESTIVE SPROUTED WILD RICE

Sprouted black long-grain wild rice has a robust taste and smell. The seeds sprout under water that you change twice a day. When the seeds are rinsed, the earthy aroma rises up. Take a deep inhalation as you pour out the water, and enjoy the scent.

Serves 4 to 6

    5 cups sprouted wild rice
    ½ onion, minced and rinsed
    1 red bell pepper, diced
    1 cup corn kernels (approximately 2 ears corn)
    5 tablespoons Bragg Liquid Aminos
    3 tablespoons paprika
    Juice of 1 orange

In a large bowl, combine the rice, onion, bell pepper, and corn. Stir in the Braggs, paprika, and orange juice. Serve.

MIDDLE EASTERN PLATE

Garbanzo beans play a major role in the cuisine of the Middle East. This Raw Experience classic uses garbanzo beans to make both the falafel-style pizza crust and the hummus spread. The falafel crusts keep quite well and any extra hummus can always be turned into falafel for later use.

Serves 4

    4 falafel crusts
    2 cups Sprouted Hummus
    1 tomato, diced
    ¼ cup minced onion, rinsed
    2 tablespoons diced cucumber
    2 tablespoons minced fresh parsley
    4 sprig of mint, for garnish
    4 olives, for garnish

Place each of the falafel crusts on an individual serving plate. Spread ½ cup of the hummus on top of each crust. Sprinkle the tomatoes, onions, cucumber, and parsley evenly over the top of each crust. Garnish with the mint and black olives.

FALAFEL

This falafel recipe can be prepared as crusts for use in the Middle Eastern Plate, or it can be made into more traditional falafel balls. To make the balls just follow the instructions below and instead of pressing into crusts, roll the mixture into 1-inch balls, then dehydrate for only 8 to 10 hours.

Makes four 8-inch crusts or eight 4-inch crusts

    6 cups sprouted garbanzo beans
    1 cup loosely packed fresh parsley leaves
    1 cup raw tahini
    1 cup freshly squeezed lemon juice
    1 onion, minced
    2 tablespoons ground cumin
    6 tablespoons Bragg Liquid Aminos,
        or 2 tablespoons sun-dried sea salt
    1 cup sesame seeds

Using a homogenizing juicer with the blank plate in place, homogenize the garbanzo beans and parsley and place in a large bowl. In a blender, blend the tahini, lemon juice, onion, cumin, and Braggs. Stir the tahini mixture into the garbanzo paste. In a spice grinder, grind the sesame seeds into a fine powder. Mix into the garbanzo paste. Press into ¼-inch-thick crusts, 4 or 8 inches in diameter. Dehydrate for 12 to 14 hours, flipping at least once during the drying time.

PESTO PIZZA & TRADITIONAL PIZZA

At the Raw Experience restaurant in San Francisco, we always came up with different pizzas as daily specials, but these two were permanently on the menu.

Serves 4

    4 8-inch Pizza Crusts (recipe follows)
    1 cup Red Sauce
    1 cup White Sauce
    1 cup Pesto
    ½ red tomato, diced
    ½ yellow tomato, diced
    1 onion, minced and rinsed
    1 small beet, shredded
    ½ cup pine nuts, ground
    5 purple basil leaves, minced
    5 green basil leaves, minced

Place each of the crusts on an individual serving plate. Spread ½ cup of the red sauce over each of two of the crusts, followed by ½ cup of the white sauce over each. Spread ½ cup of the pesto on each of the two remaining crusts. Top all four with the tomatoes, onions, beets, pine nuts, and basil.

PIZZA CRUSTS

Makes four 8-inch crusts or eight 4-inch crusts

    4 cups sprouted wheat
    1 clove garlic, pressed
    ¼ cup minced fresh parsley
    ¼ cup minced fresh cilantro
    ¼ cup minced fresh basil
    ¼ cup sprouted cumin seeds
    ¼ cup soaked flax seeds, drained
    1 beet, shredded
    2 carrots, shredded
    ½ cup minced onion
    3 tablespoons
    Bragg Liquid Aminos

Using a homogenizing juicer, homogenize the wheat sprouts with the garlic, parsley, cilantro, basil, cumin seeds, and flax seeds. Place in a large bowl and mix in the beets, carrots, onions, and Braggs. Stir until well mixed, and then press into ¼-inch thick-crusts, 4 or 8 inches in diameter. Dehydrate the crusts for 12 hours, flipping at least once during drying time.

LASAGNA

One of the claims to fame of the Raw Experience was that we could make any cooked-food dish in a raw way. We got a number of requests for a raw lasagna and created this recipe in response. For a while we called it "Living," but eventually we went back to its original name. Versions of this dish are served in raw-food and vegetarian restaurants throughout America.

Serves 4 to 8

    1 cup filtered water
    1 cup freshly squeezed lemon juice
    3 tablespoons Bragg Liquid Aminos
    1 clove garlic, pressed
    1 teaspoon dried parsley
    1 teaspoon dried basil
    1 eggplant, peeled
    2 large zucchini, peeled
    1 medium sweet onion, cut into rings
    1 cup walnuts
    4 cups Red Sauce
    2 cups White Sauce

Continued ➡

In a bowl, combine the water, lemon juice, Braggs, garlic, parsley, and basil. Using a vegetable peeler or mandoline with the thinnest blade, slice the eggplant and zucchini lengthwise into long strips. Place the eggplant, zucchini, and onions in a shallow dish and pour the lemon juice mixture over the top. Marinate overnight.

In a blender cup or coffee grinder, grind the walnuts into a fine powder. Moisten the inside of a lasagna dish with water and sprinkle the bottom and sides of the dish with 2 tablespoons of the walnut powder to coat. Cover the bottom of the dish with a layer of the marinated vegetables, and top with 1 cup of the red sauce and ½ cup of the white sauce. Repeat three times. Top with the remaining walnut powder. Serve, or dehydrate for 4 hours to concentrate the flavors then serve.

Angel Hair with Marinara

I have always been a strong believer that the key to pasta is in the sauce and not in the pasta. Spaghetti is just flour and water, much like papier-mâché. The noodles are just a carrier. Serve with a green salad and Italian dressing...

Serves 4

2 large zucchini

1 large yellow summer squash

1 large, fat carrot

1 large red beet

Pinch of sun-dried sea salt

2 cups Red Sauce

½ cup pine nuts, finely ground

½ cup pitted olives, sliced

¼ cup loosely packed fresh basil leaves, chopped

5 dry-packed sun-dried tomatoes, soaked in water until soft, drained, and finely chopped

Herbed Essence Bread, cut into triangle-shaped slices, for serving

Use a spiralizer to create spaghetti-like "pasta" or a vegetable peeler to create linguini-style "pasta" of the zucchini, squash, carrot, and beet. Rinse the vegetables well and soak in water with the salt for 1 hour. Drain. In each of four serving bowls, place one quarter of the vegetables. Pour ½ cup of the red sauce over each serving. Top each serving with some of the pine nuts, olives, basil, and sun-dried tomatoes. Serve with the bread.

Desserts

Raw Fruit Pies

No one is really certain who made the first raw fruit pie. I learned from Lenny Watson, Lenny learned from Victoras Kulvinskas, and who knows where Victoras found out about it—haven't asked him yet. All I know is that it just keeps getting better. Our pies at the Raw Experience were "to live for" and many knew us as the folks who put the pie in Paia. These pie recipes below are really just guides. Be inspired and be creative and your talent will amaze you.

Serves 8 (Makes one 9-inch pie)

Carob Almond Crust

1 cup sprouted almonds

5 seeded, soaked dates, drained

¼ teaspoon ground cinnamon

¼ teaspoon ground allspice

1 tablespoon raw carob powder

or

Walnut Zing Crust

1 cup sprouted walnuts

5 seeded, soaked dates, drained

¼ teaspoon ground cinnamon

¼ teaspoon freshly grated lemon zest

or

Praline Crust

1 cup sprouted pecans

5 seeded, soaked dates, drained

¼ teaspoon pure vanilla extract

¼ teaspoon nutmeg

or

Nut-Free Crust

1 cup dried banana pieces

5 seeded, soaked dates, drained

½ cup soaked raisins, drained

¼ teaspoon ground cinnamon

¼ teaspoon ground allspice

Oil, for greasing pan (optional)

Raw carob powder, for sprinkling

Nut Crème

5 dates, seeded

1 cup filtered water

1 cup soaked nuts (such as cashews, almonds, or hazelnuts, drained

4 cups fresh fruit pieces (such as blueberries, papaya, banana, cherimoya, sapote, or shredded coconut)

½ cup berries, for garnish

1 papaya, peeled, seeded, and sliced, for garnish

To prepare any of the four crusts, place all of the ingredients in a food processor and pulse a few times to combine. Continue grinding until the mixture forms a thick paste. Oil or moisten with water a 9-inch pie plate and sprinkle with the carob powder to coat (the carob powder helps keep the pie crust from sticking to the plate). Form the crust mixture into a ball and press it from the center of the pie plate out toward the edges, spreading as evenly as possible. Set aside.

To prepare the nut crème, place the dates in a small bowl, cover with the water, and soak for about 1 hour, or until soft. Drain, reserving ¼ cup of the liquid. Place the dates, reserved liquid, and nuts in a blender or blender cup, and grind until smooth.

To prepare the fruit, you may slice the fruit, puree the fruit, leave it whole, or any combination of the three. Fill the pie crust with the prepared fruit. Top with the nut creme and garnish with the berries and papaya slices, arranged in a sunburst formation.

Coconut Custard

This smooth and creamy dessert is a Hawaiian specialty. In old Hawaii, it was a custom to plant five coconut trees for each child born. This was to provide all of the basic food, clothing, and shelter they would need. Today there is an abundance of coconuts in Hawaii, and this custard is a true "local kine" recipe.

Serves 2 to 4

3 dates, seeded

½ cup filtered water

2 cups young coconut meat

1 teaspoon pure vanilla extract

Place the dates in a small bowl, cover with the water, and soak for about 1 hour, or until soft. In a blender cup or small food processor, blend the dates along with their soaking water, the coconut, and the vanilla into a smooth custard. Spoon into individual bowls, cover, refrigerate until chilled, and serve.

Frozen Fudge

This fudge is sweet and semiaddictive. Many of my students love this recipe and make it a daily staple in their homes. This stuff tastes so good and melts in your mouth—just be careful not to eat too much!

Serves 6 to 10

1 cup dates, seeded

1½ cups filtered water

1 tablespoon pure vanilla extract

1½ cups nut butter (such as almond or hazelnut)

1½ cups raw carob powder

½ cup dried shredded coconut

Place the dates in a bowl, cover with the water, and soak for about 1 hour, or until soft. Drain, reserving the liquid. In a blender, blend the dates and vanilla until smooth, slowly adding soaking water as needed to form a creamy consistency. Transfer the date mixture into a large bowl, add the nut butter, and stir to combine. In a separate bowl, mix the carob and coconut. Gradually add the dry carob mixture into the wet date mixture. Stir well. Press evenly into a 10 by 18-inch brownie pan, 1 inch thick, and freeze until firm, about 3 hours. To serve, cut into 1-inch squares.

Oat-Date Rawies

It's great to be able to make quick and tasty desserts. These simple treats keep well and are fabulous to break out when unexpected company stops in for a rawie and a glass of nut mylk.

Serves 4 to 6

2 cups sprouted oats

1 cup seeded, soaked dates, drained

1 cup soaked raisins, drained

1 tablespoon ground cinnamon

Using a homogenizing juicer, homogenize the oats and dates until smooth and place in a large bowl. Stir in the raisins and cinnamon. For each rawie, form 2 tablespoons of the dough into a ball, place on a drying tray, and press into a ½-inch round. Repeat for the remaining rawies. Using one of the methods described on page 405, dehydrate the rawies for 18 hours, or until dry.

—From *The Raw Truth*

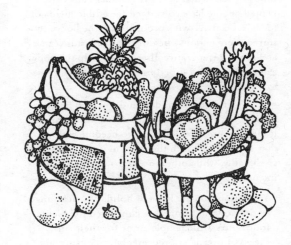

Continued →

FASTING
Jeremy Safron

What is Fasting?

Fasting allows our body to heal itself. It is the practice of cleansing through the consumption of specific substances. By putting less in, we are able to focus on healing and being, rather than eating and doing. Ingesting only pure food or water of a certain type allows the body to heal and recover faster. A massive amount of daily energy goes to processing the things we consume. When we choose to eat very simply, the body can go to work removing obstacles and clearing toxic debris.

There are actually only two types of disease—assimilation or elimination. That is to say, you are either getting less of what you need or you are holding on to unwanted material that must be removed. Certain fasting practices allow your body the opportunity to remove harmful toxic substances, while others help you obtain the necessary components to heal, rejuvenate, and function in an optimal way.

The concept of "less is best" is the faster's adage. When we do not use parts of our body, those parts are given a better opportunity to heal. Although in some beliefs fasting is the consumption of nothing at all, any abstention or austerity can be a form of fasting. Fasting brings us closer to ourselves and offers us the opportunity to press the reset button on our body and life. By fasting, we can create new beginnings. A fast is an opportunity to come into greater self-knowledge and self-discipline. By fasting, we get to know ourselves in new ways and define our future. Fasting is a time of rejuvenation and rebirth. Life is renewed and health is restored by bringing the body and its organs back into ideal functioning.

One may not reach the dawn save by the path of night.
— *The Prophet*, Khalil Gibran

Why Fast?

People fast for a variety of reasons—primarily for physical health, spiritual practice, emotional expression, and brain power. Because of the pollutants in the Western world, much of the air and food is poisoned, and many commercially corrupted people have consumed the edible media of today's society. Toxins brought into the body are stored there and may lie dormant and cause cancer and other degenerative diseases. To help the body extend its life and function more optimally, these toxins must be removed.

Many religious holidays and spiritual practices require fasting as a part of the ceremony. Spiritual leaders around the world fast to become empty so they can be filled with the spirit of god. Some fasts are lengthy, while others are short. Some examples include:

Yom Kippur is the Hebrew holiday of cleansing, where no food or drink is consumed for twenty-four hours while people atone for their sins. Pieces of bread, as a representation of sins, are cast out into flowing water to be cast out of the body and soul.

Ramadan is an Islamic holiday where only water is consumed from sunrise until sundown for thirty days.

Lent is a Christian holy time where a certain type of food is given up for six weeks to help atone for sin and to share in the events that occurred before the Resurrection.

In preparation for Native American sweat lodges, participants fast to get ready for this purification ritual.

People who find themselves in emotionally exaggerated situations choose not to eat food because so much of their energy is focused on the challenge at hand. On the other hand, when people are happy, they require less food.

Fasting can also help the mind maintain focus. By not spending extra energy to digest food, that energy can be added to our brain power to help us stay clear for such things as exams, public speaking, important meetings, or crucial events.

Planning a Fast

To properly heal and cleanse our body, it is important to properly plan a fast. Planning for a fast can be relatively simple or highly complex depending on the type and length of the fast. The first thing to do is decide what kind of fast you want to experience and how long you will remain on this fast.

Once you decide on a fast, it is important to make certain that you have all the items you need to follow the fast to completion. If you are planning to do some of the more intense fasts, make sure someone knows about it and is able to assist you if needed. For some fasts, it is important to have free time to process and cleanse, so if you choose a more rapid practice, it is beneficial to have only one obligation, healing.

Some of the fasts in this book allow you to continue with your daily life, while others require that you be at home relaxing. It is important to choose a fast that complements your current lifestyle. You will find that when healing is needed, the opportunity presents itself. If you are planning any organ cleanses or wish to gain the assistance of healers (for example, massage or colonic), be sure to schedule these in advance.

It is often beneficial to begin a fast with the new moon. The new moon is a symbol of beginnings and change. If you are creating a fourteen-day fast, it's nice to start with the new moon and to begin to eat (breakfast) on the full moon.

A fast is a time of purification. Choose to take space on your own to reflect within and gain innerstanding.

Starting and Ending a Fast

The opening and closing of a fast are crucial to how the body rejuvenates and recovers. It is very important to be gentle with your body. A good rule of thumb is to take twice as long coming out of a fast as going into one. When you begin to fast, it is often helpful to lessen the intake of food at meals and to spread your meals farther apart (possibly even cut back to one major meal a day). It is also helpful to eat food that contains a high water content. Food containing a high water content will help your body become more ready to begin your cleanse.

When concluding a fast, it is important to begin to reintroduce the proper digestive bacteria and to get your digestion flowing again. Juices and fruits are great fast breakers, and then you can move to sprouted and cultured foods to bring the digestive bacteria back in line and renew metabolic processes.

Patience is a virtue, and when we move into a cleansing process, our mind becomes resistant and attempts to reengage a pattern of imbalance. It can take a great amount of will power to begin a fast and even more to continue it, but it is ending a fast that is most challenging. It is crucial to break a fast in a slow and even way. Take your time and adjust to eating again. Many a great fast is ended incorrectly by jumping right back into food because of desire or outside influences. The breaking of a fast is sacred and, if done correctly, allows our body to heal and develop in powerful new ways.

If a fast is broken incorrectly, it can actually concentrate toxins in the body and cause further ailments. It is important to be realistic and only set goals for a fast that you know you can achieve. Start small and do a few one- to three-day fasts before beginning a lengthy fast. Be prepared and plan your fast well, and it will be a joyful and rejuvenating experience.

Length of a Fast

The length of a fast is always based on an individual's situation. The cleaner our body, the longer we can fast, and the easier it will be to fast. The question of how you know when to break your fast is very personal. When first fasting, it is best to create a fasting program that you know to be within your potential to complete. Once you have experimented with different fasts and cleanses, you can go as long as possible, or until your body has cleaned out.

One way to know that the body is clean is that a very sweet taste begins to appear in the mouth and your sweat smells very fragrant. Another great method for knowing the body is clean is that real hunger begins to surface. Real hunger is your interest in taking in nourishment through food, as opposed to false hunger, which is based on cravings due to addiction.

Long-term fasting is often used to clear away old patterns and to free the body of toxins. Some experts believe that as long as it took you to get where you are, it will take equally as long to get back. This means that, if you ate toxic foods for twenty years, it will take twenty years of eating good food for your body to naturally detoxify. Fasting gives you the ability to remove toxins at a far more rapid rate. Some of the fasts in this book remove toxins at a rate of two to one, while others are more like one hundred to one (one hundred days of toxic intake removed in one day).

Lengthy fasts can truly bring our body back to a healthy set point. From there, we can build our body into our ideal self.

Maintenance fasting is the practice of fasting for short periods of time, such as one day a week, once a month, or on the full moon. This type of fasting is used to give the body a rest and the opportunity to rejuvenate, whereas lengthy fasts put the body into rapid detox. Maintenance fasts are very useful once you have cleansed your body and help keep you functioning at an optimal level.

Short-term fasts are often used to gain focus and spiritual power or to give us the opportunity to experience ourselves. During the first day of a cleanse, you are often still processing the previous day's consumptions. Short fasts can give your body the chance to catch up and get back to empty before you start eating again.

There is great power to be gained by fasting; use it wisely.

Continued ➡

Mental and Emotional Detoxification

There are many reasons why toxins and other harmful substances stay in the body. When toxic minerals or chemicals enter your system, your body often cannot deal with processing them all at once. Your body will remove what it can and store the test away to be dealt with at a future date. Many people who live a toxic lifestyle do not give their body an opportunity to process out this old waste. Eventually, this waste builds up until the person dies of internal poisoning or the body creates a tumor or growth.

Extreme emotion can also store toxins in the body. Even the small amount of airborne toxins or toxic household items may be locked into the body by emotion. Sometimes when under stress, people consume toxic foods (junk food, meat, synthetic food). Often emotions act like glue, keeping this toxic material in the body. When fasting and cleansing, it is necessary to release these emotions. Some people fast, and, when their emotions surface, they start eating or don't deal with their emotions and are unable to release the toxic material stored in the body. Sometimes self-reassurance or affirmations can help in releasing and rebuilding our body. It is very important to go through the emotional detox when fasting. Thoughts, memories, and feelings that come up want to be processed and dealt with. It may be challenging, yet on the other side of the resurfacing issue is a healing on every level. When the feeling is recognized and transformed, it allows a great amount of toxic matter stored in the body to be released and purified out of the body. Many toxic thoughts and visual and auditory stimuli can also cause poisons around us to get stored away in the body. Cleaning up our language and making healthy choices about what we want to expose ourselves to can lead to great cleansing. By making changes in our inner self, we change what our body is made of. You are what you eat, and you are also what you think and feel.

Fasting with a Partner

It can often be helpful to have a fasting partner. This person can inspire you to be strong in times of cleansing and can be a companion to share juice or prana or whatever you might be fasting on. Fasting together is a wonderful way to bond with your mate. Fasting as a family can bring greater community to the home. Fasting partners are a bountiful source of moral support. While fasting, it is important to go through emotional cleansing. Having someone there to talk to and process with is very strengthening.

Fasting Alone

When fasting alone, it is a good idea to tell someone you are going on a fast (a friend, spouse, or family member). This person can help give you support by asking you how the fast is going and will often be inspired to fast as well (and then you have a fasting partner). By letting someone know you are fasting, you can call on him or her if you need something (like more oranges or an enema bag). This is especially helpful if you are taking quiet time while fasting and don't wish to go to town. Letting someone know you are fasting also helps hold space for your successful cleanse.

Types of Fasts and Fasting Ceremonies

The following is a collection of various fasting techniques. As with all things, use common sense and remember that it is a sign of wisdom to ask questions of those with a larger range of experience. In this part of the book, you will find explanations of certain fasts, as well as recipes and a day-by-day fasting schedule. These techniques lead you into and out of the actual fast. The "Fasting On" section contains fasts in which only certain foods are consumed. The "Fasting From" section is an austerity guide that you can use to remove items from daily intake. Feel free to use these fasts as a starting point to create your own custom-tailored fast.

Fasting On

AIR

Air or dry fasting is the consumption of no food or water whatsoever for a specified period of time. Dry fasting is often done for short periods of time. Animals in the wild when recovering from injury or in later stages of disease will dry fast. This is sometimes due to the fact that the animal cannot get to a food or water source or all the animal's energy is required for healing. We can survive for months without food, for days without water, yet only minutes without air. Air contains prana or chi, a universal energy source that can nourish a body. Many great yogis can survive purely on prana. When we are in dire need of cleansing and healing, it can be of great benefit to minimize consumption. This gives the body the opportunity to truly heal and recover. Air fasts are probably the most intense and are only recommended for the experienced faster. Be certain that you have a fasting coach or partner for this type of fast.

Dry Fast

	Breakfast	Lunch	Dinner
Day 1 in	Fruit	Smoothie	Juice
Day 2 in	Juice	Juice	Juice
Day 3 in	Consume as much water as possible before beginning dry fast.		
Day 4	Consume only air and breathe deeply. Continue for only one day.		
Day 1 out	Water (sip slowly)	Juice	Juice
Day 2 out	Juice	Juice	Juice
Day 3 out	Juice	Smoothie	Smoothie
Day 4 out	Juice	Smoothie	Fruit
Day 5 out	Begin to return to a balanced diet including sprouts and fermented foods.		

WATER

Water fasting is the process of consuming only water. When you water-fast, you are flushing out the toxins stored in the body. Water fasting is the quickest way to cleanse and purify the system. Since you will be constantly flowing water through the body to carry away toxins, it is extremely helpful to do a kidney cleanse before beginning a water fast. It is very important when you are water fasting to have a good source of water. The best water sources are reverse osmosis, charged water, and distilled water. The more alkaline the water, the greater the healing benefits. You can create alkaline water (7 pH and above) by following the recipe that follows. Water fasting is a traditional fast, since many people consider water to be the ultimate healer. Your body is more than 80 percent water, and by consuming large amounts of pure water, your body has the ability to rejuvenate faster. It is ideal to consume as much water as possible to get the greatest benefits.

CHARGED WATER

1 glass gallon jar
1 gallon distilled water (with no minerals)
1 quartz crystal (well formed and naturally grown)
7 fresh-cut blades of wheatgrass
3 teaspoons seawater or one pinch sea salt

Place all ingredients in the glass jar. Leave the jar out in the sun for at least one day. (Full moon-charged water is great too!) Your water is now charged.

Water Fast

	Breakfast	Lunch	Dinner
Day 1 in	Fruit	Smoothie	Juice
Day 2 in	Juice	Juice	Juice
Day 3 in	Water	Water	Water
Day 4	Continue on only water for as long as desired.		
Day 1 out	Juice	Juice	Juice
Day 2 out	Juice	Juice	Juice
Day 3 out	Juice	Smoothie	Smoothie
Day 4 out	Juice	Smoothie	Fruit
Day 5 out	Fruit	Fruit	Fruit
Day 6 out	Begin to return to a balanced diet including sprouts and fermented foods.		

COCONUT WATER

The water from the nut of the coconut palm is almost identical to human blood plasma (which makes up 55 percent of our blood). Coconut water is naturally filtered by a tree for more than nine months and is sealed sterile inside of the shell. Coco water fasting is easier on the body than pure water fasting because of the rich organic minerals and micronutrients contained within. Therefore, the body can go far longer on coco water than on distilled water. Coconut water is one of the highest natural sources of electrolytes and allows the body to maintain a balance of energy and exist in an alkaline environment.

Coconut Water Fast

	Breakfast	Lunch	Dinner
Day 1 in	Fruit	Smoothie	Juice
Day 2 in	Juice	Juice	Juice
Day 3	Consume as much coconut water as possible for as long as you choose.		
Day 1 out	Juice	Juice	Juice
Day 2 out	Juice	Smoothie	Smoothie
Day 3 out	Juice	Smoothie	Fruit
Day 4 out	Begin to return to a balanced diet including sprouts and fermented foods.		

GRASS

Grass fasting is the consumption of only chlorophyll-rich grasses. Grasses such as wheat, corn, rye, and oat all provide a wealth of nutrition as well as a high concentration of chlorophyll. Grass fasts are great for removing toxins from the intestinal wall and breaking up old mucoid matter. Grass fasts can also help build the body. Wheatgrass, for example, can provide all the necessary nutrition to the body

Continued →

and is considered a whole food or superfood. All amino acids and basic proteins ate contained within grasses. Grasses are also great for colonic implants. Fasting on grass can cause the body to detoxify at a more rapid rate. When undergoing a grass fast, dizziness and nausea often accompany the cleanse because of the amount of toxins released.

Grass Fast

	Breakfast	Lunch	Dinner
Day 1 in	Fruit	Blender soup	Juice
Day 2 in	Grass	Juice	Juice
Day 3 in	Grass	Grass	Grass
Day 4	Continue on only grass for as long as desired.		
Day 1 out	Grass	Juice	Juice
Day 2 out	Grass	Juice	Juice
Day 3 out	Grass	Juice	Blender soup
Day 4 out	Grass	Smoothie	Soup
Day 5 out	Grass	Smoothie	Salad
Day 6 out	Begin to return to a balanced diet including sprouts and fermented foods.		

LEMONADE OR MASTER CLEANSER

Fasting using lemonade is highly beneficial because of the enormously high alkalinity of lemons. Master Cleanser is a variation of lemonade that adds spice to induce internal cleansing and works as a vasodilator (opening veins and arteries). Both cleansers are effective.

MASTER CLEANSER

½ cup lemon juice

¼ teaspoon cayenne powder

Honey, dates, or maple syrup for sweetening

Place ail ingredients in a one-gallon glass jar and shake. Sweeten to taste with honey, dates, or maple syrup.

Makes 1 gallon

ELECTROLYTE LEMONADE

1 gallon charged water

½ cup lemon juice

¼ teaspoon sea salt

⅛ teaspoon vanilla

¼ teaspoon flax oil (butterscotch)

Honey, dates, or maple syrup for sweetening

Place all ingredients in a gallon glass jar and shake well. Sweeten to taste with honey, dates, or maple syrup.

Makes 1 gallon

JUICE

Juice fasting is one of the more traditional long-term fasts. Juice fasting is the consumption of only juice. Juice provides a wide range of nutrients to help sustain the body during periods of abstinence from food. Through juice fasting, it is possible to live your daily life and still be on a cleanse. It is important to be certain that you can get as much juice as you want. Juice fasting can only be done with fresh juices. Packaged or bottled juices often are pasteurized (no enzymes). It is important to use only organic juices. The juice of a sprayed or chemically fertilized vegetable can have five times as many toxins as its whole unjuiced counterpart.

Juice fasting is highly beneficial for cleansing the cells. Juice is essentially organic water distilled

Lemonade or Master Cleanser Fast

	Breakfast	Lunch	Dinner
Day 1 in	Fruit	Blender soup	Juice
Day 2 in	Juice	Juice	Juice
Day 3	Consume as much lemonade or master cleanser as desired for as long as you choose.		
Day 1 out	Lemonade	Juice	Juice
Day 2 out	Juice	Juice	Juice
Day 3 out	Juice	Smoothie	Blender soup
Day 4 out	Juice	Blender soup	Salad
Day 5 out	Begin to return to a balanced diet including sprouts and fermented foods.		

Mono Juice Fast

	Breakfast	Lunch	Dinner
Day 1 in	Fruit	Blender soup	Juice
Day 2 in	Juice	Blender soup	Juice
Day 3	Choose one type of juice and continue for as long as you choose.		
Day 1 out	Juice	Juice	Juice
Day 2 out	Juice	Juice	Blender soup
Day 3 out	Juice	Juice	Blender soup
Day 4 out	Juice	Smoothie	Soup
Day 5 out	Juice	Smoothie	Salad
Day 6 out	Begin to return to a balanced diet including sprouts and fermented foods.		

Multijuice Fast

	Breakfast	Lunch	Dinner
Day 1 in	Fruit	Blender soup	Juice
Day 2 in	Juice	Blender soup	Juice
Day 3	Choose from the list of combinations and continue for as long as you choose. As a general guideline, it is helpful to use fruit juices in the morning, vegetable juices in the afternoon, and return to fruit juices in the evening. If working with sugar imbalances, kidney disorders, or yeast/candida, focus mostly on nonsweet or starchy fruit and vegetable juices.		
Day 1 out	Juice	Juice	Juice
Day 2 out	Juice	Juice	Blender soup
Day 3 out	Juice	Juice	Blender soup
Day 4 out	Juice	Smoothie	Soup
Day 5 out	Juice	Smoothie	Salad
Day 6 out	Begin to return to a balanced diet including sprouts and fermented foods.		

by a plant with organic vitamins, cell salts, and minerals concentrated in it. Organic water is plant processed and filtered rather than machine filtered. Plants spend many months filtering the water that becomes stored in their leaves, stems, roots, and fruits. By providing clean water, the cells can easily release toxins and cleanse any unwanted substances from the body. Some juice fasts are done on only one type of juice (usually short term), while some are done on combinations. Traditional juice fasts are done for 7, 14, 30, 60, 90, and even 120 days. Juice will oxidize very quickly if made in a centrifugal juicer and must be consumed immediately. Juicing in a masticating or tricherating juicer will oxidize in about two to eight hours, and pressed juice will last as long as twenty-four hours before losing most of its value. The more vital the juice, the more nourishment it can provide the body. Fresh juice is rejuvenating and detoxifying on a cellular level and is a powerful way to heal and renew the body.

Jeremy's Favorite Juices and Combos

WATERMELON

Watermelons have the highest content of cellular-contained water of any fruit. This makes them ideal for fasting and cleansing. Watermelon juice is very refreshing, and its high water content helps remove toxic debris on a cellular level. Watermelon can be juiced with the rind for chlorophyll and to help cleanse the liver. Melon juice is best done separately from other juices because of the rapid rate of absorption into the body through the stomach lining. If possible, press or blend your watermelon juice to maintain integrity and reduce oxidation.

PANINI

Panini, also known as the prickly pear, is the fruit of a cactus. This fruit has similar benefits to aloe vera. The fruit comes in green and purple and is extremely sweet. It has many small seeds and juices quite well in a Champion juicer or a juice press. The panini is covered in many tiny, thorny spines, so be very careful when handling it. It is best to peel it before juicing. Cut off the top and bottom and then slice a line down one end and peel back the skin. Put the fruit through the juicer and enjoy.

GREEN PAPAYA

Green papaya contains a plethora of enzymes. This fruit is so enzymatically active that it can digest itself and many other foods including old material (especially proteins). Papaya seeds themselves are a vermifuge, an agent that causes the expulsion of worms and parasites from the body. To juice the green papaya, cut off the top where the stem is and then cut it lengthwise in half. Scoop out the seeds and save some for blending. Cut the papaya into strips for juicing or into chunks for blending. The papaya can be juiced with or without the skin. Although the skin is bitter, it has many healing benefits such as tannins (antioxidants) and extra high enzyme activity. Use caution when ingesting papaya skin, as the enzymes can actually burn your tongue.

Sweet Grass

PINEAPPLE AND WHEATGRASS

Pineapples are extremely high in bromelain, a crucial enzyme in the breaking down of foods. Bromelain can help digest food and can often settle the stomach. Wheatgrass, one of nature's simplest medicines, is a great source of chlorophyll and other vital minerals. The combination of the two is less detoxifying than straight wheatgrass but has a great taste. Combine 15 ounces of pineapple juice with one ounce of wheatgrass juice. Stir and enjoy.

Continued ➡

Volcano Blood Builder

Coconut ꞏ Wheatgrass ꞏ Beet

Coconut water is almost identical in composition to human blood plasma. You can drink it, or it can be used intravenously (plasma makes up 55 percent of our blood). Wheatgrass juice is one of the highest sources of chlorophyll. Human hemin (the source of hemoglobin, the oxygen carrier) is very similar to chlorophyll; in fact, molecularly they differ by only one molecule (magnesium in plants and iron in humans). By combining the water of one coconut and one ounce of wheatgrass juice with two ounces of beet juice (a great source of iron), a healing and rejuvenating drink can be made. This drink synthesizes almost 77 percent of human blood.

Citrus

Citrus juice is extremely helpful in digesting old material, especially plaque and calcifications. Citrus is the sun bearer and offers a wide variety of vitamins (especially rich in vitamin C). Citric acid helps in the processing of fats and oils and can assist the liver in cleansing and help break down gallstones.

Grape

Grape juice is an excellent rejuvenator. Grapes can be juiced or ground in a Vita-Mix to produce a delicious juice with a delightful texture. Grapes are best juiced with their seeds (Concord grapes are some of my favorites). The grape seed is very high in picnogynols, a powerful antioxidant.

Apple, Cucumber, and Kale

Apples are abundantly rich in pectin and are very alkaline. Cucumbers are a vine fruit with many seeds containing large amounts of silica and magnesium, as well as high concentrations of organic sodium. Kale is a dark, rich, leafy green providing tons of iron and chlorophyll. This combo is great for people working on cleansing on a cellular level who want to avoid concentrated sugars. You can drink this juice two or three times a day with mild results to the digestive system and still provide yourself with an abundance of energy and nutrition. Combine one part kale juice with two parts apple juice and two parts cucumber juice. Stir and enjoy.

Aloe, Lime, and Celery

Aloe vera is a powerful healer and a member of the succulent family (a type of cactus). Aloe is extremely high in mucopolysaccharides and saponins. Aloe has very bitter taste, though the taste varies depending on the strain. Aloe vera juice is a wonderful detoxifier and flushes toxins from the bloodstream. Aloe also helps heal the lining of the stomach, which can get damaged by extreme acidity. The cells are made more permeable and can release intercellular toxins more easily after regular use of aloe vera juice. Lime is an excellent way to increase alkalinity, and the citric acid helps break down old fats, assisting the liver and gallbladder in their functioning. Celery, like cucumber, is a fantastic source of organic sodium and contains a good amount of chlorophyll. This combo, if made properly, is delicious and a strong way to rejuvenate the body from the cells to the organs. Combine three parts celery juice with one part aloe juice and one part lime juice. Stir and enjoy.

Apple, Celery, and Ginger

Apples and celery are covered in the two previous juice combinations. Ginger is a fantastic bronchial aid and a vasodilator. That means that it helps open up the bronchi in the lungs, and the veins and capillaries are also widened. Ginger also increases internal heat and warms the body as well as helps to eliminate parasites and blood toxins. Combine four parts apple juice with four parts celery juice and one part ginger juice. Stir and enjoy.

Soup

Fasting on soup is practiced by blending everything you consume. Soup fasting is excellent because you can do it for extended amounts of time. Soup in many ways is easier for the body to digest, since it is already fully masticated (chewed). When you are doing a soup fast, it is best to have a strong blender. It is a good idea to mix soup with salivary amylase in the mouth before swallowing and follow the adage "chew your drinks and drink your food." Salivary amylase is an enzyme found in human saliva that breaks down starch to sugar. It is very easy to come off a soup fast because you always keep your body working by giving it food. If you fast on soup for an extended amount of time—six months or many years—take at least twenty-eight days to move back into eating.

Soup Fast

	Breakfast	Lunch	Dinner
Day 1 in	Fruit	Blender soup	Soup
Day 2 in	Juice	Blender soup	Soup
Day 3	Choose a variety of soups and continue for as long as you choose.		
Day 1 out	Juice	Soup	Soup with avocado chunks
Day 2 out	Papaya	Soup	Soup with avocado chunks
Day 3 out	Papaya	Soup	Paté
Day 4 out	Fruit	Paté	Paté and avocado
Day 5 out	Fruit	Paté	Salad
Day 6 out	Fruit	Paté	Salad and sprouts

Sensational Soups

To prepare the following soup recipes, place all ingredients in a blender or Vita-Mix and pulse blend until the pieces are chopped up. Then blend until smooth and serve.

Tom Yum Ghai

2 cups fresh young coconut meat

2 cups coconut water

1 small hot pepper

1 inch of ginger root

1 cup mixed herbs (oregano, cilantro, basil, parsley)

3 teaspoons shoyu or salt

Dr. Ann's Energy Soup

1 ripe avocado

1 ripe papaya

1 handful of sprouts

2 tablespoons dulse flakes

1 tablespoon spirulina

Add water to blend.

Curried Cauliflower

2 cups diced cauliflower

1 large avocado or the meat of one coconut

1 small handful of cilantro

1 heaping teaspoon tahini

1 teaspoon honey

3 teaspoons Braggs Liquid Aminos or salt

1 heaping tablespoon curry powder

Add water to blend.

Carrot-Ginger Soup

2 cups carrot juice

1 large ripe avocado

2 teaspoons Braggs or 1 teaspoon shoyu

1 small handful of parsley or cilantro

1 inch of ginger root

Pesto Soup

1 cup grated carrot and beet, mixed

1 cup tomato, diced

1 handful of dry walnuts

1 to 2 teaspoons miso

1 teaspoon nutritional yeast

2 sun-dried tomatoes, soaked

Pinch of onion

1 small clove of garlic

5 large basil leaves

Add water to blend.

Sprouts

Sprouts are one of the most powerful healers on the planet. Sprouts such as wheatgrass contain high amounts of chlorophyll and help carry oxygen throughout our body. Sprouts provide an abundant amount of life force and nutrition. It is excellent to eat sprouts that you have grown yourself. You can do a sprout fast by drinking green juice or sprout juice for two or three days, and then eat sprouts you have grown yourself to break the fast.

Sprouts are highly rejuvenating and bring vital nutrients to the cells. They also remove harmful toxins and free radicals from the body in safe and easy ways. Every seed, nut, bean, and grain is sproutable, and each sprout provides its own range of vitamins and minerals. It is a good plan to eat a variety of sprouts while fasting. Some of my favorite sprouts are Sunflower, sesame, almond, buckwheat, garbanzo, and mung. Sprouts are the beginning of life for a plant and are bioactivated seeds. The seed is the plant's potential energy, and the sprout is that life force unleashed.

Sprout Fast

	Breakfast	Lunch	Dinner
Day 1 in	Fruit	Soup	Bowl of sprouts
Day 2 in	Juice	Soup	Bowl of sprouts
Day 3	Eat a variety of sprouts for as long as two weeks at a time. Create sprout drinks, soups, and salads.		
Day 1 out	Sprout juice	Sprout soup	Bowl of sprouts
Day 2 out	Sprout juice	Soup	Bowl of sprouts
Day 3 out	Juice	Soup w/ avocado chunks	Bowl of sprouts
Day 4 out	Juice	Kim chi	Sprout paté and avocado
Day 5 out	Juice	Paté	Salad and sprouts
Day 6 out	Smoothie	Paté	Salad and sprouts

Continued ➡

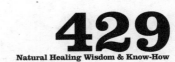

Fruit

Fruit fasting is a fun fast where only fruit is eaten. Some fruit fasts are done as mono meals, eating only one fruit at a time. Other fruit fasts use many fruits in different combinations. Fruit fasting is suggested in warm climates where fresh fruit is available. Fruit fasts can be done for extended periods to allow the body and cells to cleanse themselves by bathing in clean organic water provided by the fruit. Organic water has an easier time entering and exiting the cell, thereby bringing nourishment into the cell and removing toxins efficiently. When fasting on a variety of fruit, it is good to maintain a balance of sweet fruits such as mangoes, cherimoyas, and other tropical fruits with cucumbers, tomatoes, and melons. It is also excellent to eat fatty fruits such as olives or avocados to maintain protein and fat content while fasting. Multifruit fasts can be continued for lengthy periods such as one month to one year even if only one type of fruit is eaten at a time. Mono fruit fasts (one kind of fruit for the whole fast) are best done for three days to one month maximum. For further fruit suggestions, see my book *The Raw Truth*, (Ten Speed Press, 2003).

Fruit Fast

	Breakfast	Lunch	Dinner
Day 1 in	Fruit	Salad with avocado	Anything raw
Day 2 in	Smoothie	Fruit	Fruit salad with nuts
Day 3	Eat a variety of fruits or just one and continue for as long as you choose.		
Day 1 out	Fruit	Fruit	Fruit with nut kreme
Day 2 out	Fruit	Fruit	Fruit with nut kreme
Day 3 out	Fruit	Fruit with nut kreme	Veggie soup
Day 4 out	Fruit	Fruit with nut kreme	Veggie soup
Day 5 out	Fruit with nuts	Paté with avocado	Salad
Day 6 out	Fruit	Paté	Salad and sprouts

Nutrition (Living Food)

Fasting on nutrition is accomplished by consuming only food designed to provide the maximum amount of nutrition. Many foods these days are referred to as superfoods. These foods provide an abundance of vitamins, minerals, protein, fats, and carbs and usually have a tremendous amount of life force and energy. Sometimes the needs of your body can be met in a more efficient way. Nutritional deficiencies occur slowly as your body uses stores of nutrients. Providing concentrated nutrition lets your body store away what might be needed at a later date. Dr. Ann Wigmore is famous for saying that 85 percent of the nutritional value of food is destroyed by cooking it. That means that people eat eight to ten times as much food as they need in order to get the proper nourishment. By consuming food that provides maximum nutrition with minimum waste, you offer your body the opportunity to do less and be more effective. Some of the finest sources of nutrition are spirulina, bee pollen, kelp, hot peppers, sea vegetables, nutritional yeast, avocado, flaxseeds, hemp seeds, papaya, wheatgrass, sprouts, coconut water, green juices, and sprouted coconut.

In order to fast on nutrition, you consume only raw food. You eat as much from the above listed items as possible, and eat one to two meals a day of energy pudding. Nutritional fasting can be done for extended periods of time (one to six months).

ENERGY PUDDING

In a food processor blend: 1 to 2 avocados, 1 hot pepper, 3 teaspoons spirulina or other algae, 3 teaspoons nutritional yeast, 1 pinch of Celtic sea salt, 1 teaspoon dulse or kelp, 1 teaspoon lemon juice, 1 teaspoon flax or hemp oil, and some fresh sprouts or green herbs. This can be eaten on flax crackers (made from ground flaxseeds and fresh herbs dehydrated).

The purpose of this fast is to bring concentrated nutrition into the body, and it is an excellent way to live and rebuild between cleanses or during a time of focused healing. (In and out times are not required as you continue to eat raw food the whole time.)

Alkaline Substances

Fasting on alkaline substances is a great way to bring the body into a more balanced state. Your body's pH helps regulate the way bacteria interact with your body. Often, because of overconsumption of starches, meat, dairy, and chemicals or through inhaling smoke or harmful vapors, your body can become highly acidic. One good way of telling your acidity level is to look into the iris of the eye (iridology), and if there is a large amount of white lines or flecks, this suggests an acid condition. Another method of testing is to use pH or litmus paper. An acidic body is much more likely to hold onto toxins than an alkaline body. Acidic bodies are the breeding ground for all types of parasites and also create an environment that allows cancer and immune deficiencies to prosper. By consuming alkaline water and alkaline-forming food, your body becomes healthier. Some examples of alkaline food are dry figs, dry apricots, raisins, Swiss chard, dandelion greens, soy sprouts, cucumbers, avocados, almonds, and kale.

Acidic Substances

Sometimes the body gets into an extreme alkaline state, which can cause energy deficiencies and can even cause internal organs to become soft and wet (too yin). This can lead to degenerative diseases such as Crohn's or diabetes. Certain food can bring the body back into balance and create an ideal state of homeostasis. Acidic-forming food includes Jerusalem artichokes, walnuts, wheat, olives, filberts, blueberries, peas, and watermelon.

To create an alkaline or acidic fast, consume mostly or only food that creates the ideal condition and avoid food that supports the unwanted condition.

—From *The Fasting Handbook*

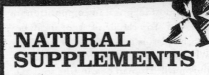

NATURAL SUPPLEMENTS
Ellen Tart-Jensen

The prime purpose of food supplements is to fill in the nutritional gaps produced by faulty eating habits and by nutritionally-inferior foods.

—Dr. Paavo Airola

In an ideal world where the topsoil layers were still deep and rich with nutrients, where foods were grown organically and free from pesticides, where air was clean and water was pure, we would not need to add supplements to our diet. Ideally, we would be able to get all of our vitamins and minerals from our foods. In today's world, however, most fruits and vegetables have been grown on very thin layers of soil, watered with polluted water, and heavily sprayed with chemicals. Most meat has high doses of antibiotics and hormones, and much of our world's water has had toxic wastes dumped into it. Even organic foods in our health food stores are many days old and the vitamin content has been significantly reduced. In addition, many families are so rushed and hurried they don't take the time to properly prepare healthy meals or don't have access to natural organic foods. Food supplements help replace important vitamins and minerals that are sorely lacking in our diets today. They also help protect us from the poisonous elements in our foods, water, and air. Supplements can help strengthen our immune systems and strengthen our bodies so they become resistant to viruses, bacteria, and fungi. The tool kits in this chapter provide you with knowledge about vitamins, minerals, and superfood supplements and the roles they play in building good health. They will help you understand symptoms you would have if these nutrients were missing and give you suggestions for foods that provide them. I am all for getting as much as we can from foods. But if eating the foods does not eliminate the health condition, these vitamins, minerals, and superfood supplements can also be purchased at most health food stores. Consult a knowledgeable nutritionist or natural health practitioner for additional guidance in using any of these supplements. Remember, more of certain nutrients might be required if you fighting an illness than if you are well. (For additional in-depth information on vitamins and minerals, I recommend the book *Encyclopedia of Nutritional Supplements* by Michael T. Murray, ND.)

Tool Kit for Buying Healthy Vitamins

Vitamins are essential for health and well-being. They work together with enzymes to release energy into our bodies. Vitamin deficiencies can cause illness. Be very careful when selecting vitamins. Many vitamins on the market today are synthetic and do not come from whole foods. These vitamins often contain fillers and food colorings that are not good for us. Natural vitamins come directly from foods. Our bodies are made to utilize elements from natural foods. Read labels and make sure the vitamins come from food sources. Some of the natural vitamins, including C and B complex, are water-soluble and others, including A, D, E, and K, are fat-soluble. The body cannot store water-soluble

Continued ➡

vitamins. They are excreted within hours of taking them in. The body can store fat-soluble vitamins within the liver and in fatty tissue. Since we can't be assured of getting all of our vitamins in our food, a good multiple vitamin can help supplement what we are missing. If you are ill or feel you need specific vitamins in addition to a good multiple, it is always best to consult with a natural health practitioner who can help you with your specific needs. Check with your doctor if you are taking a medication to make sure the supplement does not interfere.

Vitamin A: Fat Soluble

Vitamin A strengthens the immune system. It fights infections and helps prevent colds and flu. A powerful antioxidant, vitamin A fights free radicals and defends the body from cancer. It also lowers high cholesterol levels and prevents heart disease and stroke. Necessary for growing and maintaining skin tissue, vitamin A helps prevent acne and other skin disorders, keep the skin soft, and inhibit wrinkles. Vitamin A also promotes eye health and prevents night blindness.

Food Sources

Apricots, asparagus, beet greens, broccoli, butternut squash, carrots, chard, collards, dandelion greens, dulse, fish liver oils, kale, liver, mustard greens, papaya, peaches, pumpkin, spinach, sweet potatoes, turnip greens, watercress, and yellow squash.

Natural Supplement Sources

Beta-carotene, which is converted to vitamin A in the liver, and fish liver oil.

NOTE: Do not take more than 100,000 International Units (IU) of vitamin A for prolonged periods without supervision. A dosage this high could become toxic to the liver. If you have a liver disease, consult your physician before taking vitamin A. Pregnant women should not take more than 10,000 IUs of vitamin A daily as it may affect fetal development. Children should not take more than 10,000 IUs daily. Diabetics and people with hypothyroid function may have difficulty converting beta-carotene to vitamin A.

The B Vitamins: Water Soluble

Several different B vitamins often come in a combination called B complex. B vitamins help nourish and calm the nervous system and may relieve anxiety or depression. The B vitamins work together and should be taken together. If you need an additional amount of one of the B vitamins, take it along with a B complex.

VITAMIN B₁ (THIAMINE)

Vitamin B₁ helps keep the nervous system healthy. It metabolizes carbohydrates, assists in blood formation, improves circulation, and is necessary for good muscle tone. It also aids in the production of hydrochloric acid. Vitamin B₁ prevents beriberi, a disease of the nervous system.

Food Sources

Beans, brown rice, chicken, egg yolks, liver, nuts, peas, wheat germ, and whole grains.

Natural Supplement Sources

Brewer's yeast and rice bran.

VITAMIN B₂ (RIBOFLAVIN)

Vitamin B₂ assists in the formation of red blood cells and antibodies. It is needed for proteins, fats, and carbohydrates to metabolize. It also helps to prevent cataracts. Vitamin B₂ prevents inflammation of the tongue and mouth as well as cracks at the corners of the mouth.

Food Sources

Avocados, broccoli, cheese, dandelion greens, dulse, egg yolks, fish, goat's milk, nuts, poultry, spinach, watercress, whole grains, and yogurt.

Natural Supplement Sources

Rice bran and whole grains.

VITAMIN B₃ (NIACIN, NICOTENIC ACID, AND NIACINAMIDE)

Vitamin B₃ aids in good circulation, which helps prevent numbness in arms and legs and promotes good nerve and brain function. It also helps maintain healthy skin. Vitamin B₃ aids in proper digestion and helps lower cholesterol. Vitamin B₃ also relieves headaches and helps prevent cold sores. A deficiency of vitamin B₃ causes pellagra, which has symptoms of diarrhea, dermatitis, and dementia (a decline in mental ability).

Food Sources

Carrots, beef liver, broccoli, cornmeal, dandelion greens, potatoes, and wheat germ.

Natural Supplement Sources

Brewer's yeast, rice bran, and wheat germ.

VITAMIN B₅ (PANTOTHENIC ACID)

Vitamin B₅ boosts stamina and helps proteins, fats, and carbohydrates release energy. It also aids in proper metabolism and digestion. It assists in the production of adrenal hormones. Vitamin B₅ relieves stress, anxiety, and depression.

Food Sources

Avocados, beef, chicken, eggs, legumes, liver, mushrooms, nuts, potatoes, salmon, trout, vegetables, and yogurt.

Natural Supplement Sources

Brewer's yeast and royal jelly.

VITAMIN B₆ (PYRIDOXINE)

Vitamin B₆ assists in the formation of antibodies. It helps build red blood cells and prevent anemia, and it helps prevent cholesterol deposits around the heart, arteriosclerosis, and heart disease. It also aids in keeping sodium, potassium, and phosphorus in balance. In addition, it helps protein, fat, and carbohydrate metabolize. Vitamin B₆ acts as a natural diuretic for those retaining fluids, and it helps relieve nausea during pregnancy.

Food Sources

Brown rice, carrots, corn, dulse, fish, legumes, liver, peas, potatoes, sunflower seeds, and walnuts.

Natural Supplement Sources

Brewer's yeast and rice bran.

VITAMIN B₁₂ (CYANOCOBALAMIN)

Vitamin B₁₂ helps red blood cells develop in bone marrow and thereby prevents anemia. It helps maintain nerve sheaths and keep the nervous system healthy. It also helps the body metabolize protein, fats, and carbohydrates, and aids in digestion. Vitamin B₁₂ helps to produce acetylcholine, which supports learning and memory.

Food Sources

Alfalfa, beef liver, dulse, eggs, halibut, herring, kelp, mackerel, nori, salmon, and yogurt.

Natural Supplement Sources

Beef liver and brewer's yeast.

Biotin: Water Soluble

Biotin is necessary for healthy hair and skin, and it can help prevent cradle cap in infants. Shampoos that strengthen hair and prevent hair loss often contain biotin. It is important in the production of fatty acids and the utilization of other B vitamins. It helps protein, fats, and carbohydrates metabolize and aids cell growth. Biotin is necessary for healthy nerves and bone marrow, and it can relieve muscle pain.

Food Sources

Beef liver, black-eyed peas, Brazil nuts, cod, egg yolks, halibut, hazelnuts, herring, oatmeal, and yogurt. Eating raw egg whites can deplete the body of biotin. Raw egg whites contain an indigestible protein called avidin, which interferes with the absorption of biotin.

Natural Supplement Sources

Beef liver, brewer's yeast, and soy.

Choline: Water Soluble

Choline is necessary in the formation of lecithin and it helps fats and cholesterol metabolize. It also helps regulate liver and gallbladder function. Choline aids nerve impulse transmissions and proper brain function, and it is used with nervous system disorders, such as multiple sclerosis, tardive dyskenesia, and Parkinson's disease. Choline keeps the cardiovascular system healthy and prevents arteriosclerosis.

Food Sources

Beans, beef, egg yolks, goat's milk, and whole grains.

Natural Supplement Sources

Lecithin and soybeans.

Folic Acid (Folacin): Water Soluble

Folic acid ensures the formation of red blood cells and prevents anemia. It also helps with the formation of white blood cells, which strengthens immunity. It helps prevent the tongue from becoming sore or red. Folic acid feeds the brain and nervous system and it helps inhibit the formation of homocysteine, a toxic chemical that allows cholesterol to deposit around the heart.

Folic acid also supports proper cell division through the synthesis of RNA and DNA, and it is vital to the normal development of fetal nerve cells. The mother should take four hundred micrograms of folic acid prior to and throughout pregnancy to ensure proper development of fetal brain and nervous system and prevent a premature birth or anencephaly (where parts of the brain are missing).

Folic acid is best utilized if taken together with vitamin B complex, including B₁₂, and vitamin C.

Food Sources

Asparagus, barley, black beans, brown rice, garbanzo beans, green leafy vegetables, kidney beans, lima beans, liver, nuts and seeds, oranges, parsnips, salmon, and tuna.

Natural Supplement Sources

Brewer's yeast, liver, and rice bran.

Inositol: Water Soluble

Inositol is important in the formation of lecithin and the proper utilization of cholesterol and fat. It is also essential for hair growth. Inositol helps prevent hardened arteries, high cholesterol, skin eruptions, depression, anxiety, and compulsive disorders.

Continued ➡

Food Sources
Beef, blackstrap molasses, legumes, vegetables, whole grains, and yogurt.

Natural Supplement Sources
Brewer's yeast and rice bran.

Paba (Para-Aminobenzoic Acid): Water Soluble

With the assistance of intestinal bacteria, PABA is converted to folic acid, which then helps the body assimilate pantothenic acid (vitamin B_5). PABA is used in the formation of red blood cells. It also works as a coenzyme to break down and utilize proteins. It acts as an antioxidant and absorbs harmful ultraviolet-B radiation from the sun, thus protecting against sunburn and skin cancer. As an antioxidant, it also protects the body from cigarette smoke. In addition, PABA helps maintain healthy intestinal flora. Taking PABA can help restore to color gray hair, if the graying occurred as a result of B vitamin and PABA deficiency and stress. It may also help restore pigment to areas of white skin patches.

Food Sources
Blackstrap molasses, liver, mushrooms, spinach, and whole grains.

Natural Supplement Sources
Liver and whole grains.

Vitamin C (Ascorbic Acid): Water Soluble

Vitamin C strengthens the immune system by helping to produce antibodies. A powerful antioxidant, it fights free radicals that can cause damage to the cells, thus fighting infection and protecting against cancer. It assists in tissue growth and repair and helps heal wounds. Vitamin C is essential in the utilization of folic acid and the absorption of iron. It also helps the body excrete lead and other harmful heavy metals.

Vitamin C is important in maintaining healthy collagen and in forming strong connective tissue, healthy gums, and bones. It also helps prevent varicose veins, bruising, hemorrhoids, and hernias. Additionally, it assists in lowering cholesterol levels and high blood pressure. Vitamin C also helps block the release of histamines and reduce the intensity of allergic reactions. It can even help minimize the symptoms of asthma. In high doses, vitamin C can help negate the harmful effects of a black widow spider bite. The body does not manufacture vitamin C, so it must be obtained from nutritional sources. If large amounts of vitamin C are required, it is best given intravenously. Taken in large doses with aspirin, ascorbic acid can cause burning in the stomach and ulcers. Vitamin C from the sago palm tree is a mild and gentle form of vitamin C that will not burn the stomach but still should not be taken with aspirin. To learn about effective aspirin replacements, read *Beyond Aspirin* by Thomas M. Newmark and Paul Schulick.

Food Sources
Bell peppers, berries, broccoli, citrus fruits, green leafy vegetables, mangoes, melons, onions, persimmons, pineapple, potatoes, strawberries, and tomatoes.

Natural Supplement Sources
Acerola cherries, rose hips, and sago palm.

Vitamin D: Fat Soluble

Vitamin D is essential for the absorbtion of calcium and phosphorus; thus it is needed for developing bones and teeth in children and for maintaining strong bones and teeth in adults. It also helps prevent osteoporosis and osteoarthritis. Vitamin D keeps the muscles strong (including the heart) and keeps the nervous system balanced. It ensures normal blood clotting, thyroid function, and healthy immune activity. Vitamin D prevents rickets in children; rickets can lead to bone deformities and osteomalacia, a condition that softens, weakens, and demineralizes the bones. Sunshine is a wonderful source of vitamin D. People who live in regions where sunshine is limited in the winter cannot produce enough vitamin D and should take a supplement. The liver and kidneys convert the vitamin D from food supplements so it can be completely utilized. People with liver or kidney disorders, who cannot take full advantage of vitamin D supplements, are more likely to develop osteoporosis.

Food Sources
Butter, dandelion greens, eggs, feta cheese, fish liver oils, halibut, liver, oatmeal, salmon, sardines, sweet potatoes, tuna, and yogurt.

Natural Supplement Sources
Cod liver oil and fish liver oil.

Vitamin E: Fat Soluble

Vitamin E neutralizes the damaging effects of free radicals, blocks the formation of carcinogens (cancer-producing compounds), and stimulates the immune system. It also protects other fat-soluble vitamins from damage by oxygen, and it protects the body's cells, including red blood cells. It helps regulate blood pressure, strengthens arterial walls, promotes normal blood clotting, and helps wounds heal without scarring. Vitamin E promotes healthy skin, hair, and nerves. In addition, it slows the aging process and helps prevent age spots from developing. It may postpone the development of cataracts, and it may slow the progression of Parkinson's disease.

Vitamin E relieves muscular cramping, including leg cramps. It also helps regulate menstrual periods, relieve symptoms that occur with PMS such as abdominal cramping, prevent fibrocystic breast disease, and reduce hot flashes in perimenopausal women. Vitamin E can help increase the sperm cell count in men.

According to Phyllis A. Balch, CNC, and James F. Balch, MD, in *A Prescription for Nutritional Healing*, ". . . studies have shown daily use of Vitamin E to be more protective than aspirin for prevention of heart attacks, with no harmful side effects. The misuse of aspirin, in contrast, causes or contributes to an estimated 3,000 deaths in the United States each year." If you are taking blood thinners or have high blood pressure you can take vitamin E, but consult a qualified health practitioner for an appropriate dosage.

Read labels! Natural vitamin E is much more potent and better for you than a man-made form. Natural vitamin E is d-alpha-tocopheral. The label may also say d-alpha-tocopherol and mixed tocopherols of alpha, beta, gamma, and delta. Synthetic vitamin E is listed as dl-alpha-tocopherol, with an *e* after the *d*. This type may not cost as much, but it also will not provide as much healing.

When combining food supplements, avoid inorganic iron, called ferrous sulphate; it will destroy vitamin E. Natural iron or organic sources of iron, such as ferrous fumerate or ferrous gluconate, does not harm it.

Food Sources
Brown rice, cold-pressed oils, green leafy vegetables, nuts, raw milk, raw wheat germ, and seeds.

Natural Supplement Sources
Soybean oil and wheat germ oil.

Vitamin K: Not Water Soluble

The liver uses vitamin K to make prothrombin, which is needed for clotting blood. Vitamin K also prevents internal bleeding and excessive external bleeding. It is necessary for forming and repairing bones. Vitamin K works in the intestines to help convert glucose into glycogen, which is stored in the liver and is important for keeping the liver healthy.

Vitamins K_1, K_2, and K_3

There are three types of vitamin K. Vitamin K_1 (phylloquinone) is derived from plants. Vitamin K_2 (menaquinone) is made by bacteria in the intestinal tract. These two types of vitamin K are natural.

Vitamin K_3 (menadione) is a synthetic form, and it can be toxic in large doses. It can cause jaundice in infants and anemia in children and adults. Taking antibiotics can inhibit the natural production of vitamin K_2 by intestinal bacteria. Mineral oil attaches to vitamin K and carries it out of the body. Therefore, it is important to avoid taking mineral oil, which is a harsh laxative that can deplete your body's supply of vitamin K. Those taking blood thinners should not take vitamin K without the advice of a physician.

Food Sources of Vitamin K_1
Asparagus, brussels sprouts, cabbage, egg yolks, garbanzo beans, green leafy vegetables, green tea, lentils, liver, oatmeal, spinach, and turnip greens.

Natural Supplement Sources
Fermented soy, leafy greens.

Vitamin P (Bioflavonoids): Water Soluble

Vitamin P helps the body absorb vitamin C, and it is often combined with vitamin C in tablet or capsule form. Bioflavonoids and vitamin C should be taken together. Vitamin P comes in several forms, including citrin, flavones, hesperetin, hesperidin, quercetin, quercetrin, and rutin. It builds and repairs connective tissue and keeps the arterial walls strong.

Rutin (taken by itself or in addition to vitamin C) and bioflavonoids can help heal the swelling and pain of hemorrhoids. It is also very effective in reducing the severity of varicose veins. Vitamin P also helps prevent hernias and relieve pain. Acting as a natural antibiotic, when taken with vitamin C it relieves the pain and swelling of herpes sores around the mouth. It may also relieve the pain and swelling of shingles. Quercetin taken with vitamin C and bromelain from pineapple can prevent the symptoms of asthma. Vitamin P improves circulation and helps lower cholesterol levels.

Food Sources
Bell peppers, blackberries, black cherries, black currants, buckwheat sprouts, grapes, plums, and the white part of all citrus fruits (just inside the peeling).

Natural Supplement Sources
Bell peppers, cherries, and rose hips.

Continued ➡

Tool Kit for Selecting Healthy Minerals

Minerals occur naturally in the earth and are absorbed by plants and transmuted into forms we can utilize. Minerals are vital to all life. Every plant and living creature must have minerals in order to survive. In our bodies, every cell requires minerals in order to function. Minerals build strong bones, promote healthy nerve function, and help maintain proper muscle tone. Minerals support the heart muscle and cardiovascular system as well as all other bodily systems. Minerals work with vitamins and enzymes to help our bodies produce energy and heal from illness. This tool kit will teach you about the minerals, what they do for the body, and food sources they can be found in. When buying minerals, you will find they come in various forms. Liquid minerals are probably the most easily absorbed. Some minerals are chelated or bound to a protein, which enhances absorption. If you feel you need minerals, a good multimineral will often ensure that you get what you need. If you have questions about the minerals you need, consult a good natural health practitioner.

Boron, the "Maintainer"

Boron in trace amounts helps maintain strong bones. It helps with the metabolism and absorption of calcium, magnesium, and phosphorus. According to James F. Balch, MD, and Phyllis A. Balch, CNC, in *Prescription for Nutritional Healing*. "A study conducted by the U.S. Department of Agriculture indicated within eight days of supplementing their daily diet with 3 milligrams of boron, a test group of postmenopausal women lost 40 percent less calcium, one-third less magnesium, and slightly less phosphorus through their urine than they had before beginning boron supplementation." One should not take more than three milligrams of boron daily.

Natural Supplement Sources
Trace minerals and boron combined with calcium supplements.

Food Sources
Apples, carrots, green leafy vegetables, nuts and seeds, pears, and whole grains.

Calcium, the "Knitter"

Calcium is a wonderful mineral that builds strong bones, teeth, and fingernails. It is also needed to mend and repair bones, muscles, ligaments, and tissues. Calcium promotes healing during illness.

Natural Supplement Sources
Calcium citrate and gluconate. Calcium from dolomite (a type of stone) or oyster shell is difficult to absorb.

Synthetic Sources
Di-cal phosphate.

Food Sources
Almonds, beet tops, broccoli, cabbage, green leafy vegetables (such as kale, mustard greens, turnip greens), raw milk and cheese, seaweeds (such as dulse and kelp), and sesame seeds.

Carbon, the "Builder"

Carbon promotes growth. Together with oxygen, it brings heat to the body. Carbon is the basic element of cell birth and life. When there is too much carbon in the body, it leads to obesity.

Natural Supplement Sources
Trace minerals.

Food Sources
Almonds, avocados, butter, egg yolks, olive oil, raw cheese, and whole grains.

Chlorine, the "Cleanser"

Chlorine nourishes the nerves, maintains electrolyte and fluid balance, cleanses the liver, helps with tissue construction, assists in the production of hydrochloric acid, and assists in peristalsis.

Natural Supplement Sources
Trace minerals.

Food Sources
Asparagus, avocados, cabbage, celery, chard, cucumbers, goat's milk, kale, leeks, olives, saltwater fish, turnips, and watercress.

Chromium, the "Energizer"

Chromium helps balance blood sugar levels and assists in metabolizing glucose. Therapeutically, it is helpful in cases of diabetes and hypoglycemia. It helps people not to crave sweets. Chromium plays a vital role in the synthesis of fats, cholesterol, and protein. Without chromium, people become tired and fatigued.

Natural Supplement Sources
Chromium carbonate and chromium picolinate. Herbs that contain chromium are licorice root, oatstraw, and horsetail.

Food Sources
Brewer's yeast, brown rice, corn, corn oil, dried beans, eggs, mushrooms, raw cheese, and whole grains.

Fluorine, the "Decay Resistor"

Natural fluorine, from food sources, is important to the health of our bones, teeth, and hair. It helps the teeth resist decay.

Natural Supplement Sources
Multivitamins and trace minerals.

Synthetic Sources
Mouthwash and toothpastes.

Food Sources
Avocados, Brussels sprouts, cabbage, quince, raw fish, and raw goat's milk.

Iodine, the "Metabolizer"

Iodine is important to the thyroid gland's health. People who live near the ocean and eat lots of food from the sea do not get goiter. In mountainous regions where iodine is not readily available in the foods, we find a great deal of goiter and other thyroid disorders. Without iodine, the body is not able to metabolize nutrients well and the thyroid cannot manage blood circulation and body temperature.

Natural Supplement Sources
Dulse or kelp in tablets, powder, or capsules. Nova Scotia dulse, grown in the cold waters of that region, is highest in iodine.

Synthetic Sources
Potassium iodide.

Food Sources
Agar, eggplant, fish, garlic, kale, and all seaweeds.

Iron, the "Frisky Horse"

Iron builds strong blood cells and keeps people from feeling tired and anemic. Iron is called the "frisky horse" mineral because it keeps us active. Iron attracts oxygen into the cells of the body. Oxygen has been called "the giver of life"; we would die without it. Harmful bacteria cannot live in the presence of oxygen. The lungs, nerves, brain, and liver are organs that particularly need iron.

Natural Supplement Sources
Bone marrow supplements, brewer's yeast, desiccated liver, ferrous fumerate, ferrous gluconate, and iron oxide.

Synthetic Sources
Ferrous sulfate and iron peptonate.

Food Sources
Black cherries, blackstrap molasses, brewer's yeast, rice bran, dulse, figs, green vegetables, kelp, lentils, liver, raisins, prunes, and walnuts.

Magnesium, the "Relaxer"

Magnesium soothes and relaxes the muscles and helps prevent muscle cramping. It calms the nervous system and promotes rest. Magnesium also relieves and prevents constipation. Magnesium helps the heart and arteries function properly and can help prevent a heart attack. It also strengthens and builds bones and teeth. A deficiency in magnesium can cause high blood pressure.

Natural Supplement Sources
Brewer's yeast and magnesium oxide.

Synthetic Sources
Magnesium sulfate.

Food Sources
Almonds, apples, black walnuts, dulse, figs, goat's milk, green leafy vegetables (such as chard, kale, and endive), sesame seeds, sunflower seeds, turnip greens, yellow corn and cornmeal, and yellow squashes.

Manganese, the "Lover"

Manganese is important to healthy brain and nerve functioning. It helps reproduction and sex hormone production, and it is important in tissue respiration and muscle coordination. People with a hearing loss or with ringing in the ears need manganese.

Natural Supplement Sources
Manganese carbonate.

Synthetic Sources
Manganese gluconate.

Food Sources
Almonds, apricots, black walnuts, butternut squash, egg yolks, grains, green beans, peas, and spinach.

Nitrogen, the "Restrainer"

Nitrogen helps to restrain oxygen that is otherwise too volatile in the body. Nitrogen builds, preserves, and protects body tissues, also giving vitality to body tissues. It is important for skin and muscle health and elasticity.

Food Sources
Almonds, black-eyed peas, butternut squash, kidney beans, legumes, and salmon. NOTE: There are no supplement or synthetic sources of nitrogen for human consumption.

Continued ➡

Phosphorus, the "Light Bearer"

We can see phosphorescent qualities in many life forms, such as the firefly that glows in the dark on summer nights, glowworms, and certain types of eels and fish. Phosphorus is the medium for the soul's expression through brain activity. Without phosphorus, we could not think or reason, study or visualize, read or comprehend. Phosphorus helps us be intuitive and sensitive. Bones are made more dense and the nerve networks strong with phosphorus. Phosphorus is responsible for cellular repair, energy production, kidney function, metabolism, and heart muscle contraction.

Natural Supplement Sources
Bonemeal and ionic trace minerals.

Food Sources
Almonds, egg yolks, fish, goat's milk and cheese, lentils, pumpkin seeds, rice bran, and sunflower seeds.

Potassium, the "Great Alkalizer"

Potassium nourishes the muscles, including the heart, and helps keep them strong and functioning properly. It helps them contract and relax. Potassium is also important for blood, kidneys, nerve, and skin health.

Natural Supplement Sources
Potassium citrate.

Synthetic Sources
Calcium phosphate.

Food Sources
Almonds, apricots, bananas, beets, cantaloupe, grapes, organic ripe citrus fruits, parsley, parsnips, pears, potato peelings broth, potato peelings, sunflower seeds, tomatoes, and turnips.

Silicon, the "Magnet"

Silicon builds and repairs skin, teeth, hair, fingernails, and bones. It also builds connective tissue. It strengthens blood vessels and helps prevent bruising, varicose veins, hemorrhoids, and hernias. Silicon nourishes the brain and nervous system as well. It is called the "magnet" because a person with sufficient silicon in their bodies will have beautiful teeth; strong, shiny hair; good skin; and beautiful fingernails. Their brain and nerves are strong and they usually have a good personality. Because of their beauty, strength, and happy disposition, others are drawn to them.

Natural Supplement Sources
Silica capsules. Horse chestnut, horsetail, oatstraw, and shavegrass in liquids or capsules. Rice bran syrup. Horse chestnut cream used topically on varicose veins.

Food Sources
Alfalfa tea, flaxseeds, oats, oatstraw tea, onions, parsnips, red bell peppers, rice bran, rice polishings, and sunflower seeds.

Sodium, the "Fountain of Youth"

Natural sodium (not table salt) nourishes the lymph system and helps hold fluids in areas where they are needed, such as around the eyes, in the sinus cavities, mouth, and lungs, and around the joints. Sodium helps us stay limber and pliable. Babies have a lot of sodium in their bodies and are very soft. Sodium holds calcium in solution where it is needed in the tissues and bones, instead of forming crystals in the joints and stones in the kidneys and gallbladder. It normalizes glandular secretions and maintains a proper balance in blood pH as well as a balance of water in the cells. An adequate amount of sodium may help prevent cataracts as well.

Natural Supplement Sources
Dulse tablets and goat's whey capsules.

Synthetic Sources
Sodium chloride.

Food Sources
Beet tops, celery, celery juice, green leafy vegetables, goats whey, okra, parsley, seaweeds, strawberries, and turnips.

Sulfur, the "Heater"

Sulfur warms the body. It energizes each cell, enabling it to eliminate toxic substances. Because it drives toxins from tissues, it can help to heal skin disorders, such as psoriasis, eczema, and rosacea. Such protection against toxic substances, radiation, and pollution slows down the aging process. Sulfur also assists in tissue formation and repairs and restores collagen elasticity. It helps relieve the pain of arthritis, bursitis, and gout. Sulfur disinfects the blood and helps the body resist bacteria.

Natural Supplement Sources
Trace minerals, multimineral supplements, and ointments. Methyl-sulfonylmethane (MSM) is highly bioavailable and can be found in capsules, powder, lotions, creams, and facial cleansers.

Food Sources
Brussels sprouts, cabbage, celery, dried beans, eggs, fish, garlic, kale, onions, and turnips.

Zinc, the "Regulator"

Zinc ensures that the reproductive organs and prostate gland function well. It helps with collagen formation, tissue repair, and immune function. Zinc helps maintain our ability to smell and taste. It also regulates the production of oil from the oil glands and therefore is beneficial in treating skin disorders, such as oily skin and acne. Without zinc, our fingernails become thin, get ridges in them, and crack and peel. Do not take more than fifty to one hundred milligrams of zinc daily.

Natural Supplement Sources
Zinc oxide.

Synthetic Sources
Zinc sulfate.

Food Sources
Brewer's yeast, egg yolks, green leafy vegetables, lecithin, legumes, pumpkin seeds, seafood, soaked almonds and sunflower seeds, and whole grains.

Tool Kit for Choosing Superfood Supplements

Superfood supplements include a wide variety of foods or nutrients that provide supernourishment to the body and/or wonderful health benefits. Many of the superfood supplements can be used in place of food when one is traveling or in case of emergency when food is scarce. For example, if people are not eating salads, alfalfa tablets, or chlorella can give them the fiber and nutrients they are missing by not getting salad. Bee pollen is another great example of a superfood supplement because it contains 40 percent protein and all the essential components of life. It helps correct allergies, strengthen the body, and provide energy. This tool kit will provide you with information about some of the best super food supplements available.

Alfalfa

Alfalfa is a green superfood rich in vitamins, minerals, and chlorophyll. The roots of the alfalfa plant reach far into the earth to gather nourishment, sometimes as far as 120 feet! Alfalfa can be taken in liquid, tablet, or capsule form. As a liquid, it is great for people on a cleanse or fast, who are not eating solid foods. As a tablet, it helps tremendously with bowel cleansing. The fiber in the tablets helps scrub the colon wall clean. Crack alfalfa tablets with your teeth before swallowing to aid digestion. Alfalfa also helps promote good peristalsis in the bowel, because it provides the fibrous bulk the bowel needs for squeezing and pushing. It gives the bowels a great exercise workout.

Alfalfa helps cleanse and build the blood and liver and improve digestion, and it may help prevent cancer and liver disease. Alfalfa can help heal and relieve arthritis, gout, hemorrhoids, diverticulitis, intestinal ulcers, constipation, bad breath or body odor (including smelly feet), athlete's foot, and bleeding gums. It can balance blood sugar, making it beneficial for both hypoglycemics and diabetics. It even helps people who are dieting feel fuller longer and resist sweets.

Aloe Vera Juice and Gel

Aloe vera can be taken orally as a juice or gel, and it soothes the entire digestive tract. Aloe vera is a natural anti-inflammatory and helps tremendously with cases of gastritis, heartburn, acid reflux, colitis, diverticulitis, ulcers, and irritable bowel syndrome.

Irritable bowel syndrome causes people to swing from diarrhea to constipation. For relief, grind flaxseeds, soak them in aloe juice, and drink the juice twice a day. Flaxseeds are mucilaginous and very beneficial for the colon. This aloe-flaxseed combination helps relieve both constipation and diarrhea.

Aloe vera helps fight infection in the body. Aloe vera gel is reputed for its ability to heal burns and relieve dry skin. It is wonderful for acne, cuts, insect bites, skin ulcers, eczema, psoriasis, dandruff, cradle cap, and poison oak or poison ivy. Aloe vera soothes and softens the skin and can be used as a facial mask. Look for aloe vera in lotions, salves, ointments, and creams.

There are approximately two hundred species of aloe. If you like growing plants, you might enjoy growing your own aloe vera plant. When it is large enough, you may break or cut a leaf, and squeeze out the gel to treat a burn, insect bite, or wound. Properly cared for, an aloe vera plant can provide years of service. Enjoy!

Barley Grass

Barley grass is available in powder or capsule form. As a powder, it can be stirred in distilled water to provide a nutritious low-calorie drink. It is high in chlorophyll, vitamin C, protein, enzymes, and minerals, including calcium and iron. It is great for vegetarians because it also has some vitamin B_{12}. (B_{12} is predominantly found in animal products.) Barley grass nourishes the entire body. It is also an anti-inflammatory, which makes it beneficial for any inflammation of the gastrointestinal tract.

Bee Pollen

Bee pollen is a wonderful food for humans, rich in protein, vitamins, and minerals. Bee pollen is different from the pollen that many people are allergic to. Pollens that cause allergies are called

Continued ➡

anemophiles; they are very light and easily blown through the air. Bee pollen is called entomophiies, which means "friends of the insects," and it is heavy and sticky. This pollen is collected from the legs of the bees by a special device placed near the opening of the beehives. Allergies caused by bee pollen are rare, and local bee pollen can help alleviate allergies to airborne pollens. Take it six weeks prior to allergy season, starting with small amounts—one granule the first day, two the second day, and three the third day, until you are taking one-half teaspoon one to two times per day. Mankind has consumed bee pollen for centuries. It was praised in the Bible, used in ancient Chinese medicine, and prescribed by traditional doctors for its healing properties. Bee pollen contains all the known nutrients necessary for survival and has been used consistently to build energy levels. Athletes have used it since the earliest Olympic games in Greece. Bee pollen builds the blood and improves endurance and vitality, has antibiotic properties, and helps prevent colds and flu. It also has been used successfully to reduce cravings and addictions to sugar, caffeine, nicotine, and alcohol.

Royden Brown writes extensively in *The World's Only Perfect Food* about the wonderful value of consuming bee pollen. In addition to its other uses, he notes that bee pollen can help balance hormones in both men and women and restore potency. He also explains the tremendous value of using bee pollen to prevent illness, build the immune system, and promote longevity. And according to Steven R. Schechter, ND, in *Fighting Radiation and Chemical Pollutants with Foods, Herbs and Vitamins*, a study in Sarajevo, Yugoslavia, reports findings that bee pollen successfully corrected radiation sickness.

Bee Propolis

Bee propolis is a resinous substance that bees collect from the bark of trees and leaf buds. They mix it with beeswax and pollen to form a sealer that protects the hive from harmful bacteria and viruses.

Bee propolis can be taken internally in a liquid or tablet form. It is high in vitamin A (carotene), vitamin C, bioflavonoids, vitamin E, and some of the B vitamins. It also contains a large number of minerals. It is antibacterial, antiviral, and protects us from radiation. Bee propolis acts as a powerful antibiotic and immobilizes bacteria and viruses. It helps fight colds, flu, tonsillitis, and infections, including those in the mouth and throat. Propolis is also very effective when used externally in salves and ointments.

Its antibacterial properties fight infection in cuts and other wounds. Propolis can be taken on a regular basis with no side effects and be consistently effective because bacteria and viruses cannot build a tolerance to it. This differs from penicillin and other antibiotic drugs, which germs grow resistant to over time.

Beet Tablets and Beet Powder

Beets are deep red root vegetables that are rich in vitamins and minerals, especially iron. Beet juice, according to German research, can help heal anemia. Beets can also cleanse the liver, gallbladder, and kidneys. They can help reduce inflammation in the nervous system and promote good peristaltic action in the bowel. According to Steven R. Schecter, ND, in *Fighting Radiation and Chemical Pollutants with Foods, Herbs and Vitamins*, "Beets have been shown to rebuild hemoglobin of the blood after exposure to radiation. Rats fed a diet of 20 percent beet pulp were able to prevent cesium-137 absorption 97 to 100 percent more effectively than rats exposed to the same radiation but given no beets."

Beets and raw organic beet juice are available in powdered form as well as tablet form for those who don't like beets, haven't the time to juice them or prepare them, or simply want to supplement their nutritional program.

Beta-1, 3-D-Glucan

This supplement is made from the cell walls of yeast, the type used for baking. It does not, however, contain any yeast in supplement form. Beta-1,3-D-glucan works to boost the immune system by stimulating destroyer cells, or macrophages, to devour and destroy bacteria, viruses, and fungi. It has even been used to kill tumoral cells.

Bifidobacterium Bifidum (Bifidus)

Probiotics are friendly bacteria in the digestive tract that build a healthy intestinal flora and improve digestion. One type of probiotic is called bifidobacterium bifidum or bifidus. Bifidobacterium bifidum fight harmful bacteria in the gut as well as yeast infections, including those of the vaginal tract. These good bacteria promote healthy intestinal movement and help relieve constipation and gas. They provide a conducive environment in the intestines for the manufacture of B vitamins and vitamin K.

Bifidobacterium bifidum should be taken after a round of antibiotics to replace the healthy bacteria in the bowel. Antibiotics kill harmful bacteria, but they also destroy friendly bacteria. If these friendly bacteria are not replaced, yeast infections can grow rapidly and harmful bacteria can grow strong.

Ammonia is often the by-product of destructive bacteria and faulty digestion. Tears and holes can develop in the intestinal walls, resulting in leaky gut syndrome. The blood will carry toxins from the bowel to the liver, causing tremendous strain on the liver. Undigested food can cause the body to produce too much histamine, and allergies can result. Unhealthy intestinal flora can cause exhaustion, headaches, and nausea. By replenishing bifidobacterium bifidum, we can prevent or heal a lot of these problems and keep our digestive tract healthy and working smoothly.

Black Cherry Concentrate

Black cherry concentrate is a delicious syrup made from the finest black cherries. It is rich in vitamins and minerals and is a wonderful source of natural iron. You can add water to make a great juice. It can be used occasionally over yogurt as a nutritious dessert. It is even great on pancakes made from sprouted whole grains, and much better for you than a lot of commercial syrups made from sugar and water. Children love it! Incorporated into your nutritional plan, black cherry concentrate can help prevent anemia, heal gout, and dissolve kidney stones and gallstones.

Blue-Green Algae

Blue-green algae is a green freshwater algae grown in the great Klamath Lake in Oregon. It can be acquired in powder, capsule, or tablet form. Blue-green algae is filled with chlorophyll, which cleans the blood and liver, as well as with protein, vitamins, and minerals. It is a whole food that boosts energy levels because it is quickly and easily absorbed. For this reason, blue-green algae helps balance blood sugar levels and stop cravings for sweets. It nourishes the brain and nervous system and promotes clear thinking.

Chlorella

Chlorella is a single-celled alga that is grown in freshwater. One of the best sources of chlorella is grown and harvested in Japan. This nutritious green algae is over two and a half million years old, which makes it one of the most stable sources of food on the planet. Chlorella can be obtained in liquid, tablet, capsule, or powder form. When purchasing chlorella, make sure the label says that the cell wall has been pulverized. This ensures proper digestion and absorption. In fact, one of the best ways to know the chlorella cell wall has been sufficiently pulverized is to look for the DYNO-Mill name. "DYNO-Mill" refers to the machine that pulverizes the cell walls, making the chlorella over 80 percent absorbable. Most chlorella has had the cell wall broken with intense heat or chemical treatments, and is only 40 percent absorbable or less.

Chlorella is one of the most nutritious plant foods and contains the highest amount of chlorophyll in the known plant world, making it a great blood cleanser. About 58 percent of chlorella is protein, so it is especially nourishing for vegetarians.

Chlorella contains one of the highest contents of RNA and DNA of any known food substance. The RNA and DNA in chlorella provide materials for cellular repair and can protect against the effects of ultraviolet radiation, contribute to rapid healing, and promote longevity. Chlorella is rich in beta-carotene and contains all the B vitamins, including more B_{12} than liver; vitamins C and E; and rare trace minerals. In addition, one of the most important aspects is the presence of a substance called chlorella growth factor (CGF), which is often extracted and sold as a separate product. Experiments have shown that CGF increases the rate of tissue healing. Chlorella can help reduce the cellular damage that accompanies chemotherapy and radiation. Chlorella tablets taken with flaxseed oil is a wonderful stool softener and can relieve constipation.

Chlorophyll

Chlorophyll is the green juice of plants that is created during photosynthesis, their interaction with sunshine. Chlorophyll is a rich source of absorbable iron, which helps attract oxygen to cells and builds hemoglobin. It is high in potassium, which supports the muscles and heart; magnesium, which helps tone and relax the muscles; calcium, which helps build teeth and bones; and many other minerals and trace minerals. Chlorophyll is also rich in vitamins, including vitamins A and C, making it wonderful for the immune system, and some vitamin D, which helps in the absorption of calcium. Chlorophyll also contains vitamin K, which assists in normal blood clotting.

Chlorophyll benefits the body in many ways. It builds the blood, neutralizes acids, cleans and deodorizes the bowels, purifies the liver and blood, helps prevent bad breath and body odor, helps relieve sinus drainage, soothes a sore throat, reduces inflammation, soothes ulcers, regulates menstruation, and improves milk production.

Chlorophyll can be obtained in liquid form and added to water. It can be obtained from the raw juice of wheatgrass or green leafy vegetables. You can also buy green powdered drinks, such as raw powdered wheatgrass, kamut, barley grass, chlorella, and blue-green algae.

Coenzyme Q10

Coenzyme Q10 is responsible for helping the body's cells produce adenasine triphosphate (ATP), an important source of energy. When people are deficient in coenzyme Q10, they can become

Continued ➡

fatigued. The muscles may ache or feel tired. Cardiovascular disease can develop, because the heart will lack the energy necessary to perform its vital functions. Coenzyme Q10 also plays a role in metabolizing fats and carbohydrates.

Colloidal Silver

Colloidal silver is a clear golden liquid that contains the purified trace mineral silver in a water-based solution. Medical doctors in America used it to treat a variety of diseases from the late 1800s to 1938, before man-made antibiotics became available. Settlers in the Old West used to keep their milk from spoiling by putting a silver dollar in it.

Colloidal silver is a powerful germicidal agent. Silver acts by crippling the oxygen-metabolizing enzyme in single-celled organisms (germs and viruses). The organisms are suffocated in a matter of minutes, and they are carried out of the body through the elimination channels.

An article titled "Silver, Our Mightiest Germ Fighter" (*Science Digest*, 1978), reported that silver kills over 650 disease-causing organisms.

Colloidal silver is nontoxic to mammals and plants, but a powerful destroyer of bacteria, viruses, and fungi. Topically, it fights fungal infections such as athlete's foot. It works wonders on acne, boils, eczema, herpes, ringworm, staph infections, warts, and impetigo.

Colloidal silver can be used in vaginal douches to clear up yeast infections. It works well when used as eyedrops, nose drops, and throat gargle. It can be used to heal gum infections or clear up bad breath. It helps get rid of dandruff, cradle cap in infants, and bedsores in the disabled. Colloidal silver also can be mixed with distilled water in a spray bottle and sprayed through the home or office to kill airborne viruses and bacteria. It can be added to bottled water when traveling.

Internally, colloidal silver that has been formulated correctly is safe for adults as well as children. It helps heal colds and flu, pneumonia, strep throat, bladder infections, and many other internal infections.

Colostrum

Colostrum is the nourishing fluid that is secreted by the milk glands of all mammal mothers for the first few days after birth, before the milk begins to flow. This is nature's way of providing powerful immune factors, friendly bacteria, and high levels of protein to ensure good health in the newborn. The immune factors protect the body against infection and the friendly bacteria provide a healthy intestinal flora.

Colostrum (from bovine sources) can be purchased in capsule, tablet, and powder form, and both children and adults may take it. It helps build and strengthen the immune system and is especially helpful for those who were never nursed by their mothers. It may help alleviate allergies, strengthen frail children and adults, and relieve chronic fatigue, constipation, environmental illness, and fibromyalgia. Colostrum is great for dieters. It nourishes the body, reduces hunger, and helps burn fat and build lean muscle.

Dulse

Dulse is a seaweed that is sold in dried form, powder, tablets, and capsules. It is high in natural iodine and a multitude of vitamins and minerals, including calcium. Dulse from the cold ocean water of Nova Scotia is one of the best sources available. It can be very effective in treating obesity because it greatly improves metabolism. Dulse is also good for the nervous system, brain, and spinal cord. It is

beneficial in restoring hair after hair loss and strengthening the nails. Dulse and all the edible seaweeds—including kelp, hijiki, arame, and kanbu—are high in iodine. They nourish the thyroid gland and protect from the effects of radiation. They also bind with harmful heavy metals and remove them from the body or neutralize them. Dulse and kelp in powdered form can be used in a salt shaker on the table in place of salt. Both are nutritious, add a delicious salty flavor to foods, and are much more nutritious than table salt.

Essential Fatty Acids (EFAs)

Essential fatty acids have also been called vitamin F. Though our bodies cannot produce them, they are vital to good health. None of our cells can survive without fatty acids, and our bodies need them to produce new cells. We also need them to produce prostaglandins, which are similar to hormones, and to help regulate important bodily functions. EFAs keep our skin soft and our hair shiny. They protect nerve sheaths and the heart and help lower cholesterol and blood pressure. They also help keep the joints limber and prevent arthritis.

There are two categories of essential fatty acids. The omega-3 EFAs are found in fresh ocean fish, such as salmon, herring, sardines, and mackerel, as well as fish oil, flaxseed oil, and walnut oil. Omega-6 EFAs are in beans, borage oil, Brazil nuts, grape seed oil, pecans, pumpkin seeds, primrose oil, raw almonds, sesame oil, sesame seeds, and sunflower seeds.

Fiber

If you have high cholesterol, fiber can help lower it. For those with blood sugar imbalances, fiber can stabilize the blood sugar. Fiber helps keep the intestinal tract working well and promotes good peristalsis and regular bowel movements. Fiber also helps prevent and heal hemorrhoids. It relieves constipation as well as diarrhea and even helps prevent colon cancer. Most Americans are not getting nearly enough fiber. Some good sources of fiber are beans, fruits, nuts, seeds, vegetables, and whole grains. Oat bran and rice bran are options for people who are allergic to wheat. Oat bran and rice bran can be added to cereals and baked in muffins.

Another source of fiber is pectin. It is found in apples, cabbage, carrots, and okra. Apple pectin can be purchased in powdered form and stirred in water to drink. It cleans the colon, lowers cholesterol, and helps balance blood sugar.

Psyllium seed is a good source of fiber that is great for cleansing the bowel. The best way to take it is mixed in water or juice. Some people have such poor peristalsis, and they have difficulty pushing this through the bowel. The psyllium may swell in the colon and cause the abdomen to extend. If this happens, drink more water. If it doesn't work for you, use flaxseed meal, apple pectin, alfalfa tablets, or chlorella to keep the colon clean.

Flaxseeds

Flaxseeds are high in fiber, very nutritious, and have a nutty flavor. They are digested best when they have been ground. A small coffee grinder is ideal for this job. Ground flaxseeds help soften the stool and relieve constipation. They can be sprinkled on salads, cereal, soups, and yogurt, and taken in vegetable juice. They contain omega-3 essential fatty acids, protein, B vitamins, magnesium, zinc, and potassium.

Try grinding flaxseeds together with almonds, sunflower seeds, pumpkin seeds, and walnuts, and sprinkle this mixture over a bowl of hot millet or quinoa for breakfast. It tastes delicious and gives

you additional nourishment throughout the morning. Try it!

Flaxseed Oil

Flaxseed oil should be taken only if it is organic and cold-pressed. It is a rich source of omega-3 EFAs and can help reduce inflammation in the body, keep the arteries limber, and lower cholesterol and triglyceride levels. People with symptoms from arthritis, multiple sclerosis, Parkinson's disease, and fibrositis improve after taking flaxseed oil.

Flaxseed oil does not have the fiber and nutrients contained in flaxseeds, and it will not relieve constipation as well. However, you would have to eat a lot of the seeds to get the same omega-3 benefits found in one tablespoon of flaxseed oil. I recommend using both.

Garlic

Garlic is a wonderful superfood that can save a life. It helps lower cholesterol and blood pressure, and it prevents abnormal blood clotting and protects the heart. Garlic contains allicin, which is a powerful antibiotic. There are also many sulfur compounds in garlic, which give it wonderful healing properties. Taken internally, garlic can stimulate the immune system and help heal colds, flu, bronchitis, and pneumonia. It also has a cleansing effect on the colon. It even helps to prevent and fight cancer. According to James E Scheer, Lynn Allison, and Charlie Fox, in *The Garlic Cure*, "Sloan-Kettering cancer authorities, doctors John F. Pinto and Richard S. Rivlin, write that at least 20 ingredients in garlic prevent cancer or help to cope with it in as many as three ways: (1) block tumors from developing from precursor cells, (2) prevent cancer from spreading to vulnerable target cells, and (3) delay or reverse malignancy." One of the best ways to take garlic is raw, chopped in salads or with vegetables. It can also be added to olive oil and used as a salad dressing. It can be juiced with apples. Garlic oil can be taken in capsule form to protect the heart, fight bacteria and viruses, and kill parasites and Candida. Garlic oil can be used externally as an antibiotic on cuts, wounds, fungal infections, and cold sores. For ear infections, rub it inside the ear. If you don't like the taste of garlic, or to freshen the breath after eating garlic, gargle with chlorophyll or baking soda and water, or chew some fresh mint leaves or fennel seeds. Bathing in baking soda baths staves off bad breath from the garlic.

Glucosamine Sulfate

Glucosamine is produced naturally in our bodies and helps build connective tissue, tendons, ligaments, bones, skin, and nails. It cushions the joints and helps keep them functioning smoothly. It helps prevent and heal osteoarthritis and build joint cartilage.

Glucosamine sulfate can be taken in supplement form to reduce the pain of and help heal arthritis, bursitis, and osteoporosis. It is often found combined with chondroitin sulfate, which also helps build cartilage.

Goat's Milk Whey or Mineral Whey

Whey is the translucent liquid that separates from milk solids during the process of making cheese. High in minerals, goat's whey drink is prized in Europe and the Middle East as a youth elixir that promotes health and long life.

Goat's milk whey is a golden-brown powder, rich in minerals, that has been dehydrated and is free from chemical additives. A tablespoonful stirred in hot water is delicious, tasting like a slightly salty broth. It is an ideal way to correct min-

Continued ➡

eral deficiencies and the multitude of health problems that occur because of them. Goat's milk whey or mineral whey can be purchased in most health food stores.

Mineral whey is high in organic potassium, calcium, chloride, phosphorous, sodium, magnesium, zinc, and iron. It also has some manganese, chromium, silicon, and selenium. In addition, it contains many of the important trace minerals that are vital to good health. Electrolytes are plentiful in mineral whey, and they make up the electrically charged ions that help regulate acid-alkaline balance, water balance, muscle contraction, nerve impulse conduction, osmotic pressure, and the transport of nutrients into and out of the cells.

High in sodium and potassium, mineral whey can prevent or help heal conditions such as chronic indigestion, constipation, intestinal irritation, colitis, and ulcers when mineral deficiencies, acidity, and stress are the causes.

Mineral whey also replaces the sodium content that helps hold calcium in solution. This can help prevent and heal arthritis, osteoarthritis, and osteoporosis by restoring minerals to the lymph fluid, joints, and bone. Capra Mineral Whey, with its high content of potassium and sodium, can reduce muscular pain and fatigue, and help the heart beat with a normal healthy rhythm. Whey provides the nutrients necessary to keep a balanced pH. In addition to all these wonderful health benefits, mineral whey is also being used successfully to detoxify heavy metals from the body. See page 350 for a delicious warming mineral whey drink.

Grape Seed Oil

Grape seed oil is one of the richest sources of omega-6 EFAs and is the only oil with the exception of olive oil that can be heated without producing free radicals. It is delicious on salads and in cooked dishes such as stir-fried vegetables. Grape seed oil can be added to night creams and hand lotions to keep the skin soft, young, and healthy. Purchase organic grape seed oil, as grapes are one of the most chemically sprayed crops.

Gymnema Sylvestre

Gymnema sylvestre is a plant that grows in India and has been used for medicinal purposes for hundreds of years. It has been used in Ayurvedic medicine as a natural diuretic and for the relief of upset stomach. Hindus use the powdered root on snakebites while having the patient drink a decoction from it.

One of the most wonderful benefits of gymnema sylvestre is that it has blood sugar-lowering actions. Extracts from the leaves are being used successfully as a remedy for diabetes mellitus. Excessive secretion of glucose in the urine has been greatly reduced in diabetics using this botanical, without side effects. In addition, gymnema sylvestre has been shown to increase beta cells that naturally produce insulin in the islets of Langerhans within the pancreas. This activity decreases the body's requirement for additional insulin treatments. Thus gymnema sylvestre has proven to be very promising in treating and healing of type 1 and type 2 diabetes. However, it is not a panacea. Diabetics should follow a healthy nutritional plan and never lower their insulin dosages before consulting with their doctor.

Lactobacillus Acidophilus

Lactobacillus acidophilus is a friendly bacteria that helps establish a healthy flora in the colon. Taking antibiotics will kill these friendly bacteria and often cause yeast infections to develop. Lactobacillus aci-

dophilus works to prevent the overgrowth of Candida, fights fungus, inhibits pathogenic organisms, improves digestion and absorption of nutrients, helps reduce cholesterol, and prevents leaky gut syndrome. It is also involved with the digestion of proteins and the production of B vitamins and certain enzymes in the intestinal tract.

Lactobacillus acidophilus can be purchased in powder, tablets, or capsules. It is often derived from cow's milk, but there are nondairy formulas available for people allergic to dairy products. It is best to take it when the stomach is empty—first thing in the morning, between meals, and before bed. If you are taking an antibiotic, you can and should take acidophilus, but at different times during the day than when you take the antibiotic.

Lecithin

Lecithin is a lipid, or good fat, that is essential to the entire body, ensuring proper cellar functioning in the brain and nervous system. It makes up the protective sheaths of the brain and nervous system. Lecithin is an emulsifier that helps dissolve plaque in the arteries and lower cholesterol. It helps keep the arteries from hardening, and it can prevent heart disease. Lecithin helps repair damage to the liver and keeps it working well.

Lecithin often comes from soybean sprouts or eggs and contains choline (a B vitamin), inositol, and linoleic acid, which is an omega-6 EFA. Other sources of lecithin are legumes, grains, and brewer's yeast.

Methylsulfonylmethane (Msm)

MSM is organic sulfur that is found in broccoli, Brussels sprouts, cabbage, cauliflower, fish, raw cow's milk, and raw goat's milk. MSM is necessary for good health because it helps detoxify cells. It helps the body heal itself from injury, repair cellular damage, reduce inflammation, relieve pain such as that associated with arthritis or headaches, improve allergic symptoms, and strengthen the immune system. MSM also acts to heal gastrointestinal disorders and lung congestion. MSM is an important nutrient for the skin, hair, and nails.

Olive Leaf Extract

Studies have proven olive leaf extract to be extremely effective against viruses, bacteria, and fungal infections. Taken orally, this herbal extract can help heal sore throats, colds, flu, bronchial infections, sinus infections, and intestinal viruses. It can even help protect against viruses such as herpes and HIV (human immunodeficiency virus).

Oregano Oil

Oregano oil taken from wild-crafted oregano (oregano grown in the wild) is a powerful antiseptic and fights bacteria, viruses, and fungi. It contains phenols, which are natural chemicals that act as strong antiseptics that destroy harmful germs. Rubbed on the skin, oregano oil can heal cold sores and destroy fungal infections, including ringworm and athlete's foot. It can be rubbed on the gums to heal gum disease. Oregano oil has even helped heal warts, which are caused by a virus, and may even diminish moles. Oregano oil can be taken internally as well to knock out infections, viruses, and even food poisoning. For more information on this wonderful natural medicine, read *The Cure Is in the Cupboard: How to Use Oregano for Better Health* by Dr. Cass Ingram.

Policosanol

Policosanol is a natural food substance taken from the sugar cane plant that dramatically reduces elevated levels of cholesterol. Though it is from the same plant that sugar comes from, policosanol does not affect blood sugar levels. Studies have shown that it lowers cholesterol without the harmful side effects caused by drugs. In addition to reducing the LDLs (low-density lipoproteins), or bad fats, in the body, policasonol helps raise HDLs (high-density lipoproteins), or good fats, in the body. According to Raj Pal, PhD, RNC, author of *Hardening of the Arteries: Intravenous (I.V.) Chelationl Antioxidant Approach*, "Policosanol inhibits the formation of lesions in arteries, reduces inflammation-promoting thromboxane, and inhibits platelet aggregation (a cause of arterial blood clotting) and doesn't interfere with sex life."

If you would like to try policosanol but are already taking cholesterol-lowering medications, consult with your physician before discontinuing any prescription drug.

Rice Bran and Rice Bran Syrup

Rice bran syrup is concentrated from the juice of the bran, or outer husk, of brown rice. This is the nutritious part of the rice that is discarded from refined white rice. It is high in the B vitamins that keep the nervous system healthy and minerals, including silicon, which keep the hair, skin, joints, bones, and nails healthy. Rice bran syrup is high in niacin (vitamin B_3), which promotes circulation. If taken on an empty stomach, a flush will come to the cheeks. Take a spoonful after a meal to avoid the flush. It can be sprinkled on cereal or baked in breads. Rice bran is sweet so it will curb the desire for a dessert.

Royal Jelly

Royal jelly is the food that worker bees give to the queen bee to help her grow twice as large and live six times as long as all the other bees. It gives her the nourishment she needs to lay eggs and procreate. This magnificent sweet, creamy food is produced in the glands of the worker bees. It contains enzymes to aid in digestion and absorption, and eighteen amino acids, making it a good source of protein. It also contains vitamin A; all the B vitamins; vitamins C, D, and E; minerals; and hormones. Royal jelly has antibacterial components as well. It nourishes the body and helps fight bacteria and free radicals, thus strengthening the immune system. It balances hormones and promotes longevity.

Royden Brown, one of the world's leading experts on bees and bee products, said we should take royal jelly that is no more than twenty-four hours old. In *The World's Only Perfect Food* he explains that royal jelly should be freeze-dried immediately to maintain its potency. Take twenty-four-hour royal jelly to maintain youth and energy.

S-Adenosyl-L-Methionine (SAM-e)

SAM-e is a wonderful compound that contains sulfur. It acts as a powerful antioxidant, helps raise serotonin levels in the brain, and detoxifies cellular membranes. It has been used successfully in Europe to treat fibromyalgia, migraine headaches, osteoarthritis, liver disorders, and neurological problems. It also has clinical applications in depression, anxiety disorders, and ADHD. Sam-e assists the body with metabolizing neurotransmitter phospholipids such as phosphatidylcholine and phosphatidylserine. SAM-e also helps increase levels of other neurotransmitters, such as serotonin, norepinephrine, and dopamine. These neuro-

Continued ➜

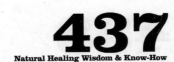

transmitters help increase brain function and prevent or relieve depression.

SAM-e also plays a key role in producing lipotropic compounds in the liver. These ensure the utilization of fats and help eliminate toxins. Thus, it has been very beneficial in promoting liver health. Liver dysfunction can cause fatigue, insomnia, weight gain, poor digestion, allergies, PMS, and hormonal imbalance. SAM-e helps increase the flow of bile in the liver that is needed to digest fat. It has even been shown to be useful in serious liver disorders such as cirrhosis.

SAM-e is produced naturally in the body and is manufactured from the amino acid methionine. When there is an illness or the absence of methionine, B_{12}, or folic acid, the synthesis of SAM-e can be compromised.

Spirulina

Spirulina is a green algae that grows in water in areas where there is a lot of sunshine. Spirulina is an excellent food that contains as much as 70 percent protein; minerals including iron; vitamins including B_{12}, RNA and DNA; and essential fatty acids. Spirulina is also high in chlorophyll. It is a powerful nutritional supplement and has been used successfully by dieters to lose weight and by hypoglycemics to balance blood sugar. Spirulina is a great cleanser for the kidneys. It helps remove heavy metals, drugs, and radiation. Spirulina can be taken in capsule form, but it makes a nice green drink when stirred in water.

Vita Biosa

Vita Biosa is an herbal drink produced in Denmark under the control of the Danish Food and Health Ministry. It was developed by Erik Nielsen, a Danish organic farmer who was inspired by the research of Japanese professor Dr. T. Higa and German herbalist Friedrich Weinkath. Vita Biosa is composed of a mixture of herbs and plants that have been fermented by lactic acid cultures. These cultures are made from friendly bacteria known as effective microorganisms (EMs), which are normally present in well-functioning healthy bowels. The herbs in Vita Biosa consist of angelica, anise, basil, chamomile, chervil, dill, elder, fennel, fenugreek, ginger, juniper, licorice root, nettle, oregano, parsley, peppermint, rosemary, sage, and thyme. The herbs supply the body with beneficial antioxidants, which counteract the development of free radicals. They are also quite beneficial to the digestive tract, helping to improve digestion.

The Vita Biosa's pH is 3.5. This low pH prevents the development of harmful bacteria both in the product and in the body. The lactic acid in the drink works together in the alimentary tract with other friendly microorganisms to abolish harmful bacteria, fungi, viruses, parasites, and yeast infections. Vita Biosa acts directly upon the mucus membranes of the intestines, helping to heal and repair leaky gut syndrome and to develop a powerful defense so harmful bacteria are killed before they can leak out of the gut and cause damage in the body and bloodstream. The effective microorganisms in Vita Biosa work amazingly well to heal Crohn's disease, ulcerative colitis, food intolerances, constipation, diarrhea, and Candida albicans.

Wheatgrass Juice

Wheatgrass juice is a bittersweet rich green juice that has been extracted from green grass grown from grains of wheat. It was made popular by Dr. Ann Wigmore, who founded the Hippocrates Institute in Boston to educate people about healing through good nutrition. Wheatgrass juice is high in chlorophyll, iron, vitamins, and minerals. Taken internally, it fights free radicals in the body and slows the aging process. Wheatgrass juice has helped heal cancerous growths. People drinking the juice report feeling greater energy and vitality. For best results, drink the juice on an empty stomach. Wheatgrass juice can be used externally as an eyewash, a throat gargle, eardrops, a vaginal douche, and a rectal implant. It can be used in the mouth to heal gum infections. Wheatgrass juice promotes healing when placed on cuts, burns, and wounds.

Whey

See "Goat's Milk Whey."

Yeast. Brewer's Yeast, and Torula Yeast

Brewer's yeast and torula yeast are nutritional yeasts, different from the yeast used for baking. Brewer's yeast is grown on the herb called hops and torula yeast is grown on wood bark or blackstrap molasses. Nutritional yeast is high in protein, B vitamins (except for B_{12}), and vitamins and minerals, including phosphorus. It is beneficial to people with hypoglycemia because it helps with sugar metabolism. High in niacin (vitamin B_3), it helps improve circulation. The cheeks may become flushed after eating nutritional yeast because more blood is flowing to the head and brain. This is good because the blood is carrying nutrients to the brain, eyes, ears, nose, and throat, and carrying away toxins. Nutritional yeast can be sprinkled on salads or taken in water or vegetable juice.

—From *Health Is Your Birthright*

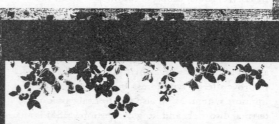

A SELECTION OF NUTRITIONAL REMEDIES
Elen Tast-Jensen

Natural remedies have been used successfully throughout time to relieve pain, heal wounds, combat illnesses, and even save lives. Natural healing techniques empower us to be ready during times of crisis. These remedies are not meant to take the place or the advice of a knowledgeable physician. If a problem persists, go for professional testing and treatment.

Acne

Take twenty-five thousand international units of vitamin A and fifty milligrams of zinc each day, and take two capsules of oregano oil twice a day. Drink yellow dock root tea three times per day.

Anemia

Drink a glass of black cherry juice daily. Drink a glass of raw vegetable juice I made from carrots and parsley; carrots, beets, and parsley; or carrots, beets, and spinach. Be sure to get into the fresh air and sunshine daily, walk, and do some deep-breathing exercises. Oxygen attracts and holds iron in the body. Yellow dock root and dandelion leaf teas are also great blood builders. Chlorophyll is like the blood of the plant and builds the blood of the body

Arthritis

According to Dr. Ruth Yale Long of the Nutrition Education Association, "Arthritis is a nutritional deficiency disease. If we all eat the nutrients we need, we can live out our lives without the misery of arthritis."

Drink eight ounces of celery juice three times per day. Celery juice is made simply by juicing four to six whole sticks of celery to make eight ounces of juice. You can add two ounces of carrot juice made with one large or two small carrots to the celery juice to improve the taste and receive the benefits of the carrot. Celery juice is high in organic sodium, which helps neutralize acidity in the body, dissolve bone spurs, and allow the calcium to go back into solution or back into your bones. Black cherry juice is also great for breaking up crystals in the joints. It helps relieve and heal arthritis as well as gout. Buy only natural black cherry juice that contains no added sugars or preservatives. For the best results, grow or purchase your own black cherries and juice them. It takes about two cups of cherries with stems and seeds removed to make one eight-ounce glass of black cherry juice. People with diabetes or hypoglycemia will need to dilute the black cherry juice (use three ounces of black cherry juice and five ounces of water) because of the fruit sugars it contains.

Vegetables and fruits contain an organic, biochemical, absorbable form of sodium. According to Dr. Bernard Jensen in *The Chemistry of Man*:

Organic sodium keeps calcium in solution in the human body. Sodium was named the "youth" element due to its properties of promoting youthful, limber, flexible, pliable joints. Joint troubles need not manifest in the individual who has a good reserve of sodium, the "youth" element in the stomach walls and the joints. Goat milk and goat whey are rich in natural sodium.

Dr. Jensen raised goats at his ranch. Rather than having to raise goats, you can drink a wonderful goat's milk whey drink daily.

Other important nutrients that help relieve and heal arthritis include; alfalfa tablets, which are high in absorbable minerals. Include essential fatty acids in your diet to relieve inflammation. Glucosamine sulfate helps form and repair bones and cartilage. Liquid minerals and trace minerals ensura absorption into the bone. Take a good multivitamin containing all the B vitamins to help nourish the body overall and reduce free radicals. Tal turmeric, which has anti-inflammatory properties. White willow bark can relieve inflammation and ease pain. This can be taken as an herbal tea or in capsule form.

Asthma

Asthma is a disease that causes the bronchi or air passages in the lungs become inflamed, congested with mucus, and constricted, blocking the flow of air and oxygen. Symptoms of asthma include wheezing, tightness of the chest, inability to breathe, and coughing. Children, teens, and adults can have asthma and it is usually caused by allergies and weakened immune system. Several triggers cause asthma including dust, mold, mites, pets, feathers, air pollution, cigarette smoke, food additives including MSG and sulfites, perfume, chemicals in cleaning solutions, and hair spray.

People with asthma may also have reactions to wheat, dairy products, and sugar, and should avoid them. Wheat and dairy products are gluey and pasty and might contribute to the mucus in the lungs. Wheat also can paste down the small villi in the intestinal tract. Many asthmatics are allergic to

Continued ➡

dairy products and notice improvement when they leave them out of the diet. Sugar and all artificial sweeteners can weaken the immune system. The nutritional plan and cleanse in this book have helped many asthmatics gain relief and begin healing because toxins are cleansed from the body and the immune system is strengthened. Consult with your doctor or health practitioner before you begin a cleanse. Eat foods that help release mucus from the body, such as turnips, lemons, limes, radishes, garlic, and onions. Add cayenne and ginger to your diet.

Atherosclerosis

In *Hardening of the Arteries, Heart Attack—Stroke*, Raj Pal, PhD, RNC, states:

Cardiovascular disease is the number one killer in the country. Deaths surpass those from all other causes combined. Atherosclerosis, or hardening of the arteries, is a contributing factor not only in heart attacks and strokes, but also in high blood pressure. It causes poor circulation, which in turn restricts the disbursement of nutrients to other parts of your body organs, tissue and skin. It contributes to providing less oxygen to the brain, thus slowing down your thinking process and memory.

Atherosclerosis allows arteries to become filled with fat and the arteria walls to harden. The heart has to pump harder to move the blood through these blocked arteries, and blood pressure goes up.

One of the main causes of atherosclerosis is damage to the arteries by free radicals. Another cause is diets high in fried foods, margarine, partially hydrogenated oils, saturated fats, and rancid oils. Smoking causes tremendous damage to the arteries.

To prevent and heal atherosclerosis, consume antioxidants that fight free radicals, such as vitamins A, B, C, and E, as well as absorbable minerals and trace minerals. Make sure you ingest essential fatty acids such as flaxseed oil. Coenzyme Q10 is a powerful antioxidant, and garlic is a wonderful agent that helps regulate fat and cleanse the arteries. Lecithin and citrus pectin emulsify fat in the arteries as well. There is a wonderful natural oral chelating agent product called A-Flow. It contains most of these nutrients and several others in a balanced ratio. It is natural, safe, and effective, but still a good idea to consult with your physician before taking. A-Flow helps to remove arterial plaque and fights the causes of plaque. It is also high in antioxidants that disarm free radicals.

Breast Ailments

For nursing mothers whose breasts are caked from milk, blend organic tomatoes and make a tomato poultice.

To promote milk flow in nursing mothers, make a tea with nettles and blessed thistle. Drink at least a few cups each day. Also, eat plenty of green leafy vegetables. Almond cream, sesame sauce, and sunflower seed sauce also help to promote a rich milk flow. Here are a couple of other recipes that help increase mother's breast milk.

Atole

4 cups purified water

3 heaping tablespoons cornmeal

1 cinnamon stick

1 cup almond milk

½ cup natural maple syrup or 5 to 10 drops of stevia

Boil 4 cups of purified water with a cinnamon stick. Take 1 cup of the boiling water and add 3 heaping tablespoons of cornmeal. Stir until smooth. Add this cup of mixture nto the pot of boiling water. Stir until smooth. Boil for 10 minutes on low. Cool. Mixture will get thick, Add one cup of homemade almond milk or almond milk from the health food store and natural maple syrup or stevia to taste. Refrigerate. Drink at least twice a day.

To supplement breast milk, the following is a nice formula to give to babies.

Natural Baby Formula

1 ounce goat milk powder

3 ounces distilled water

½ ounce pure cream

1 teaspoon milk sugar

Combine all the ingredients and stir well.

When the mother is not producing enough of her own milk, fresh raw goat milk is the best substitute. It is the nearest in composition to human milk and is very healthy for the baby. If there are no goats in the area, the natural baby formula above is also a very good substitute.

Breasts often become sore just before menstruation due to excess estrogen. When the liver has not processed the estrogen properly, the breasts can swell and ache. To help the liver process estrogen, avoid fried foods, caffeine, sugar, alcohol, and meats and milk that are high in hormones. Take four hundred international units of vitamin E three times daily, a good multivitamin/multimineral with all the B vitamins, and evening primrose oil. Get plenty of exercise, eat lots of vegetables, and make sure the bowels are moving.

Cholesterol, High

Cholesterol plays a vital role in cellular health. It is necessary for the brain and nervous system to function properly and for the manufacture of sex hormones. Cholesterol is a fat and is manufactured in the liver.

There is a lot of confusion right now about cholesterol. Many people believe that margarine is good for them and that butter is bad. This is far from the truth! Chemicals that harden margarine can also harden the arteries! A little real butter is better for you. Butter contains vitamin A, which is great for your eyes, and some protein. Hydrogenating oils keep margarine solid, even in your blood and arteries. Avoid hydrogenated oils and polyunsaturated oils. Read labels.

Many people also believe that artificial eggs are better for maintaining healthy cholesterol levels than real eggs from healthy chickens. This is not true. Fertilized eggs from healthy chickens are high in lecithin, which emulsifies cholesterol.

Refined white sugar can cause high cholesterol. The liver converts excess sugar into fat in your blood! These fats are then deposited in the arteries, creating plaque.

To lower cholesterol, eat foods high in fiber, such as whole grains—including oats, barley, millet, and quinoa—beans, steamed vegetables, and salads. Use apple pectin or citrus pectin, which binds to plaque and fat and pulls it out of the body. Use lecithin on soups, in vegetable juice, or on salads to help cleanse plaque and lower cholesterol levels. Eat lots of garlic or take garlic capsules. Policosanol, a natural food substance, has proven to be tremendously successful in lowering cholesterol. Use beets or take beet tablets. Beets help cleanse the liver and gallbladder. Eat raw grated beets and steamed beets and drink raw vegetable juice, such as carrot, celery,

parsley, beet, and ginger. Carrot juice flushes fat from the bile in the liver and helps control cholesterol, and ginger improves circulation.

Food supplements that help reduce cholesterol include alpha lipoic acid and lipotropic factors, which help prevent fat deposits. A-Flow, an oral chelation formula, and essential fatty acids, such as black currant seed, flaxseed, borage, and primrose oils, help raise the good fats or high-density lipoproteins and lower the bad fats or low-density lipoproteins. Cayenne, coenzyme Q10, and niacin help improve circulation, and glucomannan and gugolipids also reduce serum cholesterol.

Diabetes Mellitus

Diabetes mellitus is a disorder that results when the pancreas stops producing sufficient amounts of insulin. Insulin is a hormone that regulates the absorption of glucose, which produces energy in the cells; it stimulates fat cells and the liver to store reserve glucose. When there is an insufficient amount of insulin, glucose builds up in the blood, causing hyperglycemia.

High levels of glucose in the blood lead to frequent urination because of the increased volume of urine required to carry sugar out of the body. One side effect of an increase in urination is constant thirst. Excessive levels of sugar in the urine can impair the body's ability to fight infection. Sugar can even cause infections, including yeast, bladder, and skin infections. People with diabetes become weak with fatigue because their cells lack glucose (an important source of energy), which has been carried away with the constant urination. Diabetics often lose weight as their bodies strive to obtain energy by breaking down stored fat. Hyperglycemia can eventually cause damage to the blood vessels and nerves, leading to numbness of the limbs and diseases of the heart, eyes, and kidneys.

According to the American Diabetes Association:

There are 20.8 million children and adults in the United States, or seven percent of the population, who have diabetes. While an estimated 14.6 million have been diagnosed, unfortunately, 6.2 million people (or nearly one-third) are unaware that the have the disease.

There are two major types of diabetes. Type 1 diabetes, or insulin-dependent diabetes mellitus (IDDM), is the more severe type and affects 5 to 10 percent of people with diabetes. It develops rapidly, usually occurring in young people between the ages of ten and sixteen. In this type, the insulin-secreting beta cells have been destroyed (often from a virus or overactive immune response), and insulin can no longer be produced.

Type 2 diabetes, or noninsulin dependent diabetes, affects 90 to 95 percent of diabetics and usually occurs in people over the age of forty. However, there recently has been an alarming increase among teenagers and children. In this type, insulin is produced but not enough to manage the sugar levels in the blood. There are several risk factors for developing type 2 diabetes. These include a diet rich in refined carbohydrates, hydrogenated oils, processed foods, soft drinks, high fructose corn syrup, and sugar; excess weight; and lack of exercise.

Type 2 diabetes claims about a hundred million victims worldwide each year. In the United States, it is the sixth-leading cause of death and one of the primary causes of blindness, kidney disease, and amputations.

Avoid refined white sugar. Use natural sugars such as maple syrup, honey, dates, and molasses sparingly. Use stevia or agave to sweeten your food and drinks. These sweeteners actually balance the pancreas and have very few calories. Take chromium

Continued ➡

picolinate and trace minerals to help balance the pancreas and reduce sweet cravings.

Gymnema sylvestre, a wonderful herb from India, lowers high blood sugar levels and greatly reduces excessive secretion of glucose in the urine. It also increases beta cells that produce insulin, and may reduce the need for insulin treatments. Recent studies have shown that cinnamon can actually balance blood sugar levels as well. Fenugreek seeds were used in ancient Italy, Greece, and India to treat blood sugar disturbances in the body. Fenugreek seeds can help reduce insulin requirements by lowering blood glucose levels. Soak fenugreek seeds, sprout them, and put them in salads and on soups. The high fiber content delays glucose absorption.

Eye Disorders

Included below are a few simple eye remedies and suggestions. If you experiencing any eye problems, see your ophthalmologist immediately. For nutritional suggestions for strengthening the eyes, see page 364. For more in-depth eye information, read *Smart Medicine for Your Eyes* by Dr. Jeffrey Anshel.

If the eyes become dry in the wintertime, vessels in the sclera become irritated, swollen, and red. Bioflavonoids, which strengthen blood vessels, can help prevent this condition. The fluid of the eyes is part of the lymph system, so feed your lymph with the mineral whey drink described on page 350, and drink plenty of celery juice. Oils are an important lubricant too, so incorporate flax seed oil, borage oil, and pumpkin seed oil into your diet.

The eyes are vulnerable to several types of infection. A sty results when one of the small glands attached to an eye becomes infected. Iritis, an inflammation of the iris, can be caused by allergies or infection. Conjunctivitis, an inflammation of the conjunctiva, can be caused by allergies, infection, chemical burns, or injury. Pink eye is a type of conjunctivitis. A compress can be prepared that may help soothe and heal infected eyes.

GOLDENSEAL EYE COMPRESS

⅓ teaspoon goldenseal powder
1 ounce fresh cabbage juice

Boil two ounces distilled water. Turn off the heat, let cool, and add the goldenseal and juice. Goldenseal contains the alkaloid berberine, which helps fight infection; cabbage juice is high in vitamins C and A and can help fight bacteria and viruses. Stir with a sterile spoon and strain through a cheesecloth. Dip two pieces of gauze, large enough to cover each eyelid, in the solution and place over the closed eyelids. Leave for fifteen minutes to a half hour.

Cataracts are an opacification or cloudiness that occur in the lens and which block light from reaching the retina and impair vision. Most cataracts begin after age forty-five and are often caused by free-radical damage, heavy metals, eye injury, smoking, or diabetes. Vitamin B, eyebright tea, which is also rich in vitamins C and A, and bilberries and blueberries, which are rich in bioflavonoids, may help prevent cataracts. Splashing the eyes with cold water each morning also helps because it stimulates the circulation of blood through the eyes. A diet rich in vegetables, especially spinach and carrots, help maintain eye health.

Glaucoma results when fluid pressure increases inside the eyeball. This occurs when either the eye is producing too much fluid or the drainage system in the eye has broken down or is blocked. Glaucoma has many causes including eye injury, eye surgery, nutritional imbalances, and some medications such as steroids. It may also be related to high blood pressure and diabetes. To help prevent glaucoma, follow the nutritional plans in chapter 1, the cleansing program outlined in chapter 6, and the eye poultice in chapter 3. Include plenty of cold-pressed oils including flax, borage, and olive oils in your diet, as well as liquid trace minerals and zinc. Vitamin A, beta-carotene, B complex, B6, and bioflavonoids may be helpful. Vitamin C can possibly help to reduce the pressure.

Blepharitis is an inflammation of the outer edges of the eyelids that can occur when the glands in the eyelids and hair follicles become blocked with mucus and inflamed. A bacterial infection may be involved and burning, swollen eyelids can result. The eyes may also become pasted together during sleep. Drink raw juices of green leaves and carrots. Rinse your eyes with warm water and use the compress above. Include bilberry and eyebright herbs in your diet. Vitamin A, beta-carotene, vitamin C with bioflavonoids, liquid trace minerals, and zinc (no more than 50 milligrams) have traditionally been used to improve conditions. Use an air filter to remove dust, mold, and pollen from your home.

Fibromyalgia

Fibromyalgia is a rheumatic disorder that causes severe aching in the muscles, much as if one has been beaten or bruised. Approximately ten million people in the United States have been diagnosed with fibromyalgia, and that figure is rising. The etiology is still unknown and there is no known cure. Most people who have fibromyalgia have often had some type of trauma, injury, or severe stress. The immune system may be weak, and there may be a disturbance in the brain's chemistry. The Epstein-Barr virus or other viruses may be involved. People with fibromyalgia may have *Candida albicans* (a fungus) or parasites. They may be anemic and have low thyroid function and hypoglycemia. However, people can have any of these disorders and not have fibromyalgia.

The common denominators in patients with fibromyalgia are stress and sleep disturbance. Studies have shown that people deprived of sleep have muscular pain. People who have chronic stress produce high amounts of adrenaline, which can cause insomnia, poor digestion, rapid heartbeat, and even sore muscles. Nobel prize winner Hans Seyle found that stress can cause calcium leak from the bone and become deposited in tissues. He explains his research in Stress Without Distress. Nancy Selfridge, MD, conquered fibromyalgia and has worked with many others to do the same. She has written a wonderful book called *Freedom from Fibromyalgia: The 5-Week Program Proven to Conquer Pain*. Two other very informative books are *New Hope for People with Fibromyalgia* by Theresa Foy DiGeronimo, MEd and *From Fatigued to Fantastic* by Jacob Teitelbaum, MD.

People with fibromyalgia suffer from insomnia and when they don't sleep, the muscular-pain is more severe. They often feel exhausted with chronic fatigue never reaching a deep restful sleep due to the pain. Other symptoms of fibromyalgia include headaches, digestive disorders, feelings of disorientation, difficulty concentrating, depression, and bruxism (tooth grinding).

Several herbal remedies can be very effective in healing *Candida albicans* and viruses. These are, Pau d'Arco, grapefruit seed extract, and capryllic acid (made from coconut). People with fibromyalgia who have *Candida albicans* should start with small dosages and build up gradually, or they might feel much worse.

Ionic trace minerals are essential for keeping the body alkaline. Turmeric and white willow bark, two anti-inflammatory herbs, can ease discomfort.

Malic acid, found in apples, assists the cells in producing energy. CoQ10 improves tissue oxygenation. Ginkgo biloba improves brain and nerve function, and cayenne improves circulation. Glucosamine sulfate is a naturally occurring precursor for proteoglycan synthesis. Glucosamine sulfate can strengthen joints as well as connective tissue. Bioflavonoids are important components of vitamin C that help to build connective tissue. Acidophilus and Eugalan Topfer Forte (a powdered form of *Lactobacillus bifidus*) are good probiotics that soothe the digestive tract and provide friendly bacteria that keep the colon healthy. Flaxseed tea and aloe vera juice also soothe the digestive tract. Take enzymes before each meal to assist the body in breaking down and absorbing nutrients. Flaxseed oil and borage oil help provide the essential fatty acids necessary for healthy nerve functioning. Magnesium, calcium, and potassium help relax the muscles and in some cases are all a person with fibromyalgia will need to help them relax and sleep. If not, 5-hydroxytryptophan (5HTP) is a natural supplement that helps promote proper sleep cycles. Skullcap and valerian root can also help promote deep restful sleep.

A good multivitamin/multimineral with a high amount of B vitamins for the nervous system is very important. Chlorella is most effective in cleansing the colon, liver, and blood. Vitamin E improves circulation and is a powerful antioxidant. NOTE: There is a wide selection of supplements that can help with fibromyalgia. However, all people with fibromyalgia will not need to take all mentioned supplements. For specifics, it is important to work with a doctor to determine first if you have fibromyalgia. Then find out for sure if you have have *Candida albicans* or a virus. If not, you will not need the remedies suggested for these. You need to find out if you have hypoglycemia, low thyroid function, or exhausted adrenal glands. If so, bringing these areas into balance will help strengthen the body so it can rest properly. Relaxing the muscles, improving nerve function, and getting proper sleep is paramount for those suffering with the pain of fibromyalgia. Cleansing the colon and liver can also be very beneficial.

People with fibromyalgia must avoid caffeine and alcohol.

Hair Loss

Eat two organic raw egg yolks laid by free range hens daily. Wash the eggs well before cracking them open. You may add black cherry juice to the egg yolks for better flavor and blend them into a Good Morning Health Shake or Avocado Pudding (see recipes in chapter 1). Drink two cups of oatstraw tea per day and one cup of rosemary leaf tea per day. Follow the advice under scalp treatment for hair loss (see chapter 3). Poached eggs and soft-boiled eggs are also helpful. If the problem is chronic, balance the adrenal glands by taking raw organic adrenal, ashwaganda, or licorice root capsules and meditating and relaxing each day. Taking B complex and biotin has also proven to be very helpful. Put rice bran on your cereal or salads.

Herpes Simplex 1 (Hsv-1) and Herpes Simplex 2 (Hsv-2)

Herpes simplex 1 is a virus that usually causes cold sores on the mouth, skin eruptions, and eye infections. As many as 80 percent of the United States population have been infected by this virus but not all have noticeable symptoms.

Herpes simplex 2 is a virus that can cause genital blisters. Approximately thirty-five million Americans have been infected but not all are symptomatic.

Continued ➡

Both herpes viruses are contagious. People who have these viruses should follow a healthy eating regime for two weeks, as outlined in chapter 1, then do the colon and liver cleanse.

Take five hundred' milligrams of L-lysine with water twice daily on an empty stomach. L-lysine is one of the eight essential amino acids found in protein that the body does not produce on its own. It helps strengthen the immune system and has the ability to fight and prevent the herpes virus. Food sources include brewer's yeast, eggs, fish, and lima beans. Take a good multivitamin high in B complex three times daily; two thousand milligrams of vitamin C three times daily; sixty milligrams of quercetin (a bioflavonoid and powerful antioxidant) three times daily; fifty milligrams of zinc two times daily; acidophilus four times daily on an empty stomach; HPVS (an effective herbal formula) according to directions; one dropperfull of colloidal silver twice daily; and oregano oil capsules three times daily. Apply oregano oil or tea tree oil to any cold sores. Apply three parts olive oil mixed with one part oregano or tea tree oil to genital blisters. The Monastery of Herbs carries very effective herbal remedies called HPVS #1 and HPVS #2.

Hypoglycemia

Hypoglycemia means the blood sugar or glucose levels are low. This usually occurs when the pancreas is producing too much insulin. Insulin helps manage blood sugar levels by facilitating the transport of sugar to the body's cells. It is also responsible for glucose synthesis in the liver. When there is too much insulin, blood sugar is utilized too rapidly, causing a person to feel light-headed, weak, shaky, tired, dizzy, anxious, depressed, short-tempered, nervous, and hungry. These people are often hungry and crave sweets. However, if they eat sweets, they may feel better for a short while only to have their blood sugar level crash again, feeling worse than ever.

Sugar intake prompts the pancreas to produce a surge of insulin. Eating small meals of foods that break down slowly throughout the day will normalize insulin production. Eat lots of raw and steamed vegetables, beans, soaked nuts and seeds, nut butters, brown rice, lentils, baked or broiled fish, chicken, turkey, yogurt, and cottage cheese. Eat no more than two fruits per day. In addition, ground flaxseeds, oat bran, and rice bran are high in fiber and slow a hypoglycemic reaction.

Avoid sugar, fruit juice, soft drinks, caffeine, nicotine, alcohol, and refined white flour. Supplements that are very helpful include glucose tolerance factor (GTF), chromium picolinate, digestive enzymes, chlorella, spirulina, B complex, brewer's yeast, amino acids, trace minerals, and vitamin E.

Blueberry leaf, huckleberry leaf, dandelion root tea, and stevia can help balance the pancreas. Licorice root tea supports the adrenal glands. Do not use licorice root on a daily basis. Every other day or every third day is best. Do not use it at all if you have high blood pressure.

Indigestion, Burning Stomach, and Gas

Indigestion, burning stomach, and gas usually occur after eating a large meal with poor food combinations. Eugalan Topfer Forte is a wonderful product that contains a natural culture of live lactobacillus bifidus in a special food base that enhances their proliferation. It does contain some milk powder, but even people who have allergies to dairy products can usually tolerate it because of the high content (thirty million live lactobacillus bifidus organisms per one-ounce serving) of beneficial bacteria, which aid digestion. To prepare, place five level teaspoons (one ounce) of Eugalan Topfer Forte in five ounces of warm water. Stir the mixture well and drink it slowly. Children should take one teaspoon two times a day, and infants may take a half teaspoon daily. This delicious drink soothes the entire digestive tract and usually relieves indigestion, burning, and gas almost immediately. It can also benefit, people with stomach ulcers.

If you have a tendency to get indigestion with your meals, take a few plant-based digestive enzymes with some water just before eating. The enzymes will help facilitate proper food digestion. Most Americans over the age of forty have lost a lot of their digestive ability, having consumed many meals of processed foods throughout their lives.

Papaya, papaya juice, and papaya tablets can help relive indigestion, burning in the stomach, and gas. I had a client with a stomach ulcer that he believed was a result of years of chronic beer consumption. Papaya juice helped him heal the ulcer. Charcoal tablets absorb excess gas in the gut. However, they should not be used on a regular basis. Charcoal may absorb healthy nutrients from the digestive tract as well. If you are taking medications, pregnant, or nursing consult your doctor before taking charcoal.

Combine your food properly, take digestive enzymes, aloe vera juice, acidophilus, and lactobacillus bifidus to correct the problem. If indigestion and burning persist or if nausea develops, seek the advice of a knowledgeable physician.

Kidney and Bladder Infections

When suffering from a kidney or bladder infection, avoid all dairy products except natural yogurt. Avoid caffeine, alcohol, salt, pork, and red meat (which is high in uric acid). Eat lots of raw vegetables, such as asparagus, parsley, celery, cucumber, green leafy lettuce, watercress, and garlic. Drink raw vegetable juices with carrot, cucumber, and parsley. Drink parsley tea. Eat watermelon but not with other foods. Eat steamed vegetables, brown rice, quinoa, millet, lentils, and beans.

Take acidophilus, propolis, and goldenseal. Take or drink as a tea: juniper berries, corn silk, and uva ursi. Take a dropper of colloidal silver or six drops of grapefruit seed extract three to four times per day. Take lots of acidophilus between meals on an empty stomach. Drink eight glasses of distilled water with four drops of ionic trace minerals in each glass. Keep the colon clean by taking chlorella and flaxseed oil.

NOTE: When taking grapefruit seed extract, do not get it on your teeth because it can be wearing on the enamel. Put it in water and drink it with a straw.

Kidney Stones

For kidney stones, follow the program for Kidney and Bladder Infections (above). Avoid red meat and dairy products. Drink eight ounces of water with one tablespoon of raw apple cider vinegar added to it, four times per day. Drink water with freshly squeezed lemon juice. Use lemon juice and olive oil or apple cider vinegar and olive oil salad dressings. Drink raw apple juice. Apples, lemons, and asparagus are helpful. Hydrangea, gravel root, and marshmallow root tinctures, teas, or capsules can help dissolve stones and relieve pain.

Menstrual Cramping

Cramps can occur when the transverse colon has prolapsed and is pressing on the uterus. They can also occur when the liver does not process estrogen well or when minerals—especially calcium and magnesium—which keep muscles in the abdomen relaxed, are lacking. Also, clotting can occur during menstruation and cause cramping. Vitamin E and red raspberry leaf tea greatly reduce clotting and cramping. Avoid caffeine, sugar, and dairy products.

Menstruation, Irregular

Take two hundred international units of vitamin E three times per day to facilitate blood flow and circulation. Make sure the vitamin E is natural and the label says d-alphatocopherol rather than dl-alphatocopherol. Dl-alphatocopherol is the synthetic form of vitamin E. It is not utilized as well by the body and its potency is reduced compared to that of natural vitamin E. Herbs, such as dong quai, red raspberry leaf tea, and vitex can help regulate the menstrual cycle.

Morning Sickness

Pregnant mothers may take ginger tea or peppermint leaf tea to relieve morning sickness. Vitamin B6 taken with a B complex can also be very helpful as well as eating small meals throughout the day.

Osteoporosis

Osteoporosis, which means "porous bones," is a common bone disease. In old age, porous bones are brittle, and they break easily. After a fracture or break, they are slow to heal. A deficiency of vitamin D causes bones to soften. This condition is called osteomalacia in adults and rickets in children. The term used to describe a lowered bone mass which can be a precursor to osteoporosis is osteopenia. One of the best treatments for bones is raw organic vegetable juice because it is so easily absorbed. One glass of carrot juice is equal in calcium to a glass of milk and is much more absorbable. Most juices from green leafy vegetables are even higher in calcium than carrot juice.

Avoid caffeine in coffee, tea, sodas, and chocolate. Excessive caffeine contributes to osteoporosis by leaching calcium from bones and increasing urinary output of calcium. Douglas Kiel conducted a study and found that drinking two cups of coffee each day greatly increased the risk of bone fractures. A diet high in animal protein, sugar, salt, and processed foods create: acidity in the body, leading to calcium loss. An article in the *American. Journal of Clinical Nutrition*, 6, summarizes a study conducted at the University of California in San Francisco, on 9,704 postmenopausa women. It showed that those women who ate a diet high in animal food: and low in vegetables had increased acidity levels and a resultant greater risk for lowered bone density than women with normal pH levels. When the body is acidic, it will pull calcium from the bones to help neutralize acids.

The phosphoric acid found in soft drinks inhibits the body from absorbing calcium properly. Vitamin D, boron, zinc, magnesium, calcium sodium, and digestive enzymes will assist in calcium absorption. Raw vegetables and raw vegetable juices contain organic sodium, which neutralizes acids and holds calcium in the bone. Goat whey is high in absorbable minerals as well as organic sodium, and it is a great acid neutralizer.

Ulcers

A peptic ulcer is an open wound in the stomach lining or anywhere along the intestinal tract. People with peptic ulcers have intense burning or seven pain. Some may suffer from nausea and vomiting. Pain is more intense when the stomach is empty, and eating or drinking lots of water relieve the pain.

Ulcers occur as the result of ongoing stress, which causes the release of excess stomach acids.

Continued ➡

Taking antacids and certain medications such as aspirin and even vitamin C over a long period of time can contribute to ulcers. A diet high in sugar, caffeine, and processed foods can produce too much acidity and cause ulcers. Food allergies can cause an imbalance in intestinal flora. Heavy smokers and people who abuse alcohol often get ulcers as well.

To heal ulcers, avoid alcohol, caffeine, cigarette smoking, heavy use of antacids, ascorbic acid in some types of vitamin C, and many types of drugs. Food allergens must be identified and avoided. Avoid wheat, salt, sugar, fried foods, and processed foods. Eat papayas and drink papaya juice. Follow the food plans presented in chapter I. Raw cabbage juice has been tremendously successful in healing ulcers. Five cups of cabbage juice taken throughout the day can help heal some ulcers in seven to ten days. Drink slippery elm tea. Take goldenseal root or colloidal silver to help inhibit bacterial growth. Check with your physician to find out if you have the bacteria called helicobacter pylori or H. pylori. This virus may be the cause of ulcers.

—From *Health Is Your Birthright*

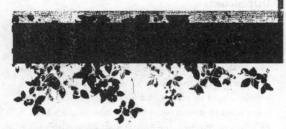

VITAMINS, MINERALS, AND AMINO ACIDS

Diane Stein

Vitamins and Minerals

Vitamins and minerals are intrinsic components of the body's chemistry, and they are necessary for life. They are essential nutrients, called micro-nutrients because of the minute amounts required. Vitamins regulate metabolism and release the energy produced by food digestion. They are coenzyme precursors, regulating and working with enzymes to catalyze all of the processes of the body. Minerals also participate in enzymatic processes. They are needed for blood and bone formation, the formation and chemistry of body fluids, and the maintenance of nerve function and the entire nervous system.

Both vitamins and minerals are primarily obtained from foods. Vitamins are either not made in the body or are made in inadequate amounts. Since water-soluble vitamins are excreted through the urine, they must be taken in daily. These vitamins include vitamin C and the full B complex. Oil-soluble vitamins are stored for a period of time in the liver and fatty tissues. Vitamins A, D, E and K are oil-soluble. Because water soluble vitamins are excreted and not stored, actual overdoses are not possible though there may be some discomfort from major excesses. Oil-soluble vitamins can be overdosed (except for vitamin E), but the extent of toxicity has been highly overemphasized by those who disparage vitamins.

Minerals come from the soil that is the body of the planet, entering plant matter first on the food chain. Herbivorous animals and human vegetarians obtain their minerals from eating plants. Meat eaters obtain their minerals from the bodies of herbivores. Thus women obtain minerals from eating plants, meat, poultry or fish. There are two types of minerals: trace minerals and macro (bulk) minerals. Trace minerals are needed in very minute quantities but those quantities are essential. They include zinc, iron, copper, boron, manganese, chromium, germanium, selenium and iodine. Macro minerals, needed in larger amounts, include calcium, magnesium, sodium, potassium, and phosphorus. The most frequent nutritional deficiencies for women are the minerals calcium and iron and the B vitamins folic acid and B_6. Minerals are stored in bone and muscle tissue, but only massive amounts taken over long periods of time will cause toxicities.

Ninety-eight percent of women (and slightly less of men) are deficient in the B complex vitamin folic acid, and ninety percent of women are deficient in vitamin B_6. Calcium deficiency affects seventy-three percent of women, zinc deficiency fifty-seven percent of women, and iron deficiency is experienced by 60 percent of women[1] Folic acid is essential for the formation of blood, as is B_6, and B_6 is vital for metabolism of amino acids and protein. Many women's premenstrual stress is caused by these vitamin deficiencies, and women on the contraceptive pill are particularly at risk. Calcium is needed for bone, muscle and nerve formation and function, as well as for milk production in lactating mothers. Calcium deficiency is also implicated in premenstrual nervous tension, water retention, muscle spasms of the legs and osteoporosis. Zinc regulates the immune system, the healing of organs and wounds, and the development of healthy skin and hair. Iron produces hemoglobin, the oxygen-carrying component of red blood cells. Women with heavy menstrual flows often have iron deficiency anemia.

Vitamin and mineral deficiencies are a major factor in women's health. Yet, if vitamins and minerals come from food, why is this so even in women who eat a healthy diet? Why is vitamin and mineral deficiency increasing as a factor in women's disease? Vitamins and minerals are nutrients essential to human life. The food chain begins with plants' absorption of minerals from the soil. The soil is the earth, the planet, that is now depleted and polluted to the crisis point. Women's vitamin and mineral deficiencies begin with the depleted earth, the nutrients that are no longer available for plants to assimilate from the soil. Depleted plant nutrition means depleted nutrition all along the food chain.

Earth's soil is mineral deficient from farming practices like overcropping and single-crop farming. Soil erosion is a worldwide crisis that continues to remove needed minerals from the soil and from food plants. Chemical replacement fertilizers are often not nutrients that can be assimilated by humans or animals eating plants grown with them. Chemicals are used by today's agribusiness farmers to stimulate plant growth, create attractive appearance, and extend shipping and shelf-life at the expense of the nutritional value (and taste) of the crops. Pesticides are highly overused on today's farms, the residues of which are present in all food and contaminate the water tables. Extended shipping time from picking to eating further depletes the vitamin content of foods, as does preservation by chemicals, dyes and additives. Irradiation reduces the vitamin content by 20 to 80 percent.

Food that was grown and eaten a hundred years ago, or even fifty years ago, contained the essential vitamins and minerals for good health. Today's chemicalized and refined food does not. Because of this, most women are vitamin and/or mineral deficient in some way, and I consider a *good* (not cheap but *good*) daily multiple vitamin and mineral supplement a *must* for everyone. This simple step alone goes a long way toward prevention of dis-ease, and often the addition of it to the diet is enough to heal many women's health problems. Choose a quality healthfood store supplement, not one from the supermarket, and take it with meals. My own choice is Schiff's Single Day, but there are many others of good quality. A balanced calcium-magnesium supplement is needed by most women, also.

Vitamins and minerals suggested for healing in this book start with the assumption that you are taking a daily multiple vitamin and mineral tablet. Many vitamins require others taken with them to work and the multiple provides these in proper balance and quantity. Calcium, for example, requires small amounts of vitamins A, C, and D, as well as iron, phosphorus and an amount of magnesium that is half the amount of the calcium. Each of the B complex vitamins requires the rest of the B complex to activate it. Vitamin E requires selenium, manganese and inositol in small amounts. Supplement amounts of a vitamin or mineral used alone can cause an imbalance that functions like the deficiency it is meant to heal. The vitamins and minerals present in a multiple prevent this. The amounts of each suggested supplement require a balance of others.

The Food and Drug Administration (FDA) has set up a list of vitamin and mineral amounts called the RDA, Recommended Dietary Allowances, and bases its watchdogging of supplements on these amounts. The figures, however, were founded on very little nutritional research and at best are only what is required to prevent a nutritional deficiency dis-ease such as scurvy or pellagra. Vitamins and minerals are needed in much greater quantities than the RDA limits for optimal health, and greater amounts yet may be needed to correct an illness or deficiency. It is also important to remember that each individual has her own body requirements that may be different from other women's or the norm. A chart is provided comparing the RDAs for the most common vitamins and minerals with the amounts recommended for women's good health. For specific dis-eases, the amounts suggested may vary from those given.

Here is a very quick run-down of vitamins and minerals and their uses in women's healing. For more complete information, see my book *All Women Are Healers* (The Crossing Press, 1990), as well as James Balch, MD, and Phyllis Balch, CNC, *Prescription for Nutritional Healing* (Avery Publishing Group, 1990) and Velma Keith and Montene Gordon, *The How-To Herb Book* (Mayfield Publishing, 1984).

Vitamin A is an antioxidant. It protects the body from pollutants, aging and cancer, and boosts the immune system. It is effective in nightblindness and eyestrain, in rough or dry skin and hair, acne, eczema, angina, recurrent colds, flus or infections, and impaired sense of smell. Vitamin A may help or heal gastric ulcers, boils, allergies, hay fever, respiratory infections, hyperthyroidism, emphysema and any dis-eases of the skin, hair, eyes, teeth and gums. It may delay heart attacks in high risk women, and is important for weight gain, children's growth and bone formation.

Beta-carotene is converted to vitamin A in the liver and the vitamin may be taken in this form. Hypothyroid or diabetic women, however, may be unable to convert beta-carotene adequately. Vitamin A should not be taken in large amounts by women with liver dis-ease, and women on the pill may need less vitamin A than others. If you are pregnant, take no more than 25,000 IU per day. Adults have taken as much as 100,000 IU a day of vitamin A, and infants up to 18,000 IU a day for many months without toxicity. Beta-carotene is water soluble and cannot be overdosed, and vitamin A also comes in a water soluble dry form.

Continued ➡

The B Complex is a group of vitamins that need to be taken together, rather than as individual vitamins used alone. In a deficiency situation, take the full B complex or a multiple vitamin that contains it, then add the individual B supplement needed. Unlike vitamin A, these are water soluble vitamins with no toxicity, but too much can result in diarrhea, constipation or nightmares (B_6) for some women. Reducing the dosage stops these side effects immediately. B vitamins are helpful for mental and nervous disorders, depression, insomnia, stress and anxiety. They are useful in premenstrual tension, migraines, epilepsy, Candida albicans, asthma, anemia and allergies. Vegetarians, women on antibiotics and women on diuretics especially need B complex. AZT, the primary drug used in AIDS, drains B vitamins from the body. B vitamins are energy balancing calmatives, useful for the skin, eyes, hair, liver and nerves.

Vitamin B_1 (Thiamine) enhances circulation, digestion, blood formation, mental attitude, heart function, the muscles and the central nervous system. It is helpful in motion sickness, dental postoperative pain, shingles, brain damage, fatigue, mental confusion, heart dis-ease, and numb hands or feet. Taken every three or four hours on camping trips, it repels mosquitos, particularly when started (in less amounts) a few weeks before. Women who are pregnant, nursing or on the pill, women with multiple sclerosis, and women who smoke or have digestive problems need more B_1. Antibiotics, sulfa drugs, caffeine, alcohol, sugar, estrogen, a high-carbohydrate diet, and heat all decrease thiamine levels in the body. B_1 is essential for anyone with central nervous system dis-ease or damage.

Vitamin B_2 (Riboflavin) is a major antistress vitamin. It is needed for red blood cell formation, the production of immune system antibodies, cell metabolism, growth, iron absorption, and the metabolism of proteins, fats and carbohydrates. Riboflavin helps prevent birth defects and is important in pregnancy, vision and eye fatigue, cataracts, anemia, digestive problems, eczema, sores on mouth, lips or tongue, oily skin, exhaustion and depression. It prevents hair loss, dandruff, and vaginal itching, is an anticancer agent and helps carpal tunnel syndrome (with B_6). Vegetarians, diabetics and women on antiulcer diets, as well as women on the pill or who take strenuous exercise need more B_2. The vitamin is destroyed by light, cooking, antibiotics and alcohol. It may decrease the effect of some cancer drugs. Cracks and sores at the corners of the mouth are an indication of riboflavin deficiency.

Vitamin B_3 (Niacin) is necessary for circulation and the function of the nervous system; it aids metabolism of carbohydrates, fats and proteins, and aids digestion by producing hydrochloric acid in the stomach. Niacin reduces cholesterol in the blood and lowers high blood pressure. Vertigo, headaches, constipation or diarrhea, backaches, bad breath, stress and insomnia are helped by B_3. Schizophrenia may be a niacin deficiency dis-ease, as well as autism in children, hostility, paranoia and personality changes.

The niacin flush—B_3's tendency to cause a temporary heating, tingling, flushing and reddening of the skin—starts about fifteen minutes after taking it and has an important use for women who have migraines. I describe the sensation as the "the hot-flash of your life," but it is harmless and short term (about 15–20 minutes). With daily use of niacin, the effect lessens in a few days and finally disappears. At the earliest start of a migraine, a dose of 50 mg niacin (nicotinic acid form) induces this flush, which dilates the blood vessels, increasing

blood circulation to the brain and head, and stops the cycle. If the first 50 mg does not cause the flush, take a second one in about fifteen minutes. One or two usually are enough.

To take B_3 without the flush use niacinamide; it is not useful for migraines but can replace niacin/nicotinic acid for other dis-eases. Women with gout, peptic ulcers, glaucoma, liver disease, diabetes or who are pregnant should use vitamin B-3 conservatively. The amino acid ltryptophan is converted to niacin in the body.

Vitamin B_5 (Pantothenic Acid) is the major antistress vitamin for women, and important help for those who are hypoglycemic or suffer from adrenal fatigue. The vitamin is needed for the production of adrenal hormones (including natural cortisone) and in the formation of immune system antibodies. It aids in the metabolism of vitamins and foods for energy and the functioning of the gastrointestinal tract. Pantothenic acid is a safe and drugless stimulant—use 500 mg twice a day with meals, increasing to up to 2000 mg a day if needed. There are no known toxicities and no side effects, but avoid at bedtime.

B_5 is concentrated in the body organs and is needed by every body cell. Indications for this vitamin include peptic or gastric ulcers, headaches, hair loss, eczema, skin disorders, respiratory disorders, impaired motor coordination, anemia, cataracts, thyroid dis-ease, depression, anxiety, fatigue and postoperative shock. A furrowed tongue is an indication of B_5 deficiency, and arthritis, sinusitis, hay fever and allergies may be deficiency dis-eases of pantothenic acid. For allergies take 1000 mg each of B_5 and vitamin C twice a day with meals.

Vitamin B_6 (Pyridoxine) is essential for both physical and mental health and is intrinsic to more body functions than any other vitamin, mineral or nutrient. Brain function, red blood cell formation, the central nervous system, absorption of fats and proteins, immune system function and the synthesis of DNA and RNA all require this vitamin. Pyridoxine is an anticancer agent and protects the heart; it reduces arteriosclerosis and kidney stones, arthritis, allergies, asthma and premenstrual syndrome. B_6 is also useful for women who have hypoglycemia, epilepsy, ulcers, anemia, AIDS, diabetes (check blood levels frequently; it may reduce insulin need), insomnia, anxiety, irritability and general or muscular weakness.

Women on the contraceptive pill need increased amounts of pyridoxine to prevent phlebitis. The vitamin is also essential in pregnancy to aid morning sickness and prevent toxemia and leg cramps. Many women's premenstrual anxiety and water retention can be reduced or eliminated with B_6, and ninety percent of both men and women in the United States are deficient in it. Carpal tunnel syndrome may be a B_6 deficiency disease, and antidepressants or estrogen increase women's need for this vitamin. (For carpal tunnel syndrome, try B_2 with B_6.) If pregnant use no more than 50 mg a day. The vitamin is water soluble and nontoxic but overuse can cause nightmares.

Vitamin B_9 (Folic Acid) is another serious deficiency for women, involving about 98 percent. Uterine cervical dysplasia (suspicious Pap smear) often responds to a supplement of folic acid. If you are a vegetarian, pregnant, anemic, insomniac or depressed, you probably need more of this vitamin. B_9 is needed for energy production and brain function, cell division, protein metabolism, embryonic and fetal development, and normal growth. Neural tube defects and spina bifida in infants can be reduced by 60 to 70 percent by the mother's use of folic acid in very early pregnancy or

at the time of becoming pregnant. The vitamin is a coenzyme in DNA synthesis. It helps in heavy menstrual bleeding and hemorrhaging in childbirth, aids nursing, helps in tissue repair, regeneration and debilitation. It increases intelligence and with vitamin B_5, can return color to greying hair. Folic acid is generally used with vitamin B_{12} and often with B_6. Oral contraceptives, estrogen, dilantin, sulfa drugs, alcohol or high use of vitamin C increases women's need for this vitamin. If you are a smoker, folic acid may decrease your risk of lung cancer; use it along with vitamin A/beta-carotene. Avoid high doses long term if you have hormone-related cancer or convulsive disorder.

Vitamin B_{12} (Cyanocobalamin) prevents nerve damage and anemia, and aids in cell and-blood formation, proper digestion, fertility and growth. Women who are long term vegans are susceptible to B_{12} deficiency. Persons with AIDS on AZT, elders, and those with digestive disorders are also often deficient. B_{12} is useful for women with menstrual difficulties, nervousness, insomnia, memory loss, depression, fatigue, some skin problems, asthma, schizophrenia, heart palpitations, abdominal difficulties, and difficulties of pregnancy or lactation. Hormone use, gout medications, anticoagulant drugs and potassium supplements may block the absorption or increase the need for this vitamin. B_{12} is taken by doctor's injections or sublingually (under the tongue) as it is not easily assimilated through the digestive tract. The symptoms of B_{12} deficiency anemia, presenting all at once, are: reduced sensory perception, jerky limb motion, arm and leg weakness, trouble walking and speaking, memory loss, hallucinations, eye disorders and digestive disorders.

Vitamin B_{13} (Orotic Acid) metabolizes B-9 and B_{12}, but is not readily used or available in the United States. Some better multiple vitamin-mineral combinations contain it. It may help multiple sclerosis.

Vitamin B_{15} (Pangamic Acid) is an antioxidant; it increases cell life and immunity, and is useful in angina, asthma, high cholesterol and fatigue. Also known as DMG (dimethyl-glycine), it is used by athletes to reduce oxygen debt The vitamin prevents some glandular and nerve disorders and is helpful for women in sobriety—it reduces alcohol cravings and protects against cirrhosis of the liver.

Vitamin B_{17} (Laetrile) is banned by the FDA, but used in Mexico and other countries. A controversial substance, it is reputed to be a cancer cure, while opponents say it is worthless. The high cyanide content of apricot pit kernels, apple seeds and other fruit seeds is the vitamin's source. Suggested use is five to thirty apricot kernels taken through the day. One in three women in the United States will die of cancer, and one in nine women will develop breast cancer in her lifetime. Cancer is big business for the medical system and drug industry, and natural cures are suppressed as not profitable. Much more research is needed on B_{17} but does not seem to be happening, and women who want laetrile treatment cannot get it here.

It should also be noted that vitamins B_{13}, B_{15}, and B_{17} are not accepted as vitamins by the establishment (which calls them "pseudovitamins"). They have been largely ignored for research, and compared to other vitamins are almost unknowns. Likewise, choline, inositol and PABA, usually listed as B complex vitamins, are not strictly vitamins, but called vitamin-like substances.

Biotin is one of the few vitamins that can be produced in the body. It is synthesized in the intestines from food, and is present in breast milk. Cell growth, fatty acid production, carbohydrate metabolism, metabolism of fats and proteins, and metab-

Continued ➡

olism of all the B complex vitamins are biotin attributes. The vitamin promotes healthy hair and skin, reduces hair loss and regulates the sweat glands, nerves and bone marrow. Seborrhea, eczema, dermatitis, dry peeling skin or cracked lips may be biotin deficiency symptoms, as well as extreme fatigue, heart dis-ease, muscle pains, depression and insomnia. Raw egg whites deplete biotin from the body, as do rancid fats, saccharine, sulfa drugs, antibiotics and estrogen. Pregnant or nursing women and women with skin problems are usually deficient.

Choline and inositol together make lecithin. Choline helps to prevent arterio- and atherosclerosis, heart failure, glaucoma, gall bladder dis-ease, circulatory problems and blood clots. It minimizes excess fat in the liver, gall bladder and heart, and aids in hormone production, brain function and memory. The vitamin is useful for nervous system dis-eases like multiple sclerosis, Parkinson's and Alzheimer's dis-ease, plus for diabetes, liver and kidney dis-ease and hepatitis. Choline is an anti-cancer agent, regulating the thymus and spleen for immune and red blood cell production.

Inositol, like choline, is also vital for preventing and aiding arterio and atherosclerosis, and in fat and cholesterol metabolism. It helps to remove fats from the liver, reduce fibroid cysts and is necessary for brain function and assimilation of vitamins C and E. Women after menopause need more inositol and choline (lecithin), particularly black women who have higher frequency of arterial dis-ease. Coffee drinkers and alcohol users need more inositol, as these substances deplete it from the body. Women with cerebral palsy, multiple sclerosis and other central nervous system dis-eases are helped by inositol, as well as women with vision and eye disorders, gall bladder dis-ease, diabetes, skin problems, eczema and psoriasis, hair loss and some forms of mental retardation.

PABA (Para-Amino Benzoic Acid) is the last of the B complex and a constituent of vitamin B_5. It is an antioxidant that helps protect the skin from sunburn and skin cancer (which has increased four-fold in the last five years as a result of global ozone layer damage). PABA also aids in protein assimilation and in the formation of red blood cells. In cases of stress or nutritional deficiency, PABA can return color to greying hair. Eczema is a PABA deficiency dis-ease, and digestive disorders, fatigue, depression and irritability may be deficiency symptoms. Infertility in women, psoriasis, vitiligo and intestinal disorders are helped by PABA. Sulfa drugs may cause a PABA deficiency, and in turn the vitamin may inactivate sulfa medications. PABA should be included in your multiple vitamin-mineral supplement; most common additional amounts are 30–100 mg taken three times a day (internally). The vitamin is often found in sunscreen lotions.

Vitamin C is the important vitamin for white blood cell and immune system building, and is a major antioxidant, antitoxin, and anticancer substance. C is required for tissue growth and repair, adrenal function and healthy gums. It protects the body against pollutants, infections, high blood pressure, cholesterol and atherosclerosis, bruising, bleeding and phlebitis. Vitamin C promotes wound healing and the production of interferon and antistress hormones. A gram (1000 mg) of vitamin C taken every hour at the start can stop a cold or bladder infection. Use a lot of water with this, and/or increase your calcium/magnesium or B_6 intake to prevent kidney stones; decrease gradually when symptoms end. C also reduces menstrual flows and heavy bleeding in menstruation (or otherwise). Megadoses of C taken intravenously have been

known to put AIDS patients into remission; HIV status has been changed from positive to negative if done early enough.[3] Schizophrenia has also been reversed with vitamin C.[4]

There are countless uses and benefits of vitamin C. Use it for bacterial and viral infections, colds, tonsillitis and ear infections, gum disease and flu. Use it for hepatitis, diabetes, cataracts and eye infections, allergies and sinus, ulcers, gallstones and burn healing. Women living in inner cities or near highways need more vitamin C, and so do women who are smokers. Vitamin C may prevent sudden infant death syndrome, and women who are pregnant, nursing or on the pill, steroids or antibiotics need more of it. Alternate aspirin with vitamin C, as aspirin depletes C in the bloodstream. The vitamin can cause false results in some laboratory tests, so doctors need to be aware of it. It can also reduce the effectiveness of sulfa drugs and diabinase (for diabetes), and should be avoided by women taking radiation or chemotherapy for cancer. Pregnant women should limit C intake to 5000 mg per day or under.

At the onset of dis-ease or for serious illness or detoxification, take vitamin C to bowel tolerance for the time necessary to clear the dis-ease, then decrease the amount gradually. To determine bowel tolerance, take one or more grams of C per hour, with a lot of water, until diarrhea develops. At that point, cut back 10 percent. The goal is to take as much C as possible without diarrhea, and this amount will vary with the individual and the state of her immune system. The amount of C that can be taken may vary from day to day, but surprisingly high amounts will be tolerated when they are needed. When using large amounts or in serious illness, try Ester-C—more is assimilated into the system. Take a calcium/magnesium tablet or 50 mg of B_6 three times daily when using C in megadoses to prevent the possibility of kidney stones. Vitamin C is water soluble and nontoxic; too much results in diarrhea or nausea that stops when the amount is decreased. Many women's dis-eases can be healed with C.

Vitamin D and calcium deficiencies are major causes of osteoporosis in women. An oil soluble vitamin, natural vitamin D may be taken in very high amounts (100,000–150,000 IU daily) longterm before toxicity results, but about 800 IU per day is recommended. D is necessary for growth and for bone and tooth formation, and in the prevention of bone dis-eases. Black women in northern climates, Islamic women and nuns whose body is kept completely covered, women who work at night, and women living in smog-laden cities are more susceptible to deficiencies. The vitamin is naturally obtained by exposure to the sun, where it forms in the skin. Supplemental D requires conversion by the kidneys and liver, and should not be taken without calcium. Women with kidney or liver dis-ease are more likely to be vitamin D deficient and to develop osteoporosis. Some cholesterol-lowering drugs interfere with absorption of vitamin D in the body, as well as antacids, mineral oil, thiazide diuretics and cortisone.

Vitamin E is essential for healing and regeneration in every part of the body, and is an antioxidant that prevents cancer and heart dis-ease. Use it for fertility, fibrocystic breasts, breast cancer, premenstrual syndrome, prevention of miscarriage, to reduce hotflashes and menopause discomfort, in pregnancy and lactation, and when on estrogen or the pill. Vitamin E is used for the healing of burns, wounds and scars and is positive before and after surgeries for internal and external regeneration. The vitamin prevents and aids cataracts, reduces blood pressure and removes cholesterol deposits from artery walls (start at 100 IU per day and

increase slowly for heart and artery dis-ease). It protects women's bodies from pollution and secondary cigarette smoke and retards aging, aids migraines and visual problems, skin, hair and muscular dis-eases. Vitamin E taken in pregnancy prevents muscular dystrophy in children, and women with muscular dystrophy need high doses. Black women are especially susceptible to keloids, high blood pressure, breast cancer and arthritis, and vitamin E is a major preventive.

To maintain vitamin E levels in the blood, zinc is required with it. While a fat-soluble vitamin, vitamin E is only stored in the body for a short time so that there are no toxicities in any amount. Iron and vitamin E should be taken eight hours apart, and women with diabetes, rheumatic hearts or overactive thyroids should not take high amounts.

Vitamin F (Essential Fatty Acids) is used with vitamin E as a factor in reducing cholesterol and heart dis-ease. It is an antioxidant that protects against x-ray damage and free radicals from saturated fats. Free radicals are atoms that damage cells, leading to cancer, leukemia, reduced immune function, cell fluid retention, infections, and a variety of dis-eases. Vitamin F helps the endocrine glands, especially the adrenals and thyroid. Skin dis-eases such as acne or eczema are vitamin F deficiencies, as are dry skin and hair, dandruff, diarrhea, gallstones, varicose veins, and the loss of beneficial bacteria in the intestines (which in turn cause Candida overrun and dis-eases such as colitis). Essential fatty acids aid respiration, the nervous system, reproduction and blood coagulation. They can cause weight loss, but in excess cause gain. The substance is best used with vitamin E and with meals. It is composed of three items—linoleic acid, linolenic acid and arachadonic acid, and though oil soluble, has no toxicities. I listed it here as a vitamin, though the FDA does not.

Vitamin K is essential for the proper coagulation of the blood, and has a role in bone formation and preventing osteoporosis. It converts glucose to glycogen for storage in the liver, and therefore is important in sugar metabolism. The vitamin is usually available by prescription only, though it is nontoxic in natural forms; in foods it is most easily found in alfalfa and yogurt. Vitamin K is used before surgery and childbirth to prevent hemorrhaging and for overly heavy menstrual flows, as well as to treat heart attacks. Deficiency symptoms include colitis, excessive diarrhea, nosebleeds and celiac dis-ease. X-rays, radiation, aspirin, air pollution, mineral oil, antibiotics and frozen or irradiated foods destroy it in the body. When synthetic vitamin K is used heavily in pregnancy, the infant may have a toxic reaction.

Vitamin P (Bioflavinoids) are several citrus factors that work synergistically with vitamin C and enhance its effects. They include rutin, hesperidin and citrin, and have particular benefit for the capillaries and in reducing pain, for blood circulation, cataracts, bile production, herpes, and in lowering cholesterol levels. Bioflavinoids are used by athletes to reduce bruising and bumps, as well as for back and leg pain, and they lessen the effects of prolonged bleeding. Bleeding gums, blood clots, hot flashes, ulcers, asthma, edema, varicose veins and inner ear problems (dizziness and vertigo) are helped by bioflavinoids. They are antibacterials that also help to fight infections. Bioflavinoids and C together are known as C complex, and there should be 100 mg of bioflavinoids for every 500 mg of vitamin C. For daily use, take 1000 mg (1 gram) vitamin C with bioflavinoids in a time-release form. There are no toxicities, but high doses may cause diarrhea. Along with vitamin U below, bioflavinoids are technically not vitamins.

Continued ➡

Vitamin U may help with ulcer healing. It is not readily available and little else is known about it. More research is needed.

Coenzyme Q10 (Ubiquinone) resembles vitamin E but is even more powerful as an antioxidant. It is not a vitamin, but is chemically similar to one. CO-Q10 retards aging and significantly boosts the immune system. It shows promise in cancer healing for reducing tumors and in leukemia for reducing the side effects of chemotherapy. Heart dis-ease and high blood pressure, high cholesterol, allergies, asthma, respiratory disease, Alzheimer's, diabetes and multiple sclerosis all respond and improve with this coenzyme. Other uses include schizophrenia, obesity, candidiasis, gum dis-ease and AIDS. It is important for healing duodenal ulcers, and helps prevent cancer. There are no side effects. Keep it away from heat and light for best potency; pure coenzyme Q10 is bright yellow and has very little taste. Prices on this vary widely, but it is expensive; watch the mg amounts on the bottle. Use 30–100 mg per day.

These are the vitamins, and information on the minerals follows. Vitamins and minerals are a complex but major method of treating women's diseases in this book, and the length of the descriptions is justified. More dis-ease prevention is possible with knowledge of vitamins and minerals than in any other form of healing. For best results, the supplements should be taken in natural forms, rather than synthetic, wherever possible. Be careful with cheap or old vitamin E's that may be rancid. Vitamins taken in capsules or gelatin soft pills are preferred over hard-pressed tablets, as some women's bodies have difficulty in dissolving the tablets. Minerals are best in chelated form, molecularly protein bonded, as more is assimilated. Because so much is lost in digestion, much higher amounts must be taken than are actually needed. 1000 mcg equals 1 mg. 1000 mg equals 1 gram.

Minerals make up the actual structures of the body, such as bones and teeth, and deficiencies can cause serious dis-eases. Some minerals make vitamin assimilation possible, a few are toxic in excess, and most require a balance of other vitamins and minerals. Some women with extensive deficiencies or digestive problems need hydrochloric acid or digestive enzyme supplements to assimilate minerals. Mineral deficiencies affect the bones and teeth, as well as cause fatigue, menstrual problems, depression, insomnia, skin and hair problems, muscle cramps and stress intolerance.

Boron is a trace mineral often not listed in mineral information but of major importance to menopausal and postmenopausal women. In a study by the U.S. Department of Agriculture, it was found that within eight days of adding 3 mg of boron to the diet, "postmenopausal women lost forty percent less calcium, one third less magnesium and slightly less phosphorus through their urine."[5] This has hopeful implications for women susceptible to osteoporosis and its resulting weakened and broken bones. Three milligrams is enough to take per day; avoid taking more.

Calcium is a bulk mineral and one of the most important for all women. It prevents osteoporosis, aids premenstrual stress, cramps and water retention, and halts insomnia and leg cramps. It is essential in regulating heartbeat, in blood clotting, as a preventive of colon cancer, in muscle growth and contraction, and in the transmission of nerve impulses. It is involved in DNA and RNA function and activates several enzymes.

Most women require supplemental calcium from menarche on. It is useful for any form of stress, for headaches and migraines, pleurisy, bone or tooth dis-ease, arthritis, and heart dis-ease. It decreases pain, lowers cholesterol and blood pressure, and is particularly useful in menstruation, menopause and postmenopause. Calcium deficiency symptoms include: charlie horses and muscle cramps or spasms, nervousness, heart palpitations, brittle nails, eczema, aching back or joints, rheumatoid arthritis, tooth decay, rickets, and numbness in arms or legs.[6]

To test absorption of your calcium supplement, place it in warm water and shake. If it does not dissolve within twenty-four hours, try a different brand. Most sources list calcium as nontoxic in any amount, but recommend doses under 2000 mg per day. Take a calcium supplement that includes half the amount of magnesium, traces of zinc, and vitamins A and D for the best possible absorption and activation. General Nutrition's Calcium Plus is a good one. Try calcium at bedtime as a relaxant, and take 1000–4000 mg after dental work to relieve pain. Women whose diets contain less protein need less calcium.

Chromium is a trace mineral also known as GTF (Glucose Tolerance Factor). It balances blood sugar levels, lowers high blood pressure and retards cholesterol buildup in the liver and arteries. Two-thirds of Americans are either diabetic or hypoglycemic because of chromium deficiency and junkfood diets. This is an important mineral for women, and is essential for women over sixty-five. Suggested dosages are 25–250 mcg per day. There are no side effects or toxicities, but diabetics need to watch blood sugar levels as less insulin may be needed while taking this supplement.

Cobalt is a part of vitamin B_{12} and longterm vegetarians (vegans) may be deficient. Obtain it through a B complex or B_{12} supplement; it helps prevent anemia.

Copper's earliest deficiency symptom is osteoporosis, a major health threat to postmenopausal women. It helps in the assimilation of iron and vitamin C, but supplements may upset the balance of zinc in women's bodies. Copper deficiencies are rare, and doses of more than 15 mg per day cause side effects. Copper aids bone, hemoglobin and red blood formation, forms elastin and is important in healing and energy, skin and hair color, the nerves and sense of taste. Get copper from a multiple vitamin-mineral supplement rather than adding it alone. Raw organic foods are high in natural copper.

Fluoride is present in fluoridated water and toothpaste, and supplements are not needed. It helps prevent tooth decay but does nothing for gum degeneration (the most frequent cause of tooth loss). Chemical fluoride may be harmful to the liver and a cause of osteoporosis. If your water is fluoridated, you are probably getting too much.

Germanium increases oxygen in the cells, tissues and organs. It is a major aid to the immune system but highly expensive. This trace mineral is important for AIDS and cancer, chronic fatigue syndrome, food sensitivities and allergic reactions, rheumatoid arthritis, high cholesterol, systemic Candida, and any infectious dis-ease or low immunity situation. It is also a relaxant, antistress factor and mood balancer, and important for women exposed to toxic chemicals and pollutants. Women in chronic pain will benefit from germanium, as well as those with asthma or respiratory problems. There are no toxicities, and plants that contain germanium include garlic, ginseng, comfrey, aloe vera, chlorella, shiitake mushrooms, onions, barley and suma. If taking germanium capsules, expect to pay about a dollar each.

Iodine deficiency may be a factor in breast cancer, and as such it is an important trace mineral for women. Use it to regulate the thyroid and help metabolize fat. It is important in mental development and a deficiency in pregnancy may cause mental retardation in the child. Goiter, slowness and obesity are iodine deficiency symptoms. If using supplements, be sure to take natural ones. Kelp tablets are the most recommended form. Find it also in Edgar Cayce's Atomidine, 636, or Lugol's Solution. Toxicities have been cited by the FDA as a reason to restrict supplemental iodine, but 2400 mg have been given daily for as long as five years with no side effects. Too much iodine results in a metallic taste, mouth sores, swollen salivary glands, diarrhea and vomiting.

Iron is one of the major mineral deficiencies for women, with heavy menstruation as its cause. Iron produces hemoglobin, the oxygen-carrying component of red blood cells, and is required for the function of many enzymes. It is necessary for dis-ease resistance and immune system health. Iron deficiency symptoms include anemia, weakness and fatigue, debility, dizziness, irritability, brittle nails with vertical ridges, pallor, gas, nausea after meals, itching, constipation or diarrhea, hair loss, heart palpitations, poor attention span, and recurrent illnesses. When using supplements, use only organic iron called hydrolized-protein chelate, and avoid synthetic iron (ferrous sulfate). Suggested daily doses are 20–60 mg a day for women, the higher amounts in menstruation or after childbirth and for elders and growing girls. Floridix is a good supplement brand.

Do not take extra iron when having an infection, as bacteria requires iron for growth and the body will store and not utilize it. Take vitamin E and zinc eight hours apart from iron, as they interfere with iron absorption. Women with chronic Candida or herpes are susceptible to iron deficiency, and those with cancer or rheumatoid arthritis will have difficulty assimilating it. Deficiencies can be caused by excessive menstrual flows, high phosphorus diet, poor digestion, ulcers, and excess use of antacids, coffee or tea. In cases of iron deficiency anemia, vitamins B_6 or B_{12} deficiency may be the cause, rather than iron itself. Women with sickle cell anemia, thalessemia or hemochromatosis should not take iron. Use it carefully in pregnancy. Most women who menstruate are iron deficient.

Magnesium is necessary for the utilization of calcium, potassium and phosphorus and most women are deficient in it. It is necessary for muscle function, nerve impulse transmission and enzyme activity, prevents kidney stones and gallstones, and helps bone, tooth and tissue growth. Magnesium increases energy, helps the nerves, insomnia and depression, lowers blood pressure and helps to prevent heart attacks.

Mental confusion, fast pulse and irregular heartbeat are magnesium deficiency symptoms, as are weakness, twitching muscles and leg cramps. It protects the artery linings, is important in mineral metabolism and regulates the acid-alkaline balance of the body. Premenstrual chocolate cravings are a sign of magnesium deficiency, as is premenstrual nervous tension. Use a calcium/magnesium tablet for indigestion, but avoid any antacid right after meals.

Women who are pregnant or lactating, on the pill or taking estrogen, and who have premenstrual or menstrual discomfort need more magnesium. Alcoholics are usually magnesium deficient, and so are women who use diuretics, have frequent diarrhea, live in fluoridated or softwater areas, or take high amounts of zinc or vitamin D. Cod liver oil, too much calcium for the amount of magnesium, or a high-fat or protein diet decrease the assimilation of this mineral. Magnesium requires twice the amount of calcium to work, as well as phosphorus

Continued ➡

and vitamins A and C. A good calcium/magnesium supplement will contain it all in one tablet, at about ten dollars for a three-month (or more) supply. There are no toxicities.

Manganese is a trace mineral needed for protein and fat metabolism, assimilation of the B vitamins, C and E, for balanced blood sugar, healthy nerves and immune system, and for production of breast milk. Deficiency symptoms include poor memory, poor muscle coordination and reflexes, bowed bones, dizziness, hearing problems, tinnitus (ear noises), and high blood sugar. Use it for multiple sclerosis and other muscular weakness diseases, epilepsy, diabetes, hypoglycemia, digestive or food assimilation disorders, fatigue, irritability, the central nervous system, and dis-eases such as Alzheimer's. Heavy milk drinkers or meat eaters may need more manganese as it is used in the production of milk and fat-digesting enzymes. Women who are pregnant or lactating will need increased amounts as well—it is essential for milk production. Use 2.5–5 mg per day; there are no toxicities. Take B complex with manganese for a feeling of rested well-being.

Molybdenum deficiency is found in women with cancer and with gum or mouth disorders. A highly refined diet of processed foods may cause it. The mineral is used by the body in minute amounts for iron and nitrogen utilization and production of uric acid, as well as in enzyme and cell reactions. It is one of the minerals suggested for AIDS and cancer, but excessive use (over 15 mg per day) may cause gout and interfere with copper assimilation. Keep supplements away from heat or dampness.

Phosphorus works in balance with calcium and magnesium and more women are overloaded than deficient in it. The mineral is used as a chemical fertilizer and food additive, and junk foods are full of it. Too much phosphorus causes the body to over-release calcium and is a factor in osteoporosis. The mineral is necessary for utilization of vitamin D, calcium and niacin (B_3), and too much iron or calcium makes phosphorus ineffective. Tooth and gum problems, poor bone growth, arthritis, kidney dis-ease, heart contraction problems, poor appetite control, and overweight or underweight are symptoms of deficiency. Most women do not need supplements, but if wishing to add phosphorus to your diet, use bonemeal with vitamin D, or use it in a balanced calcium-magnesium-phosphorus supplement.

Potassium may benefit women with edema, hypoglycemia, hypoadrenia, allergies, irregular heart rhythm or high blood pressure. Fasting, diuretics, diarrhea, kidney disorders or stress can cause a deficiency, as can coffee, alcohol, laxatives, cortisone and chocolate. Potassium helps prevent strokes, aids in muscle and heart muscle contraction, regulates blood pressure, balances the nervous system, and with sodium controls the body's water balance. Deficiency symptoms include continual thirst, tiredness, insomnia, poor reflexes, weak heart or muscles, constipation, hypoglycemia and poor breathing. Daily orange juice or bananas may prevent the need for supplements.

Selenium works with vitamin E as an antioxidant and has been called the antiaging mineral. It protects against free radicals, toxins and pollutants to boost the immune system, create antibodies and strengthen the heart. It is a DNA/RNA activator, an anticancer agent, and relieves hot flashes. Selenium deficiency may be a factor in strokes and heart dis-ease, skin problems, infertility, early aging and muscular dystrophy. Dosage is 50–200 mcg, and though no toxicities have been discovered, avoid higher amounts.

Silicon (Silica) is a trace mineral that may protect the body from aluminum poisoning; it is important in preventing Alzheimer's dis-ease and osteoporosis. Silicon helps maintain flexible arteries and protect against cardiovascular dis-ease. It is needed for calcium absorption, bone and connective tissue formation, and for healthy nails, skin and hair. Silicon is needed more by elders, as levels decrease in the body with age. There are no reported toxicities. It is found in several herbs.

Sodium (Salt) is a major contaminant of processed foods and most women are overdosed on it continually. It is necessary with potassium to maintain the water balance and pH of the cells. Too much sodium results in high blood pressure, liver and kidney dis-ease, edema, heart failure and potassium deficiency. Deficiency symptoms include confusion, low blood sugar, weakness, lethargy and heart palpitations. Except in rare cases of heat exhaustion, few or no women need supplements.

Sulfur is part of the chemistry of amino acids, and if you are getting enough protein, you are probably getting enough of this trace mineral. Sulfur protects the cells, stimulates bile, is an antibacterial, and aids oxidation reactions in the body. It protects against radiation and pollution to slow aging and lengthen life. Sulfur is needed for good skin and hair, and many skin creams contain it. Supplements are available, but the best source is in complete amino acids.

Vanadium is useful in lowering cholesterol and preventing heart attacks, as well as in reproductive difficulties and preventing infant mortality. Vanadium is needed for cell metabolism, and bone and tooth formation. This trace mineral is not easily absorbed and is rarely supplemented; take chromium and vanadium at different times. Smoking decreases uptake.

Zinc is necessary for proper functioning of the immune system and for all regeneration and healing. It regulates body processes, forms insulin and controls muscle contraction; it regulates the body's pH balance and the flow of enzymes in the cells, and is a factor in the synthesis of DNA. Use zinc for scaly dry skin or skin rashes, sores or boils, hair loss, acne, growth problems, too slow healing, dandruff and poor night vision. It is a factor in preventing diabetes, protecting the liver from chemicals, resisting infections and inflammations, and reducing senility and body odors. Use it for poison ivy, infertility, schizophrenia, AIDS, Alzheimer's dis-ease, hypoglycemia, arteriosclerosis, and loss of sense of smell.

Women with irregular menstrual cycles may benefit from zinc. Girls, pregnant women, women after surgery or heavy bleeding, and elder women need more zinc. Losses occur in sweating, pregnancy, nursing, diarrhea, kidney dis-ease, cirrhosis of the liver, and diabetes. A symptom of deficiency is white spots on the fingernails. Extra zinc may require extra copper, and doses over 100 mg a day depress the immune system, whereas doses under 100 mg enhance it. Zinc is essential for all forms of healing.

Women reading this information may find the answers to their own dis-eases right here. Vitamins and minerals are important and essential for women's well-being, and are the primary dis-ease preventive and healing method of this book. Many women's dis-eases are caused by vitamin-mineral deficiencies and are healed simply by returning the needed nutrient/s to the diet. Each of the dis-eases discussed in this book is helped by vitamins and minerals as based on the material of this section. Primary sources for vitamins in this section and throughout the section are: Balch and Balch, *Prescription for Nutritional Healing* (Avery Publishing Group, 1990), Dr. Ross Trattler, *Better Health Through*

Natural Healing (McGraw-Hill Book Co., 1985), Adele Davis, *Let's Get Well* (Signet Books, 1965), and Diane Stein, *All Women Are Healers* (The Crossing Press, 1990).

Amino Acids

In women's bodies, the muscles, ligaments, tendons, organs, glands, nails, hair, body fluids, enzymes, hormones and genes are all composed of protein, and protein is also essential for bone growth. Amino acids are the chemical components of which proteins are made. The twenty-nine known amino acids in various combinations create 50,000 different proteins and 20,000 enzymes in the body. The combinations are specific and cannot occur if even one amino acid is missing or in short supply. Amino acids are neurotransmitters or neurotransmitter precursors for the central nervous system and brain, allowing the brain to receive and send messages.[1] They comprise the nucleus of every cell. Obviously, amino acids are essential to human and mammalian life.

Of the twenty-nine known amino acids, the liver produces about 80 percent and the rest must come from diet. Essential amino acids are the ones that must be obtained from outside the body. The eight essential amino acids are: isoleucine, leucine, lysine, methionine, phenylalanine, threonine, tryptophan and valine. Cysteine and tyrosine are synthesized in the body from methionine and phenylalanine, respectively. Amino acids produced in the body from other sources are alanine, arginine, aspartic acid, glutamic acid, glutamine, histidine, glycine, ornithine, proline and serine. Amino acid supplements that come in the L (alpha) form are considered natural and are more compatible to women's body chemistry than those in the D form. The exception here is phenylalanine, which also comes as DL-phenylalanine.

The use of amino acids and proteins in the body is continuous, and a depletion or shortage of any of the essential amino acids leads rapidly to dis-ease. Deficiencies can occur from improper or imbalanced diet, long-term vegan vegetarianism, or inability to properly assimilate protein via the digestive system. Since vitamins and minerals require amino acids for their use in the body, and since protein comprises more of body weight than any other substance except water, amino acids require women's attention.

Much of my own lack of energy and too early exhaustion have been remedied by taking an amino acids combination supplement, and I believe that many more women can benefit from them. If you have any form of degenerative dis-ease, mental or nervous disorder, heart dis-ease, chronic fatigue syndrome, diabetes, epilepsy, anemia, are in recovery from alcohol or drugs, or are a long-term vegetarian who feels something missing, amino acids may be important for you. If you have herpes, you are probably already aware of L-lysine as a factor in preventing and reducing attacks.

Amino acids are available singly and in combinations. Twin Labs is a good brand. Combinations are sold as free-form amino acids, which are considered the purest and are made from a grain base. Free-form amino acids combinations and single amino acids are taken alone on an empty stomach, rather than with meals. Combination amino acids are also sold as liver extract or predigested liver amino acids. Twin Labs makes this, as does Enzymatics Therapy. These may be taken with meals and cost about $10–13 for 100 capsules; take one or two a day. Free-form amino acids are often found in the body building section of health food chains.

Continued ➡

The pictures of musclemen on the bottles may put you off, but they are fast acting and vegetarian. Some health food stores now have full sections of amino acid supplements, without the body builders.

Here is what each amino acid does; twenty-eight of them are listed here, and women will recognize their own needs immediately from the descriptions. Their uses are startling—why haven't we known about these before?—and important for many, many women. The information is primarily from James F. Balch, MD, and Phyllis A. Balch, CNC, *Prescription for Nutritional Healing*, and *The Vitamin Herb Guide* (Global Health Ltd., 1990), plus some health food store handout sheets. Little information has been readily available on amino acids, but I feel they are highly important for women's well-being.

L-Alanine is important in glucose metabolism, and is useful for women who are diabetic, hypoglycemic or have fatigue or energy problems.

L-Arginine slows tumors and cancer growth, detoxifies the liver, regulates growth hormones, aids in kidney disorders, helps wound healing, and helps to maintain the immune system. It is used by body builders to increase muscle mass and reduce fat, and is important in healing or preventing cirrhosis of the liver and fatty liver disorders. Use it with L-lysine. Avoid arginine if pregnant or nursing, or if you have herpes.

L-Asparagine balances the central nervous system, preventing both hypernervousness and overcalming. Try it for mood-swing disorders and hyperactivity in children or adults.

L-Aspartic Acid increases stamina and endurance, and prevents fatigue and exhaustion. Some forms of chronic fatigue syndrome may be aspartic acid deficiencies. It detoxifies and protects the central nervous system, liver and bloodstream, promotes RNA/DNA formation, and aids cell metabolism.

L-Carnitine prevents fat buildup in the body and arteries, helping in weight loss and prevention of heart dis-ease and atherosclerosis. It is helpful in reducing angina attacks, in heart healing, hypoglycemia, diabetes, kidney and liver dis-ease, in acclimation to cold temperatures, and in reducing ketosis (a serious acid blood condition). Carnitine converts fat to energy and enhances the antioxidant vitamins E and C. It helps in athletic performance. Vegetarians are more likely to be deficient in this than meat eaters, as well as in lysine. This is an essential nutrient for newborns.

L-Citrulline boosts the immune system, increases energy, and detoxifies ammonia (a damaging liver pollutant) in the body.

L-Cysteine is an antioxidant and free radical destroyer best used for this with selenium and vitamin E. It protects the cells from radiation, and protects the liver and brain from cigarette smoke and alcohol consumption. It breaks down mucus and is recommended in treatment of bronchitis, emphysema, tuberculosis and pneumonia. Cysteine is also recommended for rheumatoid arthritis, and detoxifies excess copper from the body. If you are having radiation therapy or are otherwise exposed to x-rays or radiation, this is a protection. If you are a smoker or exposed to secondary cigarette smoke, this amino acid is important L-cysteine changes easily to L-cystine; they both do the same things.

L-Cystine also helps to detoxify the body of heavy metals and toxins, and helps in respiratory disorders. It is necessary for the healing of burns and wounds, for skin formation, and assists in the assimilation of insulin. Use it after surgery for faster healing, for diabetes, wound healing and to protect the body from radiation, alcohol and cigarettes.

Gamma-Aminobutyric Acid (GABA) is a fully natural tranquilizer, an addiction-free, nonprescription alternative to valium or librium. Use 750 mg per day with niacin/amide and inositol (the full B complex is best) to reduce anxiety, stress and depression. The need for chemical tranquilizers can be much reduced or ended for many women with this amino acid available in health food stores.

L-Glutamic Acid (Glutamate) is a brain food and fuel that helps to correct personality disorders. It metabolizes sugars and fats.

L-Glutamine is converted to glutamic acid in the brain. It is important for reducing fatigue and depression, lessens alcohol and sugar cravings, and is helpful in epilepsy, senility, schizophrenia, mental retardation, peptic ulcers, digestive dis-eases, and for increasing intelligence. Its use increases the need for GABA. Do not substitute L-glutamine with glutamic acid for use in alcoholism; L-glutamine is more effective for this dis-ease.

L-Glutathione is an antioxidant that prptects the body from damage by cigarette smoking and radiation. Use this to reduce the side effects of chemotherapy and cancer radiation treatments. It detoxifies heavy metals, drugs and alcohol poisoning, and is used in liver and blood detoxification and dis-eases.

L-Glycine prevents central nervous system and muscular degeneration. It helps prevent epileptic seizures, boosts the pituitary and immune system, and is used to treat bipolar depression. Too much can cause fatigue; the right amount increases energy. Use glycine for muscular dystrophy, multiple sclerosis and other degenerative dis-eases.

L-Histidine is used to heal gastric ulcers, hyperacidity, digestive dis-eases, allergies, rheumatoid arthritis and anemia. It is important for tissue growth and repair, and for red and white blood cell production.

L-Isoleucine is another amino acid for regulating blood sugar and energy levels. This one is important particularly for women who are hypoglycemic. Balanced amounts of valine and leucine are needed with isoleucine, and this amino acid is also important in blood formation.

L-Leucine lowers blood sugar levels, in balance with valine and isoleucine. Use leucine for diabetes and postsurgical recovery; it is a factor in the healing of bones, skin and muscles. Too much may aggravate hypoglycemia.

L-Lysine helps calcium absorption in adults and is required for bone development and normal growth in children. Women with herpes and cold sores know this amino acid's value is healing and prevention. Lysine helps postsurgical recovery by aiding tissue and muscle regrowth, aids in antibody, hormone and enzyme production, and in collagen formation for wound healing. It lowers serum triglycerides in the blood, a factor in heart dis-ease. Deficiency symptoms include low energy, lack of alertness and concentration, irritability, bloodshot eyes, anemia, hair loss, retarded growth and reproductive disorders.

L-Methionine is important in treating toxemia of pregnancy, rheumatic fever, allergies, chemical sensitivities, chronic fatigue and osteoporosis. It is a detoxifier that helps to break down fats in the liver and arteries, aids digestion and muscle weakness, and helps in cases of brittle hair and nails. Methionine is used by the body to create choline, and must be obtained from food. Use it for atherosclerosis, high cholesterol levels, edema, fat metabolism and schizophrenia.

L-Ornithine converts fat into muscle and energy, in combination with L-arginine and L-carnitine, and is needed in immune system and liver function. It promotes wound healing and tissue growth, and detoxifies ammonia from the body. Because it releases a growth hormone, it is not for use by children without expert direction.

L-Phenylalanine controls hunger, aids in memory and learning ability, and enhances sexual arousal. It is a mood raiser useful for depression and decreases physical pain, especially in migraines, menstruation and arthritis. Do not use phenylalanine if you are pregnant or have high blood pressure, phenylketonuria (PKU), or if you have preexisting pigmented melanoma cancer.

DL-Phenylalanine works in the same ways as L-phenylalanine. Use it for chronic pain, arthritis, and Parkinson's dis-ease. It suppresses appetite, aids mental alertness, and is a strong nonaddictive antidepressant. It should be avoided by the same women that are contraindicated in the L form.

L-Proline heals and strengthens cartilage, joints, tendons, the heart, and the texture of the skin.

L-Serine is important for the immune system in the production of antibodies and immunoglobulins. It is needed for metabolism of fats and fatty acids, and for muscle growth. If you have recurrent colds or infections, a depleted immune system, or atherosclerosis, serine is indicated.

L-Taurine heals heart dis-ease, atherosclerosis, high blood pressure, hypoglycemia, and edema. Use it for epilepsy, anxiety, hyperactivity and poor brain function, as well as for the central nervous system, muscular system, the white blood cells, and bile. It aids in the digestion and assimilation of fats and fat-soluble vitamins, and is important for multiple sclerosis and other degenerative dis-eases.

L-Threonine helps to prevent and control epileptic seizures. It is important in skin formation and in the functioning of the liver, central nervous system and heart.

L-Tryptophan is converted to niacin (vitamin B_3) in the body. Find it in amino acids combinations; it is no longer available singly. A blood disorder called EMS (eosinophilia-myalgia syndrome) surfaced in 1989 and was linked by the FDA to L-tryptophan supplements made in New Mexico. It seems to have come from a tampered-with or contaminated batch. L-tryptophan was taken off the market—all of it—and is now found only in amino acids combinations, some of which substitute niacin for it. A full inquiry into EMS and its real cause was never made. Nutritionists feel that L-tryptophan will be back on the market eventually. The FDA is dragging its feet, as usual.

This amino acid is a mood stabilizer, antidepressant and stress reducer. It helps insomnia and hyperactivity, promotes children's growth, lowers pain sensitivity and helps in reducing alcohol and food cravings. A warm glass of milk before bed helps insomnia because of milk's tryptophan content.

L-Tyrosine is an antidepressant and anxiety reducer; it aids fatigue and exhaustion, and alleviates withdrawal symptoms for those coming off cocaine and other drugs. It is useful in allergies, headaches, irritability, mood disorders, and hypothyroidism. It helps to reduce body fat and suppress appetite, aids in skin and hair pigment production (for premature greying, for vitiligo and age spots), and in adrenal, thyroid and pituitary gland function. Tyrosine deficiency results in deficiency in the hormone norepinephrine, causing depression and mood swings.

L-Valine is a natural stimulant. Use it with leucine and isoleucine for muscle and tissue repair.

Continued ➡

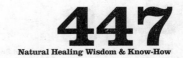

Obviously, amino acids are more than minor healing agents for women's dis-eases. They have been promoted in the health market for men's body building, but have far more serious uses that may be lifesaving for many women. They are substances that women need to know about and use. The primary sources for amino acids in this section are James F. Balch, MD, and Phyllis A. Balch, CNC, *Prescription for Nutritional Healing* (Avery Publishing Group, 1990), and Louise Tenney, MH, *Health Handbook* (Woodland Books, 1987).

Vitamin, Mineral, and Amino Acid Remedies

AIDS

Vitamins and Minerals: Holistic treatment for AIDS and HIV-positive people focuses on building the immune system. Along with a healthy lifestyle—quality food, enough sleep and exercise, reducing stress and avoiding harmful substances—the following vitamin regime is important. I have used this on HIV-positive gay men and watched their blood values normalize as long as they stayed on it. Two became HIV-negative after less than a year on the vitamins and better diet, with no other treatment. Use a high-quality daily multiple vitamin and mineral supplement and double the standard dose. If you are using Schiff's Single Day, for example, use it twice a day with meals. Along with this add a B complex-50 or -100 two or three times a day, and vitamin C to bowel tolerance. Use at least 10,000 mg (10 g) of C with bioflavinoids a day, and it can go far higher. These are essentials.

Dr. Robert Cathcart in Califomia has ample evidence of HIV remission and total disappearance on megadoses of intravenous vitamin C, using 200–500 grams a day.[3] For C by mouth, use calcium ascorbate powder (nonacid form), 1/2–3/4 teaspoon taken in water six times a day. Use a straw to bypass the teeth (this is strong enough to eventually dissolve tooth enamel), and rinse your mouth with water after each use. Take a B complex or calcium/ magnesium tablet with it at least a few times a day to prevent kidney stones from the high dose of C.

Take 50,000–75,000 IU of beta-carotene per day, 100 mg of zinc, and 400–800 IU of vitamin E with 200 mcg of selenium. Supplement folic acid to about 400 mcg, B_6 to 250–500 mg, extra B_{12} to 2000 mcg (injections are even better), extra biotin to 500 mcg, and 500–2000 mg of B_5 (pantothenic acid). B_{15}, pangamic acid, may be helpful in reducing nausea. If stopping any of these large amounts, decrease them slowly. Zinc should not exceed 100 mg total per day.

Minerals besides zinc include: copper (3 mg), manganese (10–20 mg), magnesium (500–1000 mg with double calcium), molybdenum (100 mcg), and chromium (500 mcg).[4] Germanium (200 mg), S.O.D. (an enzyme—super oxide dismutase), or coenzyme Q10 are highly recommended antioxidants. Use iron if needed. If you are on AZT, the above amounts should replace what the drug drains from the body and help in diarrhea and side effects. Egg lecithin (20 g) on an empty stomach divided through the day is also recommended, as well as essential fatty acids (evening primrose oil or black currant oil).

Herbs: Use cayenne in water daily to prevent opportunistic infections of AIDS. Take a teaspoon of dried cayenne flowers to half a gallon of water and boil for one or two minutes before shutting off the flame. Cool and strain and place in a covered bottle in the refrigerator. Build up an ability to tol-erate this—it's HOT. Start with a teaspoonful a day and work up to a juiceglass full. It may irritate the stomach.[2]

Use the herbal antibiotics, echinacea, yellow dock, goldenseal, chaparral or pau d'arco. Use blood cleansing herbs, particularly red clover with blue violet, and particularly with AIDS-related cancers. Silymarin, milk thistle extract, protects and repairs the liver and is needed if you are using doctor's medications and AIDS drugs. Dandelion also cleanses the liver. Ginseng, mullein, gingko biloba (for the brain), St. John's wort (hypericum), or Jason Winter's Tea (chaparral) are all positive. For medication side effects: use slippery elm for indigestion and diarrhea; catnip tea, chamomile, spearmint, raspberry leaf or peppermint for nausea, diarrhea and indigestion. Slippery elm can also be used as a food if nothing else will stay down, and alfalfa is an essential nutrient. For stress or insomnia, try scullcap, hops, catnip or passion flower, and for pain use valerian. Take your pick among these herbs and try one or two—do not use them all.

Amino Acids: Use a free-form amino acids combination; it offers high nutrition and immune building, plus B complex vitamins that are badly needed, and is an antioxidant besides. Single aminos include L-carnitine, cysteine, methionine and ornithine; take on an empty stomach with 500 mg vitamin C and 50 mg of B_6 (or B complex).

Arthritis

Vitamins and Minerals: Use a daily multiple vitamin and mineral supplement with vitamin C to bowel tolerance. Add a B complex-50 to -100 two or three times a day with meals, and extra B_3, B_5 and B_6 (100 mg each up to three times a day; 500 mg of B_5); PABA reduces swelling. Take 800–1200 IU of vitamin E (with selenium is best, 50–200 mcg), and 25,000–50,000 IU of vitamin A as beta-carotene. A calcium/magnesium supplement (1000 mg calcium, 500 mg magnesium) is important to prevent bone loss. Zinc (50 mg), manganese, copper, and iodine (as kelp tablets, six to eight per day) are helpful, as well as the antioxidant pain relievers coenzyme Q10 (60 mg), germanium (200 mg) or S.O.D. Do not take supplemental iron.

Amino Acids: A combination free-form amino acids is highly recommended to ease pain and rebuild tissue. Take it between meals. Single aminos include histidine, methionine, DL-phenylalanine and cystine. Tryptophan will be available again eventually.

Asthma

Vitamins and Minerals: Along with a multiple vitamin and mineral supplement, use vitamin A (15,000–25,000 IU daily) in dry form for the lungs and immune system. Use a B complex-50 or -100 two or three times a day; important individual B-vitamins include B_6 (50–250 mg total), B_5, which is a natural antihistamine and antistress factor (500–2000 mg daily), and sublingual B_{12}. Use vitamin C with bioflavonoids to bowel tolerance or at least 3000 mg per day, and vitamin E with selenium up to 1200 IU per day. Minerals are even more important, and a calcium/magnesium tablet taken every half hour can lessen or stop attacks. For daily use take 1500 mg calcium to 750 mg magnesium in a complete calcium supplement—deficiencies in these may be the cause of asthma. Zinc for immune support can be supplemented at about 50 mg per day, and 5 mg of manganese taken twice a week. Coenzyme Q10 helps lessen the body's histamine reaction and oxygenates the blood. Germanium is also an oxygenator and immune builder, or Bromelin with Quercetin C. For children, give half the amounts.

Amino Acids: Take 500 mg of L-methionine with vitamins B_6 (50 mg) and C (500 mg) twice a day on an empty stomach.

Back Pain

Vitamins and Minerals are highly important in reducing back pain. With a multiple vitamin and mineral supplement, use a B complex-50 to -100 twice a day and sublingual vitamin B_{12} (2000 mcg) daily. Minerals are essential: take a complete calcium/magnesium supplement (200 mg calcium to 100 mg magnesium daily). A complete calcium will have small amounts with it of vitamins C, D, and A and zinc. You need 50 mg daily (total) of zinc and 3 mg of boron (stop boron when healed, unless over age fifty). Manganese helps in healing cartilage in the neck and back. Use at least 3000 mg (three grams) of vitamin C daily to ease pain and for tissue repair. Vitamins A, D and E are also important. Use germanium for pain (calcium/magnesium is also a pain reliever and muscle relaxant). For disc problems, vitamin C is important, along with vitamin E and a high-protein (amino acids) diet. For sciatica, the focus is on B complex and protein.

Amino Acids: Protein is important for relieving back pain, so use a combination amino acids, either free-form or liver-based. Individual aminos include DL-phenylalanine, tryptophan and methionine. Methionine is particularly important for disc problems, phenylalanine is an analgesic for pain, and tryptophan is a relaxant.

Breast Lumps

Vitamins and Minerals: Along with a multiple vitamin and mineral supplement, add a B complex-50 to the diet to make sure there is enough folic acid and vitamin B_6 nutritionally available. More B_6, up to 200 mg per day, is helpful for hormone balancing, especially if there are menstrual problems along with the breast lumps. Vitamin E is of highest importance in reducing cystic breasts and lumps; use 1000 IU per day in gradual increases for a month, then 600–800 IU per day (use dry form). This alone may correct the condition within a few weeks. Evening Primrose Oil (gamma linolenic acid, essential fatty acids), two capsules three times a day, is a hormone balancer that may also change the condition without other help. Coenzyme Q10 is a powerful antioxidant, along with vitamin E, and May be helpful as well.

Amino Acids: Use a combination free-form amino acids. Single aminos recommended for breast lumps and cystic breasts are methionine, glutathione, and arginine (use with lysine; avoid if you have herpes).

Cancer

Vitamins and Minerals: Along with a multiple vitamin and mineral supplement, vitamins A, E and B complex are essential in both prevention and treatment. Vitamins A and E are antioxidants, and particularly use a dry-form natural E that contains selenium—up to 1600 IU of E and 200 mcg of selenium a day. Use high amounts of vitamin A (50,000–100,000 IU for ten days, decrease to up to 50,000 IU for a month, then use 25,000 IU as a maintenance dose). This is especially good in cervical dysplasia (suspicious Pap smear) for normalizing. Stomach upset and nausea indicate too much, so know when to cut back, and use vitamin A in dry form. Beta-carotene can be added to this, about 10,000 IU per day. Use vitamin C to bowel tolerance, and a B complex; niacin may be important in preventing precancerous cells from becoming malignant, as may calcium, and calcium is also a pain reliever. Germanium (200 mg) and coenzyme

Continued ➡

QIO (60 mg) both help to reduce the side effects of chemotherapy and radiation, and are pain relievers; germanium may be more important. Zinc (50 mg per day) boosts the immune system. For precancerous conditions, vitamins B_6, B_{12} and folic acid may be enough to reverse the situation. Do not take supplemental iron if you have cancer.

Amino Acids: These are listed as highly important both in preventing cancer and in cancer healing. Use a combination free-form or liver amino acids (liver-based aminos also contain B_{12} niacin and other B complex vitamins; see Twin Labs Predigested Liver Amino Acids combination). Single aminos detoxify and protect the liver from free radical formation: L-carnitine, cysteine, methionine, or taurine. For chemotherapy and x-ray side effects, use L-glutathione.

Candida Albicans

Vitamins and Minerals: Use a yeast and sugar free (most are) multiple vitamin and mineral complex, and a yeast-free B complex-50. Deficiency in vitamin B_6 is a cause of Candida albicans and extra B_{12} and biotin are needed. Use zinc for immune building, and vitamin C in high doses, with selenium 100–300 mcg per day. A major candida/yeast treatment is acidophilus, which replaces the beneficial bacteria in the gut. Use nondairy Maxidophilus, Megadophilus or Superdophilus for this. An acidophilus compound from Switzerland called Eugalen Forte, expensive and once very hard to find but becoming easier, is highly positive and worked very well for me. Essential fatty acids (evening primrose oil, salmon oil, linseed oil, omega-3 or black currant oil) can be extremely effective also. Caprylic acid is one of several things used to eliminate the yeast fungus; follow directions on the bottle. Some of these are not strictly vitamins, but seem to fall most easily into the vitamin category. Digestive enzymes like HCL can make a difference.

Amino Acids: A free-form combination amino acids is important in rebuilding the immune system and detoxifying. Use L-cystine singly.

Cataracts

Vitamins and Minerals: These go along with, but are not a substitute for, a good diet. Use a high quality multiple vitamin and mineral supplement; if you are an elder and have difficulty digesting pills and tablets, look for vitamins in soft gel or capsule form or even liquids. Major vitamin deficiencies in cataracts include vitamin C and B_2. Use at least 3000 mg per day of vitamin C with bioflavinoids, a B complex-50 three times a day, and additional B_2 (15–50 mg), B_6 (50–100 mg) and B_1 (50 mg). Use 25,000–50,000 IU of vitamin A daily in dry form, and vitamin E (increase gradually to 400–800 IU per day) with selenium (200 mcg per day). Minerals are highly important; use a calcium/magnesium tablet, 50 mg of zinc daily, and 3 mg of copper. Manganese is also helpful, and so is lecithin. Vitamin A eyedrops, called Conjunctisan A, are important.

Amino Acids: Protein deficiency is a nutritional factor in cataract formation, and a liver-based combination amino acids is highly important. Single aminos for cataract healing include: methionine, cystine, lysine and glutathione.

Chronic Fatigue Syndrome

Vitamins and Minerals: Along with a high-quality diet, use a good multiple vitamin and mineral supplement. With it use vitamin C with bioflavinoids to bowel tolerance (5–10 g daily). Use a B complex-50 to -100 three times daily, with pantothenic acid B_5.

Use vitamins A, E and coenzyme QIO as antioxidants—50,000 IU of dry-form vitamin A for a month, then decrease to 25,000 IU, use 800 IU of vitamin E and 75 mg of CO QIO. Potassium is highly important, and so are zinc, calcium and magnesium. Make sure your multiple vitamin includes the trace minerals. Because 60 percent of chronic fatigue can be traced to Candida albicans, use acidophilus to return the bacterial balance to the intestines. (See the section on Candida Albicans; all of the remedies there are also applicable.) Digestive enzymes are positive for many women with this dis-ease, and essential fatty acids (black currant oil). Egg lecithin, used by some AIDS patients, can be helpful.[1]

Amino Acids: Take a free-form amino acids combination, and consider the following singly: asparagine and aspartic acid together, or isoleucine with leucine and valine.

Colds and Sore Throats

Vitamins and Minerals: A 1000 mg (1 gram) vitamm C and bioflavinoias tablet taken hourly with lots of water or calcium/magnesium can stop a cold if used early enough, at the very first symptoms. During a cold, go to bowel tolerance but decrease slowly. Some women report the same cold-stopping effect with vitamin A, using a 25,000 IU capsule hourly (for no more than three days), then decreasing to 25,000 IU per day. The two vitamins may be used together, and most women will respond to one or the other. Again the trick is to start very early, at the first signs and symptoms. This will also work for sore throats and strep throats, and for these add zinc gluconate lozenges. Dissolve one under the tongue every three hours for three days, then every four hours for a week. Vitamin B_5, pantothenic acid, is a natural antihistamine.

Amino Acids: Use a free-form amino acid combination to detoxify and rebuild the immune system.

Constipation

Vitamins and Minerals: Avoid mineral oil laxatives as they strip the body of vitamins; take fiber bulk laxatives and cleansers at a different time than vitamin tablets, which are washed away by them. Along with a multiple vitamin and mineral supplement, take a vitamin B complex-50 with extra B_5 (500 mg) and B_{12} before meals. Lecithin or brewer's yeast can resolve many women's constipation, and high amounts of vitamin C are laxative. Vitamin E (400–800 IU), calcium and magnesium (1500 mg calcium/750 magnesium) prevent colon cancer. To these add 50 mg of zinc per day. Iron supplements may cause constipation; use only organic iron (hydrolized protein chelate), or a commercial preparation called Floradix. Digestive enzymes often solve the problem, but avoid HCL (hydrochloric acid) if you have ulcers. Some constipation is an imbalance of intestinal bacteria, and can also be caused by systemic Candida: take acidophilus as Megadophilus, Maxidophilus or Superdophilus. There may be some initial diarrhea before balance is reached.

Amino Acids: Use a liver-extract amino combination for the B complex vitamins and its detoxifying and nutritive properties.

Coughs and Flu

Vitamins and Minerals: The vitamin program is similar to that of colds and sore throats. Along with a multiple vitamin and mineral supplement, use vitamin C (1000 mg hourly) at the start to try to stop it completely. Drink a lot of water with this and decrease it slowly. Use C to bowel tolerance during

the dis-ease. Vitamin C helps to lower fever, boost the immune system, and flush toxins from the body; it is also antiviral. Vitamin A is another immune booster and antioxidant; take 25,000 IU daily and add more with beta-carotene. Zinc gluconate lozenges are used with sore throats and coughs and are highly important in flu healing. Dissolve one lozenge under the tongue every two hours. The B complex vitamin B_5 is an antihistamine, and B_6 is also important; use them with a full B complex-50. Gamma linolenic acid (black currant oil) is recommended.

Amino Acids: A free-form amino acids combination is important for its B complex vitamins, immune building factors, ability to control fevers, and ability to detoxify the body.

Depression

Vitamins and Minerals: The B complex vitamins are essential in healing depression; use a B complex-100 three times a day. Specific B-vitamins include B_1, B_3 (niacin), B_6, B_9 (folic acid) and B_{12}. Women with menstrual problems or on the pill need B_6 (250–500 mg total per day) and folic acid (400 mcg total daily). Lecithin is important for brain and nerve function but is not for use by manic depressives; niacin is a calmative and necessary for women with migraines (use 100 mg per day total). A B complex-100 will do the job without others added for most women. Use vitamin C for stress (1000–3000 mg per day or go to bowel tolerance). A complete calcium/magnesium supplement can make a great difference for many women and is recommended, in addition to a multiple vitamin—mineral supplement.

Amino Acids: These are highly important for depression, stress reduction, nutrition and brain function. Use 750 mg of GABA (Gamma-aminobutyric acid) with niacinamide and inositol as a tranquilizer. This can take the place of many medical drugs. For personality disorders, use glutamic acid, and tyrosine for brain function. Avoid phenylalanine, as many depressed women are allergic to it; if you are manic depressive avoid choline (vitamin), omathine and arginine (aminos). Try a combination amino acids otherwise, and monitor your response.

Diarrhea

Vitamins and Minerals: Persistent diarrhea causes a deficiency in every nutrient, particularly minerals. This same diarrhea may also be caused by deficiencies, particularly of the B complex vitamins folic acid, B_1, B_6 or niacin, magnesium (from taking an imbalance of too much calcium without enough matching magnesium), iron, and/or potassium. Take a full B complex-50 and up to 100 mg of potassium per day, along with a multiple vitamin and mineral supplement. If malabsorption is a problem, use a liquid B complex and/or a liquid multiple. Take acidophilus in the form of Maxidophilus or Megadophilus to replace friendly intestinal bacteria, and charcoal tablets—every four hours with water but not at the same time as other supplements or medications—until the diarrhea stops. If acidophilus aggravates the diarrhea, the cause of the diarrhea is dairy intolerance.

Amino Acids: Use a combination liver-based amino acids for B complex vitamins, tissue repair and rebuilding. They are powerful as antioxidants and nutrients.

Heart Dis-Ease

Vitamins and Minerals: Along with a multiple vitamin and mineral supplement, B complex is essential. Use 25–50 mg with each meal and extra

Continued ➡

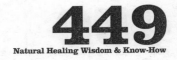

B_1, B_6, B_3 and folic acid. Vitamin B_3 (niacin) reduces incidence of angina; work slowly up to 400–500 mg a day, but only if you do not have rheumatic heart dis-ease. B_6 lowers cholesterol and prevents blood clots, and folic acid (B_9) is a vasodilator (use 75 mg per day total). Pangamic acid (B_{15}, 150 mg per day) helps heart healing, lowers cholesterol and oxygenates the blood. It also lowers the side effects of medical heart drugs. Lecithin, comprised of two B complex vitamins inositol and choline, is a fat emulsifier; take two capsules or a tablespoonful with meals. Use vitamin C with bioflavinoids (1000 mg three times a day); it lowers triglycerides, strengthens capillaries, and keeps plaque from forming on arterial walls. Take a natural vitamin E with selenium, increasing gradually from 100 IU per day, adding 100 IU weekly, to a total of 800–1000 IU daily (with 200 mcg of selenium). These are the essentials.

Beta-carotene (vitamin A, 10,000–25,000 IU per day) reduces heart attacks in high-risk patients with angina, chest pain or obstructive artery dis-ease. Use essential fatty acids (omega-3, EPA, black currant oil, primrose oil, olive oil). Calcium chelate with magnesium chelate or orotate regulates heart rhythm and decreases blood cholesterol. Most heart patients are chromium deficient (use 200 mg per day), potassium deficient (90 mg) and may be copper deficient (3 mg). Coenzyme Q10 and germanium oxygenate the blood and help to prevent additional heart damage after a heart attack, and Kyolic (odorless garlic) reduces cholesterol and lowers blood pressure.

Amino Acids: Take a free-form amino acids combination. Of single aminos, taurine corrects heart arrhythmia, carnitine (1500–3000 mg daily) decreases blood cholesterol and triglycerides and is useful in angina; take with vitamin C. Histidine and proline are also positive, as is methionine.

Immune System Dis-eases

Vitamins and Minerals: A quality multiple vitamin and mineral supplement is a basic start in replacing some of what we've lost nutritionally from food. Use 15,000–25,000 IU of vitamin A as beta-carotene (unless you are diabetic or hypothyroid, then use A itself). The B complex is essential (50–100 mg per day and more if you are ill). Most women need additional B_6 (100–250 mg) and folic acid (400 mcg), and if you are under great stress use B_5 (500–2000 mg per day total). Vitamin C (1000–5000 mg per day) with bioflavinoids and lots of water is the most significant immune building vitamin factor; with B complex and calcium/magnesium even the high doses will cause no problems. Stop at bowel tolerance. Vitamin E (400–800 IU) with selenium (200 mcg) is an important antioxidant and free radical scavenger, a protection against pollutants (with vitamins A and C).

Many women are iron deficient, but try B complex vitamins first before supplementing with iron. Zinc regulates the immune system; use 25–50 mg per day (don't go over 100 mg). Most women are calcium/magnesium deficient and require a supplement daily to prevent osteoporosis and help menstrual and menopause symptoms. Copper (1–3 mg per day) and boron (1–3 mg per day) are important and may be in your multiple vitamin. Boron prevents the body from losing needed minerals. Germanium or coenzyme Q10 are antioxidants and oxygenate the blood. Essential fatty acids (black currant oil, evening primrose oil, etc.) and acidophilus are useful, as well as combination raw glandulars or raw thymus, lymph, spleen or bone marrow. This is an overall picture that changes with

individuals and individual dis-eases but is basic for immune building.

Amino Acids: A combination free-form or liver-extract amino acids capsule is important in protein, B complex and many other nutrients and is a free radical scavenger. Single aminos include arginine (3–5 g per day unless you have herpes) or cysteine, methionine, lysine and ornithine (500 mg each twice daily).

Leg Cramps

Vitamins and Minerals: Here is where leg cramps are most easily and quickly taken care of. Along with a daily multiple vitamin and mineral supplement, a calcium/magnesium tablet is most often the quickest cure. This is particularly so for night cramps suffered by younger women and those who are pregnant. Use a complete calcium/magnesium formula, 1000–2000 mg calcium to half the amount of magnesium. The trace minerals in a complete calcium are needed for assimilation. For leg cramps while standing or walking, usually caused by poor circulation in elders, vitamin E is the answer. Start with 400 IU per day and increase up to 800–1200 IU, adding 100 IU per week. If you have rheumatic heart disease start with 100 IU per day and stop at 400 IU. For women on diuretics, or women who are athletes and perspire excessively, potassium is usually the remedy; take under 100 mg per day. For exertion with excessive perspiration in hot weather, salt loss can occur, but potassium replacement rather than salt is more usually needed. The B complex vitamins, particularly B_6 and B_3, are essential in writer's-type cramps and toe cramps and for proper circulation. Vitamin D (400 IU daily) is needed for calcium uptake, and vitamin C with bioflavinoids is needed for proper blood flow/circulation to the muscles. Vitamin A (25,000 IU), zinc (50 mg), hydrochloric acid (HCL), and/or coenzyme Q10 are all helpful. Boron (3 mg per day) significantly increases assimilation of calcium and other minerals, and some complete calciums include it. The major remedies here are calcium/magnesium, vitamin E, B_6 and/or potassium.

Amino Acids: A combination free-form or liver amino acids provides protein, B vitamins, antioxidant action and tissue regeneration. All of these are important.

Menopause

Vitamins and Minerals: A multiple vitamin and mineral supplement is important for normal hormone function. With it use a B complex-50 to -100 up to three times a day. You may also need additional B_6 (up to 50 mg three times a day), B_5 (100–500 mg two or three times a day) and/or PABA for adrenal function and stress. B_6 decreases water retention and menopause symptoms, with more needed if you are taking estrogen. B_5 aids adrenal function; estrogen production is shifted from the ovaries to the adrenals at menopause. Vitamin E, along with the B complex, is the remedy of choice for hot flashes and all menopause symptoms including emotional symptoms. Use it topically for vaginal dryness, and internally start with 400 IU per day, increasing by 100 IU weekly to 800–1600 IU, divided into several doses a day. Stop at the dose that ends the hot flashes. If you have rheumatic heart dis-ease, you are limited to 400 IU per day; if you are on estrogen, you need the higher amounts. A vitamin E with selenium (200 mcg) is recommended. Also for hot flashes, use vitamin C (from 3000 mg per day up to bowel tolerance).

Calcium/magnesium (up to 2000 mg calcium/1000 mg magnesium) helps emotional symptoms and is essential to prevent bone loss. (If this is a problem, add 3 mg of boron; see the section on Osteoporosis.) If you have cervical dysplasia (suspicious Pap smear, too often leading to hysterectomy), B vitamins including B_6 and folic acid, vitamin E with selenium, vitamin A as beta-carotene (25,000 IU per day), and vitamin D (400 IU) may be enough to change the condition within three or four months for up to 70 percent of women. Also look for low-grade cervical infections in this case. Essential fatty acids (evening primrose oil, black currant oil) act as a sedative and diuretic and aid hot flashes; these are important for estrogen production. Germanium will also help menopause symptoms; use 60 mg twice daily. Insert acidophilus capsules into the vagina at night to help prevent vaginal infections. Enzymes with hydrochloric acid (HCL) help digestion. Primary here are the B complex, E, calcium/magnesium, and essential fatty acids.

Amino Acids: L-arginine (500 mg twice daily) and lysine (500 mg per day) taken on an empty stomach detoxify the liver and aid liver function These are important in reducing menopause symptoms.

Menstruation

Vitamins and Minerals: Overall nutrition is important; use a quality multiple vitamin and mineral supplement, not something cheap from the supermarket. Add to it a complete calcium/magnesium tablet (General Nutrition's Calcium Plus is good) that contains 1000–2000 mg of calcium and half that amount of magnesium. This can be taken divided into three or four doses a day (including one at bedtime), and taken with water, or sipped with water that has a teaspoon of apple cider vinegar in it for absorption. It can also be taken hourly for acute cramps and pain, with B_6. For some women, this is enough to stop PMS and cramping. To go further, take a B-complex-50 to -100 three times a day. This is especially important for women on the pill or who are smokers. Women on the pill and women who have tension, bloating, premenstrual acne or anxiety need extra B_6 (50–400 mg per day). Vitamins B_5 and B_{12} are stress and fatigue reducers, and folic acid (25–50 mg per day)1 is important for women with suspicious Pap smears (see Menopause section). Use 1000–3000 mg of vitamin C with bioflavinoids or go to bowel tolerance to reduce heavy flows, and 400 IU per day of vitamin D (total) for calcium exudations.

Amino Acids: Take a free-form amino acids combination for eczema, acne, dermatitis or skin cancer. Single aminos for all skin dis-eases are L-cysteine and methionine together as detoxifiers and antioxidants, or taurine for skin cancer to rebuild tissues.

Obesity Affecting Health

Vitamins and Minerals: Begin with a multiple vitamin and mineral supplement of good quality; if assimilation is a problem, they come in liquid form. A high level B complex-50 is next, used twice a day, with additional B_6 (100 mg) for fluid retention and to change stored fat to energy. Additional B_5 (500 mg with each meal) doubles the rate of fat assimilation and boosts the adrenals. Lecithin taken with meals helps the body burn fat, reduces blood cholesterol and prevents or aids high blood pressure and artery dis-ease. These are essential for liver function, as well. Use vitamin C (3000–6000 mg per day) for glandular functions, and vitamin E (400–800 IU per day) doubles the rate of fat

Continued ➡

metabolism again. Start with 400 IU of E and increase by 100 IU per week; if you have rheumatic heart dis-ease you are limited to 400 IU total daily. Essential fatty acids aid in utilization of fat already in the body, suppress appetite and keep off lost weight. Use as evening primrose oil, salmon oil, black currant oil, or cod liver oil. If you are hypoglycemic, and also to reduce fluid retention, try potassium (90 mg). Chromium (200 mcg) aids weight loss by balancing blood sugar. All women need to be on a calcium/magnesium supplement; it helps water retention, is a muscle relaxant and slight carminative, and an antacid.

Amino Acids: These are important for easy-to-assimilate protein and B vitamins for obesity and hypoglycemia; use a free-form combination. Single aminos include DL-phenyalanine as an appetite suppressant (100–300 mg per day); avoid high amounts if you are diabetic or have high blood pressure. The combination of arginine, ornithine and lysine (500 mg of each) decreases body fat; avoid for diabetics and children. Carnitine aids fat assimilation and weight loss.

Sinusitis and Allergies

Vitamins and Minerals: Use a complete vitamin and mineral supplement, particularly one high in B complex vitamins. Add to it mega doses of B complex, using a B complex-100 twice daily, with extra B_6 (100 mg twice a day) and B_5 (500 mg twice a day). Use vitamin C with bioflavinoids (2000–10,000 mg per day or to bowel tolerance). In acute sinusitis attacks, take 1000 mg hourly with B_6 or a calcium/magnesium tablet. C is an anti-inflammatory, and antifungal and antibacterial; the B_6 or calcium prevent megadoses of C from causing kidney stones. Take 25,000 IU daily of vitamin A in dry form or beta-carotene, or take as much as 100,000 IU daily for up to one month, then cut back to 25,000 IU. A is a nutrient for the mucous membranes. In chronic cases, coenzyme Q10 (60 mg) or germanium (100 mg daily) increase oxygen to the cells, are free radical scavengers, and boost the immune system.

Amino Acids: Use a combination free-form or liver-based amino acids. Single aminos include lysine, histidine and tyrosine.

Skin Dis-eases

Vitamins and Minerals: Women with any form of skin dis-ease need a daily multiple vitamin and mineral supplement, a B complex-50 to -100, a complete calcium/magnesium tablet (1000–2000 mg calcium and half as much magnesium), and zinc. Add 50–250 mg of B_6 for acne, menstrually related acne, and eczema; B_3 (100 mg up to three times daily) for skin cancer and stress; PABA (under 400 IU) for eczema and as a skin cancer protection; and sublingual B_{12} (300–1000 mcg) for skin cancer and stress. Eczema may be a PABA deficiency dis-ease. Use a vitamin C with bioflavinoids for all skin dis-eases (100 mg per day and up, to bowel tolerance for skin cancer). Dry form vitamin A or beta-carotene is important for any skin dis-ease; use up to 100,000 IU daily for as long as a month, then cut back to 25,000 IU per day. Nausea and stomach upsets indicate too much; stop for a week, then start again at lower amounts. Use vitamin D (400–800 IU), vitamin E (400 IU and up—1000 IU daily with skin cancer), and add selenium to the E (100–200 mcg) with high zinc use, skin cancer or for elders. For acne in young women, take 50 mg of zinc and for adults take up to 100 mg total daily (not over).

Evening primrose oil (essential fatty acids) is vital for healing skin dis-eases. Use two capsules two or three times a day for acne, eczema, dermatitis or skin cancer. This can also be applied topically. Other forms of essential fatty acids include: salmon oil, cod liver oil, black currant oil, omega-3, sesame seed oil or linseed oil. The above will aid itching, sores, eruptions or other symptoms, prevent scarring and regenerate the skin. With skin cancer, add an antioxidant such as S.O.D., coenzyme Q10 (100 mg), or germanium (200 mg) daily. Chromium reduces skin infections, and acidophilus helps digestion. If vitamins seem not to help, add HCL or digestive enzymes; it may be an assimilation problem.

The fingernails can be an indication of what vitamins you are deficient in. Ridges indicate protein or vitamin A deficiency, and washboard ridges deficiencies in calcium, iron or zinc. Thin, brittle nails are lack of iron, calcium, vitamin D or hydrochloric acid, while splitting nails are deficient in the sulfur amino acids. Peeling nails need vitamin A and pale nail beds are anemia. White spots indicate deficiencies in zinc, hydrochloric acid or a thyroid deficiency. Poor nail growth usually means lack of zinc.[7]

Amino Acids: Tryptophan is a calmative and muscle relaxant and will be available again eventually. If you have hypoglycemia or herpes, use 500 mg of lysine starting five days before periods. L-tyrosine (500 mg twice daily) helps with anxiety, depression and premenstrual or menstrual-related headaches. A combination free-form or liver-extract amino acids is recommended for its value as a mood and hormone balancer, calmative, detoxificant, and nutrient.

Stop Smoking

Vitamins and Minerals: Smokers suffer depletion in a number of vitamins and minerals, so start with a quality multiple vitamin and mineral supplement. Use a B complex-50 to -100 in time release form up to three times a day with meals; additional B_1 (50–100 mg), B_3 (100–1000 mg two-three times a day), B12 and folic acid. Use vitamin C with bioflavinoids (3000–10,000 mg per day or to bowel tolerance) to detoxify nicotine, from the body; up to 30 g are used intravenously daily for withdrawal. With each dose of vitamin C, or at least four times a day take either a B complex capsule, B_6, or a calcium/magnesium tablet. Calcium is one of the things leached from the bones by smoking and it is a nervous system relaxant (as is B_3 and B complex) to aid in withdrawal symptoms. Use vitamin A as beta-carotene up to 100,000 IU per day for up to one month, then cut back to 25,000 IU per day; it heals the mucous membranes, is an antioxidant, and protects the lungs from cancer. Starting with 200 IU of vitamin E per day, increase by 100 IU per week until you are taking 800–1200 IU daily, preferably with selenium (200 mcg). Vitamins A, E and C are antioxidants and help the liver and other organs to detoxify. Zinc (50–80 mg per day) boosts the immune system, and coenzyme Q10 (30 mg) or germanium (30 mg) are other powerful antioxidants. Chromium is important to reduce nicotine cravings and balance blood sugar; take 300 mcg per day—cigarette withdrawal is an induced hypoglycemia. Essential fatty acids, black currant oil or fish lipid oils, may help.

Amino Acids: A complete free-form amino acids combination helps with nutrition, detoxification, free radical scavenging, and tissue repair. Single aminos include taking cysteine with vitamin C, or methionine, cysteine and cystine together.

Endnotes

1. James F. Balch, MD, and Phyllis A.Balch, *CNC Prescription for Nutritional* (Garden City, NY, Avery Publishing Group, Inc., 1990), 27. The information for this section comes primarily from this source.
2. I want to thank Laurel Steinhice for this cayenne water recipe.
3. Tom O'Connor, *Living with AIDS* (San Francisco, Corwin Publishers, 1987), 324–338.
4. Lawrence Badgley, MD, *Healing AIDS Naturally* (San Bruno, CA, Human Energy Press, 1987), 114–133. Much of the remedy information is from Badgley.
5. James Balch, MD and Phyllis Balch, CNC, *Prescription for Nutritional Healing* (Garden City Park, NY, Avery Publishing Group, Inc.., 1990), 135–136.
6. It may take a doctor's prescription to get this high amount, but it is being used by Atkin's Clinic in New York and by Dr. Ross Trattler, *Better Health Through Natural Healing* (New York, McGraw-Hill Book Co., 198S, 442), with success for cervical dysplasia.
7. Dr. Ross Trattler, *Better Health Through Natural Healing* (New York, McGraw-Hill Book Co., 1985), 450.

—From *The Natural Remedy Book for Women*

THE ENLIGHTENED DIET
Deborah Kesten, MPH, and Larry Scherwits, Ph.D.

The Seven Eating Styles

Are you a food fretter? A task snacker? An emotional eater? Or do you typically "flavor" food with all—or none—of the eating styles? The seven eating styles we discovered during our research on weight loss revealed new insights into why so many of us overeat and gain weight and what we can do about it. The eating styles are: food fretting, task snacking, emotional eating, fast foodism, solo dining, unappetizing atmosphere, and sensory disregard.[1] Throughout this book, we'll show you how to modify each eating style, so that it no longer leads to weight gain.

Here's how it works. The total eating style program in the book works by giving you the skills you need to fine-tune each of the eating styles, so that you can achieve and maintain your ideal weight. Fill out our personalized seven eating style profiles at the end of this section to find out which ones may be keeping you from staying slim. The quiz will reveal the degree to which you are practicing—or not—each eating style. In other words, you will discover how the *food choices* you most often make, and the *eating behaviors* you typically practice, work together to contribute to overeating and weight gain. Once you become aware of this, you will know the eating styles that need your attention the most, as well as those that may need minor modifications.

Once you discover your trouble spots and areas in which you can improve, each section gives you scientifically sound insights into the eating style, then a menu of choices and actions you can take that are the antidotes to overeating and weight gain. In other words, once you discover the eating styles that are holding you back, we give you an action plan that includes an abundance of personalized choices and options that you can practice and apply daily. These whole person nutrition and eating skills, tools, and insights are what you need to get slim and stay slim for life.

Continued ➔

At the same time, you will be empowered to change the way you think about food, dieting, eating, and achieving and maintaining normal weight. The end result: the experience of whole person nutrition, wellness living, and weight loss.

In short, if there's a secret to successful dieting, the Enlightened Diet is it. With clearly defined and informed recommendations based on our research and other scientific studies, the Enlightened Diet provides a total resource for creating an individualized plan that's right for you. It accomplishes this by giving you the evidence-based insights you need to modify not only what you eat, but also how, why, when, with whom—even where.

Once you understand all aspects of your relationship to food and eating (biological, psychological, spiritual, and social), you will have a high level of awareness about what's leading you to overeat and gain weight. In turn, you can use these insights and wisdom to create conscious choices that optimize your relationship with food and eating. In other words, you discover how to turn a pattern of unsustainable food restriction into whole person nutrition and weight loss as a way of life. By "setting your table" this way, you will be empowered to create an action-oriented plan that turns overeating into optimal eating—in other words, to "diet" successfully for a lifetime.

We call our newly discovered patterns of overeating "styles" because they are a unique expression of the way you, personally, live or behave in relationship to food and food-related activities, from shopping and selecting food to eating food—even the atmosphere in which you dine. Think about the eating styles in the following way: every day you make a decision to style your hair in a manner that you believe is attractive, interesting, easy, and comfortable. Ultimately, your hairstyle reflects your taste and becomes typical of you; in other words, it becomes your personal style. When you're feeling good about your hair, you might say you're having a good hair day; when it's not looking its best, you may describe it as a bad hair day. And then there are days when your hairstyle is somewhere between looking either good or bad. As with good, bad, and in between hair days, each of the seven eating styles provides insights into the spectrum of your food-related behaviors. On one end of the continuum, you are eating optimally, while the other end reveals that you are more likely to overeat and gain weight.

What does it mean to eat optimally? It means you take the time to nourish your body with a balanced intake of nutrients (biological nutrition); you get pleasure from food so that you feel satisfied (psychological nutrition); you connect to the life force in food (spiritual nutrition); and, because we're social beings, you realize you thrive when you dine with others while sharing convivial conversation in pleasant surroundings (social nutrition).

These biological, psychological, spiritual, and social nutrition facets comprise the essence of our Whole Person Nutrition Model and Program, and the comprehensive food, eating, nutrition, and lifestyle plan in this section. The more you distance yourself from these multidimensional facets of food, the more you're likely to be practicing one or more of the seven overeating styles, which in turn, leads to increased risk for becoming overweight or obese.

We realize it may be tempting to skip through this part of the chapter and, instead, to fill out the personal eating style questionnaire ("What's Your Eating Style?"), then to turn immediately to the material that most fits your profile. Taking only the first step is a good way to start, but it isn't likely to get you the results you want. That's because reaping the relationship-to-food rewards of our program asks that you "be here now," that you begin to relate to food and eating as an "in the moment" experience, and that you start—and continue—the journey by familiarizing yourself with all elements of our Whole Person Nutrition Model and Program, so that you can master the program, starting now.

With this overview of the seven eating styles, you will discover how to restyle your food life by discovering how to eat in order to lose weight and at the same time to enjoy food and the experience of eating. Each section will give you the tools, skills, and guidelines you need to accomplish this. Right now, though, we want to first shed light on the seven eating styles we've discovered that lead to overeating and weight gain, most of which have been overlooked by dieters, health professionals, and the diet industry. As you'll see, each style decodes the many reasons so many of us overeat and gain weight, while at the same time, each eating style—indeed, this entire subchapter—offers the solution to the cycle.

Food Fretting

Good food, bad food. Legal food, illegal food. Sinful food, pure food. The food fretting eating style is overly concerned about and focused on food, as well as projecting moral judgment onto what we and others *should* eat. If you are often filled with thoughts about what you or others should or shouldn't eat, traditional dieting, or the "right" way to eat, or you tend to measure your self-worth and that of others based on what or how much is eaten, the food fretting eating style is a key contributor to your overeating.

Do you see yourself in any of the following examples of food fretting?

"I was good today," you may think when you've managed to avoid unhealthful foods, stick to your diet, and eat what you think you should.

"When my food cravings become powerful and I eat foods that are bad, I feel so guilty," is typical self-think for many food fretters.

"She should resist that sinful chocolate cake. Doesn't she have any will power?" you might think as you watch a person eat what she "shouldn't."

Overcoming this eating style begins first with recognizing such judgmental, fret-filled chatter about food and eating. Being honest with yourself will be challenging, in part because being critical and feeling anxious about food has become common in our culture. The work you do to overcome this eating style is well worth the effort because it will enable you to replace fret-filled self-think with smart-think that will empower you to overcome this weight-promoting eating style.

In "Food Fretting," we'll reveal the pitfalls of the judgmental dimension of eating. For instance, as you'll see, a key underlying element of this weight-inducing eating style is traditional dieting, and then berating ourselves if we go off the diet. But the many food-fretting guidelines we provide for overcoming fret-filled thoughts and recriminating behaviors about food and food choices—for both yourself and others—show you how to identify food fretting, and then what you can do about it. In other words, we will give you the specific strategies you'll need to turn weight-inducing judgmental thoughts and activities into a whole-person, nonjudgmental eating style so that you may enjoy food in light of its being a social, ceremonial, sensual pleasure—that doesn't lead to weight gain.

Task Snacking

Some call it "multitasking"; the French call it "vagabond eating"; many others in America think it's "normal." However it's perceived, if you often eat meals or snacks while working by yourself in front of your computer, while driving, watching TV or standing at the kitchen counter, shopping with a friend, or talking on the phone, it's likely that the "task snacking" eating style is increasing your odds of becoming overweight or obese.

With this eating style, you will discover how to rearrange your environment—both internally and externally. We will show you how to work when you work, drive when you drive, and eat when you eat, rather than eating while doing other activities. At the same time, you will find that making simple choices about eating mindfully can lead to big changes in overcoming overeating.

In "Task Snacking," you will discover the complex of related busyness behaviors and how they can contribute to weight gain. The antidote is offered later in the section, where you will learn how to break the cycle of merging eating with other activities. As you'll see, eliminating task snacking completely isn't necessarily the goal; instead, we'll give you easy-to-take actions you can do right now to cut down on your food-related multitasking and, in turn, reduce your overeating . . . and weight.

Emotional Eating

Most of us are familiar with the phrase "emotional eating," a term that refers to those who turn to comfort food to soothe negative feelings, such as depression, anxiety, or loneliness, but also to enhance joyous, positive, celebratory emotions in response to, let's say, a wedding, birthday, or promotion. If you often eat to manage your feelings and to self-soothe—in other words, for reasons other than hunger— it's likely you're an emotional eater. Some health professionals describe this eating style as "compulsive overeating" or "food addiction." No matter what it's called, many of us turn to food to relieve emotional tension because it works. After all, doesn't eating certain foods or even thinking about eating serve as a distraction from emotions that may be making you feel uncomfortable?

It may not come as a surprise to you that our research revealed that emotional eating is the strongest predictor of overeating and becoming overweight and obese and, therefore, the key contributor to weight gain. What is groundbreaking, though, are the specific emotions we've identified—the family of emotions—that are strongly linked with the likelihood you'll overeat. In "Emotional Eating," we will reveal the feelings that most strongly predict overeating. We'll also give you other insights into this overeating style, such as breakthrough brain-chemistry research, which reveals how turning to certain foods may mean you're self-medicating, which, in turn, may set off a binge in order to feel better. We shed light on the foods—and specific nutrients in them—that can bust the blues, boost memory, cut carb cravings, and more; in essence, this chapter will give you the nutritional insights, skills, and tools you'll need to make feel-good food choices.

Fast Foodism

A donut or sugary cereal for breakfast; a McDonald's double-burger with fries for lunch; and a supersized pizza, perhaps placed casually onto the dining table in its cardboard box, for dinner—add several servings of soft drinks throughout the day, and you have a profile of the fast-food cuisine that is typical for many Americans. Not surprisingly, this eating style is strongly linked with overeating,

Continued ➡

overweight, and obesity—and it threatens more than your waistline.

As you will discover, we qualify the fast foodism overeating style with the phrase "as often as possible," to ensure that you don't interpret this overeating style or its solution as more dietary dogma, or as more rules and regulations for you to follow. As with all elements of the Enlightened Diet, our intention is to help you think of what and how you eat as a spectrum rather than as an all-or-nothing, black-or-white dietary dogma.

To help you accomplish this, "Fast Foodism," will reveal foods linked with overeating and ensuing weight gain; we'll also show you what's in the foods that keeps you from achieving your weight and health goals, and how such a diet and eating style threatens more than your waistline. Then we will give you the solution to changing your relationship to this overeating style by demystifying optimal eating. To jump-start you, we will also give you a plethora of practical tips, exercises, and strategies, so you can choose the foods that will help you achieve and maintain an optimal relationship to food, vitality, health, and well-being for a lifetime.

Solo Dining

The overeating style in "Solo Dining," will show you how to turn dining with others into a balm for body, heart, and soul. As your eating style shifts from a "me" mentality to a "we" awareness—and, more and more, you share food and the dining experience with others—you'll be taking yet another step toward fulfillment and weight loss.

As extraordinarily simple as the overeating style of solo dining appears, beware: it is a two-edged sword in that it can be both easy and difficult to implement. As many of you know, the demands of home, family, and work can make it challenging to carve out time to dine with others. Yet, once you learn the amazing healing possibilities of this eating style, you'll instantly begin to reap the benefits. To help you do this, "Solo Dining" will reveal the complex of related dining-alone behaviors and how they can contribute to overeating, as well as the "ingredients" and skills you need to create and enjoy dining experiences with others. With this eating style, you'll have yet another insight to eat optimally and to succeed at enhancing your relationship with food and eating.

Unappetizing Atmosphere

You may find it amazing to consider that the atmosphere in which you eat may make a difference in whether you overeat and gain weight, but it does. The unappetizing atmosphere eating style is powerful in that, once you implement it, it will provide instant gratification because it will quickly improve the quality of your life by enhancing how you feel, both physically and emotionally; it may even improve your relationships—with others as well as with food.

With this eating style, you will focus on the psychological and physical dining aesthetics of your life—from the atmosphere in your home to your surroundings at the office, in restaurants, drive-through restaurants, or at the home of family and friends. If you intend to be successful at overcoming overeating over the long term, this eating style will serve as a reminder to strengthen your resolve.

"Unappetizing Atmosphere," will reveal more about the often overlooked contribution that ambiance and your surroundings play in overeating and weight gain, while the "Rx" we offer will give you a rich repository of strategies for accessing the healing power inherent in a relaxing, delightful, aesthetically pleasing, and welcoming dining atmosphere. We'll also show you what constitutes a pleasant dining milieu, and how to create and choose one as often as possible.

Sensory Disregard

A sensory and spiritual relationship to food, eating, and the dining experience may be the most overlooked aspect of overeating and ensuing weight gain. The problem is that most of us don't even know what it means to relate to food in this way, let alone have a clue about how to turn it into a key whole person eating style. Be assured that we will demystify the sensory disregard eating style for you. As a matter of fact, of all the eating styles we've identified, sensory and spiritual eating has the largest number of food-related experiences that are linked with optimal eating and weight.

Be assured that with this eating style, we will not be suggesting that you meditate on your meals for hours each day. Rather, you will discover how implementing each of the elements of the spiritual and sensual eating style will turn your meals into a palate-pleasing adventure that nourishes both body and soul. At the same time, whether you're taking a tea break, sharing brunch with friends, or shopping for food, this groundbreaking, but age-old eating style may eliminate what isn't working for you, while turning your day-to-day dining experiences into a sensory experience that will lead to less overeating and optimal weight.

Consider this: even if this eating style is unfamiliar territory for you, it is still likely it is a major contributor to your overeating. If so, "Sensory Disregard," will give you insights into the price your mind, body, and waistline pay if you typically make meals and eat them without flavoring them with sensory and spiritual ingredients. Then we will empower you to experience food and dining as a symphonic masterpiece, for when you eat from the heart, you also reap the rewards of enjoying—indeed, savoring—your meals in a meaningful way. . . .

Making Meals Memorable

When we ask people in our workshops to share a memorable meal or dining experience, without fail, the stories they share include all elements of the Enlightened Diet: (1) they anticipated the meal and ate it with pleasure, without judgment or anxiety; (2) they focused on the food and its flavor; (3) they enjoyed, indeed relished, the food, while filled with positive feelings; (4) the meal was made with fresh ingredients; (5) they shared the food and the dining experience with others; (6) they dined in pleasing surroundings; and (7) they appreciated the meal's sensory and spiritual ingredients. In other words, their meal memories instinctively included all elements of the Enlightened Diet: pleasure, mindfulness, feel-good feelings, fresh food, social ingredients, aesthetics awareness, and eating *from* the heart.

Whether the fare is simple or sublime, it's possible for you, too, to have memorable meals and to manage your weight at the same time. How? By practicing and living the seven eating styles in a whole person nutrition way. We'll show you how to begin with the following "What's Your Eating Style?" questionnaire we've created for you. By completing each section, tallying your scores, then interpreting your results, you'll discover your strengths as well as any weaknesses that are contributing to your overeating and weight gain and, therefore, the areas that need your attention.

By becoming familiar with the overeating styles that are currently integral to your life, you'll be able to take an active role in changing what isn't working for you. Step by step, we will give you practical, specific, action-filled whole person nutrition tools, skills, and strategies to make the changes that you, personally, need to be successful in creating an optimal, positive relationship to food and eating, and a healthy weight for a lifetime.

What's Your Eating Style?

Where are you now? We created your personal eating style profile, so you can find out how much—or how little—each eating style may be contributing to your overeating and weight gain. Consider the profile to be a lighthouse that helps you get your bearings, a guide for determining your eating style whereabouts so that you can choose the direction that will lead you to the destination of your dreams.

Once you have insights into your eating styles, you can use each part of *The Enlightened Diet* as a guide to unlocking the code to your overeating. Completing the profile prior to reading our solutions will also give you a baseline you can use over time to measure improvements and changes in each eating style.

Checking the checkpoints. After you check off the boxes and tally your total score, you will have a clearer perspective about the eating styles that are working for you, as well as a better understanding of areas you may want to improve. You'll also be taking the first step toward getting acquainted with each eating style, so you can benefit from them each time you eat.

Tallying your scores. To see where you are now, complete each eating style questionnaire below by checking the boxes that best represent your current eating style. As you fill out the profile, please note that some of the eating style questionnaires have two sections. For these eating styles, score the top section by tallying all plus (+) numbers; tally the bottom section by adding all the minus (−) numbers. Then, to get your eating style score, subtract the minus subtotal from the plus subtotal and enter the result on the total line at the bottom of each eating style profile.

Interpreting your scores. At the bottom of each style profile, you will also find a scoring key that tells you whether your score ranks as "excellent," "good," "satisfactory," or "needs improvement." To discover your total Eating Style Score for all seven eating styles, add the totals from each of the seven profiles; then read the interpretation about your Eating Style Score at the end of the profile.

Getting Started

Because all of the eating styles are interrelated, each has a powerful influence on whether you overeat and how much you weigh. The good news is that regardless of your starting point, if you change one eating style, it likely will lead to changes in others. Or you may decide to make more dramatic changes by implementing each element of the Enlightened Diet all at once. Or perhaps you may choose to make changes in your eating styles by targeting specific behaviors and choices within each eating style. There's no right or wrong way to follow the Enlightened Diet. Rather, use all the insights and strategies in each section to decide what will work best for you, personally.

Continued ➜

Food Fretting Personal Profile

For each question, check the box in the column that best represents your "anxious eating" dynamic.

	Never	Rarely	Some-times	Usually	Almost always	Always
	0	–1	–2	–3	–4	–5
1. I feel anxious about the best way to eat.	❏	❏	❏	❏	❏	❏
2. I feel good or righteous when I eat what I think I should.	❏	❏	❏	❏	❏	❏
3. When I overeat, I feel:	❏	❏	❏	❏	❏	❏
bad	❏	❏	❏	❏	❏	❏
guilty	❏	❏	❏	❏	❏	❏
gluttonous	❏	❏	❏	❏	❏	❏
4. I judge others by what they eat.	❏	❏	❏	❏	❏	❏
5. I try different diets.	❏	❏	❏	❏	❏	❏
6. I count calories, fat grams, etc.	❏	❏	❏	❏	❏	❏
7. I obsess about food.	❏	❏	❏	❏	❏	❏

Total Food Fretting Score:_____

FOOD FRETTING SCORING KEY

0 to –7: Excellent
–8 to –14: Good
–15 to –21: Satisfactory
–22 or less: Needs improvement

Task Snacking Personal Profile

For each question, check the box in the column that best represents your task snacking dynamic.

	Never	Rarely	Some-times	Usually	Almost always	Always
	0	–1	–2	–3	–4	–5
1. When I eat, I am:						
walking, rushing somewhere	❏	❏	❏	❏	❏	❏
at my desk at work	❏	❏	❏	❏	❏	❏
in my car	❏	❏	❏	❏	❏	❏
at my computer	❏	❏	❏	❏	❏	❏
talking on the phone	❏	❏	❏	❏	❏	❏
driving	❏	❏	❏	❏	❏	❏
watching TV	❏	❏	❏	❏	❏	❏
reading	❏	❏	❏	❏	❏	❏

Total Task Snacking Score:_____

TASK SNACKING SCORING KEY

0 to –8: Excellent
–9 to –14: Good
–15 to –19: Satisfactory
–20 or less: Needs improvement

Emotional Eating Personal Profile

For each question, check the box in the column that best represents your emotional eating dynamic.

	Never	Rarely	Some-times	Usually	Almost always	Always
	0	+1	+2	+3	+4	+5
1. Before eating, I check my hunger level.	❏	❏	❏	❏	❏	❏
2. I eat only when I am hungry	❏	❏	❏	❏	❏	❏

Subtotal:+_____

Evaluating Your Score

Use the table on page 457 to enter your Eating Style scores

131 or more: Excellent. Congratulations! The "excellent" level is comparable to an A+. Your relationship with food is mostly satisfying and gratifying. In other words, you eat less and enjoy it more most of the time. Both what and how you eat is beneficial to your weight, your overall health, and your quality of life.

A score of "excellent" suggests that you are already practicing many of the elements of the Enlightened Diet. To reap even more benefits, look over your answers for each eating style, then target even more changes you could make that would lead to even more delightful dining. Then turn to the sections on each eating style for more insights and tips on eating even more optimally.

130 to 55: Good. You're doing fairly well! The "good" level falls between the grades of A and B+. The foods you choose, how you eat, and with whom you eat are typically positive and beneficial. You eat optimally sometimes; when you're not able to—or choose not to—you let it go.

To reap even more benefits, look over your answers for each eating style, and decide whether there are changes you would like to make that would bring you closer to the Enlightened Diet. Then turn to the sections on each eating style—particularly those to which you seem to have some resistance—for more insights and tips on eating even more optimally.

54 to –24: Satisfactory. Food and eating are often issues for you. If you ranked "satisfactory," the way you typically eat is comparable to between a grade of B and C. You may have some confusion about what and how to eat optimally, or your eating style hasn't been a priority for you so far. Your relationship to food and eating are fairly typical, which leaves lots of room for making beneficial changes.

A score of "satisfactory" suggests that you may be finding it challenging to practice many of the elements of the Enlightened Diet. To reap more benefits, look over your answers for each eating style to target specific changes you would like to make that would lead you closer to the Enlightened Diet. Then turn to the sections on each eating style for more insights and tips on eating even more optimally.

–25 or less: Needs improvement. Your overall eating style is far from optimal. Decide whether you want to take steps toward improving your relationship with food. To help you do this, first read the "Stages of Change" section in "Food Fretting." Once you're clear about wanting to make changes, get some ideas for how to begin by retaking the "What's Your Eating Style?" questionnaire, or look over the questions in each section of the questionnaire for some quick and easy ways to implement ideas and suggestions.

A score of "needs improvement" suggests that you would benefit a lot by learning about, and then living, all the elements of the Enlightened Diet. To get started, look over your answers for each eating style to target specific changes you would like to make that will bring you closer to living the Enlightened Diet. Remember, small steps can lead to big benefits. Then turn to the sections on each eating style for more insights and tips on eating even more optimally.

Continued ➡

	Never	Rarely	Some-times	Usually	Almost always	Always
	0	–1	–2	–3	–4	–5
3. I overeat.	❑	❑	❑	❑	❑	❑
4. After eating I feel stuffed.	❑	❑	❑	❑	❑	❑
5. I have food cravings.	❑	❑	❑	❑	❑	❑
6. I eat because I feel:	❑	❑	❑	❑	❑	❑
depressed	❑	❑	❑	❑	❑	❑
sad	❑	❑	❑	❑	❑	❑
anxious	❑	❑	❑	❑	❑	❑
angry	❑	❑	❑	❑	❑	❑
frustrated	❑	❑	❑	❑	❑	❑
happy	❑	❑	❑	❑	❑	❑

Total Food Fretting Score: _____

Total Emotional Eating Score: (+) or (–) _____

EMOTIONAL EATING SCORING KEY

10 to –1: Excellent   –13 to –23: Satisfactory
–2 to –12: Good   –24 or less: Needs improvement

Fast Foodism Personal Profile

For each question, check the box in the column that best represents your fast foodism dynamic.

	Never	Rarely	Some-times	Usually	Almost always	Always
	0	+1	+2	+3	+4	+5
1. I eat fresh:	❑	❑	❑	❑	❑	❑
fruits						
vegetables						
whole grains	❑	❑	❑	❑	❑	❑
legumes	❑	❑	❑	❑	❑	❑
nuts	❑	❑	❑	❑	❑	❑
seeds (e.g., sunflower, flax)	❑	❑	❑	❑	❑	❑
2. I eat meals that are homemade	❑	❑	❑	❑	❑	❑

Subtotal:+ _____

	Never	Rarely	Some-times	Usually	Almost always	Always
	0	–1	–2	–3	–4	–5
3. I eat food that is:						
fast (such as McDonald's)	❑	❑	❑	❑	❑	❑
processed (canned, packaged)	❑	❑	❑	❑	❑	❑
prepared (deli, take-out)	❑	❑	❑	❑	❑	❑
sweet (donuts, muffins)	❑	❑	❑	❑	❑	❑
fried (potato chips, chicken)	❑	❑	❑	❑	❑	❑

Subtotal: _____

Total Fast Foodism Score: (+) or (–) _____

FAST FOODISM SCORING KEY

35 to 23: Excellent   10 to –1: Satisfactory
22 to 11: Good   –2 or less: Needs improvement

Food Fretting

Rx: Perceive food and the experience of eating as a social, ceremonial, sensual pleasure.

Although dieting, a judgmental attitude, and anxiety about food may seem as if they don't have much in common, they share the distinguishing characteristics of a food fretter: apprehension about what food to eat; feeling gluttonous when eating foods you think you shouldn't; guilt when you go off your diet; and comparing yourself with others and then judging the differences. The key characteristic, though, is obsessing about food.

If you're a food fretter, you may also experience an alternating sense of righteousness or self-disdain—depending on how you're doing on your diet on a particular day. You tend to regard food with anxiety, and to judge what and how you eat as "good" or "bad" behaviors. You may even feel inadequate or envious when you see a thin person. The end result: you fill much of your day-to-day thinking and ruminating about food, "eating right," being thin—and often overeating.

De-Food Fretting Strategies

There's a lot more you can do to de-food fret and overcome your food-related anxieties, obsessing, self-recrimination, judgment, and guilt. Here is a close look at what it takes to transcend food fretting and its cycle of dieting, anxiety, and obsessing about food and weight.

Don't diet. More and more research is linking traditional dieting with increased risk of weight gain. Consider *dieting* in the best sense of the word. The word incomes from the Old French *diete* or Greek *diaeta*, which means "mode of life." Hippocrates, the father of modern medicine, used *diet* as a "prescribed mode of life," which eventually evolved into meaning "prescribed regime of food." We're suggesting that you *diet* as an expression of the ancient meaning of the word, as a way of life: you relate to eating as a social, ceremonial, and sensual delight, and to food as a gift that enhances your physical, emotional, spiritual, and social well-being.

Stop counting calories. Traditional diets that ask you to restrict calories and to eat-by-number (count calories, figure fat grams, etc.) to lose weight are no longer appropriate. To lose weight, you don't need more numbers; you need other ways of relating to food so that each time you eat you have an enjoyable experience that nourishes your entire being. Instead of staying lost in a maze of measurements, nutrients, and numbers, focus on fresh foods, their flavors, the profound pleasure of eating, and the delight you take in dining with others.

Halt judgment. In 1987, my father died abruptly of a heart attack; my mother also died of heart disease—congestive heart failure. Having worked as the nutrition educator with pioneering physician Dean Ornish on his first clinical trial for reversing heart disease and later as the director of nutrition in Europe on a similar research project, I knew a lot about nutrition, lifestyle, and health. Yet I still could not seem to find the "right" or "best" way to help my parents. I knew my parents understood the heart-healthy dietary information I'd given them, but in retrospect, I realize that the underlying message I was giving was, "You *should* be eating differently. You *should* stop eating familiar and comfortable foods. You *should* assess and analyze what you're eating." Should. It simply doesn't work—for you or others. How did I and so many of us learn to judge both ourselves and others' food choices and eating habits? I discovered that in the

Continued ➡

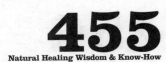

Solo Dining Personal Profile

For each question, check the box in the column that best represents your solo dining dynamic.

	Never	Rarely	Some-times	Usually	Almost always	Always
	0	+1	+2	+3	+4	+5
1. I eat with:						
friends	❏	❏	❏	❏	❏	❏
family members	❏	❏	❏	❏	❏	❏
2. I eat at home at the dining table	❏	❏	❏	❏	❏	❏
3. I enjoy preparing meals for friends.	❏	❏	❏	❏	❏	❏
4. I enjoy holiday feasts with others.	❏	❏	❏	❏	❏	❏
5. I celebrate special occaisions with others with festive foods.	❏	❏	❏	❏	❏	❏
6. I prepare and share special meals for friends and family.	❏	❏	❏	❏	❏	❏
7. When eating alone, I often think about special people in my life, or memorable meals I've enjoyed with others.	❏	❏	❏	❏	❏	❏
					Subtotal: +_____	

	Never	Rarely	Some-times	Usually	Almost always	Always
	0	−1	−2	−3	−4	−5
8. I eat alone.	❏	❏	❏	❏	❏	❏
9. I plan secret overeating.	❏	❏	❏	❏	❏	❏
10. I dine with others, then afterward binge by myself.	❏	❏	❏	❏	❏	❏
11. I stand at the counter while eating.	❏	❏	❏	❏	❏	❏
					Subtotal: −_____	
				Total Solo Dining Score: (+) or (−) _____		

SOLO DINING SCORING KEY
40 to 28: Excellent   15 to 4: Satisfactory
27 to 16: Good   3 or less: Needs improvement

Unappetizing Atmosphere Personal Profile

For each question, check the box in the column that best represents your unappetizing atmosphere dynamic.

	Never	Rarely	Some-times	Usually	Almost always	Always
	0	+1	+2	+3	+4	+5
1. The atmosphere in which I prepare food is:						
serene	❏	❏	❏	❏	❏	❏
pleasing	❏	❏	❏	❏	❏	❏
fun	❏	❏	❏	❏	❏	❏
2. After eating, I feel:						
relaxed	❏	❏	❏	❏	❏	❏
calm	❏	❏	❏	❏	❏	❏
alert	❏	❏	❏	❏	❏	❏
					Subtotal: +_____	

late 1800s, Puritan values still predominated in America, which meant that food was often perceived as sinful, or as good and bad; in other words, we projected moral values onto food—and still do. Instead, view food, eating, and the experience of dining as a celebration of life.

Give up guilt-tripping. Guilt and its relatives—self-reproach, shame, remorse, and blame—are part of a food fretter's relationship to food. It's all about what is "right" and what is "wrong." Eat something "wrong" that isn't on your diet, that you "shouldn't," that tastes "sinful," and, if you're a food fretter, you're likely to respond with guilt. The dictionary tells us that to feel guilty is to feel remorse about having done something wrong. That wrongdoing is linked with guilt has roots in the word's original meaning, derived from Old English, when it meant "crime."[1] Is eating food you "shouldn't" eat a crime? Or, as with the food fretter feeling of judgment, when you feel guilt over something you ate (or want to eat), are you projecting a moral value onto the food, and in the process making yourself miserable? Consider this: guilt isn't a real feeling. At its core lies the belief you've done something wrong, and now you must suffer for it. To break that conviction and get the upper hand over guilt, change what you choose to believe. Replace guilt-laden thoughts with a positive picture. Realize that you can't undo what was done, and . . . simply accept it. Finally, forgive yourself, for forgiveness is a necessity in any relationship—including the one you have with food.

Cease obsessing. If you're fixated on, and preoccupied with, food-related thoughts, feelings, and behaviors, if you think or worry about food or weight constantly and compulsively, you are obsessing. The way out is to step from the shade you're living in, into the sunshine. Meditation can help you do this.

Meditation and Meals

During a conversation in a cafe with a new acquaintance, I first realized the power of meditation as a path that leads to letting go of food fretting and replacing it with naturally occurring weight loss. Midway through our get-together, she told me she had lost twenty pounds as a side effect of meditating regularly. Accessing the wisdom within yourself through regular meditation is one path you can take to de-food fret and to create a more balanced relationship to food, eating, and your weight.

Meditation, and its myriad variations, has been a spiritual discipline espoused by world religions, philosophies, and traditions for thousands of years. In the East, yogis say it leads to a superconscious state that emerges from the cessation of thought; Taoists tell us it leads to a sense of harmony with all things and moments and a return to the depths of the self; while proponents of Zen perceive meditation as a path to sudden illumination. In the West, it is often linked with the mystical and monastic. The Kabbalah, Judaism's mystical teaching, turns to it to carry consciousness through various "gateways"; early Christian monks and saints used it as a stringent contemplative process to achieve spiritual exaltation; and Islam's spiritual Sufis interpret it as a way to suffuse their mind, heart, and soul with "higher things."

The ancient tradition of meditation comes from the Latin *meditari*, meaning "deep, continued reflection." Over the millennia, many types have evolved. For instance, *apophatic* meditation is designed to empty the mind by eliminating thoughts from consciousness, while the *cataphatic* focus is holding a specific image, idea, or word in the mind's eye, allowing emotions to manifest.

Continued ➔

	Never	Rarely	Some-times	Usually	Almost always	Always
	0	–1	–2	–3	–4	–5
3. The atmosphere in which I prepare food is:						
hectic	☐	☐	☐	☐	☐	☐
tense	☐	☐	☐	☐	☐	☐
Subtotal: – _____						
Total Unappetizing Atmosphere Score: (+) or (–) _____						

UNAPPETIZING ATMOSPHERE SCORING KEY

30 to 22: Excellent
21 to 14: Good

13 to 6: Satisfactory
5 or less: Needs improvement

Sensory Disregard Personal Profile

For each question, check the box in the column that best represents your sensory disregard dynamic.

	Never	Rarely	Some-times	Usually	Almost always	Always
	0	+1	+2	+3	+4	+5
1. I plan and prepare meals:						
with care	☐	☐	☐	☐	☐	☐
with appreciation	☐	☐	☐	☐	☐	☐
2. While dining, I consider my surroundings.	☐	☐	☐	☐	☐	☐
3. I express gratitude for food through prayer, blessings, heartfelt thankfulness	☐	☐	☐	☐	☐	☐
4. I honor the mystery of life in food	☐	☐	☐	☐	☐	☐
5. befor and during eating, I focus on the food's:						
color	☐	☐	☐	☐	☐	☐
aroma	☐	☐	☐	☐	☐	☐
portion size	☐	☐	☐	☐	☐	☐
flavors	☐	☐	☐	☐	☐	☐
6. I "eat" with my senses, by:						
appreciating the presentation	☐	☐	☐	☐	☐	☐
tasting textures	☐	☐	☐	☐	☐	☐
savoring scents	☐	☐	☐	☐	☐	☐
7. I focus solely on food and the experience of dining.	☐	☐	☐	☐	☐	☐
8. I appreciate the web of humanity (farmers, grocers) surrounding food.	☐	☐	☐	☐	☐	☐
9. I consider the elements of nature that create food.	☐	☐	☐	☐	☐	☐
10. I eat with loving regard for food.	☐	☐	☐	☐	☐	☐
11. After eating, I:						
savor the moment	☐	☐	☐	☐	☐	☐
reflect on the meal	☐	☐	☐	☐	☐	☐
Total Sensory Disregard Score: _____						

SENSORY DISREGARD SCORING KEY

77 to 90: Excellent
53 to 36: Good

54 to 71: Satisfactory
35 or less: Needs improvement

Your Eating Style Score

To find your Total Whole Person Nutrition Eating Style Score:

1. Enter the **positive** scores from each of the seven eating styles in the "Positive Subtotals" column.

2. Enter the **negative** scores from each of the seven eating styles in the "Negative Subtotals" column.

3. For your "Total Whole Person Nutrition Eating Style Score," subtract the total positive subtotals.

Eating Style	Positive Subtotals	Negative Subtotals
Food Fretting	_____	_____
Task Snacking	_____	_____
Emotional Eating	_____	_____
Fast Foodism	_____	_____
Solo Dining	_____	_____
Unappetizing Atmosphere	_____	_____
Sensory Disregard	_____	_____
Positive Total _____		Negative Total _____

Total Whole Person Nutrition Style _____

During the past decades, many scientific studies have verified the ways in which meditation can heal body, mind, and soul. Vipassana meditation, an ancient practice from India that was rediscovered by Gotama Buddha more than 2,500 years ago, is an especially powerful technique for food fretters. With its focus on self-transformation through self-observation, it is designed to dissolve chaotic, drifting thoughts that sabotage well-being, and instead to bring balance and peace of mind. Using the same concept of transformation through self-observation, we created a self-guided technique that we call the "food-friendly meditation." We designed it as a meditation for food fretters who are often obsessive about food and eating, and whose thoughts are filled with anxiety and judgment about food, eating, and weight. It can be a powerful tool, for meditation can change both conscious and unconscious food-related behaviors.

The Food-Friendly Meditation

Before beginning our step-by-step food-friendly meditation, look over the "What's Your Eating Style?" questionnaire, and identify the elements of food fretting with which you have the most trouble. Then, with each inhalation, imagine how each element makes you feel; with each exhalation, imagine a non-food fretting scenario. For instance:

Example: As you inhale, imagine how you feel when you are "on a diet"; exhaling, envision yourself eating tasty fresh food in a relaxed frame of mind.

Example: As you inhale, recall the guilt you feel after eating food you "shouldn't"; exhaling, delight in the flavor of a favorite food, without judgment.

Example: As you inhale, conjure up an obese person you see eating in a restaurant; exhaling, feel compassion for the person.

To obtain the full benefit, practice the following meditation fifteen to thirty minutes each day. When your mind wanders, gently bring your attention back to the imagery.

Continued ➡

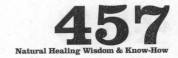

1. Set aside some time when you will not be disturbed.

2. Choose a comfortable place to sit.

3. Sit in a comfortable upright position, with relaxed shoulders.

4. Close your eyes.

5. Position your head so it is comfortably balanced between your shoulders.

6. Inhale deeply, pause for two seconds, then exhale deeply. Do this three times.

7. As you inhale, say to yourself, "I know that I am breathing in."

8. As you exhale, say to yourself, "I know that I am breathing out."

9. Identify an element of food fretting that is problematic for you, such as dieting, guilt, or judgment.

10. Inhale the problematic situation; exhale the solution.

The food-friendly meditation gives you the skills you need to let food fretting thoughts emerge, to simply observe the thoughts and behaviors, and then to let them go. The key concept: substitute the food fretting thoughts you release with opposite, positive emotions, such as acceptance, joy, pleasure, or compassion.

As you practice this meditation, keep in mind that staying focused, mindful, and in-the-moment is challenging; after all, it's easy and normal for our thoughts to wander. Because of this tendency, realize that meditation is a lifetime process. When and if you find your mind wandering, bring your thoughts back to the meditation. Your intention is to stay with the meditation as long as possible and not to perceive it as something you have to do "perfectly."

Overcoming Food Fretting

To eat—and live—optimally, consider that food is more than an amalgam of nutrients and calories that lead to weight loss—or gain. Along with healing you physically, it can improve your mood, satisfy your soul, and connect you to others and to the mystery of life. To turn food fretting—think, filled with dieting, calorie-counting, and anxious overeating, into Enlightened Diet nourishment, decide to enjoy food and the experience of eating as a social, ceremonial, sensual pleasure.

Task Snacking

Rx: Bring moment-to-moment nonjudgmental awareness to each aspect of the meal.

Some call it "multitasking"; the French call it "vagabond eating"; in America, it's a growing trend. Whatever its form, eating a meal or snacking mindlessly while working in front of your computer, driving, watching TV, shopping with a friend, or talking on the phone, the task snacking eating style puts you at risk for overeating and becoming overweight or obese. Have you ever meandered through the mall while munching? If so, you're task snacking. Do you watch TV, flip through a magazine, or study while eating? These are more task-snacking behaviors. As a matter of fact, doing other things while you're eating has become so common in our culture, it's become normal.

Consider "car cuisine," the growing tendency for drivers to eat in their cars at drive-in restaurants or while driving. As Americans continue to eat more and more meals in their cars, food makers have accommodated the trend with what they call "cup-holder cuisine": finger-friendly foods and compact "meals" that are drop-free and glop-free. Examples include cereal bars made with dry milk; salad-in-a-cup and pancakelike breakfast sandwiches with the "yummy taste of maple syrup baked right in," available at McDonald's; squeeze tubes that contain yogurt; and drinkable soups that can be sipped from a cup. Some experts say that almost 20 percent of us consume such "meals" in cars. The trend of "dashboard dining" is so entrenched in our culture that Honda provides a pop-up table in the console, and Saab sells models with refrigerated glove boxes.[1]

However, not only do most of us not pay much attention to where we're eating, and what we're doing while we're eating, but we also don't even believe that these two factors have anything to do with our weight. But they do. We link task snacking to weight gain because our eating styles research revealed that those who were overweight task snacked more often than those who did it less often or not at all.

Anatomy of Task Snacking

Sure, it's obvious that if you're a task-snacking couch potato or mouse potato, it's likely you're not moving much. And this means that, like our friend who put on twenty pounds by being stationary for months while working on his book at his computer, lack of exercise is a key contributor to weight gain. But how might task snacking, specifically, work against your waistline when you eat while working, or you munch while watching TV, or you snack while driving? In other words, how may eating in a not-too-conscious, not-too-mindful way be a recipe for weight gain? Understanding what happens when you eat while task snacking provides a clue.

Because the brain can attend to only one topic at a time, when you do multiple tasks simultaneously, the mind constantly shifts its attention. If you were to undergo a PET (positron emission tomography) scan—a powerful, noninvasive imaging technique that accurately images the cellular function of the human body—while task snacking, it would show lights blinking on and off in selected areas of the brain associated with the various tasks you're doing. To cope with your task snacking, when you eat while the mind is not focused on your food, the mind disengages from the body. In response, the digestive process is impaired, making food not nearly as nutritious as it could be. In turn, this malfunction can trigger hunger and malnutrition and the drive to eat more so you will feel satisfied via the nutrients both your mind and your body need for optimal health—nutrients that you're not metabolizing. In this way, task snacking can create a vicious cycle of poor digestion, inadequate nutrition, and overeating to compensate, to try to get the vitamins and minerals you're not metabolizing.

Task snacking works on yet another level: when the mind is not paying full attention to the sensation of food, such as its taste, scent, texture, and presentation (more about eating to satisfy the senses in "Sensory Disregard"), then eating, itself, becomes less satisfying. And a key way to compensate for getting less pleasure or gratification from food is to continue to eat. . . more and more. The bottom line? Mindless task snacking is likely to lead to eating more and enjoying it less.

In contrast, there is evidence that paying attention to food while you eat affects how your body metabolizes the food in a positive, beneficial way. Because your mind is focused solely on eating, more digestive juices, starting with your saliva, are recruited. And because eating mindfully slows down the speed with which you eat, you're also optimizing the digestive juices in your stomach; indeed, the entire digestive process is enhanced.

Can the awareness with which you eat really make a difference to your health and well-being, to the way in which you metabolize your food? Or, vice versa, does eating while task snacking actually impair your ability to absorb food?

Metabolism of Mindfulness

To find out whether eating mindfully is really beneficial to digestion, researcher Donald Morse, a physician and professor emeritus at Temple University in Philadelphia, designed a unique study to assess whether eating mindfully versus eating while distracted or stressed (task snacking) made a difference to metabolism. He designed his experiment this way: a group of female college students would meditate for five minutes before eating cereal (a food high in carbohydrates), while another group would distract themselves with mental arithmetic before eating the cereal (a form of task snacking). Afterward, when Dr. Morse and his team measured the saliva (where metabolism of food begins) of the "mindful meditators" and then compared it to that of the task snackers, he discovered, amazingly, that those who meditated mindfully before eating produced 22 percent more of the digestive enzyme alpha-amylase.

There are two interesting implications of this study. First, because alpha-amylase helps you digest and metabolize carbohydrates in carbohydrate-dense foods (such as potatoes, bread, and of course cereal), as well as B vitamins (of which there are eight), if you eat while task snacking you're likely to absorb fewer nutrients than you need for your mind-body to function optimally. It also "shows that there's a real benefit to having a leisurely meal," speculates Morse. "The decrease in alpha-amylase production is just the tip of the iceberg. When you gulp down your food, your entire digestive system is affected." And not only does task snacking have long-term implications for your digestion, but Morse's findings also imply that if you make subtle but significant changes in the awareness you bring to food and eating (meaning, when you eat, eat; when you work, work; do one thing at a time) so that you're eating mindfully, you're more likely to stop overeating and gaining weight.[2]

Meet "Tea Mind"

Molecular biologist Jon Kabat-Zinn created a mindfulness meditation model and program that, today, is used worldwide in institutions ranging from Kabat-Zinn's Stress Reduction Clinic at the University of Massachusetts Medical Center to hundreds of hospitals and clinics, corporations, sports teams, and prisons. A meditator himself since 1966, Kabat-Zinn created his technique to give people an experiential, hands-on sense of what it means to meditate mindfully. And patients, who have been referred to his clinic for ailments ranging from stress to heart disease, reap the rewards with a unique Buddhist-based meditation structured by Kabat-Zinn around the ordinary experience of eating; he calls it the "raisin meditation."

As Kabat-Zinn guides participants through his raisin meditation, they focus on all aspects of the experience of eating one simple raisin: how it looks, smells, and feels; what happens in the mouth before, during, and after eating it; the motion and movement involved; the raisin's taste and texture; swallowing; and the role of breathing throughout the experience. From start to finish, it takes ten minutes to eat the sole raisin. And then the group is ready to begin the mindfulness raisin meditation process again with the second raisin everyone is holding.[3]

Continued ➡

I'll guide you through this meditation (see "Raisin Consciousness"), but for now the key concept for you to get is the "consciousness" behind it: eating with moment-to-moment, nonjudgmental attention to each element of the entire experience. What does it mean to have such focused attention on food? Is it simply paying attention to the ordinary experience of eating? Or is it something more extraordinary? Or is it mundane? Ancient food wisdom that has served humankind for millennia offers some clues about what it means to be aware of being aware.

Raisin Consciousness

From yoga to Hinduism to Buddhism, hundreds of types of meditation from the East have evolved over the millennia. Over the past few decades, more and more of these techniques have been integrated into mind-body medicine, a growing field of Western medical care. The practice and cultivation of mindful awareness is rooted in one of Buddhism's earliest sutras, ancient Buddhist teachings. Called the Mindfulness Sutra, it describes how to cultivate judgment-free, impartial awareness of what you are doing during each moment. The raisin meditation that Jon Kabat-Zinn imparts to his patients is based on ancient Buddhist wisdom he learned from Jack Kornfield, one of the key Buddhist teachers in the West. Here is a version that you can experience for yourself. To get the most benefit from it, first read through it, then do it.

1. Sit in a comfortable chair and set a small bowl filled with raisins next to you on a table.
2. Select one raisin from the bowl.
3. Look at the raisin as if it were an alien object you had never seen before.
4. As you look at the raisin, imagine it in its original form as a grape, growing in the sunshine surrounded by air, earth, and water.
5. Continuing to look at the raisin, describe what you see: its texture, color, and shape, and anything else that comes to mind.
6. Bring the raisin up to your nose. Smell it. Describe its scent.
7. As you smell the raisin, are you experiencing any changes in your mouth, in your saliva, as you anticipate eating the raisin?
8. How does the raisin feel? Describe it.
9. Become aware of your body and the hand that is holding the raisin. Consider how your hand knows how to hold the raisin, how to bring it up toward your nose.
10. Bring the raisin toward your lips, then place it in your mouth. What motion is your tongue doing? Your jaw? Your teeth? Your cheek?
11. Now, put all your attention into your mouth. As you do, bite into the raisin ... slowly ... and begin to chew ... slowly. Stop chewing after three chews. On which side of your mouth are you chewing? What motion are your tongue, jaw, teeth, and cheek doing now?
12. Describe the taste you're experiencing.
13. Now, continue to chew, but do not swallow the raisin. Do you notice a difference in the taste? What is the texture like?
14. Are you tempted to swallow yet? Observe what is happening in your mouth as you prepare to swallow. Now, swallow the raisin. Then imagine it in your stomach, and acknowledge that your body is one raisin heavier.
15. Can you "taste" your breath now? Focus your attention on your breath, as you inhale and exhale ... slowly.

16. Remain focused on your breath as you continue to inhale and exhale. Now, simply become silent.

If your mind wanders, once you notice this is happening, bring your attention back to your breath. For the next five, ten, or fifteen minutes, or longer, continue to focus on your breathing.

Congratulations! You have just experienced mindfulness meditation. To reap the rewards, meditating twenty to thirty minutes each day is optimal. If setting aside some special time to meditate is challenging for you, consider turning each meal or snack into an opportunity to eat mindfully. Later in this book, in "Elemental Overview", I'll guide you through a step-by-step seven-eating-styles meditation that will give you the skills you need to put the Enlightened Diet into action each time you eat. But for now, take a cue from time-tested ancient food wisdom: pay attention to every food-related act, every sensation and perception, for its own sake, to stay in the moment. From planning and preparing a meal, to serving, eating, and cleanup, regardless of which stage or stages of the meal on which you choose to focus, take your actions off autopilot and, instead, commit to being fully aware of what your hands, mouth, and mind are experiencing moment to moment. For in the witnessing lies the antidote to task snacking.

Other Simple Strategies

Cultivating mindfulness—paying attention intentionally—empowers you to slow down long enough to experience the subtleties of food. This awareness is beneficial because when you focus on your food, you're not task snacking; you're simply tasting your food and savoring the experience of eating. In "Sensory Disregard," I'll tell you more about the power of the time-tested nutrition philosophy of the "six tastes" espoused by Eastern healing systems, such as India's Ayurveda medicine, traditional Chinese medicine (TCM), and Tibetan medicine. Right now, though, you can reap the rewards by focusing on the flavors in food each time you eat.

Savor flavor. The next time you eat a mixed meal, such as a salad or stew made with varied ingredients, bring your attention to your mouth; then, as you chew your food, try to identify the flavors in your food. For instance, is it mostly sweet, or is salt the major flavor? Did you experience a burst of flavor at the first bite? Are you still enjoying the taste of the food after the second and third bites?

Take tea time. Another way to approach your journey of mindfulness is to perceive tea as an opportunity to balance the five elements of metal (minerals in the soil that help create tea leaves); wood (the tea plant); water (that brews and brings tea back to life); fire (the sun that heats the water); and earth (the mother of tea and material for tea pots). Followers of Japan's Way of Tea (often called the Japanese Tea Ceremony) believe that when the elements are balanced and in harmony, they create a form of perfection. The next time you take time to savor some tea, can you see and taste each element with each sip? Consider bringing a similar tea consciousness to all beverages you consume during the day, such as water, juice, coffee, or milk.

Move into mindfulness. There are three distinct steps to take to move into mindfulness and replace task snacking with conscious, intentional awareness: (1) Intentionality: don't just think about doing it; make a decisive choice to focus on the food before you when you're eating; (2) Commitment: act on your intention, and carry it out, by gently letting go of feelings, thoughts, and activities that may be interfering with your intention and commitment to

mindfulness; and (3) Focus: with intention and commitment to mindfulness, keep your attention on the food or food-related activities.

Overcoming Task Snacking

Taking the time to enjoy food, to truly taste and savor it, is the key to overcoming task snacking and reducing the odds of weight gain. Replace eating while doing other things, such as walking, working, or watching television, with moment-to-moment nonjudgmental awareness of each aspect of your meal, and you're on the path of the Enlightened Diet.

Emotional Eating

Rx: Eat only for pleasure and when you're feeling feel-good feelings.

Feeding Negative Feelings with Food

For Ann, nighttime binge eating starts after work with a trip to the supermarket to buy bags of corn chips and chunks of her favorite chocolate. Then she heads home, changes into comfortable clothes, and turns on the TV Settling into bed surrounded by her favorite foods, she begins what she describes as "zoning out"—eating until she feels calmer—often to the point of falling in and out of sleep well before bedtime.

Although this is a typical evening for Ann, three hours after starting her binge, she is amazed to find that she has finished all the food. On a not-quite-conscious level, she senses the chips and chocolate allay her anxiety in some way. She's also concerned about these binges because she wants to lose fifty pounds and stop zoning out, but she hasn't figured out how to accomplish this. Dieting hasn't helped, nor has willpower or the techniques she's read about in self-help books. In the meantime, Ann remains vaguely depressed and distressed, and dependent on food binges to manage her darker moods

From hard-core drugs to food, theories have abounded for decades about the causes of all kinds of chemical and behavioral addictions. Cassandra Vieten, Ph.D., is a clinical psychologist and researcher who specializes in mind-body medicine and behavioral disorders at California Pacific Medical Center Research Institute in San Francisco and at the Institute of Noetic Sciences in nearby Petaluma. She believes "negative affect" may be the unifying factor in overeating, disordered eating, or a growing dependency on an addiction to food influenced by genetics, environment, brain chemistry, and family dynamics. "Negative affect is distress that can be conscious or unconscious, physiological, emotional, psychological, and/or spiritual," Vieten told me. "Distress is part of life, but some experience greater amounts of it, or are more highly sensitive to it due to their hardwiring or upbringing. Others experience stress as intolerable because they haven't developed the capacity to endure negative feelings." Indeed, our research on the Enlightened Diet, which revealed the seven eating styles that form it, showed that negative emotions—especially depression, boredom, and frustration—are the feelings that drive impulse eating and cravings; indeed, they are the strongest predictor of overeating and ensuing overweight and obesity.

Bad, worrisome, anxious, unpleasant feelings are clearly a key aspect of negative affect for many, but for others—such as Ann, who fixates on food for less conscious reasons—suppressed, unexpressed, or unidentified feelings can also be part of the negative affect picture that may manifest in

Continued ➡

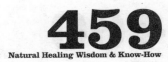

emotional eating. "Some people can't or won't express themselves even when they know they are experiencing fear or anger. Still others often feel nondescript distress, but they can't say why, nor can they put a name on it," said Vieten.

When a person experiences undifferentiated negative affect, it may convey itself through bodily sensations, such as a tight stomach or muscular tension. If ongoing or extreme, these physical feelings can translate into a sense that you're not going to survive the emotions. Unfortunately, many treat (self-medicate) these sensations by overeating certain foods that actually alter their mental state. Because overeating can halt the distress—for the moment—it can become a powerful reinforcer. But there's a caveat: it's possible to build up a tolerance, and to need more and more food to feel good again. When this happens, you're not really eating to feel better; you may be bingeing just to feel normal. The good news is there are also ways to build your tolerance to distress—ways to relate to it, contain it, and cope with it, so that you are less and less driven to engage in self-medicating behaviors.[1]

Of Food and Mood

Although the term "emotional eating" wasn't in the culture in 1960 when Overeaters Anonymous (OA) was founded, "HALT" was already in use by Alcoholics Anonymous and was borrowed by OA. An organization that offers a twelve-step recovery program for compulsive overeating and other eating disorders, OA warned its members early on against becoming too Hungry, too Angry, too Lonely, or too Tired because when you're feeling HALT emotions and you're an overeater, such emotions may trigger a binge. Feeling HALT emotions means you are more likely to seek *false* relief by abusing yourself with food: become too hungry, and too many cookies may override healthful food choices; chomping on chips may suppress anger; ice cream may soothe loneliness; or you may befriend french fries when you feel tired. Whatever the emotional upset, in place of giving (gifting?) yourself what you really need, you choose food and compulsive overeating as your solution.

OA was way ahead of its time—and science—when it linked HALT emotions with the tendency for overeaters to turn to food for comfort. Today, health professionals often use the term "self-medicate" to describe the drive behind eating to cope and to feel better when unpleasant emotions such as depression and anxiety emerge.

Transformation Strategies

Right now, you're at a turning point. You can decide to take care of your physical and symbolic hunger needs for food in an appropriate way. Or you can continue to turn to food to do the job. By choosing the path of transformation, though, you're deciding to feed your body, mind, and soul what they really need; in other words, you're giving yourself true nourishment. The following exercises may not resolve all your eating problems overnight, but they can be a helpful step toward resolving your emotional eating issue if you practice them each time the urge to splurge surfaces. The secret? Barbara Birsinger's "decoding process" shows you how to shed light on unmet intrinsic needs you may have that are rooted in disordered eating. And then, symbolically, she'll show you how to transform your craving by filling your needs with something other than food.

Birsinger has a clear and strong conviction that there's a reason and a purpose for overeating. You're trying to take care of yourself on some level, to fill a need that's not getting cared for in another

way. Food is available. It can do the job well, but it's only temporary—and there are side effects and consequences. If no effective self-care mechanisms are in place, your emotional eating isn't going to go away. The antidote? Develop the capacity to tolerate a range of unpleasant emotions. Birsinger offers the following two strategies for dealing with emotional eating: one for physical hunger; one for symbolic hunger.

Is Your Hunger Physical or Symbolic?

Overcoming overeating starts with discerning physical hunger from symbolic hunger. When you think of eating, is your desire to eat coming from physical hunger (located in your stomach) or symbolic hunger (eating for reasons other than for physical nourishment)? Check in now. Physical hunger is often experienced in the stomach, while symbolic hunger often manifests in the chest, throat, or mouth. In other words, *where* you're feeling the feeling is a clue about whether the hunger is physical or symbolic.

Physical hunger. *How hungry are you?* Imagine the following scenario: You're at your desk and you begin to think about eating. Ask yourself whether you're physically hungry in your body, or whether you have symbolic hunger. You realize you're actually hungry. Sitting at your desk and thinking of food is your cue to check in with your hunger level. On a scale of 1 to 10, identify your hunger level (1 is famished, 5 is neutral, at 10, you are way overfed). You identify that you're at level 3, which means you're identifying that you're physically hungry and you need to eat.

Decide what to eat and how much. Now, decide what you want to eat. How much of it do you want? To know what your mind-body wants to eat, develop a mind-body connection. You can do this by checking in with your body before eating. To begin, ask your body what it wants. Doing this, Birsinger claims, means eating from the neck *down*, instead of the neck *up* (all in your mind)—which is where most people make decisions about what to eat.

Do the guided imagery visualization. Birsinger developed the guided imagery visualization exercise on the next page to give you the skills you need to make the mind-body connection, which in turn can empower you to dramatically change what and how you eat forever. Practice it every time before you eat.

Symbolic hunger. Imagine the following scenario: You're at your desk and you begin to think about eating. Ask yourself whether you're physically hungry in your body, or whether you have symbolic hunger. Okay, you're feeling anxious, you realize. No. You're not hungry. Your hunger is symbolic, not literal and physical. You really want chocolate chip cookies to help you cope with uncomfortable emotions. Even though you're not hungry, you're still wanting to eat. What's going on? You can't wait until you're hungry. If you can wait, great. Many can't wait, though, because emotional eating is an ingrained habit. If so …

Birsinger suggests that you go to step 2 of the Guided Imagery Visualization Exercise. If you can have anything you want, what would it be? The intensity of the emotion will determine whether you can wait or not. If nothing else will help, you may need to eat that cookie. Keep in mind, though, that by doing this process before you eat, you're becoming conscious of your needs and eating behaviors—without judgment. And such nonjudgmental awareness is a key step that can diminish overeating.

Guided Imagery Visualization Exercise

1. Inhale deeply, pause for two seconds, and exhale deeply, bringing your awareness from your head to your body. Notice air moving through your lungs. Notice the movement of your stomach expanding and contracting.

2. Imagine that you could have anything on the planet to eat right now—without any judgment about the food's calorie, protein, or carbohydrate content. What would that be? No one needs to know. It's a private fantasy.

3. Now think of the amount you would love to have of this food. Again, don't bring judgment to your decision. How much would you really like to have? Imagine you can see the food and the amount you just visualized. It's just there in front of you. Is it in a serving dish? On a plate?

4. Now, you've eaten the food. Imagine this food is now in your stomach. How does it feel? Does the amount feel just right? Too much? Is it pushing on your stomach? Is it making you feel bloated? Does your stomach hurt?

5. Ask your body how much would be okay to eat so you feel comfortably full, alert, and energized.

6. Now imagine this food is moving down into your digestive system. Ask your body how the food feels in your digestive tract. Is there any discomfort in that part of your body as the food is being digested, such as pain, bloating, or gas?

7. Ask your body how much of this food would be okay to eat for you to feel good. Then, modify the amount you ate to fit the "feel good" amount, meaning, any symptoms of discomfort are gone.

8. Now imagine the food has been digested. The nutrients are being absorbed into your bloodstream, and they're circulating through the brain, through the muscles, the organs, the skin; all your cell tissues are now being nourished.

9. After envisioning the optimal amount of food you can eat and still feel comfortable, scan your body to see whether there are any changes in sensations or feelings.

Give Yourself Permission to Eat

Whether your hunger is physical or symbolic, if you really want to eat a cookie, that's what you ought to do: eat the cookie without judging yourself. A key reason people overeat is that they impose restrictions on themselves about what they should or shouldn't eat and then they don't eat what they really want. When you do this, though, you continue to "chase" whatever you were trying to get from the cookie.

Birsinger believes you won't overeat if you practice the above mind-body visualization "because we're born with this ability to 'know' what and how much to eat," she says, and the guided imagery technique, above, is a way to reconnect to this. In a way, it's like programming a computer: once you have the amount that feels good in your body, it doesn't matter how food is put in front of you. For instance, let's say you want a banana split, with whipped cream and hot fudge. But when you do this exercise, you realize the entire banana split is way too much for you to eat if you're to continue to feel comfortable in your body. When this happens, before eating, decide on the amount that'll feel good in your body, which may be only a couple of bites. Or not.

Continued ➜

Birsinger offers this insight: If you don't do the guided imagery visualization (left), you're more likely to sit down and eat the whole banana split; you'll overeat and then feel stuffed. Self-sabotage may take over: "Now I've really blown it. That was way too much," you might think, but this only leads to more eating later because you're likely to eat to berate yourself. And then, to feel better, you're going to have to eat again, and then restrict yourself, and then exercise, and then, on the rebound, overeat again, and so on . . . Birsinger says that "all this happens because you've lost touch with your internal cues of what, when, and how much to eat. But when you make the connection to how much you need to feel okay, your mind-body remembers it. And then you—not food—are in charge of your emotions."

Transform the Craving

Here's another technique Birsinger created to help you transform negative, unpleasant feelings that lead to emotional eating, into pleasant, sense-filled emotions that fill you without food:

- Using all your senses, find ways to evoke the sense you get doing an enjoyable activity (such as yoga or meditation or taking a walk). Have a symbol nearby of something that represents the pleasurable activity, for example, a picture of a beautiful seascape, a heart-shaped paper weight, a lucky coin. Choose anything you like as a symbol that represents the activity.

- What do you love about the particular activity? For instance, if it's a walk on the beach, do you love the sound of the ocean? The air? Putting your feet in the sand?

- Find a fragrance you love. Cinnamon? Vanilla? Musk? To transform the craving, inhale your favorite scent. By doing this, you're symbolically filling up your senses with your favorite activity. Along with scents, you can try this with textures, sounds, and so on.

The key concept: Fill your senses as much as possible with the scent until you can evoke the feeling you get when you're actually doing your favorite activity of choice. Enjoy the journey instead of food.[2]

Fine-Tune Feelings with Food

There's another way you can take charge of emotional eating. Replace unpleasant feelings that drive you to overeat with conscious food choices that hold the power to enhance your mood. The following scenario will give you an idea about how you can fine-tune your feelings to your advantage.[3]

Susan is often overwhelmed with all-day fatigue, minimal motivation, and a sluggish metabolism. Her sister, Allison, feels edgy, irritable, and nervous, symptoms that worsen because of bouts of indigestion that make it hard for her to fall or stay asleep. Their dad, Tom, who has always been a competent accountant, more and more has frequent memory lapses and trouble recalling information. Their mom is dealing with the same old symptoms: constant cravings for carbohydrates, feeling blue and bloated, and depressed about her stubborn weight gain.

Be balanced. Ann, Allison, and their parents are unaware that natural "chemical messengers" (neurotransmitters) released from foods they choose can modify their moods, alleviate anxiety, bolster brain power—even curb the urge to splurge on that donut—so they continue to consume their "routine cuisine." They are not alone in their ignorance of four key neurotransmitters— *dopamine, acetylcholine,*

gamma-aminobutyric acid (GABA), and *serotonin*— that influence everything from energy and mood to memory and metabolism. When these four hormones are in balance, your mind-body is poised for peak performance. But when one or more dip and cause an imbalance, symptoms ranging from fatigue and weight gain to confusion and depression can manifest. The good news: you can choose "designer foods" that reduce unpleasant feelings and unwelcome behaviors.

Enhance energy. Have you ever felt fatigue or lethargy throughout the day, even after a full night's sleep? If low energy is typical for you, the cause could be dopamine deficiency. From fabulous flavors to sensual scents, if your brain interprets a food (or an activity) as pleasurable, and you tend to turn to it for a pleasure hit, it may be because you're seeking the feel-good response of dopamine. In essence, dopamine works its wonders by stimulating the central nervous system (CNS), keeping energy levels, motivation, and excitement high.

Dopamine Rx. The pleasure-producing ingredients in high-protein foods are the amino acids tyrosine and *phenylalanine,* building blocks of both protein and dopamine. To elevate mood and energy, consider consuming water-packed tuna, low-fat yogurt, or lean meat.

Alleviate anxiety. If anxiety, nervousness, and irritability—with bouts of indigestion and trouble sleeping—are all too familiar symptoms, it may mean you have low levels of GABA. A nerve chemical and nerve modulator that stimulates the central nervous system, this natural sedative works its wonders by controlling brainwave rhythms, which in turn regulate behavior.

GABA Rx. Take action to produce more GABA by choosing foods high in the B vitamins, especially B_6. Although the mechanism of how B_6 affects the nervous system and brain isn't completely understood, even marginal intakes influence levels of GABA (and other mood-modifying neurotransmitters). Boost dietary intake of this B vitamin with *whole* grains, dark leafy greens, bananas, avocados, and protein-rich chicken, fish, legumes, and nuts.

Defog. Some older people call it a "senior moment"; others who find it harder and harder to recall information might say they're experiencing a memory lapse. Those who study food and mood may interpret such symptoms of "brain fog" to be a sign of acetylcholine deficiency. Produced in the brain by the fatlike substance *choline,* this nerve chemical is a building block of *myelin,* which helps CNS cells communicate.

Acetylcholine Rx. To manage general mental functioning, boost brain levels of this memory manager by consuming choline-rich foods, such as wheat germ, fish, eggs, blueberries, and peanuts, all of which are converted into acetylcholine during digestion.

Curtail cravings. Do you crave high-carbohydrate, high-salt foods, such as cookies, cake, and chips— especially when you're feeling blue? Do you feel hungry even when you're full? Is weight gain a constant? If so, your supply of serotonin may be low. Soothing serotonin is a natural antidepressant; it also contributes to stable blood sugar levels, which in turn prevents food cravings and the urge to overeat.

Serotonin Rx. To produce more serotonin, seek out foods rich in the amino acid *tryptophan,* such as avocado, poultry, and wheat germ. Other options include foods high in complex carbohydrates, such as potatoes (with the skin), beans, and whole grains.

Instead of feeding that drive to overeat, food can serve as your antiemotional eating ally with its power to bring emotional balance, enhance your energy, alleviate anxiety, and contribute to clearer thinking. Instead of caving into cravings, put yourself in the driver's seat and take your feelings where you want them to go.

"B" Wise

From dreary doldrums to a deeper depression, various B vitamins, including B_1 B_2, niacin, folic acid, and B_{12}, can help you bust the blues. To help defeat depression, "B" wise, and consider the following guidelines when deciding which foods to eat.

Choose whole foods. Fast food "is a loser when it comes to vitamins and minerals that help to boost spirit," writes nutritionist Elizabeth Somer. Indeed, folic acid, in particular (the most common nutritional deficiency in the United states), is linked to depression, as are other B-family relatives that are processed out of refined foods: B_6, niacin, and B_{12}. Some especially good vitamin B—abundant blues busters are unprocessed, unrefined grains (whole wheat, oats, millet, brown rice, etc.), fruits, vegetables, beans, nuts, and seeds. Vitamin B–rich greens, such as spinach, are especially good blues busters.

Shake the sugar habit. When you consume a lot of refined white sugar, it both damages and destroys B vitamins in the body; in this way, it contributes to deficiencies. Eliminate sugar from the diet and depression often lifts—although why this is so is not well understood. One theory is that the high derived from sugar is due to elevated glucose (blood sugar) and endorphins, which produce feelings of relaxation and euphoria. When the sugar in food is metabolized, blood sugar levels and endorphins and other hormones "crash," contributing to depression and fatigue. When a diet is rich in foods loaded with vitamin B, and low in sugar, levels of B vitamins, glucose, and endorphins remain stable, reducing the odds of depression.

Avoid or limit alcohol and caffeine. Consuming too much alcohol and caffeine can cause the loss of certain B vitamins. And deficiencies of vitamins B_6 and niacin, especially, can bring you down. Not only does excessive alcohol and caffeine consumption reduce the absorption of B vitamins, but it also contributes to protein and mineral deficiencies.[4]

Many of us have felt sad or have had the Monday morning blahs at times; still others—more than fifteen million Americans—experience serious depression during their lifetime. Include more foods high in the B vitamins, and you may improve your mood and lower the odds of depression linked to emotional eating.

Overcoming Emotional Eating

The science that studies nutrients in the foods we consume, and the way in which they influence our brain chemistry and emotions, provides a peek into how food and the mind and body work together. By being aware of this connection, each food you choose to eat may be looked at as an opportunity not only to feed your body but also to fine-tune your moods and emotions. At the same time, the key to Enlightened Diet success is making a commitment to eat only for pleasure and when you're feeling feel-good feelings.

Continued ➔

Fast Foodism

Rx: Choose fresh whole food in its natural state as often as possible.

Foodish Food

Some say it's "snack crack"; others imply it's an "industrial artifact"; corporations call it a "commodity"; my friend and colleague, naturopathic physician Bruce Milliman, calls it "ersatz food," meaning "an inferior substitute imitating an original"; the Center for Science in the Public Interest (CSPI) calls it "food porn"; I call it "foodish food.". . .

Foodish food has three attributes: it is typically fast, processed, and unhealthy. Most of you are familiar with fast food, which is inexpensive and prepared and served quickly in fast food restaurants, such as McDonald's, Burger King, Wendy's, Kentucky Fried Chicken, and Taco Bell.[1] Processed food, on the other hand, has been cooked, baked, cured, heated, dried, mixed, ground, separated, extracted, sliced, preserved, dehydrated, frozen; because processed food is often manufactured, it typically includes packaging, canning, jarring, or enclosing the processed food in some other sort of container.[2] Both fast and processed foods have one thing in common: they are junk food, a slang term that refers to fare that is typically high in calories, salt, sugar, fat, and additives, and low in nutritional value, such as fiber, vitamins, and minerals[3]; hence the term "empty calories" to suggest the lack of nutrients . . .

What does the fast foodism eating style look like? A breakfast bar for breakfast; Chicken McNuggets with a Coke for lunch; and perhaps why I believe that fast food isn't food in the classic, traditional sense of the word; rather, it is foodish food, ersatz sort-of-like-food food, but not real food—and why the modifications that make fast food, well, fast food, can contribute to your growing girth.

Eat More, Weigh Less

It really is possible to eat more and weigh less.[4] Doesn't such a suggestion go against everything we've learned about weight loss? Actually, what "eat more, weigh less" really means is that if you eat more of certain *types* of food, instead of focusing on the *amount* of food you eat—like Samuel, a morbidly obese man who lost weight following his doctor's fresh, whole food advice—you, too, are likely to lose weight. Calories from fast food, and calories from fresh, whole, lean food, are not the same. Consider this:

Fruit. An apple a day may do more than keep the doctor away; it may also keep you slim. When researchers from the State University of Rio De Janeiro in Brazil put two groups of women on a *comparable calorie diet*, those who snacked on an apple lost more weight than those who munched on oatmeal cookies. Some possible reasons: With an 85 percent water content and lots of soluble fiber, apples are filling; they also keep blood sugar levels even, which cuts cravings and signals to your brain that you're full. And because apples are fresh and whole, they supply your mind-body with the nutrients you need in the balanced ratio intended by nature.

Vegetables. Studies have linked abundant mixed salads, as well as cauliflower, with weight loss. By "abundant," I'm referring to more than the typical iceberg lettuce and tomato duo that passes for a salad for many of us; rather, I'm talking about a resplendent mix of veggies that may include mixed greens, spinach, and arugula tossed with cherry tomatoes, chopped mushrooms, sliced cucumber, chopped red and green peppers, sliced avocado, beans, lean chicken or baked tofu, a sprinkling of chopped walnuts, grated cheese, and perhaps some raisins. Not only is such a salad filling and delicious, but when researchers at Penn State University studied women who consumed a satisfying salad prior to eating a pasta lunch, they discovered that they ate less pasta than those who ate pasta only.

There are still other weight-loss benefits to fruits and vegetables: vitamin C is found in fruits and vegetables only. A study from Purdue University suggests it may be a key weight loss helper, because vitamin C helps you burn fat during physical activity; in fact, the study suggests vitamin C is a key determinant of weight loss.

Whole grains. Since whole grains were cultivated more than ten thousand years ago, they have been a boon to health. Now, recent research from Harvard, published in the *Journal of Clinical Nutrition*, reveals that they also prevent weight gain. In a twelve-year study with more than twelve thousand nurses from ages thirty-eight to sixty-three, researchers found that those who ate the most whole grain foods (such as oatmeal, popcorn, wheat germ, and multigrain breakfast cereal) weighed less than those who ate the least. And the difference was quite significant: women in the high whole-grain group had a 49 percent lower risk of gaining weight.

Legumes. It's a fact. Including dried beans, such as pintos, navy, and lima (not green beans or soybeans) in your diet can help you lose weight. When Maurice Bennink, professor of nutrition at Michigan State University, reviewed a plethora of studies that had been published on beans over a twenty-five-year period, he discovered a compelling wealth of evidence that beans work their weight loss wonders in three ways: satiety, because beans are rich in fiber, so you feel full; sustained energy, because beans have a very low glycemic index, and thus glucose is released slowly into the bloodstream, so your blood sugar stays stable over time; and lower odds that you'll eat calorie-dense fast foods, because consuming low glycemic index foods tends to lead to subsequent choices of low glycemic index foods.

Nuts and seeds. Although they look like nuts, taste like nuts, and crunch like nuts, technically, peanuts are a legume. Because most of us relate to them as nuts, I am telling you about the potential of *fresh, raw, unroasted* peanuts as part of an eating plan for weight management in the "nuts and seeds" category. Although I wouldn't call any kind of high-fat nut a weight loss food, large population studies have linked their consumption to lower weight than for nonconsumers.

To test these survey results, Richard Mattes and his team in the Department of Foods and Nutrition at Purdue University studied three groups, each of which consumed 500 calories of peanuts: people in group one, who ate the peanuts without any dietary directions, gained an average of only 2.2 pounds; those in the second group, who added the peanuts to their usual diets, gained only one pound; and the people in the third group, who were asked to follow a low-fat diet and to substitute 500 calories of peanuts for 500 calories from other foods, maintained their weight. The mechanism by which peanuts minimize weight gain or help us maintain weight isn't completely clear; what is theorized, though, is that peanuts may work by being super-filling.

Dairy. At least one type of dairy food has been linked with lower weight: low-fat yogurt. When researchers at the University of Tennessee in Knoxville put people on a twelve-week weight-loss program, those who consumed three servings of yogurt daily lost twice as much weight at the dieters who did not eat yogurt. The study's lead researcher, Michael B. Zemel, speculates that the metabolic reason for this is that the calcium *combined with the bioactive compounds in yogurt* speeds up the fat-burning process, while at the same time, decreases the production of fat.

Eggs. It was only a one-day study, which makes it hard to draw conclusions, but there seems to be something slimming about eggs. When researcher Nikhil Dhurandhar from Pennington Biomedical Research Center in Baton Rouge, Louisiana, first gave study participants two eggs for breakfast, and then later in the study, bagels, the two-egg breakfast eaters consumed as much as 400 fewer calories than when they had bagels for breakfast. A possible reason for the difference in calories: it's likely that high-protein, low-fat eggs promote satiety more than processed, white-flour bagels. (Note: Because eggs are high in *dietary* cholesterol, they can raise your blood cholesterol levels. So if you have heart disease, limit or avoid consumption of eggs.)

Fish. As with eggs, fish is high in protein and low in fat. And as with the above egg study, researchers at the Karolinska Institutet in Sweden found that when people consumed fish for lunch, in comparison to those fed a beef-based meal—with both meals containing the same number of calories—the fish eaters consumed 11 percent less for dinner. It may be the protein that's filling, or, suggests lead researcher Saeedah Borzoei, it could be the rich flavor of fish (more about the flavor of food and weight in "Sensory Disregard"). Interestingly, steamed white fish (such as halibut) ranks number one as the most filling food (out of thirty-eight foods) in the Australian Satiety Index.

Vitamins in fruits and vegetables. Bio-active compounds in yogurt, fiber in plant-based foods, whole grains and whole apples, fresh fish—what the fresh food groups have in common is that the components in each food add up to more than the sum of their parts. In other words, while scientists have isolated particular nutrients in food that are either health enhancing or health robbing, the key to optimal nourishment is not to pursue the "parts" of food by turning mostly to synthetic supplements for health and well-being. Rather, nature is the best nutritionist possible: *consume fresh whole foods in their natural state as often as possible*, and you'll be obtaining nutrients in the ratio nature intended; in turn, your mind and body are given the nutrients they need to be balanced and healthier. Why is this so? The many ingredients in fresh, whole, lean foods—many we know about, and many more that remain to be discovered—not only balance your weight and keep you lean, but they also help prevent, treat, and reverse a plethora of ailments, from heart disease and diabetes to high blood pressure, cataracts, and arthritis. In other words, you receive many, many benefits when you inversely consume food that is as close to its natural state as possible because fresh whole fruit, vegetables, grains, legumes, and nuts and seeds, low- or nonfat dairy, and lean fish, poultry, and meat, have the whole package of nutrients for optimal health and well-being.[5]

Overcoming Fast Foodism

Throughout this section, we've introduced you to the ways in which foodish food can make you fat and, in contrast, how choosing fresh whole foods in their natural state as often as possible can lead to leanness—as well as to a lifetime of delicious dining. Consuming fresh whole foods can also be antidotes to the other eating styles; for instance, it is truly satisfying, so you're less likely to overeat; it contains nutrients that enhance emotions; and it is flavor filled, making it easier to eat mindfully.

Continued →

Solo Dining

Rx: Share food-related experiences with others.

Fare for One

We are a lonely culture, and nowhere is this more evident than in the millions who eat meals alone. While a *tamada*-flavored meal includes food and friendship and a welcoming and memorable dining experience for all, more often than not, an eat-alone dining scene plays out daily for millions of Americans: children reach for a piece of packaged pizza, then eat it at the computer; single working women heat up their low-cal frozen meal in the microwave, then dine solo while watching TV; or anxious traveling salesmen are driven to dashboard dining in their cars while en route to yet another meeting. Not surprisingly, these scenarios also reflect the other eating styles: food fretting, task snacking, emotional eating, fast foodism, unappetizing atmosphere, and sensory disregard. This phenomenon isn't surprising; after all, the eating styles are an interconnected, related family of eating choices and behaviors that lead to overweight and obesity.

Not only does our research shed light on the social isolation that surrounds food and dining, but it also links eating alone more often than not with an increased likelihood of being overweight or obese. Indeed, our research on the eating styles revealed that the more often people dine alone, the higher their body mass index (BMI), which is the measure for weight levels. In contrast, we found that normal weight people typically eat with others and that they are also more likely to eat wholesome fresh food and less fast, processed, and pre-pared food (see "Fast Foodism," for more about this weight-inducing eating style). This observation is a sobering fact because it suggests that chronic social isolation while dining increases the odds that not only will you overeat but also that you'll eat more of the kinds of food that can easily add pounds.

There is yet another way to make sense of solo dining: children, t'weens, and teens who don't eat dinner with other family members, such as siblings and parents, are at high risk for supersizing themselves. The problem of solo dining and its link to increased risk of various health problems has so invaded our culture that Joseph A. Califano Jr., chairman and president of the National Center on Addiction and Substance Abuse at Columbia University and former secretary of the Department of Health, Education, and Welfare, has initiated "Family Day—A Day to Eat Dinner with Your Children."[1] For those of you who think that addiction and substance abuse have nothing to do with food and overeating, consider this: millions of Americans who overeat and zone out with fast food, do, indeed, have a substance abuse problem; while they may not literally be addicted to food, they have a strong physiological or psychological dependency on food and a habit of overeating, which ultimately damages their weight and self-esteem. Why are children and adolescents who don't eat meals with their families more prone to obesity? Some researchers have put this exact question to the test.

Recipes for Social Satisfaction

When I'm giving presentations and I'm discussing social nutrition and the solo dining eating style, I often offer the following scenario for consideration: Imagine it's wintertime at 6:30 P.M., and you're in your car, driving home from work. It's dark and cold outside, you're fairly hungry (on a 1 to 10 scale, if 1 is famished and 10 is stuffed, you're

at level 3), and you won't be home for half an hour. As you drive in rush-hour traffic, not only are you hungry, but you're also feeling alone and isolated. But then you think about the meal that awaits you. You know that your grandmother, who lives with you, your spouse, and your three adolescent children, has been making dinner for you and your family for the past few hours. You know that when you enter your home, your first greeting will be the aroma of your grandmother's freshly made meal. As you hang up your coat, you'll glance at the dining table, which, as always, is set with place settings for six; sighing with delight, you'll think about how welcoming it looks, and how lucky you are to come home to a home-cooked meal with your family. As you continue driving, somehow your reverie of what awaits you has kept your hunger in check. It is no longer gnawing at you, tempting you to stop at a fast food outlet to get something—perhaps a muffin—to appease your appetite. Somehow, just the thought of the fresh, family meal has filled you enough that your hunger isn't setting off sirens of discomfort; instead, you realize that it's merely a signal that it's time for you to eat.

When I ask people to share their reaction to this family-fare scene, I often hear sighs of satisfaction, and comments such as: "I feel peaceful," "I'm envious," or "I wouldn't fear my hunger and rush to fill it with fast food." What follows are some recipes—both literal and figurative—for starting your own social nutrition traditions—and for turning a table for one into a table for two, three, or more.

Set a Friendship-Flavored Table

In ancient Rome, after a three-course meal, the host of the evening would ask guests to chose a *magister bibendi*, a toastmaster who was responsible for each person's alcohol consumption; this honored person would also select speakers for the evening and decide on topics for convivial conversation. If we take our cue from both the ancient Romans as well as the *tamada* toast made by a host throughout a meal, it's possible to imbue your own meals with the same soul-satisfying connection to others.

In a similar spirit, when you're hosting a meal, ask one special guest to orchestrate the evening by creating a pleasurable atmosphere that ensures everyone present is honored and enjoys the occasion. An easy way for the evening's *magister bibendi* to accomplish this is to invite each guest to toast people, the food, or the event, perhaps every fifteen minutes or so, starting with the first course, then continuing through the main course and dessert. In this way, through the modern creative expression of an ancient tradition that embodies the best of friendship and shared spirits, you and your friends are creating your own time-honored ritual that encourages a welcoming and memorable meal for all. And now I would like to make another toast: to "friendship-flavored" food ... all ways.

Create Multigenerational Meal-Memories

If there's one comment about her cooking that Anita Bellandi often made, it was, "No, it's not sauce, it's tomato *gravy*." Explains her granddaughter Vinita Azarow: "During a summertime job while in college, I lived with my Italian grandmother, Nonna Anita, in her flat in San Francisco's Marina district. When I arrived home for dinner, I would sometimes be greeted by the exquisitely familiar aroma of her tomato sauce. But, ask my grandmother if she was making tomato sauce (*salsa di pomodoro*), and in her Italian accent she would often respond, 'No, I'm making tomato gravy!'"

While most of us would describe Nonna's elixir as a sauce and not gravy, perhaps she had the original meaning of "gravy" in mind— for it initially sig-

nified a sort of spiced stock-based sauce; only in the sixteenth century did its meaning as a "sauce made from meat juices" emerge. More likely, the legacy of Nonna's tomato "gravy" has its roots in Italy, where various tomato-based recipes evolved to form the base of a soup, stew, or sauce. Sometimes ingredients consisted of *soffritto* (soh-FREE-toh), which literally means "under or barely fried," to describe finely minced carrots, celery, and onion that have been sautéed in olive oil. Optional additions include garlic, parsley, and a few leaves of fresh sage; if the recipe calls for it, pancetta (pan-CHEH-tuh), Italian bacon cured with salt, pepper, and other spices, but not smoked, may be included in a *soffritto*. Or another option could be bat-tuto (bah-TOO-toh), *soffrito* without the olive oil saute.

When I asked Vinita how she knew Nonna had made tomato gravy on certain days when she came home from her summer job, her response about the sensory ways in which it filled the flat was instant: "How do you describe that wonderful smell of the sauce cooking, the herbs, the basil, the garlic that went into it? There was a full flavor to it—not like prepared store-bought sauces that are overly tomato-y. Instead, Nonna's fresh ingredients and finely diced vegetables (some grown in her garden) created a rich underbase, a layering that was part of the complexity of the flavor."

Spicing the sauce with special social occasions also added to its flavor. "Nonna would make and serve her special sauce during those times when the family would come over to her home,' reflects Vinita. "The table would glow with her best crystal, china, and hand-embroidered linen tablecloth." Clearly, her granddaughter's summer-long stay also warranted serving the special sauce. "We would sit in her dining nook and eat the sauce with other fresh food she would cook for us. The meal was served on dishes with pink roses, not far from the kitchen door that led to the garden. It's still a special memory," adds Vinita. "Unappetizing Atmosphere," offers insights into the benefits of an aesthetically set table.)[1]

As with the different generations of Italian-Americans in Roseto, Pennsylvania, eating and enjoying a meal together seemed to make a difference in the health and well-being of Nonna and her family. To create your own multigenerational memories:

- Start your own family tradition by inviting one or more family members over to enjoy a meal made with a recipe from an older member of your family—perhaps an aunt or uncle, parent, or cousin. As Nonna did during special holidays and occasions, set a glowing table with special ware.
- Create your own "family" by starting a cooking club. Invite coworkers, friends, and community members with whom you interact—such as a librarian, neighbors, and people you know who work in restaurants—to be part of your club. Rotate meals at the homes of different members. In the spirit of tamada, share meal-memories and stories as you dine.
- Make a favorite recipe, and then invite friends and family from different generations over for an informal meal.
- If you live alone, consider placing a picture of a family- or friendship-filled meal on the table as you eat; or, if there's a special meal your mother used to make that you especially enjoyed, make it for yourself on the weekend when you have some extra time, defrost it while you're at work, and then enjoy it when you get home, while, at the same time, you reflect on your family or friends as you eat.

Continued ➡

NONNA'S TOMATO GRAVY

Recipe by Anita Giovacchini Bellandi and Vinita Bellandi Azarow

Prior to the latter half of the twentieth century, recipes that parents made for their families were often learned from their parents or other family members. Create your own culinary family tree and, therefore, a connection to your roots, both people- and food-wise, by putting together recipes from your own family. Here is Nonna's Tomato Gravy, which Vinita Azarow remembers fondly as a special after-school meal made specially for her by her grandmother. Says Vinita: "These amounts are approximate; my Nonna didn't measure her ingredients. As I watched her, I guessed at the amounts she was using. Add or take away according to your taste."

To put the meal together, make a simple meal of your favorite pasta, mixed together with Nonna's tomato gravy, which has been infused with the flavor of fresh, finely diced vegetables. Finally, don't forget to sprinkle it with freshly grated cheese. "Nonna was partial to Pecorino Romano, but Parmesan is also good," Vinata says. "She always served the pasta with fresh greens dressed with red wine vinegar and extra-virgin olive oil, with salt and pepper to taste. San Pellegrino water would be on the table. And dessert might consist of an apple, with a couple of her anisette cookies."

1 to 2 tablespoons olive oil

1 small onion, finely chopped

½ stalk celery, finely chopped

1 small carrot, finely chopped

2 cloves garlic, finely chopped

1 tablespoon finely chopped fresh parsley

1 (28-ounce) can plum tomatoes

4 to 6 basil leaves, torn into smallish pieces (if using dried basil, use ½ teaspoon and add it with the parsley)

Salt and pepper

Sugar

2 tablespoons butter

To make the *soffrito*, heat the olive oil over medium heat. Lower the heat, then sauté the onion for 5 to 7 minutes, or until lightly golden. Add the celery, carrot, garlic, and parsley and cook for 5 minutes, or until lightly browned. The garlic should turn a light golden color; be careful not to brown it. (Note: Nonna often deglazed the vegetables by adding some red wine and scraping up the browned bits before she added the plum tomatoes.)

Decrease the heat to low. Break apart the plum tomatoes with your hands, then add to the *soffrito*. Simmer for about 5 minutes. Add the basil and season with salt and pepper to taste. Add a bit of sugar to adjust the acidity of the tomatoes, if needed. Continue to simmer for about 20 minutes, or until the sauce has reached the desired thickness. When it's ready, the bubbles coming up wilt be a lighter orange color than the gravy.

Just before serving, stir in the butter.

Variation: Tomato gravy with meat. Vinita told me that sometimes Nonna would make the tomato gravy with meat. To do this, "she would brown a smashed clove of garlic first in the olive oil and then remove it. Then she would brown pieces of beef (which could be ground beef, ground veal, or pieces of steak) in the garlic-flavored olive oil. At that point she would remove the meat and deglaze the pan with a little wine (Marsala, or a good red that she would have on hand). After the pan was deglazed, she would proceed to cook the vegetables as above, adding the meat back in during the final simmer."

Share Meaningful Meals ... in Spirit

It's a fact: ancient Romans followed pagan customs by feasting and eating to excess. Only the worship of their more moderate, frugal ancestors, and of their many gods, served to curtail their gorging. Pagans believed that the gods depended on humans to create lodging for them in the form of temples and to feed them through food offerings. Thinking that extravagant temples and an abundance of food kept the gods in a good mood, the Romans were eager to acknowledge their presence by inviting them to join in the meal. Only after the gods were offered the first mouthfuls of food and the first drops of poured wine, did the Romans eat.

In the tradition of the ancient Romans, even though many of us eat alone, it is still possible to share food with friends and family members ... in spirit. To make your own meaningful connection, just prior to eating, think of a family member, friend, or person you admire (living or not). Then, while thinking of this person—and perhaps also of a meaningful memory you shared—place a small portion of food from your plate on a separate, small plate positioned next to your table setting. In the spirit of honoring ancestors, also add a drop or two of your beverage of choice to the plate. Just before eating, close your eyes and inhale and exhale slowly as you reminiscence about your friend or family member. Throughout the meal, eat from your heart (see "Sensory Disregard," for more about this) by continuing to reflect on the much-valued person.

Overcoming Solo Dining

The antidote to the solo dining eating style is taking a cue from Europeans, ancient Romans, and state-of-the-art science, and deciding to dine and to share food experiences with others—either literally or in memory—as often as possible; to share a fresh meal or snack with colleagues, coworkers, family, or friends. As simple as the eating style of solo dining may seem, it is a two-edged sword in that it can be both easy and difficult to implement—especially with the demands of home, family, and career, and contending with cellular phones, pagers, and ongoing e-mail that keep us on call seemingly twenty-four hours a day. But the rewards are well worth the effort.

Unappetizing Atmosphere

Rx: Dine in psychologically and aesthetically pleasing surroundings.

Both the *psychological* and the *aesthetic* atmospheres in which you dine hold the power to influence your weight and well-being. What do we mean by psychological and aesthetic atmospheres? Have you ever eaten in an especially pleasant place, surrounded by supportive people, convivial conversation, and classy accoutrements? Perhaps it was a special occasion, and your friends took you to a welcoming restaurant for your birthday; because they had organized the meal to celebrate you, the evening crackled with joy, conversation, and laughter.

The *external* mood, tone, and ambiance that surrounds you while eating determines the psychological atmosphere. In the example of the birthday party, it is celebratory and a source of pleasure. The milieu has an agreeable effect on you psychologically, as you and your friends chat convivially over a delicious meal; in response, your heart is open, and your soul is singing.

But the psychological atmosphere can also be negative, stress-filled, and unpleasant. Have you ever eaten while being scolded or criticized? Or in your car while driving during rush hour? Or while watching a horror movie or murder mystery on TV? If so, then you have had the experience of eating in an unpleasant psychological atmosphere. The surroundings in which you ate were so hectic or unpleasant that it affected your mind or mental processes in some way—either consciously (which would happen when you're being scolded while eating, for example) or unconsciously (you might not be aware of the impact that a horror movie, for instance, is having on your psyche or digestive process).

The other key component of the unpleasant atmosphere eating style is the aesthetics that surround you when you eat. Simply put, is the place in which you're dining welcoming in appearance—or not? If you're sitting on a hard plastic bench, if you're eating on a garishly colored plastic tabletop, with damp paper plates and plastic utensils, surely your dining aesthetics are unpleasant. Or perhaps you're eating on the run in a noisy fast food restaurant, with rock music blaring and fluorescent lighting glaring overhead. These are examples of aesthetically unpleasant surroundings.

As a contrast, envision a place with an agreeable atmosphere; for instance, as you arrive at a friend's home for a meal, you're greeted by the aroma of freshly prepared food cooking in the kitchen; you take a break from work at your favorite local café to enjoy the brew that the barista makes for you, personally; or during a special celebratory occasion, you enter an upscale restaurant that glows with glistening crystal chandeliers, a crisp, white tablecloth, and the murmur of quiet conversation; or maybe the soft candlelight makes you aware that the wooden dining table has a lovely patina that peeks out from pleasing placemats that are set with cloth napkins and quality utensils.

Whether appealing or appalling, both the psychological mood and the physical accessories that surround you when you eat may influence the way in which you metabolize food and, in turn, your health and well-being. Both the psychological and the aesthetic atmospheres that surround you when you eat are externally based, and both somehow impact your psyche and the way in which you metabolize meals.

You may find it amazing to consider that the atmosphere in which you eat may make a difference in your weight, but it does. This eating style is powerful in that, once you implement its antidotes, it may quickly improve the quality of your life by enhancing how you feel— both physically and emotionally; as another side effect, it may even improve your relationships—with others as well as with food. With this eating style, you will focus on the psychological and physical aesthetics of your food life; the atmosphere in your home, in restaurants, and at drive-thru restaurants; and the quality of companionship when you dine with family, friends, and coworkers—or by yourself. By this I mean, when you eat alone, are you taking the time to set a sumptuous table, play enjoyable music, and eat with a meditative mindset? Or are you eating pizza directly out of the cardboard box in which it was delivered, with the TV blasting in the background, distracted by the details of daily life? In other words, are you providing nice company for yourself?

Continued ➡

Optimal Healing Environments

Although it's an emerging field, more and more the medical community is becoming aware that environment has a profound impact on health and healing. The movement is gaining such momentum that, at the second Symposium on Optimal Healing Environments sponsored by the Samueli Institute, physician and author Larry Dossey described the study of healing environments as a '"huge social movement' whose momentum is unstoppable." Indeed, a newsletter on the topic said that more than fifty scientists and clinicians were invited to the event to define "healing environments" and challenges related to creating them.

Intrigued, I studied the symposium's topics, which addressed environments for disciplines as diverse as nursing, integrative medicine, and health care in general, as well as for ailments ranging from chronic cardiovascular disease and chronic low-back pain to cancer and childhood obesity. Given our own research and the unappetizing atmosphere eating style we identified, the presentation that really caught my attention was the work of Marc Schweitzer and colleagues because it identified specific elements in the environment that make an impact on health. "The 'ambiance' of a space has an effect on people using the space," Schweitzer states. And then he goes on to identify elements that are integral to a healing environment: personal space; sound/ noise; temperature; fresh air and ventilation; enjoyable social interaction (social support); warm, natural light; color; a view and experience of nature; arts, esthetics, and entertainment (such as music).[1]

I was especially interested in Schweitzer's overview of the elements of a healing environment that have so far been identified, because, I'm suggesting that the atmosphere in which you eat can be healing—by increasing the odds of optimal digestion and, in turn, optimal weight and well-being—or harmful— by increasing the odds of poor digestion or overeating, thus contributing to weight gain. After all, as we have seen, throughout the day you have plenty of nonhealing opportunities to assault your psyche and system (and waistline) by eating in an abrasive atmosphere, such as in the gas station store situation I described above. If you recall, it was replete with harsh lighting, contrary people, and depressing news blaring from the TV. Add cramped quarters, stuffy and stale air, and a motley collection of disparate, disconnected, and cluttered food products and car accoutrements, and you have the antithesis of the healing environment that Schweitzer's research revealed.

Optimal Eating Atmosphere

Most of us know that eating in congenial surroundings is, at the very least, enjoyable. This is especially good news, since you can access or create delightful surroundings any time. For instance, envision a fall picnic, surrounded by the bittersweet mood of autumn, as the colors of the season materialize both in the leaves on trees and in the deep orange of pumpkin soup. Or think of the soothing serenity and comfort of a homemade stew that you eat in winter as candlelight flickers on the dining table and you're surrounded by steamed-up windows, while outside, a blanket of snow covers your yard. Or imagine an impromptu meal of improvised pasta, sauce, salad, and wine that you make with friends, when a sudden spring shower abates. Or picture a summer salad that you sprinkle with edible and organic flowers, such as squash blossoms. The possibilities are endless. Yet the role that ambiance and your surroundings play in overeating and weight gain (as well as indigestion problems) continues to be an overlooked aspect of optimal eating and well-being.

What would an optimal psychological and aesthetic eating environment look like? Here are some suggestions for creating an affable dining milieu … as often as possible.

Limit lighting. One of our favorite restaurants has low hanging lights above each booth, which we find to be harsh. Each time we eat there, we think about how much more we would enjoy the meal and the entire dining experience if, instead, it were infused with candlelight. When you eat at home, diffuse the light by turning on a favorite nearby lamp, dimming your overhead light, or eating by candlelight.

Walk away. A friend of mine told me that not too long after she read our research paper on the eating styles, she was feeling hypoglycemic (weak from low blood sugar) and hungry in the middle of the day while "choring." So she made the spontaneous decision to buy a sweet from a gourmet cookie shop to quickly appease her hunger. But the acid rock music that blasted from speakers, and the uninterested clerks who continued to talk among themselves instead of taking her order, dissuaded her from staying. She found a friendlier place down the block for a midday munch. When you eat out— whether it's a full meal or a munchie—choose an amiable place whenever possible.

Cherish china. When Oprah did a show on "anti-aging breakthroughs," a weight-loss lifestyle was one of the topics. To highlight the elements of her successful weight loss, an audience member shared her personal success story. Along with moving more and choosing fresh food, the aesthetic atmosphere she created was part of her successful twenty-two-pound weight loss. "I put my portion [of food] on beautiful plates, with great style, lovely linens, crystal, [and] china, and enjoyed every morsel," she said. "No more standing in the kitchen eating out of a little container."[2] Whenever possible, eat on quality plates, with the best utensils you have, and sit down at a dining table to enjoy your meal even more.

Rest, relax. A friend of ours who is a *yogini* (a woman who practices yoga), told us that after she shared a large lunch in the home of a revered family in India, her hosts invited her to lie down and rest so that she could digest the meal in a peaceful and quiet environment. In a time- and work-driven country like ours, this isn't a realistic option, but what we can do is a modified version: after eating, take the time to enjoy some easygoing, postprandial conversation with others, some relaxing music, or an enjoyable article.

Release emotions. Because of Candace Pert's research on emotions and digestion, it is safe to say that the psychological atmosphere in which you eat influences the way you metabolize food and, in turn, your weight and well-being. That's why you'll

---

Food Facials

Helene Silver

Yogurt Toning Mask

The Yogurt Toning Mask is a rejuvenating beauty treatment that takes only seconds to apply. You will feel its deep cleansing effect as it penetrates the pores to remove obstructing wastes. When used regularly, yogurt facials refine and smooth the texture of the skin.

Combine one-half cup of plain yogurt with a little fresh lemon juice. Apply it to your face and keep it on while you bathe, about twenty minutes. The mask will tighten and dry on your face.

The tingly, cooling sensation of the yogurt contrasts refreshingly with the heat of your bath. After your bath, remove the mask with splashes of cold water.

Cucumber Cleansing Facial

Cucumber juice is a great natural treatment for the complexion. It helps to soften hardened skin, soothes sunburn, and gently bleaches dark spots and freckles. It has an astringent effect that will leave your face feeling wonderfully cleansed and refreshed.

Apply thin slices of fresh cucumber to your face. Cover the cucumber slices with a washcloth dipped in very hot water and wrung out. Let the facial stay on for fifteen minutes, then remove the cucumber slices, splash your face with cold water, and pat dry.

A cucumber facial is one of the beauty treatments that you could spend a lot of money for in a salon, but that you can easily do at home.

Egg–Yolk Mask

Separate the yolk from the white of an egg and save the white for use in the oatmeal—egg white pack listed below. Beat the yolk until it is frothy, and dab it onto your face, allowing it to dry and harden. Rinse the dried egg yolk from your face with cold water. The egg-yolk mask helps to moisturize dry skin.

Oatmeal–Egg White Pack

Mix one handful of raw oatmeal with one egg white and a few drops of fresh lemon juice to form a paste. Spread the paste on your face and throat, rubbing it into the areas around the chin and nose. As you allow this facial mask to dry, you will feel it soothing and tightening your skin. Remove it with splashes of cold water. This facial mask helps to smooth rough, bumpy skin and tighten wrinkles and furrows.

Milk Eye Packs

Dip cotton balls in warm or cold milk and place them over your eyes while you soak in your bath. Milk helps to cleanse and nourish the delicate skin around your eyes.

Hot Olive-Oil Rejuvenating Facial

Hot olive oil applied to the face, throat, and neck helps to moisturize and rejuvenate the skin and guard against wrinkles.

Warm a quarter-cup of olive oil. Smooth it over your face and neck, all the way down to the chest.

For added benefit, wrap a hot towel around your neck, so the oil can really seep into this area, which often becomes prematurely wrinkled. Lie back in a relaxing, fragrant bath and enjoy the soothing richness of the olive oil as it penetrates your skin and refreshes your complexion. At the end of your bath, remove the olive oil with cleansing bath gel or other gentle bath soap.

—From *Rejuvenate*

Continued ➡

find it helpful to release toxic molecules of emotion when you eat. To do this, if you find that you're ruminating about something unpleasant, put your emotions on hold and press the pause button as you eat; instead, think about something agreeable. You can always return to the problem later. Or, if the people with whom you're dining are more negative than positive, try to redirect the conversation by asking them to share something that is working well or is enjoyable in their lives.

Eat outside. If there's a park near your house, some outdoor dining tables and chairs in the courtyard where you work, or a café that enables you to eat while outdoors as you enjoy some fresh air and beautiful surroundings, take advantage of the opportunity. And there's another benefit: you can get some exercise while walking to your favorite outdoor eating place.

Overcoming Unappetizing Atmosphere

I wasn't surprised when our research revealed unappetizing atmosphere as an eating style linked with overeating. What astonished me was that, as with all the eating styles, it was statistically significant; in other words, it's not due to chance. The psychological and aesthetic environments connected to food and eating may be the most overlooked aspect of weight gain, but, as we've seen throughout this chapter, it is a powerful determinant of your weight. To increase your odds of achieving and maintaining optimal weight, we've given you lots of guidelines for dining in psychologically and aesthetically pleasing surroundings that are inherently healing and healthy.

Sensory Disregard

Rx: Savor flavors when you eat.

Sensory Disregard-Spiritual Disconnection

Fresh food that has been prepared with care and savored by the diners can fill the senses and satisfy the soul—the two key ingredients lacking in the sensory disregard eating style. We are especially excited to tell you about this eating style because our research is the first to reveal the sensory and spiritual elements—which go together like twins—of eating . . . and of overeating. When you take time to experience your food through all your senses—taste (flavor), smell (aroma), sight (presentation), sound (of surroundings), and touch (kinesthetics)—and to regard the mystery of life inherent in both food and yourself, you're more likely to be truly nourished, and less likely to overeat. In other words, dining with your senses (sensory *regard*) while at the same time eating with a deep appreciation for the food before you (spiritual *connection*) are powerful ways to nurture and nourish yourself and, in turn, to feel fulfilled by the dining experience. When you take the time to do this, you're more likely to eat less and enjoy it more.

Such regard and connection to eating is the antithesis of how many who struggle with weight relate to food. What is more typical is sensory *disregard* and spiritual *disconnection*. What does this eating style look like? If you've ever eaten quickly and mindlessly (more about this in "Emotional Eating") and scarfed down food because, perhaps, you've let yourself become superhungry or, say, you're feeling depressed and your emotions are dictating what and how you're eating, then you've eaten without experiencing the color of the food, its aroma, flavors, texture, presentation, and portion size; this is sensory disregard. At the same

time, if you typically eat without reflecting on the mystery of food's ability to sustain life; if you ignore the way in which the elements, such as rain, sunshine, wind, and soil, work together to create the fruits, vegetables, whole grains, legumes, and nuts and seeds, as well as dairy, eggs, fish, poultry, and meat, that nourish you; and if you eat without savoring and appreciating, from the heart, the origins of the food before you—then you are eating with spiritual disconnection.

The idea that eating with sensory disregard and spiritual disconnection can lead to weight gain, it must be said, may seem somewhat unusual. After all, the straightforward and seemingly simple one-size-fits-all, calories in—calories out formula discussed in "Food Fretting" is the standard solution to weight loss that most health professionals stand by: just cut down on the amount of food you eat, and move more, and you'll lose weight. Eating with your senses and connecting to the meaning in meals, on the other hand, isn't so straightforward and simple. Rather, it requires you to replace calorie counting with sensory and sensual pleasure, and to transform phobic food thoughts ("I can't eat that; it's fattening") into a world filled with the wonder and delight of food and eating, and into a relationship with food that includes appreciating the meaning and mystery of life inherent in your meals.

Surely most of us don't flavor our meals with sensory and spiritual delight. And we're paying a big price for it with our growing girth. While vacationing in Mexico, Mark Morford, a columnist at the *San Francisco Chronicle*, observed many overweight Americans; he considered the sensory and spiritual starvation that is normal for many Americans, and its link with being overweight. Such thoughts prompted him to speculate about the detachment so many overweight people must feel from their body, a spiritual emptiness and lack of true nourishment—even as they're overeating.[1]

You can fill a sense of spiritual vacuity, a lack of true nourishment each time you eat, if you take the time to taste your food and to appreciate the multidimensional ways it nourishes you; in other words, if you take the time to savor the flavors in your food.

Sensory Regard Strategies

We've already discussed what it means to "eat with your senses" by taking in, for example, the color, textures, and aromas of food. But did you know that while there are five key senses (sight, smell, touch, taste, and motion or movement—or kinesthetic response), for millennia, Eastern healing systems, such as India's Ayurveda, traditional Chinese medicine (TCM), and Tibetan medicine, have turned to six flavors in food to signal optimal eating and complete nutrition? I had been familiar with the role of the six tastes in Ayurveda and TCM, but I discovered its place in Tibetan medicine during a lecture by Tibetan physician Dr. Namgyal Qusar. In response to a question from a member of the audience about optimal food preparation and nutrient preservation, Dr. Qusar responded by clarifying the Tibetan concept of "balance," consuming food from all food groups—both plant- and animal-based. Then, he added that for complete nutrition, you have to eat all six tastes: sweet, sour, salty, bitter, pungent, and astringent. In other words, Tibetan nutrition uses a finely honed sense of taste to ascertain whether a meal is balanced, and to find out, you have to focus your attention on the flavors inside your mouth as you chew.[2] The six tastes are so integral to health and well-being in Ayurveda that some ancient Ayurvedic schools encourage a sequence of tastes in a meal that progresses from

sweet to salty, sour, pungent, bitter, and then astringent.

Savor six tastes. To put the concept of the six tastes into practice, gather the ingredients to make a unique Thai appetizer salad called *miang kam*: one each lime, small red onion, and red pepper; a piece of ginger; two tablespoons of roasted coconut; some honey (perhaps ¼ cup); and about ten spinach leaves. Except for the spinach, chop each food into tiny pieces. Next, spread a thin layer of honey (perhaps a teaspoon) on one spinach leaf, then take a pinch of each ingredient and sprinkle it over the sticky honey. Now, roll up the spinach leaf, creating a small food-filled tube. With your eyes closed, take a bite and begin to chew. Focus solely on the food in your mouth. Can you taste fantastic flavors? Are you able to identify one or more of the six tastes? Simply appreciate every single flavor.

Engage your senses. Experiencing food with your senses can connect you to the sacred, to the mystery of life, to other beings (indeed, to "being"). It's possible for you to nourish yourself this way with one of humankind's most simple and basic foods—bread—whether you're having a sandwich with friends, buttering bread at a restaurant, or having friends or family members over to create communion by sharing bread, cheese, and fruit, in your home.

Making such a meaningful connection calls for engaging all your senses: sight, touch, smell, taste, and hearing. To do this, *look* at the bread you are going to eat and become aware of its texture and color. Is it smooth, rough, light, or dark? When you take the bread in your hands, what does it *feel* like? Is it soft, tough, or grainy? Next, identify the *smell* of the bread. Is it sweet? Sour? Or in between? When you take a bite of the bread, do you taste one or more flavors? (Hint: the taste of food often changes as you chew.) Finally, how does the bread you're chewing *sound*? Loud or subtle?

Each time you break bread is an opportunity to be nourished spiritually. But... the extent to which this connection is revealed to you depends on your heartfelt intention and the degree to which you are willing to infuse bread (and all food and eating) with the mystery of sensory regard.

Connection Strategies

The antidote to sensory disregard and spiritual disconnection is discovering how to "eat from a place of spirit." A phrase coined by clinical psychologist Michael Mayer, it means that when you eat, you access *chi*, a centuries-old concept from China that describes the life-force within all living things, from feelings to food. When you cultivate *chi*, "you merge with the mysterious energy source in the world that is life itself," says Mayer. And, because such a comprehensive connection soothes the soul, it holds the power to fill the sense of emptiness that drives many of us to overeat.[3]

Judaism's havdalah ceremony captures the senses as a reminder to hold on to the Sabbath's moments of sweetness and peace during the busy work week. Bringing similar attention and regard to food and eating and the entire experience of dining means you're eating *from* the heart. When you do, this might be described in Hebrew as *yetzirah*, the spiritual awareness of unity and connection. And it is this understanding, recognition, and perception that fills and nourishes heart and soul.

Eat like a yogi. Devout yogis—people who practice yoga—follow a philosophy of *Sanatana dharma*, the Sanskrit expression for the underlying, eternal, true essence of all life. Such a philosophy complements the *Bhagavad Gita*, which encourages honoring

Continued ➡

all living things— including food—as part of an interdependent oneness. Approached with such a focus, the consciousness, or mentality, you bring to food may be the most important ingredient in the meal. When preparing or cooking food, think positive, loving, appreciative thoughts. After all, such a mentality may be transferred into the food, enhance digestion, and empower the food with the ability to nourish body, mind, and soul.

Like vitamins and minerals in life-giving foods, negative, angry thoughts are believed to be metabolized, too. Because of this, do not eat when you're angry, because negative thoughts are believed to create toxins that eventually are secreted by the glands. Also, anger or stress may limit the production of digestive enzymes in our stomachs, making it difficult for food to be adequately digested (see "Unappetizing Atmosphere," for more about this).

Brahman is the Sanskrit word that attempts to describe the indescribable; "a supreme, blissful consciousness" only hints at its meaning. Such a noble frame of mind is believed to contribute to optimal digestion. Just before eating, meditate on the following verse from the Bhagavad Gita (4:24), which express *Brahman* this way:

> The process of eating is Brahman;
> The offering [of food] is Brahman.
> The person offering is Brahman,
> And the fire is also Brahman.
> Thus by seeing Brahman everywhere in action,
> He [alone] reaches Brahman.

Experience a Eucharist consciousness. Most religions and cultures intuitively have developed rituals that use food as a vehicle to connect to their deeper significance. For instance, believed to transform (either literally or symbolically, depending on the denomination) the bread and wine of the Sacrament into Jesus' body and blood, Communion provides an opportunity for believers to experience a profound spiritual connection through food. In part, the path includes connecting to the Divine here on earth through a ritual that engages all your senses: sight, hearing, touch, smell, and taste.

Spiritual connection may manifest in other ways. During the Thanksgiving holiday, millions of Americans gather together to share a meal of thanks with family and friends. As we consume the lavish meal of turkey and dressing, potatoes, cranberries, and pumpkin pie, we are honoring, and connecting with, the harvest of 1621, when about fifty settlers at the Plymouth Plantation invited approximately one hundred neighboring Native Americans to celebrate a much-appreciated crop of corn, barley, and peas. After all, these were friends who had helped them through hard times. Imagine the gratitude they held in their hearts during this meal!

Make each meal meaningful. As with the aesthetics of tea mind, the scents of the Sabbath, and living a Eucharist consciousness, it's possible to make each meal a feast for both the senses and the soul. Accomplishing this calls for "charging the *chi*" by approaching food from that "place of spirit." When you eat with such heartfelt regard, you open the door to feeling connected to yourself and others, indeed, to the entire universe. At the same time, as you become more and more connected to your true nature, you make it more and more possible for your natural, normal weight to manifest.

Grow your own food. Gardening and growing the food that you cook creates a strong connection among you, the land, and the seasons. If you don't have space to garden, consider growing your own windowsill herb garden. Or buy food from your local farmers' market to experience the sensual pleasures of sampling and buying fresh, seasonal food; at the same time, you'll get to meet and appreciate the people who grow or make it.

Overcoming Sensory Disregard

With this discussion of sensory disregard, we have revealed the spiritual ingredient of the Enlightened Diet, that is, to savor flavors when you eat, and to take the time to create a meaningful connection to the food before you by appreciating all that went into bringing the food to you.

Our research on the seven eating styles highlights the mistake many make in thinking about food, eating, and weight loss, which is the basic belief that a simple formula—eat less, move more—will cure the problem. Such a conviction, though, underestimates the complexity of people's food choices and eating behaviors. Each eating style that makes up the Enlightened Diet and our whole person nutrition program for nourishing your biological, psychological, spiritual, and social well-being reveals that we overeat and we're overweight for many reasons: too much dieting (food fretting), distraction while eating (task snacking), unpleasant feelings (emotional eating), denatured fake food (fast foodism), isolated eating (solo dining), an unsettling environment (unpleasant atmosphere), and a sensory and spiritual vacuum or spiritual disconnection (sensory disregard). In other words, our research reveals that there are many reasons so many of us find it so hard to *eat less* and that, realistically, we have many biological, psychological, spiritual, and social reasons to *eat more*.

Elemental Overview

The ultimate antidote to weight gain and related ailments is to live the Enlightened Diet each day. For many of you, this calls for *changing your relationship to food and eating*—biologically (eat fresh whole foods and don't diet), emotionally (eat for pleasure), spiritually (eat mindfully, with an aesthetic awareness), and socially (dine with others). As many of you realize by now, the Enlightened Diet reframes optimal nourishment as an eating practice for the whole person—and for a lifetime. However, reading about the Enlightened Diet, by itself, won't change what and how you eat, nor will it open the door to multidimensional nourishment and optimal weight. Rather, reaping the rewards of the Enlightened Diet calls for implementing the antidotes to each eating style on a daily basis. It's not theory, it's not wishful thinking; it's about being proactive, taking action, and making your commitment to changing your relationship to food. To reap the rewards now, here is an overview of the seven elements—the key principles—of the Enlightened Diet. Look them over carefully, and familiarize yourself with them. Having an intimate understanding of each one is pivotal to overcoming overeating, overweight, and obesity.

Each time you eat or participate in any food-related activity, remember that all seven elements of the Enlightened Diet count and that optimal nourishment includes both the familiar nutrients in food, as well as the psychological, spiritual, and social nutrients missing from the food charts. We created the elements of the Enlightened Diet to make it easy for you to practice them daily. For only by actually doing them each day will you be empowered to nourish your physical health, your emotions, your senses, and your social well-being. Also, be patient with yourself: making such sweeping changes in what, how, where, and even with whom you eat is a process. In other words, changing your relationship to food and overcoming overeating so that you may stay slim for life isn't likely to happen overnight: success takes ongoing nurturing, care, and regard . . . for yourself.

To enhance your odds for success and nutritional self-care, the following section gives you strategies for overcoming obstacles that may be keeping you from integrating the elements of the Enlightened Diet into your life.

The Enlightened Diet Antidotes to the Seven Eating Styles

Here are the elements of the Enlightened Diet, the essential antidote to each of the seven eating styles we've discussed throughout this section.

- **Food Fretting Rx:** Perceive food and the experience of eating as a social, ceremonial, sensual pleasure.
- **Task Snacking Rx:** Bring moment-to-moment nonjudgmental awareness to each aspect of the meal.
- **Emotional Eating Rx:** Eat only for pleasure and when you're feeling feel-good feelings.
- **Fast Foodism Rx:** Choose fresh whole food in its natural state as often as possible.
- **Solo Dining Rx:** Share food-related experiences with others.
- **Unappetizing Atmosphere Rx:** Dine in psychologically and aesthetically pleasing surroundings.
- **Sensory Disregard Rx:** Savor flavors when you eat.

Identifying Your Obstacles

At the beginning of this section, you filled out the What's Your Eating Style? profile. Needless to say, every person's profile is different. So, too, are the areas—and degrees—of resistance that some of you may experience in implementing the elements of the Enlightened Diet and getting the results you want—or don't want. In the profile, you identified the elements that are challenging for you, and others you already do easily and effortlessly. Look over the eating styles you pinpointed as being integral aspects of your food life and therefore hardest for you to overcome, then identify them below to discover strategies for moving closer to your biological, psychological, spiritual, and social nutrition goals.

FOOD FRETTING

Obstacle: You perceive food and the experience of eating as a social, ceremonial, sensual pleasure, but you continue to be overly concerned about food, calories, and diets.

Strategy: Because so many of us have been taught that food fretting and obsessing about calories, weight, and dieting is normal, this eating style can be particularly challenging to turn around. But it is possible—if you decide to go against the dieting and deprivation norm and, instead, change your relationship to food and eating at the core. Doing this calls for nothing less than turning diet-think into pleasure-think, each time you eat. Each time you find yourself heading back on the calorie-counting roller coaster, halt the thought by closing your eyes, inhaling deeply, then exhaling as you release the thought and the related tension that surrounds it. Now, think of food and eating as one of life's greatest gifts . . . and pleasures.

TASK SNACKING

Obstacle: You bring moment-to-moment nonjudgmental awareness to each aspect of the meal, but you find it difficult to keep focused.

Continued →

Strategy: It's natural and normal for thoughts to wander. That's why mindfulness meditation is called a practice; it's something you can practice for a lifetime. Here are three steps for bringing mindfulness to all food-related activities—from planning the meal to eating and washing dishes afterward. First, decide to focus on food and eating (or shopping or prepping, and so on). Simply become aware that you intend to do this. Second, if you find your attention wandering, gently let go of the thoughts or actions that are interfering with your intention and commitment and then refocus on food. Third, hold your intention and commitment to mindfulness and focus your attention on the food or food-related activity.

EMOTIONAL EATING

Obstacle: You eat only for pleasure and when you're feeling feelgood feelings, but your food cravings and negative emotions take over, making checking in difficult.

Strategy: Accessing the potent power that food has on your feelings—and vice versa—isn't always easy. In fact, our research on the seven eating styles revealed that emotions are more strongly related to overeating than any other element of the Enlightened Diet. The antidote: tease out the emotions that manifest before, during, and after you eat; this requires a subtle refocusing of attention—a shift of mind and heart, a new way of communicating with both yourself and your food. To accomplish this shift, prior to eating, set aside some specific time to observe and acknowledge your feelings without judgment or the impulse to act upon them. Simply be with your feelings, even if they're negative ones, even if it's uncomfortable for you.

FAST FOODISM

Obstacle: You choose fresh whole foods in its natural state as often as possible, but the carrot cake is often more tempting than the carrot.

Strategy: Keep in mind that the optimal food guideline isn't about rigid dietary dogma, or rules and regulations; this is why we've qualified this guideline with the phrase "as often as possible." Our intention is to help you think of a variety of fresh, whole food as your most-of-the-time way of eating, not as yet another diet to follow for a while before returning to your usual way of eating. If you've accomplished this, congratulate yourself, and enjoy nonwhole food if you choose it intentionally and it is no longer typical for you. On the other hand, if you want something sweet and you also want to keep it fresh and whole, consider dates, figs, or a homemade fruit smoothie.

SOLO DINING

Obstacle: You share food-related experiences with others, but you eat alone more often than not.

Strategy: If you often dine by yourself, the easiest way to change that is to bring others to your table through memory and by reflecting on past meals you shared with people you like. As you eat and think of prior dining experiences with others, consider what made the meals so memorable. Was it the people? The food? The atmosphere? The conversation? A special holiday or celebration? An outdoor picnic or an impromptu indoor meal? Once you identify the delightful elements of the shared meal, create a comparable dining event with friends, family members, or coworkers. Take pictures of the occasion, and place the photos of food and friends on your dining table; in this way, you can replicate the experience each time you eat.

UNAPPETIZING ATMOSPHERE

Obstacle: You would like to dine in psychologically and aesthetically pleasing surroundings, but you don't know where to begin.

Strategy: Both the psychological and the aesthetic surroundings in which you dine influence the meal in many ways. If you typically eat in an atmosphere that's fraught with fighting, hostility, or loud noises, here are some options for change. The most obvious action you can take is to change where you eat, or to stop dining with people who create an unpleasant atmosphere. If this isn't an option, ask others whether they can put their hostilities on hold while eating. Aesthetically, small changes can make a big difference: light some candles; play some favorite, soothing music; and use your best china. Make the atmosphere as pleasant as possible.

SENSORY DISREGARD

Obstacle: You savor flavors when you eat, but you are finding it hard to make a meaningful connection to meals.

Strategy: Receiving meals with gratitude is the secret to savoring flavors in food; indeed, it's the secret to achieving all elements of the Enlightened Diet. To accomplish this, regard and acknowledge all aspects of the meal before you—from the nature that created it to the farmer who raised the crops. Identify at least one aspect of food to appreciate (for instance, nature and the elements, such as rain, earth, air, and sunshine). Perceive food (both plant- and animal-based) as an equal, in that it contains the mystery of life as do we human beings. As you eat, consider the alchemy, the interconnection, the oneness inherent in food and eating. Then, holding appreciation in your heart, focus on the flavors in the food. Make a brief blessing of appreciation: thank you for being.

—From *The Enlightened Diet*

Endnotes

1. All seven eating styles are statistically significant in terms of predicting overeating. Here is how they ranked, beginning with the strongest predictor: emotional eating (.561); food fretting (.318); fast foodism (.224); sensory disregard (.172); task snacking (.156); unappetizing atmosphere (.119); solo dining (.028). The five statistically significant eating styles that predict overweight and obesity are: emotional eating (.295); fast foodism (.265); sensory disregard (.068); task snacking (.061); and unappetizing atmosphere (.057). This suggests that if a person typically practices all seven eating styles, she or he is likely to overeat; but practicing five of the eating styles is a strong predictor of becoming overweight or obese. Scherwitz and Kesten, "Seven Eating Styles Linked with Overeating, Overweight, and Obesity," 340–41.

FOOD FRETTING
1. *The American Heritage Dictionary of the English Language*, 4th ed. (New York: Houghton Mifflin, 2003).

TASK SNACKING
1. CBS News, Healthwatch, "Car Cuisine: Food Industry Caters to Drivers Eating Behind the Wheel," November 9, 2005, www.cbsnews.com/stories/2005/11/09/health/main 1029857.shtml (accessed October 11, 2006).
2. Deborah Kesten, *Feeding the Body, Nourishing the Soul: Essentials of Eating for Physical, Emotional, and Spiritual Well-Being* (Berkeley, CA: Conari Press, 1997).

EMOTIONAL EATING
1. Cassandra Vieten (PhD, clinical psychologist and research scientist, San Francisco and Petaluma, CA), in discussion with Deborah Kesten, February 8, 2005.
2. Barbara Birsinger, "Conversations with Bod: Discovering the Spiritual Archetypal and Symbolic Messages in Food, Eating, Body Language, and Weight" workshop, "Weekly Topics—Intended Results, Methods, and Measures," 2005.
3. Judith Wurtman, *Managing Mind and Mood Through Food* (New York: Perennial/HarperCollins, 1988).
4. Elizabeth Somer and Nancy Snyderman, *Food and Mood: The Complete Guide to Eating Well and Feeling Your Best* (New York: Henry Holt, 1996).

FAST FOODISM
1. Judith C. Rodriguez, "Fast Foods Health," *Gale Encyclopedia of Nutrition and Well Being* (New York: Gale Group, 2004), www.healthline.com/galecontent/fast-foods (accessed June 15, 2007).
2. James J. Ferguson, "Definition of Terms Used in the National Organic Program" (Gainesville: University of Florida, Institute of Food and Agricultural Sciences [UF/IFAS], Horticultural Sciences Department, Florida Cooperative Extension Service, January 2004), www.edis.ifas.ufl.edu/HS209 (accessed May 1, 2007).
3. "Junk food definition," Yourdictionary.com, www.yourdictionary.com/ahd/j/j0084300.html (accessed June 11, 2007).
4. Dean Ornish, *Eat More, Weigh Less: Dr. Dean Ornish's Life Choice Program for Losing Weight Safely while Eating Abundantly* (New York: HarperCollins, 1993).
5. Julie Meyer, "10 Best Slimming Foods," *Woman's Day* (October 3, 2006), 96.

SOLO DINING
1. Vinita Azarow, in discussion with Deborah Kesten, about her after-school meals made by Nonna, her Italian grandmother.

UNAPPETIZING ATMOSPHERE
1. Marc Schweitzer, et al., "Healing Spaces: Elements of Environmental Design That Make an Impact on Health," *The Journal of Alternative and Complementary Medicine* 10 (2004), supplement 1: S71–S83.
2. Christine Aaron in conversation with author Mireille Guiliano and Oprah Winfrey, "Anti-Aging Breakthroughs," transcript, *Oprah: The Oprah Winfrey Show*, May 17, 2005 (Livingston, NJ: Burrelle's Information Services), 21.

SENSORY DISREGARD
1. Mark Morford, "Obese American Tourists, Ho!" Notes & Errata, *San Francisco Chronicle*, February 22, 2006, www.sfgate.com/cgi-bin/article.cgi?f=/gate/archive/2006/02/22/notes022206. DTL&nl=fix (accessed June 15, 2007).
2. Namgyal Qusar, First International Conference on Tibetan Medicine, Washington, D.C., November 7-9, 1998.
3. Michael Mayer, (PhD, psychologist, Orinda, CA), in discussion with Deborah Kesten, December 5, 1996.

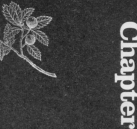

Other Healing Techniques

HOME THERAPIES

Lesley Tierra, L. Ac., Herbalist, A. H. G.

Quite often it is not enough to just take herbs internally. Rather, various therapies are needed as important supplementary healing approaches. These help correct any internal imbalances causing the illness as well as speed the healing process. Folk people and professionals alike continue to use many of these therapies in China, Korea, Japan, Indonesia, India, Malaysia, Turkey, Iran, Iraq, Greece, France and several countries in South American and Africa. Incredibly valuable and effective, these therapies have been employed around the world and by various cultures for thousands of years. Fortunately, you can learn to use them in your own home. . . .

Cupping

Cupping is an ancient technique that was (and still is in rural areas) widely used as folk medicine by people throughout Europe, the Middle East, South America, Indonesia and the Far East. I have even seen glyphs of cups on ancient Egyptian healing temple walls. Cupping is shown in the movies *Zorba the Greek* and *Dangerous Liasons*, and can be read about in the book *Every Month Was May* by Evelyn Eaton.

Cupping is the treatment of disease by suction of the skin surface. This is done by creating a vacuum in small jars and attaching them to the body surface. The vacuum draws the underlying tissues into the cups, pulling inner congestion and Heat out of the body. When effective in its job, the skin may appear reddened, or even bruised, after the cup is removed (with no discomfort). This marking can take several days to disappear, yet, relief is immediate and noticeable.

Cupping is done over areas of swelling, pain or congestion, edema, asthma, bronchitis, dull aches and pains, arthritis, abdominal pain, stomachache, indigestion, headache, low back or menstrual pain and places where bodily movement is limited and painful. I have also seen cupping relieve depression, anger and moodiness.

Technique: To do cupping, you'll need several lightweight jars or cups with even and smooth rims. Good cups to use include small votive cups easily found where candles are purchased. Yet wineglasses or other lightweight and thin glasses or bamboo cups may also be used. "Modern" plastic cups using a plunger to create suction are commonly used today. You'll also need cotton balls, tweezers or forceps, rubbing alcohol and matches (you may also use a candle instead of cotton, tweezers and alcohol).

Make sure the person is comfortable and all tools are in place before starting. Then attach cotton ball to tweezers and dip in alcohol. Hold cup so its mouth opening faces down, or the flame will burn your hand. Ignite cotton and while burning with a low to medium flame, insert into downward mouth of cup for about 2 seconds. Then *moving swiftly*, withdraw cotton and place mouth of cup firmly against skin at desired location (if using a candle, hold cup with flame inside cup, just past its rim, for a short time, then *quickly* place on skin). The flame consumes the oxygen in the cup, causing a vacuum when placed on the skin, and suction holds the cup in place. Check by lightly tugging cup to make sure it doesn't release into your hand.

It's important that you don't leave flaming cotton in the cup too long or it'll heat the cup's rim, possibly burning the skin. Conversely, if flaming cotton isn't left in long enough, a vacuum won't occur and the cup will fall off when tugged gently. Practice yields desired results, and it's actually easier to do than it may sound. How you remove the cup is quite important, too. Rather than rip it off the body, first break suction by holding the cup in one hand while gently sliding a finger from your other hand down and under the cup's rim. This breaks the seal and the cup pops off.

My favorite cupping method, native to India, requires a few pennies and some tissue along with the cups. Put one penny in a tissue and twist to form a wick (cut excess tissue, leaving 1/2 inch). Place wrapped penny on body surface where desired and light. Immediately place cup over wick. Within a sec-

Continued ➜

ond the consumed oxygen extinguishes the flame and underlying skin sucks into cup.

Cups should be retained in place 5–15 minutes, depending on the strength of suction. Especially in hot weather, or when cupping over shallow flesh, the duration of treatment should be short. Often I have seen the cups pop off for no apparent reason. If suction was good in the first place, this generally indicates that suction wasn't needed, or excessive body hair or wrong body angle doesn't allow the cups to hold. Further, several skin marks may occur that can be used for diagnosis: bruising indicates there's stagnant Blood; redness indicates Heat; water bubbles indicate Dampness; and no mark indicates stagnant Qi. Marks disappear within a few hours to several days.

Cautions: Cupping should not be done during high fever, convulsions or cramps, over allergic skin conditions, ulcerated sores, or on the abdomen or lower back of pregnant women. Cups won't hold over irregular body angles, excessive body hair, or thin muscles....

Magnets

I first learned about magnets while treating a patient with such a severely torn meniscus, his knee was swollen to twice its normal size. He could only walk with crutches and doctors warned that surgery was the only (and necessary) alternative. Since he didn't like that option, he learned about magnets from a friend and taped four large magnets together of alternating polarity, placing them over his knee for several hours every day. Within many months, his knee was normal again and he could walk without crutches.

Magnets have long been used in Japan to treat pain, eliminate scars, speed healing of broken bones and skin and eliminate tumors and cancer (in fact, almost 50 percent of the people in Japan sleep on magnetic mattresses). In our clinic, we mainly use magnets to treat pain and inflammation, and have found it extremely effective for this.

Easy to obtain and use, magnets are rated according to their gauss (strength), which has nothing to do with their size, but the materials from which they are made. Some are made of alloys of several metals, while ferrite magnets are quite powerful. Low gauss is around 300–700 g, medium around 1000–2500 and high at 7000–12,000 g. We find medium gauss to be quite sufficient and they come in tiny rounds, easy to wear under clothing.

Magnets have two poles, negative (north) and positive (south).[1] The negative polarity is dispersing, slowing cellular metabolism. It usually has a small indentation on it. The positive pole is consolidating, augmenting cellular metabolism. It normally has a smooth, unmarked side. If neither side is marked, use a compass: the end of the magnet attracted to north is the negative side and its opposite end is the positive side.

Technique: Place magnet with chosen positive or negative pole directly against skin and tape in place (purchased magnets usually already have tape on them). Keep in place until problem heals or disappears. If problem gets worse, turn magnet over so opposite polarity rests against skin. Problem should then improve (if it doesn't, remove magnet). Periodically, tap magnet for 1 minute to intensify magnetic field.

Negative Pole: Use to disperse (clear, eliminate, detoxify and cool) an area—acute pain (sharp, stabbing or burning quality) or conditions caused by

Heat, Excess and inflammation, hypertension, insomnia, nervousness, infections, arthritis, spondylitis, prostitis, lumbago, chronic and acute headaches, bruises, injuries, bacterial infections, dysentery, skin ailments, eczema, psoriasis, ringworm, tumors, cataract, glaucoma, neuralgia and initial stage of hernias. Do not use on Deficiency conditions, coldness, low metabolism, or weakness.

Positive Pole: Use to consolidate (tonify, strengthen, build or heat) an area to treat pains caused by weakness, Coldness and Deficiency (usually more chronic and "achy" in nature with accompanying weak digestion and immunity, energy and vitality), paralysis, leucoderma, alopecia, chronic hernia, asthma, tingling and numbness, comatose conditions, gastroenteritis, scars, tuberculosis, debilitating illness and to strengthen weak muscles and tissues. Avoid using on inflammatory conditions, bacterial infections, cancer and tumors.

Combined Positive and Negative Poles: Certain conditions or pains respond better to a combination of both positive and negative poles used together. Either alternate the application of these poles every 15 minutes, or apply them simultaneously on the area. This harmonizing approach is commonly used because it strengthens the magnetic field and treats a larger range of complex problems. However, quicker results occur if optimum polarity is used. If pain or the condition worsens, revert to using single polarity. Use on chronic pain, arthritis, rheumatism, speed mending of fractures or breaks and to strengthen organ systems and functions.

Cautions: Do not wear magnets if you're pregnant, wear a pacemaker or have epilepsy; do not place over the heart; use with care on small infants, children and on the eyes or brain. Be cautious with magnets around computer hard drives and discs, credit cards, recording tapes, videos, CDs, battery operated watches or clocks, hearing aids, homeopathic remedies, areas of the body with inserted metallic parts and other magnetically, battery, or energetically charged items.

Moxibustion

Pain usually results from blockage, improper flow of Qi, Blood or Fluids, or stagnation of Cold, Wind, Damp, Heat or food. Moxibustion, a method of burning herbs on or above the skin, alleviates these blockages, stimulates Qi, Blood and Fluid circulation and warms areas of Coldness. It is especially wonderful for sprains, traumas and injuries, although it treats other types of pain, such as arthritis, rheumatism, sciatica, menstrual pain and muscle aches and pains. In addition, it stimulates and supports immunity and eliminates Cold and Damp, thus promoting normal Organ functioning.

Although made from a variety of herbs, moxa (short for moxibustion) is generally made from the mugwort plant (Artemesia vulgaris). This herb has a mild heat, burns easily and penetrates deeply. It comes in a variety of forms, either as loose wool, in cones or as sticks, often called moxa cigars. Moxa sticks may be made at home by picking and drying mugwort (usually from 7 to 14 years— the older the better—although you may use it within a few months). Next, grind dried herb into a fine powder, sift and filter to remove coarse materials and repeat this entire process until fine, soft, wooly powder results. Then tightly roll in tissue paper to form a 6" long thick "cigar."

There are other uses for moxa. The ashes stop

bleeding (put 1 tsp. in water and drink for internal bleeding, or apply topically for external wounds— beware, this can tattoo the spot for several months), and the smoke beneficially treats sinus infections and blockages by closing one nostril and inhaling smoke into open nostril, alternating nostrils and repeating for about 5 minutes.

Technique: If using purchased moxa, remove commercial paper wrapper from stick (not white inner paper) and light one end. Hold about 1 inch from skin surface over chosen area, the distance varying with the person's tolerance and the amount of heat stimulation desired. There are three methods of using moxibustion: (1) either hold stick still and only move when heat tolerance is reached, returning after a few seconds and repeating process; (2) move stick in circular fashion to warm larger areas—especially good for soft tissue injuries, skin disorders and larger areas of pain; (3) rapidly "peck" moxa at one small area without touching the skin, enabling heat to penetrate deeply, beneficial when strong stimulation is desired. If several areas need treatment, alternate between them. Continue with moxa until area turns red, about 5–15 minutes. In the meantime, it's extremely important to periodically scrap ashes off stick into a container, as else they'll fall on the person's skin (or carpet, clothing, etc.) and burn. (Keep ashes as first-aid remedy to stop bleeding).

Extinguishing moxa is just as important as learning to use it, for otherwise it can easily continue smoldering and cause a fire. To do, either gently twist sick into container of uncooked rice, place in jar and screw on lid, or tightly wrap lit end in tinfoil. Sometimes the stick fits into a small-holed candleholder and placing the lit end inside effectively puts it out. Whichever you choose, do NOT put moxa in dirt, for it doesn't work but continues smoldering.

Applications: When used over the following areas, moxibustion helps the indicated conditions:

Chest: Lung congestion, cough, cold, flu, allergies, asthma, bronchitis, mucus, difficulty in breathing, other lung complaints.

Upper abdomen: Poor digestion, gas, poor appetite, nausea, vomiting, local spasms and cramps, food congestion. **Caution:** Don't use over person's right upper abdomen near rib cage as this is residence of the liver, an organ already too prone to Heat.

Middle abdomen: Poor digestion, gas, diarrhea, local cramps and spasms, weakness, low energy.

Lower abdomen: Gas, diarrhea, local cramps and spasms, bladder infections (without the appearance of blood), low energy, body coldness, lowered immunity, menstrual cramps, frequent urination, nighttime urination, weakness, leukorrhea and other discharges, poor circulation, prostate difficulty.

Upper back: Treats same conditions as listed under chest, only this area isn't as sensitive or vulnerable to treat on most people.

Middle back (waist level): Kidney and Urinary Bladder disorders, frequent and nighttime urination, low back pain, bone and disc problems, hair loss, knee and other joint pains, sciatica, lowered immunity and resistance, poor circulation, coldness, weakness, low energy. Heating this area increases immunity and energy, relieving any diseases experienced. It is also especially good for vegetarians or those with more Internal Coldness.

Lower back: Low back pain, menstrual difficulties, leukorrhea, bladder infections, diarrhea, sciatica.

Continued ➡

Joints: Local pain and swelling, arthritis, aches, soreness, local injuries, coldness, congestion, sciatica.

Other body parts: Use over any area of tension, soreness, ache, arthritis, cramps, spasms, blockage and nonhealing places.

Cautions: Do not burn the skin or use over the liver (lower right rib cage region), areas of severe inflammation or infection; over the lower backs or abdomen of pregnant women, during a fever; in the vicinity of sensory organs or mucous membranes and over areas of numbness, little feeling or poor circulation (unless with great caution and awareness, or the person can burn easily). If burning occurs, apply salve or aloe vera immediately to prevent blistering; if blister rises, dress to prevent infection.

Note: While Western medicine advocates an ice application over injuries and inflammations, TCM uses heat. In the short term, ice alleviates pain, yet in the long run, it causes stagnant Blood and Qi, eventually resulting in arthritic pain in that area later in life. As well, it slows the healing process (ice and coldness slow circulation and congeal Blood and Qi, just as cold turns water to ice). Heat, on the other hand, stimulates fresh Blood and Qi circulation, alleviating pain and quickening the healing process, especially over the long run. Although other heat applications exacerbate inflamed conditions, moxa heat is different and doesn't aggravate most of these conditions. The only time moxa should not be used is when the application of moxa doesn't feel good. Alternatively, you may interchange cold and moxa applications, using ice no more than 20 minutes at a time, and ending the session with moxa.

Although this approach sounds doubtful to most Western ears, I can only suggest you give it a try and see for yourself. I've personally seen many cases benefit from moxa where ice aggravated the condition. I've had people with three-week-old knee injuries throw away their crutches after only one moxa session. I've seen sprains heal faster than most doctors admit possible. And I've watched arthritic conditions and frozen joints (that even surgery didn't improve) disappear after regular moxa treatment. Experiment yourself and see how amazingly effective it is.

Other: If moxibustion is not available and heat is needed, a hot-water bottle, hair dryer and stones or bags of sand or salt heated in an oven or on a wood stove are useful alternatives, although they can't be used on inflamed areas like moxa can.

Nasal Wash

Nasal wash is a procedure of rinsing the entire nasal tract with a saltwater solution. Doing this clears sinus congestion and infections, allergies, stuffy nose, difficulty of breathing through the nose, sore throats and especially recurring sinus and throat infections. It may be done on a preventative basis once a day first thing in the morning, or several times a day in the case of an infection.[2]

Techniques: To do a nasal wash, you'll need a water container with a small spout, such as a netipot or small watering can (alternatively, you may use a bulb syringe, squeeze bottle or turkey baster). Fill with saltwater (about ½ tsp. salt/2 cups water) and, over a sink or tub, place end of spout in right nostril while tilting head to left. Slowly pour solution into nostril, making sure it runs out left nostril (adjust your head as needed). Now reverse sides, inserting spout into left nostril while tilting head to

right, making sure solution comes out right nostril. Continue alternating nostrils until solution is gone. You'll frequently need to blow your nose in between as fluids collect.

While it may seem difficult, if not impossible, for the solution to flow through a blocked nostril, eventually it does since salt dissolves mucus and moves congestion (if this doesn't occur in the first session, it will during the next one or two). In the meantime, continue blowing your nose. A wonderful clearing of your nasal passages occurs and you'll be amazed at how well you can breathe afterward.

For stubborn, recurring chronic sore throats, sinusitis, tonsillitis and other throat infections, pour saltwater solution alternatively through the right and left nostrils but tilt head back, allowing it to run down throat and out mouth (then spit solution out). This method of nasal wash quickly clears such infections since they recur from lingering bacteria breeding in passages between nose and throat. These bacteria cannot be reached with the traditional gargle or throat medication, but a nasal wash running down the throat effectively treats it.

Although warm saltwater solution prevents and clears infections and inflammations (as many people healing their sore throats with warm saltwater gargles can attest to), an herbal tea may be made and used as the wash instead. Good herbs to use include antibiotic, alterative and antiinflammatory herbs, such as echinacea, chaparral, red clover, dandelion and goldenseal (especially valuable since it tones the mucous membranes) and astringents, such as raspberry and partridgeberry. A small amount of demulcent may be added, like marshmallow or licorice, to soothe inflamed and irritated tissues. Make your own customized solutions and experiment to find your favorite ones.

Rituals

I frequently suggest patients perform rituals to assist and speed their healing process. Because emotional issues are so frequently involved in (and cause) disease, doing a ritual not only clears them, but also releases past issues, makes decisions, confirms your life choices, establishes a deeper relationship with yourself, ends old habits, creates a new beginning and much more. There are as many functions and benefits of rituals as there are rituals to do.

A ritual for healing differs from daily ritual routines with one important trait—intention. Drinking hot tea or reading the paper first thing every morning is a ritual habit. But if you drink your herb tea intending all the while that it heal a particular health problem, then you create meaning that gives a different energy and influence to your body-mind-spirit.

As an example, one ceremony I frequently suggest to patients for making "either/or" tough decisions is a feather ritual. Go alone into nature with a feather and when ready, say aloud the choice you can let go. Then release the feather. If that decision reflects your deeper wish, you'll be able to let the feather go and may even feel liberated seeing it fly away. If it doesn't reflect your deeper desires, then you won't be able to release the feather, or may chase after and retrieve it. Either way, it gives valuable insight to your true hidden feelings and desires, making your decision clearer and easier.

Rituals are fun to create and can be simple or quite elaborate and even involve other people. They can include such things as music, singing dancing, gestures, prayer, statements of belief, offerings and movement. Whatever ritual you create, I suggest you

begin with smudging (described later) to "set the stage." Several ritual elements to try are listed in the table Ritual Components. Combine as appropriate for your needs.

Creating talismans is a ritual using the subtle healing energies of plants. A talisman is the wearing of herbs imbued with intention for certain effects. Talismans are a known part of folk traditions worldwide and more often than not, there is solid scientific basis behind these "quaint" ways. Wearing plants such as garlic, asafoetida or camphor to ward off "evil spirits" and contagion actually works because their volatile oils either attract beneficial insects, or repulse harmful pathogens. To make a talisman, choose your desired herbs, make or purchase a little pouch and create a ritual to "empower" it (transmit your intentions into it). Select herbs based upon their properties and traditional uses.

For instance, valerian root, an herbal sedative, was traditionally used to restore peace between two people. Dried pansy or periwinkle flowers were carried as talismans of love. Angelica root, whose sweet scent was said to resemble the scent of angels, may be carried to prolong life. Mugwort in dream pillows evokes dreams when sleeping and opens intuitive knowledge of the future when worn during the day. The familiar rose increases feelings of love and devotion.

You may directly wear an herb around your neck or carry it in your pocket. As well, it may be wrapped in a special leaf, cloth or leather pouch and held in a pocket, pinned on a shirt, or worn around the neck, depending on whether you want a constant visual or tactile reminder, or a less obvious and more intimate connection with your talisman. Whatever is done, I suggest making the carrier personally meaningful, such as using a silk string, an embroidered bag or utilizing something which has been given to you. This makes the talisman that much more special to you, thus increasing its effectiveness.

Ritual, the final step for making the talisman, is one of the most important as this empowers the herbs with your intentions, resulting in a powerful magnet and transmitter of healing properties. Example rituals include lighting a candle, fasting with the plants, meditating, drumming and chanting, reciting of prayers, smudging, blowing the breath on the herbs, sprinkling them with some special water from a sacred stream or river, adding a special stone, or any other single or combination of ceremonies.

Choose what creates a relaxed and focused state of consciousness. After performing the ritual, hold the herb(s) or pouch of herbs in your hands and project your healing intentions into them verbally. This transfers your thoughts to the herbs, empowering them as talismans. Then carry your talisman until your healing intentions are realized. You may desire to periodically renew or reinforce your intentions, or refresh the herbs as needed.

Smudging, another ritual, is a Native American term for using the smoke of burning herbs to cleanse and renew. It's very similar to using incense for purification, but rather than using stick incense, loose dried herbs are burned in a container, such as a bowl or shell. The smoke is then wafted over the area to be cleansed—the body, room, car, objects or whatever you choose.

Smudging centers the body, mind and spirit, helping you focus and concentrate better. It also clears the mind of all previous activities and wholly (holy!) prepares one for the next, creating one-pointed attention to the matter at hand and funneling the mental, emotional and spiritual energies in a focused and attentive manner. Smudging calms

Continued ➡

the mind and nervous system, evens emotions and purifies the outer physical body. When done in a group, it aligns each individual's energy with the whole. It also serves as a ritual, providing a focus and preparatory rite.

Sweating

Sweating therapy is used in the early stages of acute colds, flu and fevers to stimulate elimination of toxins through skin pores, cleanse the lymphatic system and eliminate mucus conditions. It also stimulates a sluggish appetite and treats conditions such as chills, stubborn fevers, arthritis and rheumatism. When we "catch" cold, it means our immune system is weakened so Cold, Heat, Wind and/or Dampness penetrate through the skin. This invading energy stimulates the body to close its pores, locking the invading Influence into the muscles below the skin. The body's next recourse is to raise surface temperature, dilate pores, and sweat out the invading pathogens if it can.

Immunity is compromised in many ways—poor eating and lifestyle habits, mental, emotional and/or physical stress, inappropriate dress for the weather, or overexposure to the elements are some. However these pathogens intrude, sweating not only opens the pores and releases the invading Influence, it also eliminates through the skin any internally accumulated toxins.

Sweating therapy is well known and highly used throughout the world. The Native American sweat lodge incorporates sweating therapy along with spiritual renewal. Ayurvedic medicine of India performs swedan treatments, a method of sweating that consists of lying in an enclosed box (covering all but the head) under which an herbal steam cooks, causing a sweat. Traditional Swedish sweating includes sitting in a wet or dry sauna with periodic rolls in the snow for relief and further stimulation. Sweating therapies used by the European, American folk and naturopathic traditions are useful home methods you can use yourself.

There are two basic kinds of sweating therapy: (1) Sweating with fire, including saunas, hot baths, applications of dry heat with sand, poultices and fomentations (raising the temperature only in a local part of the body) and drinking hot stimulating liquids and (2) sweating without fire, including

being closed in a hot unventilated room, exercise and sun bathing. Of these two, we will learn several variations of sweating with fire: cool sponge, cold sheet and stool methods.

Whichever of these methods you use, drink hot herbal teas at the same time—warming stimulating diaphoretics for those with strong chills and low fever (such as fresh ginger, cinnamon branches, garlic, mustard, horseradish, angelica, lovage, scallion bulbs, ephedra, osha, sage and hyssop), or cooling stimulating diaphoretics for those with little to no chills and a higher fever (such as mint, lemon balm, catnip, elder, feverfew, chrysanthemum, bupleurum, yarrow and pueraria).

In undergoing sweating therapy, no heavy or solid foods should be in the stomach, or it will detract from the body's ability and energy to fight the infection. The patient should also keep feet warm, such as dipping a towel in a diluted solution of hot apple cider vinegar with grated ginger and/or garlic, wrapping around the feet, then apply a heating pad, hot water bottle, or a hot brick against feet to keep warm. This is tremendously effective in helping normalize the circulation during acute fevers.

It's important to remember that as high fevers can be dangerous, they should be reduced as quickly as possible. Be sure the person drinks plenty of liquids to prevent dehydration. After sweating therapy, keep drinking fluids, eat simple nourishing food (if at all) and rest to rebuild strength.

Cool Sponge Method

This method of sweating is a sure-fire treatment for breaking stubborn fevers, either occurring alone or with colds and flu. I have seen it break a 2–3-day-old high fever in a child when nothing else worked. It's equally effective for adults—it saved me once in Mexico from spoiling too much of my vacation.

The cold sponge method simply uses a cloth or sponge, water and lots of blankets. Completely sponge the sick person's skin off, head to toe as quickly as possible, using room to cool temperature water. Then *immediately* dress and put person in bed covered by as many blankets as can be tolerated. The body reacts by sweating, so repeat sponging every 1–2 hours until fever breaks.

It's important to do this process quickly or else a chill could set in, complicating the condition even further. This method isn't always a comfort-

able one for the patient, as the coolness of the sponge feels rather shocking to a fevered body, but it's so effective there are times its necessary. Be sure to keep the head and male genitals cool by regularly applying a cool damp cloth to those areas. Administer appropriate sweating teas throughout the day.

Cold Sheet Treatment

Here, the person removes all clothes and completely wraps in a large sheet wet with cool water. S/he is then enveloped in plastic (large cut-up garbage bags do) and immediately placed in bed under a pile of blankets. Cover head (and male genitals) with a cool cloth and let person sweat. The cool sheet wrapped by plastic causes sweating, reducing fever and releasing toxins. After sweating for 10–15 minutes, unwrap person, dress in clean dry clothes and return to a clean dry bed, covered adequately, to rest. Be sure to give plenty of fluids and simple nourishing food when appropriate. If necessary, repeat every several hours.

Foot Soak Method

Remove shoes and socks, sit on a stool or chair and stick feet in pot of hot water or herbal tea (such as ginger tea). Then drape blankets around person, head to toe, encompassing the pot of hot water and only leaving an air hole for breathing. Leave in place until sweating is induced; then sweat for 5–10 minutes. The person should then disrobe, be sponged off, dressed in clean dry clothes and put to bed.

Cautions: Keep head and male genitals cool, as too high a fever can destroy nerve cells in the brain or cause sterility in men. Do not sweat if too weak, obese, thin, severely debilitated or alcoholic, if suffering from hepatitis, jaundice or anemia, if pregnant or during menstruation (causes Deficient Blood), or in a state of shock, fright, grief, anger or other extreme emotional state. Extreme sweating and sweating to the point of exhaustion is counterproductive, especially for individuals with weakness or Deficient Blood. Further, it causes salt loss, severely depleting plasma volume and causing hypotension, weakness, fainting, Deficient Blood and lowered immunity. Thus, be sure to drink lots of fluids during and after the sweating process.

Other Therapies

There are several other techniques worth mentioning here. Various therapies strengthen an Organ system and can powerfully heal the body-mind-spirit complex. They are as follows:

Creative expression is an essential element in freeing Liver energy, helping it flow smoothly and evenly. This in turn treats as well as prevents a myriad of problems from chest and rib pain to depression, menstrual, digestive and eliminative irregularities, feelings of unhappiness, irritability, frustration, anger, loss of life direction, PMS symptoms, nausea, acid regurgitation, abdominal pain, abdominal distension and lumps (or masses) in the neck, breast, groin or flank. It doesn't matter what you choose to do, be it rearranging furniture or painting a picture, just so it creatively expresses your energy.

Similarly, exercise and movement also free stagnant Liver energy, treating these same symptoms. As well, they increase energy, stimulate metabolism, aid sleep, rejuvenate bodily functions, clear Dampness and improve digestion and elimination. Blood type O's especially need abundant and strenuous exercise—aerobics 3 times/weekly is insufficient (your ancestors walked 10–15 miles a

Ritual Components

Endings	Transition	Beginnings	Other
Cutting hair	Symbolic clothing	Hair style change	Smudging
Smashing	Solitude	Clothing style change	Journal writing
Burning	Vigils	Feasting	Dream recall
Cutting	Making vows	Tying knots	Power walks
Tearing	Wearing masks	Mending	Night walks
Burying	Period of silence	Symbol of new status	Purification
Washing	Immersion in water	Weaving	Collages
Veiling	Fasting	Unveiling	Lighting candles
Cleaning out stuff	Celibacy	Exchanging gifts	
Crossing a threshold	Staying in sacred space	Re-crossing threshold	
Stripping away		Joining together	

Continued →

day carrying extremely heavy loads!). Blood type A's need less and more relaxed exercise, such as Tai Chi or yoga. Blood type B's need something in between.

Movement may be any activity that physically moves your body. Putting on music and dancing while performing chores, walking, swimming, bicycling, wrestling with kids, any activity that physically moves your body frees stagnant Liver energy. An important note here is to make sure the exercise and movement you choose is FUN. Let it express your unique being otherwise it defeats the purpose.

Thanks to Norman Cousins, laughter therapy has been given the recognition it deserves. Not only does laughter substantially boost immunity and improve all bodily functions, but it's also the sound of the Heart, thus improving blood circulation, mental functions (memory, articulation), sleep, anxiety, palpitations and uplifting your spirit, treating lack of joy and sadness. Laughter also dispels grief, sadness and anxiety.

Singing is extremely beneficial to the Spleen, stimulating metabolism and circulation and treating digestive and eliminative disorders, such as gas, tiredness, lethargy, diarrhea or constipation, weakness, heaviness and anemia. Singing after eating especially helps digestion, but sing any time of day to improve emotions and treat health disorders. It doesn't matter if you sing a specific song; any tune you hum or chant is beneficial.

Many parts of the world incorporate siesta (or napping) into their daily schedules to rest during midday, often the hottest part of the day. In the West, it's almost inconceivable to do this since our cultural beliefs teach us to go-go-go, get more done, be productive, don't slack off. Coffee breaks are allowed, but they're just enough time to use the bathroom and get a drink, and one that usually stimulates us to keep going. This is unfortunate because resting is the best activity for replenishing the Kidneys, which revitalizes the body and prevents "burnout."

Resting also improves symptoms of low back pain, poor memory, knee weakness, lowered libido, infertility, ringing in the ears, hair loss, exhaustion, poor sleep, urinary problems, teeth issues, impaired hearing or eyesight and premature aging symptoms among many others.

Interestingly, resting actually allows you to get more done in the long run, since it replenishes the mind and energy and encourages creative ideas and solutions to emerge. If you can't sleep, take the time anyway to rest—listen to music, or daydream. So go ahead, give yourself permission to rest, even nap, during the day! Its innumerous benefits are well worth it.

Endnotes

1. There's great confusion amongst those using magnets if the south pole is actually south, or south-seeking, and if the north pole is actually north, or north-seeking. This is why I'm using the terms negative and positive, rather than north and south.

2. Called neti, nasal wash is traditionally done by yogis in India to clear air passages before performing breathing practices. The yogic methods of neti are described in *Ashtanga Yoga Primer*, by Baba Hari Dass, Sri Rama Publishing, 1981 (Box 2550, Santa Cruz, CA 95063).

—From *Healing with the Herbs of Life*

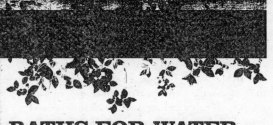

BATHS FOR WATER THERAPY

James Green, Herbalist
Illustrations by Ajana Green

I considered giving this section a controversial title, possibly incorporating terms like *passionate immersions*, or *wet bodies*, or *secrets of water erotica revealed*, for, as it is titled, on first encounter many readers might pass over it (packaging is the gist of most products these days). For the most part in our culture, we have lost appreciation for and interest in the profound therapeutic effects of simple hot, warm, and cold water applications. We have forfeited most of our conscious knowledge of how to tap into the healing energetics of water by merely varying its temperature, getting in it for a short while and back out. This is unfortunate for, with its characteristic ability to affect human circulation by transferring heat to and from the body and from here to there in the body, water therapy lies at the very heart of health maintenance and natural medicine.

Water's solvency and fluidity have been major players in most of the medicinal preparations we have discussed so far, and in many of them water is one of their primary ingredients. I am compiling this section on baths and other forms of water application, because intuitively it feels important also to explore the nature of water as an externally applied tonic and medicine. My instincts make it clear to me that simple water therapy, or hydrotherapy, is an important component of any book that promotes home-crafted medicines and independent domestic health care. I've learned a great deal by undertaking this task, as I, too, had limited exposure to and experience in using water/bath therapy. I have relied on the publications in the early 1900s of professional practitioners of hydrotherapy, such as physicians J. H. Kellogg, A. Stillé, and G. B. Wood, along with the teachings of my now deceased friend, Wade Boyle, N.D., along with other specific information that I found here and there to guide me in my own understanding and experimentation. So I offer you the following basic principles of water therapy, and, after having applied much of it myself, I wholeheartedly encourage you to work with this information to further educate yourself about the phenomenal uses and pleasures of full body and partial immersion water/bath therapy. At the very least immerse yourself in the information about the strategy of the "whole body, cold water plunge," and then do it. I'm confident you will enjoy your experiences as you experiment with these techniques on your own wet body.

You'll need a good bath thermometer.

A section on hydrotherapy has to begin by first dipping its toe in the water. Water is an enchanting phenomenon, exhibiting remarkably diverse physical properties and modifications in its chameleon-like chemical antics. In its pure state, water is a transparent liquid, lacking color, taste, and smell, pure water has been highly esteemed by science's assumption that its specific gravity is unity (1.0), and forms the term of comparison for the specific gravities of all other solids and liquids, earmarking water as the apple of gravity's eye.

Not to be totally unyielding, this provocative substance allows itself to be compressed, but only to the merest extent. When reduced to 32°F (0°C), water freezes and becomes solid, forming transparent crystals of ice, and when raised to 212°F (100°C), it boils and transforms into an elastic gas.

Water's thermo-antics have also been honored by scientists by selecting it as their standard for specific heat, marking it as the official glint in the sun's resplendent eye.

As steam, water's bulk increases nearly 1700-fold, and its celebrated liquid specific gravity diminishes to merely half that of atmospheric air where it ascends sun bound, leaving gravity to court other elements for the time being. This impetuosity is understandable, for the essence of water's parental lineage, hydrogen and oxygen, is obviously a gaseous one, and it is only judicious for an offspring to commingle with family whenever possible. Then inevitably, while frolicking with its airy kin, gaseous water condenses into minute drops (which explains why steam appears opaque). And likewise, in a bigger picture, the oversaturation of air with water vapor causes a similar condensation in the atmosphere where water makes its appearance, this time with an expansive gesture as opaque clouds, preparing for its inevitable return as rain to the patient and willful arms of Earth's gravity.

At the temperature of 39°F (4°C), pure water attains its maximum density where one cubic centimeter weighs precisely one gram, and increases its bulk and decreases its specific gravity when either heated or cooled. Therefore, as steam, water expands and rises into the air, and as ice it expands and floats upon itself.

In the world of liquids, gases, and chemical compounds, water is definitely not known as abstinent, for it is a voracious entity with the power and appetite to dissolve many salts and more or less all gases, including common air, the constituents of which are always present in natural water. Therefore, natural water is rarely found in its purest state.

Globally, water is forever uniformly present in the atmosphere in the guise of an invisible vapor, even in the driest weather, and, as we all have experienced, exerts a vital influence on comfort, and on the animal and vegetable economy of our planet. Water unites with other bodies either in liquid or solid form, producing in the former case solutions, and in the latter case hydrates; therefore, when a vegetable or animal body is deficient in water it is considered dehydrated.

Water as the universal solvent has a profound influence in the operations of nature. Water by far constitutes the major portion of the mass of all living beings, and it is as essential to their organic physical nature as it is to the molecular actions and movements by which life is manifested. Water constitutes the basis of nearly all the secretions of the body, and nine-tenths of the weight of the blood. Consequently, water can be seen as an important article of food, which not only directly supplies one constituent of the body but also supplies a means of promoting the solution of solid food in the gastrointestinal organs, facilitating its absorption. Water is also the solvent of all the body's secretions and excretions, and the vehicle by which the excretions are ushered out of the body.

But obviously not all natural water is suitable for food. The greater part of the water in the world is contained in the ocean; another large portion consists of spring and river waters, which (apart from the issue of pollution by civilized human beings) are commonly so mineralized as to be unfit for ordinary drinking; or of other water in certain sluggish rivers, stagnant ponds, and marshes, which contain too large a portion of animal and vegetable matter to be palatable or wholesome. (I would include chlorinated tap water somewhere on the "unsuitable for human consumption" list, too, and I'd place artificially fluoridated water at the very top of that list.)

Continued ➡

Sources of Water for Human Use

Common fresh water can be divided according to its source. We are aware of rain, snow, spring, river, well, lake, and marsh water. These divisions are not so useful, however, as the source of water is not always indicative of its quality. From water's extensive solvent powers, it is obvious that in its natural state it must be more or less contaminated with foreign matter. Common water from different localities and sources possesses innumerable shades of differences. What is more useful for us as consumers and manipulators of water is to view water as soft and hard.

Soft water contains only a sparse amount of impurities, ordinarily tastes good, and when used with soap readily forms lather. Hard water is impregnated with mineral salts, most commonly sulfate of lime, which often doesn't taste so good, curdles soap and is relatively unfit for most domestic purposes.

Rainwater and **snow water** are the purest kinds of natural water; in effect they are produced by natural distillation where ground water evaporates, leaving any dissolved materials behind, condenses in the atmosphere forming clouds, then returns to the earth as relatively pure rain or snow. Rainwater, however, as it lingers in its cloud form, ordinarily dissolves and thereby contains atmospheric air. It is carbonic acid that is dissolved and gives this water its lively fresh taste.

In its purest state, rainwater is best collected in large vessels away from buildings and at a time well after the rain has first begun to fall. Otherwise rainwater will be contaminated with the dust and various organic and inorganic matters that float in the atmosphere or have been dissolved in the air, and by impurities derived from rooftops, etc. Speaking of rooftops, rainwater can be collected in a relatively pure state even in cities by taking advantage of a heavy rain after it has descended for a considerable time and washed away every impurity, and is collected as it flows from roofs and spouts.

Snow water has a peculiar taste, because when water freezes the ice crystals formed are free of any and all compounds that may have been dissolved in the water. Therefore, when snow is newly melted it contains no air constituents (no dissolved carbonic acid) and this accounts for its rather stale, lifeless taste. Melting snow and exposing it to the air for some time allows it to take up the constituent gases of the atmosphere, and it will taste like other natural waters. Rain and snow water are both well used as food, and in the preparation of herbal medicines, fomentations, and baths. Water equal in purity to distilled water can be obtained by melting perfectly clear and transparent ice under conditions that protect it from dust and other impurities. Also sea water, with all its dissolved salts and minerals, can yield ice of as great a purity as river water (sea ice that is crystalline with a bluish cast has very little salt in it—gray or opaque sea ice is salty).

Spring water's purity and taste depend entirely on the strata through which it flows; it is usually found to be purest when it passes through sand or gravel. The refreshing taste of many spring waters is mainly due to the presence of the carbonic acid they have dissolved. This water usually contains a trace of common salt (sodium chloride), and generally other impurities, depending on the location of the spring. When these saline compounds (salts) are increased beyond a certain quantity, the spring is called a mineral spring where we collect various mineral waters, some of which we bottle for drinking, or sit in at spas for pleasant, healthful soaking.

River water is generally less impregnated with salt matter than spring water, due to its considerable proportion of rainwater and to the fact its volume of water is so proportionally large compared to the surface of its (mineral source) bed. However, even though river water is normally freer from saline matter, it is more apt to have certain insoluble matter of a vegetable and earthy nature mechanically suspended in it, which frequently impair its transparency.

Well water, like spring water, is liable to contain various impurities. The purity of well water is often proportional to the depth of the well and to the consistency with which the water is drawn and used. Artesian or overflowing wells and springs, because of their great depth, generally bring forth deliciously pure water.

Lake water (aside from the issue of pollution by civilized human beings) offers the human community very pure and wholesome water.

Marsh water is generally stagnant and contains vegetable remains undergoing decomposition to the delight of innumerable fascinating plants as well as a myriad of mud and muck-seeking, jumping, scooting, moist, and warty creatures. However, this water is considered unwholesome for most human beings' domestic and medicinal purposes.

Water, therefore, is known as good (for Homo sapiens' use) if it is lively, clear, without smell, and does not curdle soap; and upon being evaporated to dryness, leaves an insignificant residue. This form of water answers well for the cooking of grains and vegetables, cleaning up, satisfying thirst, hydrating one's body, and for the preparation of herbal potions and healthful baths.

Effect of Water on the Human Body as a Tonic and Restorative Agent

In general, water acts primarily as a direct means to modify the temperature of the body. Water at a temperature higher than the body is a direct stimulant of the circulation, and therefore stimulates all the body's functions. Cold water, on the other hand, diminishes a portion of the body's heat, and therefore is a direct tranquilizer or sedative to circulation and other functions. However, when applied correctly, cold can indirectly become a potent stimulant of bodily functions and a healthful tonic. This happens because a salient property of a living organism is to react against whatever tends to depress it. Ordinarily, the more vigorously and abruptly the depressing influence is exerted the more powerful the organism's reaction. (That can give wedlock a run for its money.) Therefore, cold applications to the body in a certain measure and for a given time produce a diminished activity of function, which is quickly followed by a degree of activity greater than that which originally existed. In this circumstance, the primary effect of heat and the secondary effect of cold resemble one another quite closely. However, cold and heat are relative terms; they do not designate any definite temperature. So we can use 98.6°F, the approximate temperature of the human body in health, as a standard and whatever is higher than this may be described as heat; whatever is lower as cold.

The term *bath* means the complete or partial immersion of the body in a fluid or in a vaporous medium such as steam. The effects of different baths on the system are very dissimilar according to their temperature, the area of the body being immersed, and the duration of time the individual is subjected to the bath's influence. For consistent remedial results, the original temperature of the

---

Before you read on: Briefly apply very cold water, ice, or snow to a portion of your skin. Quickly, you will feel a stimulation there that mimics the sensation of the application of heat. This happened because the interior of your body insists on maintaining a certain average temperature throughout itself, including the skin, and quickly acts to replace the lost heat by a thermic reaction where in the internal tissues generate heat and direct it to the chilly zone.

---

bath (tepid, warm, or hot) is to be maintained during the whole time the individual remains in the water. At the end of a few minutes, the temperature should be tested with a thermometer and, if required, hot water added. The sensations of the bather are usually an inaccurate thermometer.

Heat and cold, as noted before, are relative terms. Objects are recognized as cold by the body when they have a temperature less than that of the skin—and the reverse. For convenience in this discussion of the physiological effects of water, as well as for describing therapeutic application of various forms of baths, we can use the terms that have been commonly applied: very cold cold, cool, tepid, warm, hot, very hot. It is not easy, however, to fix the limits of temperature to which each term should be applied, and this seems to have given rise to much discussion in the hydrotherapy world. The following table of temperatures appears agreeable to most hydrotherapy texts and is convenient for our practical application:

Very cold	32° to 50° F
Cold	50° to 65° F
Cool	65° to 75° F
Tepid	75° to 85° F
Warm	85° to 98° F
Hot	98° to 104° F
Very hot	104° F. and above

Whole Body Baths

The Cold Bath (Quick Cold Plunge)
(approximately 32° to 65°F)

The effects of cold water on the living body are complex. They include the direct abstraction of heat, and are followed by a multitude of fascinating reflex effects due to the mutually responsive relations between the skin and the body's internal organs. The interior of a healthy body maintains a certain average temperature or within two or three degrees of it, in spite of the temperature of the surrounding medium. The loss of heat by the contact of cold water with the skin is more or less completely balanced by the generation of heat through the organic changes which are steadily active in every tissue. This immediate and powerful reaction of the body to cold, along with its efforts to replace the heat that has been lost by restoring the equilibrium of the body temperature, is referred to, in hydrotherapy circles, as a thermic reaction.

The brief application of cold to the skin is so quickly followed by thermic reaction that the effects seem to be those of direct stimulation, mimicking the body's initial reactions to the application of heat. However, when the body undergoes a continual abstraction of heat by a prolonged immersion in cold water (or any cold medium), all the vital processes are depressed; there is a diminished pro-

Continued ➡

duction of heat, the skin grows pale and shriveled, the internal organs are overloaded with blood, the pulse beats slowly, the secretions are diminished, and the muscles grow lethargic.

When a person plunges into a cold bath, she or he is first sensible of a sudden sensation of cold upon the surface, accompanied by an oppression of breathing, causing this function to be performed in convulsive gasps. This is called the shock, and is caused by a rapid contraction of the cutaneous capillaries pushing a rush of blood back to the lungs and other internal organs. In a short time the difficulty of breathing disappears, the temperature becomes agreeable, and if the person now leaves the water, a warmth of the surface of the body comes on, termed the glow or the reaction. This is followed by a sense of invigoration of the entire system and an upliftment of the mind and emotions. (Try it. you'll love the glow, invigoration, and upliftment parts.)

However, should the person remain too long in the water, for whatever reason, another train of symptoms becomes apparent. The sensation of cold soon turns to an unpleasant degree of chilliness, followed by tremors. Soon, the surface of the body shows a bluish tint as the blood accumulates in the internal organs. Upon leaving the water there is no reaction, or at best a feeble one; the surface of the body remains cold; the extremities benumbed; and headache and difficult respiration ensue with a sense of depression and lassitude.

The goal in proposing a health enhancing quick-cold (plunge) bath is the tonic influence produced by a sudden, powerful impression on the nervous system, followed by due reaction. A tonic is an agent which, systematically applied, gives tone to the tissue, aiding in the restoration and maintenance of the functions of nutrition and assimilation and increases the body's vital resistance. The tonic effect of cold water is constant and regular whenever water is applied at a temperature below that of the body.

Cold water is a physiological tonic that awakens quintessential nervous activity without putting a burden on any vital organs and without hampering the activity of any bodily function. The tissue activity set up in the heat-producing tissues of the muscles (as the result of exposure of the skin to a cold medium for a short time) is participated in by every cell and tissue in the entire body.

By quickly touching the body's whole skin surface with waters having temperatures of 90°F or below (the more below the better, short of bouncing on ice), the skin, with its vast network of sen-

sory, motor, sympathetic, vasomotor, and thermic nerves, arouses every nerve center, every sympathetic ganglion, every sensory and motor filament in the entire body to heightened life and activity. Every blood vessel and cell in the entire body is awakened and quickened with vital impulse. The reaction produced by tonic application fills the skin with blood, and if it is repeated daily the blood is finally fixed in the skin, rendering the skin vibrantly wholesome by permanently increasing its vascular activity, relieving internal congestion. Tissue building is accelerated, more blood is in circulation, more oxygen is absorbed, more CO_2 and urea are eliminated, and all the vital functions are quickened, thus causing the stream of life to flow at a more rapid rate.

Early morning baths or plunges in the sea, lake, or river, in a tub, or a naked roll in the snow are immensely invigorating; and in the summer months cold baths before bedtime are of great service by rendering sleep more sound and refreshing.

Any individual who has been wearied by laborious effort in a heated atmosphere will find her or his muscular strength immediately reinforced by a cold spray, shower, or bath. When fatigued, a quick application of cold water to the face and head has a delightfully refreshing effect. The relief, brightened expression, and increased vigor which follows this simple bathing of the head, face, and neck with cold are the results of the reflex stimulation of the nerve centers of the brain and spinal cord and the tonic reaction which follows such an application. When the whole surface of the body instead of merely a small area is acted upon, the effect is proportionally greater.

Water, by its accessibility, its convenience in use, its abundance, and its high specific heat, more readily lends itself to human beings in producing restorative and permanent tonic effects than any other agent.

However, it must be pointed out that it is essential to the efficacy and safety of a cold bath that a body's stock of vitality must be sufficient to create, immediately after its immersion in the water, those general sensations of warmth and invigoration pictured above. In other words, cold baths are always contraindicated when, from debility, the system is too weak to produce a reactive glow In all seasons, baths at a lower temperature than 50°F are considered unsafe for children and for old persons who are not in good health. Extremely feeble persons are in the greatest need of tonic treatment, and yet have the least tolerance for cold water. These folks must be attended to by an experienced hydrotherapist who knows how to employ the gentlest measures for administering tonic applications, such as cold wet-hand rubs, cold friction (rubbing the body with coarse material dipped in cool water), the salt glow (rubbing the skin with moist salt and sprayed with cool water which produces a circulatory reaction), and alternate hot and cold applications to the spine.

When there is any serious infirmity of the heart, lungs, or kidneys, or illness of any organ essential to life, the temperature of a bath should not be lower than 75°F (a cool bath). If local applications of cold water cause any chilliness at all they should be discontinued.

It is important to mention the necessity of avoiding the use of the general cold bath in cases of extreme exhaustion from violent exercise, or when, with or without exhaustion, a sensation of chilliness exists. A cold application should never be used when the surface of the skin is covered with cold perspiration, or immediately after a meal.

Some techniques and physical conditions that aid the energies of the body so that it can develop a

> The reaction produced by tonic application fills the skin with blood, and it is repeated daily the blood is finally fixed in the skin, rendering the skin vibrantly wholesome.
>
> When there is any serious infirmity of the heart, lungs, or kidneys, or illness of any organ essential to life, the temperature of a bath should not be lower than 75°F (a cool bath). If local applications of cold water cause any chilliness at all they should be discontinued.

prompt and vigorous reaction, making the toning energy of a cold bath most efficient:

Before the bath

- Wear warm clothing or expose oneself to the air of a warm room.
- Take a short hot bath or shower of some sort. If preferred, begin with a shower at about the temperature of the skin, and gradually increase it. A very high temperature may be borne this way without pain. Raising the temperature of the skin has great value as a preparation for the application of cold. The skin is not only rendered more susceptible to the influence of cold, but is prepared to react after a cold application because of the increased nervous and vascular activity, and the large amount of heat stored up. When there is rheumatism with painful joints, or the skin is cold, fatigue, neuralgia, anemia, or lack of energy, this preliminary heating of the skin is of the greatest importance and value.
- Drink hot water or some other hot beverage.
- Exercise more or less vigorously according to one's strength, but not so much as to bring on perspiration or fatigue. Vigorous exercise or a hot bath taken just prior to a cold bath increases the initial rise of temperature because muscular activity increases heat production to such a marked degree that the cold application finds the heat-producing process already in full play. Hence, it is more able to produce a strong thermic reaction.
- Friction of the skin until warm and well reddened.
- Having warm, dry, or slightly moist skin.
- Being in a state of general health and vigor.

Pertaining to the bath itself

- The water should be a low temperature (the lower the temperature the more prompt the reaction).
- Wet the head before the rest of the body.
- Immersion should be short and sudden.

After the bath to encourage reaction

- Employ heat in the form of warm clothing, or hot, dry air, and/or by drinking a hot beverage (a steaming cup of green tea or hot chai gives supreme pleasure at this time).
- Exercise vigorously.
- Brisk friction of the skin surface with the hand, rough towel, or skin brush.
- A high external temperature of whatever means available, favors reaction, both by lessening heat elimination and by increasing heat production.

Conditions to take into consideration which can prevent or delay the thermic reaction

- Old age, not necessarily referring to the number of years an individual has lived, but more

> **In my opinion,** the glow of exhilaration, and the invigoration and buoyancy of body and mind which accompany the reaction from a quick immersion in cold water, along with good food that you relish eating, pursuing enjoyable exercise and periods of repose, drinking lots of pure water, establishing and maintaining adequate intestinal flora, focusing on happy thoughts, and playing in the sunlight are the most valuable means of arousing to activity any and all flagging energies of the body. These are the most simple, inexpensive, and reliable means for individuals to prune chronic and acute disease off their limb of the family tree.
>
> The cold plunge produces a reliable tonic effect by lifting the body's whole vital economy to a higher level and increasing vital resistance to all the causes of the pathological processes.

Continued ➡

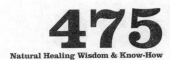

specifically to the condition of his or her arteries. Individuals with progressed hardening of the arteries react with difficulty, and thus very cold baths must be avoided unless the area of the body immersed in the bath is very small.

- Infancy, very young children react poorly.
- Exhaustion, either of a temporary nature from excessive exercise, or from lack of sleep, or of extreme nervous exhaustion due to the weak condition of the nerve centers upon which prompt reaction depends.
- Obesity, due to relative anemia of the skin
- Unhealthy or inactive skin
- Very low temperature of the skin
- Profust perspiration, but only when accompanied by great fatigue
- Extreme nervous irritability or distress
- An immediately preceding or impending chill
- Extreme aversion to cold applications

A simple method for testing a person's ability to react healthfully to a cold immersion is as follows:

- Dip the corner of a towel in ice-water.
- Hold the saturated towel against the bared forearm of the person for one minute, covering a surface of at least ten or twelve square inches.
- Do not rub the surface, simply maintain contact of the cold wet towel with the skin.
- On withdrawing the towel, dry the surface by light pressure with the dry end of the towel.
- Cover to prevent slow cooling by evaporation, and note the length of time required for the occurrence of reaction, as shown by the return of redness and natural heat.
- A good reaction should show distinct reddening of the surface within 1 or 2 minutes after the application of ice water. General chilliness produced by this application indicates an irritability of the nerve centers and of the vaso-motor nerves which regulate the contraction and expansion of the blood vessels, along with an inept activity of the reflexes. A mottled blueness shows considerable cardiac weakness.

The Cool Bath (approximately 65° to 75°F)

The actions and uses of the cool bath are similar to the cold bath, but they are less powerful. They are, therefore, better used for children, for training those individuals who have a strong aversion to cold, and for those who are somewhat debilitated.

The Tepid Bath (approximately 75° to 85°F)

The temperature of this bath is closely approaching that of the body, therefore the shock and subsequent reaction are slight. This bath is not calculated to have much modifying influence on the heat of the body; rather, its peculiar effects are employed more to soften and cleanse the skin. However, in spite of the fact that the tepid bath is generally employed for comfort and cleanliness and not as a remedial agent, for frail persons and very young children, it might be better suited than lower temperature baths.

To help bolster the health and vigor of the more delicate individual, it is best to use this bath about noon, when the first process of digestion of breakfast is over; immediately after the bath take a brisk walk in the open air. In cases of fatigue and irritation from overexertion or a long journey, this tepid bath can be quite beneficial to soothe, invigorate, and uplift the worker and traveler.

The Warm Bath (approximately 85° to 98°F)

The temperature of the warm bath, though below that of normal body heat, nevertheless produces a sensation of warmth, as its temperature is above that of the skin's surface. The warm bath cannot be deemed, strictly speaking, a stimulant. The first effect of a warm bath is to produce a sensation of warmth upon the surface of the body which diminishes any tenseness of pulse. It also diminishes the frequency of the pulse (especially if previously accelerated), slows down the respiration, lessens the heat of the body, and relaxes the skin. The circulation in the skin is noticeably affected, and the bulk of the body is increased as evidenced by the increased pressure of any snug-fitting bracelets and of rings worn on the fingers or toes (it snugs up certain body piercings as well).

With regard to using a bath to help reduce fever, a cool or cold bath is not recommended. A bath of 88° to 95°F which would produce little or no fall of temperature in a healthy person, seems to decrease temperature in one who is experiencing fever (for treating recurrent or intermittent-type fevers, see the section "Partial Body Baths; Employing Cold Water"). When a person's temperature is three or four degrees above normal body temperature, the difference in the temperature of the hot skin of his or her body and that of the bath water is much greater than ordinary, and consequently the temperature-reducing effect of the bath is proportionately greater. (A water temperature of 80° to 85°F makes an impression on the hot skin of a nervous, feverish individual similar to that produced by water at a temperature five or even ten degrees lower on a normal person's skin.) Baths of 88° to 92°F are highly effective in reducing temperature if sufficiently prolonged (30 to 45 minutes); a bath of this temperature has the advantage that it does not provoke a thermic reaction to any considerable degree and therefore does not increase heat production either during or after the bath. This bath is usually tolerated without difficulty by feeble individuals experiencing fever who would do poorly with a more intense application, and will be effective in lowering their body temperature if needed.[start Box]

The secondary effects of prolonged immersion in a warm bath are muscular relaxation, sometimes to a considerable degree. Even after leaving the bath, there is an inclination to lassitude with a tendency to perspiration which can continue for some time—a pleasant experience. This bath often acts as a soothing remedy, producing a proclivity to sleep, and helps relieve certain diseased actions and states accompanied by abnormal irritability. This makes a warm bath quite helpful in eruptive fever conditions (such as measles) in which the pulse is frequent, the skin exceptionally hot and dry, and the general condition characterized by restlessness. The restorative effects of a warm bath depend on its temperature and the time a person remains in it. Twenty to twenty-five minutes (making sure to maintain the temperature of the water at 85° to 98°F) is commonly recommended, but this is best regulated by whatever effect is being produced.

> A bath of 88° to 95°F, which would produce little or no fall of temperature in a healthy person, seems to decrease temperature in one who is experiencing fever.
>
> The secondary effects of prolonged immersion in a warm bath are muscular relaxation, sometimes to a considerable degree.

Warm baths are beneficial in the onset of any inflammation of mucous membranes, especially those of the nose and throat, in some congestion of internal organs, chronic rheumatism, and in spasmodic afflictions, especially of children. These baths are remarkably beneficial for relieving convulsions in children (convulsions may be very serious and need medical diagnosis); they not only relax spasms, but they soothe nervous irritation. If the convulsions are severe, it is helpful to also apply cold water to the head.

When a child is given a warm bath, care must be taken not to expose him or her to the cold air for the purposes of drying the body. The best technique is to envelop the child in a warm flannel sheet or warm blanket (including a huge wraparound hug with the gesture), and place him or her in bed at once. This way the child will not get chilled.

Warm baths are contraindicated in lung illness or when there is congestion or an engorgement of blood in the head.

The Hot Bath (approximately 98° to 104+°F)

Water is recognized as hot when its temperature is above the temperature of the surface of the body, or between 98° to 104°F. Above 104°F it is termed as very hot. Aside from the healthy, stimulating reaction generated by the body from a quick cold bath immersion, the hot bath is far more stimulating than the preceding baths. This is evidenced by the excitement of the pulse, the quickening of respiration, the sensation of fullness in the head, the flushing of the face, the reddening of the skin, profuse perspiration, and the throbbing of cerebral vessels. At a temperature of 120°F a full-water bath becomes unendurable and hazardous for most individuals, although small areas (as in the hand or foot bath, or in the application of a fomentation) can be gradually trained to endure a temperature of 130° to 135°F. Vapor (steam) baths, Turkish baths, and saunas can be tolerated and enjoyed at temperatures of 112° to 120°F and up to 220° or even 250°F for a short time by trained persons. I've actually met some of those puzzling individuals who enjoy that experience.

Heat is *primarily* an *excitant*. It is the most powerful of all vital excitants, as evidenced by the heat of the sun being the direct source of animal and vegetable life, stimulating all protoplasmic activity. In the human organism, heat can increase vital activity, elevate the temperature, and excite the brain and nerve centers.

The *secondary* effect of heat is depressant manifested by the body's atonic reaction to it (the reverse of the tonic reaction is discussed in the section on cold baths). This atonic reaction shows itself as lowered temperature manifested through reflex action, which produces lessened heat production and increased heat elimination with general diminished tissue activity.

A general application of heat first slows, then quickens the pulse.

Short hot applications to the skin surface cause dilation of the small veins, which draws blood from the internal parts and increases the excitability and energy of voluntary skeletal muscles. These short hot applications also powerfully excite the nerves and nerve centers, and these excitant effects are soon followed by depressant effects or atonic reaction.

Prolonged hot applications increase heat production and can give rise to mixed effects of excitation and exhaustion, either of which may predominate. Excitation may involve circulation, respiration, and heat production. Exhaustion may involve nerve impulses and muscles.

Continued →

Prolonged hot application lessens the energy and excitability of voluntary skeletal muscles. Very hot applications increase the excitability of the involuntary smooth muscles. Neutral temperatures have no influence upon the excitability of the voluntary muscles; the sedative effect produced by neutral temperatures depends rather upon the influence on the nerves of the skin.

Precautionary techniques

A hot bath should never be greatly prolonged, because baths at any temperature above that of the body cause a rapid accumulation of heat and rise of temperature. This can mimic the unpleasant symptoms and effects of sunstroke. The duration of the hot bath should be 5 to 20 minutes according to the temperature. If the intention of a hot bath is mainly to induce excitement, it should be of short duration. The bather is not to be exposed to its action long enough to cause exhaustion. When the sensation of heat is very great or one feels strong palpitations of the heart, it is time to leave the bath.

Before immersing oneself into a hot bath, the head should be rubbed with hot water. This relaxes the blood vessels of the head and lightheadedness (anemia of the brain) is avoided. While partaking in a full hot bath, care must then be taken to avoid cerebral congestion. To prevent this overengorgement of the blood vessels in the brain, apply a cold compress or ice-cap to the head when hot applications are being made to any large area of the skin. It is also important to avoid overexcitement of the heart. Therefore, in general, very hot applications are contraindicated in cases of weak heart, arteriosclerosis, advanced age if debilitated, and infancy (below seven years), and also with folks previously injured by sunstroke or heatstroke.

The hot immersion bath is probably most useful for producing powerful elimi-native effects primarily through increased sweating. This bath is taken at 104°F and above for 10 minutes. When followed by a dry pack, this bath is very efficient for promoting intense sweating. A dry pack consists of completely enveloping a person after a hot bath in a cotton sheet and warm dry blankets; the head only is excluded. A cool damp cloth should be placed on the person's forehead.

The hot bath is also a powerful derivative in that it can draw blood and other fluids from one part of the body to relieve congestion in another. I've read a number of reports where this has been used successfully in treating bronchitis and bronchial pneumonia in children; it relieves the overfilled vessels of the lungs by congesting the vessels of the skin and muscles. This effect is manifested very quickly as the child's coughing stops and the breathing becomes easier. The child is placed in a bath of 104° to 106°F and removed as soon as there is a strong reddening of the skin. This can be done 2 to 4 times within a 24-hour span as necessary. The child may be placed in the bath up to the pit of the stomach while cool water is gently poured over the upper part of the body.

The hot immersion bath has proved itself valuable in relieving suppressed menstruation and amenorrhea (the absence of the menses). This bath is administered at the time menstruation is due at 101° to 105°F for a half hour or more. This may be repeated twice a day for two or three days in succession. A hot bath taken at 102° to 112°F for 15 minutes is also an effective measure for dysmenorrhea (difficult and painful menstruation) with scanty flow. And the hot bath may also be administered in painful menstruation when the flow is profuse, but

when using it for this purpose it should be of a short duration of only 3 or 4 minutes at a temperature of 105° to 110°F.

The very hot bath above 104°F for 5 to 7 minutes followed by rubbing the chest and body with a coarse towel or some other type of friction device relieves congestion of the mucous membrane when dealing with chronic bronchitis. If this condition is complicated with asthma, this technique generally affords prompt relief. Following this, the individual should be gently cooled and oil rubbed on the skin.

For relieving the discomforts of chronic rheumatism, the hot bath at 102 to 106°F can be quite helpful. Rubbing the joints with a coarse cloth or with the hands and massaging the joints during the bath aids the circulatory reaction and increases the bath's beneficial effect. A prolonged tepid shower is recommended following this hot bath.

In muscular rheumatism, the hot bath relieves the pain by encouraging the elimination of the toxins that are the source of the condition and by relieving congestion with its derivative effects.

In gastric and intestinal colic, stomach and intestinal pain are quickly relieved by the very hot bath up to 110°F for 10 to 15 minutes.

The hot bath is also valuable as a palliative measure in cases of gallstones and kidney stones.

The pain of cystitis or inflammation of the bladder is diminished by taking a very hot bath of 104°F and above, but this condition is aggravated by cold, so the gradual cooling to a neutral temperature is imperative. Other measures (herbal nutrition and emotional upliftment) are well used concurrently to remove the causes of the inflammation.

Heat prepares the skin for cold applications, rendering them more acceptable to those individuals who feel resistance to cold applications. As discussed in the section on cold baths, an initial application of heat assists the tonic reaction one will experience from a quick cold application to the skin

Hot baths are contraindicated in cases of organic diseases of the brain or spinal cord such as sclerosis and inflammation of the spinal cord, and in cases of cardiac weakness and hypertrophy, and arteriosclerosis. In feverish disorders, as the body temperature is rapidly increased, hot baths are naturally contraindicated.

Reaction consists of a series of vital processes following the application of either a hot or cold medium to the skin or the mucous membrane. The reflex vital activities induced by cold applications are much more pronounced than those by heat, and they differ in their character, depending on a variety of circumstances as discussed in the section titled "The Cold Bath." However, the vital reactions produced by applications of heat are clearly defined and quite constant in character, and these may be advantageously utilized.

Tonic reaction of body to cold

1. Vasodilatation
2. Skin red
3. Pulse slowed
4. Arterial tension increased
5. Skin action increased
6. Temperature lowered
7. Feeling of invigoration
8. Muscular capacity increased
9. Amount of respired air increased
10. Heat production increased

Comparative Summary of the Chief Effects of Cold and Heat

From Rational Hydrotherapy *by J.H. Kellogg*

Cold

General

Primarily a depressant. Short application is an excitant by tonic reaction. Prolonged application is a depressant

Special

Skin: Action, diminished activity. Reaction, increased activity, diminished sensibility

Heart: First quickened, then slowed. Increased force

Vessels: Action, contraction. Reaction, dilation

Nerves: Benumbs and paralyzes excites by tonic reaction

Muscles: Short application increases excitability and capacity Prolonged diminishes capacity and excitability

Lungs: Slows and deepens respiration. Increases amount of respired air. Increases CO_2

Stomach: Increased HCL and motor activity

Kidneys: Congests and excites

Body heat: Short application increased heat production. Prolonged, diminished heat production

Blood: Increased blood count, especially leukocytes

Metabolism: Increased CO_2. Increased urea and improved oxidation

Heat

General

Primarily an excitant. Short application is a depressant by atonic reaction. Prolonged application is excitant and then depressant

Special

Skin: Action, increased activity. Reaction, diminished activity, diminished sensibility

Heart: First slowed, then quickened. Decreased force

Vessels: Action, contraction then dilation. Reaction, contraction

Nerves: Excites. Depresses by atonic reaction

Muscles: Short application lessens fatigue effects. Prolonged lessened excitability and capacity

Lungs: Quickens and facilitates respiration. Diminishes amount of respired air. Decreases CO_2

Stomach: Decreased HCL and motor activity

Kidneys: Renders anemic and lessens activity

Body heat: Short application diminished heat production. Prolonged, increased heat production

Blood: Decreased blood count, especially leukocytes

Metabolism: Decreased CO_2. Increased urea and general protein waste

Continued ➡

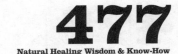

Atonic reaction of body to heat

1. Vasoconstriction
2. Skin pale
3. Pulse rate increased
4. Arterial tension diminished
5. Skin action decreased
6. Temperature lowered
7. Languor
8. Muscular capacity decreased
9. Amount of respired air decreased
10. Heat production decreased

From the above it is apparent that the general and usual reaction effects of heat are of an atonic or depressant character. For most purposes it is doubtless true that the tonic reaction effects resulting from quick cold application are to be preferred to those from hot applications; nevertheless (as discussed in the section "The Hot Bath"), the peculiar effects obtainable front heat are sometimes better suited to the case in hand than those arising from cold. Often the dread of cold water on the part of an individual can be so intense it makes its use inadmissible without a course of gradual training. In this case the effects obtainable from heat are particularly serviceable, and its employment may prevent the development of an irreversible aversion to cold.

Partial Body Baths

Employing Cold Water

A single short application of cold water brought in contact with the general surface of the body is always restorative and invigorating in its influence. According to the circumstances under which it is experienced, the actions of cold water can be stimulant, astringent, tonic, refrigerant, sedative, or debilitating. Relying on these actions, cold water can be used to refresh and invigorate after hard labor, to check feverish and inflammatory processes, to stimulate a sluggish and overburdened nervous system, to arrest spasm, to relieve congestion and pain, or to diminish excessive secretions and bleeding. A cold water bath seems to energize whatever you decide to do following its application; if you choose to be mellow, it relaxes you, if you want to be activated, it stimulates you.

Cold water is one of the best applications for a variety of local inflammations, such as *burns, scalds, chafed skin,* and the *stings* of insects. Cold is one of the most immediate and potent means of arresting bleeding, whether from the lungs, stomach, bowels (bleeding from these organs can be serious problems and need medical diagnosis), nose, uterus, or from wounds. In such cases it should be applied as near as possible to the source of bleeding. A prolonged application to the upper portion of the back relieves congestion of the nasal mucous membrane, and is therefore useful in nosebleed. A friend of mine, Dr. Don, has been a practicing physician for more years than he probably cares to mention. He uses ice as his initial first-aid treatment. He explains that the simple application of ice promotes the healing process of all forms of injury as it cleans the wound site, reduces the onset of inflammation, inhibits the action of opportunistic microorganisms, arrests bleeding, and hastens the repair of tissue. I suggest applying the ice (cold) treatment for 5 to 10 minutes. When it is removed, the body's natural thermic reaction will kick in (see discussion of thermic reaction in "Whole Body Baths"), raise the temperature of the area, and enhance vascular activity, quicken vital functions, and promote rapid delivery of the body's healing agents for efficient repair.

Cold water in the form of baths and wet wrappings is well employed in many cases of recurrent or intermittent fevers where there is a fall of temperature to normal at periodical intervals, as in malarial fevers. The use of cold water as a drink for tending to fevers is instinctual as well as reasonable.

It is possible to induce a warming reaction in cold body parts by rubbing them with snow or ice in a warm room, and you can warm cold feet by taking off shoes and stockings and rubbing your bare feet with snow, then immediately drying and dressing them again to promote a thermic reaction.

The application of cold fomentation around inflamed joints or soon after an acute injury to a joint is of great benefit as an astringent agent to help contain swelling, pain, and inflammation. To restrain local inflammatory processes, thereby relieving the pain and swelling of a sprained or strained joint, keep the sprained part raised high, and during the first 24 hours soak the joint in cold water or wrap it with a cold or iced fomentation (so as to suppress as much as possible the body's natural warming reaction to cold). Then, after the first day, use hot soaks.

The repressive power of cold water is reliable in the treatment of burns and scalds. One need apply the cold water immediately after the injury and continue this steadily. This will help remove the heat of the burn, lessen inflammation, and reduce damage to tissue.

Heatstroke or sunstroke is an emergency, and first aid measures need to be initiated as soon as possible. In this situation there is not only an excess of blood within the cranium, but the blood is excessively hot. A person who can't be taken to a hospital immediately should be wrapped in wet bedding or wet clothing and immersed in cool water or even cooled with ice friction and fanned while waiting for transportation (cool the individual until the heat of the skin and fever drops, but beware not to overcool them).

There is no better palliative for hemorrhoids than frequent cleansings (ablutions) with cold water, especially after a stool; this is most efficiently applied with a sponge.

Employing Hot Water

A short hot application over the region of the stomach diminishes the secretion of HCL, at least in cases of hyperacidity. Prolonged application of heat over the region of the stomach after eating increases the amount of hydrochloric acid secreted by the organ.

Prolonged application of heat over the region of the liver and other viscera increases their activity.

Short hot application on the abdominal region relieves visceral congestion.

Sitz Bath

The sitz bath, also called the hip bath or the sitting bath, is one of the oldest and most useful of water therapy procedures. It has fallen into disuse in our professional health care system, as has hydrotherapy in general, due most likely to its relatively labor-intensive nature. Yet, with just a little ingenuity, this process can be made a vital part of domestic health care and home therapy.

The hot and/or cold sitz bath acts simply to increase circulation to the organs of the lower abdomen and the pelvis. This in turn relieves congestion in other areas of the body such as the head and lungs. At the same time, this also tonifies the organs of digestion and the sexual organs. Hot baths relax while cold baths tonify the soft tissue

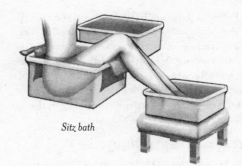

Sitz bath

structures; neutral baths have a calming effect on nervous system control of these areas. It is a valuable remedy in weaknesses and ailments of the womb, prostate region, genitals, and in irritations of the pelvic organs.

During a sitz, a hot foot bath is applied to minimize possible congestion to the pelvic region by pulling excess blood and lymphatic fluid to the lower extremities. The hot phase of a sitz bath is concluded with a cold immersion. This acts to prevent congestion of circulation and to reestablish the natural tone of (heat-generated) ultra-relaxed soft tissue.

The tub that is required for a sitting bath should be of such a form and size that the individual may be comfortably seated in it by leaving the feet outside and hanging the limbs to the floor, and the feet placed in a separate and smaller tub (foot bath) during the application. Large plastic wash tubs are just about all one can find these days to use for this. I set two of them in the bathtub, one for hot, one for cold, and extend a hose from the spigot to the tubs with which to fill them and maintain their temperatures. Obviously, the larger the bath tub, the better.

It is very important that the circulation in and to the legs not be interfered with by pressure from underneath the legs by the tub's edge. Placing a thickly folded towel on the tub's edge beneath the legs or elevating the foot bath tub sufficiently to raise up the legs avoids this problem. When using sitz tubs that have been placed in a bath tub, the bather can use the tub's sides to assist their movement. Otherwise, to make it easier for the bather to get up and down, it helps to elevate the sitz tub on blocks. For added comfort, place a folded towel on the bottom of tub along with one draped over the back and over the sides of the tub.

The physiological effects of a sitz, as in other baths, depends upon the temperature, the duration, and sometimes the mechanical effects (rubbing of the skin with hands or friction cloths) that are combined with the bath. The temperature of the sitz-bath may be cold, cool, tepid, warm, hot, or very hot depending on the purpose of the bath. The bath may be administered two or three times a day.

During a cold sitz or a prolonged tepid sitz, the bather's body should always be covered with a flannel sheet and/or blanket, or rubbed with an attendant's hands or a coarse towel to prevent chilling, and the feet are to be kept warm either by the hot foot bath (104° to 110°F) or by hot towels wrung out and placed around the feet and legs.

The materials needed for a sitz bath

- A washtub (two tubs when doing an alternate hot and cold sitz)
- A foot tub or simple dishpan
- Towels and washcloths
- Flannel sheet and/or blanket to cover the bather
- Hot water and cold water
- A bath thermometer

Continued ➔

The process

1. Assemble materials.
2. Place towels on bottom, back, sides, and front of tub.
3. Fill sitz tub and foot tub with appropriate temperature and appropriate amount of water.

In general

- If it is to be a hot sitz, use 106° to 110°F water with a 110° to 112° F. foot bath. Include enough water so level is about ½" above the navel.
- Bathe for a 3 to 8 minute duration.
- If it is to be a cold sitz, use 55° to 75°F water with a 105° to 110°F foot bath.
- Include enough water so level is about ½" below the navel.
- Bathe for a 3 to 8 minute duration.
- If it is to be a neutral sitz, use 92° to 97°F water with a 105° to 110°F foot bath.
- Include enough water so level is to the navel.
- Bathe from ¼ to 2 hours' duration.
- For an alternate hot and cold sitz, use the above temperatures.
- Bathe 2 to 5 minutes hot, 20 to 60 seconds cold. These can be repeated as desired.
- Always start with hot and end with cold.
- Assist disrobed bather in and out of tub, making sure she or he is comfortable.
- It is very important to prevent chilling of the bather. Cover her or him with a flannel sheet and/or a blanket if necessary.
- While the bather is in a hot bath, apply cold compresses or ice bag to head and back of neck to prevent cerebral congestion.
- Finish a hot sitz bath by pouring cold water over all the parts that were submerged in the hot water.
- Finish a hot foot bath by pouring cold water over the feet.
- Assist bather out of the sitz tub and dry with towels.
- Have bather lie down for at least a half hour.

Indications and Contraindications for Sitz Baths

There are certain indications and contraindications for using this water tool. Basically, the indications for the cold sitz are the same as the contraindication for the hot sitz and vice versa. Contraindications for the alternate sitz are a combination of the contraindications for both the hot and cold sitz.

Hot sitz indications: painful spasm; acute abdominal pain; intestinal pain; or painful inflammation of kidneys (a serious condition, needs medical diagnosis); uterine pain; throbbing or stabbing nerve pain from the ovaries, testicles, or intestines; sciatica; lumbago; suppressed menses; painful hemorrhoids; congestive headache.

Hot sitz contraindications: hemorrhage; excessively profuse menstruation; pelvic congestion; atonic conditions or prolapsed organs.

Cold sitz indications: incontinence; constipation; benign prostatic hypertrophy (BPH) and any incontinence due to BPH; prolapsed uterus; herniated bladder; herniated rectum; excessively profuse menstruation.

Cold sitz contraindications: acute inflammation; any painful conditions; spasms; colic; acute lung condition; and heart problems.

Alternating hot and cold sitz indications: pelvic congestion; congestive headache; prostatitis; vaginal infection; pelvic inflammatory disease (PID, a serious condition, needs medical diagnosis); chronic urinary tract infections; improving nerve pain (neuralgias); insomnia; hemorrhoids; fissures; postpartum constipation.

Alternating hot and cold sitz contraindications: see contraindications under both hot and cold sitz.

Neutral sitz indications: acute urinary tract infection (never employ a hot or cold sitz for this acute condition); intense itching of anus or vulva; to calm mental or emotional overexcitement or sexual overexcitement (that sounds like an oxymoron to me).

Quick Cold Sitz

A quick cold sitz (30 seconds to 2 minutes) produces active dilation of all vessels of the lower abdomen, increasing the movement of blood through these parts. The thermic reaction produced heightens the nutritive processes in the parts concerned. At the same time it excites contraction of the muscular structures of the viscera along with the musculo-ligamentous structures which support the abdominal and pelvic viscera. This has great influence on the bladder, all pelvic organs (male and female), and all structures that are involved in the acts of urination and defecation. It is good to note for those concerned that during the first moments of the cold sitz there is an increased activity of the heart and a temporary rise of the blood pressure.

Cold Sitz

The cold sitz (55° to 75°F, 5 to 8 minutes duration) produces a profound tonic effect on the body and must be frequently applied. The cold sitz is most frequently employed to bring about flowing effects upon the internal pelvic organs. This cold sitz is an excellent application for individuals who are at least moderately vigorous, and who suffer from congestion of the liver or spleen. It is very useful in atonic genito-urinary organs and in the nocturnal urinary incontinence of children (however, this needs to be introduced and employed in such manner that the child does not view it as punishment). It is equally valuable in chronic congestion of the prostate, in atonic weakness of seminal vessels, and in constipation, and in lack of tone of the bladder of both men and women. The cold sitz must not be used in cases of acute inflammation of the pelvic or abdominal organs, in painful conditions of the bladder or genital organs, in sciatica, or in cases of lung congestion.

Cool Sitz

A cool sitz bath (65° to 80°F) is derivative when continued for 15 to 20 minutes, or long enough to cause a decided reddening of the submerged skin which will attest to adequate dilation of the surface vessels. The special use of this bath for decongesting the internal organs lies in the persistence of a large quantity of blood that has flowed to and is fixed in the skin. This, accompanied by the contraction of the internal vessels which is produced at the same time by the irritation of the cold, aids in the decongestion of the internal parts.

Prolonged Cool Sitz

The prolonged cool sitz bath at 65° to 75°F for 15 to 40 minutes causes prolonged contractions of the vessels of the pelvic and abdominal organs. This action makes this bath an excellent measure for relieving chronic congestion in this area. A hot foot bath must always be given simultaneously and the pelvic area should be rubbed so as to maintain strong surface circulation. This friction is important to assist the deconges-tion of the pelvic organs. The prolonged cool sitz also renders excellent results, when combined with other measures of treatment, and in relieving chronic excessively profuse menstruation (when not due to endometriosis). It is also useful in any bleeding from the bladder, the intestines, the uterus, urethra, and rectum, in hemorrhoids, and chronic inflammation of the prostate.

In many cases a temperature of 75° to 80°F is preferable to a lower temperature, especially for individuals who have not been accustomed to cold water applications. In some cases it is desirable to begin the bath at a temperature of 85° to 90°F and lower it after the first few minutes to 75°F. The duration of the bath should be 1 5 to 20 minutes. This should always be accompanied by a hot foot bath of 104° to 110°F, but no hotter than this.

The cool sitz bath and the cold sitz bath are to be avoided with individuals who have any kind of heart condition that would be adversely affected by a sudden increase in arterial pressure. It is also contraindicated in all acute inflammations and infections involving the organs of the abdomen or pelvis, painful conditions of the genitourinary organs, any conditions of the pelvis accompanied by muscular spasms, spermatorrhea accompanied by frequent losses of fluid (see warm sitz), or sciatica. However, in many cases in which the cold bath is contraindicated, a sitz at 85°F, gradually cooled to 75°F, may be employed with benefit. The length of this bath should be 15 to 20 minutes.

Quick Cold-Hot Sitz

The quick cold-hot sitz bath is also referred to as a revulsive sitz. It is a very short cold sitz, a simple dip in the cold water for a few seconds followed by a very hot sitz of 115° to 120°F for 3 to 8 minutes duration. This extreme contrast of temperature is a powerful sedative measure in painful affections of the pelvic viscera. It has been used quite successfully in cases of ovarian or uterine pain that has a severe throbbing or stabbing characteristic, cramps, colic, severe pain in the intestine, often accompanied by spasmodic contraction of the muscles, and in painful conditions of the prostate, bladder, and rectum.

Warm (Neutral) Sitz

The warm (neutral) sitz bath is 92° to 97°F, and the duration may be from 15 minutes to an hour or two if you have the time There is no appreciable thermic or circulatory reaction produced, which is the beauty of this sitz. It exercises a pronounced calmative effect upon the viscera of the pelvis and lower abdomen, and the genitalia.

The neutral sitz is an exceedingly useful means of relieving nervous irritability and congestion of the pelvic viscera. It is of great service in the treatment of painful and inflammatory affections of the genito-urinary organs in both men and women, such as itching of the vulva and anus, hemorrhoids, frequent urination from irritability of the bladder, spermatorrhea arising from excessive irritability of the genito-urinary center, nervous irritability of the spermatic cord and testicles, and also chronic backache from rectal and uterine disorders.

The neutral sitz subdues inflammation and may be employed in subacute and even acute inflammatory conditions of the abdominal and pelvic regions, such as acute catarrh of the bladder and urethra, subacute inflammations of the uterus, ovaries, and tubes. It is especially helpful for relieving nervous pains of the fallopian tubes and the testicles. It is indicated as a sedative means in cases of spermatorrhea accompanied by excessive sensibility or painfulness to touch of the urethra and ejaculatory ducts.

Continued ➡

This sitz bath is highly useful in all cases of pelvic disease in which cold applications feel inappropriate on account of pain or the inflammatory conditions that may be present.

VERY HOT SITZ

The very hot sitz bath is 106° to 120°F, and the duration is 3 to 8 minutes if the bather can handle it. It is suggested to begin with a temperature of 100°F, rapidly adding hot water until the maximum temperature is reached. A hot foot bath of 110° to 120°F is taken with it. At all times, keep the head cool with cold compresses. Following this bath, cool the surface of the body gradually and be sure the bather does not experience any chilly sensations to the area being treated, for this will undo the benefits of the bath.

The general effects are essentially the same as those of the hot immersion bath. At temperatures above 110°F, especially if the bath is continued beyond 3 or 4 minutes, the effect is to excite the pelvic circulation, and to concentrate the blood in this portion of the body. This bath is an excellent means of restoring the menstrual function when it has been suspended as the result of general chill or from other causes.

The hot sitz bath is a powerful analgesic, an effective in-home, nondrug measure for the stilling of pain. For the best effects, it should be followed by a short cold application. Therefore, this bath is of great value in relieving the pain and discomfort of sciatica, and neuralgia or nerve pain of the ovaries, testicles, and the bladder. In general, this hot sitz is of great help for relieving pain in all affections of a non-inflammatory character involving the viscera of the pelvis and lower abdomen.

A shallow, very hot sitz is an excellent measure in relieving the pain of inflamed hemorrhoids.

Foot and Leg Baths

HOT FOOT BATH

This bath requires a suitable receptacle tor the feet, and a supply of very hot water, with cold water for tempering. (See also "Herbal Baths" right.)

The hot foot bath should be of as high a temperature as can be borne, so as to redden the skin of the immersed parts effectually. Ideally the vessel used should be sufficiently deep to allow the legs to be immersed in the water nearly to the knees. The temperature required for most positive effects is 104° to 122°F. The foot bath should begin at a temperature of 100° to 104°F, and should be gradually increased until 115° to 122°F, reached in about three minutes. The duration of the bath may be from 5 minutes to half an hour. The feet should be completely immersed in the water, and the effect may be intensified by increasing the depth of the water up to the knees. To produce the true revulsive effect (drawing the blood from one part of the body to another), the feet should be dipped in cold water after the hot soak. This sudden cooling of the skin will encourage a tonic circulatory reaction. At a temperature of 103° to 110°F the hot foot bath is very useful for balancing the circulation, by the dilation of the blood vessels of the legs, relieving congestion of the brain and other organs in the upper half of the body. The very hot foot and leg bath (as well as cold applications to the feet) stimulate the involuntary muscles of the uterus, intestines, bladder, and other pelvic and abdominal viscera. The hot foot and leg bath are well used in the treatment of insomnia, lung congestion, dysmenorrhea, suppressed menstruation, ovarian congestion, and pelvic pain from other causes. It is a simple and valuable remedy in the early stages of mucous membrane congestion and local congestion

of the head, chest, or abdomen. It may be made more stimulating by the addition of common salt or mustard powder. In foot baths, mustard relieves headaches and cerebral and other internal congestion, especially uterine congestion that is accompanied with dysmenorrhea.

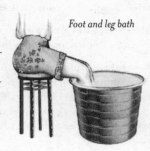
Foot and leg bath

The very hot foot bath is exceedingly useful in a case of sprained ankle joint— to be employed the day after a cold application is used first to subdue inflammation and swelling. (See below, "Cold/Cool Foot Bath"; also see above "Partial Body Baths—Employing Cold Water.")

A hot foot bath is contraindicated in any sensory loss to the feet or in cases of peripheral vascular disease.

COLD FOOT BATH (45° TO 55°F)

The cold foot bath is of great service in producing reflex, revulsive, or counterirritant, and other effects. The sole of the foot is one of the most important areas in the body, having direct connection with the nerve centers that control the circulation of the pelvic and abdominal viscera. The reflex effects cause contraction of the vessels and muscles of the uterus and the organs connected with it. The blood vessels of the brain, the stomach, the liver, the bladder, and the intestines are made to contract at the same time. Intestinal peristalsis and contraction of the bladder are also excited.

The revulsive effects of the cold foot bath are very strong and continue for a long time—longer than those obtained from hot foot baths. The short cold foot bath (duration of 20 to 60 seconds only, for it is only the primary effect that is desirable) is useful in cerebral congestion and uterine hemorrhage.

COOL FOOT BATH (60° TO 70°F)

The prolonged cool foot bath is well used as an anti-inflammatory measure in cases of injury to the feet and ankle, such as sprains, strains, and inflamed bunions. The feet must be well warmed by rubbing or by heat before the application is made.

THE ALTERNATE FOOT BATH

This foot bath is a more highly excitant measure than the cold foot bath.

In cases in which the feet are constantly cold and in cases of persistent sweating of the feet the alternate foot bath is most helpful. The feet are placed in hot water for 2 to 3 minutes, then in cold water for 20 seconds to 1 minute. They are then returned to the hot water for 2 minutes, then replaced in the cold water, this operation being repeated a number of times daily.

This alternate bath is also especially useful in treating chilblains and in eliminating any local stagnation of circulation that can lead to gangrene.

Hand Baths

Immersing the hands in very cold water exercises a powerful influence upon the cerebral vessels and vessels of the lungs. The immersion of the hands in cold water for a sufficient length of time is capable of slowing the pulse and the respiration, and lessening the pressure in the cerebral arteries. Immersing them in a hot bath produces the

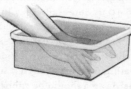
Hand Bath

opposite phenomena. The cold hand bath or simply holding cubes of ice in the hands is an excellent means of checking nosebleed, and has been used to check the bleeding in pulmonary hemorrhage very quickly.

Herbal Baths

Herbal preparations added to a bath enhance skin stimulation. At the same time the body absorbs through the skin a great number of the medicinal components of herbal formulations. The action of an herbal bath enhances the blood supply to the layers of tissue close to the skin, and the herbs' medicinal and tonic actions benefit the body organism in general. Western therapeutic science has substantiated these facts with their official experimentation and by authoritatively announcing its findings (mostly to itself) has finally caught up in this area of therapeutics with centuries-old folkloric herbal science. Further clinical data is still required, however, to convince the more resistant medical authorities and practitioners. In Europe, the work of two extraordinary herbalists, Herr Kneipp and Monsieur Messegue, made the use of medicinal herbs in baths a relatively common procedure. I suggest we lay practitioners move on with our empirical herbal research and let medical science catch up with us again later.

Possibly the best, and certainly one of the most sensually delicious ways of absorbing herbal remedies through the skin, is by bathing in a full-body herbal bath. Life in general is more fun when you're naked. A full-body herbal bath is certainly more exotic than a tincture, naughtier than an elixir, and a heck of a lot more pleasant than swallowing a capsule or a pill. Herbal bath therapy is economically administered in one's home and is practical when administered as a weekend course of treatment or as a regularly sustained system of self-pampering health care.

To prepare a herbal bath, one merely has to pour a quart of strong herbal infusion, herbal decoction, or concentrate into the bath water, swirl it around, take off the clothes, slip into the brew, lay back, and relax; high tea is served.

Often volatile oils are placed into the bath water for their aromatic and medicinal effects. Add a total of 10 to 15 drops to an already full bath. Agitate the water to thoroughly disperse the oils before getting in. It is important to bear in mind that when using essential oils, one drop goes a long way. These oils easily penetrate the skin and some may cause skin irritation or sensitivity if not properly diluted or if used in high concentrations. Some people have sensitivity reactions to essential oils; therefore, it is wise to test oneself first by applying the dilute oil to a small skin area before using on larger areas (dilute the volatile oil in a little vegetable oil).

Often a warm, sensually aromatic bath is prepared for a friend to savor and indulge. If aromatic volatile oils are used to provide the magic of the moment, it is imparative to agitate the surface of the water briskly before entering—particularly if it is a gentleman bather—for undiluted aromatic oils can burn tender, delicate skin that usually makes up one of the first parts of the male anatomy to plunge through the water's surface. This experience can radically alter the serenity of the moment for him if the oils are concentrated on the water's surface. Probably to a lesser extent, this experience can also be disturbing to a lady bather's bottom.

Continued ➡

Partial body herbal baths and herbal sitz baths are generally prepared in the same fashion. An herbal foot bath is prepared by pouring a quart of tea into a vessel that is large enough to contain the feet and to this preparation enough hot or cold water is added to cover the feet to the desired height and the desired temperature. This can range from a shallow foot bath where merely the soles of the feet are covered, to one that extends up to the knees.

Herbal hand baths are prepared by simply placing one's hands into a container of undiluted herbal infusion or decoction. When using essential oils in a foot or hand bath, put 5 to 7 drops into the container of water and disperse fully by agitating the water before getting into it.

Instead of preparing an infusion or decoction of the herbs beforehand, a couple handfuls of dried herb can be put into a cotton muslin bag and the opening of the bag held tightly around the hot water tap. Turn on the hot water and let it flow into the bag. This will make a fresh infusion as the hot water flows through the herbs into the bath. Once the tub is filled, tie off the bag and let it continue to soak in the bath water. This method is better used in partial baths and not normally in a full baths for in the latter (except for small children's little baths) it becomes quite diluted.

Of course, one can simply harvest medicinal and aromatic plants, throw them into the hot bath water, and climb in with them. Normally, this preparation is only appreciated by individuals who also enjoy swimming in fresh water ponds, or in kelp beds, and don't mind the water flora (and attendant fauna) touching their skin. My first herb teacher, Norma Myers, used to soak herself in herb and seaweed baths routinely, but she was a wild woman; she thrived in that lifestyle.

Any herb that can be taken internally can also be used in a bath. The following are some suggestions for particularly good herbs to use for special occasions:

- Relaxing herbs that help relieve tension and promote restful sleep—Lavender (*Lavandula spp.*), Linden blossoms (*Tilia spp.*), Chamomile (*Matricaria recutita*), Peppermint (*Mentha piperita*), Lemon Balm (*Melissa officinalis*), or Valerian (*Valeriana officinalis*); for children use the more gentle Red Clover (*Trifilium pratense*), Chamomile, and/or Linden blossoms.
- For relief of itchy skin—Chickweed (*Stellaria media*), Black Walnut leaves or bark (*Juglans nigra*), Hyssop (*Hyssopus officinalis*), or Chamomile; for dry itchy skin fill a sock with oatmeal and tie it at the top, steep this in the bath water for a while, then rub the skin with the bag.
- For relief of muscular tension and pain—Mugwort (*Artemisia vulgaris*), Chamomile, Horsetail (*Equisctum arvense*).
- To help circulation use any of the following stimulating herbs—Rosemary (*Rose-marinus spp.*), Yarrow (*Achillea millefolium*). Marigold (*Calendula officinalis*), Cayenne (*Capsicum minimum*), Ginger (*Zingiber officinalis*). Use small amounts of the Cayenne and Ginger.

These are only a few of the limitless possibilities one can come up with.

Summary

I'm giving you the above suggestions and precise techniques as helpful guidance If you are a water person and inclined to use the bath as a means of health care, you will need to use your intuition and good judgment as you implement these procedures in your home. And, of course, the bather will be the final judge as to how good and helpful it all feels. When the results you seek are manifested, please make notes on these successful experiences. If you make mistakes, learn from them and annotate your experiences. These notes will be invaluable to you and to others as we relearn how to employ the remarkable healing energy of hydrotherapy and simple herbal baths.

—From *The Herbal Medicine Maker's Handbook*

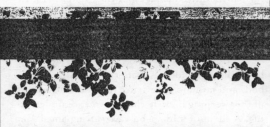

ESSENTIAL MASSAGE

Helene Silver
Illustrations by Kathleen Savage

Massage is a remarkably effective and deeply pleasurable method for moving fresh, rejuvenating fluids into the cells and pushing stale, toxin-laden fluids out. At the same time, massage is also a powerful tool for managing stress, which can age even the best-nourished complexion and mar the look of vitality in even the best-exercised body.

For many people, the idea of massage summons up images of sleazy "massage parlors" or self-indulgent pampering exclusively for the idle rich. Our society still retains many of its puritanical attitudes about the human body, clinging to the belief that anything that feels good cannot really be good for the health or the character.

I would like to dispel such negative, fearful ideas about massage once and for all. For me, massage is an essential part of my health-maintenance program. It is an effective way of releasing the stress that builds up in my daily life, and it is a very important way for me to take care of myself. If I cannot express love for myself and take care of my own body, then how can I love and take care of other people, both professionally and in my personal life?

I am not unique in this attitude. Many successful sports figures, entertainers, business people, and politicians depend on massage to improve their performance, keep them youthful and attractive, and relieve their stress. Lee Iacocca, after his retirement from the Ford Motor Company, continued to receive massages from the company masseur. Members of the U.S. Olympic Team were given massages after competing in their events in Calgary, Canada, and Seoul, Korea. Celebrities such as Bette Midler, Tina Turner, Madonna, Bob Hope, Bruce Springsteen, and Luciano Pavarotti all relied on regular massage to keep them fit, youthful, and able to manage the stress of their hectic public lives.

The use of touch to soothe physical and emotional pain is a built-in response in the human organism. Even animals lick their wounds and groom one another. Massage has a long history in the healing arts. A Chinese medical treatise recorded the use of massage as early as 3000 B.C., and the ancient Hindu literature described its therapeutic value around 1800 B.C. In ancient Greece, Hippocrates, the father of Western medicine, taught that physicians must be experienced in the healing art of rubbing. In Rome, Julius Caesar received daily massages for his neuralgia. During the Middle Ages, massage (and bathing) fell out of favor as the church encouraged a general disdain for "fleshly indulgences." With the rebirth of interest in bodily health during the Renaissance, massage again grew in popularity and began to develop as a science. Many prominent physicians subsequently included massage as part of their repertoire of healing techniques.

In this century, massage has repeatedly come in and out of fashion. During World War I, it was used to treat wounded soldiers. The human-potential movement in the 1970s brought new attention to the healing power of touch. Today, massage is becoming very respectable once again, and competent professional massage therapists are available in ever-increasing numbers.

How Massage Helps to Keep You Young

....Many people think that I look much younger than my years. I attribute much of my youthful appearance and clear complexion to massage. For me, massage has pulled all the other aspects of my self-care program together into a unique, rejuvenating combination. I first started receiving massage when I was doing competitive swimming in grammar school. I noticed that the older, more advanced swimmers were having regular massage, and so I tried it, too. I discovered that if I had a massage after a strenuous workout, I would recover faster, my pre-competition tension would be relieved, and I would be able to swim farther and faster. Later, when I became involved in dance, I used massage to help stretch my muscles and prevent injuries. I then began to study yoga, and noticed that yoga postures served as a sort of self-massage. Like massage, yoga also helped to promote my own body awareness.

Massage is a vital part of staying young. It supports the cleansing and nourishing of the cells by stimulating circulation—of lymph, of blood, and of energy. Massage causes the blood vessels to dilate, so circulation is improved and congestion is relieved. It temporarily raises the red blood cell count, by moving sedentary cells into circulation, thereby increasing the oxygen-carrying capacity of the blood. With increased oxygenation of the cells, the metabolic rate is increased, wastes are broken down more completely, and the calories in food are burned more efficiently. Massage also helps to push the lymph along in its channels, delivering nutrients, hastening the elimination of waste, and keeping the immune system healthy.

Oriental healing systems teach that massage affects an energy system in the body that flows through channels known as meridians. This meridian energy is the basis of the Chinese science of acupuncture, which holds that illness is a result of blockage or stagnation of this energy flow. In acupuncture, sterile needles are inserted into specific points along the meridians to stimulate energy flow. Oriental systems of massage such as acupressure or shiatsu, rather than using needles, simply apply pressure to these very same points to unblock the flow of energy.

Massage helps you to get the greatest possible benefit from your exercise program. By stimulating the circulation of blood and lymph, massage helps to bring fuel— oxygen and nutrients—to the muscles. At the same time, it carries away metabolic waste. Lactic acid, which is produced as a metabolic by-product of exercise, causes muscle soreness and a feeling of fatigue. Massage helps to move this lactic acid out of the muscles, speeding recovery time after strenuous exercise.

Massage also preserves muscle tone. If injury, illness, or an overly demanding schedule force you to be physically inactive for some time, massage can help to compensate for the lack of exercise. I

Continued ➡

became aware of the toning and conditioning benefits of massage during the years when an increasingly busy professional life caused me to drop exercise from my daily activities. If it weren't for the regular massages I had during this period, I probably would not have maintained the muscle tone that I still enjoy today.

Because it promotes body awareness, massage can also help prevent injuries. So often we tend to disregard the messages from our bodies. We may push ourselves beyond the limit of some part of our body that is tense or sore or weak. Having a regular massage helps you tune in to these problem areas, so you can work with them before they break down or become injured.

If you should happen to be injured, massage also helps to promote rapid healing. It reduces swelling by carrying fluid away from the injured area. It keeps muscle fibers from developing adhesions or fibrosis. Massage has even been shown to speed the healing of fractures by influencing metabolism and encouraging the retention of minerals needed for the bone repair.

For me, the psychological benefits are probably the most important aspect of massage. We live in a society that is starved for touch. It is a perfectly natural thing to touch a child, a friend, or even a stranger to comfort or soothe them. Sometimes a wordless hand on the shoulder, a hug, or a stroke on the back can be the most healing thing we can do for another person. Research at the University of Miami Medical School showed that premature infants who were massaged for fifteen minutes three times a day gained weight 47 percent faster than babies who were left alone in their incubators, as was the usual practice. The massaged infants showed more rapid development of their nervous systems and were able to leave the hospital six days earlier than other premature infants who were not massaged. Skin-to-skin touch is essential for all babies, premature or not. Infants receiving more touch have been shown to have a six-month advantage in their mental development. As a result of such findings, American parents are now learning techniques for massaging their infants—an activity that is a natural part of child care in many other parts of the world.

Adults as well as infants require physical touch. I find that getting a massage is one of the most effective ways to nurture and take care of myself. Many people seek out sexual contacts simply because they need to be touched, and do not realize that they can get touch in other ways as well.

Anita, one of my clients, was typical of such people. A successful artist, she worked alone in her studio, and she lived alone as well. During the time I worked with Anita on a cleansing program, she confided to me that she was having a lot of trouble with her relationships. She would get sexually involved with one man after another, and never seemed to find the love or satisfaction she was looking for. As we talked, it became clear that she was really hungry for touch. I suggested that she try massage, and she discovered that receiving a massage once a week helped her to place sex in the proper perspective and enabled her to be more discriminating in her relationships.

For me, massage is essential for stress management. Stress can have a very aging effect on the appearance, causing furrowing of the brow and worry lines around the mouth and between the eyebrows. I remember one massage therapist who would always point out when I was frowning. I had never realized until then how much tension I was holding in my face. A very important part of stress management is being aware of your stress-warning signals. Being touched by another person helps you to tune into every part of your body and to see where you are holding stress and tension. Over time, such stress held in the body can lead to real physical symptoms. Massage helps call attention to these warning signs before they reach the danger point.

Massage is becoming so widely accepted as a stress reliever today that many major corporations, such as Apple Computer and AT&T, now sponsor regular in-office massages for their employees. In cities across the United States, therapists are providing on-site massages that generally take about fifteen minutes.

....Sometimes massage is just what is needed to break through old stress patterns and allow your body and mind to experience the dramatic benefits of the sweeping lifestyle changes you are undertaking. A client of mine, a busy executive named Alan, is a perfect example of the hard-driving, Type A personality. He was having trouble with his digestion, and he was constipated most of the time. Although he denied it initially, it was obvious to me that a great deal of his problem was due to stress. He worked hard at changing his diet, took all the recommended supplements, adhered faithfully to his exercise, and cooperated in the cleansing program, but he was still holding a lot of stress in his body, particularly in his abdominal organs. Finally, I persuaded Alan to set up a series of appointments for massage. For the first time, Alan allowed someone to do something for him, rather than insisting on controlling what was happening to him. With regular weekly massage sessions, Alan finally learned how to let go and relax. He began to respond better to the cleansing program, and he also began to understand what I meant when I suggested he use his exercise period as a time to relax and breathe and open himself up to the beauty of the outdoors, rather than feeling compelled to push himself through a strenuous daily regimen. All the components of his cleansing program began to fall into place once he learned to relax and tune in to the stress signals his body was sending him.

I often find that tension held in the abdomen can be the principal cause of problems with digestion and elimination. Stress can cause clenching of the muscles along the intestinal tract, inhibiting peristalsis and preventing proper digestion and bowel movement. Massage is a great tool for helping people to recognize these muscular holding patterns and learn to release them.

Which Massage Is Right for You?

Essentially, massage can be divided into four main categories: Swedish, Oriental or shiatsu, reflexology, and sports massage. Each type of massage is used for different purposes, and has a different "feel." It is very common for massage therapists to combine elements of different techniques into a more eclectic approach.

My own personal health-maintenance program includes at least one professional massage per week. Every other week, I receive an eclectic bodywork type of massage that works at a very deep tissue level, not only moving the blood and lymph but also producing intense emotional release. On the alternating weeks, I have a Swedish type of massage that helps to keep my lymph moving, relaxes me and relieves my stress, and is wonderfully nurturing. Whenever I am out of balance or feeling emotionally vulnerable, I have an additional Swedish massage during the bodywork week.

Swedish massage, introduced by Peter Ling of Sweden in the nineteenth century, combines traditional techniques brought back from China with a Western understanding of anatomy and physiology. Swedish massage works with the body's muscular and skeletal structure to promote circulation, soothe the nervous system, and promote a feeling of well-being. It consists of long, gliding strokes and a variety of kneading, friction, squeezing, tapping, and shaking movements. Swedish massage is given on a table, with the client partially or completely undressed, since the massage therapist works directly on the bare skin, using oil for lubrication. A less vigorous variant of Swedish massage, known as Esalen massage, uses gentle, rhythmic movements that many people find to be a good introduction to the nurturing, relaxing benefits of massage.

Shiatsu massage, also known as acupressure, is an Oriental technique based on the acupuncture theory of meridian energy. By applying pressure rather than needles to specific points along the meridians, this form of massage is believed to unblock the circulation of the life energy, helping to promote self-healing and prevent illness. Therapists who use these Oriental techniques work with their fingers, hands, elbows, and knees on points along the energy pathways. The deep pressure of shiatsu massage may feel painful when applied to sore, tense muscles; while some people enjoy this intense stimulation, others may find it too much for them. Oriental massage tends to produce an energized feeling rather than relaxation, and is helpful for relieving tension in specific areas of the body. It is usually performed on a mat on the floor, with the client wearing loose, comfortable clothing.

Reflexology is a form of acupressure that concentrates on the feet and sometimes, the hands. It is based on the theory that every organ, muscle, and gland in the body corresponds to a specific area on the feet. By manipulating the appropriate part of the feet, the masseur can relieve tension in the corresponding distant part. I have found, for example, that clients with elimination or digestion problems are able to relax in their abdominal organs when I massage the colon point in the middle of the sole of the foot. Introduced relatively recently, in the early 1900s, reflexology is based on ancient Chinese, Japanese, and Egyptian techniques. You can do this particular kind of massage for yourself, or a massage therapist can give you a reflexology foot or hand massage while you are lying on a table or sitting in a reclining chair. Try massaging your feet as a pleasant, effective way to induce relaxation.

Sports massage is a rapidly growing subspecialty in the United States today. It caters specifically to serious athletes, but is becoming increasingly popular among amateurs as well. Sports massage consists of a combination of Swedish-massage strokes and pressure-point techniques derived from shiatsu, as well as specific manipulations to prevent injury, improve performance, and aid recovery. If you are actively engaged in a sport that places stress on certain joints or muscles, you may find that sports massage, focused on those parts of your body, can be a valuable part of your training program. Sports massage tends to be brisk, vigorous, and more energizing than a relaxing full-body Swedish massage.

Other forms of massage include Rolfing, which works on deep tissues to release tension patterns stored in the muscles and joints, and provides a release of emotions held in the body. Bodywork techniques such as the Trager and Feldenkreis methods and Polarity therapy use movement and manipulation to balance the body energies and release physical and emotional patterns. These emotional-release forms of massage are really in the realm of psychotherapy.

Continued ➡

How to Choose a Massage Therapist

Your massage therapist will be providing a very personal service for you, and you want to be sure you will feel comfortable with the person you select. Begin by asking your friends if they have a favorite massage therapist. A personal referral helps to ensure that the therapist is ethical and experienced. Sometimes, it can be difficult to differentiate the legitimate massage therapist among the listings in the telephone yellow pages or the classified ads in a newspaper. If there is an alternative publication such as Common Ground in your area, you will find qualified massage therapists listed there. You can also call the American Massage Therapy Association at 847-864-0123 for referrals to massage therapists in your area.

Some states require a license to practice massage therapy. If your state requires a license, make sure your therapist has one. Ask what kind of training the therapist has had; ideally, select someone who has gone through an extensive formal training program, including the study of anatomy and physiology. Experience is just as important as training. I recommend that you look for a therapist who has been in practice for at least one year.

It is not unusual to feel self-conscious about your body or anxious about what will happen at your first session with a massage therapist. You may feel apprehensive about being naked or about having a stranger touch you. A good massage therapist is sensitive to your feelings and will not push you to do anything that you don't want to. If you are not comfortable removing all your clothes, leave on your underwear. Once you are on the massage table, the therapist will drape you with sheets and towels, both to respect your modesty and to keep your body warm.

At your first meeting, the massage therapist should ask you about your physical condition and your personal needs. You will be asked whether you have any medical problems, are pregnant, on medication, or menstruating, and whether you have had any recent surgery. The answers to these questions will determine what kind of massage you will receive.

Do not hesitate to discuss the cost of the massage when you first call the therapist on the phone. In most parts of the country, rates generally average in the thirty-dollar to fifty-dollar range for a one-hour massage. If there is a massage school in your area, and you are willing to allow a beginner to work on you, call and inquire whether the school offers sessions with apprentices. The rates will be considerably lower.

While I recommend a professional massage on a regular, once-a-week basis, this is more than some people can afford. An alternative is to pay for a professional massage as often as you can and on other weeks call on a friend. You may both need instruction to make the exchange of massage as beneficial as possible. See if massage classes are offered in your area. If you don't have time for a class, some excellent self-teaching materials are available. Exchanging massage with a mate or a friend can be a pleasant and meaningful way to share healing, loving energy. Not only is it wonderful to receive a massage, but it is a very satisfying experience to know how to give one to someone close to you.

Make Your Own Aromatherapy Massage Oil

Massaging the skin with essential oils is an ideal way to get the healing properties of aromatic plant essences into the body. The herbal essences are absorbed even more readily through the skin than through inhalation. Try rubbing some essential oil on the palm of your hand; you should be able to taste it in your mouth in a couple of minutes. The nurturing touch of massage enhances the relaxing, soothing, and stimulating properties of the oils themselves.

You can prepare your own massage oil to use regularly for all the massage activities in this program.

In an eight-ounce container, place the following vegetable oils, which will serve as the base for the essential oils:

3 ounces of olive oil

3 ounces of peanut oil

3 ounces of almond oil

Olive oil moisturizes and softens the skin, soothes irritation, and alleviates dryness of cuticles and nails. Almond oil is an excellent moisturizer that imparts its fragrance to many fine cosmetics. Peanut oil is believed to be very beneficial for the joints and is used frequently in natural remedies applied externally for arthritis.

To the base mixture, add essential oils to make your own personalized massage oil formula. A good general-purpose combination is:

12 drops of eucalyptus oil

15 drops of chamomile oil

15 drops of lavender oil

12 drops of rosemary oil

These essential oils have a pleasant sedative effect, promote circulation, and relax the muscles. . . .

Oil for Varicose Veins

Prepare a small batch of the following special massage oil to help increase circulation and improve the tone of the veins.

1 ounce of olive oil

8 drops of cypress essential oil

Massage with this oil only above the area affected with varicose veins, never below—that is, massage between the varicosities and the heart. Use this oil only for those parts of your body, such as your legs, that have the varicose veins, and use your regular massage oil for the other body areas.

Self-Massage

While nothing can equal the relaxation and sense of being cared for that you derive from receiving a professional massage, you can experience many of the benefits of massage by doing it for yourself. Through self-massage, you can develop a better understanding of your own body. Because you are getting your own feedback, you will know exactly how much pressure to apply without causing pain, and you will discover what feels best to you. Self-massage allows you to tune in to areas where you are holding tension in your body, to relieve aching muscles, and release energy blockages. Whenever you feel tense and under pressure, use these massage techniques, drawn from Swedish and Oriental massage, to relax and nurture yourself.

Antigravity Facial Massage

Massaging your face on a slant board is particularly beneficial because the antigravity position brings the blood supply to the face, so this massage is beautifying as well as relaxing. You can use the same facial-massage techniques whenever you are under stress. In the privacy of your office, in the bathroom at work, or while commuting by bus, train, or car, you can do a one-minute version of this facial massage for a quick relaxer and youth restorer.

Set up the slant board. Relax for a few minutes in the antigravity position, with your feet above your head. Breathe in through your nostrils and out through pursed lips to calm and center yourself. Before you begin, dab a little massage oil or cream of your choice on your fingertips. If you have never been introduced to castor oil, this is a good time to try it; an occasional facial massage with castor oil is very rejuvenating to the skin. Castor oil is a popular folk remedy for all sorts of skin problems, and it is an ingredient in many cosmetics because of its hydrating and soothing properties. You may also use your own massage oil or plain vegetable oil. . . .

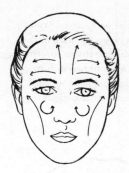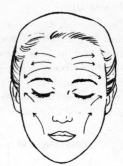

Facial massage

Now, with your fingertips, gently massage your temples in a circular motion. Move all around the temple area. If you find a sensitive spot, do not avoid it, but bring your attention to that spot and gently massage the tenderness away. Continue your conscious breathing as you feel the relaxation spread through the muscles of your face.

Next, use your fingertips to gently massage between your eyebrows in a circular motion. Then stroke your fingertips across your forehead, moving out from the center toward the temples. Use gentle but firm pressure, as much pressure as feels comfortable to you. Work your way up and down the forehead, stroking across in this manner, so that you cover the entire forehead. Then place the fingertips of each hand along the corresponding eyebrow and with firm but gentle pressure slide the fingertips from the eyebrows into the hairline. Cover the entire forehead with this sliding motion, to relax the forehead and smooth out the wrinkles in your brow.

Massage your cheeks by sliding the fingers upward on each side, from the chin up over the cheeks, out to the temples, and into the hairline. Repeat this movement several times, covering the sides of the face completely. Then massage in a circular motion over the cheekbones, beginning below the outer corners of the eyes, moving across the cheek and down to the base of your nose. Massage in a circular motion back out and down to the hinge of the jaw. Spend some time massaging here, noticing any tender spots. Many people hold a lot of tension in the jaw.

As you massage your face, feel the muscles relax and the blood flow into all the tissues, nourishing them and bringing a glow to your complexion. This facial massage is also helpful for freeing the sinuses of congestion.

Finish your facial massage by placing your thumbs under your chin and pulling them up, first on one side and then the other, along the jawline toward the ears. The longer you continue this alternate chin stroking, the greater will be the toning effect if you have a tendency to a sagging chin line.

Continue your facial massage for a full five minutes. Then, still lying on the slant board, use your fingertips to massage your scalp. Use the pads of the fingers, being careful not to damage the scalp with your nails. If you find tender spots, concentrate on those. Massage in a circular motion over

Continued ➡

the entire scalp, being sure to go all the way down to the neck and behind the ears. This scalp massage encourages hair growth and improves scalp problems. Keep up the scalp massage for two to three minutes. It is a very relaxing and pleasant way to enhance your natural beauty.

Quick Oriental Massage Remedies

Pressure-point massage techniques are derived from shiatsu and acupressure. . . . Try these massage remedies for drugless first aid the next time you have the indicated problem.

HEADACHE

Press your left thumb onto the back of your right hand, in the: web of flesh between the base of the thumb and the bone that connects to the forefinger. Hold firmly for five seconds to two minutes, and you should feel your headache pain subside. This acupressure point was known in ancient times as the "Great Eliminator."

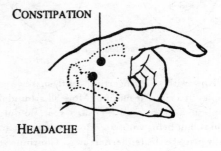

Hand pressure points

CONSTIPATION

Move your left thumb just up from the Great Eliminator point, so that you are pressing with the thumb into the inside edge of the metacarpal bone of the right index finger, just beyond the V where this bone meets the bone from the thumb. Hold this point firmly while attempting to move the bowels, to ease tension in the large intestine.

LOW ENERGY

Massaging specific points in the abdomen and the chest is a great substitute for coffee, whenever you are groggy and want to stay awake—while driving, working, or dozing off at a concert. The first points, used to stimulate the adrenal glands, are located two and one-half inches above and one inch to either side of the navel. Hold your hands with the palms across the abdomen, with the fingertips pointing toward each other. Now using; a circular motion, massage with the fingertips of each hand deep into the abdomen in this area, just below the rib cage. Do not massage these points too close to bedtime, as you may not be able to go to sleep.

The second set of points that stimulate the brain is located on each side of the chest, running from a point on the collarbone directly below the ears vertically down to the armpit. Use your thumbs or fingers to massage with firm pressure in a circular motion all the way down this line. These points may feel rather sensitive or painful at first, but as the massaging takes effect, the tenderness will decrease, and you will become more alert.

SLEEPLESSNESS OR EMOTIONAL UPSET

Place the tips of the four fingers of each hand over the frontal eminence on each side of the forehead. This is the slight bulge on either side of the forehead, between the eyebrows and the hairline. Feel for a faint pulse in this area, and hold with gentle fingertip pressure on these points for two to five minutes. Usually, within a few minutes you will begin to feel relaxed enough to sleep, or your troubling thoughts will begin to melt away. Pressing

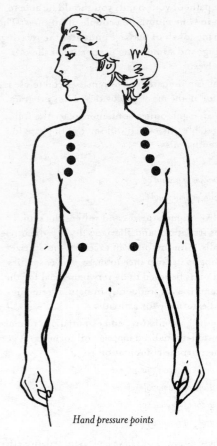

Hand pressure points

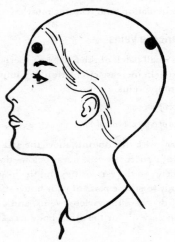

Head pressure points

these points helps to normalize the adrenal glands after an upsetting event.

Another point for sedating the adrenal glands is located on the posterior fontanel on the top rear of the head—the "soft spot" on the back of a baby's head. Feel for the slight pulse, and hold for two to ten minutes, to calm upset or ease yourself into sleep.

Warm Soak and Stroke

A wonderful way to relax before bedtime is to do a self-massage in your bath. You can use these self-massage techniques anywhere, at any time during the day, to work on easily reached trouble spots that accumulate tension.

Be sure that your bathroom is nice and warm when you begin. Add one pound of Epsom salts. Periodically add a little hot water if necessary to maintain the temperature for twenty to thirty minutes. The Epsom salts promote the eliminative activity of the skin, carrying through on the work of elimination begun by stimulating the circulation of blood and lymph with massage. You do not need to use oil for this massage, since the bath water will provide lubrication.

Sitting up in the tub, begin with the neck. Using the thumb and fingers, grasp the muscle on either side of the spine at the back of the neck. Move gradually up and down each side of the spine, pinching and releasing the muscle, going down as far as you can and up to the base of the skull. Concentrate on the areas that feel tight and sore. Bend your neck back and hang your head forward as you continue to pinch and knead the muscles. Do some neck rolls to the sides to loosen up the neck, then massage the neck muscles some more.

From the neck, move out toward the shoulders. Rest the heels of the hands on the tops of the shoulders against the neck, with the fingers curled over the back of the shoulders. Now, slide your hands forward with a firm, smooth, sliding pressure, so your elbows come down over the chest. Repeat this sliding movement, gradually working out from the neck to the shoulder, pressing as hard as you wish. Feel the heat in your skin as you slide your hands firmly over the muscles.

Now, work on one shoulder at a time with the opposite hand, squeezing all around the shoulder joint. Begin with gentle squeezing, then increase until you are squeezing as hard as is comfortable.

Next, work on the arms, always moving toward the heart. Work on one hand and arm and then switch to the other. Begin by massaging each finger from the tip up to the palm. Take the time to squeeze, stroke, and shake each of the fingers and the thumb, working the blood and lymph back toward the heart. Now, squeeze and massage the hands, stroking firmly along the bones, always moving toward the heart to flush out the wastes and stagnant blood. Work your way up the arm, kneading and squeezing the muscles. Work around the elbow, massaging any tender spots you find, and moving up toward the armpits. Finish with strong upward strokes, using the whole opposite hand, with the fingers wrapped around the arm, to push the blood and lymph back toward the heart. If you feel tender spots, you may be encountering areas of congested lymph. Work on them, and then move everything onward, squeezing and stroking toward the heart. Take the time to do some shoulder rolls to loosen up your shoulders as you work.

Next, massage your legs. Use both hands to work on one foot and calf, then go on to the other. Bend one knee so that you can rest the foot on the opposite thigh. Squeeze and massage the toes from the tip toward the foot, to force the blood back toward the heart. Slide your index finger back and forth between the toes, feeling the wonderful relaxation spreading through your body. Grasp all your toes with one hand, and with the other hand bend the foot back and forth. Massage along the bones on the top of the foot and knead deeply into the sole, gently moving up toward the leg.

Keeping your knee bent with the foot resting on the opposite thigh, massage the calf, kneading and squeezing. Then use strong, firm strokes with both hands to move the circulation up the calf into the thighs. When you have finished one calf, work on the other foot and calf.

Now, straighten the legs in front of you to work on the knees and thighs. Work on one knee at a time, squeezing and kneading with both hands behind and around the sides of the knee. Next, grasp the top of one thigh between thumb and fingers, squeeze, and let the muscle slip out of your hand. Work your way all over the thighs in this manner to stimulate the circulation. Then stroke strongly up the thigh with both hands curved around the leg. Finish by stroking the insides of both thighs, up toward the groin. Remember that massaging toward the heart helps to flush the veins, promoting circulation and cleansing.

Continued ➡

After your massage, get out of the bath and dry briskly with a coarse towel. Wrap in a robe or towel and get into bed and relax for fifteen minutes, or prepare for sleep. The skin-cleansing properties of the Epsom salts, activated by the self-massage, will continue to draw wastes out of your skin through the night. . . .

Lymphatic Massage

. . . .An excellent way to continue lymphatic stimulation is through massage. I am going to show you how to do a lymphatic massage, to stimulate lymph flow in your lower body. Remember that the lymph flows toward the heart—up from the feet and down from the head.

Lower-Body Lymphatic Massage

Massage one leg at a time. Using one or two hands, begin by massaging at the base of each toe and between the toes. Massage gently in a circular motion; imagine yourself loosening the toxins and debris from all the tiny lymph vessels between your toes.

After you have gently massaged the base of each toe, stroke upward with both hands, drawing the lymph up and toward the ankles with a gentle, feathery, upward stroking motion. Move up to the ankle; gently massage in a circular motion all around the ankle, and then lightly stroke upward, drawing the lymph up the calf until you get to the knee.

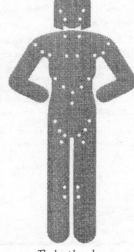

Massage with both hands all around the knee, over the lymph nodes behind the knee, and around the kneecap, in circular motions. Use light pressure; this is the best way to stimulate the lymph. Remember that the lymph vessels are close to the surface of the skin.

The lymph nodes

Draw the lymph up along the thighs, using the fingertips or the palms of the bands. At the back of the thigh, massage gently at the base of the buttock, in a gentle circular motion; this is one of the areas where the toxic waste of cellulite tends to accumulate.

Stroke upward, along the thigh, and bring it all around and back into the groin. After you have completed one leg, work on the other leg.

In the groin area, work on both sides at once. Stroke upward and diagonally across the groin area with the flat of the hand on each side, moving the hands toward each other so they come together over the abdomen. Repeat this upward stroking all along the groin area; there are many lymph nodes in this area.

As you stroke gently upward and into the abdominal area, picture all the debris and waste being moved along, to be absorbed and eliminated through your colon.

When you do a lymphatic massage, you may notice that some areas react painfully to pressure. Most people, for example, if they press hard between their breasts, will feel a very sensitive spot. This is one of the areas where lymph congestion can produce tenderness. If you find such a sensitive spot, do not be afraid to touch it; continue to gently massage it with a light, circular motion, and then with a feathery touch move it onward—up from the legs, down from the head. As you progress in your rejuvenation program, you will notice that there is less and less lymphatic congestion and that you have fewer sensitive spots.

Spend about ten minutes on the lymphatic massage. Proper lymphatic functioning produces clear, glowing skin, and, because lymph is a vital part of your immune system, it helps to promote your resistance to disease.

As you fall asleep tonight, imagine the lymph flowing freely beneath your skin, carrying away wastes and toxins. Know that even as you sleep, your program of diet, exercise, cleansing, and massage is promoting the growth of clean, clear new cells in the bottom layer of your skin, building the foundation for a fresh, youthful complexion. . . .

Upper-Body Lymph Massage

This gentle upper-body self-massage, which you will perform this evening, helps to flush congested lymph out of the extremities and toward the heart, where it joins the main lymph drainage of the body. Combined with skin brushing and detoxifying baths, lymph massage also assists in rejuvenating the complexion.

Begin your massage at the neck, under the chin, in the areas where you may have sometimes noticed swollen lymph glantls. Massage with the fingertips from ear to ear in a gentle circular motion, then gendy stroke from the ears under the chin toward the center. Now, with your fingertips, gently stroke downward, from under the chin down the neck. Use these gentle downward stroking movements all around the neck, moving the lymph from beneath the chin and the base of the skull down into the top of your chest.

Next, using your left hand, work on the right arm, beginning at the wrist. Use your fingers to repeatedly smooth and stroke the inside of the arm, from the wrist up to the inner elbow. When you reach the inside of the elbow, gently massage with a circular motion, then continue with a light, feathery, stroking movement up the inside of the arm to the underarm. In the armpit area, gently squeeze with thumb and fingers, releasing the lymph and moving it up and out of the arm. This is another area where many lymph nodes are located, and where you may have noticed swelling when you have been sick. Stroke from the armpit up over the top of the right breast, using light, feathery strokes to bring the lymph out of the armpit and around toward the center of the chest. Guide the lymph from the right shoulder, the right arm area, and the neck, all down toward the middle of the chest.

Now, use the right hand and repeat this process, bringing the lymph up the left arm and into the armpit. Concentrate a little longer on the left side, to work the lymph out of the armpit and along the extensive lymph drainage around the heart. Draw it all in toward the center of the chest, into the area between the breasts. Now, rub in a gentle circular motion between the breasts. It is quite possible that you will feel some tenderness in this area; this simply means that there is some lymph congestion here. Do not be alarmed; just continue to gently massage, and over time the congestion will begin to be relieved. Now, massage beneath the breasts, about an inch or so below each breast, stroking gently around the bottom of the breasts toward the middle, bringing it all down into the abdomen. Stroke gently downward all the way across your chest beneath your breasts, moving the lymph into the abdomen, where the waste will be eliminated by the colon.

—From *Rejuvenation*

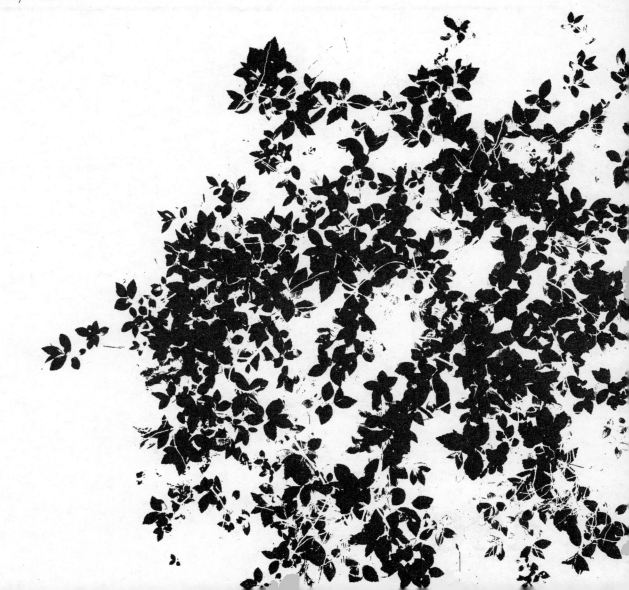

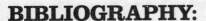

BIBLIOGRAPHY:

Works Excerpted and/or Reprinted in this Book

Bauer, Catherine. *Pocket Guide to Acupressure Points for Women*. Crossing Press, 1997.

Boice, Judith. *Pocket Guide to Naturopathic Medicine*. Crossing Press, 1996.

Burke, Adam. *Self-Hypnosis: New Tools for Deep and Lasting Transformation*. Ten Speed Press, 2004.

Cantin, Candis. *Pocket Guide to Ayurvedic Healing*. Crossing Press, 1996.

Crawford, Amanda McQuade. *The Herbal Menopause Book: Herbs, Nutrition and Other Natural Therapies*. Crossing Press, 1996.

Craydon, Deborah, and Warren Bellows. *Floral Acupuncture: Applying the Flower Essences of Dr. Bach to Acupuncture Sites*. Celestial Arts, 2005.

Evelyn, Nancy. *Pocket Guide to Herbal First Aid*. Crossing Press, 1998.

Ferré, Carl. *Pocket Guide to Macrobiotics*. Crossing Press, 1997.

Gardner, Joy. *Pocket Guide to Chakras*. Crossing Press 1998.

——. *Vibrational Healing Through the Chakras*. Celestial Arts, 2006.

Green, James. *The Herbal Medicine–Maker's Handbook: A Home Manual*. Crossing Press, 2000.

——. *The Male Herbal: The Definitive Health Care Book for Men & Boys*. 2nd ed. Crossing Press, 2007.

Hasnas, Rachelle. *Pocket Guide to Bach Flower Essences*. Crossing Press, 1997.

Kesten, Deborah, and Larry Scherwitz. *The Enlightened Diet: Seven Weight-Loss Solutions that Nourish Body, Mind, and Soul*. Celestial Arts, 2007.

Keville, Kathi. *Pocket Guide to Aromatherapy*. Crossing Press, 1996.

Knight, Sirona. *Pocket Guide to Crystals & Gemstones*. Crossing Press, 1998.

Lark, Susan. *Dr. Susan Lark's the Menopause Self Help Book: A Woman's Guide to Feeling Wonderful for the Second Half of Her Life*. 4th ed. Celestial Arts, 1990.

Mason, L. John. *Guide to Stress Reduction*. Celestial Arts, 2001.

Milburn, Michael P. *The Future of Healing: Exploring the Parallels of Eastern and Western Medicine*. Crossing Press, 2001.

Picozzi, Michele. *Pocket Guide to Hatha Yoga*. Crossing Press, 1998.

Safron, Jeremy A. *The Fasting Handbook: Dining from an Empty Bowl*. Celestial Arts, 2005.

——. *The Raw Foods Resource Guide*. Celestial Arts 2005.

——. *The Raw Truth: The Art of Preparing Living Foods*. Celestial Arts, 2003.

Schoenbart, Bill. *Pocket Guide to Chinese Patent Medicines*. Crossing Press, 1999.

Silver, Helene. *Rejuvenate: The 21-Day Natural Detox Program for Optimal Health*. Crossing Press, 1998.

St. Claire, Debra. *Pocket Herbal Reference Guide*. Crossing Press, 1992.

Stein, Diane. *Healing With Gemstones and Crystals*. Crossing Press, 1996.

——. *The Natural Remedy Book for Women*. Crossing Press, 1992.

Tart-Jensen, Ellen. *Health Is Your Birthright: How to Create the Health You Deserve*. Celestial Arts, 2006.

Tierra, Lesley. *Healing With the Herbs of Life*. Crossing Press, 2003.

Wauters, Ambika. *Homeopathic Color & Sound Remedies*. Crossing Press, 2007.

——. *Homeopathic Medicine Chest*. Crossing Press, 2000.

The Crossing Press and Celestial Arts are imprints of Ten Speed Press, located in Berkeley, California. For more information on these publishers or any of their titles, visit www.tenspeed.com.

Author Web Sites

For more information from the following authors, their books, and their work, please visit their Web sites.

Candis Cantin, *Pocket Guide to Ayurvedic Healing* www.evergreenherbgarden.org

L. John Mason, *Guide to Stress Reduction* www.dstress.com

Debra St. Claire, *Pocket Herbal Reference Guide* www.stclaires.com*

*Editor's note: This Web site, supplied by this author, does not contain information about the author or her book, but sells St. Claire's Organic Candies.

Diane Stein, *Healing with Gemstones & Crystals and The Natural Remedy Book for Women* www.dianestein.net

Ellen Tart-Jensen, *Health Is Your Birthright* www.bernardjensen.com

Continued ➔

INDEX

Continued ➡

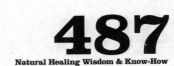

Continued ➡

Continued →

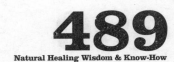

Continued →

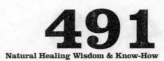

Continued ➜

Continued ➡

Continued ➡

Continued ➡

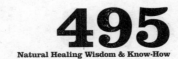